Contraceptive Technology

Contraceptive Technology

Twentieth Revised Edition

Robert A. Hatcher, MD, MPH

James Trussell, PhD

Anita L. Nelson, MD

Willard Cates Jr., MD, MPH

Deborah Kowal, MA, PA

Michael S. Policar, MD, MPH

ARDENT MEDIA, INC.

ISSN 0091-9721

ISBN 978-1-59708-004-0 (Paperback with Single-User CD-ROM and ebook)
ISBN 978-1-59708-005-7 (Hardcover with Single-User CD-ROM and ebook)

TRADEMARKS: All brand and product names are trademarks or registered trademarks of their respective companies. It has been attempted throughout this text to distinguish proprietary trademarks from generic or descriptive terms by following the capitalization style used by the manufacturer; however, the publisher cannot attest to the accuracy of this information. Use of a term in this text should not be regarded as affecting the validity of any trademark or service mark.

1 3 5 7 9 10 6 4 2

The paper used in this publication meets the minimum requirements of American National Standard for Information Sciences — Permanence of Paper for Printed Library Materials, ANSI Z39.48-1984. Printed in USA.

DISCLAIMER

The information contained herein is intended to be used by physicians and other qualified healthcare professionals. The information is not intended to \e used for medical diagnosis or treatment by persons who are not qualified h\ealthcare professionals. Such persons should not rely upon or use the information contained herein in place of a visit, call, or consultation with, or the advice of their personal physician or other qualified healthcare provider.

Physicians and other qualified healthcare professionals should recognize that this book is to be used only as a reference aid, and that this book is not intended to be a substitute for their exercise of professional judgment. Since medical science is always changing, physicians and other qualified healthcare professionals users are advised to confirm the information contained herein with an independent source. The authors and reviewers are not liable for errors and omissions.

Credits:

Executive and Managing Editor: Deborah Kowal, MA, PA
Composition: DataStream Content Solutions, LLC
Manufacturing Coordination: Stan Redfern
CD-ROM Preparation: Jason Blackburn, Digital Impact Design
Indexer: WordCo Indexing Services, Inc.
Cover artist: KC Hatcher
Proofreader: Kelly Cleland, MPA, MPH

Dedication

This 20th edition of *Contraceptive Technology* is dedicated to the Fellowship in Family Planning, the only fellowship in the nation that trains contraception and abortion specialists in high-level research and clinical skills. Working with respected and innovative leaders in the field, Fellows receive training in clinical and epidemiologic research, develop clinical and teaching skills, have opportunities to work internationally, and connect to a rapidly expanding network of family planning experts. During the two-year program, Fellows have the option of pursuing a master's degree in either Public Health or Science. Here we profile twelve current or former Fellows who are authors of chapters in this edition of *Contraceptive Technology*.

Deborah Bartz, MD, MPH, is an Instructor in the Department of Obstetrics, Gynecology and Reproductive Biology at Harvard Medical School. She graduated from medical school at the University of Wisconsin-Madison and completed her residency in Obstetrics and Gynecology at Indiana University, Indianapolis. She obtained her MPH at Harvard School of Public Health while completing a Fellowship in Family Planning under the mentorship of Alisa Goldberg at Brigham and Women's Hospital.

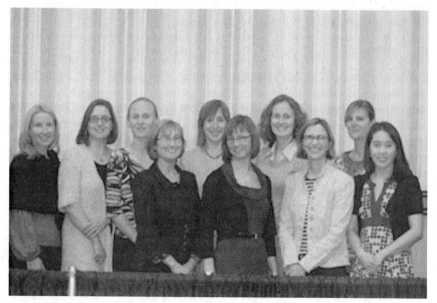

Source: Beth Robbins

v

Anne Burke, MD, MPH, is an Assistant Professor in the Department of Gynecology and Obstetrics and the Department of Population, Family, and Reproductive Health in addition to being the Director of the Family Planning Fellowship at The Johns Hopkins University School of Medicine. She received an MD from the University of Pittsburgh School of Medicine and completed her residency in Obstetrics and Gynecology at Pennsylvania Hospital. She completed her Fellowship in Family Planning at Hopkins under the mentorship of Paul Blumenthal and received her MPH from the Johns Hopkins University Bloomberg School of Public Health.

Carrie Cwiak, MD, MPH, is an Assistant Professor in the Department of Gynecology and Obstetrics at Emory University School of Medicine. She is the Director of the Family Planning Division and the Family Planning Fellowship, and the Acting Director of Grady Memorial Hospital Generalist Division. She completed her Fellowship in Family Planning and her MPH in Epidemiology at Emory, under the mentorship of Bob Hatcher and Mimi Zieman. She attended the St. Louis University School of Medicine and completed her residency in Obstetrics and Gynecology at the University of Connecticut Health Center.

Anne Davis, MD, MPH, is an Associate Professor of Clinical Obstetrics and Gynecology in the Department of Obstetrics and Gynecology at Columbia University Medical Center. She received an MD from Columbia College of Physicians and Surgeons and an MPH from the Mailman School of Public Health at Columbia University. After residency in Obstetrics and Gynecology at the University of Washington Medical Center, she completed the Fellowship in Family Planning and Contraceptive Research at Columbia; she now co-directs that Fellowship with Dr. Carolyn Westhoff, who was her mentor. Dr. Davis serves as the Medical Director of Physicians for Reproductive Choice and Health.

Gillian Dean, MD, MPH, is an Assistant Professor in the Department of Obstetrics, Gynecology and Reproductive Science at Mount Sinai School of Medicine and the Associate Medical Director of Clinical Research and Training at Planned Parenthood of New York City. She graduated from Harvard Medical School and completed her residency in Obstetrics and Gynecology at the University of California, San Francisco. After residency, she completed the fellowship in Family Planning at UCSF under the mentorship of Dr. Philip Darney. She received an MPH from the Mailman School of Public Health at Columbia University.

Alison Edelman, MD, MPH, is an Associate Professor in the Department of Obstetrics and Gynecology at Oregon Health & Science University (OHSU). She is also the Assistant Director of OHSU's Family Planning Fellowship and is on the editorial board of *Contraception*. Her medical training and residency in Obstetrics and Gynecology were completed at OHSU, as was her Family Planning Fellowship under the direction of Mark Nichols and Jeffrey Jensen. She received her MPH from the University of Washington, Seattle.

Alisa Goldberg, MD, MPH, is an Associate Professor of Obstetrics, Gynecology and Reproductive Biology at Harvard Medical School. She is Director of the Division of Family Planning at Brigham and Women's Hospital, Director of the Harvard Family Planning Fellowship Program, and Director of Clinical Research and Training at Planned Parenthood League of Massachusetts. After graduating from Harvard Medical School, she completed her residency in Obstetrics and Gynecology at Brigham and Women's Hospital and then completed the Family Planning Fellowship at University of California, San Francisco under the mentorship of Philip Darney. She received her MPH degree from the University of California, Berkeley.

Bryna Harwood, MD, is an Associate Professor (with tenure) in the Department of Obstetrics and Gynecology at the University of Illinois at Chicago, where she is Director of both the Section of Family Planning and the Family Planning Fellowship. After graduating from the University of Chicago Pritzker School of Medicine, she completed her residency in Obstetrics and Gynecology at the Kaiser Foundation Hospital in San Francisco. She then completed a Fellowship in Contraceptive Research and Family Planning and a Master degree program in Epidemiology under the direction of Daniel Mishell at the University of Southern California.

Melody Hou, MD, MPH, is an Instructor in the Department of Obstetrics and Gynecology at Boston University School of Medicine/Boston Medical Center. She graduated from Harvard Medical School and completed her residency in Obstetrics and Gynecology at Beth Israel Deaconess Medical Center in Boston. She obtained her MPH at the Harvard School of Public Health while completing a Fellowship in Family Planning under the mentorship of Alisa Goldberg at Brigham and Women's Hospital.

Danielle Roncari, MD, is a Family Planning Fellow in the Department of Obstetrics and Gynecology at Boston Medical Center under the mentorship of Lynn Borgatta and Karen Lifford. She is also enrolled in an MPH program at Boston University School of Public Health. After graduating from the University of Miami School of Medicine, she completed her residency in Obstetrics and Gynecology at Tufts Medical Center in Boston.

Jill Schwartz, MD, is currently an Associate Research Professor in the Department of Obstetrics and Gynecology at Eastern Virginia Medical School and the Medical Director of CONRAD, a nonprofit organization. After graduating from the Mount Sinai School of Medicine, she completed her residency in Obstetrics and Gynecology at George Washington University Hospital in Washington, DC. She then completed a

Fellowship in Contraceptive Research and Family Planning under the direction of Mitchell Creinin at the University of Pittsburgh.

Tara Stein, MD, MPH, is currently an Assistant Professor in the Department of Family and Social Medicine (DFSM) at the Albert Einstein College of Medicine in the Bronx, NY. She is working in the Montefiore Medical Center School-Based Health Program in partnership with the DFSM and the NYC Department of Health as a Clinician Educator for their long-acting contraceptive program. She graduated from Brown University School of Medicine and completed her residency in Family Medicine at the Columbia University Medical Center/NY Presbyterian Hospital. She obtained her MPH at Columbia University's Mailman School of Public Health while completing a Fellowship in Family Planning under the direction of Marji Gold at the Albert Einstein College of Medicine.

These are fabulous women with whom to collaborate, and we are profoundly grateful for their scholarship, their energy, their enthusiasm, and their deep commitment to research on and provision of contraception and abortion. They are the legacy of the inestimable clinician and researcher, the late Felicia Stewart, MD, editor-author of *Contraceptive Technology* for 11 editions. We remaining editor-authors are not getting any younger—each of us will be aged 60 or older and our average age 65 when this edition is published—and we (and Felicia) are delighted that there is a *next* generation of *Contraceptive Technology* authors, and that they and their colleagues in the Fellowship are the next generation not only of authors but also of providers and scholars of contraception and abortion. They make us proud!

Ward Cates
Bob Hatcher
Debbie Kowal
Anita Nelson
James Trussell
Michael Policar

July, 2011
Atlanta, Georgia

Table of Contents

17 **Female and Male Sterilization** **435**
Danielle Roncari, MD
Melody Y. Hou, MD, MPH, FACOG

18 **Postpartum Contraception and Lactation** **483**
Kathy I. Kennedy, DrPH, MA
James Trussell, PhD

List of Tables

xix

List of Figures

Foreword

Felicia H. Stewart, MD, (1943–2006) was a respected and beloved co-author of Contraceptive Technology *for eleven editions. What made her so special? She was an original and creative thinker, intellectually curious and scrupulously honest, absolutely fearless, an inspirational leader, an effective activist, a gifted writer, a terrific speaker, and a skilled clinician. She performed abortions from the beginning, at a time hardly anyone else did, and she continued to do so throughout her professional life. She was an articulate spokesperson for reproductive health and reproductive rights. She inspired a generation of young clinicians, researchers, and activists to strive to be like her. Above all else, she was very wise. Although she is not listed on the cover of this 20th edition, her vision permeates the chapters and her writing continues to reflect our own principles. This Foreword, inspired by Felicia Stewart and incorporating some of her writing, articulately expresses why we find the work of reproductive health care so satisfying and rewarding.*

Professionals in our field, familiar with its amazing scientific and medical advances, are comfortable explaining the research evidence and science involved. Many of us, however, are less accustomed to the other important dimension of this work—its *moral* value. For most of us, this dimension is why working in reproductive health care is so compelling. When we counsel patients about birth control, help patients make decisions about an unintended pregnancy, help women plan for pregnancy and safely traverse its nine months, work to shape public policy for the health of future generations, or contribute to reproductive health research, whether or not we are aware of it, we are engaged in a critically important and deeply moral undertaking.

For some areas in clinical medicine, the *why* seems hardly to need articulating. Becoming an expert on heart disease management has self-evident value, and is not controversial. The value of work as a heart disease clinician is not likely to be attacked as immoral, and heart problems are not likely to be carved out for special scrutiny as expenditures by public health services. The local town council or school board is not likely to ask the local heart specialist to testify about proposed local policies. Unfortunately, this is not true for clinicians working in the field of family planning services and reproductive health.

As the health reform debates of 2010 showed, basic reproductive choices remain under attack.[1] Emergency contraception, intrauterine contraceptives, and oral contraceptives continue to be challenged by arguments based on questionable evidence. Common ground on abortion seems impossible to achieve. Debate over whether it makes sense to provide insurance coverage for contraception is suggestive of the second-class status of women in this country. In the face of these challenges to individual freedoms, we need to rededicate ourselves to the goal that a woman does have the right to control her own fertility and that she needs access to information, services, and psychological support for her decisions. And we need to remember that fertility control improves pregnancy outcomes and the health of future generations.

As scientists, clinicians, and educators, we may not be accustomed to talking about values. For many of us, however, the moral importance of our work is fundamental and helps sustain us in the face of political challenges that threaten to silence science. As we work with colleagues and policymakers, we need to convey not only the science of reproductive health, but also why it is of vital importance in people's lives. If we fail to do so, we are abdicating the moral high ground to those who oppose women's rights to self-determination and the efforts to provide reproductive health care.

When we perform our work in clinics, hospitals, laboratories, and offices, we are engaged in a critically important and *deeply moral* undertaking. Reproductive health care enables individuals and couples to make and implement some of the most important decisions that shape their lives, and in turn shape society.

Reproductive health care reflects a deep commitment to parenthood and children. Our work helps ensure that every pregnancy is intended and as safe as possible, and that children are born when their parents are best able to provide the love and support they need to thrive. Reproductive health care makes an essential contribution to the human infrastructure we count on for our society to thrive. Our participation in strengthening individuals, families, and the community provides each of us—including those who write this book—with a foundation for our own unique moral code, which brings meaning to our lives.

In addition, reproductive health care, especially family planning, has an impact on global health and development. All eight of the Millennium Development Goals (MDGs) are affected by the informed reproductive choices provided by accessible family planning services.[2] In short, family planning is one of the most cost-effective development investments.[3]

Let's examine each Millennium Development goal separately:

1) **Eradicate extreme poverty and hunger.** Per capita Gross National Product is correlated with the prevalence of modern contraceptive methods. Family planning reduces the aggregate demand for increasingly scarce food products.
2) **Achieve universal primary education.** Girls often have to drop out of school due to an unintended pregnancy. Family planning prolongs education for young women.
3) **Promote gender equality and empower women.** Unplanned pregnancies divert women from other life plans. Empowering

women in achieving their desired family size is the most important driver of modern development efforts.

4) **Reduced child mortality.** About 1.2 million infant deaths are averted globally each year by preventing unintended pregnancies. If we could meet all demands for contraception, another 64,000 newborn deaths would be prevented. Family planning increases child survival.

5) **Improved maternal health.** Preventing unintended pregnancy reduces the subsequent risk of unsafe abortion or childbearing. Wider family planning access is a cost-effective method of decreasing maternal mortality.

6) **Combat HIV/AIDS, malaria, and other diseases.** Women with HIV who have unintended pregnancies run the risk of transmitting the virus to their children. Preventing unintended pregnancies among HIV-positive women reduces the number of HIV-positive births to a greater extent than providing antiretroviral treatment to mothers during pregnancy, birth, and breastfeeding.

7) **Ensure environmental sustainability.** A family with fewer children needs less food, land, and water and puts less pressure on a country's forests and tillable land. Moreover, family planning is five times less expensive than conventional green technologies for reducing atmospheric carbon dioxide that leads to climate change.

8) **A global partnership for development.** Four decades of global investment in family planning programs have contributed to strong collaborative partnerships among international agencies, governmental ministries, multinational organizations, and local community groups.

Health reform within the United States, and a renewed commitment to health and development globally, has built new momentum for family planning and accessible contraceptive technologies. Achieving universal access to family planning is within our grasp. We hope that the evidence-based recommendations contained within *Contraceptive Technology*, 20th edition, will expand commitment to family planning, health, and development worldwide.

The Authors

REFERENCES

1. National Partnership for Women & Families. The nation examines debate over contraception, prevention. Women's Health Policy Report. 2011 [cited 2011 Mar 3]: about 1 page. Available from: http://www.nationalpartnership.org/site/News2abbr=daily2_&page=NewsArticle&id=27441
2. Cates W Jr. Family planning: the essential link to achieving all eight Millennium Development Goals. Contraception. 2010; 81: 460–461.
3. Disease Control Priorities Project. Why contraception is considered a best buy: family planning saves lives and spurs development, fact sheet. Washington, DC: Disease Control Priorities Project, 2007.

Let's Get Serious

My first day working in family planning was July 1, 1966. I was an Epidemic Intelligence Officer for the Centers for Disease Control, soon to be providing pills, fitting diaphragms, giving away condoms, and placing IUDs at the Muscogee County Health Department in Columbus, Georgia. On that day, I learned that about half of all pregnancies in the United States were unintended.

Today, more than four decades later, not much has changed. About half of all pregnancies are unintended.[1] Close to half of those unintended pregnancies lead to abortions.[1] What we have been doing simply has not been working. If we as a nation want to avoid the consequences of unintended and unwanted pregnancies, we will need to approach sex and contraception differently. Otherwise, we risk Albert Einstein's definition of insanity: "doing the same thing over and over again and expecting different results."

So what can we do different to decrease the number of unintended pregnancies? Here are four possibilities, beginning with the three that must be accomplished by those of us in our society providing contraceptive and reproductive health services (readers of this 20th edition of *Contraceptive Technology*):

1. Women, after counsel from clinic staff and their clinicians, can choose for ongoing contraception one of the three "you can't forget me" methods—a copper T 380A IUD (ParaGard), a levonorgestrel IUD (Mirena), or an implant (Implanon). For these methods, the inherent efficacy is so high and correct and consistent use is so nearly guaranteed that extremely low pregnancy rates are found in all studies.[2] If the "Contraceptive Choice Project" in St. Louis can provide Mirena IUDs, ParaGard IUDs, or Implanon implants to 70% of the first 6,000 women entered into their program (ages 14 to 45),[3] all of us can learn from the many things they did to make the "you-can't-forget-me" methods an attractive option for women.
2. When a woman has had unprotected sex, we can offer her an intrauterine contraceptive rather than emergency contraceptive pills. Placement of the IUD within several days of unprotected sex reduces a woman's risk of pregnancy to about 1 in 1,000 *and* provides her with 10 to 12 years of highly effective, fully reversible contraception if she tolerates her IUD well and wants to continue contraception.[4] The effectiveness of the copper T 380-A (ParaGard) is almost as high as the effectiveness of female sterilization. Our educational materials and counseling must move beyond the knee-

jerk reaction to offer emergency contraceptive pills. We can do so much better.

3. Within 10 minutes of the delivery of the placenta, whether delivery is by caesarean section or vaginally, a copper T IUD or a levonorgestrel IUD may be placed. This has been accomplished for 4,000 women delivering vaginally using a sponge forceps that is longer so that it reaches all the way to the top of the fundus. The expulsion rate was 1.6% and the cost of the sponge forceps is $7.[5]

4. And finally, our society must move away from abstinence-only sex education. The data are in: it just doesn't work.

These four changes in how we do business need to move to the top of the list of priorities if we want to get serious about

- Reducing unintended pregnancies
- Reducing abortions
- Reducing teen pregnancies

Robert A. Hatcher, MD, MPH

REFERENCES

1. Finer and Henshaw. Disparities in rates of unintended pregnancy in the United States, 1994 and 2001. Perspect Sexual Reprod Health. 2006;38: 90-6
2. Trussell J, Guthrie KA. Choosing a contraceptive: efficacy, safety, and personal considerations. In: Hatcher RA, Trussell J, Nelson A, Cates W, Kowal D (editors). Contraceptive Technology, 20th edition. New York: Ardent Media, 2011.
3. Piepert J. Personal communication. September 22, 2010.
4. Sivin I. Utility and drawbacks of continuous use of a copper T IUD for 20 years. Contraception. Jun 2007;75(6 Suppl):S70-75.
5. Smith, J. Personal communication. April 21, 2010.

Author-Editors

Robert A. Hatcher, MD, MPH
Professor Emeritus of Gynecology and Obstetrics
Emory University School of Medicine

James Trussell, PhD
Professor of Economics and Public Affairs
Director, Office of Population Research
Princeton University
Visiting Professor
The Hull York Medical School

Anita L. Nelson, MD
Professor, Obstetrics and Gynecology
David Geffen School of Medicine at UCLA
Medical Director, Women's Health Care Programs
Harbor-UCLA Medical Center

Willard Cates, Jr., MD, MPH
President, Research
FHI 360

Deborah Kowal, MA, PA
President and CEO
Contraceptive Technology Communications, Inc.
Adjunct Assistant Professor, Department of International Health
Rollins School of Public Health
Emory University

Michael S. Policar, MD, MPH
Clinical Professor, Obstetrics, Gynecology and Reproductive Sciences
University of California, San Francisco, School of Medicine

Chapter Authors

Susie Baldwin, MD, MPH
Health Assessment Unit Chief, Office of Health Assessment and Epidemiology
Los Angeles County Department of Public Health
Medical Director, California Family Health Council, Clinical and Community Health Programs

Deborah Bartz, MD, MPH
Instructor, Obstetrics, Gynecology & Reproductive Biology
Harvard Medical School & Brigham and Women's Hospital

Anne E. Burke, MD, MPH
Assistant Professor
Department of Gynecology and Obstetrics
Department of Population, Family, and Reproductive Health
The Johns Hopkins University School of Medicine

Kathryn M. Curtis, PhD
Epidemiologist, Division of Reproductive Health
Centers for Disease Control and Prevention

Carrie Cwiak, MD, MPH
Associate Professor, Department of Gynecology and Obstetrics
Director, Division of Family Planning
Director, Family Planning Fellowship
Emory University School of Medicine

Anne R. Davis, MD, MPH
Associate Professor of Clinical Obstetrics and Gynecology in the Department of Obstetrics and Gynecology
Co-Director, Fellowship in Family Planning and Contraceptive Research
Columbia University Medical Center

Gillian Dean, MD, MPH
Assistant Professor, Department of Obstetrics, Gynecology and Reproductive Science
Mount Sinai School of Medicine
Associate Medical Director of Clinical Research and Training
Planned Parenthood of New York City

Alison Edelman, MD, MPH
Associate Professor, Department of Obstetrics and Gynecology
Co-Director, Family Planning Fellowship
Oregon Health & Science University

Mary Fjerstad, NP, MHS
Director of Medical Affairs and Pharmacovigilance
WomanCare Global

Henry L. Gabelnick, PhD
Executive Director
CONRAD

Alisa B. Goldberg, MD, MPH
Associate Professor, Obstetrics, Gynecology & Reproductive Biology
Harvard Medical School
Director, Division of Family Planning and Family Planning Fellowship
Brigham and Women's Hospital
Director, Clinical Research and Training
Planned Parenthood League of Massachusetts

Katherine A. Guthrie, FRCOG, FFSRH
Consultant Gynecologist
Hull Community Health Care Partnership, UK
Clinical Director
Hull and East Riding Sexual and Reproductive Healthcare Partnership, UK

Bryna Harwood, MD, MS
Associate Professor, Department of Obstetrics and Gynecology
Director, Section of Family Planning
Director, Family Planning Fellowship
University of Illinois at Chicago

Jenny A. Higgins, PhD, MPH
Assistant Professor
Department of Gender and Women's Studies
University of Wisconsin-Madison

Melody Y. Hou, MD, MPH, FACOG
Assistant Professor
Department of Obstetrics and Gynecology
Boston University School of Medicine/Boston Medical Center

Victoria H. Jennings, PhD
Professor, Obstetrics and Gynecology,
Georgetown University Medical Center
Director, Institute for Reproductive Health
Georgetown University

Kathy I. Kennedy, DrPH, MA
Associate Clinical Professor of Community and Behavioral Health,
Colorado School of Public Health
University of Colorado Denver
Director, Regional Institute for Health and Environmental Leadership
University of Denver

Jeanne M. Marrazzo, MD, MPH
Professor, Division of Allergy and Infectious Diseases
University of Washington
Medical Director, Seattle STD/HIV Prevention Training Center

Kavita Nanda, MD, MHS
Medical Scientist, Clinical Sciences Department
FHI 360
Consulting Associate, Department of Obstetrics and Gynecology
Duke University Medical Center

Maureen Paul, MD, MPH, FACOG
Associate Clinical Professor, Department of Obstetrics, Gynecology, and
Reproductive Sciences
Mt. Sinai School of Medicine
Chief Medical Officer, Planned Parenthood of New York City

Herbert B. Peterson, MD
Kenan Distinguished Professor and Chair,
Department of Maternal and Child Health,
UNC Gillings School of Global Public Health
Professor, Department of Obstetrics and Gynecology
UNC School of Medicine,
The University of North Carolina at Chapel Hill

Elizabeth G. Raymond, MD, MPH
Senior Medical Associate
Gynuity Health Projects

Danielle Roncari, MD
Instructor
Department of Obstetrics and Gynecology
Boston University School of Medicine/Boston Medical Center

John Santelli, MD, MPH
Harriet and Robert H Heilbrunn Professor
Chair, Heilbrunn Department of Population and Family Health
Mailman School of Public Health
Columbia University

Jill Schwartz, MD
Medical Director, CONRAD
Associate Research Professor, Obstetrics and Gynecology
Eastern Virginia Medical School

Eleanor Bimla Schwarz, MD, MS
Associate Professor, Department of Medicine, Epidemiology
Obstetrics, Gynecology, and Reproductive Sciences
Clinical and Translational Science Institute
University of Pittsburgh

Lee P. Shulman, MD
The Anna Ross Lapham Professor in Obstetrics and Gynecology
Chief, Division of Clinical Genetics
Co-Director, Northwestern Ovarian Cancer Early Detection and
Prevention Program
Director, Cancer Genetics Program
Feinberg School of Medicine of Northwestern University

Adjunct Professor, Department of Medicinal Chemistry and
Pharmacognosy
University of Illinois at Chicago College of Pharmacy

Tara Stein, MD, MPH
Assistant Professor, Department of Family and Social Medicine
Albert Einstein College of Medicine

Primary Care Provider, School Health Program
Montefiore Medical Center

Markus J. Steiner, PhD, MSPH
Senior Epidemiologist
FHI 360

Lee Warner, PhD, MPH
Associate Director for Science
Division of Reproductive Health
Centers for Disease Control and Prevention

Erin Wheeler, MPH
Heilbrunn Department of Population and Family Health
Mailman School of Public Health
Columbia University

Reviewers

Rebecca H. Allen, MD, MPH
Assistant Professor of Obstetrics and Gynecology
The Warren Alpert Medical School of Brown University

Paul Blumenthal, MD, MPH
Professor of Obstetrics and Gynecology
Stanford University School of Medicine

Lynn Borgatta, MD, MPH
Professor, Obstetrics and Gynecology
Boston University School of Medicine

Talcott Camp, JD
Deputy Director
ACLU Reproductive Freedom Project

Kelly Cleland, MPA, MPH
Office of Population Research
Princeton University

Eve Espey, MD, MPH
Professor and Associate Dean of Students
Department of OB-GYN
University of New Mexico

Mary Fjerstad, NP, MHS
Director of Medical Affairs and Pharmacovigilance
WomanCare Global

Maria F. Gallo, PhD
Senior Service Fellow
Division of Reproductive Health
Centers for Disease Control and Prevention

Marji Gold, MD
Professor, Family and Social Medicine
Director, Family Planning Fellowship
The Center for Reproductive Health Education in Family Medicine
Albert Einstein College of Medicine/Montefiore Medical Center

Cynthia A. Graham, PhD
Lecturer
Department of Psychology
Brunel University
Research Fellow
The Kinsey Institute for Research in Sex, Gender, and Reproduction

Michael J. K. Harper, PhD, ScD
Professor Emeritus Dept of Ob-Gyn
Eastern Virginia Medical School

Jenny A. Higgins, PhD, MPH
Assistant Professor
Heilbrunn Department of Population and Family Health
Columbia University, Mailman School of Public Health

Melody Hou, MD, MPH
Instructor
Department of Obstetrics and Gynecology
Boston University School of Medicine/Boston Medical Center

Rachel K. Jones, Ph.D
Senior Research Associate
Guttmacher Institute

Tjeerd Korver, PhD
Head Global Clinical Research Contraception
Organon Biosciences/MSD
Oss, The Netherlands

Miriam Labbok, MD, MPH, IBCLC, FABM
Professor, Department of Maternal and Child Health
Director, Carolina Global Breastfeeding Institute
Gillings School of Global Public Health
University of North Carolina-Chapel Hill

E. Steve Lichtenberg, MD, MPH
Associate Professor of Clinical OB-GYN
Northwestern University Feinberg School of Medicine

Kathleen A. Marinelli, MD, IBCLC, FABM, FAAP
Lactation Services, Connecticut Children's Medical Center
Neonatology, Connecticut Children's Medical Center
Associate Professor of Pediatrics, University of CT School of Medicine

Elizabeth Raymond, MD, MPH
Senior Medical Associate
Gynuity Health Projects

Matthew Reeves, MD, MPH
Vice President, Medical Affairs
WomanCare Global

Sharon Schnare, MSN, FNP, CNM, FAANP
Clinical Instructor, Department of Family and Child Nursing
University of Washington School of Nursing

Markus Steiner, PhD, MSPH
Senior Epidemiologist
FHI 360

Katherine M. Stone, MD
Medical Epidemiologist

Phillip Stubblefield, MD, PhD
Emeritus Professor of Obstetrics and Gynecology
Boston University School of Medicine

Lee Warner, PhD, MPH
Associate Director for Science
Division of Reproductive Health
Centers for Disease Control and Prevention

Kimberly Workowski, MD
Professor of Medicine, Emory University
Division of Infectious Diseases

Team Lead, Guidelines Unit, Epidemiology and Surveillance Branch
Division of STD Prevention, CDC

Contraceptive Technology

Sexuality and Contraception

Jenny A. Higgins, PhD, MPH
Anne R. Davis, MD, MPH

- The overwhelming majority of people, including adolescents, have sexual experiences, and the range of normal sexual behaviors is large.

- Sexuality is culturally situated; even innate aspects of sexuality (for example, libido) are strongly influenced by social factors.

- Gender influences sexual behaviors and attitudes, including definitions and treatments of sexual "problems" within the reproductive health field.

- Surprisingly, research rarely considers how contraception affects sex for women. Some studies do explore how contraceptive methods (especially combined oral contraceptives [COCs]) influence sexual experience. During COC use, some women experience a decreased interest in sex, although whether COCs cause that decrease remains unclear. Other women experience increases in sexual desire and enjoyment while using COCs or other methods.

- Clients want practitioners to be more open with them about sexuality.

Sex is primary to our work—indeed, the reproductive health field would be non-existent without it. Yet many of us remain under-informed about sexual functioning, including contraception's impact on sex, and sex's impact on contraception. Sexual messages saturate our culture, but dialogue about sexuality remains virtually nonexistent in the exam room. Few of us feel sexually fluent, able to speak with our clients and colleagues about sex in a respectful but comfortable way.[1] Continuing medical education offers few tools to improve clinicians' sexual fluency. Even practitioners well-versed in sexuality research may become nervous speaking with clients about sex; we eagerly assume that people prefer privacy. Contraceptives are designed to be used specifically in and for the sexual experience, yet our contraceptive research often excludes sexually relevant outcomes.

As individuals, we focus on sex's potential for pleasure, forming relationships, and building identity. But our professional roles redirect our focus to the negative consequences of sex: the risk and threat of exposure to conception, disease, or violence.[2,3] The perceived dangers of sexuality (versus its healthy pleasures) become even more pronounced in our work with adolescents. This *pleasure deficit*[4] characterizes contraceptive research and development, acceptability studies, and marketing. Additionally, we maintain different standards by gender. We would find incomplete, even invalid, a study of hormonal-based contraception for men that ignored effects on erectile functioning or orgasm. Yet contraceptive methods developed for women rarely receive similar consideration regarding sexual functioning and enjoyment, whether currently on the market or in the research and development phase.

A positive and proactive approach to women's sexuality should matter greatly to family planning practitioners and researchers. First, in a practical way, understanding the sexual context informs clinical conversations that help couples choose suitable contraceptive methods. Addressing the notion that *the way sex feels matters to women* could have extraordinarily positive, even revolutionary, impact on contraceptive practices; it would also acknowledge women as sexual agents rather than merely as "targets" of contraceptive programs.

Second, clients *want* us to care about sexuality. Most women wish to discuss sexual concerns but report that most providers neither inquire about nor follow up on sexual issues.[5] In one study of 1,500 routine gynecologic patients, 78% said they wanted to discuss their sexual concerns, but 70% of these women reported feeling too embarrassed to bring up the topic with their physician. The overwhelming majority (89%) said they would have discussed sexual concerns had their physician initiated the topic.[6]

A final reason to promote positive sexuality concerns a potential direct impact on unintended pregnancy and sexually transmitted infections (STIs). Cross-cultural comparisons between Western European nations and the United States indicate that greater candidness about sexuality in the former relates to an improved overall sexual experience,[7] which may contribute to increased contraceptive use, reduced STI acquisition, and lower rates of unintended pregnancy.[8-10] As family planning practitioners, we have the opportunity to be pioneers of greater sexual openness and improved sexual and reproductive health at the national level.

In this chapter, we first review epidemiological and theoretical highlights from the sexuality field. Then, we describe burgeoning research that examines connections between women's sexual experience and contraceptive acceptability and practices. We conclude with resources to assist practitioners in addressing sexuality during clinical encounters.

Please note three important caveats to this chapter. We do not include a comprehensive discussion of the sexual response cycle and sexual dysfunction, as authoritative guides on those topics can be found elsewhere.[11] Second, we refer you to Chapter 5 for a discussion of sexual abstinence. In the current chapter we focus on vaginal intercourse, since this sexual behavior is most pertinent to contraception and the acquisition of STIs and is the most common sexual behavior, by far, among heterosexual couples.[12] Finally, although the term *sex* can refer to many activities (both with and without a partner),[13] here we—like our clients—generally use this term as a euphemism for vaginal intercourse.

SEXUALITY 101: SEXUAL BEHAVIOR IN SOCIAL CONTEXTS

Although sex appears to be a biological and physical activity, it is deeply set in our social and cultural context, and it becomes symbolic of the various attitudes and values to which our culture subscribes.[14] Behaviors that we consider second nature are also *social* in nature. Even practices like kissing, primal to sexual expression in the West, are not uniformly practiced across cultures. Sexual normalcy varies greatly, not only across the globe but also across socio-demographic groups within our society. In this section, we review some typical sexual behavior patterns, linking them to contraceptive practice wherever possible, but we remind readers that any single sexual behavior is ensconced in multiple layers of social meaning.

Gender in particular influences virtually all aspects of sexual attitudes and experiences.[15] Social movements in the 20th century, including the sexual revolution and the feminist movement, transitioned women and men into more egalitarian relationships and roles in virtually all spheres of our society. Women now enjoy more sexual autonomy and, arguably, more sexual satisfaction than at any other moment in U.S. history. But many women still cannot capitalize on their right to enjoyable sex.[16] Girls are socialized to protect and preserve their sexuality; by contrast, boys learn that they have the right to pleasurable sex.[17,18] Some young women report that unprotected intercourse "just happened"; preparing for sex would mean acknowledging they are sexual.[19] In order to justify their sexual interests, women may also feel the need to be swept away by passionate, romantic feelings,[20] a phenomenon that can also undermine successful contraceptive use. More concerning, women's risks of sexual harm, (which include harm from STIs and unintended pregnancy as well as damage to one's reputation, sexual manipulation and coercion, and

Table 1–1 Statistics on sexual violence and coercion in the United States

	Men	Women
Ever raped* and/or physically assaulted by a current or former partner.[22]	7.5%	25.0%
Ever physically assaulted** by intimate partner.[23]	7.4%	22.1%
Stalked sometime during life.[23]	2.2%	8.1%
Proportion of murder victims killed by an intimate partner.[24]	4.0%	33.0%

* Rape was defined as penetration of vagina, anus or mouth without the victim's consent
** Physical assault was defined as behaviors that threaten, attempt, or actually inflict physical harm.

outright assault and incest), far outweigh those faced by men (see Table 1–1). Men may also sabotage women's contraceptive attempts, another form of sexual coercion.[21] These gender inequalities dramatically shape women's sexual interest, enjoyment, and motivations to use contraception.

Despite these discouraging gender disparities regarding sexual violence and coercion, we need to remember that women, too, are sexual beings who want to enjoy sex. We would be remiss to ignore how gender inequality and sexual violence drastically undermine women's sexual health; however, we would be equally remiss to ignore the positive aspects of women's sexual experiences and factors contributing to optimal sexual functioning. (For example, a number of women may regularly experience multiple orgasms during sexual activity—a phenomenon not generally experienced by men.) Furthermore, as practitioners, we have the opportunity to promote better sexual well-being not only as a desirable outcome in itself, but also for its connection to better contraceptive use. Preliminary research links some forms of sexual expression with other health indicators. Young women who masturbate, for example, are more likely to report consistent contraceptive use and positive communication with their partners than those who have not masturbated.[25] In a recent nationally representative internet-based survey, women who used vibrators currently or in the past were significantly more likely to have had a gynecological exam during the past year than women who had never used vibrators.[26] In other words, there are good clinical reasons to invest in women's pleasure.

"TYPICAL" SEXUAL BEHAVIORS

Unfortunately, research on sexuality remains underfunded. Very few nationally representative, population-based surveys inform our knowledge of sexual behavior, and research on sexuality can be even more socially biased than other types of behavioral research. Before the recent nationally representative sexuality study by researchers at Indiana University,[1-10] the last such U.S. study, the National Health and Social Life Survey (NHSLS) of 3,400 men and women aged 18 to 59 years, was conducted in 1994,[12] before the dawn of text messaging and Facebook, let alone sexual technologies such as Viagra or the HPV vaccine. The NHSLS found, surprisingly, that Americans reported less sex and fewer partners than widely believed.[27,28] The overwhelming majority of respondents (83%) had either no partner or 1 partner in the previous year, and most people had engaged in partnered sexual activity only a few times in the last month. One half of both men and women reported 3 or fewer partners in their lifetime, and though men reported more lifetime partners, the gender difference was relatively small. Thus, at least based on NHSLS data, most Americans' sex lives occur in the context of monogamous, long-term relationships. Vaginal intercourse occurred in nearly all adult heterosexual encounters, indicating an ongoing risk of pregnancy in most fertile couples. Unfortunately, this survey did not include adolescents, who may differ in important ways from adults.[29]

Indiana University's more recent National Survey of Sexual Health and Behavior (NSSHB)[1-10] showed enormous variability in the sexual repertoires of U.S. adults. Adult respondents described more than 40 combinations of sexual activity at their most recent sexual event, and most respondents engaged in at least two sex acts.[9] Although the largest proportion of adults reported vaginal intercourse in the past month, investigators noted that most Americans' reproductive years hardly focused on vaginal intercourse alone. Sizeable proportions of 18 to 49-year-old respondents reported solo masturbation, partnered masturbation, oral sex, and anal sex. Compared to the NHSLS data, more men and women had engaged in oral sex and a significantly greater portion had engaged in anal sex—most of whom were represented in the younger cohorts. The NSSHB also found that a decreasing proportion of men reported engaged in vaginal intercourse across the life span, which may indicate growing incidence of erectile dysfunction related to cardiovascular disease or diabetes. Women also reported decreasing sexual activity across the life span, which may reflect intercourse-related pain, lower libido, or other sexual health concerns.

Sexual frequency. Clients sometimes worry that their personal sexual frequency is not normal. Some will be relieved to know roughly equal proportions of Americans reported sex with a partner at least twice a week, a few times a month, or only a few times a year, if at all. For example, among married couples, 13% reported having sex a few times per year, 45% reported a few times per month, and 41% reported 2 or more times per week. Among nonmarried women, 32% reported they had not had sex in the past year, 25% reported only a few times in the past year, 26% reported a few times in the past month, and 26% reported two or more times per week. In other words, wide variation exists in sexual frequency, and frequent activity is as common as little or no sexual activity. Age can also influence sexual frequency. A 1998 study indicated that 18- to 29-year-olds have sex an average of 112 times per year, 30- to 39-year-olds an average of 86 times per year, and 40- to 49-year-olds an average of 69 times per year.[30] Consider sexual frequency when matching clients with contraceptives. Condom use may be ideal for those with infrequent, irregular sexual activity. Adolescents and younger adults in particular may have very short sexual relationships and also benefit from reduced STI acquisition from condom use.

Onset of sexual activity. Adolescence brings sexual desires and experiences for most young people. The vast majority of U.S. adolescents are involved in dating relationships with at least some physical component: 85% have had a boyfriend or girlfriend, 85% to 90% have kissed someone, and 79% have engaged in "deep kissing."[31,32] The median age at first vaginal intercourse is 17.3 years for young men and 17.5 years for young women (remarkably similar to those in other industrialized countries),[33] and 7 in 10 U.S. adolescents have had vaginal intercourse by age 19.[34] Unfortunately, we have few reliable data on the age of first same-sex sexual experiences.

Unlike the NHSLS, the far more recent NSSHB did include adolescents. Investigators found that, at any given point in time, most U.S. adolescents were not engaging in partnered sexual behavior. Data indicated that young people who did engage in partnered sexual activity used condoms frequently. Among 14- to 17-year-olds in the survey, rates of condom use for vaginal intercourse in the last 90 day were 80% for young men and 69% for young women.[5]

Adolescent sexual activity is discouraged by many policy makers and professionals. Adolescents themselves, however, assign great meaning, importance, and positivity to their first intercourse experience.[35-37] Moreover, most sexually active adolescents are using contraception relatively well compared with adults. In 2002, at most recent sex, 83% of teen girls and 91% of teen boys reported using contraceptives.[34] These proportions represent a marked improvement; in 1995, only 71% of girls and 82% of boys had used a contraceptive method at last sex.[34] That said, compared to adults, adolescents engage in shorter-term relationships that may make effective contraceptive use more challenging. Many young women discontinue their hormonal method after a breakup, for example, when they do not anticipate being reunited with their partner. For young women, highly effective, long-acting reversible contraceptives (LARC) such as implants or intrauterine contraceptive may be ideal.[38] Clinicians should always speak with young people about condoms—not only for STI prevention, but also because condoms are overwhelmingly the method of choice for first intercourse experiences (66% of young women and 71% of young men reported condom use at first vaginal intercourse).[34] Water- or glycerin-based lubricants, either with or without condoms, may help overcome the discomfort and lackluster sexual satisfaction that young women in particular may experience.[39]

Same-gender sexual behavior. Alternative sexual relationships and identities are an important consideration for sexual and reproductive health practitioners. National estimates of same-gender behavior are elusive, due in part to variability in which questions and which persons are asked. The NSSHB found that about 7% of adult women and 8% of men identify as gay, lesbian, or bisexual, although the proportion who had engaged in same-gender interactions at some point in their lives was much higher.[9] In the NHSLS, 9% of men and 4% of women said they had a same-gender sexual partner at least once since puberty, but a greater proportion of women (5.5%) said they found the thought of having sex with a same-gender partner very appealing or appealing.[12] These figures are certainly lower than those of the non-random, controversial samples of Alfred Kinsey, in which 37% of the total male population had had at least one same-gender sexual experience and 10% of males had had exclusively same-gender relationships for at least 3 years.[40] (Kinsey never published comparable figures for women.)

Not all clients are heterosexually inclined, nor are they necessarily *homosexually* inclined if they do not identify as heterosexual. The sexuality field has increasingly embraced Lisa Diamond's notion of *sexual fluidity*. In this model, emotional connection, rather than gender, drives relationships; women in particular may flow in and out of sexual relationships with both men and women.[41] Young women may engage in sexual activity with other women at one point in their lives (e.g., during their university years), but chose men as their primary sexual partners at another life stage. Before making any contraceptive assumptions or recommendations, you may better serve clients by refraining from asking if they identify as heterosexual, homosexual, or some other orientation. Rather, ask about the gender(s) of the clients' current sexual partner(s), and whether they tend to be in relationships more with men, women, or both.

REASONS FOR WANTING—AND NOT WANTING—TO HAVE SEX

Many of us assume that most people want have sex for one reason only—because it feels good. But sexual researchers have been documenting an enormous array of sexual motivations, from relationship-building to stress-relieving to identity-building.[42] In their recent analysis of college students, Meston and Buss ranked the strength and intensity of 50 different sexual motivations (e.g., "I wanted to show my affection to the person," "I realized I was in love," "The person really desired me").[43] (The top three reasons were "I was attracted to the person," "I wanted to experience physical pleasure," and "It feels good".) Of course, these motivations are likely to change over one's relationship and life course. Another study tried to document some of the different varieties of sexual pleasures that people seek in sex, such as the pleasures of physical-erotic sensation, pleasing one's partner, spontaneity, and close, skin-on-skin contact.[44] In both studies, gender significantly shaped people's sexual motivations and types of pleasure-seeking.

Research must explore how sexual motivations and pleasures influence contraceptive practices. For example, women who are highly focused on men's pleasure are less likely to promote male condom use.[44] If a woman has sex to test her fertility (among other reasons), the motivation to use contraception will be minimal. At the very least, practitioners should recognize that clients have a range of motivations for engaging in sexual behaviors, which may be very different from those the provider personally experiences or endorses. Similarly, patients' sexual experiences with contraception may not match the expectations of providers. For example, a provider may insist that the woman or her partner will not notice a string from an intrauterine contraceptive during intercourse, but the woman may insist that the string is bothersome and request a change in method because of this discomfort.

There are also many reasons why people *do not* want to have sex. Several studies have thoroughly presented information on the dual responses of sexual excitation and sexual inhibition among women.[45-47] For example, fear of pregnancy often sexually inhibits women, and sometimes their male partners as well. Focus group participants in one study indicated that fears of pregnancy had a very negative impact on sexual arousal, especially when the partner did not share this concern.[48] Another recent study surveyed 5,609 adults about the degree to which the "risk of unwanted pregnancy" leads to loss of arousal. Just over half (53%) of women agreed that it did, although this proportion was greater among younger women and women in short-term relationships.[49] Notably, 37% of men in this study also said that the risk of unwanted pregnancy causes them to lose their arousal. Men whose ability to be aroused is affected by the risk of pregnancy may hold a key to effective contraceptive use. Indeed, practitioners are advised to promote the sexual benefits of contraceptives to *all* clients. Protection from pregnancy could be promoted as a way to enhance a couple's enjoyment of sex, especially among those whose arousal is diminished by pregnancy risk. Indeed, some women report enjoying sex more after menopause, when the threat of pregnancy is no longer a concern.

That said, some women (and men) may be sexually turned on by the idea of conceiving a baby with one's partner, even if a child isn't fully desired.[50] Others may be afraid that they can't get pregnant, and take deliberate risks of becoming pregnant even though they don't currently want a child. A recent nationally representative report from the National Campaign to Prevent Teen and Unplanned Pregnancy found that an astonishing percentage of 18- to 30-year-olds expressed concern about infertility: 59% of women and 47% of men reported at least some concern, and 19% of women and 14% of men reported *extreme* concerns.[51] Thus, while some might not be able to enjoy sex unless completely protected against unintended pregnancy, others may take deliberate procreative risks related to their confusion and anxiety about infertility. Discuss patients' concerns about fertility and thoughts about having a baby with their current partners.

SEXUAL PROBLEMS

Despite our interest in promoting positive sexuality, we recognize that many clients, if they bring up sexuality at all, are most likely to bring up sexual concerns or problems. See Table 1–2 for prevalence estimates of several sexual problems from two different U.S. studies. Prevalence estimates from the nationally-representative National Health and Social Life Survey (NHSLS),[12] presented in *JAMA* in 1999, were striking: 43% of women and 31% of men reported at least one sexual problem in the previous year.[52] The sexual problems measured included lack of interest in sex, inability to achieve orgasm, reports of sex not being pleasurable, anxiety about performance, trouble lubricating (women only), pain during sex (women only), climaxing too early (men only), and trouble achieving or maintaining an erection (men only). Sexual problems were most common among young women, older men, and nonmarried and poorly educated respondents. Importantly, respondents did not indicate whether these problems were persistent or distressing for them. The media have widely cited the 43% and 31% figures, which may dramatically overstate the prevalence of sexual "problems" in the United States. Many NHSLS respondents rated their relationships positively: nearly half of respondents described their relationships as "extremely" emotionally and physically satisfying.[12] The *Diagnostic and Statistical Manual of Mental Disorders, 4th Edition*, or *DSM IV*, stipulates a diagnosis of sexual dysfunction must include both personal distress and a disturbance in interpersonal relationships, neither of which was measured by the NHSLS. A national probability study in Britain, which compared the prevalence of short-term sexual problems with persistent problems (defined as lasting 6 months or more), found much lower rates of persistent problems than the NHSLS.[53]

Similar patterns were found in a more recent nationally representative study of sexual problems among women, and this study ascertained if women themselves were *distressed* by sexual problems.[54] Using a panel

Table 1–2 Prevalence estimates of common sexual problems in the United States

	NHSLS*		Shifren et al.**	
			Women	
				Distressed by
	Men	Women	Women	Problem
Lack of Interest in sex/low desire	16%	33%	39%	10%
Low arousal or arousal problems			26%	5%
Unable to achieve orgasm	8%	24%	21%	5%
Experienced pain during sex	3%	14%		
Sex not pleasurable	8%	21%		
Pain during sex	3%	14%		
Anxious about performance	18%	12%		
Climax too early	28%	10%		
Trouble lubricating		19%		
Unable to keep an erection	11%			
Premature ejaculation	29%			

* National Health and Social Life Survey (1994)[12,52,60]
**Shifren et al. (2008)[54]

study of 31,640 women, aged 18 to 102 (mean age of 49 years), researchers assessed measures related to desire, arousal, and ability to reach orgasm; they also used the Female Sexual Distress Scale (FSDS) to determine women's comfort or discomfort with their sexual functioning. The age-adjusted sexual problem prevalence was 42%, almost identical to the previously cited study in *JAMA*,[52] and approximately half of those women (22% overall) reported sexually related personal distress. The women most likely to report distressing sexual problems were poorly educated, ranked poorly on self-assessed health, and were more likely to have depression, anxiety, thyroid conditions, and urinary incontinence. A separate analysis of these data found that among those 10,429 women who reported "low sexual desire," fewer than 1 in 3 (27.5%), or 10% of the entire sample, reported sexual distress.[55] These sizeable gaps between the prevalence of sexual problems and the prevalence of any distress associated with those problems are important reminders of how the nature of a sexual problem depends on whom you ask, when, and in what context.[56,57]

Although they are legitimately distressing to certain individuals, reports of sexual problems must be considered within their social and cultural context. What we think of as sexually ideal for women and men has shifted over time, and it will continue to shift. For example, climaxing too early is considered a problem for men, but rarely for women; climaxing quickly may not have been a problem at all 150 years ago in our country, nor is it a problem in all other societies. Similarly, women's lack of orgasm has not always been considered dysfunctional.[61] Current social constructions of gender also shape how we think about low or high sexual desire. Today, female hypoactive sexual desire disorder (HSDD) is perceived as a problem, when decades ago, women were not expected to express or require desire.[62]

SEXUAL DESIRE

Over the decades, thousands of pages have been devoted to the topic of sexual desire, including renewed interest during the last couple of years—perhaps due to popular features in the *New York Times*[63] and the rise of investigational drugs to treat HSDD and low sexual desire in women. Researchers differ widely in their approaches to gender differences in sexual desire, with some positing biological and hormonal causes (including Masters and Johnson),[64] others adopting evolutionary models,[65,66] others social constructionist models,[67] and others integrative approaches of the three.[15] Still more recent research explores both biological and social aspects of the importance of *being* desired to women's (but not men's) interest in sex.[56,68]

Regardless of theoretical approach, most sexologists agree the relationship between arousal and desire for women is complex. Most men experience a relatively clear and direct sequence of desire and physical arousal, with interest in sex leading to physical changes that prepare one's body for sex (e.g., increased heart rate, respiration rate, and flow of blood to the penis). But for many women, no connection exists between physical arousal and their sexual desire, or *vice versa*. A woman may report that she is interested in sex, but without any physiological manifestations of such desire, or her body may indicate sexual arousal without any attendant interest in sex. For these reasons, Basson proposed that women's sexual response is more *cyclical* than *linear* in nature.[69] Unlike men, women may not necessarily experience desire before arousal. The incentive motivation model is similarly based on the notion that the experience of desire may follow rather than precede sexual excitement, and suggests that desire emerges following sexual arousal initiated by a sexually meaningful stimulus.[70] Women may not be thinking about sex at all, but once they are approached and sexually stimulated by their partner, they may become aroused and desire may then result. Women with such a sexual response profile who wish to experience sexual desire more regularly may want to consider the use of vibrators or erotic media to jump-start the connection between arousal and desire.

Not just the direction of sexual response, but also the question of who has more desire, men or women, has long been central to sexuality research. As measured by frequency of fantasy, masturbation, and sexual activity, current models suggest women have lower desire for sex compared with men. However, who has *more* desire may be less salient than the *quality* and *characteristics* of those desires, or how physiological responses interact with social context and relationship issues to shape sexual desire in various contexts.[71] Moreover, recent evidence suggests that women are aroused by a wider range of stimuli than are men—for example, women are aroused by pictures of women, men, and both heterosexual and same-sex couples, whereas men are most likely to be aroused by pictures of women and heterosexual couples only.[72] From this perspective, perhaps men are simply more sexually inhibited![63]

Scholarship on the history of sexuality challenges the notion that men's greater libido is an unchanging biological fact.[67,71] In certain historical moments and cultural settings, society portrayed *women* as having greater sexual appetites than men.[67] Women of color, historically and presently, have been depicted as more sexually animalistic than white women,[73,74] and therefore have been particularly affected by this perception. Such scholarship provides further indication that sexuality, including sexual desire, is shaped by social influences, and not merely biology or hormones.

We fully support developing effective treatment approaches for women who wish to increase their libido or arousal. However, we also question why male norms define what is considered low sexual desire in our culture. Imagine a different scenario: experts were concerned about men's pathologically high libidos, or drug and behavioral therapies were designed to help men recalibrate their desire to be more in line with women's. Perhaps we should accept a range of sexual desires instead of pathologizing one particular variety. Doing so would certainly alleviate much of women's distress over their sexual drive compared to men.

H OW CONTRACEPTIVES INFLUENCE SEXUALITY (AND *VICE VERSA*)

Given that contraception is expressly designed for sexual activity, we know astonishingly little about how contraception affects sexual functioning and enjoyment, and vice versa. Most sexual activity occurs during times when women wish to avoid pregnancy; women who wish to have only one or two children in their lifetime will need to use contraception for up to 30 years of their sexual lives. A vital area of understanding and expertise for family planning practitioners involves how women's sex lives can be changed in both negative and positive ways by contraceptive practices.

Unfortunately, a lack of attention to pleasure and positive sexuality undermines current understandings of the interplay between sexuality and contraceptive use.[4] Even though sexuality is a critical issue in research on the acceptability of contraception and STI prevention,[75] few systematic studies explore current methods' effect on women's libido, enjoyment, lubrication, or orgasm, or how such effects shape the uptake, continuation, and consistency of use. Researchers have thoroughly explored contraceptive side effects such as weight gain and vaginal bleeding, but rarely are such side effects explored as possible *sexual* detractors—despite their influence on women's experiences of their bodies, desires, and sexual selves. Moreover, though some sexual studies of individual methods exist (described below), few have examined multiple forms of contraception simultaneously, and despite exceptions,[44,76] even fewer have gone beyond individual experience to examine the cultural and social dimension of contraceptives and of what makes sex enjoyable.

The inattention to how women's contraceptive methods may affect sexuality is striking when juxtaposed with hormonal methods under development for men. Research on male-based methods is highly marked by concern for their effects on men's sex drive, orgasmic ability, and other sexual functions, with an implicit recognition that acceptability will be limited if men's sexual well-being is compromised.[77–79] The value placed on men's pleasure-seeking is also visible in research and programming on male condoms, the only reversible male method, other than withdrawal, currently available. Empirical literature reasonably suggests that many men do not like using condoms because they curtail sensation.[80–82] Severy and Spieler have described research efforts to develop latex and nonlatex condoms that make sex more pleasurable for men.[83] Until very recently, researchers have rarely considered the possibility that condoms may affect women's pleasure.

Yet an emerging body of literature has begun to explore how pleasure and sexual side effects can and do influence contraceptive practices for women. For example, in a study of the features most likely to shape contraceptive method choice, women ranked "lack of interference with sexual pleasure" as a "very important" consideration as often as men did (30% of men and 28% of women).[84] Similarly, in qualitative research on sexual pleasure and contraceptive use, the way contraceptives altered sexual aesthetics (sensation, libido, lubrication, spontaneity, and other sexual attributes) mattered strongly to both women and men and shaped both the choice of method and how they used their method.[44] However, gender influenced these sexual aesthetics in striking ways. For example, women reported disliking male condoms because they diminished their *partner's* pleasure, and thus their own. Women were often concerned about the sexual side effects of male condoms for their partners, whereas men expressed comparatively little concern about the sexual side effects of women's methods.

CONDOMS

Research increasingly demonstrates that the ways male condoms feel sexually matter to women as well as men. A 14-country study by the Joint United Nations Programme on HIV/AIDS found that men's most frequently reported reason for not using condoms was reduced sexual pleasure.[85] Comparatively, in an exploratory study of 189 U.S. women, 1 in 4 (23%) who had used condoms in the past month report decreased pleasure due to this method.[86] Moreover, studies from both the United Kingdom[87] and the United States[88] demonstrate that those women who felt that condoms undermined their sexual pleasure were less likely to use them than women who did not report condom-related reductions in pleasure. Furthermore, women's attitudes on whether condoms diminish arousal may influence use patterns more than men's attitudes do. In one recent survey of 5,600 adults in the United States and Canada, men were slightly but significantly more likely than women to report that "using condoms causes me to lose my arousal."[49] But *women* who reported condom-associated arousal loss were more likely than men to have had unprotected sex in the last 12 months.[49] Sexual health counselors and clinicians should acknowledge the importance of how condoms feel sexually to women.

Female condoms have been more widely studied than male condoms in regard to how they affect sexual experience for women. Some women enjoy the better heat transfer facilitated by the polyurethane female condom compared with the latex of male condoms, while other women have reported clitoral stimulation from the outer ring.[89–91] The greater attention paid to how female condoms affect sexual pleasure is not surprising, given that this technology originated from efforts to create female-controlled HIV prevention strategies rather than from purely family planning objectives.[92] (Theorists within the HIV field long ago developed models that acknowledged the role of pleasure for both partners in shaping behavior.[93]) Microbicide development has also taken women's sexual acceptability into consideration.[94–97]

COMBINED ORAL CONTRACEPTIVES

Combined oral contraceptives (COCs) entered the cultural marketplace 50 years ago and have been hailed as a key factor in facilitating this country's sexual revolution.[98] Since the approval of COCs, studies have explored if, and how, COCs affect sexual desire, enjoyment and functioning. (See reviews by Davis and Castaño[99] and Schaffir.[100]) Unfortunately, the impact of COCs, if any, remains poorly understood due not only to widely variable study methodology and quality, but also to confusion regarding the pathways of action. For example, sexual effects could result from hormonally mediated physiological changes in women's bodies, psychological changes (e.g., feeling more protected against pregnancy and thus less sexually inhibited, or feeling sure that the pill will lower one's sex drive), or a combination of physiological and psychological effects.[100] Furthermore, the majority of studies on pill use and sexuality have been cross-sectional in nature, an inherent limitation if one wants to understand the effects of the pill on sexual functioning and enjoyment over time.

Most research on COCs and sexuality examines libido. Oral contraceptives with estrogen reduce testosterone, and this change has been cited as a biological mechanism for reduced libido. A recent review assessed 30 different studies of this topic.[99] Most studies were retrospective and uncontrolled (n=17); these showed that a majority of women reported increased libido during COC use. Four small and uncontrolled, prospective studies showed little change in libido, and four prospective and cross-sectional controlled studies showed that compared with nonusers, women using COCs reported both increased and decreased libido. A prospective study following new COC users for 1 year (n=100) demonstrated that decreased sexual thoughts and decreased psychosexual arousability were strong predictors of COC discontinuation.[101] Among those 47% who discontinued COCs over the course of the study, these sexual side effects were the strongest predictors of discontinuation. This study cannot establish the mechanisms through which COCs may have contributed to lower libido, but it does highlight the importance of lowered libido to this sample of women using hormonal contraception and its effect on discontinuation.

Five randomized, placebo-controlled studies examined libido in COC users. None met every single standard for high quality reporting of randomized clinical trials (CONSORT guidelines[102]). Results were mixed, showing variable effects of COCs on libido. The most recent and well-conducted trial demonstrated a decrease in libido in COC users compared with placebo in a sample of women in Scotland (baseline libido was high), but not in a sample of women in the Philippines (baseline libido was low). All of these women or their partners were surgically sterile, so these results may not apply to women who use COCs for contraception.[103]

Overall, it appears as if COC users experience positive effects, negative effects, as well as no effect on libido. Nonetheless, in a minority of women, COCs seem to be associated with diminished sexual desire. Additional well-designed studies are needed to establish the independent, causal effects of COCs themselves, if any. Future research should also explore if differences in COC hormonal composition influence sexual functioning in diverse ways. Two prospective studies found differing effects of two formulations containing different doses of estrogen and types of progestins, one with decreased sexual desire, activity, and enjoyment[104] and one with improved lubrication, arousal, and dyspareunia.[105] Such differences should be explored in a randomized trial.

It would be unwise to base our understandings of the sexual side effects of COCs on any one of the above studies alone, given differences in study design, study population, and COC composition.[99,100] However, at least one consistent finding of *variability* emerges—women clearly vary in their sexual responses to COCs, and we understand little about the reasons for this variability. Individual women have different sexual responses and preferences, and COCs affect myriad facets of the sexual experience. For example, one recent study of condoms and hormonal methods found that while COC users were the least likely to report diminished sexual pleasure due to their contraceptive method, they also reported greater dissatisfaction with their sexual interest and had significantly lower sexual satisfaction levels than did other women, even when controlling for age, relationship length, and other factors.[86] Further research on this topic is certainly needed. We remain unsure of the precise mechanism through which COCs may affect libido. In a minority of women, COCs seem to be associated with a reduction in sexual interest. That said, since many women may experience reductions in desire *regardless of their contraceptive method,* providers should explore all possible reasons for problems with libido.

OTHER HORMONAL METHODS

Few data describe how use of rings, patches, injectables, and implants affects women's sexual functioning. Potential mechanisms for COC-mediated sexual effects (i.e., physiological and psychological) could be similar for newer hormonal methods that also combine estrogen and progestin. The ring is unique as the only hormonal vaginal contraceptive method. Data from clinical trials show that most couples find it comfortable during sexual activity, and for those who do not, the ring can be removed and replaced a few hours later without risking pregnancy. Some women may be hesitant to place a ring in their vagina due to concerns about correct placement or discomfort. Once placed, however, even women who do not use tampons or masturbate find the ring comfortable.[106] A study of Chinese women using four different forms of contraception (COCs, injectables, intrauterine contraception, and female sterilization) found that injectables were not related to sexual functioning or overall quality of life.[107]

Several studies have compared combined hormonal methods in regard to their effect on sexual functioning. Two small randomized studies that compared sexual functioning in ring versus COC users found improvements in sexual desire and satisfaction in ring users but not COC users.[108,109] In another recent study, COC users were randomized to either ring or patch use, and the Female Sexual Function Index, or FSFI, which includes domains on desire, arousal, lubrication, orgasm, satisfaction, and pain, was measured at baseline and after 3 months. Patch users experienced slight increases in overall FSFI scores. Contrary to prior literature and the study hypotheses, contraceptive ring users experienced modest decreases in FSFI scores, especially relating to arousal, lubrication, and pain.[110] Notably, despite sexual functioning changes, ring users in this study were much more satisfied with their method than patch users, indicating that sexual effects constitute only one part of overall acceptability.

Combined hormonal methods could improve sexual functioning via noncontraceptive health effects. As Davis and Castaño point out,[99] hormonal methods that inhibit ovulation can improve painful gynecologic conditions (e.g., endometriosis, dysmenorrhea, and ovarian cysts) as well as acne. Decreased pain and improved physical appearance could certainly improve sexual functioning, although these positive effects remain unstudied. Severy and Spieler have also suggested that contact between the penis, the ring, and the vagina or cervix may serve as a sexual stimulus to some couples.[83]

Changes in bleeding patterns due to any contraceptive method can also affect women's sexual expression, either positively (i.e., with a decrease in bleeding) or negatively (with an increase). For both personal and cultural reasons (e.g., religious proscriptions), some women avoid vaginal intercourse and to a lesser extent other genital contact when they are bleeding or spotting.[111] Such changes may reduce interest in sex and contribute to method discontinuation. And many women lose their arousal when the risk of pregnancy is present,[49] especially when partners are not equally committed to pregnancy prevention.[48] The excellent efficacy offered by implants in particular may very well lead to improvements in sexual confidence and disinhibition for many women, although few empirical data exist to prove this assertion.

INTRAUTERINE CONTRACEPTION

The high efficacy of intrauterine contraception (IUC, though often referred to as IUD, for intrauterine device) is also likely to influence sexual enjoyment, but few large studies document this or other sexual changes with IUC. A small randomized study found that, compared to other IUC users and women who used no contraception, Mirena users reported significant increases in sexual desire and arousal as well as significant decreases in pain during intercourse (dyspareunia).[112] Other studies have found no sexual changes, positive or negative, with IUC use. A prospective study in Spain found that sexual desire did not change with either use of COCs or IUCs, although it did diminish with age.[113] And a Chinese study found that IUC had no overall impact on sexual function. Neither study specified the types of IUC studied.[107] Finally, studies have demonstrated no change in lubrication during use of the levonorgestrel-releasing IUC.[114]

STERILIZATION

Surprisingly few studies assess the sexual acceptability of female and male sterilization, despite sterilization's rank as the second most commonly used contraceptive method in the United States. The bulk of studies on the sexual acceptability of vasectomy were conducted several decades ago, with most studies showing high sexual satisfaction among both sterilized men and their partners,[115, 116] but with others raising questions about the possible adverse sexual[117] and psychological[118] effects on men. A 2010 population-based study in Australia (N=3,390) found that sexual problems were equally common in men who had had a vasectomy and those who had not.[119] Men with a vasectomy (34%) were just as likely as other men (33%) to be extremely satisfied sexually; however, those with a vasectomy were slightly but significantly more satisfied with their relationships overall (48% vs. 43%).

Two informative studies of tubal ligation were conducted recently. In one large U.S. study, over 80% of the 4,576 women participants reported no consistent change in either sexual interest or pleasure after interval tubal sterilization.[120] Among the minority of respondents who did report consistent change, positive changes in sexual interest or pleasure were reported 10 to 15 times as often as negative effects. The women most likely to report negative changes were those who experienced poststerilization regret or postprocedure bleeding problems.

A more recent study of tubal ligation among a cohort of Australian women (N=447) found a similar relationship, and also highlighted a number of possible sexual benefits to sterilization—perhaps due to its wider measurement range of sexual effects.[121] Having a tubal ligation was not associated with any specific sexual problem, such as physical pain during sex or an inability to reach orgasm. In fact, sterilized women were significantly less likely than nonsterilized women to lack interest in having sex, to take "too long" to reach orgasm, to experience vaginal dryness during sex, and to find sex unpleasurable. Sterilized women were also more likely to experience extremely high levels of sexual satisfaction, relationship satisfaction, and sexual pleasure.

These two studies are reassuring for clinicians who provide sterilization. Overall, most women experience sexual benefits after tubal ligation. Sexual problems are uncommon and may be related to regret; women need to be sure they want permanent contraception before undergoing sterilization. Clinicians and counselors can highlight the possible sexual benefits of sterilization to their clients who are otherwise good candidates for this method.

WITHDRAWAL

Clinicians and clients alike tend not to think of withdrawal as a contraceptive method. However, researchers suspect that far more people are using withdrawal than captured by nationally representative datasets such as the National Survey of Family Growth (NFSG).[122,123] Further, the typical use failure rate for withdrawal (22%) is comparable to the typical use failure rate for male condoms (18%).[124,125] Most couples probably use withdrawal in conjunction with other coitus-dependent methods.[122,126] In keeping with the family planning field's general dismissal of this method, no studies to our knowledge have assessed the sexual effects of withdrawal among actual users. However, preliminary qualitative data indicate that some couples prefer withdrawal to condoms because it is easier to transition between various sexual activities (e.g., oral sex, vaginal sex, and back to oral) without having to apply or remove a condom or because of the taste of latex.[127] Other ethnographic work from both Italy[128,129] and Turkey[130] demonstrates how, in certain cultural locations and moments, "pulling out" successfully becomes an important badge of masculinity. Recognize that some clients may be using withdrawal even if not reporting it, and offer information about the method.

SUMMARY

On the one hand, the above review has underscored a dearth of literature and lack of attention to women's sexuality in the majority of contraceptive research. More research on the sexual acceptability of contraceptive methods is clearly needed, with equal concern for women's *and* men's sexual functioning for new and existing methods.[78] On the other hand, we have highlighted the growing number of research studies that do consider sexual aspects of various contraceptive methods for women. We strongly encourage practitioners to familiarize themselves with existing literature and help clients find a good fit with their sexual preferences and contraceptive method.

We would applaud more research of the sexual acceptability of IUCs and hormonal methods, but we also hope for a more innovative approach that taps into the sexual-improvement potential in contraceptive marketing and counseling. What if clinicians and contraceptive marketers were to tout the potential sexual benefits of methods? Existing contraceptive advertisements often portray women as empowered medical consumers but not as sexual agents. Ads promote convenience, efficacy, and noncontraceptive benefits (e.g., menstrual timing and regulation, acne improvement), but not their potential catalysis of pleasurable, worry-free sex. Sexual and reproductive health clients could be well served by investigations of the feasibility and benefits of eroticizing of contraceptives.[83] This trend can be seen globally in pleasure-centered sexual health promotion efforts, including the eroticization of safer-sex campaigns[131,132] (see also www.thepleasureproject.org). The contraceptive field should follow suit.

TOOLS & FURTHER RESOURCES
HOW CLINICIANS CAN HELP THEIR CLIENTS LEAD HEALTHY AND SATISFYING SEX LIVES

Include sexuality in discussions about contraception. Consider the sexual effects of methods, both positive and negative, when recommending them to clients. Identify sexual problems and explore whether sexual side effects led to discontinuation of methods in the past. Some clinicians may be reluctant to bring up sexual health if they feel unprepared to adequately handle patient concerns. An open conversation to identify problems may in itself naturally provide education and simple suggestions that help.

Clinicians who are not experts in sexual medicine *can* help women who experience sexual problems or dysfunction.[58] Treatment begins with an open, non-judgmental conversation. One sex therapy approach used by many nontherapist clinicians is called PLISSIT, which represents the four basic forms for sex therapy: permission, limited information, specific suggestions, and intensive therapy (explored more below).[59] The PLISSIT model gives patients permission to discuss the problem, validates their concerns as legitimate, and provides limited information and suggestions. The following simple educational interventions may be very helpful: normalizing sexual frequency, understanding a mismatch between the partners' libidos, suggesting use of lubricants, or explaining anatomy and relevant sexual responses. Primary care providers can use published algorithms for screening and treatment of sexual problems (for example, algorithms for Screening and Treating FSD, www.sexualhealthfundamentals.org). Women who need more indepth counseling for treatment can be referred to a qualified sex therapist; such therapists can be located via the American Association of Sexuality Educators (www.aasect.org). No FDA-approved medications are currently available for the treatment of sexual problems in women, although some are under investigation.

Clients report that practitioners rarely ask them about sex, despite the evidence suggesting that discussions about positive sexual experiences and satisfaction (and not merely sexual risk) yield significant benefits.[6,133]

Table 1–3 Questions clinicians may wish to ask clients about sexuality*

1. Sexual health is important to overall health; therefore, I always ask patients about it. Is it okay with you if I ask you a few questions about sexual matters now?
2. Have you been sexually involved with anyone in the past 6 months? *If yes*: With men, women, or both?
3. What kinds of things should I know about your sexual relationship or your sexual preferences so that I can provide the best care for you?
4. On a scale of 1 to 10, with 10 being the best, how might you rank your sex life right now? What do you think would have to change to bring it up to a 10?
5. How satisfied are you with your and your partner's sexual functioning?
6. Has there been any change in your or your partner's sexual desire or the frequency of sexual activity?
7. Is your current contraceptive method meeting your sexual needs? If not, why not?
8. Would you say that your current contraceptive method has improved your sex life, detracted from your sex life, or both or neither? How so?
9. What sexual concerns do you or your partner(s) have, if any?

* Some of these questions are taken from Nusbaum and Hamilton (2002).[133]

Some sexual health advocates have suggested medical schools should revamp their training in sexuality.[134,135] In the meantime, Table 1–3 contains some helpful questions to get you started. The Association of Reproductive Health Professionals (ARHP) has also created a series of resources on "sexual health fundamentals for patient care" (www.sexualhealthfundamentals.org), including guidelines on talking with patients about sexuality and sexual health (www.arhp.org/Publications-and-Resources/Clinical-Fact-Sheets/SHF-Talking).

To learn more about talking about with clients about sexual problems and solutions, refer to the following resources:

- The *PLISSIT model,* first developed in 1976 by psychologist Jack Annon.[59] The acronym PLISSIT represents the four basic forms of sex therapy: Permission, Limited Information, Specific Suggestions, and Intensive Therapy. The model, which suggests that most people with sexual problems do not need an intensive course of therapy, has been used by many clinicians over the years.[136]

- ARHP's guide on "Sex Therapy for non-Therapists" (www.arhp.org/Publications-and-Resources/Clinical-Fact-Sheets/SHF-Therapy).

- Sandra Leiblum's *Principles and practice of sex therapy.* 4th edition.[58]

- Maurice and Bowman's *Sexual medicine in primary care.*[5]

- Kinseberg et al.'s "Books helpful to patients with sexual and marital problems."[137]

To locate a trained, qualified sex therapist:

- American Association of Sexuality Educators Counselors and Therapists (www.aasect.org)

Other sex-positive educational and erotic resources:

- www.thepleasureproject.org
- www.goodvibrations.com
- www.evesgarden.com

REFERENCES

1. Pliskin KL. Verbal intercourse and sexual communication: Impediments to STD prevention. Med Anthropol Q. 1997;11:89–109.
2. Moore K, Helzner JF. 'What's sex got to do with it?': challenges for incorporating sexuality into family planning programs. New York: The Population Council; 1996.
3. Dixon-Mueller R. The sexuality connection in reproductive health. Stud Fam Plann. 1993;24:269–282.
4. Higgins JA, Hirsch JS. The pleasure deficit: revisiting the "sexuality connection" in reproductive health. Perspect Sex Reprod Health. 2007;39:240–247.
5. Maurice WL, Bowman MA. Sexual medicine in primary care. St. Louis: Mosby Year Book; 1999.
6. Nusbaum MRH, Gamble GR, Pathman DE. Seeking medical help for sexual concerns: Frequency, carriers, and missed opportunities. J Fam Practice. 2002;51:1–5.
7. Schwartz IM. Affective reactions of American and Swedish women to their 1st premarital coitus: a cross-cultural comparison. J Sex Res. 1993;30:18–26.
8. Schalet A. Adolescent sexuality viewed through two cultural lenses. In: Kuriansky J, Tepper MS, Owens AF, eds. Sex, love, and psychology: Sexual health (Vol. 3). Westport, CT: Praeger; 2007.
9. Schalet A. Raging hormones, regulated love: adolescent sexuality and the constitution of the modern individual in the United States and the Netherlands. Bod Soc. 2000;6:75–105.
10. Dodge B, Sandfort TG, Yarber WL, de Wit J. Sexual health among male college students in the United States and the Netherlands. Am J Health Behav. 2005;29:172–182.
11. Bancroft J. Human sexuality and its problems. 3rd ed. Edinburgh; New York: Churchill Livingstone/Elsevier; 2009.
12. Laumann EO. The social organization of sexuality: sexual practices in the United States. Chicago: University of Chicago Press; 1994.
13. Wynn LL, Foster AM, Trussell J. Would you say you had unprotected sex if . . .? Sexual health language in emails to a reproductive health website. Cult Health Sex. 2010;12:499–514.
14. Millett K. Sexual politics. 1st ed. Garden City, NY: Doubleday; 1970.
15. Schwartz P, Rutter V. The gender of sexuality. Thousand Oaks, CA: Pine Forge Press; 1998.
16. Reiss IL, Reiss HM. An end to shame: shaping our next sexual revolution. Buffalo, N.Y.: Prometheus Books; 1990.
17. Fields J. Risky lessons: sex education and social inequality. New Brunswick, NJ: Rutgers University Press; 2008.
18. Fine M. Sexuality, schooling, and adolescent females: the missing discourse of desire. Harvard Educ Rev. 1988;58:29–53.
19. Tolman DL. Dilemmas of desire: teenage girls talk about sexuality. Cambridge, MA: Harvard University Press; 2002.

20. Cassell C. Swept away: why women fear their own sexuality. New York: Simon & Schuster; 1984.
21. Moore AM, Frohwirth L, Miller E. Male reproductive control of women who have experienced intimate partner violence in the United States. Soc Sci Med.70:1737–1744.
22. Tjaden P, Thoennes N, U.S. Department of Justice. Extent, nature, and consequences of intimate partner violence: Findings from the National Violence Against Women Survey (www.ncjrs.gov/pdffiles1/nij/181867.pdf). Washington, DC: U.S. Department of Justice; 2000.
23. Tjaden P, Thoennes N, U.S. Department of Justice. Full report of the prevalence, incidence, and consequences of violence against women: Findings from the National Violence Against Women Survey. Washington, DC: U.S. Department of Justice; 2000.
24. Rennison CM, U.S. Department of Justice. Bureau of Justice statistics crime data brief: Intimate partner violence, 1993–2001. Washington, DC: U.S. Department of Justice; 2003.
25. Hogarth H, Ingham R. Masturbation among young women and associations with sexual health: an exploratory study. J Sex Res. 2009;46:558–567.
26. Herbenick D, Reece M, Sanders S, Dodge B, Ghassemi A, Fortenberry JD. Prevalence and characteristics of vibrator use by women in the United States: results from a nationally representative study. J Sex Med. 2009;6:1857–1866.
27. Davidson JK, Sr., Moore NB, eds. Speaking of Sexuality. Los Angeles: Roxbury; 2005.
28. Adelson J. Sex among the Americans. In: Davidson JK, Sr, Moore NB, eds. Speaking of sexuality. Los Angeles: Roxbury; 2005:40–45.
29. Ott MA, Shew ML, Ofner S, Tu W, Fortenberry JD. The influence of hormonal contraception on mood and sexual interest among adolescents. Arch Sex Behav. 2008;37:605–613.
30. Piccinino LJ, Mosher WD. Trends in contraceptive use in the United States: 1982–1995. Fam Plann Perspect. 1998;30:4–10, 46.
31. Coles R, Stokes F. Sex and the American teenager. New York: Harper and Row; 1995.
32. Haffner DW, Stayton WR. Sexuality and reproductive health. In: Hatcher RA, ed. Contraceptive technology. 17th rev. ed. New York: Ardent Media; 1998:13–41.
33. Wellings K, Collumbien M, Slaymaker E, Singh S, Hodges Z, Patel D, et al. Sexual behaviour in context: a global perspective. Lancet. 2006;368:1706–1728.
34. Abma JC. Teenagers in the United States: sexual activity, contraceptive use, and childbearing, 2002. Vital and Health Statistics. 2004;23.
35. Hawes ZC, Wellings K, Stephenson J. First heterosexual intercourse in the United Kingdom: a review of the literature. J Sex Res. 2010;47:137–152.
36. Carpenter LM. Gender and the meaning and experience of virginity loss in the contemporary United States. Gender & Society. 2002;16:345–365.
37. Carpenter LM. Virginity lost: an intimate portrait of first sexual experiences. New York: New York University; 2005.
38. Trussell J, Schwarz EB, Guthrie K. Research priorities for preventing unintended pregnancy: moving beyond emergency contraceptive pills. Perspect Sex Reprod Health. 2010;42:8–9.
39. Higgins JA, Trussell J, Moore NB, Davidson JK. Virginity lost, satisfaction gained? Physiological and psychological sexual satisfaction at heterosexual debut. J Sex Res. 2010:1–11.
40. Kinsey AC, Pomeroy WB, Martin CE. Sexual behavior in the human male. Philadelphia: W. B. Saunders Co.; 1948.
41. Diamond LM. Sexual fluidity: understanding women's love and desire. Cambridge, MA: Harvard University Press; 2008.
42. Meston CM, Buss DM. Why women have sex: understanding sexual motivations, from adventure to revenge (and everything in between). 1st ed. New York: Times Books; 2009.
43. Meston CM, Buss DM. Why humans have sex. Arch Sex Behav. 2007;36:477–507.

44. Higgins JA, Hirsch JS. Pleasure, power, and inequality: incorporating sexuality into research on contraceptive use. Am J Public Health. 2008;98:1803–1813.
45. Graham CA, Sanders SA, Milhausen RR. The sexual excitation/sexual inhibition inventory for women: psychometric properties. Arch Sex Behav. 2006;35:397–409.
46. Carpenter D, Janssen E, Graham C, Vorst H, Wicherts J. Women's scores on the sexual inhibition/sexual excitation scales (SIS/SES): gender similarities and differences. J Sex Res. 2008;45:36–48.
47. Milhausen RR, Graham CA, Sanders SA, Yarber WL, Maitland SB. Validation of the Sexual Excitation/Sexual Inhibition Inventory for Women and Men. Arch Sex Behav. 2009. 2010;39:1091–104.
48. Graham CA, Sanders SA, Milhausen RR, McBride KR. Turning on and turning off: a focus group study of the factors that affect women's sexual arousal. Arch Sex Behav. 2004;33:527–538.
49. Higgins JA, Tanner AE, Janssen E. Arousal loss related to safer sex and risk of pregnancy: implications for women's and men's sexual health. Perspect Sex Reprod Health. 2009;41:150–157.
50. Higgins JA, Hirsch JS, Trussell J. Pleasure, prophylaxis and procreation: a qualitative analysis of intermittent contraceptive use and unintended pregnancy. Perspect Sex Reprod Health. 2008;40:130–137.
51. Kaye K, Suellentrop K, Sloup C. The fog zone: how misperceptions, magical thinking, and ambivalence put young adults at risk for unplanned pregnancy. Washington, DC: The National Campaign to Prevent Teen and Unplanned Pregnancy; 2009.
52. Laumann EO, Paik A, Rosen RC. Sexual dysfunction in the United States: prevalence and predictors. JAMA. 1999;281:537–544.
53. Mercer CH, Fenton KA, Johnson AM, Wellings K, Macdowall W, McManus S, et al. Sexual function problems and help seeking behaviour in Britain: national probability sample survey. BMJ. 2003;327:426–427.
54. Shifren JL, Monz BU, Russo PA, Segreti A, Johannes CB. Sexual problems and distress in United States women: prevalence and correlates. Obstet Gynecol. 2008;112:970–978.
55. Rosen RC, Shifren JL, Monz BU, Odom DM, Russo PA, Johannes CB. Correlates of sexually related personal distress in women with low sexual desire. J Sex Med. 2009;6:1549–1560.
56. Brotto LA. The DSM diagnostic criteria for hypoactive sexual desire disorder in women. Arch Sex Behav. 2010;39:221–239.
57. Carvalheira AA, Brotto LA, Leal I. Women's motivations for sex: Exploring the diagnostic and statistical manual, fourth edition, text revision criteria for hypoactive sexual desire and female sexual arousal disorders. J Sex Med. 2010;7:1454–1463.
58. Leiblum SR. Principles and practice of sex therapy. 4th edition. ed. New York, N.Y.,: The Guilford Press; 2007.
59. Annon J. The PLISSIT model: a proposed conceptual scheme for the behavioral treatment of sexuality problems. J Sex Educ Ther. 1976;2:1–15.
60. Michael RT, Gagnon JH, Laumann EO, Kolata G. Sex in America: A definitive survey. New York, NY: Warner Books; 1994.
61. Heiman J. Orgasmic disorders in women. In: Leiblum SR, ed. Principles and practice of sex therapy. 4th edition. ed. New York, NY: The Guilford Press; 2007:84–123.
62. Jutel A. Framing disease: the example of female hypoactive sexual desire disorder. Soc Sci Med. 2010;70:1084–1090.
63. Bergner D. What do women want? Discovering what ignites female desire. New York Times. January 25, 2009: MM26.
64. Masters WH, Johnson VE, Kolodny RC. Human sexuality. 5th ed. New York: HarperCollins; 1995.
65. Buss DM. The evolution of desire: strategies of human mating. New York: Basic Books; 1994.

66. Fisher HE. Why we love: the nature and chemistry of romantic love. 1st ed. New York: H. Holt; 2004.
67. Laqueur TW. Making sex: body and gender from the Greeks to Freud. Cambridge, MA: Harvard University Press; 1990.
68. Meana M. Elucidating women's (hetero)sexual desire: definitional challenges and content expansion. J Sex Res.47:104–122.
69. Basson R. Women's sexual dysfunction: revised and expanded definitions. CMAJ. 2005;172:1327–1333.
70. Laan E, Both S. What makes women experience desire? Fem Psychol. 2008;18:505–514.
71. Tolman DL, Diamond LM. Desegregating sexuality research: cultural and biological perspectives on gender and desire. Annu Rev Sex Res. 2001;12:33–74.
72. Chivers ML, Seto MC, Lalumiere ML, Laan E, Grimbos T. Agreement of self-reported and genital measures of sexual arousal in men and women: a meta-analysis. Arch Sex Behav. 2010;39:5–56.
73. Hill Collins P. Black feminist thought: knowledge, consciousness, and the politics of empowerment. Rev. 10th anniversary ed. New York: Routledge; 2000.
74. Hooks B. Black looks: race and representation. Boston, MA: South End Press; 1992.
75. Severy LJ, Newcomer S. Critical issues in contraceptive and STI acceptability research. J Soc Issues. 2005;61:45–65.
76. Thompson M, Russell A, Sobo EJ, eds. Contraception across cultures: technologies, choices, constraints. New York: Berg; 2000.
77. Solomon H, Yount KM, Mbizvo MT. 'A shot of his own': the acceptability of a male hormonal contraceptive in Indonesia. Cult Health Sex. 2007;9:1–14.
78. Oudshoorn N. The male pill: a biography of a technology in the making. Durham, NC: Duke University Press; 2003.
79. WHO. Hormonal contraception for men: acceptability and effects on sexuality. World Health Organization Task Force on Psychosocial Research in Family Planning, Special Programme of Research, Development and Research Training in Human Reproduction. Stud Fam Plann. 1982;13:328–342.
80. Khan SI, Hudson-Rodd N, Saggers S, Bhuiyan MI, Bhuiya A. Safer sex or pleasurable sex? Rethinking condom use in the AIDS era. Sex Health. 2004;1:217–225.
81. Thomsen S, Stalker M, Toroitich-Ruto C. Fifty ways to leave your rubber: how men in Mombasa rationalise unsafe sex. Sex Transm Infect. 2004;80:430–434.
82. Crosby RA, Graham CA, Yarber WL, Sanders SA. If the condom fits, wear it: a qualitative study of young African-American men. Sex Transm Infect. 2004;80:306–309.
83. Severy LJ, Spieler J. New methods of family planning: Implications for intimate behavior. J Sex Res. 2000;37:258–265.
84. Grady WR, Klepinger DH, Nelson-Wally A. Contraceptive characteristics: the perceptions and priorities of men and women. Fam Plann Perspect. 1999;31:168–175.
85. Joint United Nations Programme on HIV/AIDS (UNAIDS). Men and AIDS - a gendered approach. Geneva: UNAIDS;2000.
86. Higgins JA, Hoffman S, Graham CA, Sanders SA. Relationships between condoms, hormonal methods, and sexual pleasure and satisfaction: an exploratory analysis from the Women's Well-Being and Sexuality Study. Sex Health. 2008;5:321–330.
87. Holland J, Ramazanoglu C, Sharpe S, Thomson R. The male in the head: young people, heterosexuality and power. London: Turfnell Press; 1998.
88. Ehrhardt A, Exner TM, Hoffman S, Silberman I, Yingling S, Adams-Skinner J, et al. HIV/STD risk and sexual strategies among women family planning clients in New York: Project FIO. AIDS Care. 2002;6:1–12.
89. Kaler A. The future of female-controlled barrier methods for HIV prevention: female condoms and lessons learned. Cult Health Sex. 2004;6:501–516.
90. Neilands TB, Choi KH. A validation and reduced form of the female condom attitudes scale. Aids Educ Preven. 2002;14:158–171.

91. Artz L, Macaluso M, Brill I, Kelaghan J, Austin H, Fleenor M, et al. Effectiveness of an intervention promoting the female condom to patients at sexually transmitted disease clinics. Am J Public Health. 2000;90:237–244.

92. Kaler A. The female condom in North America: Selling the technology of 'empowerment'. J Gender Stud. 2004;13:139–152.

93. Catania JA, Kegeles SM, Coates TJ. Towards an understanding of risk behavior: an AIDS risk reduction model (ARRM). Health Educ Q. 1990;17:53–72.

94. Bentley ME, Fullem AM, Tolley EE, Kelly CW, Jogelkar N, Srirak N, et al. Acceptability of a microbicide among women and their partners in a 4-country phase I trial. Am J Public Health. 2004;94:1159–1164.

95. Mantell JE, Myer L, Carballo-Dieguez A, Stein Z, Ramjee G, Morar NS, et al. Microbicide acceptability research: current approaches and future directions. Soc Sci Med. 2005;60:319–330.

96. Severy LJ, Tolley E, Woodsong C, Guest G. A framework for examining the sustained acceptability of microbicides. AIDS Behav. 2005;9:121–131.

97. Tanner AE, Zimet G, Fortenberry JD, Reece M, Graham C, Murray M. Young women's use of a vaginal microbicide surrogate: the role of individual and contextual factors in acceptability and sexual pleasure. J Sex Res. 2009;46:15–23.

98. Gibbs N. The pill at 50: sex, freedom and paradox www.time.com/time/health/article/0,8599,1983712,00.html#ixzz0mnCmwRoc. Time Magazine. 2010. Accessed May 2, 2010.

99. Davis AR, Castano PM. Oral contraceptives and libido in women. Annu Rev Sex Res. 2004;15:297–320.

100. Schaffir J. Hormonal contraception and sexual desire: a critical review. J Sex Marital Ther. 2006;32:305–314.

101. Sanders SA, Graham CA, Bass JL, Bancroft J. A prospective study of the effects of oral contraceptives on sexuality and well-being and their relationship to discontinuation. Contraception. 2001;64:51–58.

102. Moher D, Schulz KF, Altman DG. The CONSORT statement: revised recommendations for improving the quality of reports of parallel-group randomised trials. Lancet. 2001;357:1191–1194.

103. Graham CA, Ramos R, Bancroft J, Maglaya C, Farley TM. The effects of steroidal contraceptives on the well-being and sexuality of women: a double-blind, placebo-controlled, two-centre study of combined and progestogen-only methods. Contraception. 1995;52:363–369.

104. Caruso S, Agnello C, Intelisano G, Farina M, Di Mari L, Cianci A. Sexual behavior of women taking low-dose oral contraceptive containing 15 microg ethinylestradiol/60 microg gestodene. Contraception. 2004;69:237–240.

105. Caruso S, Agnello C, Intelisano G, Farina M, Di Mari L, Sparacino L, et al. Prospective study on sexual behavior of women using 30 microg ethinylestradiol and 3 mg drospirenone oral contraceptive. Contraception. 2005;72:19–23.

106. Schafer JE, Osborne LM, Davis AR, Westhoff C. Acceptability and satisfaction using Quick Start with the contraceptive vaginal ring versus an oral contraceptive. Contraception. 2006;73:488–492.

107. Li RH, Lo SS, Teh DK, Tong NC, Tsui MH, Cheung KB, et al. Impact of common contraceptive methods on quality of life and sexual function in Hong Kong Chinese women. Contraception. 2004;70:474–482.

108. Guida M, Di Spiezio Sardo A, Bramante S, Sparice S, Acunzo G, Tommaselli GA, et al. Effects of two types of hormonal contraception–oral versus intravaginal–on the sexual life of women and their partners. Hum Reprod. 2005;20:1100–1106.

109. Sabatini R, Cagiano R. Comparison profiles of cycle control, side effects and sexual satisfaction of three hormonal contraceptives. Contraception. 2006;74:220–223.

110. Gracia CR, Sammel MD, Charlesworth S, Lin H, Barnhart KT, Creinin MD. Sexual function in first-time contraceptive ring and contraceptive patch users. Fertil Steril. 2010;93:21–28.

111. Davis AR, Nowygrod S, Shabsigh R, Westhoff C. The influence of vaginal bleeding on the sexual behavior of urban, Hispanic women and men. Contraception. 2002;65:351–355.
112. Skrzypulec V, Drosdzol A. Evaluation of the quality of life and sexual functioning of women using a 30-mu g ethinyloestradiol and 3-mg drospirenone combined oral contraceptive. Eur J Contracept Repr. 2008;13:49–57.
113. Martin-Loeches M, Orti RM, Monfort M, Ortega E, Rius J. A comparative analysis of the modification of sexual desire of users of oral hormonal contraceptives and intrauterine contraceptive devices. Eur J Contracept Repr. 2003;8:129–134.
114. Suhonen S, Haukkamaa M, Jakobsson T, Rauramo I. Clinical performance of a levonorgestrel-releasing intrauterine system and oral contraceptives in young nulliparous women: a comparative study. Contraception. 2004;69:407–412.
115. Ferber AS, Tietze C, Lewit S. Men with vasectomies - a study of medical sexual and psychosocial changes. Psychosom Med. 1967;29:354-&.
116. Freund M, Davis JE. Follow-up study of effects of vasectomy on sexual behavior. J Sex Res. 1973;9:241–268.
117. Rodgers DA, Ziegler FJ, Altrocchi J, Levy N. A longitudinal study of the psychosocial effects of vasectomy. J Marriage Fam. 1965;27:59–64.
118. Wiest WM, Janke LD. Methodological critique of research on psychological effects of vasectomy. Psychosom Med. 1974;36:438–449.
119. Smith A, Lyons A, Ferris J, Richters J, Pitts M, Shelley J. Are sexual problems more common in men who have had a vasectomy? A Population-Based Study of Australian Men. J Sex Med. 2010;7:736–742.
120. Costello C, Hillis SD, Marchbanks PA, Jamieson DJ, Peterson HB. The effect of interval tubal sterilization on sexual interest and pleasure. Obstet Gynecol. 2002;100:511–517.
121. Smith A, Lyons A, Ferris J, Richters J, Pitts M, Shelley J. Are sexual problems more common in women who have had a tubal ligation? A population-based study of Australian women. BJOG. 2010;117:463–468.
122. Jones RK, Fennell J, Higgins JA, Blanchard K. Better than nothing or savvy risk-reduction practice? The importance of withdrawal. Contraception. 2009;79:407–410.
123. Rogow D, Horowitz S. Withdrawal: a review of the literature and an agenda for research. Stud Fam Plann. 1995;26:140–153.
124. Hatcher R, Trussell J, Nelson AL, Cates W, Jr., Kowal D, Policar M. eds. Contraceptive Technology, 20th Edition. New York, NY: Ardent Media; 2011.
125. Kost K, Singh S, Vaughan B, Trussell J, Bankole A. Estimates of contraceptive failure from the 2002 National Survey of Family Growth. Contraception. 2008;77:10–21.
126. Gray A, Chowdhury JH, Caldwell B, al-Sabir A. Coitus-dependent family planning methods: observations from Bangladesh. Stud Fam Plann. 1999;30:43–53.
127. Fennell J. Trying to plan for the future: understanding the contraceptive decisions of American couples. Providence, RI: Sociology, Brown University; 2009.
128. Schneider J, Schneider PT. Festival of the poor: fertility decline & the ideology of class in Sicily, 1860–1980. Tucson: University of Arizona Press; 1996.
129. Schneider PT, Schneider J. Coitus interruptus and family respectability in Catholic Europe: a Sicilian case study. In: Ginsburg FD, Rapp R, eds. Conceiving the new world order: the global politics of reproduction. Berkeley, CA: University of California Press; 1995:177–194.
130. Kulczycki A. The determinants of withdrawal use in Turkey: a husband's imposition or a woman's choice? Soc Sci Med. 2004;59:1019–1033.
131. Scott-Sheldon LA, Johnson BT. Eroticizing creates safer sex: a research synthesis. J Primary Prevent. 2006;27:619–640.
132. Philpott A, Knerr W, Boydell V. Pleasure and prevention: when good sex is safer sex. Reprod Health Matters. 2006;14:23–31.
133. Nusbaum MR, Hamilton CD. The proactive sexual health history. Am Fam Physician. 2002;66:1705–1712.

134. Rosen R, Kountz D, Post-Zwicker T, Leiblum S, Wiegel M. Sexual communication skills in residency training: The Robert Wood Johnson model. J Sex Med. 2006;3:37–46.
135. Wimberly Y, Moore S. Sexual history talking should be taught in medical school. Am Fam Physician. 2003;68:223–223.
136. Taylor B, Davis S. Using the extended PLISSIT model to address sexual healthcare needs. Nurs Stand. 2006;21:35–40.
137. Kingsberg S, Althof SE, Leiblum S. Books helpful to patients with sexual and marital problems. J Sex Marital Ther. 2002;28:219–228.

LATE REFERENCES

138. Sanders SA, Reece M, Herbenick D, Schick V, Dodge B, Fortenberry JD. Condom use during most recent vaginal intercourse event among a probability sample of adults in the United States. J Sex Med. 2010;7 Suppl 5:362-373.
139. Herbenick D, Reece M, Schick V, Sanders SA, Dodge B, Fortenberry JD. An event-level analysis of the sexual characteristics and composition among adults ages 18 to 59: results from a national probability sample in the United States. J Sex Med. 2010;7 Suppl 5:346-361.
140. Dodge B, Reece M, Herbenick D, Schick V, Sanders SA, Fortenberry JD. Sexual health among U.S. black and Hispanic men and women: a nationally representative study. J Sex Med. 2010;7 Suppl 5:330-345.
141. Schick V, Herbenick D, Reece M, Sanders SA, Dodge B, Middlestadt SE, et al. Sexual behaviors, condom use, and sexual health of Americans over 50: implications for sexual health promotion for older adults. J Sex Med. 2010;7 Suppl 5:315-329.
142. Fortenberry JD, Schick V, Herbenick D, Sanders SA, Dodge B, Reece M. Sexual behaviors and condom use at last vaginal intercourse: a national sample of adolescents ages 14 to 17 years. J Sex Med. 2010;7 Suppl 5:305-314.
143. Reece M, Herbenick D, Schick V, Sanders SA, Dodge B, Fortenberry JD. Sexual behaviors, relationships, and perceived health among adult men in the United States: results from a national probability sample. J Sex Med. 2010;7 Suppl 5:291-304.
144. Herbenick D, Reece M, Schick V, Sanders SA, Dodge B, Fortenberry JD. Sexual behaviors, relationships, and perceived health status among adult women in the United States: results from a national probability sample. J Sex Med. 2010;7 Suppl 5:277-290.
145. Reece M, Herbenick D, Schick V, Sanders SA, Dodge B, Fortenberry JD. Condom use rates in a national probability sample of males and females ages 14 to 94 in the United States. J Sex Med. 2010;7 Suppl 5:266-276.
146. Herbenick D, Reece M, Schick V, Sanders SA, Dodge B, Fortenberry JD. Sexual behavior in the United States: results from a national probability sample of men and women ages 14-94. J Sex Med. 2010;7 Suppl 5:255-265.
147. Reece M, Herbenick D, Schick V, Sanders SA, Dodge B, Fortenberry JD. Background and considerations on the National Survey of Sexual Health and Behavior (NSSHB) from the investigators. J Sex Med. 2010;7 Suppl 5:243-245.

The Menstrual Cycle

Lee P. Shulman, MD

The menstrual cycle represents a complex interaction of disparate organic functions, resulting in specific end-organ actions that permit and facilitate conception and allow for continuing human development. Until relatively recently, the menstrual cycle represented a poorly understood process replete with superstitious beliefs and ill-founded concepts that served to stigmatize women and encourage widely-held beliefs that women were, at best, inferior to men, and at worst, nonhuman and to be treated like animals. For example, Galen and Soranus, two well known Greco-Roman physicians whose writings form the basis for the development of modern medicine, viewed the need for a separate field of medicine for women because women were different from men (e.g., menstruation) and, in a concept similar to veterinary medicine, required a field of research and academic pursuits that would focus on the essentially nonhuman (i.e., nonmale) nature of female physiology and medicine so as to not sully the overall pursuit of medical knowledge for mankind.

Our ability to understand the process by which an ovum is made ready for conception and the resulting events that occur if conception occurs or does not occur is also seminal to the development of effective contraception, either by altering the cycle to prevent ovulation or by ensuring that a released and potentially fertilizable ovum is not fertilized. In addition, knowledge of the physiological processes that result in cyclical menstrual events is also necessary to develop approaches to contraception and to treat female infertility associated with deviations or abnormalities in various aspects of the cycle. This chapter presents an overview of the dynamics of the menstrual cycle as well as the physiological processes that allow most women to be able to conceive on a monthly basis and are the basis for developing effective and reversible contraceptive options.

THE NORMAL MENSTRUAL CYCLE

Menses involves the sloughing of a proliferated endometrial lining after the ovum fails to become fertilized. The menstrual cycle is comprised of four phases:

- Follicular phase, in which a single follicle becomes dominant and thereby available to undergo ovulation

- Ovulation, which serves to release an ovum ready for fertilization

- Luteal phase, in which progesterone is produced to support an early conceptus or, if conception does not occur, to begin the process of readying the various organs of conception for another attempt

- Menstruation, which is the sloughing of the endometrial lining and the bridge to the next cycle.

Variations in cycle length typically represent differences in the length of the follicular phase, which is dependent on the rate and quality of follicular growth and development. Variations in follicular growth occur in all women and are responsible for even small changes in the length of menstrual cycles from one cycle to another. Although the 28-day cycle is the most commonly reported cycle length and is usually mentioned as the prototype for all menstrual cycles, only 9% to 15% of menstrual cycles are 28 days in length, with differences observed in disparate racial, ethnic and socioeconomic groups.[1-3] Cycles are between 25 and 28 days long in over 40% of women aged 25 and in over 60% of women between the ages of 25 to 35.[4] Even in women who claim to have regular cycles, variations in the length of cycles and menstrual periods occur often, with 46% of respondents in a study (2004) reporting a range of 7 days or more. While there is considerable variation in cycle length, less than 1% of women have a regular cycle length of less than 21 days or more than 35 days.[2] In general, menstrual cycle lengths are shortest and have the least variability for women in their late 30s, which is likely the result of accelerated follicular growth resulting from changes in follicle stimulating hormone (FSH) and inhibin-B.[4] The cycle length begins to lengthen as women enter their 40s, likely the result of increasing follicle loss. Once the supply of follicles is depleted, menopause occurs and menstrual cyclicity ends, along with the ability to conceive. Menopause is defined as the permanent end of menstruation, and thus ovulation, occurring as result of the biologic process of gradual follicular depletion and its associated physiologic changes, or abruptly after surgical removal of the ovaries, or from the effect of certain chemotherapies on ovarian function.

THE BRAIN

Because the menstrual cycle involves a complex array of hypothalamic, anterior pituitary, ovarian and endometrial events, along with cervical and other organic changes, it is best to begin the review of this process by evaluating the organs, beginning with the brain. A visual overview of this process is found in Figure 2–1.

Hormone signaling within the brain stimulates production and release of gonadotropins that give rise to the menstrual cycle and fertility. The two gonadotropins most familiar to clinicians are FSH and LH (luteinizing hormone), which ultimately promote the appropriately timed production of *estradiol*, one of the estrogen hormones, and *progesterone*, a steroid hormone secreted by the ovary. Primarily responsible for follicular development, FSH activates the granulosa cells that line each follicle and causes them to proliferate and produce estradiol. LH causes ovarian theca cells to produce androgenic sex steroids (testosterone and androstenedione).

Hypothalamus

The hypothalamus enters the complex array of events leading to the menstrual cycle by secreting a neurohormone called gonadotropin-releasing hormone (GnRH). Synthesized in the hypothalamus and transported to the anterior pituitary by a network of dense capillaries that originate in the hypothalamus and drain into the portal vessels that empty into the anterior pituitary, GnRH is secreted in a pulsatile fashion every 60 to 90 minutes, stimulating cells in the anterior pituitary (gonadotropes) to produce the gonadotropins FSH and LH. Because there is no direct connection between the hypothalamus and anterior pituitary, any disruption of the blood flow between the two organs will prevent the pulsed production and secretion of gonadotropins.

In addition to the effect of GnRH on the production of gonadotropins in the anterior pituitary, hormones and proteins produced in the hypothalamus have positive effects on the production of thyroid-stimulating hormone (TSH), adrenocorticotropic hormone (ACTH), and growth hormone.[4] It is this neurohormonal milieu that provides us with the ability to clinically assess other physiologic processes (e.g., thyroid function) to determine if the hypothalamic function is providing an appropriate and properly timed production of necessary neurohormonal factors needed for the menstrual cycle. For example, thyroid abnormalities can be the result of hypothalamic dysfunction and be associated with menstrual irregularities and female infertility.[5] Drugs used to treat conditions such as epilepsy and bipolar disease can alter hypothalamic function and disrupt normal menstrual cyclicity.[6] In addition to its effect on the anterior pituitary, GnRH, being found in neural and non-neural tissues with receptors present in organs other than the pituitary, has autocrine-paracrine functions throughout the body.

Anterior Pituitary

The pulsatile secretion of GnRH stimulates gonadotropes found in the anterior pituitary to produce FSH and LH, two distinct compounds pro-

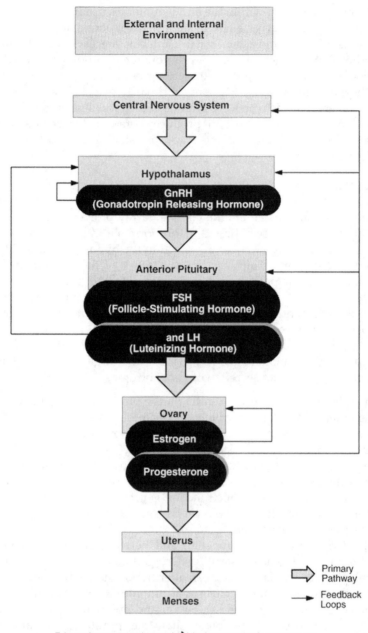

Primary hormone pathways (⇨) in the reproductive system are
modulated by both negative and positive feedback loops (➔).
Prostaglandins, secreted by the ovary and by uterine endometrial
cells, also play a role in ovulation, and may modulate hypothalamic
function as well.

Figure 2–1 Regulation of the menstrual cycle

duced by the same cell. GnRH activity causes only positive activity in the anterior pituitary, specifically, synthesis and secretion of gonadotropins. As one would expect from the pulsed secretion of GnRH, FSH and LH are also secreted in a pulsatile fashion, though not in the same pattern associated with the secretion of GnRH. Pulse frequency and gonadotropin levels are regulated by a complex system of sex steroid hormones, peptide hormones, neuroendocrine factors, and neurotransmitters that drive the positive and negative feedback mechanisms regulating the physiologic and clinical manifestations of the menstrual cycle and promoting conception and pregnancy.

THE REPRODUCTIVE SYSTEM

Ovary

At the early stage of the menstrual cycle, FSH stimulates the production of estradiol within the inner granulosa cells of the follicle, and LH stimulates the production of androgens by the ovarian theca cells. The androgens are then converted to estradiol by aromatase, which is produced by the granulosa cells. Appropriate androgen production serves as an important and vital source of estradiol during this early stage of follicular development. The production of ovarian estradiol from androgens is an interactive and intricately timed process: theca cells produce androgenic sex steroids, which then stimulate the granulosa cells to produce the aromatase that converts the androgens to estradiol, thus creating a positive feedback mechanism that provides essential levels of estradiol for follicular development and ovulation.[7]

Excess androgen production or failure to convert androgens to estradiol results in increased follicular atresia, which can prevent ovulation and result in changes in the menstrual cycle. Indeed, it is an ovarian androgenic milieu resulting from conditions such as polycystic ovarian syndrome (PCOS) which is associated with the commonly observed clinical presentation of anovulation and the characteristic lengthy and irregular menstrual cycles.[8]

The estradiol produced by the ovaries as result of FSH and LH secretion creates a negative feedback mechanism, suppressing further production of FSH and LH. However, once a particular level of estradiol is reached and maintained during the midportion of the cycle, the negative feedback mechanism changes to a positive feedback mechanism, initiating the preovulatory surges of FSH and LH, which are needed for ovulation to occur. While progesterone is mostly produced by the corpus luteum after ovulation, low levels of progesterone acting at the level of the anterior pituitary enhance the LH response to GnRH and are also integral to the FSH surge at midcycle. While the gonadotropes are the main cells involved in this dual mechanistic process, studies suggest that the hypothalamus and a variety of ovarian hormones influence this process, which seemingly has little tolerance for variation.[4]

The ovaries produce a variety of peptide hormones, many of which help regulate folliculogenesis, follicular atresia, and the feedback mechanisms involving estradiol and androgens. Activin and inhibin, produced by ovarian granulosa cells, are intimately involved in the regulation of FSH and thus the menstrual cycle. Expression of these peptide hormones is found in a variety of tissues, where they serve as autocrine-paracrine regulators of numerous physiological processes.[4] *Activin* stimulates release of FSH in the anterior pituitary and augments FSH activity within the ovary. Activin is also present in pituitary gonadotropes and consists of two subunits that are identical to the beta subunits of inhibin A and inhibin B. *Inhibin* suppresses the secretion of FSH, which serves to increase the production of inhibin, thus creating a simple negative feedback relationship. Inhibin also consists of two dissimilar peptides (known as the α- and β-subunits) linked by disulfide bonds. Two forms of inhibin (inhibin-A and inhibin-B) exist with identical α-subunits but different β-subunits; inhibin-B appears to be the predominant form of inhibin secreted by the granulosa cells. *Follistatin*, another ovarian peptide hormone, also serves to suppress FSH activity by binding to activin and reducing its ability to stimulate FSH.[4]

Other peptide hormones and neuroendocrine factors also influence the production, secretion, and function of inhibin, and thus play indirect though important roles in the regulation of FSH and the menstrual cycle. GnRH and epidermal growth factor (EGF) diminish the FSH stimulation of inhibin secretion. Conversely, insulin-like growth factor-1 (IGF-1), which mediates the growth-promoting actions of growth hormone, enhances inhibin production in the ovary. IGF-1 also amplifies LH-stimulated androgen production in the theca cells and thus may serve as a major regulator of theca and granulosa cell activities. It is postulated that increasing serum levels of inhibin-B further amplify the withdrawal of FSH from most follicles, thus creating an environment for an emerging follicle to become the dominant follicle. A plethora of hormones and neuroendocrine and growth factors is associated with the development of a dominant follicle and the ovulatory process (a more detailed description of the molecular and endocrine mechanisms is beyond the scope of this chapter). Nonetheless, it is clear that the process by which ovulation occurs is a complex, and perhaps wondrous, interaction of disparate neurological, gonadal, and end-organ processes that allow for the development and presentation of an ovum for fertilization.

Endometrium and Cervix

The endometrium responds predominantly to cyclic changes in estradiol levels. Proliferation of the endometrial lining is initiated by increasing serum levels of estradiol, a process by which a supportive environment for the implantation and development of the early embryo is begun. Estradiol increases blood flow to the endometrium and stimulates the formation of progesterone receptors on endometrial cells; the receptors are needed to commence the cellular differentiation necessary for the successful maintenance and development of the early conceptus. Indeed, much of this cellular differentiation is under the influence of progesterone, which counters the proliferative effects of estradiol on the endometrium by down-regulating estradiol receptors in the endometrium. The effect of progesterone thus serves to differentiate the proliferated endometrial cells and produce the necessary proteins and factors required for successful pregnancy.

Exogenous progestins mimic the physiologic effect of endogenous progesterone on the endometrium and can be used to develop clinical approaches to prevent and treat endometrial hyperplasia and abnormal uterine bleeding.

The increasingly estrogenic milieu in the time prior to ovulation influences the cervix and cervical mucus so as to facilitate the passage of sperm into the uterus by rendering the cervical mucus less thick and tenacious. Indeed, some women may mistakenly think the more watery cervical mucus is a discharge. It is also during this time that the cervix swells and softens as result of an increase in the production of endogenous prostaglandins. In addition, endogenous prostaglandins also lead to the dilation of the cervical os, which further facilitates the ability of sperm to pass through the cervix and into the uterine cavity, where capacitation occurs so that fertilizable sperm are available in the fallopian tubes for conception.[9] At other times of the cycle, the less estrogenic (and more progestogenic) milieu results in thicker cervical mucus that is less likely to allow for passage of sperm or microorganisms into the uterine cavity.

Exogenous prostaglandins are commonly used to soften the cervix and dilate the cervical os for a variety of clinical applications ranging from facilitating the onset and progress of labor to the insertion of an intrauterine contraceptive to the successful completion of an endometrial biopsy in a postmenopausal woman. In addition, the progesterone-mediated thickening of cervical mucus is the basis for one of the important mechanisms of progestin-only contraceptives.

PHASES OF THE MENSTRUAL CYCLE

The aforementioned physiological processes are geared to promoting ovulation, conception and maintenance and development of an early pregnancy. In women who are unable to conceive, evaluation of these pathways is critical to discovering an etiology for infertility. Conversely, the development of effective and reversible contraception has targeted specific pathways of the menstrual cycle to reversibly disrupt the overall process and prevent ovulation and pregnancy. The aforementioned processes lead to a sequence of distinct clinical events that either promote the implantation and support the development of an embryo or prepare the uterus and genital tract for another attempt at pregnancy in the next cycle. A visual overview of the phases and corresponding events of the menstrual cycle is found in Figure 2–2.

FOLLICULAR PHASE

In women not using hormonal contraceptives, the follicular phase begins after menses (which signals the completion of the previous cycle) and initiates a sequence of events in which a follicle becomes dominant and available for ovulation and conception and in which the endometrium develops and differentiates to become a suitable site for implantation and early embryonic development. In general, variations in the cycle length reflect variations in the follicular phase, as the length of the luteal phase (13 to 15 days) becomes relatively constant soon after menarche. Differences in the length of the follicular phase, which can range from 10 to 17 days in women with ovulatory cycles, have been associated with a disparate array of factors, including age, weight, and emotional distress.[2] At age 25, over 40% of women have cycles that range from 25 to 28 days, increasing to over 60% by age 35. Despite the widespread use of a 28-day cycle as the prototype for a normal menstrual cycle, only 1 in 8 to 9 menstrual cycles are actually 28 days in length.[4]

In the early part of the follicular phase (days 1 to 5), the increasing estradiol production in the ovary causes the stimulation, or recruitment, of several follicles. Ultimately, one follicle is selected to become dominant and undergo ovulation—becoming the selected follicle is based on its ability to produce the most estradiol. In a stereotypic 28-day cycle, the increasing levels of estradiol serve to recruit potential follicles; the selection of a dominant follicle occurs during days 5 to 7. At this time, FSH levels begin to decline as a result of the negative feedback mechanism associated with *increasing* estradiol levels, and all but one of the candidate follicles undergo atresia because of the subsequent *declining* levels of estradiol. The maturation of the remaining dominant follicle continues in the context of surrounding follicular atresia because of its ability to continue to produce high local levels of estradiol into the latter portion of the follicular phase. During the late follicular phase, an increase in LH

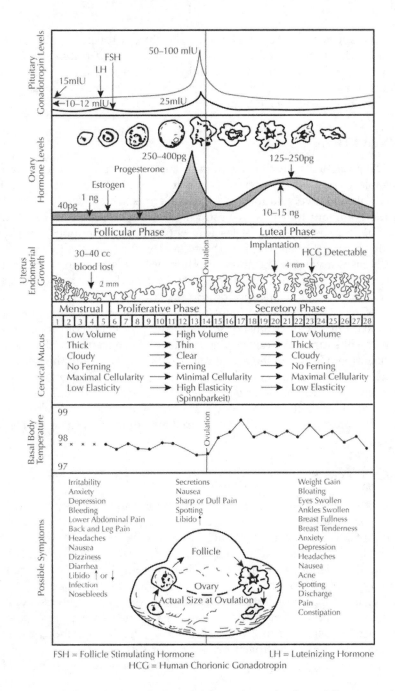

Figure 2–2 Menstrual cycle events: hormone levels, ovarian, and endometrial patterns and cyclic temperature and cervical mucus changes

activity spurs an increase in production of androgens in the ovarian stroma. Theoretically, this increase in androgens just prior to ovulation may serve to increase interest in sex in the woman and thus increase the likelihood of sexual activity at a time when a woman is most fertile, thereby increasing the likelihood of conception.[10]

OVULATION

The process by which conception occurs relies on the release of a fertilizable ovum, which occurs as result of ovulation. Ovulation is the result of a relatively sudden change in the mechanistic feedback control of the dominant follicle. Once estradiol reaches a specific elevated level (200 pg/ml sustained for at least 50 hours[4]), most commonly and optimally during the last days of the follicular phase, a positive feedback mechanism involving the anterior pituitary results in a surge of LH and FSH. It is this surge in gonadotropins that leads to a constellation of events that in the availability of a fertilizable ovum, including resumption of meiosis in the dominant follicle and luteinization of granulosa cells that initiate the extensive and requisite production of progesterone, which will support the development of an early conceptus in the event of fertilization. However, the actual release of the ovum from the follicle requires a series of other events, including the production of prostaglandins and proteolytic enzymes and the contraction of smooth muscle cells within the follicle. The oocyte and follicular fluid exude about 32 to 44 hours after the onset of the LH surge and 10 to 12 hours after the LH peak.

PREGNANCY

Conception occurs after ovulation if sperm capable of fertilization are present in the upper reproductive tract of the woman and an ovum capable of fertilization is available within the fallopian tube lumen. Because the ovum retains the potential for fertilization for only 12 to 24 hours, the likelihood of fertilization is increased if sperm are present in the upper reproductive tract when ovulation occurs; sperm remain viable and capable of fertilization for approximately 72 hours. Accordingly, fertilization is most likely to occur if semen enters the female reproductive system during the 2 to 3 days prior to ovulation, which is why an increase in androgen production at this time may be an important biosignal for sexual activity to occur and improve the likelihood of conception.[10]

Spermatozoa released into the vagina after ejaculation pass into the cervical mucus, a process that occurs in the first few minutes after ejaculation. Up to several hundred thousand spermatozoa can reside in the mucus found in cervical canal, which allows for the progression of spermatozoa through the uterine cavity. Capacitation, which incorporates the spermatic hyperactivation process necessary for sperm penetration, is needed for the development of fertilizable sperm from spermatozoa and thus is essential for fertilization. After ejaculation, thousands of sperm can soon be found in the fallopian tubes and upper uterus if there is no barrier to their ascent; however, this number represents only a relatively tiny fraction of the total number of spermatozoa deposited in the vagina after ejaculation. The process of sperm capacitation is estimated to be relatively brief (several minutes to 1 to 2 hours) but is asynchronous and transient, thus providing for an ongoing supply of fertilizable sperm after only a single intravaginal ejaculation.[11]

The ovum is released following ovulation, where it is gathered by the fimbria of the tube and swept into the tubal lumen within minutes to hours. Fertilization typically occurs here, specifically within the ampullary section of the fallopian tube, with the early conceptus remaining in the fallopian tube for 2 to 3 days before it passes into the uterine cavity. Fertilization in places other than the ampullary portion of the fallopian tube, as well as changes in the precise timing of this process, can lead to ectopic pregnancy. However, in situations not altered from the aforementioned process, implantation of the early conceptus (blastocyst) into the endometrium occurs 6 to 7 days following fertilization.

ANOVULATION

The awesome complexity of ovulation makes for a veritable myriad of potential deviations that can prevent ovulation. Indeed, systemic conditions such as obesity, anorexia, endocrinopathy, psychiatric illness, and medication use can prevent ovulation by interfering with pulsatile GnRH secretion, inhibiting gonadotrope activity, and altering the estrogenic and androgenic hormonal milieu. These numerous etiologies can also result in disease not related to ovulation; for example, women with polycystic ovarian syndrome (PCOS) are also at increased risk for metabolic syndrome and diabetes.[8] Accordingly, evaluating the cause(s) of anovulation can be tedious and difficult, leading some women who seek to become pregnant or obtain relief from the sequelae of anovulation to bypass the correction of specific abnormalities. Women who want to become pregnant may use medical or surgical interventions to obtain a fertilizable ovum (or ova). Women who want to have menstrual bleeding may choose to undergo an exogenous, hormonally mediated imitation of a normal menstrual cycle, or a cycle with unique characteristics (e.g., few to no regular withdrawal bleeding episodes) not typically found in normally cycling women.

LUTEAL PHASE

In the absence of fertilization, another process ensues to prepare the ovary and endometrium for the next follicular phase. After the rupture of the follicle and release of the ovum, granulosa and theca cells take up steroids and lutein pigment to give the corpus luteum, or "yellow body," its characteristic yellow appearance. The development of the corpus luteum shifts the cycle from an estradiol-dominant to a progesterone-dominant process. The considerable levels of progesterone suppress follicular growth and initiate secretory changes in the endometrium necessary for implantation and early development of the conceptus. Peak progesterone production occurs 7 to 8 days after the LH surge, which is roughly the time of implantation if fertilization has occurred. As opposed to the variable length of the follicular phase, the length of the luteal is relatively fixed at 14 days after ovulation, unless pregnancy occurs. One event that occurs as result of progesterone production is a rise in the basal body temperature, which is used to clinically predict whether ovulation has occurred.

MENSTRUATION

In the absence of pregnancy, menstruation—the sloughing of the endometrial lining—serves to create a new template for a new endometrial thickness appropriate for implantation of a conceptus and support of early embryonic development. Without pregnancy, the corpus luteum declines rapidly 9 to 11 days after ovulation, resulting in a commensurate rapid decline in progesterone and estradiol levels. The withdrawal of these hormones reduces blood flow to the endometrium, which serves to decrease the thickness of the endometrium. As the hormone levels decline, blood flow to the endometrium is further reduced by rhythmic contraction of the spiral arterioles. The resulting ischemia, interstitial hemorrhage, and loss of overall tissue integrity, along with increasing intrauterine prostaglandin levels, result in the commencement of uterine contractions and the expulsion of the sloughed endometrial lining, or *menstruum*. Thrombin-platelet plugs eventually reduce and eliminate the ongoing blood loss, along with the prostaglandin-produced uterine contractions, which serve to contract the spiral arterioles within the uterus and staunch the further loss of blood. However, in case of anovulation, this sloughing process may not be as complete as when there is ovulation, so anovulatory cycles result in prolonged and heavier bleeding.

The blood loss experienced by women varies greatly from individual to individual and from cycle to cycle. The average duration of menses is 4 to 6 days, with an average blood loss of 20 to 80 ml,[12] although more recent studies suggest that there is considerable variation in the length and volume of menstruation among women using no hormone therapies.[13] Hormonal (levonorgestrel intrauterine system) and nonhormonal (tranexamic acid) interventions, along with surgical interventions (e.g., endometrial ablation), have been approved for use in women with heavy menstrual bleeding, a diagnosis dependent on the perception of the woman (see Chapter 20 on Menstrual Disorders). The potential impact of persistent heavy blood loss during menses can have an impact on the hematologic system (i.e., anemia) and other organic function.[14,15]

CONTRACEPTION AND THE MENSTRUAL CYCLE

Vaginal intercourse occurring during the 2 to 3 days prior to ovulation results in the highest likelihood of pregnancy. In women with regular cycles, it is this fundamental concept that is used to promote contraception through timed sexual activity, or periodic abstinence during the most fertile days of the cycle. This is not a highly effective approach to contraception because of the vagaries of menstrual cycle length (and the follicular phase in particular) and the potential for prolonged viability of ejaculated sperm. However, periodic abstinence is practiced by millions of couples worldwide and represents the most direct and simple use of the menstrual cycle for preventing pregnancy.

Male- and female-centered barrier methods—used by millions of couples worldwide—prevent the union of sperm and ova but are associated with considerable failure rates.

Highly effective reversible contraceptives are currently available only for women. These methods—ranging from COCs to injectable or implantable progestin-only regimens—interfere with ovulation, the hormonal milieu, and some aspect of sperm capacitation. The contraceptive mechanism of intrauterine contraceptives, including progestin-releasing and copper-releasing methods, is not well delineated but likely involves interference with the sperm capacitation process. The progesterone-releasing intrauterine methods also create a progestogenic environment that serves to thicken cervical mucus and impede the transport and capacitation of spermatozoa. The majority of reversible contraceptives involve oral or systemic use of a progestin-only or progestin-estrogen combination. For these methods, ovulation inhibition and contraception result from the creation of a pseudopregnancy state in which the requisite LH and FH surges fail to occur because of a lack of appropriate positive and negative feedback mechanisms.

Maximal contraceptive effectiveness is achieved with consistent and correct use; however, many users find it challenging to use their methods consistently and correctly. Accordingly, many regimens either require minimal user interaction to achieve highly effective contraception (e.g., the combination vaginal ring, intrauterine contraception) or provide important noncontraceptive benefits—such as the treatment of acne, heavy menstrual bleeding, and emotional symptoms—to encourage consistent and correct use. However, these same regimens can cause adverse events such as bloating, mood changes, acne, and thromboembolic events, all of which can adversely influence consistent, correct, and continued use. Certain regimens have been shown both to exacerbate and to ameliorate the same symptoms. Thus, as a clinician, you must provide effective counseling so that women will have realistic expectations when they start a contraceptive regimen and also recognize the expected, and mostly short-term, changes caused by the regimens. Encourage women to continue to use their method correctly and consistently and to be in contact a health care provider if they cannot.

It is critical for women and their clinicians to recognize that effective prevention of pregnancy must involve the use of some contraceptive method with every act of intercourse regardless of cycle day. While certain times of the cycle are associated with a greater or reduced likelihood of ovulation, it is important to understand that ovulation, and therefore pregnancy, can occur on any cycle day. For the sexually active woman not using effective contraception, this basic premise can result in an unintended or unplanned pregnancy, placing her at risk for the spectrum of increased morbidities and mortality associated with such pregnancies.

REFERENCES

1. Jeyaseelan L, Antonisamy B, Rao PS. Pattern of menstrual cycle length in south Indian women: a prospective study. Soc Biol. 1992;39:306–9.
2. Münster K, Schmidt L, Helm P. Length and variation in the menstrual cycle—a cross-sectional study from a Danish county. Br J Obstet Gynaecol. 1992;99:422–9.
3. Ouyang F, Wang X, Arguelles L, et al. Menstrual cycle lengths and bone mineral density: a cross-sectional, population-based study in rural Chinese women ages 30–49 years. Osteoporosis Int. 2007;18:221–33.
4. Speroff L, Spitz MA. Clinical gynecologic endocrinology and infertility. 7th ed. Philadelphia: Lippincott, Williams & Wilkins; 2005.
5. Poppe K, Velkeniers B, Glinoer D. Thyroid disease and female reproduction. Clin Endocrinol (Oxf). 2007;66:309–21.
6. Joffe H, Hayes FJ. Menstrual cycle dysfunction associated with neurologic and psychiatric disorders: their treatment in adolescents. Ann N Y Acad Sci. 2008;1135: 219–29.
7. Enea C, Biosseau N, Diaz V, Dugué B. Biological factors and the determination of androgens in female subjects. Steroids. 2008;73:1203–16.
8. Shayya R, Chang RJ. Reproductive endocrinology of adolescent polycystic ovarian syndrome. BJOG. 2010;117:150–5.
9. Lobo RA. Reproductive endocrinology: neuroendocrinology, gonadotropins, sex steroids, prostaglandins, ovulation, menstruation, hormone assay. In: Katz VL, Lentz GM, Lobo RA, Gershenson DM (eds). Comprehensive gynecology, 5th edition. Philadelphia: Mosby Elsevier 2007, 73–120.
10. Stuckey BG. Female sexual function and dysfunction in the reproductive years: the influence of endogenous and exogenous sex hormones. J Sex Med. 2008;5:2281–90.

11. Baldi E, Luconi M, Bonaccorsi L, et al. Human sperm activation during capacitation and acrosome reaction: role of calcium, protein phosphorylation, and lipid remodelling pathways. Front Biosci 1996;1:d189–205.

12. Hatcher RA, Namnoum AB. The menstrual cycle. In: Hatcher RA, Trussell J, Nelson AL, Cates Jr, W, Stewart FH, Kowal D (editors). Contraceptive technology. New York: Ardent Media 2007, 7–17.

13. Mikolajczyk RT, Louis GM, Cooney MA, et al. Characteristics of prospectively measured vaginal bleeding among women trying to conceive. Paediatr Perinat Epidemiol. 2010;24:24–30.

14. Munro MG. Management of heavy menstrual bleeding: is hysterectomy the radical mastectomy of gynecology? Clin Obstet Gynecol. 2007;50:324–53.

15. Kaunitz AM, Meredith S, Inki P, et al. Levonorgestrelpreleasing intrauterine system and endometrial ablation in heavy menstrual bleeding: a systematic review and meta-analysis. Obstet Gynecol. 2009;113:1104–6.

Choosing a Contraceptive: Efficacy, Safety, and Personal Considerations

James Trussell, PhD
Katherine A. Guthrie, FRCOG, FFSRH

- Use of the top-tier reversible contraceptives—the two intrauterine contraceptives and the contraceptive implant—entails the lowest risk of pregnancy.

- Correct and consistent use of most contraceptive methods results in a low risk of pregnancy.

- The simultaneous use of methods dramatically lowers the risk of pregnancy.

- Emergency contraception provides a last chance to prevent pregnancy after unprotected intercourse or when the extent of contraceptive protection is unclear.

- Most contraceptives pose little risk to most users' health, although personal risk factors should influence personal choice.

- Half of all pregnancies are unintended: 3.1 million each year; more than 4 in 10 unintended pregnancies end in an induced abortion and half of all unintended pregnancies result from contraceptive failure.

Choosing a method of contraception is an important decision. A method that is not effective for an individual can lead to an unintended pregnancy. A method that is not safe for the user can create significant negative medical and social consequences. A method that does not fit the individual's personal lifestyle is not likely to be used correctly or consistently. Individuals themselves must make the decision about the contraceptive method they use, taking into consideration the feelings and attitudes of their partners. The best method of contraception for an individual or couple is one that is safe and that will actually be used correctly and consistently.

Because most people will use a variety of contraceptive methods throughout their lives, they should be knowledgeable about various contraceptive methods. The patient's choice of a contraceptive method depends on several major factors: efficacy, safety, cost, noncontraceptive benefits, and personal considerations. Through counseling, you can help your patient choose the most suitable contraceptive method. You also can influence the user's motivation and ability to use the method correctly.[1] Encourage clients to educate themselves about the various methods available. Direct clients toward available resources.

Information on levels and trends in contraceptive use in the United States is based on the National Survey of Family Growth (NSFG), periodic surveys conducted by the National Center for Health Statistics in which women ages 15 to 44 are interviewed about topics related to childbearing, family planning, and maternal and child health. Among the 61.9 million women of reproductive age (ages 15 to 44) in 2006–2008, about 62% (38.2 million) were using some method of contraception, according to the 2006–2008 NSFG. Among the 38% (23.6 million) who were not currently using a method, only about one fifth were at risk of pregnancy. The remaining four-fifths were not at risk because they had been sterilized for noncontraceptive reasons, were sterile, were trying to become pregnant, were pregnant, were interviewed within 6 weeks after the completion of a pregnancy, or did not have intercourse during the 3 months prior to the survey.[2]

Almost 90% of the women at risk for an unintended pregnancy were using a contraceptive method, but 10.6% of all women at risk of unintended pregnancy were not using any contraceptive method. Today, the most popular contraceptive methods are oral contraceptive pills (10.7 million), female sterilization (10.3 million), male condoms (6.2 million), and male sterilization (3.8 million).[2] See Table 3–1 for information on contraceptive method use by age of woman.

Use of the male condom and withdrawal is higher than indicated in Table 3–1, because some women are protected by dual methods. In the 2006–2008 NSFG, women were asked to report all contraceptive methods used in the current month for any reason (for protection against either pregnancy or STIs). When more than one method was reported, only the most effective method is coded as the current method. When the data in Table 3–1 are recoded to capture all use of the male condom, the fraction using male condoms among all women at risk rises by 39%, from 14.5% to 20.1%. Increases are greatest among women ages 15 to 24 (a 56% increase, from 20.2% to 31.4%) and among women ages 25–34 (a 40% increase, from 18.4% to 25.9%). When the data in Table 3–1 are recoded to capture all use of withdrawal, the fraction using withdrawal among all

Table 3–1 Percent and number of women at risk[1] and percent at risk currently using various methods from the 2006–2008 National Survey of Family Growth

Contraceptive method	Percent Using Among Women at Risk[1]						
	15–44	15–19	20–24	25–29	30–34	35–39	40–44
Oral contraceptive pill	25.0	43.8	41.0	31.0	23.0	17.3	10.2
Female sterilization	24.2	*	2.0	13.2	27.3	33.9	46.4
Condom	14.5	18.5	21.0	18.0	15.9	10.1	8.1
No method	10.6	18.7	14.3	11.8	7.0	9.6	7.6
Male sterilization	8.8	0.0	0.6	2.9	7.7	14.9	18.2
Intrauterine contraception	4.9	2.9	5.0	5.5	6.2	5.3	3.8
Withdrawal	4.6	3.2	4.4	7.0	4.9	5.2	3.0
Three-month injectable	2.9	7.5	4.4	4.5	2.1	0.8	1.1
Ring	2.2	2.9	5.3	2.7	2.2	0.8	0.4
Implant or patch	1.0	1.4	1.3	1.8	1.2	0.4	*
Fertility awareness-based methods	0.9	*	0.3	1.0	1.7	1.1	0.6
Calendar rhythm	0.7	*	0.3	1.0	0.9	1.1	0.6
Other methods[2]	0.4	*	*	0.5	0.9	*	*
Number of Women in Cohort, Percent and Number at Risk[1]							
Number (thousands) of Women	61,864	10,431	10,140	10,250	9,587	10,475	10,982
Percent at Risk[1]	69.1	34.7	63.8	72.8	75.6	83.0	84.2
Number (thousands) at Risk[1]	42,756	3,618	6,475	7,468	7,245	8,701	9,251

Source: Mosher et al. (2004).

Notes:
Percents may not add to 100 due to rounding

[1] At risk = those who *either* are current contraceptive users *or* are nonusers who have had sex in the past three months and are not trying to become pregnant, are not pregnant, or were not interviewed within two months after the completion of a pregnancy and are not sterile. Percentages may not add to 100 due to rounding.

[2] Other methods = diaphragm (with or without jelly or cream), emergency contraception, female condom or vaginal pouch, foam, cervical cap, Today® sponge, suppository or insert, jelly or cream (without diaphragm), and other methods.

* Figure does not meet standard of reliability or precision

women at risk rises by 94%, from 4.6% to 9.0%. Increases are greatest among women ages 15 to 24 (a 179% increase, from 3.9% to 10.8%) and among women ages 25 to 44 (a 91% increase, from 6.4% to 12.3%).[2]

The mix of methods shown in Table 3–1, including the 10.6% of women at risk who do not use any method, resulted in a staggering 3.1

million unintended pregnancies in 2001, the latest year for which data are available.[3] Nearly half (48%) of unintended pregnancies result from contraceptive failure.[3] Nearly half (49%) of the 6.4 million pregnancies and one-third (34% or 1.4 million) of the 4.0 million births were unintended.[3] Every night in the United States, about 9.7 million couples at risk of unintended pregnancy have intercourse; among these, about 29,000 experience a condom break or slip (assuming a 1.5% breakage/slippage rate), and over 1 million are not protected against pregnancy at all.[2,4] (See Table 3–1 and Chapter 26 on Contraceptive Efficacy.)

EFFICACY: "WILL IT WORK?"

"Is the condom really effective?"
"Which would be the most effective method for me?"
"Why did one magazine say diaphragms are 94% effective and another say they're 84% effective?"
"Can you still get pregnant if you take your pills every day on schedule?"

"Will it work?" is the question usually asked first and most frequently about any method of contraception.[5] Although this question cannot be answered with certainty for any particular couple, clinicians and counselors can try to help patients understand something of the difficulty of quantifying efficacy.

It is useful to distinguish between measures of contraceptive effectiveness and measures of the risk of pregnancy during contraceptive use. Many persons, including clinicians and clients, prefer positive rather than negative statements; instead of the negative statement that 20% of women using a method become accidentally pregnant during their first year of use, they prefer the alternative positive statement that the method is 80% effective. However, it does not follow that the method is 80% effective, because it is not true that 100% of these women would have become pregnant if they had not been using contraception. If 90% of these method users would have become pregnant had they used no method, then the use of the method reduced the number of accidental pregnancies from 90% to 20%, a reduction of 78%. In this sense, the method could be said to be 78% effective at reducing pregnancy in the first year. But if only 60% of these women would have become pregnant if they did not use contraception, then the method would be only 67% effective. Because no study can ascertain the proportion of women who would have become pregnant had they not used the contraceptive method under investigation, it is simply not possible to measure effectiveness directly. Therefore, we focus attention entirely on pregnancy rates or probabilities of pregnancy during contraceptive use, which are directly measurable. However, we continue to use the term effectiveness in its loose everyday sense of how well a method works throughout this book, and we use the terms effectiveness and efficacy interchangeably. We also provide estimates of the proportion of women who would become pregnant if they did not use contraception, so that the reader may calculate rough effectiveness rates if they are needed.

THE RISK OF PREGNANCY DURING TYPICAL AND PERFECT USE

Four pieces of information about contraceptive efficacy would help couples to make an informed decision when choosing a contraceptive method:

- Pregnancy rates during *typical use* show how effective the different methods are during actual use (including inconsistent *or* incorrect use).

- Pregnancy rates during *perfect use* show how effective methods can be, where perfect use is defined as following the directions for use.

- Pregnancy rates during *imperfect use* show how ineffective methods will be if they are used incorrectly or inconsistently. Pregnancy rates can be computed separately for different categories of imperfect use to reveal which types of imperfect use are most risky.[6]

- The percentage of *perfect users* or percentage of months during which a method is used perfectly reveals how hard it is to use a method correctly and consistently.

The difference between pregnancy rates during *imperfect use* and pregnancy rates during *perfect use* reveals how forgiving of *imperfect use* a method is. The difference between pregnancy rates during *typical use* and pregnancy rates during *perfect use* reveals the consequences of *imperfect use*; this difference depends both on how unforgiving of *imperfect use* a method is and on how hard it is to use that method perfectly. Only the first two pieces of information are currently available. Our current understanding of the literature on contraceptive efficacy is summarized in Table 3–2.[7,8]

TYPICAL USE

In the second column, we provide estimates of the probabilities of pregnancy during the first year of typical use of each method in the United States. This information is shown graphically in Figure 3–1 in a way that clients may find more useful.[9-11] The four methods in the top section of that Figure are sometimes called "forgettable"[12] or "top-tier" methods. The two reversible methods in the top tier have been called

Table 3–2 Percentage of women experiencing an unintended pregnancy during the first year of typical use and the first year of perfect use of contraception, and the percentage continuing use at the end of the first year. United States.

Method (1)	% of Women Experiencing an Unintended Pregnancy within the First Year of Use		% of Women Continuing Use at One Year[3]
	Typical Use[1] (2)	Perfect Use[2] (3)	(4)
No method[4]	85	85	
Spermicides[5]	28	18	42
Fertility awareness-based methods	24		47
Standard Days method[6]		5	
TwoDay method[6]		4	
Ovulation method[6]		3	
Symptothermal method[6]		0.4	
Withdrawal	22	4	46
Sponge			36
Parous women	24	20	
Nulliparous women	12	9	
Condom[7]			
Female (fc)	21	5	41
Male	18	2	43
Diaphragm[8]	12	6	57
Combined pill and progestin-only pill	9	0.3	67
Evra patch	9	0.3	67
NuvaRing	9	0.3	67
Depo-Provera	6	0.2	56
Intrauterine contraceptives			
ParaGard (copper T)	0.8	0.6	78
Mirena (LNg)	0.2	0.2	80
Implanon	0.05	0.05	84
Female sterilization	0.5	0.5	100
Male sterilization	0.15	0.10	100

Emergency Contraception: Emergency contraceptive pills or insertion of a copper intrauterine contraceptive after unprotected intercourse substantially reduces the risk of pregnancy.[9] (See Chapter 6.).

Lactational Amenorrhea Method: LAM is a highly effective, *temporary* method of contraception.[10] (See Chapter 18.)

Source: See Chapter 26.
(continued)

Table 3–2 Percentage of women experiencing an unintended pregnancy during the first year of typical use and the first year of perfect use of contraception, and the percentage continuing use at the end of the first year. United States—*(cont'd)*

Notes:

[1] Among *typical* couples who initiate use of a method (not necessarily for the first time), the percentage who experience an accidental pregnancy during the first year if they do not stop use for any other reason. Estimates of the probability of pregnancy during the first year of typical use for spermicides, withdrawal, fertility awareness-based methods, the diaphragm, the male condom, the oral contraceptive pill, and Depo-Provera are taken from the 1995 National Survey of Family Growth corrected for underreporting of abortion; see the text for the derivation of estimates for the other methods.

[2] Among couples who initiate use of a method (not necessarily for the first time) and who use it *perfectly* (both consistently and correctly), the percentage who experience an accidental pregnancy during the first year if they do not stop use for any other reason. See the text for the derivation of the estimate for each method.

[3] Among couples attempting to avoid pregnancy, the percentage who continue to use a method for 1 year.

[4] The percentages becoming pregnant in columns (2) and (3) are based on data from populations where contraception is not used and from women who cease using contraception in order to become pregnant. Among such populations, about 89% become pregnant within 1 year. This estimate was lowered slightly (to 85%) to represent the percentage who would become pregnant within 1 year among women now relying on reversible methods of contraception if they abandoned contraception altogether.

[5] Foams, creams, gels, vaginal suppositories, and vaginal film.

[6] The Ovulation and TwoDay methods are based on evaluation of cervical mucus. The Standard Days method avoids intercourse on cycle days 8 through 19. The Symptothermal method is a double-check method based on evaluation of cervical mucus to determine the first fertile day and evaluation of cervical mucus and temperature to determine the last fertile day.

[7] Without spermicides.

[8] With spermicidal cream or jelly.

[9] ella, Plan B One-Step and Next Choice are the only dedicated products specifically marketed for emergency contraception. The label for Plan B One-Step (one dose is 1 white pill) says to take the pill within 72 hours after unprotected intercourse. Research has shown that all of the brands listed here are effective when used within 120 hours after unprotected sex. The label for Next Choice (one dose is 1 peach pill) says to take 1 pill within 72 hours after unprotected intercourse and another pill 12 hours later. Research has shown that both pills can be taken at the same time with no decrease in efficacy or increase in side effects and that they are effective when used within 120 hours after unprotected sex. The Food and Drug Administration has in addition declared the following 19 brands of oral contraceptives to be safe and effective for emergency contraception: Ogestrel (1 dose is 2 white pills), Nordette (1 dose is 4 light-orange pills), Cryselle, Levora, Low-Ogestrel, Lo/Ovral, or Quasence (1 dose is 4 white pills), Jolessa, Portia, Seasonale or Trivora (1 dose is 4 pink pills), Seasonique (1 dose is 4 light-blue-green pills), Enpresse (one dose is 4 orange pills), Lessina (1 dose is 5 pink pills), Aviane or LoSeasonique (one dose is 5 orange pills), Lutera or Sronyx (one dose is 5 white pills), and Lybrel (one dose is 6 yellow pills).

[10] However, to maintain effective protection against pregnancy, another method of contraception must be used as soon as menstruation resumes, the frequency or duration of breastfeeds is reduced, bottle feeds are introduced, or the baby reaches 6 months of age.

highly effective reversible (HER) methods[13] (partly to distinguish them from long term reversible contraceptives (LARC), which also include Depo-Provera)[14]. It is clear that the incidence of unintended pregnancy in the United States will not be reduced unless many more women adopt HER methods.[13]

For most methods, these estimates were derived from the experience of women in the 1995 NSFG or the 1995 and 2002 NSFGs, so that the information pertains to nationally representative samples of users.[15] For the other methods, we based the estimates on evidence from surveys and clinical investigations. See Chapter 26 on Contraceptive Efficacy for more complete explanations and for tables summarizing the efficacy literature for each method.

Pregnancy rates during typical use reflect how effective methods are for the average person who does not always use methods correctly or

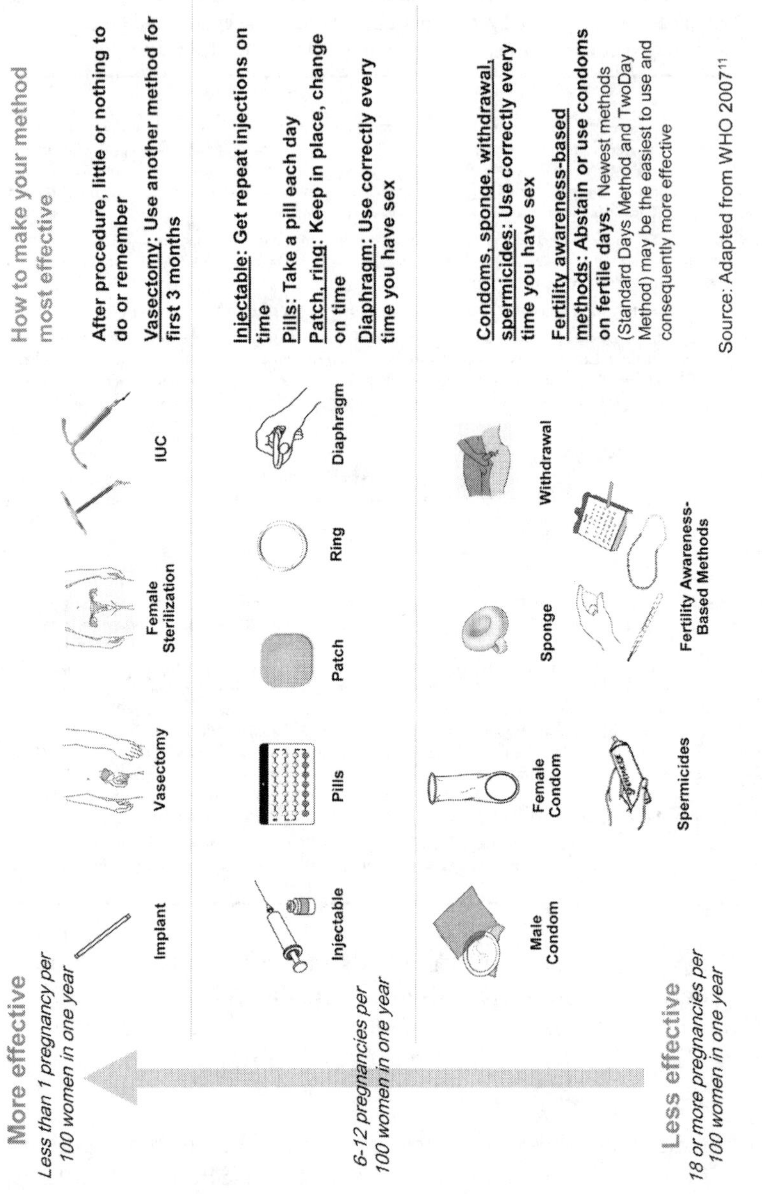

How to make your method most effective

After procedure, little or nothing to do or remember

Vasectomy: Use another method for first 3 months

Injectable: Get repeat injections on time

Pills: Take a pill each day

Patch, ring: Keep in place, change on time

Diaphragm: Use correctly every time you have sex

Condoms, sponge, withdrawal, spermicides: Use correctly every time you have sex

Fertility awareness-based methods: Abstain or use condoms on fertile days. Newest methods (Standard Days Method and TwoDay Method) may be the easiest to use and consequently more effective

Source: Adapted from WHO 2007[11]

IUC

Diaphragm

Female Sterilization

Ring

Withdrawal

Vasectomy

Patch

Sponge

Fertility Awareness-Based Methods

Implant

Injectable

Pills

Female Condom

Spermicides

Male Condom

More effective
Less than 1 pregnancy per 100 women in one year

6-12 pregnancies per 100 women in one year

Less effective
18 or more pregnancies per 100 women in one year

Figure 3–1 Comparing typical effectiveness of contraceptive methods

consistently. Typical use does not imply that a contraceptive method was always used. In the NSFG and in most clinical trials, a woman is 'using' a contraceptive method if she considers herself to be using that method. So typical use of the condom could include actually using a condom only occasionally, and a woman could report that she is 'using' the pill even though her supplies ran out several months ago. In short, *use*—which is identical to *typical use*—is a very elastic concept that depends entirely on an individual woman's perception.

PERFECT USE

In the third column, we provide our best guess of the probabilities of *method* failure (pregnancy) during the first year of perfect use. A method is used perfectly when it is used consistently according to a specified set of rules. For many methods, perfect use requires use at every act of intercourse. Virtually all method failure rates reported in the literature have been calculated incorrectly and are too low (see the discussion of methodological pitfalls below). Hence, we cannot empirically justify our estimates except those for four fertility awareness-based methods,[6,16-18] the diaphragm,[19] the sponge,[19] the male condom,[20-22] the female condom,[23] spermicides,[24] and methods for which there are extensive clinical trials with very low pregnancy rates. (See Chapter 26 on Contraceptive Efficacy.) Even the estimates for the fertility awareness-based methods, female condom, diaphragm, spermicides, and sponge are based on only one or two studies. Our hope is that our understanding of efficacy during perfect use for these and other methods will be enhanced by additional studies.

CONTINUATION

The fourth column displays the first-year probabilities of continuing use. They are based on the same sources used to derive the estimates in the second column (typical use). (See Chapter 26 on Contraceptive Efficacy.)

COMPARISON WITH PREGNANCY RATES AMONG WOMEN USING ISOTRETINOIN (ACCUTANE)

It is interesting to compare these estimates with pregnancy rates observed among women using isotretinoin, which is effective in treating severe acne but is also teratogenic. To minimize pregnancies among women undergoing treatment, the manufacturer and the U.S. Food and Drug Administration (FDA) implemented a pregnancy prevention program. Among 76,149 women who reported using contraception, 268 became pregnant, yielding a rate of 3.6 per 1,000 20-week courses of therapy;[25] this rate, if constant for a year, would be equivalent to an annual probability of pregnancy of 0.9%. The estimated annual probabil-

ities of pregnancy were 0.8%, 2.1%, and 2.6% among women who reported using oral contraceptives, diaphragms, and condoms, respectively. Thus, women using diaphragms achieved lower rates of
pregnancy than we estimate would occur during perfect use, and those
using condoms and oral contraceptives experienced about the same
pregnancy rates that would be expected during perfect use. Pregnancy
rates for women using any of these three methods, however, were substantially below rates generally observed during typical use; this finding
would appear to indicate that users' understanding of the teratogenic
risks of isotretinoin substantially enhanced correct and consistent use. It
is also possible that women in this study had lower than average fecundity, (because acne is a marker for excess androgen production associated with anovulation[26]), that they lowered their coital frequency during
treatment, or that they under-reported their number of pregnancies (and
abortions).

SIMULTANEOUS USE OF METHODS

Using two methods at once dramatically lowers the risk of unintended
pregnancy, provided they are used consistently. If one of the methods is
a condom or vaginal barrier, protection from disease transmission is an
added benefit. For example, the probabilities of pregnancy during the
first year of perfect use of male condoms and spermicides are estimated
to be 2% and 18%, respectively, in Table 3–2. It is reasonable to assume
that during perfect use the contraceptive mechanisms of condoms and
spermicides operate independently, since lack of independence during
typical use would most likely be due to imperfect use (either use both
methods or not use either). The annual probability of pregnancy during
simultaneous perfect use of condoms and spermicides would be 0.03%,
about the same as that achieved by the Implanon (0.05%) and much
lower than that achieved by the combined pill (0.3%), Depo-Provera, and
levonorgestrel (LNg) intrauterine contraceptive (0.1%) during perfect
use.[27]

EFFICACY OVER TIME

We confine attention to the first-year probabilities of pregnancy solely
because probabilities for longer durations are generally not available.
There are three main points to remember about the effectiveness of contraceptive methods over time. First, the risk of pregnancy during either
perfect or typical use of a method should remain constant over time *for
an individual woman* with a specific partner, providing that her underlying fecundity and frequency of intercourse do not change (although it
is possible that the risk for a woman could decline during typical use of
certain methods because she learns to use her method correctly and con-

sistently). Second, in contrast, the risk of pregnancy during typical use of a method will decline over time *for a group of users*, primarily because those users prone to fail do so early, leaving a pool of more diligent contraceptive users or those who are relatively infertile or who have lower coital frequency. This decline will be far less pronounced among users of those methods with little or no scope for imperfect use. The risk of pregnancy during perfect use for a group of users should decline as well, but this decline will not be as pronounced as that during typical use, because only the relatively more fecund and those with higher coital frequency are selected out early. For these reasons, the probability of becoming pregnant during the first year of use of a contraceptive method will be higher than the probability of becoming pregnant during the second year of use. Third, probabilities of pregnancy cumulate over time. Suppose that 15%, 12%, and 8% of women using a method experience a contraceptive failure during years 1, 2, and 3, respectively. The probability of not becoming pregnant within 3 years is calculated by multiplying the probabilities of *not becoming pregnant* for each of the 3 years: 0.85 times 0.88 times 0.92, which equals 0.69. Thus, the percentage becoming pregnant within 3 years is 31% (= 100% - 69%).

The lesson here is that the differences among probabilities of pregnancy for various methods will increase over time. For example, suppose that each year the typical proportion of women becoming pregnant while taking the pill is 8% and while using the diaphragm is 16%. Within 5 years, 34% of pill users and 58% of diaphragm users will become pregnant.

CONTRACEPTIVE FAILURES IN A LIFETIME

Data from the 1995 NSFG have been used to estimate age-specific contraceptive failure rates to produce a total lifetime contraceptive failure rate: the number of contraceptive failures that the typical woman would experience in a lifetime if she used reversible methods of contraception continuously (except for the time spent pregnant after a contraceptive failure) from exact age 15 to exact age 45. This estimate is based on the standard synthetic-cohort assumption: that the typical woman uses at each age the same mix of methods observed at each age in the NSFG and experiences the same rate of contraceptive failure observed at that age. The typical woman who uses reversible methods of contraception continuously from age 15 to age 45 would experience 1.8 contraceptive failures. If we consider both reversible methods and sterilization, the typical woman would experience only 1.3 contraceptive failures from age 15 to age 45.[28]

FACTORS THAT INFLUENCE REPORTED EFFICACY

Our understanding of the efficacy of contraceptive methods is entirely dependent on results published in the literature and is influenced by three primary factors (1) the inherent efficacy of the method when used correctly and consistently (perfect use) and the technical attributes of the method that facilitate or interfere with proper use, (2) characteristics of the user, and (3) the quality of published evidence.

INHERENT METHOD EFFICACY

For some methods, such as sterilization, implants, levonorgestrel and the copper-T intrauterine contraceptives (IUCs), the inherent efficacy is so high and correct and consistent use is so nearly guaranteed that extremely low pregnancy rates are found in all studies, and the range of reported pregnancy rates is quite narrow. For other methods such as the pill and injectable, inherent efficacy is high, but there is still room for potential misuse (e.g., forgetting to take pills or failure to return on time for injections), so that the second factor can contribute to a wider range of reported probabilities of pregnancy. In general, the studies of sterilization, injectable, implant, pill, patch, ring, and IUC use have been competently executed and analyzed. Studies of fertility awareness-based methods, spermicides, and the barrier methods display a wide range of reported probabilities of pregnancy because the potential for misuse is high, the inherent efficacy is relatively low, and the competence of the investigators is mixed.

USER CHARACTERISTICS

Characteristics of the users can affect the pregnancy rate for any method under investigation, but the impact will be greatest when the pregnancy rates during typical use are highest, either because the method has less inherent efficacy or because it is hard to use consistently or correctly.

Imperfect use. The most important user characteristic is imperfect use of the method. The importance of perfect use is demonstrated in the few studies where the requisite information on quality of use was collected. For example, in a World Health Organization (WHO) study of the ovulation method, the proportion of women becoming pregnant among those who used the method perfectly during the first year was 3.1%, whereas the corresponding proportion failing during a year of imperfect use was 86.4%.[6] In a large clinical trial of the cervical cap conducted in Los Angeles, among the 5% of the sample who used the method perfectly, the fraction failing during the first year was 6.1%. Among the remaining 95% of the sample who at least on one occasion used the cap imperfectly, the first-year probability of pregnancy was nearly twice as high (11.9%).[29]

Frequency of intercourse. Among those who use a method consistently and correctly (perfect users), the most important user characteristic that determines the risk of pregnancy is frequency of intercourse. For example, in a study in which users were randomly assigned to either the diaphragm or the sponge, diaphragm users who had intercourse 4 or more times a week became pregnant in the first year twice as frequently as those who had intercourse fewer than 4 times a week.[30] In that clinical trial, among women who used the diaphragm at every act of intercourse, only 3.4% of those who had intercourse fewer than 3 times a week became pregnant in the first year, compared with 9.7% of those who had intercourse 3 or more times per week.[19]

Age. A woman's biological capacity to conceive and bear a child declines with age. This decline is likely to be pronounced among those who are routinely exposed to STIs such as chlamydia and gonorrhea. Among those not exposed, the decline is likely to be moderate until a woman reaches her late thirties.[31] Although many investigators have found that contraceptive failure rates decline with age,[32–35] this effect almost surely overstates the pure age effect because age in many studies primarily captures the effect of coital frequency, which declines both with age and with marital duration.[36] User characteristics such as race and income seem to be less important determinants of contraceptive failure.

Regular cycles. Women with regular cycles were 7.2 times as likely as were women with irregular cycles (one or more cycles <17 days or >43 days) to become pregnant while using the Reality female condom.[37]

QUALITY OF PUBLISHED EVIDENCE

The errors committed by investigators range from simple arithmetical mistakes to improper design or execution or analysis of studies to outright fraud.[7]

Fraud. One well-documented instance of fraud involved the Dalkon shield. In a two-page article published in the *American Journal of Obstetrics and Gynecology*, a first-year probability of pregnancy of 1.1% was presented and the claim made that "only the combined type of oral contraceptive offers slightly greater protection."[38] It was not revealed by the researcher that some women had been instructed to use spermicides as an adjunctive method to reduce the risk of pregnancy, nor that he was part-owner of the Dalkon Corporation. Furthermore, he never subsequently revealed (except to the A.H. Robins Company, which bought the shield from the Dalkon Corporation but did not reveal this information either) that as the original trial matured, the first-year probability of pregnancy more than doubled.[39]

What gets published. The incentives to conduct research on contraceptive failure vary widely from method to method. Many studies of the pill and IUC exist because companies wishing to market them must conduct clinical trials to demonstrate their efficacy. In contrast, few studies of withdrawal exist because there is no financial reward for investigating this method. Moreover, researchers face differing incentives to report unfavorable results. The vasectomy literature is filled with short articles by clinicians who have performed 500 or 1,000 or 1,500 vasectomies. When they report pregnancies (curiously, pregnancy is seldom mentioned in discussions of vasectomy "failures," which focus on the continued presence of sperm in the ejaculate), their pregnancy rates are invariably low. Surgeons with high pregnancy rates simply do not write articles calling attention to their poor surgical skills. Likewise, drug companies do not commonly publicize their failures. Even if investigators prepared reports describing failures, journal editors would not be likely to publish them.

Analytical pitfalls. Several analytical pitfalls can snare investigators. Three of the most common are (1) use of a misleading measure of contraceptive failure called the Pearl-index, (2) the incorrect calculation of method failure rates, and (3) failure to follow up subjects in a trial. Other, more technical, errors that have biased reported results are discussed elsewhere.[7,40,41]

Pearl index. The Pearl index is obtained by dividing the number of unintended pregnancies by the number of years of exposure to the risk of unintended pregnancy contributed by all women in the study. This measure can be misleading when one wishes to compare pregnancy rates obtained from studies with different average amounts of exposure. The likelihood of pregnancy declines over time because those most likely to become pregnant do so at earlier durations of contraceptive use and exit from observation. Those still using contraception after long durations are unlikely to become pregnant, so that an investigator could (wittingly or unwittingly) drive the reported pregnancy rate toward zero by running the trial "forever." Two investigators using the NSFG could obtain Pearl-index pregnancy rates of 7.5 and 4.4 per 100 women-years of exposure for the condom.[42] One (who got 4.4) allowed each woman to contribute a maximum of 5 years of exposure while the other (who got 7.5) allowed each woman to contribute only 1 year. Which investigator is incorrect? Neither. The two rates are simply not comparable. Life-table measures of contraceptive failure are easy to interpret and control for the distorting effects of varying durations of use. Another problem occurs when deciding which pregnancies to count. Most studies count only the pregnancies observed and reported by the women. If, on the other hand, a pregnancy test were administered every month, the number of pregnancies (and hence the pregnancy rate) would increase because early fetal losses not observed by the woman would be added to the number of observed pregnancies. Such routine pregnancy testing in the more recent contraceptive trials has resulted in higher pregnancy rates than would otherwise have been obtained and makes the results not comparable to those from other trials.

Incorrect calculation of method failure rates. Unfortunately, nearly all investigators who have attempted to calculate "method" and "user" failure rates have done so incorrectly. Investigators routinely separate the unintended pregnancies into two groups. By convention, pregnancies that occur during a month in which a method was used improperly are classified as user failures (even though, logically, a pregnancy might be due to failure of the method, if it was used correctly on some occasions and incorrectly on others), and all other pregnancies are classified as method failures. But investigators do not separate the exposure (the denominator in the calculation of failure rates) into these two groups.

For example, suppose that 2 method failures and 8 user failures occur during 100 women-years of exposure to the risk of pregnancy. Then the common calculation is that the user failure rate is 8% and the method failure rate is 2%; the sum of the two is the overall failure rate of 10%. By definition, however, method failures can occur only during perfect use and user failures cannot occur during perfect use. If there are 50 years of perfect use and 50 years of imperfect use in the total of 100 years of exposure, then the method failure rate would be 4% and the user failure rate would be 16%. The difference between the two rates (here 12%) provides a measure of how forgiving of imperfect use the method is. However, since investigators do not generally inquire about perfect use except when a pregnancy occurs, the proper calculations cannot be performed.

Loss to follow-up. The standard assumption made at the time of analysis is that women who are lost-to-follow-up (LFU) experience unintended pregnancy at the same rate as those who are observed. This assumption is probably innocuous when the proportion LFU is small. But in many studies the proportion LFU may be 20% or higher, so that what really happens to these women could drastically affect the estimate of the proportion becoming pregnant. Our strong suspicion is that women LFU are more likely to experience a contraceptive failure than are those who remain in the trial. For example, one study found that the pregnancy rate for calendar rhythm rose from 9.4 to 14.4 per 100 women-years of exposure as a result of resolution of cases LFU.[43]

GOALS FOR COMMUNICATING ABOUT EFFICACY

Keep these thoughts in mind when counseling about contraceptive efficacy:

1. **Emergency contraception provides a last chance to prevent pregnancy after unprotected intercourse.** Insertion of a copper

IUC is the most effective option and provides up to 20 years of protection. Emergency contraceptive pills (ECPs) are an especially important second method for those relying on condoms, in cases of breakage or slippage, for those who do not actually use their ongoing method for whatever reason, and those who are forced to have unprotected intercourse.

2. **What matters most is correct and consistent use.** For example, an 8% probability of pregnancy during the first year for typical use of the pill will not protect the careless user. The 16% probability of pregnancy during the first year of typical diaphragm use need not overly discourage a careful and disciplined woman who has infrequent intercourse from using a diaphragm.

3. **Methods that protect a person for a long time and do not require daily or coital adherence** (sterilization, implants, IUCs, and long-acting injections) **tend to be associated with lower pregnancy rates,** primarily because they allow little scope for user error.

4. **Abstinence is always available as an option, as are outercourse and withdrawal.**

5. **Using two methods at once dramatically lowers the risk of unintended pregnancy,** provided they are used consistently. If one of the methods is a condom, protection from disease transmission is an added benefit.

6. **Make sure your staff provides consistent and correct information.** One study of the information provided by family planning staff indicated that providers tended to give the lowest reported probabilities of pregnancy for pills and IUCs, probabilities of pregnancy during typical use for diaphragms and spermicides, and higher-than-typical probabilities of pregnancy for condoms.[44] Thus, family planning providers may extensively bias their patient education in favor of methods they provide most frequently. Condoms and withdrawal get an undeserved low efficacy score within many family planning clinics and offices. You can avoid unintentional bias by deciding carefully what pregnancy rates your clinic or staff members are going to use.

7. **Technology fails people just as people fail technology.** Patients are sometimes told that unintended pregnancies are their own fault because they did not use their method correctly or carefully. Contraceptive methods are imperfect and can fail even the most diligent user.

S AFETY: "WILL IT HURT ME?"

"I smoke. Won't the pill give me a heart attack?"
"Could the IUC puncture my womb?"
"Will I be able to get pregnant after stopping my method?"
    In general, contraceptives pose few serious health risks to users. Moreover, the use of contraceptive methods is generally far safer than pregnancy. Unintended pregnancies unnecessarily place women at risk. Women in many developing countries will experience an even greater advantage in using contraceptive methods—in comparison with pregnancy-related mortality—than women in the developed world. Nonetheless, use of some contraceptive methods may entail potential risks.

- Use of the method may lead to serious outcomes such as death, hospitalization, surgery, medical side effects, infections, loss of reproductive capacity, or pain.

- Contraceptive failure (pregnancy) is associated with risk: a woman must assess the likelihood of contraceptive failure and the dangers that a pregnancy would pose.

MAJOR HEALTH RISKS

    When it comes to the most serious outcome of all—death—the absolute level of risk is extraordinarily low for most women. Table 3–3 puts into perspective some of the mortality risks of everyday life in the United States.[45–53] Other major health risks from contraceptive use are not only uncommon, but they are also most likely to occur in women who have underlying medical conditions.

Cardiovascular Disease

    Use of combined oral contraceptive pills (COCs) (and presumably the patch and ring as well) is associated with an increased risk of myocardial infarction (MI) and stroke. Smoking definitely increases the risk of MI, especially in women over age 35. However, nonsmoking, normotensive, nondiabetic women of any age who use COCs are not at increased risk for MI. The risk of stroke in nonsmoking women under age 35 is not increased by use of COCs with less than 50 mcg estrogen.[54] The risk of venous thromboembolism is increased by COC use, but the absolute risk is quite low among women who use COCs with less than 50 mcg estrogen, ranging from 9 events per 100,000 women-years of exposure among those aged 20 to 24 to 18 events per 100,000 women-years of exposure among those aged 40 to 44.[54]

Table 3–3 Voluntary risks in perspective

Activity	Risk of Death	Source
Risk per year		
While skydiving	1 in 1,000	Laudan (1994)[45]
From an accident	1 in 2,900	
From an automobile accident	1 in 5,000	
From a fall	1 in 20,000	
From a fire	1 in 50,000	
From riding your bicycle	1 in 130,000	
In an airplane crash	1 in 250,000	
From being struck by lightning	1 in 2,000,000	
Risk per year for women preventing pregnancy		
Using combined oral contraceptives (and presumably the patch and ring as well)		Schwingl et al. (1999)[46]
Nonsmoker		
Aged 15–34	1 in 1,667,000	
Aged 35–44	1 in 33,300	
Smoker		
Aged 15–34	1 in 57,800	
Aged 35–44	1 in 5,200	
Undergoing tubal sterilization	1 in 66,700	Escobedo et al. (1989)[47]
Risk per year from using tampons	1 in 5,734,000	Hajjeh et al. (1999);[48] U.S Census Bureau (2003)[49]
Risk from pregnancy	1 in 6,900	Berg et al. (2010)[50]
Risk from spontaneous abortion	1 in 142,900	Saraiya et al. (1999)[51]
Risk from legal induced abortion		
Mifepristone/misoprostol	1 in 200,000	Karnovsky (2011)[52]
Surgical	1 in 142,900	Bartlett et al. (2004)[53]
≤ 8 weeks	1 in 1,000,000	
9–10 weeks	1 in 500,000	
11–12 weeks	1 in 250,000	
13–15 weeks	1 in 58,800	
16–20 weeks	1 in 29,400	
≥ 21 weeks	1 in 11,200	

Cancer

Use of COCs (and presumably the patch and ring as well) protects users against cancers of the endometrium and ovary.[54] A comprehensive review concluded that use of COCs is associated with an increased risk of cancer of the cervix and liver, an increased risk of breast cancer in young women, and a decreased risk of colorectal cancer.[54] The risk of death is lower among ever-users of COCs than never-users for colorectal,[55] uterine, and ovarian cancer.[55,56] Recent evidence suggests no association between current or former COC use and breast cancer (with one exception, where current but not former users had a marginally significant higher risk[57] or breast cancer mortality.[55,56,58–60] Regardless, the net effect of COC use on cancer is negligible,[54,58] and ever-users of COCs have a significantly lower death rate from all cancers than do never-users.[55]

Persistent infection with certain types of human papillomavirus (HPV) is the most important cause of cervical cancer (see Chapter 21 on Reproductive Tract Infections). However, the incidence of cervical cancer is increased in women using COCs, particularly long-term users, among women who test positive for HPV; this risk increases as duration of use increases.[61] Results from limited data also suggest a slight increase in the risk of cervical cancer among women who use injectable contraceptives for 5 years or longer. Results from one large cohort study in the UK found that ever users of COCs had a significantly higher risk of death from cervical cancer than did never users.[56] However, oral contraceptive use had neither a harmful nor a beneficial effect on cervical cancer mortality in an even larger UK cohort study.[55]

Analysis of pooled data from 54 epidemiologic studies conducted in 25 countries found that women face a slightly increased risk (about 25% higher) for having breast cancer diagnosed while they are using COCs. Cancers diagnosed in these women are less advanced clinically than those diagnosed in women of the same age who have never used COCs.[62] The increased risk is apparent soon after pill use begins but does not increase with duration of use, declines after use ceases, and does not persist beyond 10 years after exposure ceases. These patterns are not typical for a carcinogenic agent but would be consistent with promotion of already existing tumors or with earlier diagnosis of breast cancer in women who have used COCs. However, recent studies in the United States and United Kingdom found that current or former COC use is not associated with an increased risk of diagnosis of breast cancer (with one exception, where current but not former users had a marginally significant higher risk[57]).[58,59] Moreover, COC use has neither a harmful nor a beneficial effect on breast cancer *mortality*.[55,56,60]

SIDE EFFECTS

Often, the minor side effects of contraceptive methods, in addition to the more serious complications, influence whether an individual selects a certain method. "What physical changes will I undergo?" "Will I be annoyed by spotting, cramping, or the sensation or messiness of using a given method?" Do not dismiss the important role that side effects play when an individual must repeatedly assess whether to continue using a method or whether to use it consistently.

Side effects can be hormonally, chemically, or mechanically induced. Headaches, nausea, dizziness and breast tenderness can be side effects of hormonal methods. Menstrual changes such as spotting and decreased or increased bleeding can be caused by hormonal methods and IUCs. Physical sensations such as decreased penile sensitivity, pressure on vaginal walls, or uterine cramping may be caused by mechanical methods. Other chemically-induced side effects include allergic reactions to latex and to copper.

With the great majority of these side effects, instruction and patient education can help users accept and understand what is happening. The appearance of side effects that are not serious is not a medical reason to preclude use of a method.

GOALS FOR COMMUNICATING ABOUT SAFETY

1. **Try to educate the patient about misconceptions.** People who are afraid do not respond well to rational reasoning. Many patients hold certain irrational opinions about contraceptive methods—that the pill is very dangerous even to healthy, nonsmoking young women or that injectables lead to permanent sterility. If you see that you are getting nowhere, stop. Help each client select a method that can be used correctly and consistently without fear, and support her in *her* choice.

2. **Make sure that you and your staff know all about the major side effects** of contraceptive methods and can communicate these clearly, such as the relation between pill use and blood clots or reproductive cancers.

3. **Tell patients what they need to know** even if they do not ask. Patients do not always ask the questions they need answered. Often, they do not know what they don't know.

4. **Compare risks of using contraception with pregnancy risks.** In general, the risks of pregnancy, abortion, and delivery are far greater than those for using a contraceptive method.

5. **Start with a sexual health assessment, so that if warranted you can help patients make a contraceptive method choice that will protect them from both STIs and pregnancy.** Safety concerns often overlap with worries about infections. With the exception of abstinence, currently available methods (male and female condoms) that protect against infection are not those that provide greatest protection against pregnancy. Con-

versely, the most highly effective methods of contraception provide *no* protection against infection. Therefore, highly effective protection against both risks requires use of two methods. Even "abstinence" has different rules for protection against pregnancy and protection against infection: oral and anal intercourse can result in STI transmission but not in pregnancy.

6. **Teach patients the danger signals** of the method they select. If a danger signal does appear, the informed user can quickly seek help.

7. **Use language that is appropriate for the client.**

8. **Answer any questions truthfully.**

NONCONTRACEPTIVE BENEFITS

Although the noncontraceptive benefits provided by certain methods are not generally the major determinant for selecting a contraceptive method, they certainly can help patients decide between two or more suitable methods. (See Table 3–4.) Awareness that a method of contraception is having major noncontraceptive benefits (cancer prevention, protection of future fertility or diminished menstrual cycle symptoms) may also increase the likelihood of continuing to use that method. Make it a practice to tell your patients about the noncontraceptive benefits of the various methods. If patients have additional reasons for using the contraceptive method, their motivation to use the method correctly and consistently will probably be improved.

Reducing the user's risk of STIs may weigh as heavily as preventing pregnancy. Any sexually active person who may be at risk of acquiring STIs should consider condoms (see Chapter 13 on Male Condoms and Chapter 21 on Reproductive Tract Infections), either alone, or preferably with another method more effective in preventing pregnancy. Because condoms reduce the risk of STIs that cause PID and thus lead to infertility, they protect future fertility.

Fertility awareness methods educate women about their menstrual physiology. This knowledge can also help couples achieve a planned pregnancy.

Mirena (LNg-IUC) markedly reduces menstrual blood loss (thereby reducing anemia) and cramping; it can be used to treat menorrhagia and endometriosis and to provide progestin in hormone therapy.[63]

Combined oral contraceptives protect against ectopic pregnancy, symptomatic pelvic inflammatory disease (PID), and ovarian and endometrial and colorectal cancer, and may improve bone health in women

Table 3–4 Major methods of contraception and some related safety concerns, side effects, and noncontraceptive benefits

Method	Dangers	Side Effects	Noncontraceptive Benefits
Combined hormonal contraception (pill, and presumably Evra patch, and NuvaRing.)	Cardiovascular complications (stroke, heart attack, blood clots, high blood pressure), depression, hepatic adenomas, increased risk of cervical and possibly liver cancers, earlier development of breast cancer in young women	Nausea, headaches, dizziness, spotting, weight gain, breast tenderness, chloasma	Decreases dysmenorrhea, menorrhagia, anemia and cyclic mood problems (PMS); protects against ectopic pregnancy, symptomatic PID, and ovarian, endometrial, and possibly colorectal cancer; reduces acne
Progestin-only pill	May avoid some dangers of combined hormonal contraceptives	Less nausea than with combined pills	Lactation not disturbed
IUD	Infection post insertion, uterine perforation, anemia	Menstrual cramping, spotting, increased bleeding with non-progestin-releasing IUDs	Mirena decreases menstrual blood loss and menorrhagia and can provide progestin for hormone replacement therapy
Male condom	Anaphylactic reaction to latex	Decreased sensation, allergy to latex	Protects against STIs, including HIV; delays premature ejaculation
Female condom	None known	Aesthetically unappealing and awkward to use for some	Protects against STIs
Implanon	Infection at implant site; may avoid some dangers of combined hormonal contraceptives	Headache, acne, menstrual changes, weight gain, depression, emotional lability	Lactation not disturbed; decreases dysmennorhea
Depo-Provera	Depression, allergic reactions, pathologic weight gain, bone loss; may avoid some dangers of combined hormonal contraceptives	Menstrual changes, weight gain, headache, adverse effects on lipids	Lactation not disturbed; reduces risk of seizures; may protect against ovarian and endometrial cancers

(continued)

Table 3–4 Major methods of contraception and some related safety concerns, side effects, and noncontraceptive benefits—*(cont'd)*

Method	Dangers	Side Effects	Noncontraceptive Benefits
Sterilization	Infection; possible anesthetic or surgical complications; if pregnancy occurs after tubal sterilization, high risk that it will be ectopic	Pain at surgical site, psychological reactions, subsequent regret that the procedure was performed	Tubal sterilization reduces risk of ovarian cancer and may protect against PID
Abstinence	None known		Prevents STIs, including HIV, if anal and oral intercourse are avoided as well
Diaphragm, Sponge	Vaginal and urinary tract infections, toxic shock syndrome; possible increase in susceptibility to HIV/AIDS acquisition if exposed to positive partner	Pelvic discomfort, vaginal irritation, vaginal discharge if left in too long, allergy	
Spermicides	Vaginal and urinary tract infections; possible increase in susceptibility to HIV/AIDS acquisition if exposed to positive partner	Vaginal irritation, allergy	
Lactational Amenorrhea Method (LAM)			Provides excellent nutrition for infants under 6 months old

with low estrogen levels. High-dose pills, but not low-dose pills, protect against functional ovarian cysts. High-dose pills protect against benign breast disease, and low-dose pills may also offer protection. Some combined oral contraceptives protect against acne, a key concern among youth. The pill reduces dysmenorrhea, menorrhagia, and anemia, and is effective in treating dysfunction uterine bleeding. All these benefits presumably accrue to users of the Evra patch and NuvaRing.[54]

PERSONAL CONSIDERATIONS

The best method of contraception for patients is one that will be in harmony with their wishes, fears, preferences, and lifestyle: a method that will be used correctly.

A typical woman in the United States spends about 39 years—almost half of her lifespan of 80 years—at potential biological risk of pregnancy, during the time from menarche (at age 12.6) to natural menopause (at age 51.3).[64,65] What matters most to a woman when she considers a contraceptive method will ordinarily change over the course of her reproductive lifespan. Different reproductive stages are associated with distinct fertility goals and sexual behaviors (Table 3–5).[66] From menarche to first birth, the primary fertility goal is to postpone pregnancy and birth. Between the first birth and the time when a woman intends to have no more children, the primary goal is to space pregnancies leading to births. Between the time when a woman intends to have no more children and menopause, the goal is to cease childbearing altogether. The biggest demands on a contraceptive method are generated during the period between first intercourse and first birth, when the typical woman may have several sexual partners with periods of high coital frequency; the typical woman may attach great importance to preventing pregnancy and STIs and to a method's reversibility and ease of use. In the last stage of her reproductive lifespan, from the time when a woman intends to have no more children to menopause, the most important factor is a method's efficacy at preventing pregnancy.

More than half the entire reproductive lifespan—20.4 years or 53% of the reproductive span of 38.7 years—is spent trying to avoid further childbearing, in the stage from the time when a woman intends to have no more children to menopause.[64,65] The typical woman accomplishes this goal via female or male sterilization. A further 13.4 years or 35% of the reproductive span, from menarche to the first birth, is characterized by no desire to become pregnant. Thus, of a total reproductive span of 38.7 years during which a woman is potentially biologically at risk of conception, only 4.9 years (13% of the total), from the first birth to the time when a woman intends to have no more children, is characterized by any desire to become pregnant. Even this figure is exaggerated since a

Table 3–5 The stages of reproductive life

	Adolescents/Young Adults		Later Reproductive Years	
	Menarche to First Intercourse	First Intercourse to First Birth	First Birth to Intend No More Children	Intend No More Children to Menopause
Fertility goals				
Births	postpone	postpone	space	stop
Ability to have children	preserve	preserve	preserve	irrelevant
Sexual behavior				
Number of partners	none	multiple?	one?	one?
Coital frequency	zero	moderate to high	moderate	moderate to low
Coital predictability	low	moderate to high	high	high
Importance of method characteristics				
Pregnancy prevention		high	moderate	high
PID prevention		high	moderate	low
Not coitus-linked		high	low	moderate
Reversibility		high	high	low
Most common methods				
Most common		pill	pill	sterilization
Next most common		condom	condom	pill, condom

Source: Forrest (1993).[66]

great fraction of this stage is spent in the pregnant or lactating state or trying to postpone the next pregnancy.

Pattern of sexual activity. In choosing their contraceptive method, women and men should consider their number of partners and their frequency of intercourse.

The number of partners affects the risk of exposure to STIs. In more obvious cases, the individual will have more than one partner at any given time. Less obvious are the individuals who practice serial monogamy. That is, they have only one partner at a time; however, the relationships are not permanent, so at the end of one relationship, the individual will move on to a new partner. Indeed, having more than one partner in a lifetime is the norm, and it is not uncommon for unmarried men and women to have more than 1 partner per year. The practitioner recommending the use of male or female condoms must be prepared to take the time required to discuss risks of STIs, encourage behavioral change, and teach skills.

The frequency of intercourse also has bearing on a person's contraceptive method choice. For example, the woman who has infrequent intercourse may not wish to use a method that requires daily medication or continuous exposure to possible side effects posed by hormonal methods or IUCs. On the other hand, infrequent intercourse may also indicate that a client is at risk of intercourse at unpredictable times. These clients may need skills in "expecting the unexpected."

Pattern of childbearing. Couples should choose their contraceptive method based on the number of children they desire and the timing of those births. For example, couples who plan on having a few children or having children early in their reproductive life cycle may have more flexible requirements about the spacing before and between pregnancies and may be more willing to risk a mistimed, but not unwanted, pregnancy. Such flexibility may mean that contraceptive method choices would not be limited to those with highest efficacy.

On the other hand, the couples who want only one child or want to delay childbearing until the woman is in her late 30s or early 40s may be less willing to choose any but the most highly effective methods. Among these couples, the reversible long-term methods may be more appealing than they would be for couples for whom a several-year span of protection is not an absolute necessity.

Access to medical care. Some people in our society have difficulty gaining access to the health care system: they do not understand the system or cannot afford it or find that it shuns them. Others may find their access hampered by too long a wait at the clinic. Studies in other nations have shown that access has great bearing on contraceptive method compliance and choice.[67] Presumably, the degree of access can also influence women in the United States. Access can be eased for all clients by providing a full year's supply of contraceptives. While many clinicians do provide 13 cycles of pills, for example, most do not offer sufficient quantities of condoms.

Intimate partner violence. Women at risk of intimate partner violence probably cannot rely on their partners to use withdrawal or a male condom. A noncoitally dependent or a female-controlled coital method would probably be a better choice.

GOALS FOR COMMUNICATING ABOUT PERSONAL CONSIDERATIONS

Key concepts for discussing and teaching about contraceptive method choice and personal considerations include these:

1. **The patient decides which personal considerations matter.** Only the potential user can weigh all the elements for personal

choice, and the clinician will not be able to predict what matters. Privacy? Lubrication? Light periods? What big sister uses? Do not guess; ask.

2. **It is a long way from the exam room to the bedroom.** We offer methods as medicines in a clinical setting, and then our patients go home and use them in a sexual setting, be it a bedroom, motel room, car seat, or tent. Remember to help your patient think through the sexual aspects of contraception.

3. **Give patients permission to make a second (or third) contraceptive method choice.** They may not like the first method at all and will need to know it is acceptable to come back and try something else. Besides, it is always good to know how to use several methods.

4. **Encourage your patients to talk about contraceptive issues with their partners.** How can one person decide if a method of contraception will be compatible with a couple's personal and sexual styles? Help your clients practice discussing contraception with their partners if this is new territory for them.

5. **Personal considerations change over time.** Teenagers and 35-year-olds will use different criteria as they evaluate their contraceptive method choices. Encourage patients to rethink their contraceptive method needs as life and sex and bodies change over time.

SUGGESTED READING

Brown SS, Eisenberg L. The best intentions: unintended pregnancy and the well-being of children and families. Washington DC: National Academy Press, 1995.

Harrison PF, Rosenfield A. Contraceptive research and development: looking to the future. Washington DC: National Academy Press, 1996.

REFERENCES

1. Gallen M, Lettenmaier C. Counseling makes a difference. Popul Rep. 1987;J(35):1–31.
2. Mosher WD, Jones J. Use of contraception in the United States: 1982–2008. National Center for Health Statistics. Vital Health Stat. 2010; 23(29); [cited 2010 Jun 7]. Available from: http://www.cdc.gov/NCHS/data/series/sr_23/sr23_029.pdf
3. Finer LB, Henshaw SK. Disparities in rates of unintended pregnancy in the United States, 1994 and 2001. Perspect Sex Reprod Health. 2006;38:90–6.
4. Smith, TW. (National Opinion Research Center, Chicago, IL). Conversation with: James Trussell (Office of Population Research, Princeton University, Princeton, NJ). 1993 Dec 13.
5. Grady WR, Klepinger DH, Nelson-Wally A. Contraceptive characteristics: the perceptions and priorities of men and women. Fam Plann Perspec. 1999;31:168–75.
6. Trussell J, Grummer-Strawn L. Contraceptive failure of the ovulation method of periodic abstinence. Fam Plann Perspec. 1990;22:65–75.

7. Trussell J, Kost K. Contraceptive failure in the United States: a critical review of the literature. Stud Fam Plann. 1987;18:237–83.
8. Trussell J, Hatcher RA, Cates W, Stewart FH, Kost K. Contraceptive failure in the United States: an update. Stud Fam Plann. 1990;21:51–4.
9. Steiner MJ, Trussell J, Mehta N, Condon S, Subramaniam S, Bourne D. Communicating contraceptive effectiveness: a randomized controlled trial to inform a World Health Organization family planning handbook. Am J Obstet Gynecol. 2006;195: 85–91.
10. Steiner MJ, Trussell J, Johnson S. Communicating contraceptive effectiveness: an updated counseling chart. Am J Obstet Gynecol. 2007;197:118.
11. World Health Organization. Comparing typical effectiveness of contraceptive methods. Geneva: World Health Organization, 2007; [cited 2010 Jun 7]. Available from: http://www.fhi.org/nr/shared/enFHI/Resources/EffectivenessChart.pdf
12. Grimes DA. Forgettable contraception. Contraception. 2009;80:497–9.
13. Trussell J, Schwarz EB, Guthrie K. Research priorities for preventing unintended pregnancy: moving beyond emergency contraceptive pills. Perspect Sex Reprod Health. 2010;42:8–9.
14. National Collaborating Centre for Women's and Children's Health. Long-acting reversible contraception: the effective and appropriate use of long-acting reversible contraception London: RCOG Press; 2005; [cited 2010 Jun 7]. Available from: http://www.nice.org.uk/CG030
15. Trussell J. Estimates of contraceptive failure from the 1995 National Survey of Family Growth. Contraception. 2008;78:85.
Kost K, Singh S, Vaughan B, Trussell J, Bankole A. Estimates of contraceptive failure from the 2002 National Survey of Family Growth. Contraception. 2008;77:10–21.
16. Arévalo M, Jennings V, Sinai I. Efficacy of a new method of family planning: the Standard Days Method. Contraception. 2002;65:333–8.
17. Arévalo M, Jennings V, Nikula M, Sinai I. Efficacy of the new TwoDay Method of family planning. Fertil Steril. 2004;82:885–92.
18. Frank-Herrmann P, Heil J, Gnoth C, Toledo E, Baur S, Pyper C, Jenetzky E, Strowitzki T, Freundl G. The effectiveness of a fertility awareness based method to avoid pregnancy in relation to a couple's sexual behaviour during the fertile time: a prospective longitudinal study. Hum Reprod. 2007;22:1310–9.
19. Trussell J, Strickler J, Vaughan B. Contraceptive efficacy of the diaphragm, the sponge and the cervical cap. Fam Plann Perspect. 1993;25:100–5, 135.
20. Frezieres RG, Walsh TL, Nelson AL, Clark VA, Coulson AH. Evaluation of the efficacy of a polyurethane condom: results from a randomized controlled clinical trial. Fam Plann Perspect. 1999;31:81–7.
21. Walsh TL, Frezieres RG, Peacock K, Nelson AL, Clark VA, Bernstein L. Evaluation of the efficacy of a nonlatex condom: results from a randomized, controlled clinical trial. Perspect Sex Reprod Health. 2003;35:79–86.
22. Steiner MJ, Dominik R, Rountree RW, Nanda K, Dorflinger LJ. Contraceptive effectiveness of a polyurethane condom and a latex condom: a randomized controlled trial. Obstet Gynecol. 2003;101:539–47.
23. Farr G, Gabelnick H, Sturgen K, Dorflinger L. Contraceptive efficacy and acceptability of the female condom. Am J Public Health. 1994;84:1960–4.
24. Raymond EG, Chen PL, Luoto J. Contraceptive effectiveness and safety of five nonoxynol-9 spermicides: a randomized trial. Obstet Gynecol. 2004;103:430–9.
25. Mitchell AA, Van Bennekom CM, Louik C. A pregnancy-prevention program in women of childbearing age receiving isotretinoin. N Engl J Med. 1995;333:101–6.
26. Speroff L, Glass RH, Kase NG. Clinical gynecologic endocrinology and infertility. 6th ed. Baltimore (MD): Williams & Wilkins; 1999.
27. Kestelman P, Trussell J. Efficacy of the simultaneous use of condoms and spermicides. Fam Plann Perspect. 1991;23:226–7, 232.

28. Trussell J, Vaughan B. Contraceptive failure, method-related discontinuation and resumption of use: results from the 1995 National Survey of Family Growth. Fam Plann Perspect. 1999;31:64–72, 93.

29. Richwald GA, Greenland S, Gerber MM, Potik R, Kersey L, Comas MA. Effectiveness of the cavity-rim cervical cap: results of a large clinical study. Obstet Gynecol. 1989;74:143–8.

30. McIntyre SL, Higgins JE. Parity and use-effectiveness with the contraceptive sponge. Am J Obstet Gynecol. 1986;155:796–801.

31. Menken J, Trussell J, Larsen U. Age and infertility. Science. 1986;233:1389–94.

32. Grady WR, Hayward MD, Yagi J. Contraceptive failure in the United States: estimates from the 1982 National Survey of Family Growth. Fam Plann Perspect. 1986;18:200–9.

33. Schirm AL, Trussell J, Menken J, Grady WR. Contraceptive failure in the United States: the impact of social, economic, and demographic factors. Fam Plann Perspect. 1982;14:68–75.

34. Sivin I, Schmidt F. Effectiveness of IUDs: a review. Contraception. 1987;36:55–84.

35. Vessey M, Lawless M, Yeates D. Efficacy of different contraceptive methods. Lancet. 1982;1:841–2.

36. Trussell J, Westoff CF. Contraceptive practice and trends in coital frequency. Fam Plann Perspect. 1980;12:246–9.

37. Steiner MJ, Hertz-Picciotto I, Raymond E, Trussell J, Wheeless A, Schoenbach V. Influence of cycle variability and coital frequency on the risk of pregnancy. Contraception. 1999;60:137–43.

38. Davis HJ. The shield intrauterine device: a superior modern contraceptive. Am J Obstet Gynecol. 1970;106:455–6.

39. Mintz M. At any cost: corporate greed, women, and the Dalkon shield. New York: Pantheon Books; 1985.

40. Trussell J. Methodological pitfalls in the analysis of contraceptive failure. Stat Med. 1991;10:201–20.

41. Trussell J, Hatcher RA, Cates W, Stewart FH, Kost K. A guide to interpreting contraceptive efficacy studies. Obstet Gynecol. 1990;76:558–67.

42. Trussell J, Menken J. Life table analysis of contraceptive failure. In: Hermalin AI, Entwisle B, (eds). The role of surveys in the analysis of family planning programs. Liege (Belgium): Ordina Editions; 1982. p. 537–71.

43. Tietze C, Poliakoff SR, Rock J. The clinical effectiveness of the rhythm method of contraception. Fertil Steril. 1951;2:444–50.

44. Trussell TJ, Faden R, Hatcher RA. Efficacy information in contraceptive counseling: those little white lies. Am J Public Health. 1976;66:761–7.

45. Laudan, L. The book of risks: fascinating facts about the chances we take every day. New York: J. Wiley & Sons; 1994.

46. Schwingl PJ, Ory HW, Visness CM. Estimates of the risk of cardiovascular death attributable to low-dose oral contraceptives in the United States. Am J Obstet Gynecol. 1999;180:241–9.

47. Escobedo LG, Peterson HB, Grubb GS, Franks AL. Case-fatality rates for tubal sterilization in U.S. hospitals, 1979–1980. Am J Obstet Gynecol. 1989;160:147–50.

48. Hajjeh RA, Reingold A, Weil A, Shutt K, Schuhat A, Perkins BA. Toxic shock syndrome in the United States, 1979–1996. Emerg Infect Dis. 1999;5:807–10.

49. US Bureau of the Census. Statistical abstract of the United States: 2003. Washington (DC): Government Printing Office; 2003. Table 11, Resident population by age and sex: 1980–2002. p. 13.

50. Berg CJ, Callaghan WM, Syverson C, Henderson Z. Pregnancy-related mortality in the United States, 1998 to 2005. Obstet Gynecol. 2010;116:1302–9.

51. Saraiya M, Green CA, Berg CJ, Hopkins FW, Koonin LM, Atrash HK. Spontaneous abortion-related deaths among women in the United States–1981–1991. Obstet Gynecol. 1999;94:172–6.

52. Karnovsky, R. (Danco Laboratories, New York, NY). Email to: James Trussell (Office of Population Research, Princeton University, Princeton, NJ). 2011 Jul 18.

53. Bartlett LA, Berg CJ, Shulman HB, Zane SB, Green CA, Whitehead S, Atrash HK. Risk factors for legal induced abortion-related mortality in the United States. Obstet Gynecol. 2004;103:729–37.

54. Burkman R, Schlesselman JJ, Zieman M. Safety concerns and health benefits associated with oral contraception. Am J Obstet Gynecol. 2004;190 Suppl 4:S5–22.

55. Hannaford PC, Iversen L, Macfarlane TV, Elliott AM, Angus V, Lee AJ. Mortality among contraceptive pill users: cohort evidence from Royal College of General Practitioners' oral contraception study. BMJ. 2010;340:c927.

56. Vessey M, Yeates D, Flynn S. Factors affecting mortality in a large cohort study with special reference to oral contraceptive use. Contraception. 2010;82:221–9.

57. Hunter DJ, Colditz GA, Hankinson SE, Malspeis S, Spiegelman D, Chen W, Stampfer MJ, Willett WC. Oral contraceptive use and breast cancer: A prospective study of young women. Cancer Epidemiol Biomarkers Prev. 2010;19:2496–502.

58. Hannaford PC, Selvaraj S, Elliott AM, Angus V, Iversen L, Lee AJ. Cancer risk among users of oral contraceptives: cohort data from the Royal College of General Practitioner's oral contraception study. BMJ. 2007;335:651.

59. Marchbanks PA, McDonald JA, Wilson HG, Folger SG, Mandel MG, Daling JR, Bernstein L, Malone KE, Ursin G, Strom BL, Norman SA, Wingo PA, Burkman RT, Berlin JA, Simon MS, Spirtas R, Weiss LK. Oral contraceptives and the risk of breast cancer. N Engl J Med. 2002;346:2025–32.

60. Wingo PA, Austin H, Marchbanks PA, Whiteman MK, Hsia J, Mandel MG, Peterson HB, Ory HW. Oral contraceptives and the risk of death from breast cancer. Obstet Gynecol. 2007;110:793–800.

61. Smith JS, Green J, Berrington de Gonzalez A, Appleby P, Peto J, Plummer M, Franceschi S, Beral V. Cervical cancer and use of hormonal contraceptives: a systematic review. Lancet. 2003;361:1159–67.

62. Collaborative Group on Hormonal Factors in Breast Cancer. Breast cancer and hormonal contraceptives: collaborative reanalysis of individual data on 53,297 women with breast cancer and 100,239 women without breast cancer from 54 epidemiological studies. Lancet. 1996;347:1713–27.

63. Faculty of Family Planning and Reproductive Health Care Clinical Effectiveness Unit. FFPRHC Guidance (April 2002). The levonorgestrel-releasing intrauterine system (LNg-IUS) in contraception and reproductive health. J Fam Plann Reprod Health Care. 2004;30:99–108.

64. The Alan Guttmacher Institute. Fulfilling the promise: public policy and U.S. family planning clinics. New York: The Alan Guttmacher Institute; 2000.

65. Finer LB, Darroch JE. Special tabulations of the 1995 National Survey of Family Growth. New York: The Alan Guttmacher Institute; 2001.

66. Forrest JD. Timing of reproductive life stages. Obstet Gynecol. 1993;82:105–10.

67. Tsui AO, Ochoa LH. Service proximity as a determinant of contraceptive behaviour: evidence from cross-national studies of survey data. In: Philips JF, Ross JA, (eds). Family planning programmes and fertility. Oxford (England): Clarendon Press; 1992. p. 222–56.

U.S. Medical Eligibility Criteria

Kathryn M. Curtis, PhD*
Herbert B. Peterson, MD

- Evidence-based medical eligibility criteria for contraceptive use are necessary to improve safe access to and quality of family planning services.

- The World Health Organization's (WHO) medical eligibility criteria are developed through a consensus process by an expert working group of international family planning experts, following a review of the best available evidence.

- The Centers for Disease Control and Prevention adapted the WHO guidance to create the *U.S. Medical Eligibility Criteria for Contraceptive Use, 2010*, for use by health care providers in the United States.

While most women can safely use any method of contraception, some women have health conditions that preclude the safe use of certain methods. Evidence-based guidelines regarding which women are medically eligible for contraceptive methods will help to assure that women are not exposed to inappropriate risks, while at the same time not denied access to methods that are medically appropriate. This, in turn, will improve access to and quality of family planning services. Past experience suggests that in the absence of such guidelines, unnecessary restrictions to contraceptive access may be imposed.

In 1994, the World Health Organization (WHO) initiated a process to develop appropriate medical eligibility criteria for widely used contraceptive methods. This process involved comparing existing eligibility criteria for contraceptive use from different agencies, preparing summaries of published medical and epidemiological literature relevant to medical eligibility criteria, and developing a draft classification framework. Two Expert Working Group meetings were convened by WHO in 1994 and

* The findings and conclusions in this report are those of the authors and do not necessarily represent the official position of the Centers for Disease Control and Prevention.

1995 to review the scientific evidence and to formulate recommendations. Publication of the first edition of *Improving Access to Quality Care in Family Planning: Medical Eligibility Criteria for Contraceptive Use* followed in 1996. The WHO Medical Eligibility Criteria for Contraceptive Use (MEC) is currently in its fourth edition and contains recommendations for 16 contraceptive methods and more than 60 medical conditions.[1] The Centers for Disease Control and Prevention (CDC), through close collaboration with WHO, has contributed substantially during the last 15 years to the creation of WHO's global family planning guidance. CDC has served as the lead for establishing the evidence base and presenting the evidence to WHO for use during its expert working group meetings to create and update the guidance.[3]

WHO has always intended for its global guidance to be adapted at the local level. The United Kingdom has gone through an adaptation process to create national versions of the guidance,[2] and CDC has recently adapted the WHO MEC for use by U.S. health care providers. While CDC made the decision to accept most of the WHO guidance, a small number of WHO recommendations were adapted for the United States, and recommendations were developed for several additional medical conditions. The modifications to existing WHO MEC recommendations included changes for women who are postpartum, including those who are breastfeeding, and for the medical conditions of deep vein thrombosis/pulmonary embolism, valvular heart disease, ovarian cancer, and uterine fibroids. New recommendations were developed for women with history of bariatric surgery, peripartum cardiomyopathy, rheumatoid arthritis, endometrial hyperplasia, inflammatory bowel disease, and solid organ transplantation. The U.S. MEC is intended to assist health care providers when they counsel women, men, and couples about contraceptive method choice. These recommendations are meant to serve as a source of general clinical guidance. Health care providers should always consider the individual clinical circumstances of each person seeking family planning services.

METHODOLOGY

WHO guidance is used widely around the world, including in the United States, and currently contains approximately 1,800 separate recommendations. However, the WHO MEC needed modification to account for new scientific evidence and for the context in which U.S. family planning services are provided. Consequently, CDC undertook the following steps:

- Met with partners and U.S. family planning experts in June 2008 to determine the scope of a U.S. adaptation.[4]

- Contacted numerous professional and service organizations and individual providers to identify areas in which WHO guidance was inconsistent with current U.S. practice.

- Identified specific WHO recommendations for which a compelling reason existed to consider modification.

- Assessed the need for adding recommendations for medical conditions not currently included in the WHO MEC.

CDC conducted systematic reviews of the scientific evidence to identify direct evidence of the safety of contraceptive method use by women with selected conditions (e.g., risk for disease progression or other adverse health effects in women with rheumatoid arthritis who use combined oral contraceptives). Information about indirect evidence or theoretical considerations was obtained when direct evidence was not available. The strength and quality of the evidence was graded using the system of the U.S. Preventive Services Task Force.[5] The systematic reviews then underwent peer-review by U.S. experts prior to their use for the adaptation.

In February 2009, CDC held a meeting of 31 experts including a wide range of health care providers, epidemiologists, and others with experience in family planning services and translation of evidence into guidance. CDC gathered the input from the experts during the meeting and finalized the recommendations in this document, which appear in the *U.S. Medical Eligibility Criteria for Contraceptive Use, 2010*.[6,9] Research gaps were noted on contraceptive safety for women with medical conditions and other characteristics.

HOW TO USE THE RECOMMENDATIONS

Four numeric categories are used to classify conditions affecting eligibility for the use of each contraceptive method:

- **Category 1.** A condition for which there is no restriction for the use of the contraceptive method.

- **Category 2.** A condition for which the advantages of using the method generally outweigh the theoretical or proven risks. (The method can generally be used, but careful follow-up may be required.)

- **Category 3.** A condition for which the theoretical or proven risks usually outweigh the advantages of using the method. (Use of that method is not usually recommended unless other more appropriate methods are not available or acceptable. Provision of a contraceptive method to a woman with a condition classified as a Category 3 requires careful clinical judgment and access to clinical services. The severity of the condition and the availability, practicality, and acceptability of alternative methods should be taken into account. Careful follow-up will be required.)

- **Category 4**. A condition that represents an unacceptable health risk if the contraceptive method is used.

USING THE CATEGORIES IN PRACTICE

Table 4–1 shows an example of how the categories may be put into practice. For example, a smoker who is less than age 35 can generally use combined oral contraceptives (COCs) (Category 2). However, for a woman who is 35 years or older and who smokes less than 15 cigarettes per day, the use of COCs usually is not recommended unless other methods are not available or acceptable to her (Category 3). A woman who is 35 years or older and smokes 15 or more cigarettes per day should not use COCs (Category 4). The programmatic implications of these categories may depend on the circumstances or protocols of particular professional or service organizations (e.g., in some settings, a Category 3 may mean that special consultation is warranted).

Table 4–1 Example of medical eligibility criteria for smoking and combined oral contraceptive (COC) use

Smoking	COC
a) Age < 35	2
b) Age ≥ 35	
(i) < 15 cigarettes/day	3
(ii) ≥ 15 cigarettes/day	4

The tables at the end of this chapter present a summary of the U.S. medical eligibility criteria for hormonal contraception, intrauterine contraception, and barrier methods (Table 4–2) and fertility awareness-based methods (Table 4–3). Information about the lactational amenorrhea method, coitus interruptus, and male and female sterilization can be found in the complete U.S. MEC document at: www.cdc.gov/reproductivehealth/UnintendedPregnancy/USMEC.htm.

Classification of Conditions for Fertility Awareness-based Methods

The classification of conditions for fertility awareness-based methods is different from the numeric classification described above. While there are no medical conditions that are worsened with use of fertility awareness-based methods, some conditions or characteristics may make the use of these methods more difficult. In such cases, the use of these methods may better be delayed until the condition is resolved or that special training is needed for correct use of the method. The following classification framework applies to fertility awareness-based methods:

A = Accept: There is no medical reason to deny the particular fertility awareness-based method to a woman in this circumstance.

C = Caution: The method is normally provided in a routine setting, but with extra preparation and precautions. This usually means that special counseling may be needed to ensure correct use of the method by a woman in this circumstance.

D = Delay: Use of this method should be delayed until the condition is evaluated or corrected. Alternative temporary methods of contraception should be offered.

NA = Not applicable

Contraceptive Method Initiation and Continuation

The recommendations address medical eligibility criteria for initiating and continuing use of all contraceptive methods evaluated. Continuation criteria are clinically relevant whenever a woman develops a health condition while she is using a contraceptive method. If the recommendations for initiation and continuation differ, these differences are noted in the columns 'Initiation' and 'Continuation'; otherwise, the category is the same for initiation and continuation of use.

Screening for Presence of Conditions

Conditions listed in the U.S. MEC represent either a person's characteristics (e.g., age, parity) or a known pre-existing medical or pathological condition (e.g., diabetes, hypertension). Whether screening for conditions is needed and how such screening should be conducted will be determined by national disease screening guidelines and institutional health and service delivery environments. In many cases, client history will be an appropriate approach.

Clarification of the Recommendations, Comments, and Citation of Scientific Evidence

In some cases, the numeric classification did not capture the complete recommendation, so additional narrative clarification was needed. Recommendations with a clarification are noted by an asterisk in the summary tables included in this chapter. The clarifications themselves can be found on the U.S. MEC Web site. The complete text of the U.S. MEC document also contains a brief summary and complete citation of all the evidence for each recommendation that is based on a systematic review, as well additional comments for selected recommendations.

MEDICAL ELIGIBILITY CRITERIA AND CONTRACEPTIVE CHOICE

Medical eligibility is just one element that needs to be considered by a woman, man, or couple at any given point in their lifetime when choosing the most appropriate contraceptive method. Other important elements include effectiveness, availability (including accessibility and affordability), and acceptability. For example, the classification of "Category 1" from the U.S. MEC means that the method can be used in that circumstance with no restrictions with regard to safety, but it does not necessarily imply that the method is the best choice for that person; effectiveness, availability, acceptability, and sexually transmitted infection risk also may play a key role in determining the most appropriate choice. For example, women with peripartum cardiomyopathy are at high risk of death should they experience a subsequent pregnancy. Contraceptive methods that are not highly effective are classified as "Category 1" for this condition because they do not worsen the condition or otherwise increase adverse health events. However, because of their relatively lower effectiveness, these methods are clearly not the best contraceptive option for most women with peripartum cardiomyopathy. Voluntary, informed choice of contraceptive methods is an essential guiding principle, and contraceptive counseling, where applicable, may be an important contributor to the successful use of contraceptive methods.

In choosing a method of contraception, the patient and the clinician must consider the risk for sexually transmitted infections (STIs), including human immunodeficiency virus (HIV). Although hormonal and intrauterine contraceptives are highly effective at preventing pregnancy, they do not protect against STIs. Consistent and correct use of the male latex condom reduces the risk for STIs.[7] When a male condom cannot be used properly for infection prevention, a female condom should be considered.[8] Women who use contraceptive methods other than condoms should be counseled about the use of condoms and the risk for STIs, including HIV infection.[8]

KEEPING CRITERIA UP TO DATE

A key component of evidence-based guidance is keeping the guidance up to date and based on the best available evidence. CDC will continue to work with WHO to identify and critically appraise new evidence relevant to the guidance as it becomes available and will use this process to update guidance when warranted. In general, CDC will make sure that the WHO MEC updates are appropriate for the U.S. context. Updates to the U.S. MEC can be found at: www.cdc.gov/reproductive health/UnintendedPregnancy/USMEC.htm

REFERENCES

1. World Health Organization. Medical eligibility criteria for contraceptive use. 4th edition [Internet]. Geneva: WHO; 2009 [cited 2010 May 3]. Available from http://www.who.int/reproductivehealth/publications/family_planning/9789241563888/en/index.html
2. Faculty of Family Planning and Reproductive Health Care, Royal College of Obstetricians and Gynecologists. UK medical eligibility criteria for contraceptive use, 2005–2006. London: Faculty of Family Planning and Reproductive Health Care; 2006.
3. Mohllajee AP, Curtis KM, Flanagan RG, Rinehart W, Gaffield ME, Peterson HB. Keeping up with evidence a new system for WHO's evidence-based family planning guidance. Am J Prev Med. 2005;28:483–90.
4. Curtis KM, Jamieson DJ, Peterson HB, Marchbanks PA. Adaptation of the World Health Organization's Medical Eligibility Criteria for Contraceptive Use for use in the United States. Contraception. 2010;82:3–9.
5. Harris RP, Helfand M, Woolf SH, Lohr KN, Mulrow CD, Teutsch SM, Atkins D, for the Methods Work Group, Third U.S. Preventive Services Task Force. Current methods of the U.S. Preventive Services Task Force: a review of the process. Am J Prev Med. 2001;20:21–35.
6. Centers for Disease Control and Prevention. U.S. Medical Eligibility Criteria for Contraceptive Use, 2010. MMWR. 2010;59(No.RR-4):1–85.
7. Centers for Disease Control and Prevention. Condom fact sheet in brief [Internet; cited 2010 May 3]. Available from http://www.cdc.gov/condomeffectiveness/docs/Condom_fact_Sheet_in_Brief.pdf.
8. Centers for Disease Control and Prevention. Sexually Transmitted Diseases Treatment Guidelines, 2010. MMWR. 2010; 59(RR no. 12).

LATE REFERENCE

9. Centers for Disease Control and Prevention. Update to CDC's U.S. Medical Eligibility Criteria for Contraceptive Use, 2010: revised recommendations for the use of contraceptive methods during the postpartum period. MMWR 2011;60:878–883.

Table 4-2 Summary tables: hormonal contraception, intrauterine contraception, and barrier methods

KEY:
COC Combined Oral Contraceptives
P/R Patch or Ring
POP Progestin-Only Pill
DMPA Depot Medroxyprogesterone Acetate
Cu IUC Copper Intrauterine Contraceptive
LNg IUC Levonorgestrel Intrauterine Contraceptive

C Male latex condoms, male polyurethane condoms, female condoms
S Spermicide (film, tablets, foam, gel)
D Diaphragm (with spermicide), cervical cap
I = Initiation, C = Continuation

PERSONAL CHARACTERISTICS AND REPRODUCTIVE HISTORY

CONDITION	COC/P/R	POP	DMPA	Implants	LNg IUC	Cu IUC	C	S	D
PREGNANCY	NA*	NA*	NA*	NA*	4*	4*	NA*	NA*	NA*
AGE	Menarche to <40=1 ≥40=2	Menarche to <18=1 18–45=1 >45=1	Menarche to <18=2 18–45=1 >45=2	Menarche to <18=1 18–45=1 >45=1	Menarche to <20=2 ≥20=1	Menarche to <20=2 ≥20=1	Menarche to <40=1 ≥40=1	Menarche to <40=1 ≥40=1	Menarche to <40=1 ≥40=1
PARITY									
a) Nulliparous	1	1	1	1	2	2	1	1	1
b) Parous	1	1	1	1	1	1	1	1	2*
BREASTFEEDING (see also Postpartum)									
a) < 1 mo postpartum	3*	2*	2*	2*					
b) 1 mos to < 6 months	2*	1*	1*	1*					
c) ≥ 6 months postpartum	2*	1*	1*	1*					

* Please consult the full text of the U.S. Medical Eligibility Criteria for a clarification to this classification.

(continued)

Table 4–2 Summary tables: hormonal contraception, intrauterine contraception, and barrier methods—*(cont'd)*

CONDITION	COC/P/R	POP	DMPA	Implants	LNg IUC	Cu IUC	C	S	D
POSTPARTUM (see also Breastfeeding)									
a) < 21 days	4	1	1	1					
b) 21 days to 42 days									
i. With other risk factors for VTE	3*	1	1	1					
ii. Without other risk factors for VTE	2	1	1	1					
c) > 42 days	1	1	1	1					
POSTPARTUM (breastfeeding or non-breastfeeding women, including post-Caesarean section)									
a) < 10 min after delivery of the placenta					2	1			
b) 10 min after delivery of the placenta to < 4 wks					2	2			
c) ≥ 4 wks					1	1			
d) Puerperal sepsis					4	4			
POSTPARTUM									
a) < 6 weeks							1	1	N/A*
b) ≥ 6 weeks							1	1	1
POST-ABORTION									
a) First trimester	1*	1*	1*	1*	1*	1*	1	1	1
b) Second trimester	1*	1*	1*	1*	2	2	1	1	1*
c) Immediate post-septic abortion	1*	1*	1*	1*	4	4	1	1	1

* Please consult the full text of the U.S. Medical Eligibility Criteria for a clarification to this classification.

(continued)

Table 4-2 Summary tables: hormonal contraception, intrauterine contraception, and barrier methods—*(cont'd)*

CONDITION	COC/P/R	POP	DMPA	Implants	LNg IUC	Cu IUC	C	S	D
PAST ECTOPIC PREGNANCY	1	2	1	1	1	1	1	1	1
HISTORY OF PELVIC SURGERY (see postpartum, including Caesarean section)	1	1	1	1	1	1	1	1	1
SMOKING									
a) Age <35	2	1	1	1	1	1	1	1	1
b) Age ≥35									
(i) <15 cigarettes/day	3	1	1	1	1	1	1	1	1
(ii) ≥15 cigarettes/day	4	1	1	1	1	1	1	1	1
OBESITY									
a) ≥ 30 kg/m² (BMI)	2	1	1	1	1	1	1	1	1
b) Menarche to <18 yrs and ≥30 kg/m² BMI	2	1	2	1	1	1	1	1	1
HISTORY OF BARIATRIC SURGERY§									
a) Restrictive procedures: decrease storage capacity of the stomach (vertical banded gastroplasty, laparoscopic adjustable gastric band, laparoscopic sleeve gastrectomy)	1	1	1	1	1	1	1	1	1

* Please consult the full text of the U.S. Medical Eligibility Criteria for a clarification to this classification.

(continued)

Table 4–2 Summary tables: hormonal contraception, intrauterine contraception, and barrier methods—*(cont'd)*

CONDITION	COC/P/R	POP	DMPA	Implants	LNg IUC	Cu IUC	C	S	D
b) Malabsorptive procedures: decrease absorption of nutrients and calories by shortening the functional length of the small intestine (Roux-en-Y gastric bypass, biliopancreatic diversion)	COCs: 3 P/R: 1	3	1	1	1	1	1	1	1
CARDIOVASCULAR DISEASE									
MULTIPLE RISK FACTORS FOR ARTERIAL CARDIOVASCULAR DISEASE (such as older age, smoking, diabetes and hypertension)	3/4*	2*	3*	2*	2	1	1	1	1
HYPERTENSION									
a) Adequately controlled hypertension	3*	1*	2*	1*	1	1	1	1	1
b) Elevated blood pressure levels (properly taken measurements)									
(i) systolic 140–159 or diastolic 90–99	3	1	2	1	1	1	1	1	1
(ii) systolic ≥160 or diastolic ≥100	4	2	3	2	2	1	1	1	1
c) Vascular disease	4	2	3	2	2	1	1	1	1

* Please consult the full text of the U.S. Medical Eligibility Criteria for a clarification to this classification.

(continued)

Table 4–2 Summary tables: hormonal contraception, intrauterine contraception, and barrier methods—*(cont'd)*

CONDITION	COC/P/R	POP	DMPA	Implants	LNg IUC	Cu IUC	C	S	D
HISTORY OF HIGH BLOOD PRESSURE DURING PREGNANCY (where current blood pressure is measurable and normal)	2	1	1	1	1	1	1	1	1
DEEP VENOUS THROMBOSIS (DVT)/ PULMONARY EMBOLISM (PE)									
a. History of DVT/PE, not on anticoagulant therapy									
i. Higher risk for recurrent DVT/PE (≥1 risk factors)	4	2	2	2	2	1	1	1	1
History of estrogen-associated DVT/PE									
Pregnancy-associated DVT/PE									
Idiopathic DVT/PE									
Known thrombophilia, including antiphospholipid syndrome									
Active cancer (metastatic, on therapy, or within 6 mos after clinical remission), excluding non-melanoma skin cancer									
History of recurrent DVT/PE									

(continued)

* Please consult the full text of the U.S. Medical Eligibility Criteria for a clarification to this classification.

CONTRACEPTIVE TECHNOLOGY

Table 4–2 Summary tables: hormonal contraception, intrauterine contraception, and barrier methods—(cont'd)

CONDITION	COC/P/R	POP	DMPA	Implants	LNg IUC	Cu IUC	C	S	D
ii. Lower risk for recurrent DVT/PE (no risk factors)	3	2	2	2	2	1	1	1	1
b. Acute DVT/PE	4	2	2	2	2	2	1	1	1
c. DVT/PE and established on anticoagulant therapy for at least 3 mos									
i. Higher risk for recurrent DVT/PE (≥1 risk factors) Known thrombophilia, including antiphospholipid syndrome Active cancer (metastatic, on therapy, or within 6 mos after clinical remission), excluding non-melanoma skin cancer History of recurrent DVT/PE	4*	2	2	2	2	2	1	1	1
ii. Lower risk for recurrent DVT/PE (no risk factors)	3*	2	2	2	2	2	1	1	1
d. Family history (first-degree relatives)	2	1	1	1	1	1	1	1	1
e. Major surgery									
i. With prolonged immobilization	4	2	2	2	2	1	1	1	1

* Please consult the full text of the U.S. Medical Eligibility Criteria for a clarification to this classification.

(continued)

Table 4–2 Summary tables: hormonal contraception, intrauterine contraception, and barrier methods—(cont'd)

CONDITION	COC/P/R	POP	DMPA	Implants	LNg IUC	Cu IUC	C	S	D
ii. Without prolonged immobilization	2	1	1	1	1	1	1	1	1
f. Minor surgery without immobilization	1	1	1	1	1	1	1	1	1
KNOWN THROMBOGENIC MUTATIONS (e.g. Factor V Leiden; Prothrombin mutation; Protein S, Protein C and Antithrombin deficiencies)	4*	2*	2*	2*	2*	1*	1*	1*	1*
SUPERFICIAL VENOUS THROMBOSIS									
a) Varicose veins	1	1	1	1	1	1	1	1	1
b) Superficial thrombophlebitis	2	1	1	1	1	1	1	1	1
CURRENT AND HISTORY OF ISCHAEMIC HEART DISEASE	4	I=2 / C=3	3	I=2 / C=3	I=2 / C=3	1	1	1	1
STROKE (history of cerebrovascular accident)	4	I=2 / C=3	3	I=2 / C=3	2	1	1	1	1
KNOWN HYPERLIPIDAEMIAS	2/3*	2*	2*	2*	2*	1*	1*	1*	1*
VALVULAR HEART DISEASE									
a) Uncomplicated	2	1	1	1	1	1	1	1	1

* Please consult the full text of the U.S. Medical Eligibility Criteria for a clarification to this classification.

(continued)

Table 4-2 Summary tables: hormonal contraception, intrauterine contraception, and barrier methods—(cont'd)

CONDITION	COC/P/R	POP	DMPA	Implants	LNg IUC	Cu IUC	C	S	D
b) Complicated (pulmonary hypertension, atrial fibrillation, history of subacute bacterial endocarditis)	4	1	1	1	1	1	1	1	2
PERIPARTUM CARDIOMYOPATHY[§]									
a. Normal or mildly impaired cardiac function (New York Heart Association Functional Class I or II: patients with no limitation of activities or patients with slight, mild limitation of activity)(1)									
i. <6 mos	4	1	1	1	2	2	1	1	1
ii. ≥6 mos	3	1	1	1	2	2	1	1	1
b. Moderately or severely impaired cardiac function: (New York Heart Association Functional Class III or IV: patients with marked limitation of activity or patients who should be at complete rest) (1)	4	2	2	2	2	2	1	1	1

RHEUMATIC DISEASES

SYSTEMIC LUPUS ERYTHEMATOSUS (SLE)[§]

CONDITION	COC/P/R	POP (I / C)	DMPA (I / C)	Implants	LNg IUC	Cu IUC (I / C)	C	S	D
a. Positive (or unknown) antiphospholipid antibodies	4	3 / 3	3 / 3	3	3	1 / 1	1	1	1

(continued)

* Please consult the full text of the U.S. Medical Eligibility Criteria for a clarification to this classification.

Table 4–2 Summary tables: hormonal contraception, intrauterine contraception, and barrier methods—(cont'd)

CONDITION	COC/P/R	POP	DMPA	Implants	LNg IUC	Cu IUC	C	S	D
b. Severe thrombocytopenia	2	2	3	2	2*	I 3* / C 2*	1	1	1
c. Immunosuppressive treatment	2	2	2	2	2	2	1	1	1
d. None of the above	2	2	2	2	2	1	1	1	1
RHEUMATOID ARTHRITIS									
a. On immunosuppressive therapy	2	1	2/3*	1	I 2 / C 1	I 2 / C 1	1	1	1
b. Not on immunosuppressive therapy	2	1	2	1	1	1	1	1	1

NEUROLOGIC CONDITIONS

HEADACHES (I = Initiation, C = Continuation)

CONDITION	COC/P/R	POP	DMPA	Implants	LNg IUC	Cu IUC	C	S	D
a) Non-migrainous (mild or severe)	I 1* / C 2*	1*	1*	1*	1*	1*	1		
b) Migraine									
(i) without aura									
Age <35	I 2* / C 3*	I 1* / C 2*	2*	2*	I 2* / C 2*	1*	1	1	1
Age ≥35	I 3* / C 4*	I 1* / C 2*	2*	2*	I 2* / C 2*	1*	1	1	1
(ii) with aura (at any age)	I 4* / C 4*	I 2* / C 3*	3*	3*	I 2* / C 3*	1*	1	1	1
EPILEPSY	1*	1*	1*	1*	1	1	1	1	1

*Please consult the full text of the U.S. Medical Eligibility Criteria for a clarification to this classification.

(continued)

Table 4–2 Summary tables: hormonal contraception, intrauterine contraception, and barrier methods—(cont'd)

CONDITION	COC/P/R	POP	DMPA	Implants	LNg IUC	Cu IUC	C	S	D
DEPRESSIVE DISORDERS									
DEPRESSIVE DISORDERS	1*	1*	1*	1*	1*	1*	1	1	1
REPRODUCTIVE TRACT INFECTIONS AND DISORDERS									
VAGINAL BLEEDING PATTERNS									
a) Irregular pattern *without* heavy bleeding	1	2	2	2	I 1 / C 1	1			
b) Heavy or prolonged bleeding (includes regular and irregular patterns)	1*	2*	2*	2*	1* 2*	2*			
UNEXPLAINED VAGINAL BLEEDING (suspicious for serious condition)									
Before evaluation	2*	2*	3*	3*	I 4* / C 2*	I 4* / C 2*	1*	1*	1*
ENDOMETRIOSIS	1	1	1	1	1	2	1	1	1
BENIGN OVARIAN TUMOURS (including cysts)	1	1	1	1	1	1	1	1	1
SEVERE DYSMENORRHOEA	1	1	1	1	2	2	1	1	1
GESTATIONAL TROPHOBLASTIC DISEASE									
a) Decreasing or undetectable B-hCG levels	1	1	1	1	3	3	1	1	1

* Please consult the full text of the U.S. Medical Eligibility Criteria for a clarification to this classification.

(continued)

Table 4-2 Summary tables: hormonal contraception, intrauterine contraception, and barrier methods—(cont'd)

CONDITION	COC/P/R	POP	DMPA	Implants	LNg IUC	Cu IUC	C	S	D
b) Persistently elevated B-hCG levels or malignant disease	1	1	1	1	4	4	1	1	1
CERVICAL ECTROPION	1	1	1	1	1	1	1	1	1
CERVICAL INTRAEPITHELIAL NEOPLASIA (CIN)	2	1	2	2	2	1	1	1	1*
CERVICAL CANCER (awaiting treatment)	2	1	2	2	I 4 / C 2	I 4 / C 2	1	2	1*
BREAST DISEASE									
a) Undiagnosed mass	2*	2*	2*	2*	2	1	1	1	1
b) Benign breast disease	1	1	1	1	1	1	1	1	1
c) Family history of cancer	1	1	1	1	1	1	1	1	1
d) Cancer									
(i) current	4	4	4	4	4	1	1	1	1
(ii) past and no evidence of current disease for 5 years	3	3	3	3	3	1	1	1	1
ENDOMETRIAL HYPERPLASIA	1	1	1	1	1	1	1	1	1
ENDOMETRIAL CANCER	1	1	1	1	I 4 / C 2	I 4 / C 2	1	1	1
OVARIAN CANCER	1	1	1	1	1	1	1	1	1

(continued)

* Please consult the full text of the U.S. Medical Eligibility Criteria for a clarification to this classification.

Table 4–2 Summary tables: hormonal contraception, intrauterine contraception, and barrier methods—*(cont'd)*

CONDITION	COC/P/R	POP	DMPA	Implants	LNg IUC	Cu IUC	C	S	D
UTERINE FIBROIDS	1	1	1	1	2	2	1	1	1
ANATOMICAL ABNORMALITIES									
a. Distorted uterine cavity (any congenital or acquired uterine abnormality distorting the uterine cavity in a manner that is incompatible with IUD insertion)					4	4	1	1	NA*
b. Other abnormalities (including cervical stenosis or cervical lacerations) not distorting the uterine cavity or interfering with IUD insertion					2	2	1	1	NA*
PELVIC INFLAMMATORY DISEASE (PID)					I C	I C			
a) Past PID (assuming no current risk factors of STIs)									
(i) with subsequent pregnancy	1	1	1	1	1 1	1 1	1	1	1
(ii) without subsequent pregnancy	1	1	1	1	2 2	2 2	1	1	1
b) PID - current	1	1	1	1	4 2*	4 2*	1	1	1

* Please consult the full text of the U.S. Medical Eligibility Criteria for a clarification to this classification.

(continued)

Table 4-2 Summary tables: hormonal contraception, intrauterine contraception, and barrier methods—*(cont'd)*

CONDITION	COC/P/R	POP	DMPA	Implants	LNg IUC I	LNg IUC C	Cu IUC I	Cu IUC C	C	S	D
STIs											
a) Current purulent cervicitis or chlamydial infection or gonorrhoea	1	1	1	1	4	2*	4	2*	1	1	1
b) Other STIs (excluding HIV and hepatitis)	1	1	1	1	2	2	2	2	1	1	1
c) Vaginitis (including trichomonas vaginalis and bacterial vaginosis)	1	1	1	1	2	2	2	2	1	1	1
d) Increased risk of STIs	1	1	1	1	2/3*	2	2/3*	2	1	1	1
HIV/AIDS											
HIGH RISK OF HIV	1	1	1	1	2	2	2	2	1	4	4
HIV-INFECTED	1	1	1	1	2	2	2	2	1	3	3
AIDS	1*	1*	1*	1*	3	2*	3	2*	1	3	3
Clinically well on ARV therapy	See ANTIRETROVIRAL THERAPY below										
OTHER INFECTIONS											
SCHISTOSOMIASIS											
a) Uncomplicated	1	1	1	1	1	1	1	1	1	1	1
b) Fibrosis of the liver	1	1	1	1	1	1	1	1	1	1	1

* Please consult the full text of the U.S. Medical Eligibility Criteria for a clarification to this classification.

(continued)

Table 4–2 Summary tables: hormonal contraception, intrauterine contraception, and barrier methods—*(cont'd)*

CONDITION	COC/P/R	POP	DMPA	Implants	LNg IUC I	LNg IUC C	Cu IUC I	Cu IUC C	C	S	D
TUBERCULOSIS											
a) Non-pelvic	1*	1*	1*	1*	1	1	1	1	1	1	1
b) Known pelvic	1*	1	1	1	4	3	4	3	1	1	1
MALARIA	1	1	1	1	1		1		1	1	1
HISTORY OF TOXIC SHOCK									1	1	3
URINARY TRACT INFECTION									1	1	2
ENDOCRINE CONDITIONS											
DIABETES											
a) History of gestational disease	1	1	1	1	1		1		1	1	1
b) Non-vascular disease											
(i) non-insulin dependent	2	2	2	2	2		1		1	1	1
(ii) insulin dependent	2	2	2	2	2		1		1	1	1
c) Nephropathy/retinopathy/ neuropathy	3/4*	2	3	2	2		1		1	1	1
d) Other vascular disease or diabetes of >20 years' duration	3/4*	2	3	2	2		1		1	1	1
THYROID DISORDERS											
a) Simple goitre	1	1	1	1	1		1		1	1	1
b) Hyperthyroid	1	1	1	1	1		1		1	1	1
c) Hypothyroid	1	1	1	1	1		1		1	1	1

(continued)

* Please consult the full text of the U.S. Medical Eligibility Criteria for a clarification to this classification.

Table 4–2 Summary tables: hormonal contraception, intrauterine contraception, and barrier methods—(cont'd)

CONDITION	COC/P/R	POP	DMPA	Implants	LNg IUC	Cu IUC	C	S	D
GASTROINTESTINAL CONDITIONS									
INFLAMMATORY BOWEL DISEASE (IBD) (ulcerative colitis, Crohn disease)	2/3*	2	2	1	1	1	1	1	1
GALL-BLADDER DISEASE									
a) Symptomatic									
(i) treated by cholecystectomy	2	2	2	2	2	1	1	1	1
(ii) medically treated	3	2	2	2	2	1	1	1	1
(iii) current	3	2	2	2	2	1	1	1	1
b) Asymptomatic	2	2	2	2	2	1	1	1	1
HISTORY OF CHOLESTASIS									
a) Pregnancy-related	2	1	1	1	1	1	1	1	1
b) Past COC-related	3	2	2	2	2	1	1	1	1
VIRAL HEPATITIS	I C								
a) Acute or flare	3/4* 2	1	1	1	1	1	1	1	1
b) Carrier	1	1	1	1	1	1	1	1	1
c) Chronic	1	1	1	1	1	1	1	1	1
CIRRHOSIS									
a) Mild (compensated)	1	1	1	1	1	1	1	1	1
b) Severe (decompensated)	4	3	3	3	3	1	1	1	1

* Please consult the full text of the U.S. Medical Eligibility Criteria for a clarification to this classification.

(continued)

Table 4–2 Summary tables: hormonal contraception, intrauterine contraception, and barrier methods—(cont'd)

CONDITION	COC/P/R	POP	DMPA	Implants	LNg IUC	Cu IUC	C	S	D
LIVER TUMORS									
a) Benign									
i. Focal nodular hyperplasia	2	2	2	2	2	1	1	1	1
ii. Hepatocellular adenoma§	4	3	3	3	3	1	1	1	1
b. Malignant§ (hepatoma)	4	3	3	3	3	1	1	1	1
ANAEMIAS									
THALASSAEMIA	1	1	1	1	1	2	1	1	1
SICKLE CELL DISEASE	2	1	1	1	1	2	1	1	1
IRON-DEFICIENCY ANAEMIA	1	1	1	1	1	2	1	1	1
SOLID ORGAN TRANSPLANTATION									
SOLID ORGAN TRANSPLANTATION§					I C	I C			
a. Complicated: graft failure (acute or chronic), rejection, cardiac allograft vasculopathy	4	2	2	2	3 2	3 2			1
b. Uncomplicated	2*	2	2	2	2	2	1	1	1

* Please consult the full text of the U.S. Medical Eligibility Criteria for a clarification to this classification.

(continued)

Table 4-2 Summary tables: hormonal contraception, intrauterine contraception, and barrier methods—*(cont'd)*

Drug Interactions

CONDITION	COC/P/R	POP	DMPA	Implants	LNg IUC		Cu IUC		C	S	D
					I	C	I	C			
ANTIRETROVIRAL THERAPY											
a. Nucleoside reverse transcriptase inhibitors (NRTIs)	1*	1	1	1	2/3*	2*	2/3*	2*	1	3*	3*
b. Non-nucleoside reverse transcriptase inhibitors (NNRTIs)	2*	2*	1	2*	2/3*	2*	2/3*	2*	1	3*	3*
c. Ritonavir-boosted protease inhibitors	3*	3*	1	2*	2/3*	2*	2/3*	2*	1	3*	3*
ANTICONVULSANT THERAPY											
a. Certain anticonvulsants (phenytoin, carbamazepine, barbiturates, primidone, topiramate, oxcarbazepine)	3*	3*	1	2*	1		1		1	1	1
b. Lamotrigine	3*	1	1	1	1		1		1	1	1
ANTIMICROBIAL THERAPY											
a. Broad-spectrum antibiotics	1	1	1	1	1		1		1	1	1
b. Antifungals	1	1	1	1	1		1		1	1	1
c. Antiparasitics	1	1	1	1	1		1		1	1	1
d. Rifampicin or rifabutin therapy	3*	3*	1	2*	1		1		1	1	1

ALLERGIES

CONDITION	COC/P/R	POP	DMPA	Implants	LNg IUC	Cu IUC	C	S	D
ALLERGY TO LATEX							3*	1	3*

* Please consult the full text of the U.S. Medical Eligibility Criteria for a clarification to this classification.

Contraceptive Technology

Table 4–3 Fertility awareness-based methods

KEY:

SYM Symptoms-based methods	**A** Accept
CAL Calendar-based methods	**C** Caution
	D Delay
	NA Not applicable

Women with conditions which make pregnancy an unacceptable risk should be advised that fertility awareness-based methods may not be appropriate for them because of their relatively-higher typical-use failure rates.

	CATEGORY	
CONDITION	**SYM**	**CAL**

PERSONAL CHARACTERISTICS AND REPRODUCTIVE HISTORY

	SYM	CAL
PREGNANCY		NA*
LIFE STAGE		
a) Post-menarche	C*	C*
b) Peri-menopause	C*	C*
BREASTFEEDING		
a) < 6 weeks postpartum	D	D
b) ≥ 6 weeks postpartum	C	D
c) After menses begin	C	C
POSTPARTUM (in non-breastfeeding women)		
a) < 4 weeks	D	D
b) ≥ 4 weeks	A	D
POST-ABORTION	C	D

REPRODUCTIVE TRACT INFECTIONS AND DISORDERS

	SYM	CAL
IRREGULAR VAGINAL BLEEDING	D	D
VAGINAL DISCHARGE	D	A

OTHER

	SYM	CAL
USE OF DRUGS WHICH AFFECT CYCLE REGULARITY, HORMONES AND/OR FERTILITY SIGNS	C/D	C/D
DISEASES WHICH ELEVATE BODY TEMPERATURE		
a) Chronic diseases	C	A
b) Acute diseases	D	A

* Please consult the full text of the U.S. Medical Eligibility Criteria for a clarification to this classification.

Abstinence, Noncoital Sex, and Nonsense: What Every Clinician Needs to Know

John Santelli, MD, MPH
Deborah Kowal, MA, PA
Erin Wheeler, MPH

- Abstinence can be a wise and healthy *choice* at any life stage (particularly when a person does not feel ready for sexual involvement or a relationship). Sexual activity should always be mutually agreed upon; sexual coercion is unhealthy at any age.

- In real-life practice, abstinence from penile-vaginal sexual intercourse appears to be relatively ineffective against pregnancy (and sexually transmitted infections), as abstinence intentions often fail. A back-up method should always be planned.

- Engaging in noncoital sexual behaviors may effectively prevent an unwanted pregnancy but has implications for preventing sexually transmitted infections (STIs).

- The health care provider's role should be supportive: assessing relationship history and sexual practices, screening for sexual coercion, providing counseling about pregnancy and STI risk, and providing support for patient choices and the development of healthy sexuality. Health care practice should be based on science and avoid simple (and nonsensical) solutions based on ideological beliefs.

This chapter addresses several subjects: definitions of abstinence, the practice of abstinence within the development of healthy sexuality, the contraceptive importance of abstinence and other sexual behaviors, the scientific data on sexual behaviors, and the importance of clinician counseling in fostering healthy choices and effective contraception. Women and men at every age may pass through periods of voluntary or involuntary abstinence from sexual intercourse. Likewise, women in particular experience sexual coercion at every age, which has implications for the ability to rely on abstinence to prevent pregnancy and STIs. Thus, be alert to these realities and ready to provide education, counseling, support and referrals, as needed.

D EFINITIONS AND DEMOGRAPHICS: ABSTINENCE AND NONCOITAL SEX

In the United States of the 21st century, there is a lack of consensus about what abstinence does, and does not, entail. Some people define abstinence as refraining from all sexual behavior, including masturbation. Some people define abstinence as refraining from sexual behavior involving genital contact. Others define it as refraining from penetrative sexual practices. Still others would offer different definitions. Federal policy from 1998 to 2008 focused on abstinence—generally including all sexual behaviors—until marriage.[1] Understanding how clients view abstinence has important clinical implications. Notably, clients will use a variety of terms for abstinence and sexual activity, so these terms need careful exploration when a client uses them.

Persons who are abstinent from penile-vaginal intercourse may engage in a variety of other sexual behaviors. In a study of high-school students who consider themselves virgins, 30% had engaged in heterosexual masturbation of or by a partner, 9% had engaged in fellatio (oral-penile contact) with ejaculation, and 10% had engaged in cunnilingus (oral-female genital contact).[2] More than half (59%) of college undergraduates in another study responded that oral-genital contact did not constitute having "had sex" with a partner, and 19% said the same about penile-anal intercourse.[3]

While allowing that individuals have personal definitions regarding what is meant by abstinence, it is important to also understand specifically the client's risk for pregnancy and sexually transmitted infections (STIs). For purposes of contraception, abstinence may be defined as refraining from penile-vaginal intercourse. For purposes of protection from STIs, abstinence should be defined as refraining from those acts that result in transmission of an STI and development of disease or continued transmission. These other sexual acts (particularly oral and anal sex) vary greatly in their STI risk (see below).

Abstinence can be primary or secondary [and voluntary or involuntary]. *Primary abstainers* have never had sexual intercourse with another person. First penile-vaginal intercourse generally occurs between ages 12 and 25,[4] so that primary abstinence is common among younger teens and not uncommon among young adults. At age 12, 97% of girls and boys report primary abstinence from penile-vaginal intercourse. This decreases to 84% at age 15, 23% at age 20, and 5% at age 25. By age 44, only

1% report primary abstinence. Abstinence until marriage is extremely rare (by age 44, only 3% have delayed sex until marriage). From the mid 1960s through about 1990, sexual activity among teens increased—with the median age for first sex declining from age 19 to age 17.[4] The median age for first penile-vaginal intercourse in much of the developed world today is between 17 and 17.5 years.[5] Among young women age 18 to 24 years who first had sex as a teenager, 10% reported that their first sex was not voluntary, 13% reported that they did not want it to happen at the time, and 52% reported having mixed feelings.[6]

Initiation of oral sex is closely linked in time with initiation of penile-vaginal intercourse;[7] presumably oral sex commonly occurs with the same sexual partner with whom one initiates penile-vaginal intercourse. Oral sex is slightly more common than penile-vaginal intercourse among teens, suggesting that some teens may be using oral sex as an alternative to penile-vaginal intercourse. Almost 90% of 25 to 44 year olds and 55% of 15 to 19 year olds have had oral sex with an opposite sex partner.[8] Despite concerns expressed in the popular media, the prevalence of oral sex did not change from the early 1990s to 2002.[8]

Heterosexual anal sex is less common than oral sex and penile-vaginal intercourse and generally initiated later.[7] Among 25 to 44 year olds, anal sex with an opposite sex partner is reported by 35% of women and 40% of men; among 15 to 19 year olds, this percentage is 11%.[8]

Most gay, lesbian, bisexual, transgendered and questioning (GLBTQ) youth also initiate sexual activity in their teens and early 20s. Because the development of sexual identity may be gradual and nonheterosexual identity is often highly stigmatized, GLBTQ youth may engage in heterosexual activities including penile-vaginal intercourse.[9] Many GLBTQ young women are at risk of unintended pregnancy because of engagement in heterosexual activity.

Secondary abstainers are sexually experienced but for various reasons no longer engage in behaviors they consider as "having sex." Among sexually experienced women age 15 to 44 years, 4% to 9%, depending on age group, report that they had not had sexual contact with a man in the 12 months prior to the interview (Table 5–1). Among men, those percentages are 5% to 7%.[8] (See Table 5–2.) Many of these secondary abstainers are not currently in a relationship for a variety of reasons. While some may choose long-term abstinence, many desire a new relationship or sexual activity outside the context of a monogamous relationship. With re-initiating activity, they are potentially at risk for unintended pregnancy and STIs. Thus, clinical counseling among secondary abstainers should address formation of new relationships, renewed sexual activity, contraception, and protection from STIs.

Table 5-1 Percentage of U.S. women age 15-44 who report primary abstinence, secondary abstinence and ever having oral, anal or vaginal sex with an opposite sex-partner, 2002

Age	15–19	20–24	25–29	30–34	35–39	40–44	15–44
Primary Abstinence (Never had sexual contact, not oral, vaginal or anal sex)	36.7	8.7	2.5	1.8	1.0	1.3	8.4
Secondary Abstinence (Has had sexual contact, but not in the 12 months prior to the interview)	8.1	4.7	4.4	6.1	8.2	9.1	6.9
Ever had vaginal sex	53.0	87.3	97.2	98.1	98.7	98.6	89.2
Ever had oral sex	54.3	83.0	87.8	89.3	88.2	88.0	82.0
Ever had anal sex	10.9	29.6	32.8	37.8	34.3	33.8	30.0

Source: Mosher, et al. (2005).[8]

Table 5-2 Percentage of U.S. men age 15–44 who report primary abstinence, secondary abstinence and ever having oral, anal or vaginal sex with an opposite sex-partner, 2002

Age	15–19	20–24	25–29	30–34	35–39	40–44	15–44
Primary Abstinence (Never had sexual contact, not oral, vaginal or anal sex)	40.3	9.0	4.7	2.7	1.9	1.8	10.0
Secondary Abstinence (Has had sexual contact, but not in the 12 months prior to the interview)	5.9	6.6	6.7	4.7	7.4	7.2	6.4
Ever had vaginal sex	49.1	87.6	95.3	96.9	98.1	98.1	87.6
Ever had oral sex	55.1	82.2	88.7	90.3	91.1	90.3	83.0
Ever had anal sex	11.2	32.6	36.5	41.1	42.1	39.9	34.0

Source: Mosher, et al. (2005).[8]

INDICATIONS FOR ABSTINENCE

Logic suggests that all women and men abstain from all or some sexual activities at some time in their lives, both as primary and later as secondary abstainers. Many women and men may plan to abstain for a given period of time or within given relationships, although many may find it challenging to follow through on these plans.

Primary abstainers tend to be young and may choose to avoid certain sexual activities because of their youth, personal beliefs that suggest it is unhelpful or perhaps wrong to have a sexually intimate relationship until a given set of conditions is achieved, a desire to abide by the wishes of their adult guardians, a lack of interest, or for any number of acceptable and healthy reasons.

For sexually experienced persons, short-term abstinence may also make sense, for variety of reasons. The idea of abstinence "for a while" may be useful until effective contraception is achieved, until the couple feels a mutual trust is reached in a relationship, while waiting for tests for STIs and agreement about protection, or during the 2 to 6 weeks postpartum. Short-term abstinence is also common among sexually experienced adolescents, who may engage in sex intermittently.

For many individuals, abstinence "right now, tonight or today" is the ever-available back-up method of contraception and protection. However, short-term intentions to use abstinence are likely to fail, particularly if partners are not supportive. Women and men who intend to be abstinent should be encouraged to have a back-up contraceptive or protective method, such as condoms, just in case their resolve changes. For couples, engagement in a variety on noncoital behaviors such as kissing, mutual masturbation, outercourse (nonpenetrative sexual stimulation), or oral sex may also be appropriate. For individuals, masturbation with or without sex toys is suitable; in some cases, clients may hold personal qualms based on misinformation they have heard or read. Clinical counseling should address these options.

For those who deliberately choose to abstain, your role as care provider is to understand the individual's long- and short-term goals, to support her or his healthy choices and counsel about risky choices, to teach negotiation and planning skills to achieve her or his goals, and to provide counseling and referrals as needed—certain individuals may require help if they feel abstinence stems from a dysfunction.

People may practice short-term abstinence for a range of reasons and might benefit from counseling:

- Relationship status not conducive to sexual intimacy (not currently in a relationship, unhappiness within a relationship, or in an estranged relationship)
- Fear of STI or pregnancy
- Pain with intercourse or other problems having pleasurable sex
- Depression or mental health issues
- Situational factors such as lack of privacy at home
- Poor general health, illness, or injury or fear that sexual intercourse will be unsafe because of medical reasons
- Pregnancy or recent childbirth

Counsel patients who abstain, whether voluntarily or involuntarily, that they are still sexual human beings, and explore with them the range of sexual expression (see section on sexual expression). Because opportunities may arise for having sex and because resolve may weaken, educate all abstemious persons about the other methods of contraception and safer sex available to them, including the following:

- Effective over-the-counter products

- Prescription methods

- Emergency contraception options

- Safer-sex practices

- Options for managing an unintended pregnancy

EFFECTIVENESS

As an action, abstinence prevents pregnancy or STI at the moment of abstaining. As a method, abstinence should *in theory* be highly effective; *in reality*, however, abstinence intentions often fail.[10] Many primary abstainers do not anticipate first penile-vaginal intercourse; many report, "It just happened." Programs to promote abstinence until marriage among youth are generally not effective (see below). Abstinence intentions among youth (*primary abstainers*) as exemplified by virginity pledging generally provide, at best, short-term benefits in delaying initiation of penile-vaginal intercourse and may increase initiation of non-coital activity.[11] Likewise, *secondary abstainers* may see intentions to abstain derailed by situational factors such as the development of a new romantic relationship. Clinician counseling should address these issues, and a back-up method to prevent pregnancy should always be planned.

SEXUAL RIGHTS AND SEXUAL EXPRESSION

Although abstinence has become associated with saying "no," viewed from another perspective, abstinence can mean saying "yes" to a number of other sexual activities. For some people, only penile penetration of the vagina equals intercourse. Most people, however, have a more expansive view of sexual expression, and other activities give them pleasure and meaning. Holding hands, kissing, massage, solo masturbation, mutual masturbation, dancing, oral-genital sex, fantasy, and erotic books and movies all fit along the sexual continuum, as do many other activities. Taste, smell, vision, and hearing may matter as much as touch for erotic pleasure. All human beings need touching—for nurture, for solace, for communication, for simple affection. Most human beings enjoy erotic touching, a specialized language of sexual gratification, and more intimate forms of affection.

A large group of experts convened by the World Health Organization and the World Association for Sexology to address the state of sexual health globally suggested that "Sexual health is a state of physical, emotional, mental and social well-being in relation to sexuality; it is not merely the absence of disease, dysfunction or infirmity. Sexual health requires a positive and respectful approach to sexuality and sexual relationships, as well as the possibility of having pleasurable and safe sexual experiences, free of coercion, discrimination and violence. For sexual health to be attained and maintained, the sexual rights of all persons must be respected, protected and fulfilled."[12]

Sexual rights must also include the right to be abstinent, and to feel comfortable about that choice. In our culture of highly sexualized media messages and a changing environment that has become not only more accepting but also more vocal about who is doing what with whom, some clients may benefit from counseling that explores abstinence as a healthy personal choice. An abstinent individual does not lose his or her sexuality and should be encouraged to explore the range of sexual expression he or she finds acceptable and pleasurable.

CLINICAL ASSESSMENT AND COUNSELING REGARDING ABSTINENCE OR OTHER FORMS OF SEXUAL EXPRESSION

Consider discussing abstinence even with patients who currently engage in intercourse and other sexual behaviors. At some point in their lives, they may choose to become abstinent, removing themselves at least for a while from the health risks of intercourse. You can help people learn that the door between abstinence and sexual activity opens in both directions.

Contraception. When the only goal of abstinence is to avoid unwanted pregnancy, then all forms of sexual expression are available to a couple except for penile-vaginal intercourse.

STI protection. Engaging in noncoital sexual behaviors effectively prevents pregnancy but may have implications for STI prevention. The most important risk factor for becoming infected with an STI is having sexual contact with an infected partner. A person's history of multiple sexual partners and the history of one's partner(s) having multiple partners are predictors of being infected.

In considering STI risk, it is important to understand that most people engage in a variety of coital and noncoital behaviors with the same partner. These practices include mutual masturbation, oral-genital sex, and anal intercourse. Among these noncoital behaviors, anal intercourse carries considerably greater risk for transmission of HIV. For HIV, oral sex is generally safer than vaginal sex, which in turn is safer than anal sex. However, herpes and HPV infection are commonly transmitted via oral-genital contact, and HPV may cause oral cancer. Herpes is also readily transmitted via kissing. HPV may be transmitted via digital-genital contact. Other infections such as chlamydia and gonorrhea generally do not cause pathology in the oral cavity and are not readily transmitted from the oral cavity back to the genitals. (See Chapter 21 on Reproductive Tract Infections.)

In clinical assessment and counseling, consider infection risk from partner factors (e.g. multiple partners) and the community prevalence of specific STIs, such as HIV.[13] Because most people engage in noncoital sex with the same partner with whom they engage in penile-vaginal intercourse, evaluate whether noncoital behaviors add additional risk beyond that posed by penile-vaginal intercourse. Clinical counseling should focus on reducing STI risks such as multiple partners, which may be more effective than discouraging noncoital sex.[13] Also suggest the use of condoms, latex dams, or other barriers to inhibit STI transmission during oral and anal sex. The care provider's role is to offer factual, explicit guidance on safer-sex options.

Lack of partner. Patients may be abstinent if they lack a partner or their partner becomes celibate, for any number of reasons. Give these individuals permission to engage in auto-gratification or, if needed, refer them for counseling if they are dissatisfied with their celibacy. (For more information, see Chapter 1 on Sexuality and Contraception.)

Medical reasons. In some situations insertive sex may be ill advised and clinician-client discussion is warranted:

- Known or suspected STI (also avoid other sexual practices that transmit body fluids such as semen, cervical-vaginal secretions, and blood)
- Post-operative pain or tenderness, such as from episiotomy, hemorrhoidectomy, vasectomy, and other procedures
- Pelvic, vaginal, or urinary tract infection
- Gastrointestinal illness or infection
- Dyspareunia or other pelvic pain
- Undiagnosed postcoital bleeding
- Certain late-term pregnancy conditions such as placenta previa and pre-term labor
- Postpartum (generally 6 weeks) or postabortion (1 week after a medical abortion or 1st trimester surgical abortion and 2 weeks after a 2nd trimester surgical abortion)
- Post myocardial infarction
- Certain disabling physical conditions

- Known or suspected allergic sensitization to a partner's semen

Sex therapy. Therapy for a variety of sexual problems may include exploration of avenues of sexual gratification other than intercourse. Temporarily forbidding intercourse takes performance pressure off couples struggling with erection difficulty, orgasm difficulty, or rapid ejaculation.

CLINICIAN ROLES IN COMPREHENSIVE SEXUALITY EDUCATION PROGRAMS

Sexuality education is important for promoting sexual health and an informed use of abstinence. Thus, as a clinician, you have an important role to play in supporting young people's access to medically accurate, developmentally appropriate, and evidence-based sexuality education. Professional associations have been crucial supporters of sex education through the public schools.[10,14] Clinicians have been strong and steady supporters of comprehensive sexuality education as they often see the consequences of sexual ignorance and misinformation. Informed patients are better able to understand medical advice and to practice effective pregnancy and STI prevention.

Comprehensive sexuality education has been shown to have multiple positive behavioral outcomes, including helping youth delay initiation of intercourse, reduce STI risk, and improve contraceptive use.[15,16] In contrast, abstinence-only until marriage programs have generally been a colossal failure, providing virtually no behavioral benefit.[17] Two recent meta-analyses of abstinence interventions and comprehensive intervention by the CDC-sponsored Task Force on Community Preventive Services found "insufficient evidence" for the effectiveness of abstinence interventions. The Task Force found evidence of effectiveness and recommended comprehensive risk-reduction interventions for adolescents to promote behaviors that prevent or reduce the risk of pregnancy, HIV, and other STIs. Moreover, abstinence-only-until-marriage programs often promote misinformation about sexual health and contraception.[18] States such as California that have refused federal abstinence money and that have emphasized contraceptive access have been more effective in reducing teen pregnancy than states such as Texas that focused on abstinence promotion.[19] By restricting access to health promoting and life saving information, abstinence-until-marriage programs violate the principles of medical ethics and human rights. Clinicians should support science-based policies and oppose nonsensical policies promoting ideas that are medically inaccurate and ineffective.

Comprehensive sexuality education should contain clear messages about the health benefits and health risks of both abstinence and sexual activity. Young people who are not ready for sexual intercourse need the social skills to refuse unwanted sexual advances—information they can use to protect themselves throughout their adult lives, including during periods of abstinence and sexual activity.

The Internet has become an important new source for information on sexual health. Help guide patients to websites that provide accurate and useful information by providing information in the office about these and providing social endorsement for their use. See Appendix 4 for a listing of helpful websites.

U SER INSTRUCTIONS FOR ABSTINENCE—FOR CONTRACEPTION OR STI PROTECTION

1. *Planned abstinence.* Decide what you want to do about sex at a time when you feel clear-headed, sober, and good about yourself. If you have a partner, decide together at a time when you feel close to each other but not sexual. For example, try talking while you take a walk and hold hands.

2. *Spontaneous abstinence.* The wrong partner? The wrong situation? Abstain now—today, tonight—for whatever reason.

3. Decide in advance what sexual activities you will say "yes" to and discuss these with your partner.

4. Tell your partner, very clearly and in advance—not at the last minute, if possible—what activities you will not do.

5. Avoid high-pressure sexual situations; do not get drunk or high.

6. You can choose abstinence even if you have had sex in the past. You can choose abstinence even if you have had sex in the past with a partner who may expect that your past actions dictate your current actions.

7. If you say "no," say it so it is clear that you mean it. This advice is meant to help you communicate more effectively; it is not meant to suggest you are to blame if a partner claims not to have understood what you were saying. Under no circumstances is it acceptable for a partner to pressure or force you to have sex.

8. Learn more about your body, sexual health, contraception, and how to keep yourself healthy. Good resources for young people can be found at:

   — www.goaskalice.columbia.edu

   — www.sexetc.org

— www.scarleteen.com

— www.isis-inc.org

Good resources for adults include:

— www.webmd.com/sex-relationships/default.htm

— www.cdc.gov/sexualhealth

9. Learn about contraception and safer sex, so you will be ready if you change your mind. Always keep condoms on hand.

10. Refrain from intercourse if you do not have a contraceptive method available. Learn about emergency contraception in case you have intercourse when you do not expect it or you experience a contraceptive failure. If you need information about emergency contraception, see www.NOT-2-LATE.com or ec.princeton.edu.

> **Emergency Contraception:** Emergency contraceptive pills or insertion of a copper intrauterine contraceptive after unprotected intercourse substantially reduces the risk of pregnancy. (See Chapter 6 for more information.)

RECOMMENDED READINGS ABOUT SEXUALITY EDUCATION FOR PROFESSIONALS

Guide to Community Preventive Services. Prevention of HIV/AIDS, other STIs and pregnancy: Group-based comprehensive risk reduction interventions for adolescents. www.thecommunityguide.org/hiv/riskreduction.html. Last updated: May 3, 2010.

Guide to Community Preventive Services. Prevention of HIV/AIDS, other STIs and pregnancy: Group-based abstinence education interventions for adolescents. www.the communityguide.org/hiv/abstinence_ed.html. Last updated: May 3, 2010.

Kirby, D. Emerging Answers 2007: Research findings on programs to reduce teen pregnancy and sexually transmitted diseases. Washington, DC: The National Campaign to Prevent Teen and Unplanned Pregnancy, 2007.

Ott MA and Santelli JS. Abstinence and abstinence-only education. Curr Opin Obstet Gynecol. 2007; 19(5): 446–452.

Santelli JS, Ott M, Lyon M, Rogers J, Summers D, Schleifer R. Abstinence and abstinence-only education: A review of US Policies and Programs. J Adolesc Health. 2006; 38: 72–81.

Santelli JS. Medical accuracy in sexuality education: Ideology and the scientific process. Am J Public Health. 2008; 98 (10): 1786–1792.

REFERENCES

1. Santelli JS, Ott MA, Lyon M, et al. Abstinence-only education policies and programs: a position paper of the Society for Adolescent Medicine. J Adolesc Health. 2006; 38:83–87.

2. Schuster MA, Bell RM, Kanouse DE. The sexual practices of adolescent virgins: genital sexual activities of high school students who have never had vaginal intercourse. Am J Publ Health. 1996; 86:1570–1576.

3. Sanders SA, Reinisch JM. Would you say you "had sex" if …? JAMA. 1999; 281:275–277.

4. Finer LB. Trends in premarital sex in the United States, 1954–2003. Public Health Rep. 2007; 122:73–8.

5. Teitler JO. Trends in youth sexual initiation and fertility in developed countries: 1960–1995. Ann Am Acad Pol Soc Sci. 2002; 580:134–152.

6. Abma JC, Martinez, GM, Mosher, WD, Dawson, BS. Teenagers in the United States: Sexual activity, contraceptive use, and childbearing, 2002. National Center for Health Statistics. Vital Health Stat. 2004; 23(24).

7. Lindberg LD, Jones R, Santelli JS. Noncoital sexual activities among adolescents. J Adolesc Health. 2008; 43: 231–238.

8. Mosher WD, Chandra A, Jones J. Sexual behavior and selected health measures: men and women 15–44 years of age, United States, 2002. National Center for Health Statistics. Adv Data Vital Health Stat. 2005; 362.

9. Coker TR, Austin B, Schuster MA. The health and health care of lesbian, gay, and bisexual adolescents. Annu Rev Public Health. 2010; 31:457–77.

10. Santelli JS, Ott M, Lyon M, Rogers J, Summers D, Schleifer R. Abstinence and abstinence-only education: A review of US policies and programs. J Adolesc Health. 2006; 38:72–81.

11. Bearman PS and Bruckner H. Promising the Future: Virginity Pledges and First Intercourse. Am J Sociol 2001; 106:859–912.

12. World Health Organization. Defining sexual health: report of a technical consultation on sexual health, 28–31 January 2002, Geneva: WHO, 2006.

13. ACOG Committee Opinion No. 417: Addressing health risks of noncoital sexual activity. Obstet Gynecol. 2008; 112:735–737.

14. Ott MA and Santelli JS. Abstinence and abstinence-only education. Curr Opin Obstet Gynecol. 2007; 19:446–452.

15. Kirby D. Emerging Answers 2007: research findings on programs to reduce teen pregnancy and sexually transmitted diseases. Washington, DC: The National Campaign to Prevent Teen and Unplanned Pregnancy, 2007.

16. Guide to Community Preventive Services. Prevention of HIV/AIDS, other STIs and pregnancy: Group-based comprehensive risk reduction interventions for adolescents. www.thecommunityguide.org/hiv/riskreduction.html. Last updated: May 3, 2010.

17. Guide to Community Preventive Services. Prevention of HIV/AIDS, other STIs and pregnancy: Group-based abstinence education interventions for adolescents. www.thecommunityguide.org/hiv/abstinence_ed.html. Last updated: May 3, 2010.

18. Santelli JS. Medical accuracy in sexuality education: Ideology and the scientific process. Am J Public Health. 2008; 98:1786–1792.

19. Santelli JS, Kirby D. State Policy Effects on Teen Fertility and Evidence-Based Policies. J Adolescent Health. 2010; 46(6): 515–516.

Emergency Contraception

James Trussell, PhD
Eleanor Bimla Schwarz, MD, MS

- Emergency contraception substantially reduces a woman's chance of pregnancy after an episode of unprotected intercourse.

- Insertion of a copper-releasing intrauterine contraceptive within 5 days after unprotected intercourse reduces the risk of pregnancy by more than 99%.

- Emergency contraceptive pills (ECPs) taken within 5 days of unprotected intercourse are effective but less effective than insertion of a copper-releasing intrauterine contraceptive; from most to least effective these pills contain:

  — 30 mg ulipristal acetate

  — 1,500 mcg levonorgestrel

  — A combination of ethinyl estradiol and either levonorgestrel or norgestrel.

- There are no medical contraindications to emergency insertion of a copper-releasing intrauterine contraceptive except pregnancy and a high risk of STIs at the time of insertion. There are no medical contraindications to use of ECPs at any age, except pregnancy; if a woman is already pregnant, treatment is ineffective but will not harm a pregnancy.

Emergency contraceptives are methods women can use after intercourse to prevent pregnancy.[1] Three dedicated emergency contraceptive pills (ECPs) are currently available for use in the United States:

- ella (a single 30 mg ulipristal pill) was approved by the FDA in 2010.

- Plan B One-Step (a single 1,500 mcg levonorgestrel pill) replaced the previously available Plan B (two 750 mcg tablets of levonorgestrel) product in 2009.

- Next Choice, a generic version of Plan B, was approved by the FDA in 2009.

Plan B One-Step and Next Choice are available without prescription from U.S. pharmacists to women (and men) aged 17 and over. There are no contraindications to use of any emergency contraceptive pills by females younger than 17 years of age, although a prescription is required. A prescription is still required in order for women of any age to use ella. Insertion of a copper-releasing intrauterine contraceptive (IUC) has also proved highly effective as emergency contraception.[2,3]

Less-effective options for emergency contraception include use of combined oral contraceptive pills containing ethinyl estradiol and either norgestrel or levonorgestrel, sometimes called the Yuzpe regimen. (See Table 6–1 for a list of pills that can be used for emergency contraception.) Preven, a dedicated product containing two doses of 100 mcg ethinyl estradiol and 500 mcg levonorgestrel, was approved for use in 1998 but withdrawn from the market in 2004, due to the availability of safer and more effective emergency contraceptives. Emergency use of combined pills containing norethindrone was found in one study to have an efficacy slightly lower than that for combined pills containing levonorgestrel.[4] No published studies are available for emergency contraceptive use of combined pills containing gestodene, etonorgestrel, or other progestins; such pills should therefore not be used for emergency contraception.

In China, Vietnam, and Russia mifepristone is also available as an ECP. However, in the United States, access to mifepristone remains constrained by individuals who seek to limit access to abortion services. Mifepristone, which blocks the effects of progesterone by binding to its receptors, works by preventing ovulation and disrupting luteal-phase events and endometrial development, depending on whether the drug is administered before or after ovulation.[5] A single 10 mg dose of mifepristone, initiated within 120 hours after unprotected intercourse,[6-9] is highly effective in preventing pregnancy. Mifepristone is more effective and causes less nausea and vomiting and fewer side effects than the Yuzpe regimen.[3,10-12] In contrast, 10 mg mifepristone and 1500 mcg levonorgestrel have equivalent efficacy and side effects, except that the next period is more often delayed after mifepristone treatment.[6,8,9] A recent meta-analysis of Chinese randomized trials found that a mid-level dose (25 mg or 50 mg) of mifepristone had a lower failure rate than did levonorgestrel, and the delay in menses for the two regimens was similar.[3] Another Chinese trial found that the antiprogestin gestrinone was as effective as 10 mg mifepristone.[13]

Meloxicam (a COX-2 inhibitor) given for 5 consecutive days in the late follicular phase at a dose of 30 mg may also be an effective option for emergency contraception. This regimen does not alter the endocrine pro-

Table 6-1 Pills that can be used for emergency contraception in the United States[a]

Brand	Company	Pills per Dose[b]	Ethinyl Estradiol per Dose (μg)	Levonorgestrel per Dose (mg)[c]
		Antiprogestin pills: take one pill		
ella[d]	Watson	1 white pill	0	0
		Progestin-only pills: take one dose[b]		
Plan B One-Step	Teva	1 white pill	0	1.5
Next Choice	Watson	2 peach pills	0	1.5
		Combined progestin and estrogen pills: take two doses 12 hours apart		
Aviane	Teva	5 orange pills	100	0.50
Cryselle	Teva	4 white pills	120	0.60
Enpresse	Teva	4 orange pills	120	0.50
Jolessa	Teva	4 pink pills	120	0.60
Lessina	Teva	5 pink pills	100	0.50
Levora	Watson	4 white pills	120	0.60
Lo/Ovral	Akrimax	4 white pills	120	0.60
LoSeasonique	Teva	5 orange pills	100	0.50
Low-Ogestrel	Watson	4 white pills	120	0.60
Lutera	Watson	5 white pills	100	0.50
Lybrel	Wyeth	6 yellow pills	120	0.54
Nordette	Teva	4 light-orange pills	120	0.60
Ogestrel	Watson	2 white pills	100	0.50
Portia	Teva	4 pink pills	120	0.60
Quasense	Watson	4 white pills	120	0.60
Seasonale	Teva	4 pink pills	120	0.60
Seasonique	Teva	4 light-blue-green pills	120	0.60
Sronyx	Watson	5 white pills	100	0.50
Trivora	Watson	4 pink pills	120	0.50

Notes:

[a] ella, Plan B One-Step, and Next Choice are the only dedicated products specifically marketed for emergency contraception. Aviane, Cryselle, Enpresse, Jolessa, Lessina, Levora, Lo/Ovral, LoSeasonique, Low-Ogestrel, Lutera, Lybrel, Nordette, Ogestrel, Portia, Quasense, Seasonale, Seasonique, Sronyx and Trivora have been declared safe and effective for use as ECPs by the United States Food and Drug Administration. Outside the United States, more than 100 emergency contraceptive products are specifically packaged, labeled, and marketed. Levonorgestrel-only ECPs are available either over-the-counter or from a pharmacist without having to see a clinician in 60 countries. Plan B One-Step and Next Choice are available over-the counter to women and men aged 17 and older.

[b] The label for Plan B One-Step says to take the pill within 72 hours after unprotected intercourse. Research has shown that that all of the brands listed here are effective when used within 120 hours after unprotected sex. The label for Next Choice says to take one pill within 72 hours after unprotected intercourse and another pill 12 hours later. Research has shown that that both pills can be taken at the same time with no decrease in efficacy or increase in side effects and that they are effective when used within 120 hours after unprotected sex.

[c] The progestin in Cryselle, Lo/Ovral, Low-Ogestrel and Ogestrel is norgestrel, which contains two isomers, only one of which (levonorgestrel) is bioactive; the amount of norgestrel in each tablet is twice the amount of levonorgestrel.

[d] ella contains 30 mg ulipristal acetate

file of the cycle and causes no menstrual disturbance.[14,15] However, the effectiveness of meloxicam has yet to be compared with other EC options in a randomized controlled fashion, and it is not sold as an emergency contraceptive.

Older methods of emergency contraception, which are no longer recommended, include the following:

- High-dose estrogen. Ethinyl estradiol, 5 mg to 10 mg given daily for 5 days, provides efficacy similar to the Yuzpe method[16,17] but with a high incidence of nausea and vomiting.

- Danazol. Studies of danazol, an androgenic and progestogenic steroid, were initially promising,[18] but this approach was abandoned when a subsequent study found an unacceptably low efficacy.[11]

- Diethylstilbestrol (DES), 25 mg to 50 mg.

BARRIERS TO USE

Until the fall of 1998, the lack of a product specifically packaged, labeled, and marketed as an emergency contraceptive was a major obstacle to more widespread use of emergency contraception in the United States. In 1998, Preven was approved, and in 1999, a second dedicated emergency contraceptive pill, Plan B, was approved. In 2009, a one-pill version of Plan B (Plan B One-Step) and a generic version of Plan B (Next Choice) were approved. Unfortunately, the pharmaceutical companies initially distributing these dedicated products were very small and were not able to promote the products on the same scale as most pharmaceuticals. Although Plan B was acquired from the tiny Women's Capital Corporation by Barr Pharmaceuticals in February 2004 and by Teva Pharmaceuticals in 2008, none of these companies (nor Watson Pharmaceuticals, the maker of the generic Next Choice and ella) have made significant investments in direct-to-consumer advertising.

Without commercial marketing, many women still do not know that emergency contraception is available, effective, and safe. Nevertheless, among women aged 15–44 who have ever had intercourse, the fraction who had ever used ECPs increased from 2% in 2002 to 10% in 2006–2008.[19]

Even when a woman has been raped, many hospital emergency departments do not provide emergency contraceptive services,[20–23] despite the fact that legal precedent indicates that this constitutes inadequate care and provides grounds to sue the hospital.[24] It is estimated that as many as 22,000 pregnancies resulting from rape each year could be prevented by use of EC.[25] However, the Department of Justice made no mention of emergency contraception in its 130-page *National Protocol for*

Sexual Assault Medical Forensic Examinations.[26] Of further concern, levonorgestrel ECPs were not consistently available to American soldiers when serving overseas. This is particularly disturbing because one-quarter of women veterans report experiencing military sexual trauma.[27] Although the Department of Defense Pharmacy and Therapeutics Committee added Plan B to the Basic Core Formulary (BCF) of medications which must be stocked at every full-service Medical Treatment Facility (MTF) in April 2002, one month later, in May 2002, Plan B was removed from the BCF[28] in response to complaints from conservative members of Congress,[29] and the decision of whether to stock EC was left to the discretion of each MTF until February 3, 2010, when Next Choice was finally added to the BCF.[30]

POPULATION IMPACT OF ECPS

No published study has demonstrated that increasing access to ECPs reduces pregnancy or abortion rates at the population level,[31,32] although one demonstration project[33] and three clinical trials[34-36] were specifically designed to address this issue. One explanation for this result is that even when provided with ECPs in advance of need, most women use ECPs too rarely after risky incidents to result in a substantial population impact. In the San Francisco trial, 45% of the women in the advance provision group who had unprotected intercourse during the study period did not use ECPs.[34] In the Nevada/North Carolina trial, 33% of women in the advance provision group had unprotected intercourse at least once without using ECPs.[36] In the Nevada/North Carolina trial, increased access to EC increased use of ECPs most among women who were at lower baseline risk of pregnancy.[37] This may explain in part why increased access to EC has increased use of EC without measurable effect on pregnancy rates in clinical trials.

One concern often voiced about making ECPs more widely available has been that women who know they can use ECPs may become less diligent with their ongoing contraception. However, to date, 15 studies have demonstrated that making ECPs more widely available did not increase sexual risk-taking.[34-36,38-50] In the four studies that examined the impact of easier access to ECPs on rates of sexually transmitted infections (STIs), access to ECPs did not affect incidence of STIs.[34,36,42,50] Another study demonstrated that educating teens about ECPs did not increase their level of sexual activity or use of EC but did increase their knowledge about proper administration of ECPs.[51] Reanalysis of one randomized trial suggested that easier access to ECPs may have increased the frequency of coital acts with the potential to lead to pregnancy.[52] This reanalysis found that women with increased access to ECPs were significantly more likely to report that they had used emergency contraception because they did not want to use either condoms or another contraceptive method.[53] Even if ECP availability did adversely affect regular contraceptive use, women would have the right to be fully informed about all available contraceptive options and make their own decisions about which they wanted to use.[54]

If used as a sole method, repeated use of ECPs is far less effective than most other contraceptive methods. For a typical woman who repeatedly used progestin-only ECPs, the chance of pregnancy after 1 year would be 20%; with repeated use of combined ECPs, the chance of pregnancy after 1 year would exceed 35%.[55] Therefore, for most women, repeated ECP use would not be an optimal contraceptive strategy.

PROMOTING AWARENESS AND USE

Many initiatives have been undertaken to encourage greater awareness and use of emergency contraception. To help educate people about emergency contraception, the Association of Reproductive Health Professionals in Washington, D.C. and the Office of Population Research at Princeton University sponsor the Emergency Contraception Website (www.not-2-late.com), which was launched in October 1994. Detailed information about EC is available on the Emergency Contraception Website, which now receives more than 200,000 visitors each month. The Website is completely confidential, available 24 hours a day, and offers names and telephone numbers of providers of emergency contraception located near the user's zip code (in the United States and parts of Canada). The Website is available in English, Spanish, French and Arabic. In several cities in 1997 and 1998, public service announcements advertising the hotline were the first ads about contraception to be shown on broadcast television.[56] Subsequently, a public education media campaign in Philadelphia and Seattle resulted in significant increases in knowledge about emergency contraception.[57]

Making Plan B available Over-the-Counter (OTC)

There are no medical reasons for levonorgestrel ECPs to require a prescription.[58,59] They have been available over-the-counter (OTC), without age restrictions, in Norway (since 2000), Sweden (since 2001), the Netherlands (since 2004), India (since 2005) and certain provinces of Canada (since 2005). In the United States, levonorgestrel ECPs have been available OTC with age restrictions since August 2006. In many other countries, levonorgestrel ECPs can be obtained directly from a pharmacist without a prescription: Antigua, Aruba, Australia, Austria, Bahamas, Belarus, Belgium, Belize, Benin, Bulgaria, Burkina Faso, Cameroon, China, Congo, Denmark, Estonia, Finland, France, French Polynesia, Gabon, Ghana, Guinea-Conakry, Iceland, Iran, Israel, Ivory Coast, Jamaica, Latvia, Lesotho, Lithuania, Luxembourg, Mali, Mauritania, Mauritius, New Zealand, Niger, Portugal, Romania, Senegal, Slovakia, Slovenia, South Africa, Spain, Sri Lanka, St. Lucia, Surinam, Switzerland, Tajikistan, Thailand, Togo, Tunisia, the United Kingdom, Uzbekistan, and Vietnam.

Changing Plan B from prescription to OTC in the United States was a long and politically charged process. Following recommendations by respected reproductive health leaders[60,61] and endorsements by many professional organizations including the American College of Obstetricians and Gynecologists and the American Medical Association,[62] in December 2003, an FDA advisory committee voted 23 to 4 to approve a switch for Plan B from prescription to OTC. Unfortunately, despite this recommendation, the FDA rejected an OTC switch in May 2004 in unprecedented disregard for such an overwhelmingly positive advisory committee recommendation. Subsequently, the independent Government Accountability Office concluded that this decision process was highly unusual and that the decision was made with atypical involvement from top agency officials and may well have been made months before it was formally announced.[63] In July 2004, Barr Laboratories submitted an amended application to make Plan B a prescription drug for females younger than 16 years and OTC for women and men 16 and older. On August 26, 2005, the FDA announced that Plan B was safe for OTC use by women age 17 and older, but the FDA announced an indefinite delay in reaching a decision, citing three concerns: (1) Can Plan B be both prescription-based and OTC depending on age? (2) Can prescription and OTC versions of the same drug be marketed in the same package, and (3) Can an age restriction be enforced? In addition, at that time, the FDA failed to articulate clear criteria or an explicit timetable for a final decision. This indefinite delay was heavily criticized,[64] and finally, on August 24, 2006, the FDA approved the nonprescription sale of Plan B to U.S. women and men age 18 and older. This age cutoff was not chosen based on any medical evidence that young women could not use emergency contraceptive pills safely or correctly, but rather, according to the FDA's Steven Galson, because it was easy for pharmacists to remember and enforce, since it is the same age limit placed on tobacco and nicotine-replacement products.

In March 2009, the U.S. District Court for the Eastern District of New York ordered the agency to reconsider its decision. It also ordered the FDA to act within 30 days to extend OTC access to 17-year-olds. Judge Edward R. Korman stated bluntly that the FDA had "acted in bad faith and in response to political pressure" and "repeatedly and unreasonably delayed issuing a decision on Plan B." He further charged that the FDA's denial of nonprescription access to 17-year-olds "lacks all credibility" and was based on "fanciful and wholly unsubstantiated 'enforcement' concerns."[65] On April 22, 2009, the FDA announced that it would clear the way for Plan B's manufacturer to make it available without a prescription to 17-year-olds, and on July 13, 2009, the FDA approved Plan B One-Step as a nonprescription drug for women and men aged 17 and over. Next Choice, a generic version of Plan B, was approved in August 2009. However, younger women still need a prescription to buy levonorgestrel ECPs, and packages are kept behind the pharmacy counter, not on the shelf.

This means that access to ECPs remains limited by whether the pharmacist on duty is willing to dispense ECPs. In addition, some women may feel too embarrassed to ask a pharmacist for ECPs. Two other predictable, but unintended, negative outcomes of OTC access to emergency contraception in the United States include the loss of opportunities for physicians to counsel patients about use of more effective, longer-term contraceptive methods when they present for emergency contraception,[66] and an increase in price, from about $25 per treatment to about $45, coupled with a loss of insurance coverage for ECPs for most Americans whose drug insurance covers only prescription drugs.

Cost Effectiveness

Studies based on economic models have shown that emergency contraception has the potential to be cost-effective. Use of combined or progestin-only ECPs reduces expenditures on medical care by preventing unintended pregnancies, which are very costly. In the United States, insertion of a copper T IUC is cost-saving as long as the IUC is used as an ongoing method of contraception for at least 4 months after emergency insertion. Because the copper IUC can provide continuous contraceptive protection for up to 20 years,[67] emergency placement of intrauterine contraception has the potential to produce considerable savings from the societal perspective.[68] EC pills have also been shown to be cost effective regardless of whether they are provided when the emergency arises or provided in advance of need, as a routine preventive measure.[69-75] However, all of the above studies have assumed that ECPs would actually be used after unprotected intercourse. Unfortunately, studies have not yet demonstrated that increasing access to ECPs reduces pregnancy or abortion rates at the population level. Therefore, at the population level, advance provision of ECPs has not been demonstrated to be cost effective.

Mechanism of Action
Copper-Releasing IUCs

When used as a regular or emergency method of contraception, copper-releasing IUCs act primarily to prevent fertilization. Emergency insertion of a copper IUC is significantly more effective than use of ECPs, reducing the risk of pregnancy following unprotected intercourse by more than 99%.[2,3] This very high level of effectiveness implies that emergency insertion of a copper IUC must prevent some pregnancies after fertilization. (See Chapter 7 on Intrauterine Contraception.)

Emergency Contraceptive Pills

To make an informed choice, women must know that ECPs—like the birth control pill, patch, ring, shot, and implant,[76] and even like breast-feeding[77]—prevent pregnancy primarily by delaying or inhibiting ovulation and inhibiting fertilization, but may at times inhibit implantation of a fertilized egg in the endometrium. However, women should also be informed that the best available evidence indicates that ECPs prevent pregnancy by mechanisms that do not involve interference with post-fertilization events.

ECPs do not cause abortion[78] or harm an established pregnancy. Pregnancy begins with implantation according to medical authorities such as the U.S. FDA, the National Institutes of Health[79] and the American College of Obstetricians and Gynecologists (ACOG).[80]

Ulipristal acetate (UPA). One study has demonstrated that UPA can delay ovulation.[81] In this study, 34 women were treated when the size of the leading follicle was 18 to 22 mm. Each woman contributed one cycle treated with placebo and another with UPA. Follicular rupture failed to occur within 5 days following UPA treatment in 20 (59%) subjects while normal ovulation was observed in all women within 5 days after placebo intake. Follicular rupture failed to occur within 5 days after treatment with UPA in all women treated before onset of the LH surge, in 79% of women treated after the onset of the LH surge but before the LH peak, and in 8% of women treated after the LH peak. Another study found that UPA altered the endometrium, but whether this change would inhibit implantation is unknown.[82]

Progestin-only emergency contraceptive pills. Early treatment with ECPs containing only the progestin levonorgestrel has been shown to impair the ovulatory process and luteal function.[83–87] No effect on the endometrium was found in two studies,[84,85] but in another study levonorgestrel taken before the LH surge altered the luteal phase secretory pattern of glycodelin in serum and the endometrium.[88] (Glycodelin is a protein that the endometrium produces that reduces sperm capacitation and inhibits sperm-egg binding.[89]) However, this finding was not confirmed in two later studies explicitly designed to assess endometrial glycodelin expression.[90,91] The second of these studies also found no effect on other endometrial receptivity biomarkers or progesterone receptors. In another study levonorgestrel taken before the LH surge increased prematurely serum and intrauterine concentrations of glycodelin at the time of ovulation; this result may indicate an additional mechanism of action when ovulation is not inhibited.[92] Levonorgestrel does not impair the attachment of human embryos to in vitro endometrial constructs and has no effect on the expression of endometrial receptivity markers.[93,94] In a study conducted more than 30 years ago, levonorgestrel was found to interfere with sperm migration and function at all levels of the genital tract;[95] however, another study designed to assess this issue found that 1,500 mcg levonorgestrel had no effect on the quality of cervical mucus or on the penetration of spermatozoa in the uterine cavity,[90] and a recent study found an effect on sperm function only with much higher levels of levonorgestrel than are used for emergency contraception.[96]

The reduced efficacy with a delay in treatment, even when use is adjusted for cycle day of unprotected intercourse,[97] suggests that interference with implantation is likely not an important effect of ECPs. If ECPs did prevent all implantations, then delays in use should not reduce their efficacy as long as they are used before implantation.[98] Results of a simulation model demonstrated that, without a post-fertilization effect, the levonorgestrel regimen could not be effective when started after 96 hours, because with increasing delay, a greater proportion of women would be too near to ovulation.[99]

Studies in the rat and the Cebus monkey demonstrate that levonorgestrel administered in doses that inhibit ovulation has no post-fertilization effect that impairs fertility.[100–102] However, the extent to which these results can be extrapolated to women is unknown.

Croxatto and colleagues have argued that most, if not all, of the contraceptive effect of levonorgestrel-only ECPs can be explained by inhibited or dysfunctional ovulation, based on the existing animal and human studies, including two human studies comparing observed and expected pregnancies when levonorgestrel-only ECPs were administered before and after ovulation. In the first study, no pregnancies were observed when levonorgestrel-only ECPs were taken before the day of ovulation (in contrast to the 4 pregnancies that would have been expected without use of ECPs), whereas 3 pregnancies occurred when ECPs were taken after the day of ovulation (versus 3.5 expected pregnancies).[103] In a follow-up study no pregnancies were observed when levonorgestrel-only ECPs were taken before the day of ovulation (in contrast to the 13 pregnancies that would have been expected without use of ECPs, whereas when ECPs were taken on or after the day of ovulation, 6 pregnancies occurred (versus 7 expected pregnancies).[104] While some find the existing human and animal studies adequate to conclude that ECPs have no post-fertilization effect,[105,106] others may always feel that this question has not been unequivocally answered.

Combined emergency contraceptive pills. Several clinical studies have shown that combined ECPs containing ethinyl estradiol and levonorgestrel can inhibit or delay ovulation.[107–110] This mechanism of action may explain the effectiveness of combined ECPs when used during the first half of the menstrual cycle, before ovulation has occurred. Some studies have shown histologic or biochemical alterations in the endometrium after treatment with the regimen, leading to the conclusion that combined ECPs may act by impairing endometrial receptivity to subsequent implantation of a fertilized egg.[108,111–113] However, other more recent studies have found no such effects on the endometrium.[107,114,115] Additional possible mechanisms include interference with corpus luteum function; thickening of the cervical mucus resulting in trapping of sperm; alterations in the tubal transport of sperm, egg, or embryo; and direct inhibition of fertilization.[100,116–118] No clinical data exist regarding the last three of these possibilities. Nevertheless, statistical evidence on the effectiveness of combined ECPs suggests that that if the regimen is as effective as was initially claimed, it must have a mechanism of action other than delaying or preventing ovulation.[119] However, as it now appears that the effectiveness of combined ECPs was initially overestimated, there is less concern that ECPs do more than delay or prevent ovulation.[120] Nevertheless, the important point is that effectiveness and mechanism of action are not independent.[99] For example, a regimen without a post-fertilization effect could not be 100% effective in typical populations, which inevitably include some women who take ECPs after fertilization has already occurred.

EFFECTIVENESS
INTRAUTERINE DEVICES

More than 12,000 postcoital insertions of copper-bearing IUCs are known to have been carried out since the practice was introduced in 1976. With only 12 failures, this approach has a pregnancy rate of 0.1%.[2,3] The effectiveness of using a levonorgestrel-releasing IUC (LNg-20) for emergency contraception has not been studied and is not recommended. However, some clinicians do place levonorgestrel IUCs on the same day that a woman has taken ECPs.

EMERGENCY CONTRACEPTIVE PILLS

The effectiveness of a preventive therapy is best measured by comparing the probability that the condition will occur if the therapy is used to the probability that it will occur without treatment. For many preventive therapies, effectiveness is determined by randomized clinical trials comparing treatment to a placebo. In the case of emergency contraception, however, efficacy was demonstrated initially by noncomparative observational studies, and, thereafter, use of a placebo was felt to be unethical. Therefore, the chance that pregnancy would occur in the absence of emergency contraception is estimated indirectly using published data on the probability of pregnancy on each day of the menstrual cycle.[121,122] This estimate is compared with the actual number of pregnancies observed after treatment in observational treatment trials. Effectiveness is calculated as 1-[O/E], where O and E are the observed and expected number of pregnancies, respectively.

Calculation of effectiveness involves many assumptions that are difficult to validate, including accurate estimates of timing of intercourse and cycle day (which affects estimates of the timing of ovulation). One study compared self-report of cycle day with urinary pregnanediol concentrations to demonstrate that over 30% of women presenting for ECPs had inaccurately dated their own menstrual cycles, believing themselves to be in the fertile phase of their cycle when they were not.[123] Another study found that 99 women were between 5 days before and 1 day after the day of ovulation, which was estimated as usual cycle length minus 13 days. However, hormonal data indicated that only 51 of these 99 (56%) were in fact in this fertile window.[124] In another recent study, cervical smears showed that more than one-third of women requesting ECPs had no sperm present in the vagina, and those with sperm present had fewer sperm than women attempting to become pregnant.[125] Thus, the risk of pregnancy for women requesting ECPs appears to be lower than initially assumed in estimates of ECP efficacy, which are consequently likely to be overestimates. Yet, precise estimates of efficacy may not be highly relevant to many women who have had unprotected intercourse, since ECPs are often the only available treatment. A more important consideration for most ECP clients may be the fact that data from both clinical trials and studies on the mechanism of action clearly show that both levonorgestrel and ulipristal ECPs are more effective than doing nothing.[126]

Ulipristal acetate. The antiprogestin ulipristal acetate (30 mg in a single dose) is the most effective ECP option, with reported estimates of effectiveness ranging from 62% to 85%.[127–129] Two randomized trials compared the efficacy of levonorgestrel and ulipristal acetate, one up to 72 hours after unprotected intercourse[128] and the second up to 120 hours after intercourse.[127] When these two studies were combined in a meta-analysis, ulipristal acetate was found to have a pregnancy rate 42% lower than levonorgestrel up to 72 hours and 65% lower in the first 24 hours.[127] In the second randomized study, ulipristal acetate prevented significantly more pregnancies than did levonorgestrel in the 72 to 120 hour subgroup. The reason seems to be that ulipristal acetate is more effective than levonorgestrel in postponing imminent ovulation. Levonorgestrel is no more effective than a placebo in preventing ovulation when the leading follicle reaches 15–17 mm.[87] In contrast, by the time the follicle reaches 18 to 20 mm (which indicates that ovulation should occur within the next 48 hours) and the probability of conception without medication is > 30%, ulipristal acetate delayed ovulation for at least 5 days in 59% of cycles (versus 0% for the placebo).[81]

Progestin-only and combined regimens. Eleven studies of the levonorgestrel regimen, which together included a total of more than 13,000 women, reported estimates of effectiveness between 52% and 100%; that is, this regimen reduced a woman's chance of pregnancy by that amount.[6,8,9,127,128,130–137] A meta-analysis of eight studies of the combined regimen, which in total included more than 3,800 women, concluded that the regimen prevents about 74% of expected pregnancies; the proportion ranged from 56% to 89% in the different studies.[138] A more recent analysis using possibly improved methodology found an effectiveness of 53% and 47% in two of the largest trials of the combined regimen.[120] Combined data from two randomized trials that directly compared the two regimens showed a relative risk of pregnancy of 0.51 (95% confidence limits 0.31, 0.83), indicating that the chance of pregnancy among women who received the levonorgestrel regimen was about half the chance among those who received the combined regimen.[126,132,133] This estimate makes *no* assumption about the number of pregnancies that would have been observed in the absence of treatment. The results imply that (1) if the Yuzpe regimen is completely inefficacious, then the levonorgestrel regimen has an efficacy of 49% and (2) for every additional 2 percentage points of efficacy of the Yuzpe regimen, 1 percentage point of efficacy is added to the levonorgestrel regimen.

Several studies have indicated that both regimens are more effective the sooner after sex the pills are taken.[8,12,97,130,133,136,139] Other studies have not found that delays in use have this effect,[4,6,9,131,132,135,140–142] although sample sizes were often small. The initial studies showed that these regimens are effective when used up to 72 hours after intercourse.[133,143] Consequently, some product package instructions, including those for Plan B One-Step and Next Choice, advise use only within that time frame. However, more recent studies indicate that the regimens continue to be moderately effective if started between 72 and 120 hours.[8,131,136,141,142] No data are available establishing efficacy if ECPs are taken more than 120 hours after intercourse.

Studies have shown that a single dose of 1,500 mcg levonorgestrel is as effective as (and causes no more side effects than) taking two 750 mcg doses 12 hours apart.[8,130] Another study found that two 750 mcg doses taken 24 hours apart were just as effective as two 750 mcg doses taken 12 hours apart.[131] A pilot study of 41 women found that adding a COX-2 inhibitor (meloxicam 15 mg) to 1,500 mcg levonorgestrel significantly increased the proportion of cycles with no follicular rupture or with ovulatory dysfunction (88% vs. 66%, p=0.012), and that COX-2 inhibitors can disturb the ovulatory process after the onset of the LH surge.[144]

A DVANTAGES AND INDICATIONS

Emergency contraceptives can prevent pregnancy after unprotected sexual intercourse or after a contraceptive "accident." This makes emergency contraception an essential part of treatment following sexual assault.[145] Emergency contraception may also be appropriate in the following circumstances[78,146]

- No contraceptive was used at the time of intercourse.

- A male condom slipped, broke, or leaked.

- A female condom, diaphragm, or cervical cap was inserted incorrectly, dislodged during intercourse, removed too early, or found to be torn.

- A woman missed too many combined oral contraceptive pills (e.g. 3+ consecutive pills containing 30 to 35 mcg ethinyl estradiol or 2+ consecutive pills containing 20 mcg or less ethinyl estradiol). Note: Missed pills during the first week of a pill pack pose the greatest risk of pregnancy.

- A breastfeeding woman has had her menstrual period return, is feeding her baby anything other than breastmilk, or is more than 6 months postpartum even if she remains amenorrheic.

- A woman was late in using her contraceptive:

  — 3 or more hours late taking a progestin-only pill.

  — More than 14 days late in getting a Depo-Provera injection, or does not know the date or type of the previous injection.

  — 2 or more days late starting a new vaginal ring cycle.

  — 2 or more days late starting a new patch cycle.

- A female condom was inserted or removed incorrectly leading to spillage of semen, or the penis was inserted mistakenly between the female condom and the vaginal wall resulting in intravaginal ejaculation.

- An attempt at coitus interruptus resulted in ejaculation in the vagina or on external genitalia.

- A couple, attempting to practice periodic abstinence, inadvertently had intercourse on a fertile day of the cycle.

- A woman cannot feel her IUC string, or her IUC was removed less than 8 days after her last act of intercourse.

- A woman was exposed to a possible teratogen such as isotretinoin when she was not protected by effective contraception.

The copper IUC may be an especially useful option for women who present 4 or 5 days after unprotected intercourse, because it provides extremely high emergency contraceptive efficacy for at least 5 days after intercourse, and it is an excellent choice for women who wish to continue using an IUC as a long-term method of contraception.

SIDE EFFECTS
COPPER-RELEASING IUC

Side effects after emergency insertion of an IUC are similar to those seen after routine insertion at other times and may include abdominal discomfort and vaginal bleeding or spotting. (See Chapter 7 on Intrauterine Contraception.)

HORMONAL METHODS

Nausea and vomiting. These side effects affect about 13 to 29% of women treated with progestin-only ECPs or UPA;[134,135] the incidence of nausea was significantly higher with UPA than levonorgestrel in one randomized trial[135] but not in the other.[134] In contrast, following treatment with combined estrogen-progestin ECPs, nausea occurs in about 50% of women, and vomiting in about 20%. Other reported complaints include fatigue, breast tenderness, headache, lower abdominal pain, dizziness, and diarrhea. Side effects are similar for the levonorgestrel and ulipristal acetate regimens.[134,135] Side effects subside within a day or two after treatment is completed. Routine use of the anti-nausea medication meclizine 1 hour before the first ECP dose may help reduce nausea and vomiting,[147] but is generally considered unnecessary with use of progestin-only or ulipristal acetate ECPs.

There is no research to indicate whether it is necessary to repeat the ECP dose if the woman vomits within 2 hours after taking ECPs. Some practitioners take the view that a replacement dose should be given orally, or in the opinion of some, vaginally to prevent the tablets from being vomited a second time. Other providers, believing that nausea and vomiting are evidence of an estrogen-mediated effect on the central nervous system and thus of absorption of the drugs, conclude that a replacement dose is not necessary unless an ECP tablet is visible in the vomitus.

Effects on future fertility and inadvertently exposed pregnancies. There is no evidence that ECPs have any long-term or adverse effects on a woman's fertility. One study of 332 pregnant women who had used levonorgestrel-only ECPs in the conception cycle found no increased risk of birth defects.[148] Moreover, two observations provide reassurance for any concern about birth defects.[116] First, in the event of treatment failure, ECPs are taken long before organogenesis starts, so they should not have a teratogenic effect. Second, studies that have examined births to women who inadvertently continued to take combined oral contraceptives (including high-dose formulations) without knowing they were pregnant have found no increased risk of birth defects.[149–151] For this reason, the FDA removed warnings about adverse effects of combined oral contraceptives on the fetus from contraceptive package inserts years ago.[152]

Available evidence suggests that ECPs do not increase the chance that a pregnancy following ECP use will be ectopic; moreover, like all contraceptive methods, ECPs reduce the absolute risk of ectopic pregnancy by preventing many pregnancies.[153,154] However, ectopic pregnancy can occur following ECP treatment, and it is important to keep this possibility in mind whenever a treatment failure occurs.

Menstrual changes. Three studies have been specifically designed to assess the effects of levonorgestrel ECPs on bleeding patterns. Outcomes examined included length of the treatment and post-treatment cycles (where the first day of bleeding is cycle day 1), duration of bleeding during the menstrual period, and intermenstrual bleeding. All three found that the length of the treatment cycle can be shortened when treatment occurs early in the cycle.

The first study found that when taken in the first 3 weeks of the cycle, 1,500 mcg levonorgestrel in a single dose significantly shortened that cycle as compared both to the usual cycle length and to the cycle length in a comparison group of similar women who had not taken ECPs. The magnitude of this effect was greater the earlier the pills were taken. However, when this regimen was taken later in women's cycles it had no effect on cycle length, but it did cause prolongation of bleeding during the next menstrual period. The ECPs had no effect on the length of the post-treatment cycle, but bleeding during the second period was prolonged. Intermenstrual bleeding was uncommon after ECP use, although more common than among women who had not taken ECPs.[155]

The second study compared the baseline cycle with the treatment and post-treatment cycles when 1,500 mcg levonorgestrel was administered in a single dose. Cycle length was significantly shortened by 1 day when ECPs were taken in the preovulatory phase of the cycle and was significantly lengthened by 2 days when ECPs were taken in the postovulatory phase. No difference in cycle length was observed for women who took ECPs during the periovulatory phase of the cycle (from 2 days before to 2 days after the expected day of ovulation). In both the treatment and post-treatment cycles, the duration of bleeding during the menstrual period increased significantly when ECPs were taken in the periovulatory or postovulatory phase. The length of the post-treatment cycle remained significantly longer when ECPs were taken in the postovulatory phase. During the treatment cycle, 15% of women experienced intermenstrual bleeding; this was significantly more common when ECPs were taken in the preovulatory phase.[156]

The third study examined the effects of two levonorgestrel pills taken 12 hours apart.[157] When taken in the follicular phase, ECPs significantly shortened the cycle when compared with usual cycle length; no effect on cycle length was found when ECPs were taken in the periovulatory or luteal phase. The post-treatment cycle length was the same as the usual cycle length.

CAUTIONS

There are no medical contraindications to the use of combined or progestin-only ECPs, with the exception of pregnancy; the U.S. Medical Eligibility Criteria for Contraceptive Use does not include ulipristal acetate yet.[158] In the United States, the labeling for Plan B One-Step, Next Choice and ella includes only one contraindication: known or suspected pregnancy.

The reason ECPs should not be used in pregnancy is not because they are harmful, but because they are ineffective. The advantages of ECP use generally outweigh the risks even for women who have one or more contraindications to the ongoing use of estrogen-containing contraceptives, such as vascular disease, migraine with aura, or severe liver disease. For such women, use of ulipristal acetate or progestin-only ECPs, however, is preferable to use of combined estrogen-progestin ECPs.

Few adverse events have been reported for women using emergency contraception. The Committee on Safety of Medicines in the United Kingdom reviewed all problems reported during the first 13 years of use of the combination estrogen-progestin ECP product available there (called PC4). Among 4 million uses, the review found 61 pregnancies, 3 cases of venous thrombosis (including 1 death), and 3 cases of cerebrovascular disorder. The Committee concluded that none of the 6 vascular cases could be definitely linked to ECP use because of the significant delay between ECP use and the onset of symptoms.[116]

Breastfeeding women. During the first 6 months postpartum, women who are fully breastfeeding and amenorrheic have little risk of pregnancy. There are no restrictions on use of combined or progestin-only ECPs by breastfeeding women.[158] Only one study has examined levonorgestrel pharmacokinetics in plasma and milk of lactating women who take 1,500 mcg for emergency contraception. The authors conclude that to limit infant exposure to the period of maximum levonorgestrel excretion in milk, mothers may consider avoiding nursing for the 8 hours after they take ECP,[159] but resumption of breastfeeding within 24 hours of ECP use is recommended for any mother who chooses to take this precaution. The label for ella states "It is not known if ulipristal acetate is excreted in human milk. However, ulipristal acetate is detected in milk of lactating rats. Because many drugs are excreted in human milk, risk to the breast-fed child cannot be excluded. Use of ella by breastfeeding women is not recommended."[160]

Drug interactions. Although medications such as phenytoin or rifampin that induce hepatic enzymes could theoretically reduce the effectiveness of ECPs, whether such medications actually reduce the effectiveness of ECPs has not been studied. No significant interactions have been found with concurrent use of other antibiotics (see Chapter 11 on Combined Oral Contraceptives).

Ulipristal acetate is an antiprogestin. The implications for immediately starting hormonal contraceptives after taking UPA are unknown; specifically, it is not known whether the regular instructions for abstaining or using condoms for the first 7 days of using a routine hormonal contraceptive (or during the first 2 days for progestin-only pills) are conservative enough. Our conservative recommendation is to use condoms for 2 weeks unless the woman abstains from intercourse.

Eligibility criteria and contraindications for emergency insertion of an IUC are the same as for all IUC insertions. (See Chapter 7 on Intrauterine Contraception.) A particular concern is the risk of pelvic inflammatory disease for women requesting emergency contraception after unprotected intercourse with a new sexual partner and for victims of sexual assault, when the risk of STIs may be high. Testing for STIs should occur at the time of IUC insertion, and if clinical suspicion of infection is high, empiric antibiotics may be given. Women who are found to harbor an STI after an IUC has been placed can be successfully treated with antibiotics with the IUC in place.

PROVIDING EMERGENCY CONTRACEPTION

Although pregnancy can result from intercourse only during the fertile phase of a woman's cycle, any woman requesting emergency contra-

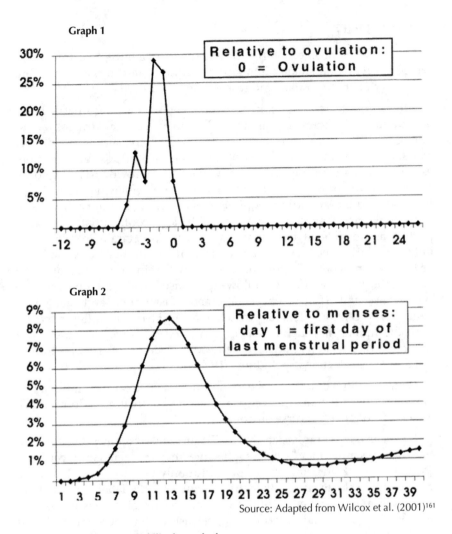

Figure 6–1 Pregnancy probability by cycle day

ception after unprotected intercourse should be offered treatment within 120 hours of intercourse.[8,131,141,142]

It is important to remember that determining pregnancy risk is not always straightforward. The risk is low except for the 5 days just before ovulation and on the day of ovulation (see Figure 6–1, graph 1).[161] The problem is that neither the woman nor her clinician is likely to know for sure which day ovulation occurs. What may be known is menstrual period dates. Plotting the probability of pregnancy versus menstrual period dates (see Figure 6–1, graph 2) shows that late (or early) ovulation is common enough that pregnancy risk is above 1% beginning as early as cycle day 7 and continuing until at least day 39.[161]

COUNSELING

In counseling women who seek emergency contraceptive treatment, remember that women are often facing a difficult and stressful situation. Be respectful of the woman and responsive to her needs.

After unprotected intercourse, some women may feel particularly anxious about becoming pregnant. They may feel embarrassed about failing to use regular contraception effectively. Rape survivors will feel traumatized. Women may be very concerned about possible infection, especially in cases of rape. Counsel women and provide STI diagnostic services (or referrals) and information about preventive measures. If appropriate, explain reporting requirements regarding statutory rape; reassure the woman that all information will be kept confidential. Be as supportive as possible of the woman's choices and refrain from making judgmental comments or indicating disapproval through body language or facial expressions. Supportive attitudes will help improve compliance and set the stage for effective follow-up counseling about regular contraceptive use and STI prevention. Women must understand that emergency contraception offers no protection against STIs, including infection with the human immunodeficiency virus (HIV). Therefore, emergency treatment of infections may also be needed. (See Chapter 21 on Reproductive Tract Infections, including HIV/AIDS.)

Women who would not have an abortion if EC treatment fails can be reassured that pregnancies occurring despite EC treatment do not have an increased risk of adverse outcome.

Frequent use. Emphasize that ECPs are not recommended for routine use, because they are less effective than regular contraceptives. (Note that repeated combined or progestin-only ECP use is not known to pose health risks to users other than pregnancy; the label for ella states that "Repeated use of ella within the same menstrual cycle is not recommended, as safety and efficacy of repeat use within the same cycle has not been evaluated."[160]

Use after 72 hours. Although most studies of ECP treatment have specified that treatment be administered within 72 hours, more recent studies have demonstrated efficacy of giving ECPs up to 120 hours after unprotected intercourse.[8,131,141,142] ella is labeled for use up to 120 hours after intercourse.[129,134,160]

Use after multiple acts of unprotected intercourse. If more than 120 hours have elapsed since the time of the first unprotected act of intercourse, ECPs may be less effective in preventing pregnancy that resulted from that first exposure. Providing ECPs, however, would not be expected to disrupt or harm subsequent pregnancy development and would reduce the risk that pregnancy would result from later acts of intercourse that occurred within the preceding 120 hours.

Ongoing contraception. Women requesting emergency contraception should be offered information and services for regular contraception. However, not all women will want extensive contraceptive counseling. Thus, while counseling about regular contraceptives is recommended, adoption of a regular method of contraception should not be a prerequisite for providing EC. If the reason for requesting emergency contraception is that the regular contraceptive method failed, discuss reasons for failure and how they might be prevented in the future.

BEFORE PROVIDING EMERGENCY CONTRACEPTIVE TREATMENT

Make certain the woman does not want to become pregnant and understands there is still a chance of pregnancy after treatment. Describe common side effects; advance counseling about possible side effects helps women know what to expect and may lead to greater tolerance. If the patient has no option but to use a combined estrogen-progestin ECP, recommend she take 50 mg meclizine (2 Antivert, Bonine, D-Vert, or Dramamine II tablets) 1 hour before starting ECP treatment.[55]

A pregnancy test may be helpful if there is some doubt about whether the woman may have become pregnant after unprotected sex earlier in the month. If this is not the case, pregnancy testing is unnecessary. If the woman is pregnant, ECP treatment will not be effective. Women with negative pregnancy tests can use ECPs to reduce their risk of becoming pregnant. Women who do not have a period within 3 weeks of taking ECP should be instructed to take a pregnancy test to see if they have become pregnant.[162]

Make sure the woman understands that ECPs will not protect her from pregnancy if she engages in unprotected intercourse in the days or weeks following treatment, as this is a common misperception. Because ECPs, especially UPA, can delay ovulation, a woman could be at risk of pregnancy if she has unprotected intercourse within the first few days of ECP treatment. Women should therefore abstain from having intercourse or use an effective method of contraception for the remainder of their menstrual cycle. If the woman wishes to use COCs as an ongoing method, she can take 1 oral contraceptive tablet the day after taking ECPs and then continue with daily pills. A woman can also begin using the levonorgestrel IUC, the implant, the injectable, the vaginal contraceptive ring, or patches immediately after ECP treatment, or she can use a barrier method, such as condoms, for the remainder of her cycle (see Table 6–2). If she starts using a hormonal method immediately after ECP treatment, a pregnancy test 3 weeks later should be performed to rule out pregnancy that may have resulted from ECP failure.

Table 6–2 Initiating ongoing contraception after ECP use

Because ECPs can delay ovulation, a woman could be at risk of pregnancy until the next menstrual period after treatment. Women should use an effective method of contraception for the remainder of the treatment cycle and thereafter.

Method	When to Initiate
Condom	Can be used immediately
Diaphragm	Can be used immediately
Spermicide	Can be used immediately
Sponge	Can be used immediately
Combined Oral Contraceptives (COCs)	Initiate a new pack the day after ECP treatment is completed or according to manufacturer's instructions after beginning the next menstrual cycle. Women using Cryselle, Enpresse, Jolessa, Levora, Lo/Ovral, Low-Ogestrel, Nordette, Portia, or Quasence for emergency contraception can continue taking one pill per day from the same pack; women using other brands can begin a new pack the day after ECP treatment is completed; abstain from intercourse or use back-up protection for the first 7 days.
Progestin-only Pills	Initiate a new pack the day after ECP treatment is completed or according to manufacturer's instructions after beginning the next menstrual cycle. If starting immediately after ECP use, abstain from intercourse or use back-up protection in addition to POPs for the first 2 days of the POP pack.
Vaginal Ring	Initiate the day after ECP treatment is completed or within 5 days of beginning the next menstrual period. If starting immediately after ECP use, abstain from intercourse or use back-up protection in addition to the ring for the first 7 days.
Contraceptive Patch	Initiate the day after ECP treatment is completed or within 5 days of beginning the next menstrual period. If starting immediately after ECP use, abstain from intercourse or use back-up protection in addition to the patch for the first 7 days.
Three-Month Injectable	Initiate the day ECP treatment is initiated or the day after ECP treatment is completed or within 7 days of beginning the next menstrual period. If starting immediately after ECP use, abstain from intercourse or use back-up protection for the first 7 days.
Implants	Initiate the day ECP treatment is initiated or the day after ECP treatment is completed or within 7 days of beginning the next menstrual period. If starting immediately after ECP use, abstain from intercourse or use back-up protection for the first 7 days.
Intrauterine Contraception	A copper-releasing IUC can be used for emergency contraception treatment. Insert the levonorgestrel IUD the day ECP treatment is initiated or the day after ECP treatment is completed or within 7 days of beginning the next menstrual period. If starting immediately after ECP use, abstain from intercourse or use back-up protection for the first 7 days.
Fertility Awareness Methods	Initiate after onset of the next normal menstrual period and after the patient has been trained in using the method
Sterilization	Perform the operation any time after pregnancy has been ruled out.

Notes:

ella is an antiprogestin. When starting hormonal contraception immediately after using ella, it is not known whether the instructions above for abstaining or using back-up contraception are conservative enough. Our conservative recommendation is to abstain or use condoms for 2 weeks.

If starting hormonal methods immediately after ECP treatment, a pregnancy test 3 weeks later should be performed to rule out pregnancy that may have resulted from ECP failure.

EMERGENCY CONTRACEPTION TREATMENT REGIMENS

Emergency contraceptive pills. For maximum effectiveness, ECP treatment should be started as soon as possible after unprotected intercourse, and within 120 hours. Treatment with ulipristal acetate (one 30 mg tablet) is the most effective ECP option. Progestin-only ECP treatment (either one 1,500 mcg levonorgestrel tablet or two tablets of 750 mcg levonorgestrel taken together as one 1,500 mcg dose) is more effective and causes significantly less nausea and vomiting than treatment with combined estrogen-progestin ECP options (e.g., 100 to 120 mcg ethinyl estradiol and 500 to 600 mcg levonorgestrel in each dose). The addition of meloxicam or another nonsteroidal anti-inflammatory agent may increase the efficacy of these ECP regimens.[144]

Combined estrogen-progestin treatment involves two doses taken 12 hours apart. If necessary, adjust the timing for the second dose by a few hours to avoid a middle-of-the-night dose. Drugs and doses are shown in Table 6–1.

Intrauterine devices. Implantation occurs 6 to 12 days following ovulation.[163] Therefore, a copper IUC can be inserted as a method of emergency contraception up to 5 days after ovulation. Thus, if a woman had unprotected intercourse 3 days before the day ovulation is estimated to have occurred, the IUC could, in principle, be inserted up to 8 days after intercourse. Most family planning providers, however, limit insertion to the first 5 days after intercourse because it is difficult to reliably estimate the day of ovulation. If emergency IUC insertion is planned, but cannot be carried out immediately, provide ECP treatment immediately. If possible, ulipristal acetate should be offered as it is the most effective ECP, especially if the interval since unprotected intercourse is longer than 72 hours. However, even if ulipristal acetate is not available, levonorgestrel ECPs should still be used, as they may help reduce the risk of pregnancy.

AFTER PROVIDING EMERGENCY CONTRACEPTIVE TREATMENT

Review all available contraceptive options, highlighting the potential benefits of using a highly effective reversible method such as an IUC or implant. If the woman wishes to continue to use a previously selected method of routine contraception, no follow-up is needed unless she does not have a normal menstrual period within 3 weeks, suspects she may be pregnant, or has other reasons for concern. If there is any concern of pregnancy, perform a pregnancy test.

If emergency contraception has failed and the woman is pregnant, provide appropriate services or referrals. If she decides to continue the pregnancy, reassure her that there is no evidence of any teratogenic effect following the use of ECPs. Pregnancy following emergency insertion of a copper IUC should be managed with prompt removal of the IUC, as is recommended for the rare cases in which pregnancy occurs following insertion of an IUC (see Chapter 7 on Intrauterine Contraception).

ADVANCE PRESCRIPTION OF ELLA

Provide a prescription in advance of need to every woman and have her take it to a pharmacist to keep on file for use up to a year later.

ADDITIONAL INFORMATION AND MATERIALS

Additional information and materials are available from the following sources:

- Information about emergency contraception method options worldwide and access to the U.S. directory of providers via internet: www.NOT-2-LATE.com or ec.princeton.edu.

- ACOG Practice Bulletin No. 112: Emergency Contraception. *Obstet Gynecol.* 2010;**115**:1100–9.

USER INSTRUCTIONS FOR EMERGENCY CONTRACEPTION

Women provided with ECPs should receive medication labeling that identifies the specific product prescribed and the number of tablets needed for each dose (see Table 6–1). Give the following instructions to women to ensure correct use.

1. **Take your emergency contraceptive pill as directed:**

   a. **ella.** Swallow the tablet as soon as possible within 120 hours after unprotected sex.

   b. **Progestin-only ECPs.** Swallow the one *Plan B One-Step* tablet OR the two *Next Choice* tablets as one dose as soon as possible within 120 hours after unprotected sex. Consider taking a dose of meloxicam, ibuprofen, or naprosyn at the same time. Taking more pills will not make you less likely to become pregnant.

   c. **Combined estrogen-progestin ECPs.** Swallow the first dose as soon as possible within 120 hours after unprotected sex. Do not take any extra pills. Taking more pills will not make you less likely to become pregnant but may make you more nauseated and may make you vomit.

Swallow the second dose 12 hours after taking the first dose. If necessary, you can delay the second dose by a few hours to avoid having to take your second dose in the middle of the night.

Consider taking anti-nausea medication (two 25 mg tablets of Antivert, Bonine, D-Vert, or Dramamine II) 1 hour before the first dose. About one half of women who use combined ECPs have temporary nausea. It is usually mild and should stop in a day or so. If you vomit within 2 hours after taking a dose, call your clinician. You may need to repeat a dose of ECP.

2. **If your period does not start within 3 weeks, take a pregnancy test and/or see your clinician.** Your next period may start a few days earlier or later than usual. If you think you may be pregnant, see your clinician as soon as possible, whether or not you plan to continue the pregnancy.

3. **Do not have intercourse until you start another method of birth control.** ECPs will not protect you from more than one episode of unprotected intercourse. If you start using hormonal contraception immediately after taking ella, abstain or use condoms for the first 2 weeks. For the other ECPs, abstain or use condoms for 7 days (2 days when starting progestin-only pills).

4. **Discuss with your clinician which birth control method may work best for you over the long term and when you can start it.**

Instructions for women who have emergency insertion of an IUC are the same as for all women who have an IUC placed (see Chapter 7 on Intrauterine Contraception).

REFERENCES

1. Consensus statement on emergency contraception. Contraception. 1995;52:211–3.
2. Trussell J, Ellertson C. Efficacy of emergency contraception. Fertility Control Reviews. 1995;4:8–11.
3. Cheng L, Gülmezoglu AM, Piaggio GGP, Ezcurra EE, Van Look PPFA. Interventions for emergency contraception. Cochrane Db Syst Rev 2008, Issue 2. Art. No.: CD001324. DOI: 10.1002/14651858.CD001324.pub3.
4. Ellertson C, Webb A, Blanchard K, Bigrigg A, Haskell S, Shochet T, Trussell J. Modifying the Yuzpe regimen of emergency contraception: a multi-center randomized, controlled trial. Obstet Gynecol. 2003;101:1160–7.
5. Van Look PF, von Hertzen H. Clinical uses of antiprogestogens. Hum Reprod Update. 1995;1:19–34.
6. Wu S, Wang C, Wang Y, Cheng W, Zuo S, Li H Xu X, Wang R, Dong J. A randomized, double-blind, multicenter study on comparing levonorgestrel and mifepristone for emergency contraception. [Sheng Zhi Yi Xue Za Zhi] J Reprod Med. 1999;8 Suppl 1:S43–6. English.

7. Task Force on Postovulatory Methods of Fertility Regulation. Comparison of three single doses of mifepristone as emergency contraception: a randomised trial. Lancet. 1999;353:697–702.

8. von Hertzen H, Piaggio G, Ding J, Chen J, Song S, Bártfai G, Ng E, Gemzell-Danielsson K, Oyunbileg A, Wu S, Cheng W, Lüdicke F, Pretnar-Darovec A, Kirkman R, Mittal S, Khomassuridze A, Apter D, Peregoudov A. Low dose mifepristone and two regimens of levonorgestrel for emergency contraception: a WHO multicentre randomised trial. Lancet. 2002;360:1803–10.

9. Hamoda H, Ashok PW, Stalder C, Flett GM, Kennedy E, Templeton A. A randomized trial of mifepristone (10 mg) and levonorgestrel for emergency contraception. Obstet Gynecol. 2004;104:1307–13.

10. Glasier A, Thong KJ, Dewar M, Mackie M, Baird DT. Mifepristone (RU 486) compared with high-dose estrogen and progestogen for emergency postcoital contraception. N Engl J Med. 1992;327:1041–4.

11. Webb AM, Russell J, Elstein M. Comparison of Yuzpe regimen, danazol, and mifepristone (RU486) in oral postcoital contraception. BMJ (Clinical Research Ed.). 1992;305:927–31.

12. Ashok PW, Stalder C, Wagaarachchi PT, Flett GM, Melvin L, Templeton A. A randomised study comparing a low dose of mifepristone and the Yuzpe regimen for emergency contraception. BJOG. 2002;109:553–60.

13. Wu S, Dong J, Cong J, Wang C, VonHertzen H, Godfrey EM. Gestrinone compared with mifepristone for emergency contraception: a randomized controlled trial. Obstet Gynecol. 2010;115:740–4.

14. Hester KE, Harper MJK, Duffy DM. Oral administration of the cyclooxygenase-2 (COX-2) inhibitor meloxicam blocks ovulation in non-human primates when administered to simulate emergency contraception. Hum Reprod. 2010;25:360–7.

15. Jesam C, Salvatierra AM, Schwartz JL, Croxatto HB. Suppression of follicular rupture with meloxicam, a cyclooxygenase-2 inhibitor: potential for emergency contraception. Hum Reprod. 2010;25:368–73.

16. Morris JM, Van Wagenen G. Postcoital oral contraception. In: Hankinson R, Kleinman R, Esckstein P, Romero H, (eds). Proceedings of the Eighth International Conference of the International Planned Parenthood Federation: 1967 Apr 9–15; Santiago, Chile. London: International Planned Parenthood Federation; 1967.

17. Van Look F. Postcoital contraception: a cover-up story. In: Diczfalusy E, Bygdeman M, (eds). Fertility regulation today and tomorrow. Serono symposia publications; vol 36. New York: Raven Press 1987.

18. Zuliani G, Colombo UF, Molla R. Hormonal postcoital contraception with an ethinylestradiol-norgestrel combination and two danazol regimens. Europ J Obstet Gynecol Reprod Biology. 1990;37:253–60.

19. Mosher WD, Jones J. Use of Contraception in the United States: 1982–2008. National Center for Health Statistics. Vital Health Stat. 2010; 23(29); [cited 2010 Jun 7]. Available from: http://www.cdc.gov/NCHS/data/series/sr_23/sr23_029.pdf

20. Harrison T. Availability of emergency contraception: a survey of hospital emergency department staff. Ann Emerg Med. 2005;46:105–10.

21. Patel A, Panchal H, Piotrowski ZH, Patel D. Comprehensive medical care for victims of sexual assault: a survey of Illinois hospital emergency departments. Contraception. 2008;77:426–30.

22. Kavanaugh ML, Saladino RA, Gold MA. Emergency contraception services for adolescents: a National Survey of Children's Hospital Emergency Department Directors. J Pediatr Adolesc Gynecol. 2009;22:111–9.

23. Goyal M, Zhao H, Mollen C. Exploring emergency contraception knowledge, prescription practices, and barriers to prescription for adolescents in the emergency department. Pediatrics. 2009;123:765–70.

24. Goldenring JM, Allred G. Post-rape care in hospital emergency rooms. Am J Public Health. 2001;91:1169–70.

25. Stewart FH, Trussell J. Prevention of pregnancy resulting from rape: a neglected preventive health measure. Am J Prevent Med. 2000;19:228–9.
26. Littel K. National Protocol for Sexual Assault Medical Forensic Examinations: Adults/Adolescents. Washington (DC): US Dept of Justice, Office on Violence Against Women; 2004 Sep.
27. McCall-Hosenfeld JS, Liebschutz JM, Spiro A, Seaver MR. Sexual assault in the military and its impact on sexual satisfaction in women veterans: a proposed model. J Womens Health. 2009;18:901–9.
28. Department of Defense Pharmacy and Therapeutics Committee. Minutes of the Department of Defense (DoD) Pharmacy and Therapeutics (P&T) Committee Meeting, 2002 May 8. [cited 2010 Jun 7]. Available from: http://www.tricare.mil/pharmacy/PT_Cmte/PT_C/May_02_PT_Minutes.pdf
29. Maze R. Emergency contraception still available. Marine Corps Times 2007 Apr 30. [cited 2010 Jun 7]; Available from: http://www.marinecorpstimes.com/news/2007/04/military_emergency_contraceptives_070430w/.
30. Department of Defense Pharmacy and Therapeutics Committee. Minutes of the Department of Defense (DoD) Pharmacy and Therapeutics (P&T) Committee Meeting, 2009 November. [cited 2010 Jun 7]. Available from: http://www.tricare.mil/Pharmacy/PT_Cmte/2010/PT%20Minutes%20-%20Nov%202009%20-%20signed.pdf
31. Raymond EG, Trussell J, Polis C. Population effect of increased access to emergency contraceptive pills: a systematic review. Obstet Gynecol. 2007;109:181–8.
32. Polis CB, Grimes DA, Schaffer K, Blanchard K, Glasier A, Harper C. Advance provision of emergency contraception for pregnancy prevention. Cochrane Database of Systematic Reviews 2010, Issue 3. Art. No.: CD005497. DOI: 10.1002/14651858.CD005497.pub2.
33. Glasier A, Fairhurst K, Wyke S, Ziebland S, Seaman P, Walker J, Lakha F. Advanced provision of emergency contraception does not reduce abortion rates. Contraception. 2004;69:361–6.
34. Raine TR, Harper CC, Rocca CH, Fischer R, Padian N, Klausner JD, Darney PD. Direct access to emergency contraception through pharmacies and effect on unintended pregnancy and STIs: a randomized controlled trial. JAMA. 2005;293:54–62.
35. Hu X, Cheng L, Hua X, Glasier A. Advanced provision of emergency contraception to postnatal women in China makes no difference in abortion rates: a randomized controlled trial. Contraception. 2005;72:111–6.
36. Raymond EG, Stewart F, Weaver M, Monteith C, Van Der Pol B. Randomized trial to evaluate the impact of increased access to emergency contraceptive pills. Obstet Gynecol. 2006;108:1098–106.
37. Baecher L, Weaver MA, Raymond EG. Increased access to emergency contraception: why it may fail. Hum Reprod. 2009;24:815–9.
38. Glasier A, Baird D. The effects of self-administering emergency contraception. N Engl J Med. 1998;339:1–4.
39. Raine T, Harper C, Leon K, Darney P. Emergency contraception: advance provision in a young, high-risk clinic population. Obstet Gynecol. 2000;96:1–7.
40. Hazari K. Use of emergency contraception by women as a back-up method. Health Popul. 2000;23:115–122.
41. Jackson RA, Schwarz EB, Freedman L, Darney P. Advance supply of emergency contraception: effect on use and usual contraception—a randomized trial. Obstet Gynecol. 2003;102:8–16.
42. Gold MA, Wolford JE, Smith KA, Parker AM. The effects of advance provision of emergency contraception on adolescent women's sexual and contraceptive behaviors. J Pediatr Adolesc Gynecol. 2004;17:87–96.
43. Lo SS, Fan SYS, Ho PC, Glasier AF. Effect of advanced provision of emergency contraception on women's contraceptive behavior: a randomized controlled trial. Hum Reprod. 2004;19:2404–10.

44. Belzer M, Sanchez K, Olson J, Jacobs AM, Tucker D. Advance supply of emergency contraception: a randomized trial in adolescent mothers. J Pediatr Adolesc Gynecol. 2005;18:347–54.
45. Trussell J, Raymond E, Stewart FH. Letter to the editor. J Pediatr Adolesc Gynecol. 2006;19:251. Comment on: Advance supply of emergency contraception. J Pediatr Adolesc Gynecol. 2005 Oct;18(5):347–54.
46. Walsh TL, Frezieres RG. Patterns of emergency contraception use by age and ethnicity from a randomized trial comparing advance provision and information only. Contraception. 2006;74:110–7.
47. Marston C, Meltzer H, Majeed A. Impact on contraceptive practice of making emergency hormonal contraception available over the counter in Great Britain: repeated cross sectional surveys. BMJ. 2005;331(7511):271–3.
48. Moreau C, Bajos N, Trussell J. The impact of pharmacy access to emergency contraceptive pills in France. Contraception. 2006;73:602–8.
49. Schwarz EB, Gerbert B, Gonzales R. Computer-assisted provision of emergency contraception: a randomized controlled trial. J Gen Intern Med. 2008;23:794–9.
50. Ekstrand M, Larsson M, Darj E, Tydén T. Advance provision of emergency contraceptive pills reduces treatment delay: a randomised controlled trial among Swedish teenage girls. Acta Obstet Gynecol Scand. 2008;87:354–9.
51. Graham A, Moore L, Sharp D, Diamond I. Improving teenagers' knowledge of emergency contraception: cluster randomized controlled trial of a teacher led intervention. BMJ. 2002;234(7347):1179–84.
52. Raymond EG, Weaver MA. Effect of an emergency contraceptive pill intervention on pregnancy risk behavior. Contraception. 2008;77:333–6.
53. Weaver MA, Raymond EG, Baecher L. Attitude and behavior effects in a randomized trial of increased access to emergency contraception. Obstet Gynecol. 2009;113:107–16.
54. Shelton JD. Repeat emergency contraception: facing our fears. Contraception. 2002;66:15–7.
55. Trussell J, Ellertson C, Stewart F, Raymond EG, Shochet T. The role of emergency contraception. Am J Obstet Gynecol. 2004;190:S30–8.
56. Trussell J, Bull J, Koenig J, Bass M, Allina A, Gamble VN. Call 1–888-NOT-2-LATE: promoting emergency contraception in the United States. J Am Med Wom Assoc. 1998;53 Suppl 2:S247–50.
57. Trussell J, Koenig J, Vaughan B, Stewart F. Evaluation of a media campaign to increase knowledge about emergency contraception. Contraception. 2001;63:81–7.
58. Ellertson C, Trussell J, Stewart F, Winikoff B. Should emergency contraceptive pills be available without prescription? J Am Med Wom Assoc. 1998;53 Suppl 2:S226–9, 232.
59. Grimes DA, Raymond EG, Scott Jones B. Emergency contraception over-the-counter: the medical and legal imperatives. Obstet Gynecol. 2001;98:151–5.
60. Grimes DA. Emergency contraception and fire extinguishers: a prevention paradox. Am J Obstet Gynecol. 2002;187:1536–8.
61. Grimes DA, Raymond EG, Scott Jones B. Emergency contraception over-the-counter: the medical and legal imperatives. Obstet Gynecol. 2001;98:151–5.
62. Association of Reproductive Health Professionals. ARHP sign-on letter: switch status of emergency contraceptive from Rx to OTC; [cited 2010 Jun 7]. Available from: http://arhp.org/uploadDocs/ec_signon.pdf.
63. United States. Food and Drug Administration Decision Process to Deny Initial Application for Over-the-Counter Marketing of the Emergency Contraceptive Drug Plan B Was Unusual : Report to Congressional Requesters. Washington (DC): U.S. Government Accountability Office, 2005. [cited 2010 June 7]. Available from: http://purl.access.gpo.gov/GPO/LPS66189
64. Wood AJJ, Drazen JM, Greene MF. A sad day for science at the FDA. N Engl J Med. 2005;353:1197–8.

65. Tummino v. Torti, 260 F. R. D. 27 (E.D.N.Y. 2009). [updated 2009 Aug 27; cited 2010 Jun 7]. Available from: http://www.nyed.uscourts.gov/pub/rulings/cv/2005/05cv366mofinal.pdf

66. Trussell J, Guthrie KA. Talking straight about emergency contraception. J Fam Plan Reprod Health Care. 2007;33:139–42.

67. Sivin I. Utility and drawbacks of continuous use of a copper T IUD for 20 years. Contraception. 2007;75:Suppl S70–5.

68. Trussell J, Leveque JA, Koenig JD, London R, Borden S, Henneberry J, LaGuardia KD, Stewart F, Wilson TG, Wysocki S, Strauss M. The economic value of contraception: a comparison of 15 methods. Am J Public Health. 1995;85:494–503.

69. Trussell J, Koenig J, Ellertson C, Stewart F. Preventing unintended pregnancy: the cost-effectiveness of three methods of emergency contraception. Am J Public Health. 1997;87:932–7.

70. Trussell J, Koenig J, Stewart F, Darroch JE. Medical care cost savings from adolescent contraceptive use. Fam Plann Perspect. 1997;29:248–55, 295.

71. Trussell J, Wiebe E, Shochet T, Guilbert É. Cost savings from emergency contraceptive pills in Canada. Obstet Gynecol. 2001;97:789–93.

72. Trussell J, Shochet T. Cost-effectiveness of emergency contraceptive pills in the public sector in the USA. Expert Rev Pharmacoeconomics Outcomes Res. 2003;3:433–40.

73. Trussell J, Calabretto H. Cost savings from use of emergency contraceptive pills in Australia. Aust N Z J Obstet Gynaecol. 2005;45:308–11.

74. Foster DG, Rostovtseva DP, Brindis CD, Biggs MA, Hulett D, Darney PD. Cost savings from the provision of specific methods of contraception in a publicly funded program. Am J Public Health. 2009;99:446–51.

75. Foster DG, Raine TR, Brindis C, Rostovtseva DP, Darney PD. Should providers give women advance provision of emergency contraceptive pills? A cost-effectiveness analysis. Womens Health Issues. 2010;20:242–7.

76. Statement on Contraceptive Methods. Washington (DC): American College of Obstetricians and Gynecologists; July 1998.

77. Díaz S, Cárdenas H, Brandeis A, Miranda P, Salvatierra AM, Croxatto HB. Relative contributions of anovulation and luteal phase defect to the reduced pregnancy rate of breastfeeding women. Fertil Steril. 1992;58:498–503.

78. Levonorgestrel for emergency contraception [Fact sheet]. Geneva (Switzerland): World Health Organization; 2005 March.

79. Protection of Human Subjects, 45 C.F.R. Sect. 46.202 (2009).

80. Hughes EC (ed). Committee on Terminology, The American College of Obstetricians and Gynecologists, Obstetric-Gynecologic Terminology. Philadelphia (PA): F.A. Davis Company; 1972.

81. Brache V, Cochon L, Jesam C, Maldonado R, Salvatierra AM, Levy DP, Gainer E, Croxatto HB. Immediate preovulatory administration of 30 mg ulipristal acetate significantly delays follicular rupture. Hum Reprod. 2010;25:2256–63

82. Stratton P, Levens ED, Hartog B, Piquion J, Wei Q, Merino M, Nieman LK. Endometrial effects of a single early luteal dose of the selective progesterone receptor modulator CDB-2914. Fertil Steril. 2010;93:2035–41.

83. Hapangama D, Glasier AF, Baird DT. The effects of peri-ovulatory administration of levonorgestrel on the menstrual cycle. Contraception. 2001;63:123–9.

84. Durand M, del Carmen Cravioto M, Raymond EG, Durán-Sánchez O, De la Luz Cruz-Hinojosa L, Castell-Rodríguez A, Schiavon R, Larrea F. On the mechanisms of action of short-term levonorgestrel administration in emergency contraception. Contraception. 2001;64:227–34.

85. Marions L, Hultenby K, Lindell I, Sun X, Ståbi B, Gemzell Danielsson K. Emergency contraception with mifepristone and levonorgestrel: mechanism of action. Obstet Gynecol. 2002;100:65–71.

86. Marions L, Cekan SZ, Bygdeman M, Gemzell-Danielsson K. Effect of emergency contraception with levonorgestrel or mifepristone on ovarian function. Contraception. 2004;69:373–7.

87. Croxatto HB, Brache V, Pavez M, Cochon L, Forcelledo ML, Alvarez F, Massai R, Faundes A, Salvatierra AM. Pituitary-ovarian function following the standard levonorgestrel emergency contraceptive dose or a single 0.75-mg dose given on the days preceding ovulation. Contraception. 2004;70:442–50.

88. Durand M, Séppala M, del Carmen Cravioto M, Koistinen H, Koistinen R, González-Macedo J, Larrea F. Late follicular phase administration of levonorgestrel as an emergency contraceptive changes the secretory pattern of glycodelin in serum and endometrium during the luteal phase of the menstrual cycle. Contraception. 2005;71: 451–7.

89. Seppälä M, Taylor RN, Koistinen H, Koistinen R, Milgrom E. Glycodelin: a major lipocalin protein of the reproductive axis with diverse actions in cell recognition and differentiation. Endocr Rev. 2002;23:401–30.

90. do Nascimento JA, Seppala M, Perdigao A, Espejo-Arce X, Munuce MJ, Hautala L, Koistinen R, Andrade L, Bahamondes L. In vivo assessment of the human sperm acrosome reaction and the expression of glycodelin-A in human endometrium after levonorgestrel-emergency contraceptive pill administration. Hum Reprod. 2007;22: 2190–5.

91. Palomino WA, Kohen P, Devoto L. A single midcycle dose of levonorgestrel similar to emergency contraceptive does not alter the expression of the L-selectin ligand or molecular markers of endometrial receptivity. Fertil Steril. 2010;94:1589–94.

92. Durand M, Koistinen R, Chirinos M, Rodríguez JL, Zambrano E, Seppälä M, Larrea F. Hormonal evaluation and midcycle detection of intrauterine glycodelin in women treated with levonorgestrel as in emergency contraception. Contraception. 2010;82:526–33.

93. Lalitkumar PG, Lalitkumar S, Meng CX, Stavreus-Evers A, Hambiliki F, Bentin-Ley U, Gemzell-Danielsson K. Mifepristone, but not levonorgestrel, inhibits human blastocyst attachment to an in vitro endometrial three-dimensional cell culture model. Hum Reprod. 2007;22:3031–7.

94. Meng CX, Andersson KL, Bentin-Ley U, Gemzell-Danielsson K, Lalitkumar PG. Effect of levonorgestrel and mifepristone on endometrial receptivity markers in a three-dimensional human endometrial cell culture model. Fertil Steril. 2009;91: 256–64.

95. Kesserü E, Garmendia F, Westphal N, Parada J. The hormonal and peripheral effects of d-norgestrel in postcoital contraception. Contraception. 1974;10:411–24.

96. Yeung WS, Chiu PC, Wang CH, Yao YQ, Ho PC. The effects of levonorgestrel on various sperm functions. Contraception. 2002;66:453–7.

97. Piaggio G, von Hertzen H, Grimes DA, Van Look PFA. Timing of emergency contraception with levonorgestrel or the Yuzpe regimen. Lancet. 1999;353:721.

98. Davidoff F, Trussell J. Plan B and the politics of doubt. JAMA. 2006;296:1775–8.

99. Mikolajczyk RT, Stanford JB. Levonorgestrel emergency contraception: a joint analysis of effectiveness and mechanism of action. Fertil Steril. 2007;88:565–71.

100. Croxatto HB, Devoto L, Durand M, Ezcurra E, Larrea F, Nagle C, Ortiz ME, Vantman D, Vega M, von Hertzen H. Mechanism of action of hormonal preparations used for emergency contraception: a review of the literature. Contraception. 2001;63:111–21.

101. Müller AL, Llados CM, Croxatto HB. Postcoital treatment with levonorgestrel does not disrupt postfertilization events in the rat. Contraception. 2003;67:415–19.

102. Ortiz ME, Ortiz RE, Fuentes MA, Parraguez VH, Croxatto HB. Postcoital administration of levonorgestrel does not interfere with post-fertilization events in the new-world monkey Cebus apella. Hum Reprod. 2004;19:1352–6.

103. Novikova N, Weisberg E, Stanczyk FZ, Croxatto HB, Fraser, IS. Effectiveness of levonorgestrel emergency contraception given before or after ovulation—a pilot study. Contraception. 2006;74:349–50.

104. Noé G, Croxatto HB, Salvatierra AM, Reyes V, Villarroel C, Muñoz C, Morales G, Retamales A. Contraceptive efficacy of emergency contraception with levonorgestrel given before or after ovulation. Contraception. 2010;81:414–20.
105. Emergency contraception's mode of action clarified. Popul Briefs. 2005;11:3. [cited 2010 Jun 7]. Available from: http://www.popcouncil.org/pdfs/popbriefs/pbmay05.pdf
106. Gemzell-Danielsson K. Mechanism of action of emergency contraception. Contraception. 2010;82:404–9.
107. Swahn ML, Westlund P, Johannisson E, Bygdeman M. Effect of post-coital contraceptive methods on the endometrium and the menstrual cycle. Acta Obstet Gynecol Scand. 1996;75:738–44.
108. Ling WY, Robichaud A, Zayid I, Wrixon W, MacLeod SC. Mode of action of dl-norgestrel and ethinylestradiol combination in postcoital contraception. Fertil Steril. 1979;32:297–302.
109. Rowlands S, Kubba AA, Guillebaud J, Bounds W. A possible mechanism of action of danazol and an ethinylestradiol/norgestrel combination used as postcoital contraceptive agents. Contraception. 1986;33:539–45.
110. Croxatto HB, Fuentalba B, Brache V, Salvatierra AM, Alvarez F, Massai R, Cochon L, Faundes A. Effects of the Yuzpe regimen, given during the follicular phase, on ovarian function. Contraception. 2002;65:121–8.
111. Kubba AA, White JO, Guillebaud J, Elder MG. The biochemistry of human endometrium after two regimens of postcoital contraception: a dl-norgestrel/ethinylestradiol combination or danazol. Fertil Steril. 1986;45:512–6.
112. Ling WY, Wrixon W, Zayid I, Acorn T, Popat R, Wilson E. Mode of action of dl-norgestrel and ethinylestradiol combination in postcoital contraception. II. Effect of postovulatory administration on ovarian function and endometrium. Fertil Steril. 1983;39:292–7.
113. Yuzpe AA, Thurlow HJ, Ramzy I, Leyshon JI. Post coital contraception—a pilot study. J Reprod Med. 1974;13:53–8.
114. Taskin O, Brown RW, Young DC, Poindexter AN, Wiehle RD. High doses of oral contraceptives do not alter endometrial a1 and anb3 integrins in the late implantation window. Fertil Steril. 1994;61:850–5.
115. Raymond EG, Lovely LP, Chen-Mok M, Seppälä M, Kurman RJ, Lessey BA. Effect of the Yuzpe regimen of emergency contraception on markers of endometrial receptivity. Hum Reprod. 2000;15:2351–5.
116. Glasier A. Emergency postcoital contraception. N Engl J Med. 1997;337:1058–64.
117. Ling WY, Wrixon W, Acorn T, Wilson E, Collins J. Mode of action of dl-norgestrel and ethinylestradiol combination in postcoital contraception. III. Effect of preovulatory administration following the luteinizing hormone surge on ovarian steroidogenesis. Fertil Steril. 1983;40:631–6.
118. Croxatto HB, Ortiz ME, Müller AL. Mechanisms of action of emergency contraception. Steroids. 2003;68:1095–8.
119. Trussell J, Raymond EG. Statistical evidence concerning the mechanism of action of the Yuzpe regimen of emergency contraception. Obstet Gynecol. 1999;93:872–6.
120. Trussell J, Ellertson C, von Hertzen H, Bigrigg A, Webb A, Evans M, Ferden S. Leadbetter C. Estimating the effectiveness of emergency contraceptive pills. Contraception. 2003;67:259–65.
121. Dixon GW, Schlesselman JJ, Ory HW, Blye RP. Ethinyl estradiol and conjugated estrogens as postcoital contraceptives. JAMA. 1980;244:1336–9.
122. Wilcox AJ, Weinberg CR, Baird DD. Timing of sexual intercourse in relation to ovulation. Effects on the probability of conception, survival of the pregnancy, and sex of the baby. N Engl J Med. 1995;333:1517–21.
123. Stirling A, Glasier A. Estimating the efficacy of emergency contraception-how good are the data? Contraception. 2002;66:19–22.

124. Espinos JJ, Rodriguez-Espinosa J, Senosiain R, Aura M, Vanrell C, Gispert M, Vega C, Calaf J. The role of matching menstrual data with hormonal measurements in evaluating effectiveness of postcoital contraception. Contraception. 1999;60:243–7.

125. Espinos-Gomez JJ, Senosiain R, Mata A, Vanrell C, Bassas L, Calaf J. What is the seminal exposition among women requiring emergency contraception? A prospective, observational comparative study. Eur J Obstet Gynecol Reprod Bio. 2007;131:57–60.

126. Raymond E, Taylor D, Trussell J, Steiner MJ. Minimum effectiveness of the levonorgestrel regimen of emergency contraception. Contraception. 2004;69:79–81.

127. Glasier AF, Cameron ST, Fine PM, Logan SJ, Casale W, Van Horn J, Sogor L, Blithe DL, Scherrer B, Mathe H, Jaspart A, Ulmann A, Gainer E. Ulipristal acetate versus levonorgestrel for emergency contraception: a randomised non-inferiority trial and meta-analysis. Lancet. 2010;375:555–62.

128. Creinin MD, Schlaff W, Archer DF, Wan L, Frezieres R, Thomas M, Rosenberg M, Higgins J. Progesterone receptor modulator for emergency contraception: a randomized controlled trial. Obstet Gynecol. 2006;108:1089–97.

129. Fine P, Mathé H, Ginde S, Cullins V, Morfesis J, Gainer E. Ulipristal acetate taken 48–120 hours after intercourse for emergency contraception. Obstet Gynecol. 2010;115:257–63.

130. Arowojolu AO, Okewole IA, Adekunle AO. Comparative evaluation of the effectiveness and safety of two regimens of levonorgestrel for emergency contraception in Nigerians. Contraception. 2002;66:269–73.

131. Ngai SW, Fan S, Li S, Cheng L, Ding J, Jing X, Ng EHY, Ho PC. A randomized trial to compare 24h versus 12h double dose regimen of levonorgestrel for emergency contraception. Hum Reprod. 2004;20:307–11.

132. Ho PC, Kwan MS. A prospective randomized comparison of levonorgestrel with the Yuzpe regimen in post-coital contraception. Hum Reprod. 1993;8:389–92.

133. Task Force on Postovulatory Methods of Fertility Regulation. Randomised controlled trial of levonorgestrel versus the Yuzpe regimen of combined oral contraceptives for emergency contraception. Lancet. 1998;352:428–33.

134. Glasier AF, Cameron ST, Fine PM, Logan SJ, Casale W, Van Horn J, Sogor L, Blithe DL, Scherrer B, Mathe H, Jaspart A, Ulmann A, Gainer E. Ulipristal acetate versus levonorgestrel for emergency contraception: a randomised non-inferiority trial and meta-analysis. Lancet. 2010;375:555–62.

135. Creinin MD, Schlaff W, Archer DF, Wan L, Frezieres R, Thomas M, Rosenberg M, Higgins J. Progesterone receptor modulator for emergency contraception: a randomized controlled trial. Obstet Gynecol. 2006;108:1089–97.

136. Dada OA, Godfrey EM, Gilda Piaggio G, von Hertzen H. A randomized, double-blind, noninferiority study to compare two regimens of levonorgestrel for emergency contraception in Nigeria. Contraception. 2010;82:373–8.

137. Farajkhoda T, Khoshbin A, Enjezab B, Bokaei M, Karimi Zarchi M. Assessment of two emergency contraceptive regimens in Iran: levonorgestrel versus the Yuzpe. Niger J Clin Pract. 2009;12:450–2.

138. Trussell J, Rodríguez G, Ellertson C. Updated estimates of the effectiveness of the Yuzpe regimen of emergency contraception. Contraception. 1999;59:147–51.

139. Kane LA, Sparrow MJ. Postcoital contraception: a family planning study. N Z Med J. 1989;102:151–3.

140. Trussell J, Ellertson C, Rodríguez G. The Yuzpe regimen of emergency contraception: how long after the morning after? Obstet Gynecol. 1996;88:150–4.

141. Rodrigues I, Grou F, Joly J. Effectiveness of emergency contraception pills between 72 and 120 hours after unprotected sexual intercourse. Am J Obstet Gynecol. 2001;184:531–7.

142. Ellertson C, Evans M, Ferden S, Leadbetter C, Spears A, Johnstone K, Trussell J. Extending the time limit for starting the Yuzpe regimen of emergency contraception to 120 hours. Obstet Gynecol. 2003;101:1168–71.

143. Yuzpe AA, Lancee WJ. Ethinylestradiol and dl-norgestrel as a postcoital contraceptive. Fertil Steril. 1977;28:932–6.
144. Massai MR, Forcelledo ML, Brache V, Tejada AS, Salvatierra AM, Reyes MV, Alvarez F, Faúndes A, Croxatto HB. Does meloxicam increase the incidence of an ovulation induced by single administration of levonorgestrel in emergency contraception? A pilot study. Hum Reprod. 2007;22:434–9.
145. Feldhaus KM. A 21st-century challenge: improving the care of the sexual assault victim. Ann Emerg Med. 2002;39:653–5.
146. Selected practice recommendations for contraceptive use. 2nd ed. Geneva (Switzerland): World Health Organization; 2005.
147. Raymond EG, Creinin MD, Barnhart KT, Lovvorn AE, Rountree RW, Trussell J. Meclizine for prevention of nausea associated with use of emergency contraceptive pills: a randomized trial. Obstet Gynecol. 2000;95:271–7.
148. Zhang L, Chen J, Wang Y, Ren F, Yu W, Cheng L. Pregnancy outcome after levonorgestrel-only emergency contraception failure: a prospective cohort study. Hum Reprod. 2009;24:1605–11.
149. Raman-Wilms L, Tseng AL, Wighardt S, Einarson TR, Koren G. Fetal genital effects of first-trimester sex hormone exposure: a meta-analysis. Obstet Gynecol. 1995;85:141–9.
150. Bracken MB. Oral contraception and congenital malformations in offspring: a review and meta-analysis of the prospective studies. Obstet Gynecol. 1990;76:552–7.
151. Simpson JL, Phillips OP. Spermicides, hormonal contraception and congenital malformations. Adv Contracept. 1990;6:141–67.
152. Food and Drug Administration. Prescription drug products; certain combined oral contraceptives for use as postcoital emergency contraception. Federal Regist. 1997;62:8610–2.
153. Trussell J, Hedley A, Raymond E. Ectopic pregnancy following use of progestin-only ECPs [letter]. J Fam Plann Reprod Health Care. 2003;29:249.
154. Cleland K, Raymond E, Trussell J, Cheng L, Haoping Z. Ectopic pregnancy and emergency contraception: a systematic review. Obstet Gynecol. 2010;115:1263–6.
155. Raymond EG, Goldberg A, Trussell J, Hays M, Roach E, Taylor D. Bleeding patterns after use of levonorgestrel emergency contraceptive pills. Contraception. 2006;73:376–81. Erratum in: Contraception. 2006;74:349–50. Erratum in: Contraception. 2007;75:476–7.
156. Gainer E, Kenfack B, Mboudou E, Doh AS, Bouyer J. Menstrual bleeding patterns following levonorgestrel emergency contraception. Contraception. 2006;74:118–24.
157. Tirelli A, Cagnacci A, Volpe A. Levonorgestrel administration in emergency contraception: bleeding pattern and pituitary-ovarian function. Contraception. 2008;77;328–32.
158. Centers for Disease Control and Prevention. U.S. Medical Eligibility Criteria for Contraceptive Use, 2010. MMWR 2010;59:(No. RR-4):1–85.
159. Gainer E, Massai R, Lillo S, Reyes V, Forcelledo ML, Caviedes R, Villarroel C, Bouyer J. Levonorgestrel pharmacokinetics in plasma and milk of lactating women who take 1.5 mg for emergency contraception. Hum Reprod. 2007;22:1578–84.
160. Available from http://www.accessdata.fda.gov/drugsatfda_docs/label/2010/022474s000lbl.pdf. Accessed 17 August 2010.
161. Wilcox AJ, Dunson DB, Weinberg CR, Trussell J, Baird DD. Likelihood of conception with a single act of intercourse: providing benchmark rates for assessment of postcoital contraceptives. Contraception. 2001;63:211–5.
162. Grimes DA, Raymond EG. Bundling a pregnancy test with the Yuzpe regimen of emergency contraception. Obstet Gynecol. 1999;94:471–3.
163. Wilcox AJ, Baird DD, Weinberg CR. Time of implantation of the conceptus and loss of pregnancy. N Engl J Med. 1999;340:1796–9.

Intrauterine Contraceptives (IUCs)

Gillian Dean, MD, MPH
Eleanor Bimla Schwarz, MD, MS

- The Copper T 380A and levonorgestrel-releasing intrauterine contraceptives (IUC) are similar to surgical sterilization in efficacy.
- Intrauterine contraception is safe for most women, including teens and HIV-positive women.
- Few contraindications exist to the use of either IUC.
- Satisfaction and continuation rates are high compared with other reversible contraceptives.
- Intrauterine contraception provides long-term pregnancy protection yet is promptly reversible.
- Intrauterine contraception is private, coitus-independent, and low maintenance.
- IUCs have several noncontraceptive heath benefits.
- IUCs are among the most cost-effective contraceptive methods available.
- Postabortal placement of IUCs is safe and increases IUC usage compared to delayed placement.
- Placement of a Copper T 380A is the most effective way to provide emergency contraception.

Intrauterine contraceptives (IUCs) are among the safest and most effective methods of contraception available today. The IUC is the most commonly used reversible method of contraception worldwide, eclipsing oral contraceptives by a large margin.[1] In the United States, an IUC renaissance is underway, but much work remains to be done to ensure that all women who may benefit from an IUC are aware of this option. IUCs are used by over 50% of contraceptive users in parts of Asia[2,3] and 6% to 27% of contraceptive users in Europe.[4,5] The United States has been slower to adopt modern intrauterine contraception; in

2002, only 2% of U.S. contraceptive users chose an IUC.[6] However, in 2006–2008, this number had grown to 5%.[7] Surveys reveal that 99% of these IUC users reported being "very" or "somewhat satisfied" with the method.[8]

Factors limiting widespread use of IUC in the United States include a history of negative publicity; misinformation about the risks of ectopic pregnancy, infection, and subsequent infertility; misconceptions about the mechanism of action; lack of clinician training; and clinicians' fears of litigation.[9] In the 1970s, IUCs were used by 10% of U.S. contraceptive users.[10] Unfortunately, one of the devices introduced in the 1970s, the Dalkon Shield, was linked to pelvic inflammatory disease (PID).[11] The multi-filamented threads attached to the Dalkon Shield may have contributed to infections by acting as a wick that allowed bacteria to ascend to the upper genital tract. Another important factor in this tragedy was the fact that in the 1970s it was not possible to test for asymptomatic chlamydia. As a result, many women developed severe pelvic infections with the Dalkon Shield, IUC-related litigation increased, and IUC use fell in the United States.

In contrast, modern IUCs have monofilament threads and have not been associated with infections or litigation against health care providers or IUC manufacturers.[12,13] In 2005, the U.S. Food and Drug Administration approved liberalized package labeling for the Copper T 380A, removing any proscription against use in nulliparous women or in those with more than one sexual partner. The labeling also supports placement immediately after an abortion or delivery. Much of the scientific evidence supporting the safety and efficacy of modern IUCs is summarized in two important reviews.[14,15] An important responsibility for health care providers and the media is to provide correct information to consumers and professionals. This, in turn, will increase the availability and use of this excellent method.

OPTIONS IN THE UNITED STATES

Two highly effective intrauterine contraceptives are available in the United States: the Copper T 380A (ParaGard, Teva Women's Health, Inc., Israel) and the levonorgestrel (LNg) intrauterine system (Mirena, Bayer HealthCare Pharmaceuticals, Wayne, New Jersey). See Figure 7–1. The term intrauterine contraception can be applied to any intrauterine method of contraception, whether the device is inert (plastic only) or medicated (containing copper or a progestin). Modern IUCs have a polyethylene frame with copper or LNg added to improve their contraceptive efficacy. The term intrauterine device (IUD) is a commonly used synonym. The LNg IUC is also sometimes referred to as an intrauterine system (IUS).

Copper T 380A IUD   **Levonogestrel IUS**

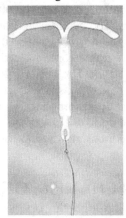

Figure 7–1 Two IUCs available in the United States

Copper T 380A. Introduced in the United States in 1988, the Copper T 380A (TCu380A) is made of polyethylene with barium sulfate added to create x-ray visibility. Fine copper wire is wound around the vertical stem of the T. Each of the two horizontal arms has a sleeve of copper. The combined copper surface area of the wire and sleeves is 380 +/− 23 mm². Serum copper levels are higher in TCu380A users compared with non-users and above the normal blood copper level range;[16] however, an increase in circulating copper has not been shown to have an adverse clinical effect. The device is latex-free; clinically relevant allergy to copper is extremely rare.[17] The device measures 36 mm tall and 32 mm wide. The bottom of the vertical stem has a 3 mm bulb into which a monofilament polyethylene thread is tied; these two threads enable easy removal of the device. Throughout the world, tens of millions of TCu380A IUCs have been distributed in 70 countries. The approved duration of use of the device is 10 years, although data indicate high effectiveness for 12 years,[18] and these devices have been safely used for up to 20 years.[19] Of note, inert IUCs and nonprogestin IUCs with less than 380 mm² of copper are less effective than those containing 380 mm² or more of copper and are no longer available in the United States.[20,21]

Levonorgestrel. The LNg IUC was approved for use in the United States in 2000 and first sold in 2001. However, several million women have used the LNg IUC since it became available in Europe in the early 1990s. The LNg IUC contains 52 mg of levonorgestrel, which is released directly into the endometrial cavity at an initial rate of 20 mcg per day. The approved lifespan of the LNg IUC is 5 years, although some studies have shown reasonable contraceptive efficacy to 7 years.[22-25] A large study of the efficacy of the LNg IUC at 7 years is currently underway.

The product is based on a Nova-T polyethylene frame, with a cylinder of a polydimethylsiloxane-levonorgestrel mixture molded around its vertical arm. The cylinder is coated with a membrane that regulates the release of the hormone. Measuring 32 mm in both height and width, the T-shaped frame contains barium sulfate for visibility on X-ray and contains no latex. The base of the vertical stem has monofilament polyethylene threads to assist with removal. Small amounts of levonorgestrel are systemically absorbed and some systemic side effects can occur. However, the daily dose of levonorgestrel is about 10% that of an oral contraceptive containing 150 mcg of levonorgestrel.

MECHANISM OF ACTION

Although the precise mechanism of action is not known, currently available IUCs work primarily by preventing sperm from fertilizing ova.[26] In other words, IUCs are not abortifacients: they do not interrupt an implanted pregnancy.[27] Pregnancy is prevented by a combination of the "foreign body effect" of the plastic or metal frame and the specific action of the medication (copper or levonorgestrel) that is released. Exposure to a foreign body causes a sterile inflammatory reaction in the intrauterine environment that is toxic to sperm and ova and impairs implantation.[28,29] The production of cytotoxic peptides and activation of enzymes lead to inhibition of sperm motility, reduced sperm capacitation and survival, and increased phagocytosis of sperm.[30,31] The TCu380A causes an increase in copper ions, enzymes, prostaglandins, and white blood cells (macrophages) in uterine and tubal fluids; these impair sperm function and prevent fertilization. The progestin in the LNg IUC enhances the contraceptive action of the device by thickening cervical mucus, suppressing the endometrium, and impairing sperm function. In addition, ovulation is often impaired as a result of systemic absorption of levonorgestrel.[23]

Three lines of evidence indicate that IUCs work early in the reproductive process.[27] First, human chorionic gonadotropin assays for early pregnancy do not reveal "chemical pregnancies."[32-34] Second, and more compelling, are tubal flushing studies in women undergoing tubal sterilization at mid-cycle. When the fallopian tubes were flushed and the fluid examined with a microscope to look for sperm and fertilized eggs, no fertilized, normally-dividing eggs were recovered from women using IUCs; in contrast, eggs were recovered from about half of the women not using contraception.[35] And third, IUC users have a markedly decreased risk of ectopic pregnancy, which implies that IUCs inhibit fertilization.

EFFECTIVENESS

Both IUCs available in the United States rank in the top tier of contraceptive effectiveness (along with surgical sterilization and implants).[36] See Figure 3–1 in Chapter 3 on Choosing a Contraceptive.

Copper T 380A (TCu380A)(ParaGard). The first-year pregnancy rate for the TCu380A is between 0.5% to 0.8%[27,37]; the cumulative pregnancy rate is 1.4% to 1.6% at 7 years,[22,38] and 2.2% at both 8 and 12 years.[39]

Levonorgestrel (LNg) IUC (Mirena). The probability of pregnancy in the first year of LNg IUC use is 0.1% to 0.2%.[40, 41] At 5 years of continuous use, the cumulative pregnancy rate is 0.5% to 1.1%.[42,43] With 7 years of continuous use, the cumulative pregnancy rate does not appear to increase over the 5-year rate.[22,44]

In contrast, the overall pregnancy rate with all methods of tubal sterilization in the United States is 1.3% at 5 years and 1.9% at 10 years.[45] Thus, the effectiveness of the TCu380A is comparable to tubal sterilization, while the LNg IUC appears to be superior.

Continuation Rates

Both IUCs have high continuation rates (about 85% to 90%) at 1 year.[44,46–48] This translates into superior long-term protection against unintended pregnancy.

ADVANTAGES

- High effectiveness
- Good safety record
- Few contraindications to use; not estrogenic
- Long-term protection
- Rapid reversibility
- Cost-effectiveness
- Convenient and private
- High user satisfaction
- Easy placement and removal
- Protection against ectopic pregnancy
- Immediate placement after end of pregnancy (post abortion, miscarriage, or delivery)
- Reduced risk of endometrial cancer
- Emergency contraception (TCu380A)

- Multiple noncontraceptive health benefits from LNg IUC
- Safely visible on X-ray, ultrasound, and MRI.

Intrauterine contraception is an excellent option for most women (including teens) because it is highly effective, safe, long-acting, and rapidly reversible. IUCs are coitus-independent, private, and easily inserted and removed by a clinician. IUCs offer several noncontraceptive health benefits. For women who want or need to avoid exogenous estrogen, IUC enables users to avoid the side effects and frequent attention required by most other reversible methods of contraception. IUCs are as effective as surgical sterilization and can usually be used by women who are poor surgical candidates for sterilization; there are few absolute contraindications to intrauterine contraception.[49–51] Modern IUCs have an impressive safety record and patient satisfaction and continuation rates are high.[46,47]

Cost-effectiveness

One office visit for IUC placement can provide a decade or more of superb contraception at a low daily cost. Although the initial cost of an IUC is high, the overall cost decreases with each year of use.[52] By 5 years of use, the IUC is one of the two most cost-effective methods of reversible contraception available, the other being Implanon.[53]

Ectopic Pregnancy Prevention

Women with a past history of ectopic pregnancy can safely use copper or LNg intrauterine contraception.[54] In fact, because the IUC works by preventing fertilization as well as implantation, the incidence of ectopic pregnancy is lower in IUC users than in women who use no contraception. Women using no contraception are 10 times as likely as IUC users to develop an ectopic pregnancy.[55]

Emergency Contraception

The TCu380A can be inserted within 120 hours of unprotected intercourse for emergency contraception and then left in place to provide ongoing contraception. In a cohort of 1,963 women using the Copper T 380A for emergency contraception, none became pregnant. In the 12 months after these women requested emergency contraception, there were only 0.23 pregnancies per 100 women.[56]

Cancer Protection

Both IUCs are associated with a reduction in the risk of endometrial cancer. Although the mechanism of action in the copper IUC is unknown, it may relate to alterations in the endometrium.[57,58] Similarly, progestin-releasing intrauterine contraception has also been shown to protect against endometrial cancer,[59] as is true of contraceptives that deliver a progestin systemically.[60] Indeed, the LNg IUC has been used to prevent development of endometrial hyperplasia in women using estrogen therapy in the peri- and postmenopause.[61-63] While the TCu380A is generally preferred for women with recent breast cancer, the LNg IUC is used at times for women treated with tamoxifen to protect the endometrium.[59,64,65] Moreover, the LNg IUC has been used for the treatment of nonatypical endometrial hyperplasia. It may also be effective for atypical hyperplasia and grade 1 stage I endometrial cancer.[66-69]

Noncontraceptive Health Benefits of the LNg IUC

Topical delivery of progestin to the uterine cavity has exciting therapeutic uses aside from contraception.[70] Some are well established and approved indications, while others are still being explored. The LNg IUC reduces dysmenorrhea and menstrual blood loss from a variety of causes. Overall blood loss drops about 90%, and at least 20% of women stop bleeding altogether. This translates into clinically important increases in hemoglobin and iron stores. The reduction in menstrual blood loss occurs both in women with normal coagulation parameters and in those with bleeding diatheses, including those using anticoagulant therapy.[71-73] Some evidence supports a benefit in treating heavy bleeding associated with adenomyosis[74] and leiomyomas with the LNg IUC.[75] Trials have compared this approach to treatment with an oral progestin, a nonsteroidal anti-inflammatory drug, or mefenamic acid (which is not available in the United States)[72] and found the LNg IUC superior to the other alternatives. In addition, the LNg IUC is an acceptable and cost-effective alternative to endometrial ablation or hysterectomy.[76-79] The LNg IUC may also decrease the risk of pelvic inflammatory disease (PID), similar to other progestin-containing contraceptives.[80,81] By thickening cervical mucus, progestin may provide a barrier to ascending infection.

D ISADVANTAGES AND CAUTIONS

COMMON BUT BENIGN SIDE EFFECTS

- Menstrual disturbances

- Cramping and pain

- Expulsion of the IUC

- Actinomyces-like organisms seen on Papanicolaou smear

RARE BUT SERIOUS HEALTH RISKS

- Infection
- Pregnancy complications
- Uterine perforation

MENSTRUAL DISTURBANCES

Changes in menstrual patterns are the most common side effects of intrauterine contraception. Irregular bleeding is common in the early months of use and a frequent cause of discontinuation. Thus, anticipatory counseling about expected menstrual changes is very important. Complaints about menstrual disturbances are less common in women older than 30 years of age, and after the first year of IUC use.[44,82]

TCu380A. Women using a copper IUC may find their menses become heavier, longer, or more uncomfortable, particularly in the first several cycles of TCu380A use. In the first year of use, heavy menses and dysmenorrhea are the most frequent reasons for copper IUC removal.[83] Although these side effects may decrease over time,[84] approximately 2 of every 100 users discontinue use in subsequent years due to bleeding and pain.[44,48] Average monthly menstrual blood loss may be increased by up to 55% throughout the duration of copper IUC use; however this rarely leads to anemia.[85]

LNg IUC. For women using the LNg IUC, irregular but light bleeding or spotting is the norm in the early months of use because endometrial suppression takes several months to achieve. Thereafter, a marked decrease in bleeding occurs. Overall, LNg IUC use is associated with a reduction in menstrual blood loss compared with women using no contraception and women using copper IUCs.[44] The proportion of LNg IUC users with amenorrhea increases with duration of use.[82] At 24 months of use, 50% have amenorrhea and 25% have oligomenorrhea.[86] Most LNg IUC users experience an increase in hemoglobin levels with time.[37,44] Amenorrhea with LNg IUC use is due to endometrial decidualization and atrophy. The majority of LNg IUC users has ovulatory cycles and may continue to experience other cyclic symptoms (e.g. acne or mood changes) while remaining amenorrheic.[44,82,87] Other side effects that may lead to early discontinuation of the LNg IUC include hormonal side effects, such as breast tenderness, mood changes, hair loss, and acne,[44,46,81] although the progestin effect is primarily local.[88] The plasma concentration of levonorgestrel is far lower than the endometrial concentration and varies among patients. Within the first few weeks of use, plasma concentration reaches 150 to 200 pg/mL,[89] a level half that seen with progestin implants and much less than that associated with progestogen-only pills, but high enough to cause systemic side effects in some users.[12] Over time, plasma levels of levonorgestrel gradually decline.[89]

CRAMPING AND PAIN

Most women experience one or two minutes of discomfort at the time of IUC placement. Immediately following IUC placement, some women may experience 10 to 30 minutes of uterine cramping accompanied by nausea or feeling faint. Some clinicians offer oral nonsteroidal anti-inflammatory drugs taken an hour prior to placement, local anesthesia, or both as preventive therapy, although most women do not require either. In the first few cycles of use, dysmenorrhea may occur with the TCu380A IUC. Along with unscheduled bleeding, dysmenorrhea is one of the primary reasons for discontinuation of use of a TCu380A IUC.[83,84] When pelvic pain develops after the day of IUC placement, consider whether the IUC may be partially expelled or dislodged. In addition, evaluate for infection or pregnancy.

EXPULSION OF THE IUC

Within the first year of IUC use, 2% to 10% of IUC users spontaneously expel their IUC. Nulliparity, age less than 20, menorrhagia, severe dysmenorrhea, and placement immediately postpartum increase the chance of expulsion.[83,90,91] However, a woman who has expelled one IUC has only a 30% chance of subsequent expulsions[91] if she decides to have another IUC placed. The companies that manufacture the devices available in the United States frequently replace expelled devices at no cost when patients seek reinsertion. The symptoms of IUC expulsion include unusual vaginal discharge, cramping or pain, intermenstrual or post-coital spotting, dyspareunia, absence or lengthening of the IUC thread, and presence of the hard plastic of the IUC at the cervical os or in the vagina.[92] However, some IUC expulsions are asymptomatic, so IUC expulsion can occur without the woman detecting it. Because women who experience asymptomatic IUC expulsion may not present for evaluation, it is important to teach all IUC users to check their IUC threads (see section on User Instructions).

ACTINOMYCES-LIKE ORGANISMS SEEN ON PAPANICOLAOU SMEAR

Several decades ago, a pseudo-epidemic of genital actinomycosis occurred among IUC users. Cytologists and cytopathologists[93] began reporting Actinomyces-like organisms on routine cytology smears, creating alarm and confusion. However, the presence of Actinomyces-like organisms on Papanicolaou smear is an invalid test for Actinomyces and so does not predict clinical illness. Actinomyces species are normal inhabitants of the female genital tract; vaginal culture is not helpful in diagnosing actinomycosis.[94] An asymptomatic IUC user who has "Actinomyces-like organisms" reported on Papanicolaou smear should be informed of the finding and of its lack of clinical significance; the IUC may be left safely in place. If she is symptomatic (pelvic pain, fever), the device should be removed and a course of oral antibiotics given. The reason for removal is that, unlike usual gynecological pathogens, this genus of bacterium preferentially grows on foreign bodies. Actinomyces species are sensitive to a variety of antibiotics, including penicillin.

PELVIC INFLAMMATORY DISEASE (PID)

Flaws in early research led to exaggerations in estimates of the risk of upper-genital-tract infection associated with use of IUC. Rigorous studies[95,96] and reviews of the literature[97] have now established that the risk of infection and infertility among IUC users is very low. Both epidemiological[13] and bacteriological evidence[98] indicates that the placement process, and not the device or its thread, poses a small transient risk of infection. No procedure that requires traversing the cervical canal can be devoid of all pathogenic organisms. Although sterile technique should be used, endocervical bacteria are routinely introduced to the endometrial cavity regardless of technique.[98] However, antibiotic prophylaxis should not be routinely used before placement.[99] A large randomized controlled trial in Los Angeles County that evaluated the potential benefit of prophylactic azithromycin given before IUC placement found no benefit.[95] More importantly, this study found that salpingitis was rare with or without prophylaxis: only one women out of about a thousand in each group developed salpingitis in the early months of IUC use. International experience with IUCs has been similarly favorable. In large trials sponsored by the World Health Organization (WHO), the risk of upper-genital-tract infection was limited to the first 20 days after placement.[96] Afterwards, the risk returned to a low level and remained there for years. Both a randomized controlled trial and cohort studies have revealed that the monofilament thread does not increase the risk of upper genital-tract infection.[97]

Early assessments of the risk of tubal infertility among IUC users appear to have exaggerated risks as well.[100,101] Recent studies of IUC users have found no significant differences in return to fertility, whether the IUC was removed because of a desire for pregnancy or because of problems with the IUC.[102,103] Indeed, in a Mexican case-control study,[104] prior use of a copper IUC was not significantly related to tubal pathology, whereas the presence of chlamydia antibodies was. Again, this underscores that sexually transmitted diseases, not contraception, cause salpingitis.

Little is known about the potential effect of an IUC on acquiring a cervical or vaginal sexually transmitted infection. Fair evidence refutes an increased risk of chlamydial infection, but no evidence is available concerning gonorrhea.[97] Women who harbor sexually transmitted infections in their cervices have an increased risk of upper-genital tract infection, regardless of their IUC status.

PREGNANCY

Pregnancy of any kind is rare with an IUC in place. However, when a woman does conceive with an IUC in place she is at increased risk of having an ectopic pregnancy. It is estimated that among women using no contraception, 2% of pregnancies are ectopic; among women using IUC, 6% to 50% of pregnancies are ectopic.[105,106] Nonetheless, a woman is much less likely to develop an ectopic pregnancy while using an IUC than while using less-effective or no contraception. IUCs protect women from ectopic pregnancy.

PERFORATION

Perforation of the uterus can occur at the time of IUC placement; no evidence supports the notion that IUCs can migrate outside the uterus thereafter. The most important determinant of the risk of perforation is the skill of the person placing the IUC. In experienced hands, the risk of perforation is 1 per 1,000 placements or less.[27]

PROVIDING INTRAUTERINE CONTRACEPTION

Most teens and women are good candidates for intrauterine contraception. IUCs can be used safely by nulliparous women, women with multiple partners, women who have had ectopic pregnancies, and women with a history of PID as long as they have no cervical infection at the time of IUC placement.

CHOOSING WHICH IUC

Most women can safely use either the copper or levonogestrel IUC. When counseling a patient about choice of IUC, it is helpful to know her menstrual history, her medical history, her desire for lighter or less painful menses, and her feelings about amenorrhea, unscheduled bleeding, or spotting. A current history of dysmenorrhea or menorrhagia is a relative contraindication to use of the TCu380A IUC.

CONTRAINDICATIONS TO IUC USE

Few absolute contraindications exist to IUC placement or continued use. The 2010 WHO Medical Eligibility Criteria for Contraceptive Use offers clinicians guidelines for determining safe candidates for IUC use (see Chapter 4). The vast majority of women worldwide are good candidates for an IUC. However, intrauterine contraception is contraindicated in women with active pelvic infection, including PID, endometritis, mucopurulent cervicitis, and pelvic tuberculosis, because the presence of a foreign body may impede resolution of the infection. Do not place the IUC in women with known or suspected pregnancy. The IUC should not be newly inserted in women with cervical or endometrial cancer but may be continued in these patients. Evaluate abnormal uterine bleeding before placing an IUC, so the abnormal bleeding will not be erroneously attributed to the IUC rather than to the pre-existing pathology. Placement of an IUC may be difficult and expulsion may be more likely in women with severe uterine distortion from anatomic abnormalities such as bicornuate uterus, cervical stenosis, or fibroids severely distorting the uterine cavity. However, nondistorting fibroids are not a contraindication to intrauterine contraception. The IUC should not be used in women with gestational trophoblastic neoplasia who have persistently elevated hCG levels. The TCu380A should not be used in women with Wilson's disease or copper allergy.[49]

SPECIAL POPULATIONS

Women Who Have Not Been Pregnant

After reviewing the available evidence, WHO concluded that the benefits of IUC use generally outweigh the potential or known risks for nulliparous women.[49] The American Congress of Obstetricians and Gynecologists supports the use of intrauterine contraception by nulliparas and adolescents, noting that there is no increased risk of infection with IUC use.[107] Most women, including nulliparas, have a rapid return of fertility after IUC removal.[108,109] IUC placement is well tolerated by most nulliparous women.[110] When necessary, cervical dilation with a 13 to 15 Fr Pratt dilator can be performed at the time of the placement. Alternatively, cervical priming with misoprostol 400 mcg, either for a few hours or the night before placement can open the canal. Similarly, one or more osmotic dilators, such as laminaria, when left in overnight can gently dilate the canal to a small diameter. Prophylaxis with an oral nonsteroidal anti-inflammatory drug and paracervical[111] or intrauterine anesthesia[15] may help as well. However, a recent meta-analysis of four trials including a total of 2,204 participants did not find nonsteroidal anti-inflammatory drugs (of varying types and doses) effective for reducing pain during IUC placement.[150] Misoprostol for cervical ripening did not reduce pain with IUC placement in nulliparous women.[151] One poorly controlled trial suggested that topical lidocaine gel may reduce placement-related pain and may warrant further study.[112]

Women Who Are Breastfeeding

The TCu380A IUC can be placed immediately after delivery of the placenta. For an LNg IUC, however, consider delaying placement until 6 to 8 weeks postpartum, because earlier placement may result in premature discontinuation of breastfeeding.[113] Although the U.S. Medical Eligibility Criteria grades immediate postpartum use of a LNg IUC as a 2,[51] the WHO rates LNg IUC placement within 4 weeks of delivery as category 3 (risks outweigh benefits) because of concern about neonatal exposure to hormones.[49] In one randomized study, immediate post-placental placement of a LNg IUC was significantly associated with a decreased likelihood of breastfeeding at 6 months postpartum when compared with women who delayed LNg IUC insertion.[113] Because the risk of perforation may be increased during lactation, be careful when placing an IUC for a breastfeeding mother.[114] However, the absolute risk of perforation remains rare, and breastfeeding is not a contraindication to IUC placement.[49,115]

Women Who Are Immunocompromised

IUC use appears safe and effective for women who are immunosuppressed due to organ transplantation,[116] autoimmune disease,[117] or infection with human immunodeficiency virus (HIV).[118] WHO states that for all of these women, the benefits of IUC use generally outweigh the potential or known risks.[49] HIV-positive IUC users appear to have a risk of complications, including infection, that is equivalent to the risk in HIV-negative IUC users.[119,120] Moreover, IUC use has been shown not to increase HIV viral shedding, and clinical HIV disease progression was slower among women using the TCu380A than among women using hormonal contraception.[121] A recent randomized controlled trial found that HIV-positive women assigned to intrauterine contraception were half as likely to become pregnant as were those assigned to hormonal contraception.[121]

Women With Heart Valve Abnormalities or Shunts

Intrauterine contraception may be used safely in women with cardiac disease and structural abnormalities.[49] The risk of infectious complications, such as bacterial endocarditis, following IUC placement or removal is unknown but presumably negligible, even among women with heart valve abnormalities or shunts. No evidence suggests that antibiotic prophylaxis is warranted. Whether bacteremia may result from removal of an infected IUC is controversial; prophylaxis may therefore be reasonable for women with prosthetic heart valves, a history of infective endocarditis, a subset of congenital heart diseases, or a history of cardiac transplantation with development of cardiac valvulopathy.[122] Should antibiotic use be warranted, patients should receive an agent active against enterococci, such as penicillin, ampicillin, piperacillin, or vancomycin 1 hour before the IUC removal.[122]

Women With Diabetes Mellitus

Intrauterine contraception is a great option for women with diabetes mellitus who face increased rates of adverse birth outcomes if they conceive while glycemic control is poor,[49] and increased risk of vascular disease with use of estrogen-containing contraceptives. Good evidence supports the use of copper IUC by women with either Type 1 or Type 2 diabetes.[123-126] A recent rigorous trial of LNg IUC use by women with Type 1 diabetes confirmed no adverse effect on glucose metabolism or insulin requirements.[127]

Women With a History of Breast Cancer

The TCu380A IUC is generally the preferred contraceptive option for women with a history of breast cancer. However, the LNg IUC may be preferable for women being treated with tamoxifen.[49,65]

Women at Risk of Sexually Transmitted Infections

Women who are at risk of acquiring STIs should be advised to use condoms but are generally still good candidates for IUC.[49]

Women With a History of Venous Thromboembolism

Both IUCs may be used safely in women with a history of deep venous thrombosis and pulmonary embolism.[49] The LNg IUC is preferred for women currently on chronic anticoagulation therapy to treat or prevent menorrhagia.[71-73] The LNg IUC, unlike hormonal contraception containing estrogen, is not associated with an increased risk of venous thrombosis.[128]

Women With a History of Cesarean Section or Other Uterine or Cervical Surgery

Both IUCs may be used safely in women with a history of cesarean section or other uterine or cervical surgery.[51]

COUNSELING ABOUT THE IUC

Make all presentations, counseling, and educational materials (handouts, flipcharts, and posters) compatible with the patient's language, culture, and education. Manufacturers have Patient Package Inserts available in Spanish and several other foreign languages. Let women handle and examine sample IUCs. Many are surprised at how small and flexible IUC are. Be aware of the local myths and misconceptions about IUCs (e.g., that the IUC can "float off" and lodge in distant parts of the body, such as heart and brain). Address these sensitively but directly (see the box on Myths and Misconceptions). Use a standard checklist to remember to share important information with women. Ask the woman to repeat important information back to you to confirm her understanding. Give each woman an identification card with the name of her IUC, date of placement, and date recommended for removal.

PROVIDER TRAINING

With appropriate training, clinical personnel including physicians, nurses, nurse-midwives, physician assistants, and paramedical personnel can safely place both types of IUC. Because the LNg IUC has a different placement process than the TCu380A, clinicians should receive formal training for each. IUC placement should first be practiced with a model and then an adequate number of IUCs should be placed under supervision to demonstrate proficiency. Rather than an absolute number of placements, certification should be based on a level of proficiency in different uterine positions and varying placement situations.

PLACEMENT TIMING

IUC may be inserted at any time during the menstrual cycle, provided reasonable assurance exists that the woman is not pregnant. Testing for chlamydia can be performed at the time of the placement visit. As such, requiring that women make two clinic visits to obtain IUC is unnecessary. In addition, no scientific reason supports limiting IUC placement to periods of menstrual bleeding, although in the past, these misconceptions constrained women's access to IUCs.[27,129] The inconvenience and cost to women caused by such policies can be substantial. Allowing placement during the entire menstrual cycle gives the woman and her provider more flexible appointment times.

Extensive experience has shown the safety and feasibility of IUC placement immediately after abortion or delivery. A recent systematic review of randomized controlled trials of immediate postabortal placement showed low rates of perforation and pelvic inflammatory disease.[130] Immediate placement after first-trimester abortion is not associated with an increased rate of expulsion; however, continuation rates of IUCs at 6 months were significantly higher among women who had im-

Table 7-1 Myths and Misconceptions about IUCs

Myth	Fact
IUCs are abortifacients.	IUCs prevent fertilization and thus are true contraceptives.
IUCs increase the risk of ectopic pregnancy.	IUCs significantly reduce a woman's risk of an ectopic pregnancy compared with her risk if not using contraception. The risk is reduced because IUCs prevent conception.
IUCs expose the provider to medico-legal risk.	In past decades, product liability suits against manufacturers alleged inherently unsafe products and/or failure to warn of risks. Both currently available IUCs have been judged safe by the Food and Drug Administration using more rigorous standards than those used in the 1970s. Package inserts and patient brochures provide extensive information about risks and benefits. Hence, litigation related to IUCs has virtually disappeared.
IUCs increase the risk of PID.	The IUC itself appears to have no effect on the risk of upper-genital-tract infection. Rather, the placement process carries a small, transient risk of postprocedure infection. The risk of PID in appropriately selected IUC candidates is so small that prophylactic antibiotics are not warranted.
IUCs should not be used in women who have not had a child.	The IUC is safe for nulliparous women. Most women, including nulliparas, have a rapid return of fertility after IUC removal. Sexually transmitted diseases, not contraception, cause salpingitis and infertility.
IUCs increase the risk of sexually transmitted infections.	IUC users are not at increased risk of sexually transmitted infections. Women who are at risk of acquiring sexually transmitted diseases should be advised to use condoms but are generally still good candidates for IUC.

mediate postabortal placement compared with women who delayed (94% vs 83%).[131] Placement of IUCs after second-trimester abortion was associated with a slightly higher expulsion rate (7%). Of note, however, 54% of women scheduled to return for delayed placement after a second-trimester abortion did not return.[132] The provision of postabortal IUCs is associated with a decreased risk of repeat induced abortion[133] and significantly decreases the number of unwanted pregnancies and repeat induced abortions in the United States.[134]

Placement of IUCs immediately after delivery is popular in many countries, including China, Mexico, and Egypt. Expulsion rates are lowest when the IUC is placed within 10 minutes of the expulsion of the placenta, often referred to as postplacental placement.[135] However, expulsions appear to be higher with postplacental placement than with interval placements (24% versus 4%). Whether placement was done by hand or by instrument made little difference in subsequent outcomes. Postplacental placement of the TCu380A is safe and practical. Advantages of this practice include convenience, high motivation, and assurance that the woman is not pregnant. In contrast, in a recent randomized trial, users who had the LNg IUC placed postplacentally were more likely to discontinue breastfeeding than were mothers who delayed placement until 6 to 8 weeks postpartum.[113] Thus, for breastfeeding mothers who desire immediate postplacental IUC placement, the TCu380A may be preferable to the LNg IUC.

PLACEMENT TECHNIQUE

Review the IUC placement procedure with the woman. Perform a careful pelvic examination to confirm the direction of the uterus and its axial length. In general, a length of 6 cm to 9 cm leads to successful IUC use; a shorter length may increase the risk of expulsion and other mechanical problems. *Always place the IUC slowly and gently.* Read and follow the manufacturer's instructions on placement. Detailed handbooks and videos are available from manufacturers on placement, removal, and management techniques.

General Preparation

1. Many clinicians provide a nonsteroidal anti-inflammatory medication, either ibuprofen or naproxen, prior to IUC placement. Use of these medications, however, has not been shown to decrease pain during or after placement.[112]
2. Perform a careful bimanual examination to exclude pelvic infection and to identify the position of the uterus. An unrecognized retroflexed uterus increases the possibility of uterine perforation at the time of the IUC placement.
3. Most clinicians wash the cervix and vagina with an antiseptic, such as povidone-iodine or chlorhexidine. However, no evidence

supports this practice, and its effect on bacterial colony counts in the endocervix is minimal.[136]

4. A paracervical block is generally not indicated and has not been shown to reduce the overall pain of IUC placement.[137] A paracervical block may be useful in women with a history of difficult or painful placements and in women who require cervical dilation to facilitate placement. If lidocaine is used, the upper limit should be 2 mg per pound (or 4.5 mg per kg), not to exceed 300 mg of lidocaine. If bupivacaine is used, a common dose is 20 cc of 0.25% bupivacaine. An alternative is to instill lidocaine into the uterine cavity.[137]

5. Apply a tenaculum to the anterior or posterior lip of the cervix and apply gentle traction to the tenaculum to straighten the axis of the uterus.

6. Sound the uterus prior to placing the IUC.

CAUTION

Instrumentation of the cervical os may result in vasovagal reactions, including fainting. Have the patient remain supine after placement until she feels well, and have her get up with caution.

COPPER T 380A (PARAGARD) PLACEMENT INSTRUCTIONS

© 2006 Teva Women's Health, Inc. All rights reserved.

The following insertion instructions for the ParaGard IUC are reproduced from the package insert with permission.

The placement technique for ParaGard is different from that used for other IUDs. Therefore, the clinician should be familiar with the following instructions.

ParaGard may be placed at any time during the cycle when the clinician is reasonably certain the patient is not pregnant. For information about timing of postpartun and postabotion insertions, see **Precautions.**

A single ParaGard should be placed at the fundus of the uterine cavity. ParaGard should be removed on or before 10 years from the date of insertion.

Before Placement:

1. Make sure that the patient is an appropriate candidate for Para-Gard and that she has read the Patient Package Insert.

2. Use of an analgesic before insertion is at the discretion of the patient and the clinician.

3. Establish the size and position of the uterus by pelvic examination.

4. Insert a speculum and cleanse the vagina and cervix with an antiseptic solution.

5. Apply a tenaculum to the cervix and use gentle traction to align the cervical canal with the uterine cavity.

6. Gently insert a sterile sound to measure the depth of the uterine cavity.

7. The uterus should sound to a depth of 6 to 9 cm except when inserting ParaGard immediately post-abortion or post-partum. Insertion of ParaGard into a uterine cavity measuring less than 6 cm may increase the incidence of expulsion, bleeding, pain, and perforation. If you encounter cervical stenosis, avoid undue force. Dilators may be helpful in this situation.

HOW TO LOAD AND PLACE PARAGARD:

Do not bend the arms of ParaGard earlier than 5 minutes before it is to be placed in the uterus. Use aseptic technique when handling ParaGard and the part of the insertion tube that will enter the uterus.

STEP 1. Load ParaGard into the insertion tube by folding the two horizontal arms of ParaGard against the stem and push the tips of the arms securely into the inserter tube.

If you do not have sterile gloves, you can do STEPS 1 and 2 while ParaGard is in the sterile package. First, place the package face up on a clean surface. Next, open at the bottom end (where arrow says OPEN). Pull the solid white rod partially from the package so it will not interfere with assembly. Place thumb and index finger on top of package on ends of the horizontal arms. Use other hand to push insertion tube against arms of ParaGard (shown by arrow in Fig. 7–2). This will start bending the T arms.

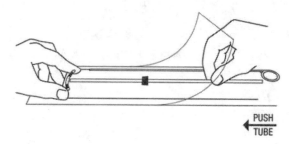

PUSH
TUBE

Figure 7–2 Step 1

STEP 2. Bring the thumb and index finger closer together to continue bending the arms until they are alongside the stem. Use the other hand to withdraw the insertion tube just enough so that the insertion tube can be pushed and rotated onto the tips of the arms. Your goal is to secure the tips of the arms inside the tube (Fig. 7–3). Insert the arms no further than necessary to insure retention. Introduce the solid white rod into the insertion tube from the bottom, alongside the threads, **until it touches the bottom of the ParaGard.**

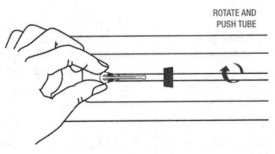

ROTATE AND
PUSH TUBE

Figure 7–3 Step 2

STEP 3. Grasp the insertion tube at the open end of the package; adjust the blue flange so that the distance from the top of the ParaGard (where it protrudes from the inserter) to the blue flange is the same as the uterine depth that you measured with the sound. Rotate the insertion tube so that the horizontal arms of the T and the long axis of the blue flange lie in the same horizontal plane (Fig. 7–4). Now pass the loaded insertion tube through the cervical canal until ParaGard just touches the fundus of the uterus. The blue flange should be at the cervix in the horizontal plane.

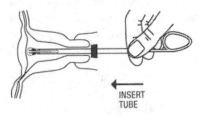

INSERT
TUBE

Figure 7–4 Step 3

STEP 4. To release the arms of ParaGard, hold the solid white rod steady and withdraw the insertion tube no more than one centimeter This releases the arms of ParaGard high in the uterine fundus (Fig. 7–5).

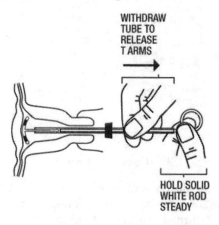

Figure 7–5 Step 4

STEP 5. Gently and carefully move the insertion tube upward toward the top of the uterus, until slight resistance is felt. This will ensure placement of the T at the highest possible position within the uterus (Fig. 7–6).

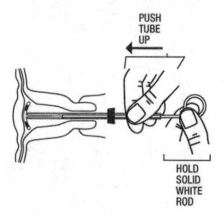

Figure 7–6 Step 5

STEP 6. Hold the insertion tube steady and withdraw the solid white rod (Fig. 7–7).

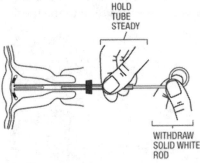

Figure 7–7 Step 6

STEP 7. Gently and slowly withdraw the insertion tube from the cervical canal. Only the threads should be visible protruding from the cervix. (Fig. 7–8). Trim the threads so that 3 to 4 cm protrude into the vagina. Note the length of the threads in the patient's records.

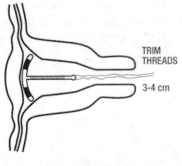

Figure 7–8 Step 7

If you suspect that ParaGard is not in the correct position, check placement (with ultrasound, if necessary). If ParaGard is not positioned completely within the uterus, remove it and replace it with a new ParaGard. Do not reinsert an expelled or partially expelled ParaGard.

LEVONORGESTREL IUC (MIRENA) INSERTION INSTRUCTIONS

©*Used under license from Bayer. 2010.*

The following insertion instructions for the Mirena IUC are reproduced from the package insert with permission. The package insert calls for the use of sterile gloves. However, the Mirena inserter obviates the need for direct handling of the IUC or any part of the inserter that will contact the uterus and cervix, therefore non-sterile gloves may be used.

NOTE: Mirena should be inserted by a trained healthcare provider. Healthcare providers are advised to become thoroughly familiar with the insertion instructions before attempting insertion of Mirena.

Mirena is inserted with the provided inserter (Figure 7–9) into the uterine cavity within seven days of the onset of menstruation or immediately after a first trimester abortion by carefully following the insertion instructions. It can be replaced by a new Mirena at any time during the menstrual cycle.

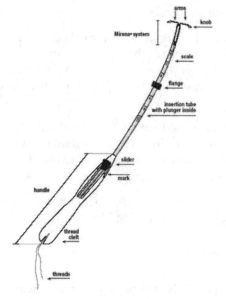

Figure 7–9 Mirena and inserter

Preparation for insertion

- Ensure that the patient understands the contents of the Patient Information Booklet and obtain consent. A consent form that includes the lot number is on the last page of the Patient Information Booklet.

- Confirm that there are no contraindications to the use of Mirena.

- Perform a urine pregnancy test, if indicated.

- With the patient comfortably in lithotomy position, gently insert a speculum to visualize the cervix and rule out genital contraindications to the use of Mirena.

- Do a bimanual exam to establish the size and position of the uterus, to detect other genital contraindications, and to exclude pregnancy.

- Thoroughly cleanse the cervix and vagina with a suitable anti-septic solution. Perform a paracervical block, if needed.

- Prepare to sound the uterine cavity. Grasp the upper lip of the cervix with a tenaculum forceps and apply gentle traction to align the cervical canal with the uterine cavity. If the uterus is re-troverted, it may be more appropriate to grasp the lower lip of the cervix. Note that the tenaculum forceps should remain in position throughout the insertion procedure to maintain gentle traction on the cervix.

- Gently insert a uterine sound to check the patency of the cervix, measure the depth of the uterine cavity, confirm its direction and exclude the presence of any uterine anomaly. If you encounter cervical stenosis, use dilatation, not force, to overcome resistance.

- The uterus should sound to a depth of 6 to 10 cm. Insertion of Mirena into a uterine cavity less than 6 cm by sounding may increase the incidence of expulsion, bleeding, pain, perforation, and possibly pregnancy.

- After ascertaining that the patient is appropriate for Mirena, open the carton containing Mirena.

Insertion Procedure

Ensure use of sterile technique throughout the entire procedure.

Step 1—Opening of the sterile package

- Open the sterile package completely (Figure 7–10).

- Place sterile gloves on your hands.

- Pick up the handle of the inserter containing Mirena and carefully release the threads so that they hang freely.

- Place your thumb or forefinger on the slider. Make sure that the slider is in the furthest position away from you, for example, at the top of the handle towards the insertion tube (Figure 7–10).

- **NOTE:** Keep your thumb or forefinger on the slider until insertion is complete.

- With the centimeter scale of the insertion tube facing up, check that the arms of Mirena are in a horizontal position. If they are not, align them on a flat, sterile surface, for example, the sterile package (Figures 7–10 and 7–11).

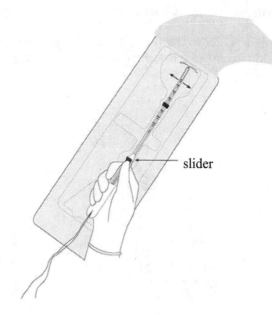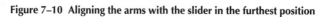

slider

Figure 7–10 Aligning the arms with the slider in the furthest position

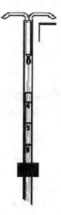

Figure 7–11 Checking that the arms are horizontal and aligned with respect to the scale

Step 2—Load Mirena into the insertion tube

- Holding the slider in the furthest position, pull on both threads to load Mirena into the insertion tube (Figure 7–12).

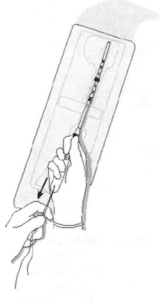

Figure 7-12 Loading Mirena into the insertion tube

- Note that the knobs at the ends of the arms now meet to close the open end of the insertion tube (Figure 7–13).

If the knobs do not meet properly

If the knobs do not meet properly, release the arms by pulling the slider back to the mark (raised horizontal line on the handle) (Figure 7–17). Re-load Mirena by aligning the open arms on a sterile surface (Figure 7–10). Return the slider to its furthermost position and pull on both threads. Check for proper loading (Figure 7–13).

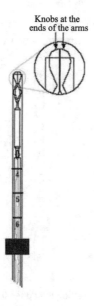

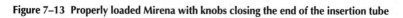

Figure 7–13 Properly loaded Mirena with knobs closing the end of the insertion tube

Step 3—Secure the threads.   Secure the threads in the cleft at the bottom end of the handle to keep Mirena in the loaded position (Figure 7–14).

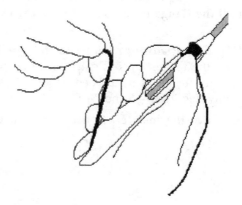

Figure 7–14 Threads are secured in the cleft

Step 4—Setting the flange. Set the upper edge of the flange to the depth measured during the uterine sounding (Figure 7–15).

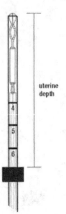

Figure 7–15 Setting the flange to the uterine depth

Step 5—Mirena is now ready to be inserted

- Continue to hold the slider with the thumb or forefinger firmly in the furthermost position. Grasp the tenaculum forceps with your other hand and apply gentle traction to align the cervical canal with the uterine cavity.

- While maintaining traction on the cervix, gently advance the insertion tube through the cervical canal and into the uterine cavity **until the flange is 1.5 to 2 cm from the external cervical os.**

- **CAUTION: do not advance flange to the cervix at this step.** Maintaining the flange 1.5 to 2 cm from the cervical os allows sufficient space for the arms to open (when released) within the uterine cavity (Figures 7–16 and 7–18).

NOTE! Do not force the inserter. If necessary, dilate the cervical canal.

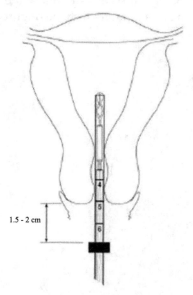

Figure 7–16 Advancing insertion tube until flange is 1.5 to 2 cm from cervical os

1.5 - 2 cm

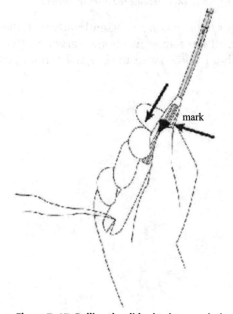

mark

Figure 7–17 Pulling the slider back to reach the mark

Step 6—Release the arms
- While holding the inserter steady, release the arms of Mirena by pulling the slider back until the top of the slider reaches the mark (raised horizontal line on the handle) (Figure 7–17).

- Wait approximately 10 seconds to allow the horizontal arms of Mirena to open and regain its T-shape (Figure 7–18).

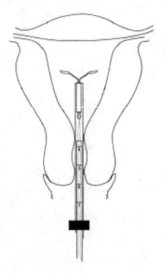

Figure 7–18 Releasing the arms of Mirena

Step 7—Advance to fundal position. Gently advance the inserter into the uterine cavity until the flange meets the cervix and you feel fundal resistance. Mirena should now be in the desired fundal position (Figure 7–19).

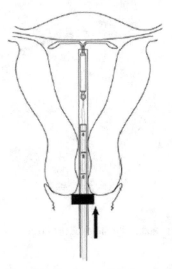

Figure 7–19 Mirena in the fundal position

Step 8—Release Mirena and withdraw the inserter

- While holding the inserter steady, pull the slider all the way down to release Mirena from the insertion tube (Figure 7–20). The threads will release automatically from the cleft.

- Check that the threads are hanging freely and gently withdraw the inserter from the uterus. Be careful not to pull on the threads as this will displace Mirena.

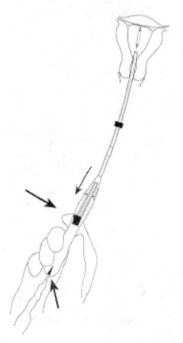

Figure 7–20 Releasing Mirena from the insertion tube

Step 9—Cut the threads

- Cut the threads perpendicular to the thread length, for example, with sterile curved scissors, leaving about 3 cm visible outside the cervix (Figure 7–21).
  NOTE: Cutting threads at an angle may leave sharp ends.

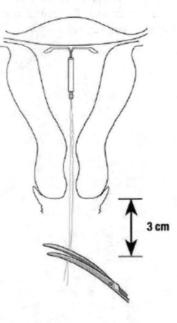

Figure 7–21 Cutting the threads

Mirena insertion is now complete.

Important information to consider during or after insertion

- If you suspect that Mirena is not in the correct position, check placement (for example, with transvaginal ultrasound). Remove Mirena if it is not positioned completely within the uterus. A removed Mirena must not be reinserted.

- If there is clinical concern and/or exceptional pain or bleeding during or after insertion, appropriate and timely measures and assessments, for example ultrasound, should be performed to exclude perforation.

IUC REMOVAL

When removing an IUC, apply gentle, steady traction and remove the IUC slowly. If you cannot remove the IUC with gentle traction, a paracervical block may make the removal easier and less painful. After placing the block, use a tenaculum to steady the cervix and straighten the anteversion or retroversion of the uterus and try again. If this technique does not work, dilate the cervix with a small amount of misoprostol, osmotic dilators, or rigid dilators.

MANAGING PROBLEMS AND FOLLOW-UP

Offer a follow-up visit approximately 1 month after IUC insertion to check that the IUC is still in place and that no signs of infection are evident. Further routine visits are not required;[138,139] however, encourage women to return at any time that they have problems, questions, or concerns. In particular, encourage a woman to visit when she cannot feel her IUC threads, the threads seem too long, or the IUC (and not just the thread) is palpable in the cervix. The 1-month visit can also help identify women who may decide to remove their IUC prematurely because they are bothered by intermenstrual bleeding or spotting or excessive menstrual flow.[140] Counseling women about the expected changes in bleeding patterns prior to insertion may enhance tolerance of the method. Unexpected changes in bleeding patterns or changes that are not tolerable to the patient should be evaluated.

INTERMENSTRUAL BLEEDING, SPOTTING, OR EXCESSIVE MENSTRUAL FLOW

Use of nonsteroidal anti-inflammatory medications can reduce excessive menstrual flow as well as dysmenorrhea.[141] Trials have not demonstrated the superiority of one product over another. Because local prostaglandin production is involved with excessive bleeding, any prostaglandin synthetase inhibitor should help; in contrast, aspirin and acetaminophen do not. Starting the medication in advance of menses does not give better results than starting with the onset of flow. If hemoglobin levels drop, consider oral iron supplementation. Alternatively, remove the copper IUC removed and insert an LNg IUC. Other therapies that have been helpful in managing irregular bleeding induced by progestin-only contraceptives include estrogen (or the addition of a combined hormonal contraceptive), tamoxifen, tranexamic acid, mifepristone combined with an estrogen, and doxycycline.[142]

Persistent abnormal bleeding requires clinical evaluation because not all nuisance bleeding can be attributed to IUC. Other gynecologic disorders, such as cervicitis or endometrial polyps, may be responsible. Alternatively, an accidental pregnancy (including an ectopic pregnancy) can present with bleeding. In addition, bleeding may accompany endometritis. If there is concern of endometrial hyperplasia, biopsy the endometrium, using a small catheter with the IUC left in place.

WOMEN WHO ACQUIRE A CHLAMYDIA OR GONORRHEA INFECTION

If an IUC user acquires an infection with chlamydia or gonorrhea, standard treatment for her and her partner(s) is indicated.[143,144] No evidence suggests that an IUC should be removed in this setting.[145]

PELVIC INFLAMMATORY DISEASE (PID)

Upper genital tract infections need prompt treatment and follow-up, although accurate diagnosis is often difficult. Widely used diagnostic criteria for acute salpingitis[146] have been found invalid,[147] and salpingitis may more commonly be atypical. Hence, *when in doubt, treat*. The Centers for Disease Control and Prevention has published recommendations for both inpatient and outpatient therapy of upper-genital tract infection (Chapter 21 on Reproductive Tract Infections).[143,144] All involve two antibiotics in order to provide an adequate spectrum of coverage. Male partners of women thought to have salpingitis should be examined and treated presumptively according to guidelines. Women may be treated for salpingitis with the IUC in place; one small randomized controlled trial showed no benefit of IUC removal as an adjunct to antibiotic therapy.[145]

ACTINOMYCES-LIKE ORGANISMS SEEN ON PAPANICOLAOU SMEAR

An asymptomatic IUC user who has "Actinomyces-like organisms" reported on Papanicolaou smear should be informed that this is a common finding of limited clinical significance.[94] If she is asymptomatic, nothing more need be done. If she is symptomatic, the device should be removed and a course of oral antibiotics given. The reason for removal is that, unlike usual gynecological pathogens, this genus of bacterium preferentially grows on foreign bodies. Pelvic actinomycosis is a very rare, serious, and poorly understood infection. Actinomyces species are sensitive to a variety of antibiotics, including penicillin.

THREAD PROBLEMS

Missing threads may signal an unsuspected perforation or spontaneous expulsion; alternatively, some threads ascend into the endometrial cavity and descend without known explanation. Ultrasound examination can quickly confirm the presence of the IUC within the endometrial cavity. An IUC that is in the endometrial cavity may be left in place even if the threads are not palpable or visible. If the IUC is not visible in the uterus with ultrasound, perform an abdominal X-ray to determine whether the IUC has been expelled or has migrated into the peritoneal cavity.

To remove an IUC when the threads are not visible, begin by using a cotton swab, Papanicolaou brush, or endometrial biopsy instrument to tease the threads from the cervix or endometrium to the endocervix. Removal of a T-shaped device without visible threads has two prerequisites: the patient's comfort and cervical dilation. A paracervical block or intrauterine instillation of anesthetic administered before manipulation, supplemented by an oral analgesic, can decrease the pain associated with the procedure. If this is insufficient to control pain and admit instruments, consider osmotic dilators left in the os overnight or misoprostol 400 mcg (vaginally or orally) to dilate the cervix. Gentle exploration with an alligator forceps usually yields the device quickly; if not, manual vacuum aspiration or ultrasound guidance may be helpful. Rarely are the expense and inconvenience of hysteroscopy required for IUC removal.

If the male partner complains of penile discomfort from the thread being cut too short, one option is to cut the threads off even shorter within the endocervical canal. This may eliminate the barb-like sensation and obviate the need to replace the IUC. If the threads initially are too long, simply trim them. If the threads become longer at a later time, check for partial expulsion of the IUC.

PERFORATION

If a copper IUC is found outside the endometrial cavity, it should be removed promptly, because copper in the peritoneal cavity induces adhesion formation, which may involve the adnexa, omentum, and bowel. Laparoscopy is the preferred approach for removal. In contrast, nonmedicated and progestin-bearing devices do not evoke similar intraperitoneal adhesions. No clear medical indication exists for removal of IUC that do not contain copper,[148] although this is commonly done.

PREGNANCY

If a woman becomes pregnant with an IUC in place, confirm that the pregnancy is intrauterine and not ectopic. Remove the device promptly, regardless of her plans for the pregnancy. Early removal reduces the risk of spontaneous miscarriage or preterm delivery should the woman desire to continue the pregnancy.[27,149] If the woman plans to continue the pregnancy, she should be advised that symptoms of an influenza-like syndrome might be manifestations of a septic spontaneous abortion. An IUC left in place during pregnancy carries no known risk of teratogenesis. If the woman plans to have an induced abortion, remove the device promptly rather than wait for removal at the time of abortion; as the uterus grows, the threads may disappear and complicate IUC removal.

USER INSTRUCTIONS FOR INTRAUTERINE CONTRACEPTION

BOTH PARAGARD AND MIRENA

- Some have dizziness and/or cramps after insertion. This is normal. If you want to take something for pain, go ahead. Products that contain ibuprofen or naproxen are best.

- Expect minimal spotting in the first day or two after insertion. This is normal.

- Don't put anything in your vagina for the next 24 hours (not a tampon, not a finger, not a penis—nothing).

- Check to make sure that you can feel your IUC threads about once a month and whenever you have had a heavy period.

- If you are concerned that your IUC has fallen out, be sure to use another method of birth control until you can come back to your health care provider.

- When you resume sexual activity, remember to use condoms for protection from sexually transmitted infections and HIV.

- Call your health care provider right away if you

  — Notice any change in the length of the thread or can feel part of the IUC

  — Have pain or bleeding with sex

  — Have unusually heavy bleeding from the vagina

  — Think you are pregnant

  — Have been, or might have been, exposed to an STI

  — Have unusual pelvic pain, cramping, or soreness in your abdomen

  — Have unexplained fever or chills

PARAGARD ONLY

- ParaGard is effective against pregnancy immediately.

- During the first 1 to 3 months that you use ParaGard, you may have some irregular bleeding or spotting and your next few menstrual periods may be longer, heavier, and with more cramping than usual.

- Call your health care provider right away if you are late for your period and think you might be pregnant.

- Discuss with your healthcare provider the pros and cons of replacing your ParaGard after 12 years.

MIRENA ONLY

- Mirena is effective against pregnancy right away if it is inserted within 7 days after the start of your period. If Mirena is inserted at any other time in your menstrual cycle, use another method of birth control for 7 days if you have sex. Protection against pregnancy will begin after 7 days.

- You may have some irregular bleeding or spotting in addition to your monthly period while you use Mirena, especially during the first 3 to 6 months. About 1 in 5 women stop having periods after the first year—this is a safe condition. It doesn't mean that you are pregnant.

- Side effects are most common during the first 3 months of Mirena use and usually subside over time. You may experience any or none of the following: menstrual changes, lower abdominal pain, back pain, breast tenderness, headache, mood changes, nausea, and acne.

- Discuss with your healthcare provider the pros and cons of replacing your Mirena after 5 years.

REFERENCES

1. Family Planning Worldwide. 2002 data sheet. 2002. http://www.prb.org/pdf/FamPlanWorldwide_Eng.pdf Accessed Feb 1, 2011.
2. United Nations. World contraceptive use 2005. In: Department of Economic and Social Affairs Population Division. Available at http://www.un.org/esa/population/publications/contraceptive2005/2005_World_Contraceptive_files/WallChart_WCU2005.pdf. Accessed 3/1/2011.
3. d'Arcangues C. Worldwide use of intrauterine devices for contraception. Contraception. Jun 2007;75(6 Suppl):S2–7.
4. Bayer Schering Pharma. 2006 Pan EU Study on Female Contraceptives. 2007.

5. Guttmacher Institute. Guttmacher Policy Review. Fall 2007, vol 10, number 4. Popularity Disparity: Attitudes About the IUD in Europe and the United States http://www.guttmacher.org/pubs/gpr/10/4/gpr100419.html. Accessed Feb 1, 2011.

6. Mosher WD, Martinez GM, Chandra A, Abma JC, Willson SJ. Use of contraception and use of family planning services in the United States: 1982–2002. Adv Data. Dec 10 2004(350):1–36.

7. Mosher WD, Jones, J. Use of Contraception in the United States: 1982–2008. Vital Health Stat. 2010;23(29).

8. Forrest JD. U.S. women's perceptions of and attitudes about the IUD. Obstet Gynecol Surv. Dec 1996;51(12 Suppl):S30–34.

9. Stanwood NL, Garrett JM, Konrad TR. Obstetrician-gynecologists and the intrauterine device: a survey of attitudes and practice. Obstet Gynecol. Feb 2002;99:275–280.

10. Hubacher D, Cheng D. Intrauterine devices and reproductive health: American women in feast and famine. Contraception. 2004;69:437–446.

11. Sivin I. Another look at the Dalkon Shield: meta-analysis underscores its problems. Contraception. Jul 1993;48:1–12.

12. Speroff L, Darney P. A Clinical Guide for Contraception. 3rd ed. Philadelphia: Lippincott Williams & Wilkins; 2001.

13. Lee NC, Rubin GL, Ory HW, Burkman RT. Type of intrauterine device and the risk of pelvic inflammatory disease. Obstet Gynecol. 1983;62:1–6.

14. ACOG practice bulletin. Clinical management guidelines for obstetrician-gynecologists. Number 59, January 2005. Intrauterine device. Obstet Gynecol. 2005;105: 223–232.

15. Penney G, Brechin S, de Souza A, et al. FFPRHC Guidance (January 2004). The copper intrauterine device as long-term contraception. J Fam Plann Reprod Health Care. 2004;30:29–41; quiz 42.

16. De la Cruz D, Cruz A, Arteaga M, Castillo L, Tovalin H. Blood copper levels in Mexican users of the T 380A IUD. Contraception. 2005;72:122–125.

17. Hostynek JJ, Maibach HI. Copper hypersensitivity: dermatologic aspects. Dermatol Ther. 2004;17:328–333.

18. World Health Organization Special Program of Research Development and Research Training in Human Reproduction. Long-term reversible contraception. Twelve years of experience with the TCu380A and TCu220C. Contraception. 1997;56:341–352.

19. Sivin I. Utility and drawbacks of continuous use of a copper T IUD for 20 years. Contraception. 2007;75(6 Suppl):S70–75.

20. O'Brien PA, Kulier R, Helmerhorst FM, Usher-Patel M, d'Arcangues C. Copper-containing, framed intrauterine devices for contraception: a systematic review of randomized controlled trials. Contraception. 2008;77:318–327.

21. French R, Cowan F, Mansour D, et al. Hormonally impregnated intrauterine systems (IUSs), versus other forms of reversible contraceptives as effective methods of preventing pregnancy. Cochrane Database Syst Rev. 2004:CD001776.

22. Sivin I, Stern J, Coutinho E, et al. Prolonged intrauterine contraception: a seven-year randomized study of the levonorgestrel 20 mcg/day (LNg 20) and the Copper T 380Ag IUDS. Contraception. 1991;44:473–480.

23. Barbosa I, Olsson SE, Odlind V, Goncalves T, Coutinho E. Ovarian function after seven years' use of a levonorgestrel IUD. Adv Contracept. 1995;11:85–95.

24. Xiao B, Zeng T, Wu S, Sun H, Xiao N. Effect of levonorgestrel-releasing intrauterine device on hormonal profile and menstrual pattern after long-term use. Contraception. 1995;51:359–365.

25. Hidalgo MM, Hidalgo-Regina C, Bahamondes MV, Monteiro I, Petta CA, Bahamondes L. Serum levonorgestrel levels and endometrial thickness during extended use of the levonorgestrel-releasing intrauterine system. Contraception. 2009;80:84–89.

26. Rivera R, Yacobson I, Grimes D. The mechanism of action of hormonal contraceptives and intrauterine contraceptive devices. Am J Obstet Gynecol. 1999;181:1263–1269.
27. World Health Organization. Mechanism of action, safety and efficacy of intrauterine devices: technical report series 753. Geneva: World Health Organization; 1987.
28. El-Habashi M, El-Sahwi S, Gawish S, Osman M. Effect of Lippes loop on sperm recovery from human fallopian tubes. Contraception. 1980;22:549–555.
29. Ortiz ME, Croxatto HB, Bardin CW. Mechanisms of action of intrauterine devices. Obstet Gynecol Surv. 1996;51(12 Suppl):S42–51.
30. Sagiroglu N. Phagocytosis of spermatozoa in the uterine cavity of woman using intrauterine device. Int J Fertil. 1971;16:1–14.
31. Ammala M, Nyman T, Strengell L, Rutanen EM. Effect of intrauterine contraceptive devices on cytokine messenger ribonucleic acid expression in the human endometrium. Fertil Steril. 1995;63:773–778.
32. Segal SJ, Alvarez-Sanchez F, Adejuwon CA, Brache de Mejia V, Leon P, Faundes A. Absence of chorionic gonadotropin in sera of women who use intrauterine devices. Fertil Steril. 1985;44:214–218.
33. Wilcox AJ, Weinberg CR, Armstrong EG, Canfield RE. Urinary human chorionic gonadotropin among intrauterine device users: detection with a highly specific and sensitive assay. Fertil Steril. 1987;47:265–269.
34. Videla-Rivero L, Etchepareborda JJ, Kesseru E. Early chorionic activity in women bearing inert IUD, copper IUD and levonorgestrel-releasing IUD. Contraception. 1987;36:217–226.
35. Alvarez F, Brache V, Fernandez E, et al. New insights on the mode of action of intrauterine contraceptive devices in women. Fertil Steril. 1988;49:768–773.
36. Steiner MJ, Dalebout S, Condon S, Dominik R, Trussell J. Understanding risk: a randomized controlled trial of communicating contraceptive effectiveness. Obstet Gynecol. 2003;102:709–717.
37. Sivin I, Schmidt F. Effectiveness of IUDs: a review. Contraception. 1987;36:55–84.
38. The TCu380A, TCu220C, multiload 250 and Nova T IUDS at 3, 5 and 7 years of use–results from three randomized multicentre trials. World Health Organization. Special Programme of Research, Development and Research Training in Human Reproduction: Task Force on the Safety and Efficacy of Fertility Regulating Methods. Contraception. 1990;42:141–158.
39. Long-term reversible contraception. Twelve years of experience with the TCu380A and TCu220C. Contraception. 1997;56:341–352.
40. Luukkainen T, Allonen H, Haukkamaa M, et al. Effective contraception with the levonorgestrel-releasing intrauterine device: 12-month report of a European multicenter study. Contraception. 1987;36:169–179.
41. Sivin I, Stern J, Diaz J, et al. Two years of intrauterine contraception with levonorgestrel and with copper: a randomized comparison of the TCu 380Ag and levonorgestrel 20 mcg/day devices. Contraception. 1987;35:245–255.
42. Sivin I, el Mahgoub S, McCarthy T, et al. Long-term contraception with the levonorgestrel 20 mcg/day (LNg 20) and the copper T 380Ag intrauterine devices: a five-year randomized study. Contraception. 1990;42:361–378.
43. Andersson K, Odlind V, Rybo G. Levonorgestrel-releasing and copper-releasing (Nova T) IUDs during five years of use: a randomized comparative trial. Contraception. 1994;49:56–72.
44. Sivin I, Stern J. Health during prolonged use of levonorgestrel 20 micrograms/d and the copper TCu 380Ag intrauterine contraceptive devices: a multicenter study. International Committee for Contraception Research (ICCR). Fertil Steril. 1994;61:70–77.
45. Peterson HB, Xia Z, Hughes JM, Wilcox LS, Tylor LR, Trussell J. The risk of pregnancy after tubal sterilization: findings from the U.S. Collaborative Review of Sterilization. Am J Obstet Gynecol. 1996;174:1161–1168; discussion 1168–1170.

46. Backman T, Huhtala S, Blom T, Luoto R, Rauramo I, Koskenvuo M. Length of use and symptoms associated with premature removal of the levonorgestrel intrauterine system: a nation-wide study of 17,360 users. BJOG. 2000;107:335–339.
47. Jensen JT, Nelson AL, Costales AC. Subject and clinician experience with the levonorgestrel-releasing intrauterine system. Contraception. 2008;77:22–29.
48. Hubacher D, Reyes V, Lillo S, et al. Preventing copper intrauterine device removals due to side effects among first-time users: randomized trial to study the effect of prophylactic ibuprofen. Hum Reprod. 2006;21:1467–1472.
49. World Health Organization. Medical eligibility criteria for contraceptive use 4th ed. Geneva: World Health Organization; 2009.
50. Gaffield ME, Culwell KR. New recommendations on the safety of contraceptive methods for women with medical conditions. International Planned Parenthood Federation (IPPF) Medical Bulletin. 2010;44(1). http://www.ippf.org/NR/rdonlyres/D67E0B0E-39C9-4A0A-99E7-44AD870C5058/0/MedBullEnglishMar2010.pdf. Accessed Feb 1, 2011.
51. Centers for Disease Control and Prevention. U S. Medical Eligibility Criteria for Contraceptive Use, 2010. MMWR 2010;59(No. RR-4):1–85.
52. Foster DG, Rostovtseva DP, Brindis CD, Biggs MA, Hulett D, Darney PD. Cost savings from the provision of specific methods of contraception in a publicly funded program. Am J Public Health. 2009;99:446–451.
53. Chiou CF, Trussell J, Reyes E, et al. Economic analysis of contraceptives for women. Contraception. 2003;68:3–10.
54. Ory HW. Ectopic pregnancy and intrauterine contraceptive devices: new perspectives. The Women's Health Study. Obstet Gynecol. 1981;57:137–144.
55. Sivin I. Dose- and age-dependent ectopic pregnancy risks with intrauterine contraception. Obstet Gynecol. 1991;78:291–298.
56. Wu S, Godfrey EM, Wojdyla D, Dong J, Cong J, Wang C, von Hertzen H. Copper T 380A intrauterine device for emergency contraception: a prospective, multicentre, cohort clinical trial. BJOG. 2010;117:1205–10.
57. Guleria K, Agarwal N, Mishra K, Gulati R, Mehendiratta A. Evaluation of endometrial steroid receptors and cell mitotic activity in women using copper intrauterine device: Can Cu-T prevent endometrial cancer? J Obstet Gynaecol Res. 2004;30:181–187.
58. Curtis KM, Marchbanks PA, Peterson HB. Neoplasia with use of intrauterine devices. Contraception. 2007;75(6 Suppl):S60–69.
59. Gardner FJ, Konje JC, Bell SC, et al. Prevention of tamoxifen induced endometrial polyps using a levonorgestrel releasing intrauterine system long-term follow-up of a randomised control trial. Gynecol Oncol. 2009;114:452–456.
60. Depot-medroxyprogesterone acetate (DMPA) and risk of endometrial cancer. The WHO Collaborative Study of Neoplasia and Steroid Contraceptives. Int J Cancer. 1991;49:186–190.
61. Suvanto-Luukkonen E, Kauppila A. The levonorgestrel intrauterine system in menopausal hormone replacement therapy: five-year experience. Fertil Steril. 1999;72:161–163.
62. Suhonen S, Holmstrom T, Lahteenmaki P. Three-year follow-up of the use of a levonorgestrel-releasing intrauterine system in hormone replacement therapy. Acta Obstet Gynecol Scand. 1997;76:145–150.
63. Varila E, Wahlstrom T, Rauramo I. A 5-year follow-up study on the use of a levonorgestrel intrauterine system in women receiving hormone replacement therapy. Fertil Steril. 2001;76:969–973.
64. Gardner FJ, Konje JC, Abrams KR, et al. Endometrial protection from tamoxifen-stimulated changes by a levonorgestrel-releasing intrauterine system: a randomised controlled trial. Lancet. 2000;356:1711–1717.
65. Schwarz EB, Hess R, Trussell J. Contraception for cancer survivors. J Gen Intern Med. 2009;24 Suppl 2:S401–406.

66. Buttini MJ, Jordan SJ, Webb PM. The effect of the levonorgestrel releasing intrauterine system on endometrial hyperplasia: an Australian study and systematic review. Aust N Z J Obstet Gynaecol. 2009;49:316–322.
67. Dhar KK, NeedhiRajan T, Koslowski M, Woolas RP. Is levonorgestrel intrauterine system effective for treatment of early endometrial cancer? Report of four cases and review of the literature. Gynecol Oncol. 2005;97:924–927.
68. Varma R, Soneja H, Bhatia K, et al. The effectiveness of a levonorgestrel-releasing intrauterine system (LNg-IUS) in the treatment of endometrial hyperplasia–A long-term follow-up study. Eur J Obstet Gyn RB. 2008;139:169–175.
69. Bahamondes L, Ribeiro-Huguet P, de Andrade KC, Leon-Martins O, Petta CA. Levonorgestrel-releasing intrauterine system (Mirena) as a therapy for endometrial hyperplasia and carcinoma. Acta Obstet. Gynecol. Scand. 2003;82:580–582.
70. ACOG committee opinion. No. 337: Noncontraceptive uses of the levonorgestrel intrauterine system. Obstet Gynecol. 2006;107:1479–1482.
71. Kadir RA, Chi C. Levonorgestrel intrauterine system: bleeding disorders and anticoagulant therapy. Contraception. 2007;75(6 Suppl):S123–129.
72. Kilic S, Yuksel B, Doganay M, et al. The effect of levonorgestrel-releasing intrauterine device on menorrhagia in women taking anticoagulant medication after cardiac valve replacement. Contraception. 2009;80:152–157.
73. Lukes AS, Reardon B, Arepally G. Use of the levonorgestrel-releasing intrauterine system in women with hemostatic disorders. Fertil Steril. 2008;90:673–677.
74. Fedele L, Bianchi S, Raffaelli R, Portuese A, Dorta M. Treatment of adenomyosis-associated menorrhagia with a levonorgestrel-releasing intrauterine device. Fertil Steril. 1997;68:426–429.
75. Grigorieva V, Chen-Mok M, Tarasova M, Mikhailov A. Use of a levonorgestrel-releasing intrauterine system to treat bleeding related to uterine leiomyomas. Fertil Steril. 2003;79:1194–1198.
76. Brown P, Farquhar C, Lethaby A, Sadler L, Johnson N. Cost-effectiveness analysis of levonorgestrel intrauterine system and thermal balloon ablation for heavy menstrual bleeding. BJOG. 2006;113:797–803.
77. Shaw RW, Symonds IM, Tamizian O, Chaplain J, Mukhopadhyay S. Randomised comparative trial of thermal balloon ablation and levonorgestrel intrauterine system in patients with idiopathic menorrhagia. Aust. N. Z. J. Obstet. Gynaecol. 2007; 47:335–340.
78. Hurskainen R, Teperi J, Rissanen P, et al. Clinical outcomes and costs with the levonorgestrel-releasing intrauterine system or hysterectomy for treatment of menorrhagia: randomized trial 5-year follow-up. JAMA. 2004;291:1456–1463.
79. Busfield RA, Farquhar CM, Sowter MC, et al. A Randomized Trial Comparing the Levonorgestrel Intrauterine System and Thermal Balloon Ablation for Heavy Menstrual Bleeding. Obstet Gynecol Surv 2006;61:444–445.
80. Toivonen J. Intrauterine contraceptive device and pelvic inflammatory disease. Ann Med. 1993;25:171–173.
81. Toivonen J, Luukkainen T, Allonen H. Protective effect of intrauterine release of levonorgestrel on pelvic infection: three years' comparative experience of levonorgestrel- and copper-releasing intrauterine devices. Obstet Gynecol. 1991; 77:261–264.
82. Ronnerdag M, Odlind V. Health effects of long-term use of the intrauterine levonorgestrel-releasing system. A follow-up study over 12 years of continuous use. Acta Obstet Gynecol Scand. 1999;78:716–721.
83. Rivera R, Chen-Mok M, McMullen S. Analysis of client characteristics that may affect early discontinuation of the TCu-380A IUD. Contraception. 1999;60:155–160.
84. Hubacher D, Chen PL, Park S. Side effects from the copper IUD: do they decrease over time? Contraception. 2009;79:356–362.
85. Milsom I, Andersson K, Jonasson K, Lindstedt G, Rybo G. The influence of the Gyne-T 380S IUD on menstrual blood loss and iron status. Contraception. 1995;52:175–179.

86. Hidalgo M, Bahamondes L, Perrotti M, Diaz J, Dantas-Monteiro C, Petta C. Bleeding patterns and clinical performance of the levonorgestrel-releasing intrauterine system (Mirena) up to two years. Contraception. 2002;65:129–132.
87. Nilsson CG, Lahteenmaki PL, Luukkainen T. Ovarian function in amenorrheic and menstruating users of a levonorgestrel-releasing intrauterine device. Fertil Steril. 1984;41:52–55.
88. Xiao BL, Zhou LY, Zhang XL, Jia MC, Luukkainen T, Allonen H. Pharmacokinetic and pharmacodynamic studies of levonorgestrel-releasing intrauterine device. Contraception. 1990;41:353–362.
89. Nilsson CG, Lahteenmaki PL, Luukkainen T, Robertson DN. Sustained intrauterine release of levonorgestrel over five years. Fertil Steril. 1986;45:805–807.
90. Zhang J, Feldblum PJ, Chi IC, Farr MG. Risk factors for copper T IUD expulsion: an epidemiologic analysis. Contraception. 1992;46:427–433.
91. Bahamondes L, Diaz J, Marchi NM, Petta CA, Cristofoletti ML, Gomez G. Performance of copper intrauterine devices when inserted after an expulsion. Hum Reprod. 1995;10:2917–2918.
92. Gruber A, Rabinerson D, Kaplan B, Pardo J, Neri A. The missing forgotten intrauterine contraceptive device. Contraception. 1996;54:117–119.
93. Gupta PK, Hollander DH, Frost JK. Actinomycetes in cervico-vaginal smears: an association with IUD usage. Acta Cytol. 1976;20:295–297.
94. Lippes J. Pelvic actinomycosis: a review and preliminary look at prevalence. Am J Obstet Gynecol. 1999;180:265–269.
95. Walsh T, Grimes D, Frezieres R, et al. Randomised controlled trial of prophylactic antibiotics before insertion of intrauterine devices. IUD Study Group. Lancet. 1998;351:1005–1008.
96. Farley TM, Rosenberg MJ, Rowe PJ, Chen JH, Meirik O. Intrauterine devices and pelvic inflammatory disease: an international perspective. Lancet. 1992;339:785–788.
97. Grimes DA. Intrauterine device and upper-genital-tract infection. Lancet. 2000;356:1013–1019.
98. Mishell DR, Jr., Bell JH, Good RG, Moyer DL. The intrauterine device: a bacteriologic study of the endometrial cavity. Am J Obstet Gynecol. 1966;96:119–126.
99. Grimes DA, Schulz KF. Prophylactic antibiotics for intrauterine device insertion: a metaanalysis of the randomized controlled trials. Contraception. 1999;60:57–63.
100. Daling JR, Weiss NS, Metch BJ, et al. Primary tubal infertility in relation to the use of an intrauterine device. N Engl J Med. 1985;312:937–941.
101. Cramer DW, Schiff I, Schoenbaum SC, et al. Tubal infertility and the intrauterine device. N Engl J Med. 1985;312:941–947.
102. Wilson JC. A prospective New Zealand study of fertility after removal of copper intrauterine contraceptive devices for conception and because of complications: a four-year study. Am J Obstet Gynecol. 1989;160:391–396.
103. Skjeldestad F, Bratt H. Fertility after complicated and non-complicated use of IUDs. A controlled prospective study. Adv Contracept. 1988;4:179–184.
104. Hubacher D, Lara-Ricalde R, Taylor DJ, Guerra-Infante F, Guzman-Rodriguez R. Use of copper intrauterine devices and the risk of tubal infertility among nulligravid women. N Engl J Med. 2001;345:561–567.
105. Furlong LA. Ectopic pregnancy risk when contraception fails. A review. J Reprod Med. 2002;47:881–885.
106. Backman T, Rauramo I, Huhtala S, Koskenvuo M. Pregnancy during the use of levonorgestrel intrauterine system. Am J Obstet Gynecol. 2004;190:50–54.
107. Increasing use of contraceptive implants and intrauterine devices to reduce unintended pregnancy. ACOG Committee Opinion No. 450, American College of Obstetricians and Gynecologists. Obstet Gynecol. 2009;114:1434–8.
108. Huggins GR, Cullins VE. Fertility after contraception or abortion. Fertil Steril. 1990;54:559–573.

109. Hov GG, Skjeldestad FE, Hilstad T. Use of IUD and subsequent fertility–follow-up after participation in a randomized clinical trial. Contraception. 2007;75:88–92.
110. Brockmeyer A, Kishen M, Webb A. Experience of IUD/IUS insertions and clinical performance in nulliparous women–a pilot study. Eur J Contracept Reprod Health Care. 2008;13:248–254.
111. Thiery M. Pain relief at insertion and removal of an IUD: a simplified technique for paracervical block. Adv Contracept. 1985;1:167–170.
112. Allen RH, Bartz D, Grimes DA, Hubacher D, O'Brien P. Interventions for pain with intrauterine device insertion. Cochrane Database Syst Rev. 2009:CD007373.
113. Chen B, Creinin M, Reeves M, Schwarz E. Breastfeeding continuation among women using the levonorgestrel-releasing intrauterine device after vaginal delivery. Contraception. 1980:204–205 and Chen B, Creinin M, Reeves M, Schwarz EB. Postplacental or delayed levonorgestrel intrauterine device insertion and breastfeeding duration. Contraception 2011.
114. Andersson K, Ryde-Blomqvist E, Lindell K, Odlind V, Milsom I. Perforations with intrauterine devices. Report from a Swedish survey. Contraception. 1998;57:251–255.
115. Chi IC, Wilkens LR, Champion CB, Machemer RE, Rivera R. Insertional pain and other IUD insertion-related rare events for breastfeeding and non-breastfeeding women–a decade's experience in developing countries. Adv Contracept. 1989;5: 101–119.
116. Browne H, Manipalviratn S, Armstrong A. Using an intrauterine device in immunocompromised women. Obstet Gynecol. 2008;112:667–669.
117. Culwell KR, Curtis KM, del Carmen Cravioto M. Safety of contraceptive method use among women with systemic lupus erythematosus: a systematic review. Obstet Gynecol. 2009;114(2 Pt 1):341–353.
118. Curtis KM, Nanda K, Kapp N. Safety of hormonal and intrauterine methods of contraception for women with HIV/AIDS: a systematic review. AIDS. 2009;23 Suppl 1:S55–67.
119. Sinei SK, Morrison CS, Sekadde-Kigondu C, Allen M, Kokonya D. Complications of use of intrauterine devices among HIV-1-infected women. Lancet. 1998;351: 1238–1241.
120. Morrison CS, Sekadde-Kigondu C, Sinei SK, Weiner DH, Kwok C, Kokonya D. Is the intrauterine device appropriate contraception for HIV-1-infected women? BJOG. ug 2001;108:784–790.
121. Stringer EM, Kaseba C, Levy J, et al. A randomized trial of the intrauterine contraceptive device vs hormonal contraception in women who are infected with the human immunodeficiency virus. Am J Obstet Gynecol. 2007;197:144 e141–148.
122. Wilson W, Taubert KA, Gewitz M, et al. Prevention of infective endocarditis: guidelines from the American Heart Association: a guideline from the American Heart Association Rheumatic Fever, Endocarditis, and Kawasaki Disease Committee, Council on Cardiovascular Disease in the Young, and the Council on Clinical Cardiology, Council on Cardiovascular Surgery and Anesthesia, and the Quality of Care and Outcomes Research Interdisciplinary Working Group. Circulation. 2007;116: 1736–1754.
123. Kjos SL, Ballagh SA, La Cour M, Xiang A, Mishell DR, Jr. The copper T 380A intrauterine device in women with type II diabetes mellitus. Obstet Gynecol. Dec 1994;84:1006–1009.
124. Skouby SO, Molsted-Pedersen L, Petersen KR. Contraception for women with diabetes: an update. Baillieres Clin Obstet Gynaecol. 1991;5:493–503.
125. Kimmerle R, Heinemann L, Berger M. Intrauterine devices are safe and effective contraceptives for type I diabetic women. Diabetes Care. 1995;18:1506–1507.
126. Petersen KR, Skouby SO, Jespersen J. Contraception guidance in women with preexisting disturbances in carbohydrate metabolism. Eur J Contracept Reprod Health Care. 1996;1:53–59.

127. Rogovskaya S, Rivera R, Grimes DA, et al. Effect of a levonorgestrel intrauterine system on women with type 1 diabetes: a randomized trial. Obstet Gynecol. 2005;105:811–815.
128. Lidegaard O, Lokkegaard E, Svendsen AL, Agger C. Hormonal contraception and risk of venous thromboembolism: national follow-up study. BMJ. 2009;339:b2890.
129. White MK, Ory HW, Rooks JB, Rochat RW. Intrauterine device termination rates and the menstrual cycle day of insertion. Obstet Gynecol. 1980;55:220–224.
130. Grimes D, Schulz K, Stanwood N. Immediate postabortal insertion of intrauterine devices. Cochrane Database Syst Rev. 2002:CD001777.
131. Bednarek PA, Creinin MD, Reeves MF, Cwiak CA, Espey E, Jensen JT. Immediate intrauterine device insertion following suction aspiration between 5–12 weeks of gestation increases rates of insertion and utilization compared to scheduled delayed insertion [abstract]. Contraception. 2009;80:203.
132. Hohmann HL, Reeves MF, Chen BA, Perriera L, Hayes JL, Creinin MD. Immediate versus delayed insertion of the levonorgestrel-releasing intrauterine device following dilation and evacuation: a randomized controlled trial [abstract]. Contraception. 2009;80:209.
133. Goodman S, Hendlish SK, Reeves MF, Foster-Rosales A. Impact of immediate postabortal insertion of intrauterine contraception on repeat abortion. Contraception. 2008;78:143–148.
134. Reeves MF, Smith KJ, Creinin MD. Contraceptive effectiveness of immediate compared with delayed insertion of intrauterine devices after abortion: a decision analysis. Obstet Gynecol. 2007;109:1286–1294.
135. Eroglu K, Akkuzu G, Vural G, et al. Comparison of efficacy and complications of IUD insertion in immediate postplacental/early postpartum period with interval period: 1 year follow-up. Contraception. 2006;74:376–381.
136. Osborne NG, Wright RC. Effect of preoperative scrub on the bacterial flora of the endocervix and vagina. Obstet Gynecol. 1977;50:148–151.
137. Tangsiriwatthana T, Sangkomkamhang US, Lumbiganon P, Laopaiboon M. Paracervical local anaesthesia for cervical dilatation and uterine intervention. Cochrane Database Syst Rev. 2009(1):CD005056.
138. Hubacher D, Fortney J. Follow-up visits after IUD insertion. Are more better? J Reprod Med. 1999;44:801–806.
139. Janowitz B, Hubacher D, Petrick T, Dighe N. Should the recommended number of IUD revisits be reduced? Stud Fam Plann. 1994;25:362–367.
140. Stanback J, Grimes D. Can intrauterine device removals for bleeding or pain be predicted at a one-month follow-up visit? A multivariate analysis. Contraception. 1998;58:357–360.
141. Ylikorkala O. Prostaglandin synthesis inhibitors in menorrhagia, intrauterine contraceptive device-induced side effects and endometriosis. Pharmacol Toxicol. 1994;75 Suppl 2:86–88.
142. Abdel-Aleem H, d'Arcangues C, Vogelsong KM, Gulmezoglu AM. Treatment of vaginal bleeding irregularities induced by progestin only contraceptives. Cochrane Database Syst Rev. 2007:CD003449.
143. Centers for Disease Control and Prevention. Sexually transmitted disease treatment guidelines, 2006. In: MMWR, ed. Vol 552006.
144. Centers for Disease Control and Prevention. Sexually Transmitted Diseases: Updated recommended treatment regimens for gonococcal infections and associated conditions. United States, April 2007. Accessed July 20, 2010 from: http://www.cdc.gov/std/treatment/2006/updated-regimens.htm.
145. Soderberg G, Lindgren S. Influence of an intrauterine device on the course of an acute salpingitis. Contraception. 1981;24:137–143.
146. Hager WD, Eschenbach DA, Spence MR, Sweet RL. Criteria for diagnosis and grading of salpingitis. Obstet Gynecol. 1983;61:113–114.

147. Hadgu A, Westrom L, Brooks CA, Reynolds GH, Thompson SE. Predicting acute pelvic inflammatory disease: a multivariate analysis. Am J Obstet Gynecol. 1986;155:954–960.
148. Adoni A, Ben Chetrit A. The management of intrauterine devices following uterine perforation. Contraception. 1991;43:77–81.
149. Foreman H, Stadel BV, Schlesselman S. Intrauterine device usage and fetal loss. Obstet Gynecol. 1981;58:669–677.

LATE REFERENCES

150. Dijkhuizen K, Dekkers OM, Holleboom CA, de Groot CJ, Hellebrekers BW, van Roosmalen GJ, Janssen CA, Helmerhorst FM. Vaginal misoprostol prior to insertion of an intrauterine device: an RCT. Hum Reprod. 2011;26:323–9.
151. Sääv I, Aronsson A, Marions L, Stephansson O, Gemzell-Danielsson K. Cervical priming with sublingual misoprostol prior to insertion of an intrauterine device in nulliparous women: a randomized controlled trial. Hum Reprod. 2007;22:2647–52.

Contraceptive Implants

Elizabeth G. Raymond, MD, MPH

- Implants are thin rods or tubes containing a progestin hormone. They are inserted under the skin of a woman's arm.

- Marketed implants provide contraception for at least 3 years. Their efficacy is comparable to that of sterilization.

- Implants cause menstrual cycle irregularities in most users.

- Implants are particularly suitable for women who desire safe, extremely effective, long-term, maintenance-free, reversible contraception.

- Like other progestin-only contraceptives, implants may be of special interest to women who cannot use a contraceptive that contains estrogen.

- As of September 2010, the only implant available in the United States is Implanon, a single rod that provides contraception for at least 3 years.

Contraceptive implants consist of one or more thin rods or tubes containing a progestin hormone. They are inserted just under the skin of a woman's arm and provide effective contraception for at least 3 years. Currently available implants are not biodegradable, and therefore removal is generally recommended when the period of efficacy expires. They may be removed earlier if the patient desires fertility or another contraceptive method. Contraceptive implants are now approved in more than 60 countries and have been used by at least 11 million women worldwide.[1,2]

As of this writing (September 2010), the only implant available in the United States is a single rod implant called Implanon, manufactured by Merck (formerly Organon). Implanon has been used in Asia, Europe, Africa, and Australia since 1998. The Implanon rod is 4 cm long and 2 mm in diameter. It contains 68 mg etonogestrel (also called 3-keto-desogestrel), which is the main active metabolite of desogestrel, a progestin used in many oral contraceptive pills. Implanon is labeled to provide contraception for 3 years after insertion.

In Europe, Merck markets an implant (Nexplanon) that is identical to Implanon except that the rods are radioopaque and the inserter has been improved.[3] This new product may be introduced to the United States in the future.

Two other implants have been approved by the U.S. Food and Drug Administration (FDA) but are not currently being distributed in the United States:

- *Norplant.* The Norplant system consists of 6 flexible tubes containing a total of 216 mg levonorgestrel. Each tube is 3.4 cm long and 2.4 mm in diameter. It provides highly effective contraception for at least 7 years after insertion. First approved in Finland in 1983,[4] Norplant was approved by the FDA in 1990 and marketed in the United States until 2002. In that year, the U.S. distributor stopped selling it, citing limitations in product component supplies. A Chinese implant system (Sinoplant I) designed to be identical to Norplant has been used in China.

- *Jadelle.* Jadelle consists of two rods 4.3 cm long and 2.5 mm in diameter, each containing 75 mg levonorgestrel. Jadelle is effective for at least 5 years. It was approved by the FDA in 1996 but has never been sold in this country. It is available elsewhere in the world, however. A 4-year Chinese version of Jadelle (Sinoimplant (II)) is currently used in several countries in Asia and Africa.[2]

Several other progestin-releasing implants are in various phases of development, including a one-year implant containing nomegestrol acetate (Uniplant) invented in Brazil[5] and a two-year implant containing nestorone being studied by the Population Council for use during lactation.

Because Implanon is the only implant now available in the United States, it is the focus of this chapter.

M ECHANISM OF ACTION

Small studies have shown that Implanon suppresses ovulation in almost all users throughout the first 3 years after insertion. One study of 244 ultrasound scans in 188 women who had had Implanon inserted 0 to 20 months (median 3 months) earlier found one ovulation at 16 months;[6] a smaller study documented two ovulations in 1 of 16 women at 30 and 33 months after insertion.[7] Implanon also alters endometrial structure, and it changes cervical mucus in a way that may impede sperm penetration.[6] These mechanisms may contribute to the method's protective effect if ovulation does occur.

On average, estradiol levels in Implanon users tend to decrease to the range of the early follicular phase immediately after implant insertion and then rise slowly, reflecting increasing follicular activity. Among individual women, however, one study found that levels of estradiol varied substantially over time. No woman was found to have consistently low or high levels.[7]

EFFECTIVENESS

Implants are among the most effective of the available contraceptive methods; they are in the top tier of effectiveness. (See Figure 3–1 in Chapter 3 on Choosing a Contraceptive.) From a clinical viewpoint, their efficacy is indistinguishable from that of sterilization and intrauterine devices.[8] To date, no pregnancies have been observed in prospective or retrospective cohort studies of Implanon, which included a total of more than 4,500 women and more than 7,000 women-years of exposure.[9-23] However, pregnancies in Implanon users have been reported to regulatory authorities and Merck, and in case reports in the medical literature.[24] Of 173 classifiable Implanon failures reported to the Therapeutic Goods Administration in Australia, 49% were attributed to non-insertion of the implant, 27% were apparently conceived before the women had Implanon inserted, 11% were ascribed to insertion outside the recommended time in the menstrual cycle, 2% occurred after expulsion of the implant, and 12% were true product failures.[25] In a much larger number of classifiable pregnancies reported to Merck (which may have included most of the Australian pregnancies), half had no implant present, and 38% were true product failures.[9] In both series, a quarter to a third of the true method failures occurred in women taking possibly interacting drugs. Based on Implanon sales data, authors have estimated an approximate failure rate of 0.5 to 1 pregnancy/1,000 Implanon insertions.

Whether user characteristics, such as body weight, might reduce the efficacy of Implanon is unknown. Serum etonogestrel levels appear inversely related to body weight,[26] although no evidence has been found of a relationship between weight and ovulation or pregnancy rates.[9] The number of obese women included in prospective and retrospective studies was relatively small.

Implanon is marketed with a duration of action of 3 years. However, pharmacokinetic data from Implanon users show stable serum concentrations of etonogestrel out to 36 months, suggesting that the method is effective for longer than that. (See Figure 8–1.) Three studies in which a total of 275 women used Implanon for longer than 3 years found no pregnancies during the fourth year of use.[10,11,27]

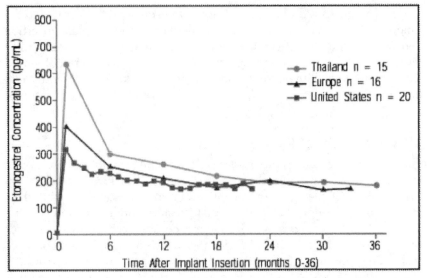

Source: Merck, with permission.

Figure 8–1 Serum etonogestrel concentrations in Implanon users

ADVANTAGES

Implants have many advantages for many women.

1. **High efficacy.** See above.

2. **Ease of use.** Once implants are inserted, no attention is required on the part of the user until the time of removal. Implants are thus an excellent contraceptive option for women who have difficulty using a contraceptive at the time of intercourse or adhering to a regular schedule independent of intercourse.

3. **Discreetness.** Implant users need keep no contraceptive supplies at home and do not require resupply or follow-up clinical care until removal. In most users, the rods are not visible under the skin. These features may be attractive to women who desire privacy about their use of contraception. However, insertion leaves a small scar, and subdermal implants can usually be detected by palpation. In some cases, side effects such as irregular vaginal bleeding may be a clue that a woman is using reproductive hormones.

4. **No adverse effect on acne.** In one study of women using Implanon for up to 2 years, 61% of those with acne at baseline reported decreased acne, whereas only 16% of those with no acne at baseline developed acne.[28]

5. **Relief of dysmenorrhea.** In one analysis of 315 women, 48% reported decreased dysmenorrhea after Implanon insertion, whereas only 8% reported increased dysmenorrhea.[28,29] The improvement in dysmenorrhea is likely related to the reduction in ovulatory bleeding induced by Implanon.

6. **Relief of pelvic pain due to endometriosis or other causes.** Implanon, like other hormonal contraceptives, may be effective in reducing pelvic pain associated with endometriosis[30,31] or other causes.[32,33]

7. **Few clinically significant metabolic effects.** Implanon appears not to be associated with clinically important adverse changes in blood pressure, liver function, hemostasis, carbohydrate metabolism, lipid levels, or thyroid function.[34-42] One study suggested that Implanon use was associated with increased insulin resistance in women who are at risk for diabetes due to polycystic ovarian disease,[43] but another study found no such impact in women with frank diabetes.[44]

8. **Reduced risk of ectopic pregnancy.** Because implants, like all contraceptives, prevent pregnancy, they also prevent ectopic pregnancy. However, some data suggest that in the extremely unlikely event that a pregnancy occurs during Implanon use, Implanon may increase the chance that it will be ectopic.[9]

9. **No estrogen.** Implants do not contain estrogen and thus may not be associated with rare but serious complications attributable to estrogenic agents, such as thrombophlebitis, pulmonary embolism, and cardiovascular effects.[45] Women with certain medical conditions that may be exacerbated by estrogen-containing methods may be eligible to use implants.

10. **Reversibility.** After Implanon removal, etonogestrel becomes undetectable in most users within a week, and most users ovulate within 6 weeks.[7,46] Data on pregnancy rates in women after removal of Implanon are scant. In one study of 46 women who discontinued Implanon and did not subsequently use any contraception, 11 (24%) became pregnant within 4 months.[28] This proportion is considerably lower than that expected among women who had never used contraception. However, this difference could have explanations other than a prolonged effect of Implanon on fertility after removal (for example, lower than usual coital frequency).

11. **High acceptability and continuation rates.** In general, users' satisfaction with this method is high. Clinical trials and observational studies have shown continuation rates of 65 to 91% at one year and 30 to 83% at 3 years.[10,18,41]

12. **Cost effectiveness.** An analysis of 2003 data from California's publically funded family planning program found that implants and intrauterine devices were the most cost effective methods, saving more than $7 for every $1 spent in services and supplies.[47] Another analysis found that in the United States, implants are less cost effective than copper or hormonal intrauterine devices and vasectomy but more cost-effective than other hormonal methods.[48]

D ISADVANTAGES AND CAUTIONS

1. **Uterine bleeding abnormalities.** Like all progestin-only methods, Implanon causes vaginal bleeding changes in a large proportion of women. These changes may include amenorrhea, infrequent bleeding, irregular bleeding, or less often, prolonged or frequent bleeding, and they are the most common reason for discontinuation of Implanon use. However, the irregular bleeding is rarely clinically significant, and many women consider amenorrhea and infrequent bleeding, if these occur, to be benefits. A combined analysis of 11 clinical trials that included a total of 923 Implanon users showed that the bleeding pattern in the first 3 months tended to predict the pattern in subsequent months, although this finding should be interpreted with caution because women whose bleeding patterns deteriorate over time tend to stop use of the method.[29] After Implanon removal, menses return to normal in most women within 3 months.[28] Researchers have evaluated various drugs to prevent or treat bleeding irregularities caused by progestin-only methods, but to date, none have been proven to provide medium or long-term benefit.[49] The best approach to reducing the impact of this side effect is to forewarn women about it, emphasizing that it is generally not dangerous.[50]

2. **Rare insertion and removal complications.** Complications of implant insertion and removal are very rare, occurring in less than 1% of patients in most studies. Infection, bruising, skin irritation, or pain occasionally occur after insertion, but they almost always resolve without treatment. Removal of implants is sometimes difficult particularly if the implant is malpositioned.[51] Implants may migrate slightly within the subdermal tissue after insertion, but deep migration has not been documented.[52] Ulnar nerve damage during insertion or removal of Implanon has been reported.[53] Breakage of implants in situ or

during removal occurs rarely.[22,54] Expulsion of implants has occurred in association with infection.[55]

3. **Possible weight gain.** In 11 clinical trials that included 942 women, the median gain was less than 5.6 pounds in a period of up to 3 years.[41] Whether this weight gain can be attributed to Implanon is not known.[11,27]

4. **Other adverse symptoms.** Headache, emotional lability, breast pain, abdominal pain, nausea, loss of libido, vaginal dryness, and other symptoms have been reported by women in trials of Implanon and other implants. Whether these symptoms are actually caused by the implants is unknown.[28]

5. **Ovarian cysts.** Progestin implants do not totally suppress ovarian activity, and persistent follicles or "ovarian cysts" have been reported in a small proportion of users of Implanon, Norplant, and Jadelle. Some studies have suggested that the incidence of ovarian cysts is higher among implant users than among users of nonhormonal contraceptives. Implant-associated cysts or follicles usually resolve without treatment. Intervention is not indicated unless a cyst becomes symptomatic or fails to regress.[55,56]

6. **Clinician-dependency.** Implants must be inserted and removed by a trained clinician. Compared with other methods, they may thus be less available and offer women less control over their contraceptive. Removal of implants requires a minor surgical procedure.

7. **Lack of protection against sexually transmitted infections (STI).** Like other hormonal contraceptives, implants offer no protection from STIs, including that associated with human immunodeficiency virus (HIV). Some but not all studies have suggested an increased risk of infection among users of injectable progestin-containing contraceptives, but no causal association has been proven. However, implants may be associated with a decreased risk of bacterial vaginosis.[57]

8. **Drug interactions.** No published studies have rigorously evaluated interactions between Implanon and other drugs. In one case report, a woman taking the anticoagulant warfarin required an increase in dose while using Implanon.[58] Pregnancies have been reported in Implanon users who are taking other drugs, including antiretroviral agents, antiepileptics, and rifampicin. Because etonogestrel levels in Implanon users are so low, a deleterious effect of other drugs on contraceptive

efficacy may be more of a concern for Implanon than for other hormonal methods.

9. **Possible decrease in bone density.** Some data suggest that Implanon may be associated with a reduction in bone density of the distal radius.[59,60] However, other data have not shown this effect.[61,62] Whether any changes caused by Implanon are clinically significant and whether they resolve after implant removal are unknown.

10. **Possible increased risk of thromboembolic conditions.** Etonogestrel, the progestin in Implanon, is a metabolite of desogestrel, which has been implicated by some studies as associated with an increased risk of thromboembolic conditions in users of combined oral contraceptives containing desogestrel. (see Chapter 11, Combined Oral Contraceptives). Currently available data offer no suggestion that Implanon itself may increase this risk, but no study of sufficient size to detect a significant increase in such rare conditions has yet been conducted. Serum etonogestrel levels in Implanon users are substantially lower than those in users of desogestrel-containing combined oral contraceptives,[26] and Implanon does not contain estrogen. Implanon does not have substantial effects on serum clotting factors.[42] Neither the World Health Organization's *Medical Eligibility Criteria for Contraceptive Use* (WHO *MEC*)[63] nor the corresponding United States document (U.S. *MEC*)[64] makes any distinction between etonogestrel implants and progestin-only methods containing other progestins with respect to risk for thromboembolic conditions.

SPECIAL ISSUES

Effect on pregnancy if inadvertently inserted during pregnancy. In general, hormonal contraceptives are not dangerous for either a pregnant woman or a developing fetus. No information is available specifically about Implanon in pregnancy. If a woman using Implanon is found to be pregnant and wishes to continue the pregnancy, Implanon should be removed, but no other special evaluation or care is needed.

Effect on lactogenesis. In general, progestin-releasing implants have no known clinically important effect on breastfeeding or infant development.[65] Published studies of Implanon in breastfeeding showed no evidence of deleterious effects on either maternal or neonatal health.[66–68] Etonogestrel does transfer to breast milk in low concentrations and is orally active.[65]

PROVIDING THE METHOD

Both the WHO *MEC* and the U.S. *MEC* list only a few medical conditions that contraindicate use of implants (Category 3 or 4):

	WHO	US
Breastfeeding women less than 6 weeks postpartum	x	
Current deep venous thrombosis or pulmonary embolus	x	
Unexplained, unevaluated abnormal vaginal bleeding	x	x
Systemic lupus erythematosus with positive or unknown antiphospholipid antibodies	x	x
Severe (decompensated) cirrhosis	x	x
Benign or malignant liver tumor	x	x
Current or past breast cancer	x	x
Use of ritonavir-boosted protease inhibitors, certain anticonvulsants, (phenytoin, carbamazepine, barbiturates, primidone, topiramate, oxcarbazepine), rifampicin or rifabutin	x	x

In addition, both the WHO *MEC* and the U.S. *MEC* note that the rods should be removed if a user develops ischemic heart disease, stroke, or migraine with aura while using implants.

Notably, neither set of criteria includes any restrictions based on age, smoking, hypertension, migraine without aura, uterine fibroids, diabetes, gallbladder disease, or sickle cell disease. No examinations or laboratory tests are needed to determine whether a woman is eligible to receive implants, except in women with lupus.

Implants are not a good choice for women who cannot tolerate irregular bleeding or amenorrhea.

Counseling. Women considering implants should be advised about their advantages and disadvantages, described above. Experience with Norplant particularly suggests that the quality of counseling before insertion can improve a patient's satisfaction with implants and reduce the likelihood she will discontinue them because of side effects.[69]

Timing of insertion. Implant insertion should be timed to minimize the possibility that a woman is pregnant or that she might become pregnant between insertion and the initiation of the implant's contraceptive effect. Precisely when the contraceptive effect begins is unknown. The recommendations provided in Table 8–1 are conservative; insertion may be acceptable at other times if reasonable evidence exists that the patient is not pregnant. Backup contraception (such as condoms) after insertion is not needed if Implanon is inserted as in Table 8–1.

Insertion procedure. Because it consists of only one rod, Implanon is easier to insert and remove than Norplant. It is distributed in a specially

Table 8–1 When to insert implants

Previous Method	When to Insert Implants
None	Days 1–5 of menstrual cycle
Combined oral contraceptive pills	While taking active pills or within 7 days after the last active pill
Progestin-only pills	While taking active pills
Injectables	Day next injection is due
Implants or intrauterine contraception	Day of removal of device
First-trimester abortion	Within 5 days after procedure
Second-trimester abortion or delivery, if not breastfeeding	Days 21–28 after end of pregnancy
Postpartum, breastfeeding	At least 6 weeks after delivery; must meet other criteria, above

designed, preloaded applicator. Insertion is usually quite simple; in research studies, the mean time for insertion was 0.5 to 1 minute.[10,17,22,28] Insert Implanon at the inner side of the upper arm in the groove between the biceps and triceps muscles. If a patient has had implants previously, place the new implants in the opposite arm. Inject a local anesthetic along the intended insertion track, and then insert the implant in the subdermal tissue. Insertion deeper than that can hamper removal later. The Implanon inserter works like an inserter for intrauterine contraceptives: the obturator is held stable while the cannula is withdrawn, and then the cannula is withdrawn leaving the implant in place.

After insertion, *confirm the presence of the implant in the arm* by palpation or, if necessary, other means such as ultrasound or magnetic resonance imaging (MRI). Unrecognized failure to insert the implant is the leading cause of pregnancy among Implanon users.[9,25]

MANAGING PROBLEMS AND FOLLOW-UP
No specific clinical follow-up is needed after insertion as long as the patient is not having any problem.

Abnormal vaginal bleeding. Implant users can be reassured that bleeding due to implants is generally not dangerous. If the implants are in place, were inserted at the recommended time of the woman's cycle, and are not outdated, pregnancy is so unlikely that a pregnancy test or evaluation for pregnancy is not mandatory unless the patient has other signs of an abnormal pregnancy (such as abdominal or pelvic pain) or risk factors for ectopic pregnancy. Prostaglandin inhibitors and supplemental estrogen have been effective acute treatments for abnormal bleeding caused by other hormonal contraceptives and may be worth trying in implant users. Remove the implants if the patient so desires.

Removal. Implant removal is usually accomplished easily through a minor surgical procedure. Inject a local anesthesia under the distal end of the implant (to avoid skin swelling over the implant, which might cause difficulty locating the implant). Make a small longitudinal incision in the skin. If a fibrous sheath has formed around the implant, the sheath must be incised. Locate and grasp the implant, then remove it with forceps. In research studies, the mean time for removal was between 2.2 and 3.5 minutes.[10,17,22,28] Removal may be more difficult if the implant is deeply placed. Rods that are not palpable may be located through ultrasound or magnetic resonance imaging. If implants cannot be seen using these modalities, consider the possibility that the implants were never inserted initially (see above). Serum etonogestrel levels have been useful in confirming whether or not implants are present.[70,71] No data are available on the risks of leaving implants in place for longer than the recommended duration of efficacy; if a woman does not desire pregnancy and is not planning to use another hormonal method of contraception, removal may not be necessary.

USER INSTRUCTIONS FOR CONTRACEPTIVE IMPLANTS

1. Contact a clinician if you develop symptoms of infection at the insertion site (tenderness, redness, swelling, discharge).
2. Record the date when the implant(s) should be removed. After that date, do not rely on the implant(s) for contraception.

REFERENCES

1. Meirik O, Fraser IS, d'Arcangues C. Implantable contraceptives for women. Hum Reprod Update. 2003;9:49–59.
2. Steiner MJ, Lopez LM, Grimes DA, et al. Sino-implant (II)–a levonorgestrel-releasing two-rod implant: systematic review of the randomized controlled trials. Contraception. 2010;81:197–201.
3. Mansour D, Mommers E, Teede H, et al. Clinician satisfaction and insertion characteristics of a new applicator to insert radiopaque Implanon: an open-label, noncontrolled, multicenter trial. Contraception. 2010;82:243–9.
4. Sivin I. Risks and benefits, advantages and disadvantages of levonorgestrel-releasing contraceptive implants. Drug Saf. 2003;26:303–35.
5. Barbosa IC, Maia H Jr, Coutinho E, et al. Effects of a single Silastic contraceptive implant containing nomegestrol acetate (Uniplant) on endometrial morphology and ovarian function for 1 year. Contraception. 2006;74:492–7.
6. Van den Bosch T, Donders GG, Riphagen I, et al. Ultrasonographic features of the endometrium and the ovaries in women on etonogestrel implant. Ultrasound Obstet Gynecol. 2002;20:377–80.

7. Makarainen L, van Beek A, Tuomivaara L, Asplund B, Coelingh Bennink H. Ovarian function during the use of a single contraceptive implant: Implanon compared with Norplant. Fertil Steril. 1998;69:714–21.

8. Steiner MJ. Contraceptive effectiveness: what should the counseling message be? JAMA. 1999;282: 1405–7.

9. Graesslin O, Korver T. The contraceptive efficacy of Implanon: a review of clinical trials and marketing experience. Eur J Contracept Reprod Health Care. 2008;13 Suppl 1:4–12.

10. Zheng SR, Zheng HM, Qian SZ, Sang GW, Kaper RF. A randomized multicenter study comparing the efficacy and bleeding pattern of a single-rod (Implanon) and a six-capsule (Norplant) hormonal contraceptive implant. Contraception. 1999;60:1–8.

11. Zheng SR, Zheng HM, Qian SZ, Sang GW, Kaper RF. A long-term study of the efficacy and acceptability of a single-rod hormonal contraceptive implant (Implanon) in healthy women in China. Eur J Contracept Reprod Health Care. 1999;4:85–93.

12. Arribas-Mir L, Rueda-Lozano D, Agrela-Cardona M, Cedeno-Benavides T, Olvera-Porcel C, Bueno-Cavanillas A. Insertion and 3-year follow-up experience of 372 etonogestrel subdermal contraceptive implants by family physicians in Granada, Spain. Contraception. 2009;80:457–62.

13. Yildizbas B, Sahin HG, Kolusari A, Zeteroglu S, Kamaci M. Side effects and acceptability of Implanon: a pilot study conducted in eastern Turkey. Eur J Contracept Reprod Health Care. 2007;12:248–52.

14. Gezginc K, Balci O, Karatayli R, Colakoglu MC. Contraceptive efficacy and side effects of Implanon. Eur J Contracept Reprod Health Care. 2007;12:362–5.

15. Harvey C, Seib C, Lucke J. Continuation rates and reasons for removal among Implanon users accessing two family planning clinics in Queensland, Australia. Contraception. 2009;80:527–32.

16. Lakha F, Glasier AF. Continuation rates of Implanon in the UK: data from an observational study in a clinical setting. Contraception. 2006;74:287–9.

17. Thamkhantho M, Jivasak-Apimas S, Angsuwathana S, Chiravacharadej G, Intawong J. One-year assessment of women receiving sub-dermal contraceptive implant at Siriraj Family Planning Clinic. J Med Assoc Thai. 2008;91:775–80.

18. Agrawal A, Robinson C. An assessment of the first 3 years' use of Implanon in Luton. J Fam Plann Reprod Health Care. 2005;31:310–2.

19. Lipetz C, Phillips C, Fleming C. Actual cost of providing long-acting reversible contraception: a study of Implanon cost. J Fam Plann Reprod Health Care. 2009;35:75–9.

20. Rai K, Gupta S, Cotter S. Experience with Implanon in a northeast London family planning clinic. Eur J Contracept Reprod Health Care. 2004;9:39–46.

21. Booranabunyat S, Taneepanichskul S. Implanon use in Thai women above the age of 35 years. Contraception. 2004;69:489–91.

22. Flores JB, Balderas ML, Bonilla MC, Vazquez-Estrada L. Clinical experience and acceptability of the etonogestrel subdermal contraceptive implant. Int J Gynaecol Obstet. 2005;90:228–33.

23. Smith A, Reuter S. An assessment of the use of Implanon in three community services. J Fam Plann Reprod Health Care. 2002;28:193–6.

24. Reader CA. Pregnancy at time of change of Implanon implant. J Fam Plann Reprod Health Care. 2009;35:265; author reply 265.

25. Harrison-Woolrych M, Hill R. Unintended pregnancies with the etonogestrel implant (Implanon): a case series from postmarketing experience in Australia. Contraception. 2005;71:306–8.

26. Bennink HJ. The pharmacokinetics and pharmacodynamics of Implanon, a single-rod etonogestrel contraceptive implant. Eur J Contracept Reprod Health Care. 2000;5 Suppl 2:12–20.

27. Kiriwat O, Patanayindee A, Koetsawang S, Korver T, Bennink HJ. A 4-year pilot study on the efficacy and safety of Implanon, a single-rod hormonal contraceptive implant, in healthy women in Thailand. Eur J Contracept Reprod Health Care. 1998;3:85–91.

28. Funk S, Miller MM, Mishell DR Jr, et al. Safety and efficacy of Implanon, a single-rod implantable contraceptive containing etonogestrel. Contraception. 2005;71:319–26.

29. Mansour D, Korver T, Marintcheva-Petrova M, Fraser IS. The effects of Implanon on menstrual bleeding patterns. Eur J Contracept Reprod Health Care. 2008;13 Suppl 1:13–28.

30. Ponpuckdee J, Taneepanichskul S. The effects of implanon in the symptomatic treatment of endometriosis. J Med Assoc Thai. 2005;88 Suppl 2:S7–10.

31. Yisa SB, Okenwa AA, Husemeyer RP. Treatment of pelvic endometriosis with etonogestrel subdermal implant (Implanon). J Fam Plann Reprod Health Care. 2005;31:67–70.

32. Walch K, Unfried G, Huber J, et al. Implanon versus medroxyprogesterone acetate: effects on pain scores in patients with symptomatic endometriosis–a pilot study. Contraception. 2009;79:29–34.

33. Shokeir T, Amr M, Abdelshaheed M. The efficacy of Implanon for the treatment of chronic pelvic pain associated with pelvic congestion: 1-year randomized controlled pilot study. Arch Gynecol Obstet. 2009;280:437–43.

34. Egberg N, van Beek A, Gunnervik C, et al. Effects on the hemostatic system and liver function in relation to Implanon and Norplant. A prospective randomized clinical trial. Contraception. 1998;58 :93–8.

35. Dorflinger LJ. Metabolic effects of implantable steroid contraceptives for women. Contraception. 2002;65:47–62.

36. Nasr A, Nafeh HM. Effect of etonogestrel contraceptive implant (Implanon) on portal blood flow and liver functions. Contraception. 2009;79:236–9.

37. Inal MM, Yildirim Y, Ertopcu K, Avci ME, Ozelmas I, Tinar S. Effect of the subdermal contraceptive etonogestrel implant (Implanon) on biochemical and hormonal parameters (three years follow-up). Eur J Contracept Reprod Health Care. 2008;13: 238–42.

38. Merki-Feld GS, Imthurn B, Seifert B. Effects of the progestagen-only contraceptive implant Implanon on cardiovascular risk factors. Clin Endocrinol (Oxf). 2008;68: 355–60.

39. Taheri M, Rahimi M, Naderi M, et al. Effects of a subdermal levonorgestrel contraceptive implant (Norplant) on serum cholesterol, triglycerides, ALT and AST in Iranian women. Contraception. 2006;73:56–8.

40. Biswas A, Viegas OA, Roy AC. Effect of Implanon and Norplant subdermal contraceptive implants on serum lipids–a randomized comparative study. Contraception. 2003;68:189–93.

41. Blumenthal PD, Gemzell-Danielsson K, Marintcheva-Petrova M. Tolerability and clinical safety of Implanon. Eur J Contracept Reprod Health Care. 2008;13 Suppl 1:29–36.

42. Vieira CS, Ferriani RA, Garcia AA, et al. Use of the etonogestrel-releasing implant is associated with hypoactivation of the coagulation cascade. Hum Reprod. 2007;22: 2196–201.

43. Meyer C, Talbot M, Teede H. Effect of Implanon on insulin resistance in women with Polycystic Ovary Syndrome. Aust N Z J Obstet Gynaecol. 2005;45:155–8.

44. Vicente L, Mendonca D, Dingle M, Duarte R, Boavida JM. Etonogestrel implant in women with diabetes mellitus. Eur J Contracept Reprod Health Care. 2008;13:387–95.

45. Chakhtoura Z, Canonico M, Gompel A, Thalabard JC, Scarabin PY, Plu-Bureau G. Progestogen-only contraceptives and the risk of stroke: a meta-analysis. Stroke. 2009;40:1059–62.

46. Davies GC, Feng LX, Newton JR, Van Beek A, Coelingh-Bennink HJ. Release characteristics, ovarian activity and menstrual bleeding pattern with a single contraceptive implant releasing 3-ketodesogestrel. Contraception. 1993;47:251–61.
47. Foster DG, Rostovtseva DP, Brindis CD, Biggs MA, Hulett D, Darney PD. Cost savings from the provision of specific methods of contraception in a publicly funded program. Am J Public Health. 2009;99 :446–51.
48. Trussell J, Lalla AM, Doan QV, Reyes E, Pinto L, Gricar J. Cost effectiveness of contraceptives in the United States. Contraception. 2009;79:5–14.
49. Abdel-Aleem H, d'Arcangues C, Vogelsong KM, Gulmezoglu AM. Treatment of vaginal bleeding irregularities induced by progestin only contraceptives. Cochrane Database Syst Rev. 2007;CD003449.
50. Archer DF, Philput CB, Levine AS, et al. Effects of ethinyl estradiol and ibuprofen compared to placebo on endometrial bleeding, cervical mucus and the postcoital test in levonorgestrel subcutaneous implant users. Contraception. 2008;78:106–12.
51. Vidin E, Garbin O, Rodriguez B, Favre R, Bettahar-Lebugle K. Removal of etonogestrel contraceptive implants in the operating theater: report on 28 cases. Contraception. 2007;76:35–9.
52. Ismail H, Mansour D, Singh M. Migration of Implanon. J Fam Plann Reprod Health Care. 2006;32:157–9.
53. Osman N, Mirlesse V. [A new complication of contraceptive hormonal implant: about two cases of lesions of the ulnar nerve at the arm level]. Gynecol Obstet Fertil. 2005;33:322–5.
54. Agrawal A, Robinson C. Spontaneous snapping of an Implanon in two halves in situ. J Fam Plann Reprod Health Care. 2003;29:238.
55. Brache V, Faundes A, Alvarez F, Cochon L. Nonmenstrual adverse events during use of implantable contraceptives for women: data from clinical trials. Contraception. 2002;65:63–74.
56. Hidalgo MM, Lisondo C, Juliato CT, Espejo-Arce X, Monteiro I, Bahamondes L. Ovarian cysts in users of Implanon and Jadelle subdermal contraceptive implants. Contraception. 2006;73:532–6.
57. Riggs M, Klebanoff M, Nansel T, Zhang J, Schwebke J, Andrews W. Longitudinal association between hormonal contraceptives and bacterial vaginosis in women of reproductive age. Sex Transm Dis. 2007;34:954–9.
58. Zingone MM, Guirguis AB, Airee A, Cobb D. Probable drug interaction between warfarin and hormonal contraceptives. Ann Pharmacother. 2009;43:2096–102.
59. Pongsatha S, Ekmahachai M, Suntornlimsiri N, Morakote N, Chaovisitsaree S. Bone mineral density in women using the subdermal contraceptive implant Implanon for at least 2years. Int J Gynaecol Obstet. 2010;109:223–5.
60. Monteiro-Dantas C, Espejo-Arce X, Lui-Filho JF, Fernandes AM, Monteiro I, Bahamondes L. A three-year longitudinal evaluation of the forearm bone density of users of etonogestrel- and levonorgestrel-releasing contraceptive implants. Reprod Health. 2007;4:11.
61. Beerthuizen R, van Beek A, Massai R, Makarainen L, Hout J, Bennink HC. Bone mineral density during long-term use of the progestagen contraceptive implant Implanon compared to a non-hormonal method of contraception. Hum Reprod 2000;15:118–22.
62. Bahamondes L, Monteiro-Dantas C, Espejo-Arce X, et al. A prospective study of the forearm bone density of users of etonorgestrel- and levonorgestrel-releasing contraceptive implants. Hum Reprod. 2006;21:466–70.
63. World Health Organization. Medical Eligibility Criteria for Contraceptive Use. 4. Geneva: World Health Organization, 2009.
64. Centers for Disease Control and Prevention. U. S. Medical Eligibility Criteria for Contraceptive Use, 2010. MMWR. 2010;59 (No. RR-4):1–85.
65. Diaz S. Contraceptive implants and lactation. Contraception. 2002;65:39–46.

66. Reinprayoon D, Taneepanichskul S, Bunyavejchevin S, et al. Effects of the etonogestrel-releasing contraceptive implant (Implanon) on parameters of breastfeeding compared to those of an intrauterine device. Contraception. 2000;62:239–46.

67. Brito MB, Ferriani RA, Quintana SM, Yazlle ME, Silva de Sa MF, Vieira CS. Safety of the etonogestrel-releasing implant during the immediate postpartum period: a pilot study. Contraception. 2009;80 :519–26.

68. Taneepanichskul S, Reinprayoon D, Thaithumyanon P, Praisuwanna P, Tosukho-wong P, Dieben T. Effects of the etonogestrel-releasing implant Implanon and a nonmedicated intrauterine device on the growth of breast-fed infants. Contraception. 2006;73:368–71.

69. Chikamata DM, Miller S. Health services at the clinic level and implantable contraceptives for women. Contraception. 2002;65:97–106.

70. Singh M, Mansour D, Richardson D. Location and removal of non-palpable Implanon implants with the aid of ultrasound guidance. J Fam Plann Reprod Health Care. 2006;32:153–6.

71. Shulman LP, Gabriel H. Management and localization strategies for the nonpalpable Implanon rod. Contraception. 2006;73:325–30.

Injectable Contraceptives

Deborah Bartz, MD, MPH
Alisa B. Goldberg, MD, MPH

- Injectable contraceptives are effective birth control.
- Progestin-only injections are an important contraceptive option for women who cannot use estrogen.
- Injections provide a highly private and convenient method of contraception.
- Counseling women about the menstrual cycle changes associated with injectable contraceptives can substantially lower discontinuation rates.
- Progestin-only injectable contraceptives have not been associated with an increased risk of fragility fractures; therefore, concerns about skeletal health should not limit their use in most women.

Depo-Provera (DMPA-IM) 150 mg/1 ml. The most commonly used injectable contraceptive is depot medroxyprogesterone acetate (DMPA), marketed as Depo-Provera, given in a deep intramuscular (IM) injection of 150 milligrams (mg) every 12 weeks (or 3 months). DMPA is extremely effective, in part because it is forgiving for women who return up to 4 weeks late for an injection.[1]

Depo-subQ Provera 104 (DMPA-SC) 104 mg/0.65 ml. This formulation of DMPA has been dose-adjusted to be given subcutaneously every 12 weeks (or 3 months). Its efficacy and side effect profile are similar to that of DMPA-IM.[2,3]

Short-term injectable contraceptives. Although not available in the United States, these short-term injectables are popular methods in China, Eastern Asia, and Latin America; they are not discussed further in this chapter.

1. Lunelle (medroxyprogesterone acetate 25 mg and estradiol cypionate 5 mg). This highly effective combined IM monthly inject-

able is associated with better bleeding patterns than progestin-only injectables.

2. Mesigyna (norethindrone ethanate 50 mg and estradiol valerate 5 mg). This IM monthly injectable has a better bleeding profile than Lunelle, with better efficacy and faster return to fertility.

3. Dihydroxyprogesterone acetophenide (150 mg) and estradiol enanthate (10 mg). This monthly IM injectable has bleeding patterns similar to Lunelle.

4. Norethindrone ethanate (200 mg). This bimonthly IM injectable has the same mechanism of action and advantages and disadvantages as DMPA.

MECHANISM OF ACTION

DMPA prevents pregnancy primarily by inhibiting ovulation.[4] The dose of DMPA provided in each injection suppresses levels of follicle stimulating hormone (FSH) and luteinizing hormone (LH) and eliminates the LH surge. The pituitary gland remains responsive to gonadotropin-releasing hormone (GnRH), which suggests that the site of action of DMPA is the hypothalamus and the primary mechanism of action is inhibition of GnRH pulsatility.[5] After a woman discontinues DMPA, there is a great deal of variability noted in time to ovulation postinjection, with most women resuming ovulation 15 to 49 weeks from the last injection.[6]

DMPA also prevents pregnancy by thickening and decreasing cervical mucus, an anti-estrogenic effect that prevents sperm penetration.[7,8]

DMPA alters the endometrium, making it atrophic and not receptive to implantation; however, given the effectiveness of DMPA at inhibiting ovulation and thickening the cervical mucus, it is unclear if this endometrial atrophy significantly contributes to the contraceptive effect of DMPA.[8,9]

EFFECTIVENESS

DMPA-IM (150 mg)

DMPA-IM is highly effective (see Figure 3–1). With correct and consistent use, the probability of pregnancy is only 0.2%. With typical use, the failure rate is 6%. These estimates apply to an 11 to 13 week regimen, with each injection providing 150 mg of DMPA per 1 cc. (For a comparative view of first-year contraceptive failure rates, see Table 26–1 in Chapter 26 on Contraceptive Efficacy.) Efficacy is not compromised by greater body weight. Because DMPA avoids first-pass metabolism, its efficacy is unaffected by a woman's use of other medications that may increase hepatic enzyme activation.[2]

DMPA-SC (104 mg)

In two large, open-label, phase 3 studies of DMPA-SC, there were no reported pregnancies in a total of 16,023 woman-cycles of use.[3] In a recent large randomized study, the cumulative pregnancy rate over the 2-year study period was 0% in DMPA-SC users compared with 0.8% in the DMPA-IM group.[10]

CONTINUATION RATES

In the largest U.S. study of DMPA use, reported in 1973, continuation rates were 59.4% at 1 year, 41.5% at 2 years, 30.2% at 3 years, and 24.1% at 4 years.[11] More recent studies report lower continuation rates: from 26% to 53% at 1 year, with the most common reasons for discontinuation relating to a lack of adequate user education regarding bleeding disturbances including amenorrhea.[12–15] In the past decade, concern about DMPA's effect on skeletal health has probably also becomes a primary reason for the patient to discontinue the method or for the physician to suggest discontinuation. (See section on Bone Density in Special Issues.) Counseling about the expected hormonal effects can improve DMPA continuation rates.[13,16,17] In rural Mexico, 175 women received detailed, structured counseling about the hormonal effects of DMPA at both pretreatment and each injection visit, while 175 received routine counseling and information. Over 12 months, only 8% of women who received structured counseling discontinued use due to amenorrhea or irregular or heavy bleeding, compared with 32% of women who received routine counseling. The cumulative life table discontinuation rate was 17% among women receiving structured counseling versus 43% among women receiving routine counseling.[16] Simply encouraging women to come in for a visit if they are having a problem with DMPA can also improve continuation rates.[17]

Upon discontinuing DMPA, many women do not switch to another highly effective contraceptive method. Two studies of low-income, urban women reported unintended pregnancy rates of 20% to 22% within 9 months of stopping DMPA.[18,19]

While not FDA-approved for at-home administration, the potential for self-administration of DMPA-SC could positively influence DMPA continuation rates due to greater convenience. In one survey study of 176 women who were currently using DMPA, 67% expressed an interest in self-administration of their DMPA at home.[20] In a follow-up survey of 313 users of other contraceptive methods, 64% reported they would like fewer clinic visits relating to contraceptive needs, while 26% of never-DMPA users and 40% of ex-DMPA users reported they would consider using DMPA if self-administration were possible.[20]

A DVANTAGES

Advantages of DMPA Injectables

1. **No estrogen.** Because DMPA injections contain no estrogen, they do not appear to cause the rare but serious complications attributable to exogenous estrogen (including venous thrombo-embolism, myocardial infarction, or stroke). Studies thus far have not shown that serious cardiovascular effects are associated with use of progestin-only contraceptives.[9,21,22] In 2006, the American College of Obstetricians and Gynecologists released a Technical Bulletin that states DMPA is an appropriate contraceptive option for women with known risk factors for or subsequent diagnosis of venous thromboembolism, coronary artery disease, congestive heart failure, or cerebrovascular disease.[23] In a recent systematic review, DMPA been shown to be safe and beneficial in anticoagulated patients with current venous thrombosis, improving symptoms associated with hemorrhagic cysts and men-orrhagia while not putting them at risk for further thrombotic events.[24]

2. **Reversibility.** DMPA is reversible once the effect of the last injection wears off. DMPA does not cause long-term loss of fertility; however, ovulation may not return until 9 to 10 months after the last dose.[1]

3. **Intermediate-term effective contraception, even for obese women.** DMPA provides 3 months of highly effective contraception per injection. There is no decrease in the efficacy of DMPA among overweight or obese women.[3]

4. **Infrequent dosing.** Because the efficacy of DMPA does not require frequent dosing or partner cooperation, this method is ideal for populations that may have contraceptive adherence difficulties, such as adolescents. Compared with adolescent users of oral contraceptive pills, teenagers using DMPA have higher continuation rates and lower repeat pregnancy rates.[25,26] Other high-risk populations may benefit from the ease of adherence with DMPA.

5. **Reduced risk of ectopic pregnancy.** Compared with women using no contraceptive at all, women who use DMPA have a reduced risk for having an ectopic pregnancy. Although the

overall risk of pregnancy and thus ectopic pregnancy is lowered by DMPA, the possibility of an ectopic pregnancy should be excluded if a woman using DMPA becomes pregnant. One study showed that 1.5% of women who got pregnant on DMPA had an ectopic pregnancy, the same ectopic rate as women who conceived while not using contraception.[27]

6. **Absence of menstrual bleeding.** DMPA causes women to have very light periods or to miss periods entirely. These patterns of bleeding are considered by many women to be an advantage, provided they have an opportunity to discuss these changes at counseling sessions. During the first year of DMPA use, approximately 10% to 30% of women are amenorrheic after one injection and 40% to 50% are amenorrheic after four injections.[11,28] By the end of the fifth year of use, approximately 80% of women are amenorrheic. In a study of teenagers, nearly two thirds of DMPA users reported amenorrhea at 6 months.[29] Similar amenorrhea rates are reported with DMPA-SC.[30] Although clinicians and some women may consider the absence of menstrual bleeding an advantage of using DMPA, others may not.

7. **Improvement of menstrual symptoms.** DMPA is associated with a decrease in ovulation pain, cyclic menstrual cramps, mood changes, headaches, breast tenderness, and nausea.[31]

8. **Culturally acceptable.** In some cultures, a woman may consider medication by injection desirable. Some women wish to use a contraceptive without their partner's knowledge. Many couples find DMPA use attractive because it is not intrusive in a relationship. Disrupted menstrual bleeding patterns may also have positive or negative cultural implications for some women, depending on the bleeding pattern.[32] Inform women about the expected hormonal effects of DMPA.

9. **Minimal drug interactions.** There has been no demonstrated interaction between DMPA and antibiotics, antiretrovirals, or enzyme-inducing drugs.[33,34] The only drug that decreases the effectiveness of DMPA is aminoglutethimide, which is used to suppress adrenal function in some women with Cushing's disease.[35]

10. **Fewer seizures.** DMPA has been found to decrease the frequency of grand mal seizures.[36,37] Improvement in seizure control is probably due to the sedative properties of progestins, and this effect may be mediated through gamma-aminobutyric acid (GABA) receptors in the hippocampus.[38] Taking anti-seizure medicine has no impact on the efficacy of DMPA.

11. **Fewer sickle cell crises.** DMPA may stabilize the membrane of red blood cells, making cells less prone to sickling and reducing the frequency of resultant pain crises. In a randomized trial, DMPA use was associated with a greater reduction in the frequency of sickle cell crises than were COC use or no intervention. After 1 year of DMPA use, 70% of women were pain-free (compared with 50% of women not using hormones), and of the women who had continuing crises, only 16% reported the ongoing pain as intense.[39]

12. **Less pain from endometriosis.** DMPA has been shown to reduce pain associated with endometriosis.[40,41] A recent randomized, blinded trial compared DMPA-SC to leuprolide for management of the pain associated with endometriosis. This trial found equivalent pain reduction with both treatment options and less bone mineral density loss with DMPA-SC.[42] In 2005, the FDA approved use of DMPA-SC for this indication.

13. **Benefits for women with myomas.** DMPA has been used effectively to decrease the bleeding associated with myomas and improve hemoglobin levels.[43,44] DMPA use may also shrink myomas[44]; however, the evidence on this is conflicting.[43] Studies have shown that DMPA use is associated with a lower risk of recurrent myomas after myomectomy.[45]

14. **Decreased risk of pelvic inflammatory disease.** Thickened cervical mucous may prevent ascent of pathogens to the upper genital tract.[46]

15. **Decreased risk of endometrial cancer.** The reduction in endometrial cancer is similar to that seen in women taking oral contraceptive pills, as much as an 80% reduction in risk.[47,48]

Potential Additional Advantages of DMPA-SC

1. Subcutaneous injections may be less painful than IM injections.

2. Although not FDA-approved, self-administration of DMPA-SC may be acceptable to many women.[20] Self-injection may improve adherence with the method by eliminating the need for women to periodically return to a health care provider for injections.[49]

DISADVANTAGES AND CAUTIONS

Adverse Effects of DMPA

1. **Menstrual cycle disturbances.** Bleeding patterns with DMPA use are unpredictable, with the majority of women experiencing

infrequent but prolonged episodes of bleeding or spotting.[28] The overall incidence of irregular bleeding is 70% in the first year, with a decrease in irregular bleeding with each reinjection, and rates as low as 10% after the first year.[50] Many women experience either an increased number of days of light bleeding or amenorrhea. Amenorrhea becomes more common over time among DMPA users. Approximately 40% to 50% of users experience amenorrhea after 1 year of use and 80% after 5 years of use.[11,28] Similar patterns have been observed with DMPA-SC, with 55% of women achieving amenorrhea after 1 year of use.[3,30] Rarely do women using DMPA experience an increased number of days of heavy bleeding. Menstrual irregularity is the most common reason for discontinuation of DMPA. Approximately 20% to 25% of women will discontinue DMPA within the first year because of menstrual disturbances.[12,14,15,29] Of those who discontinue for menstrual disturbances, the majority discontinue for either prolonged bleeding or amenorrhea.[51] The irregular bleeding associated with progestin-only contraception has been associated with an increased fragility of endometrial capillaries.[52]

2. **Weight gain.** Weight gain is common in many women using DMPA; however, this effect is not consistent for all women. In one study of adults, Brazilian women using DMPA for 5 years gained an average of approximately 9 pounds, significantly more than the 5 pounds gained by IUD users over the same time interval.[53] Another large study of DMPA use in Chinese women showed no weight gain over 1 year of use.[54]

However, the only randomized trial assigned women to DMPA versus placebo and then measured food intake, energy expenditure, and weight gain over 3 months found no difference between groups.[55] All women in this trial were of normal weight. It is possible that certain women are more likely to gain weight with DMPA use than others. A recent systematic review of the literature concluded that among adult women, baseline weight or body mass index does not have an effect on resulting weight gain in adult DMPA users.[56]

This topic has also been addressed in the literature specifically pertaining to adolescents. One study showed that 56% of teen DMPA users either lost weight or gained less than 5% of their baseline weight, and 25% gained more than 10% of their baseline weight. The teens who gained more than 5% of their baseline weight in the first 3 months of use were highly likely to gain more weight with continued use.[57] Two other studies in adolescents showed that at 12 and 18 month follow-up, overweight and obese DMPA users had gained more weight compared with adolescents of normal weight.[58,59] Consequently, the World Health Organization (WHO) established a new subcategory within the eligibility criteria for DMPA use for obese adolescents, with a rating of category 2 for DMPA initation.[60] However, the finding that girls with a higher baseline weight may gain more weight on DMPA[58–61] has not been consistent.[57,62] One study found greater weight gain among black adolescents on DMPA compared with white adolescents on DMPA.[61] In the trials of DMPA-SC, the median weight gain over 1 year of use was approximately 3.5 pounds, and 4% to 8% of women reported weight gain as an adverse effect.[3,63]

Among women who gain weight while on DMPA, the weight gain has been demonstrated to be due to increases in fat deposition, not fluid retention.[61,64] It had been presumed that the observed increase in fat deposition was probably due to increased appetite,[64] but a recent study of adolescent DMPA users that measured appetite in a standardized fashion found DMPA to be associated with decreased appetite, despite increases in total body fat.[61] Weight gain is commonly cited as a reason for discontinuation of DMPA, with 12% to 19% discontinuing for this reason.[12,14,15]

3. **Depression.** Individual women may experience an increase in depression when they use DMPA. However, data evaluating the impact of DMPA on mood are limited and conflicting. One recent study showed a slight increase in the likelihood of depression in DMPA users, but other studies have shown no association.[65–68] A history of depression is not a contraindication to DMPA use. The WHO medical eligibility criteria rate DMPA use in women with a history of depression as category 2 (benefits usually outweigh the risks).[60] If depression occurs or worsens in a woman following a DMPA injection, her symptoms may persist for the duration of the injection because it is not possible to discontinue DMPA immediately.[69] Clinical management of depression must take this into account. Use caution in providing DMPA postpartum for a woman with a history of severe postpartum depression, and consider waiting until 6 weeks postpartum for the first injection. If prescribing DMPA for a woman with current depression, ensure that she has adequate mental health care and follow-up.

4. **Bone density decrease.** Long-term DMPA users may develop temporary and usually reversible decreased bone density. (See section on bone density in Special Issues.)

5. **Allergic reactions.** Although rare, severe allergic reactions may occur.[70] Some programs encourage women to remain in the

vicinity of the clinic for 20 minutes after an injection. To prevent severe allergic reactions, ask women if they have experienced significant itching or redness at the site of previous DMPA injections and do not repeat DMPA dosing if allergic reaction is suspected.

6. **Metabolic effects.** There appears to be no clinically significant change in lipoprotein profiles while on DMPA, possibly due to the avoidance of first-pass metabolism. A multicenter clinical trial by WHO did find a transient increase in total cholesterol and low-density lipoprotein cholesterol accompanied by a brief decrease in high-density lipoprotein cholesterol in the first weeks following injection when serum hormone levels were the highest.[71] Other studies have demonstrated similar results.[72] However, the clinical significance of these findings is unclear. DMPA has not been shown to affect carbohydrate metabolism or coagulation factors.

7. **Other adverse effects.** In one of the largest studies of DMPA users, 17% of the 3,875 women complained of headaches, 11% of nervousness, 5% of decreased libido, 3% of breast discomfort.[11]

Disadvantages of DMPA

1. **Not possible to discontinue immediately.** Weight gain, depression, breast tenderness, allergic reactions, and menstrual irregularities may continue until DMPA is cleared from a woman's body, about 6 to 8 months after her last injection. Clearance is slower in heavier women. Approximately half of women who discontinue DMPA will have resumption of normal menses 6 months after the last injection, while 25% will wait a year before a normal bleeding pattern returns.[50]

2. **Delay in return of fertility.** After discontinuing DMPA, the median delay to conception is 9 to 10 months after last injection, which is longer than with other hormonal contraceptive methods.[1,11] A recent systematic review demonstrated there is a wide range in resumption of ovulation, anywhere from 15 to 49 weeks from the last injection, making fertility prediction difficult following DMPA discontinuation.[6]

3. **Return visits required every 3 months.** For some women, visits for repeated injections of DMPA are unacceptable. Approximately 20% to 50% of women continue to use DMPA at 1 year, and many who discontinue do so because of the difficulty in returning for injections.[12,15,17] Home visits for injections have been scheduled for some wheelchair-bound patients. Convenient access to DMPA injections through flexible and expanded clinic

hours or pharmacist-administered injections may improve continuation rates.[73] With DMPA-SC, self-injection may be possible, which may decrease the need for return visits.

PRECAUTIONS

Two documents—the 2009 World Health Organization (WHO) Medical Eligibility Criteria (MEC) and the 2010 adaptation of these guidelines by the Centers of Disease Control and Prevention (CDC) for the United States (U.S. MEC)—guide health care providers in determining who can safely use various contraceptive methods. (See Chapter 4 for a full discussion.) Compared with estrogen-containing methods, DMPA has only one absolute contraindication (category 4): current breast cancer.[60,74] There are several conditions listed as category 3 (risks usually outweigh benefits). Generally these conditions include evidence of current cardiovascular disease, women with abnormal liver function or liver tumors, women with a history of breast cancer, and women with unexplained vaginal bleeding prior to evaluation (see Chapter 4). Providing DMPA in these circumstances requires careful clinical judgment and access to clinical services.[60,74]

S PECIAL ISSUES

BREASTFEEDING WOMEN

Some experts have voiced concern that progestin-only methods may thwart lactation if they are initiated before the postdelivery decline in natural progesterone, which functions as the trigger for milk synthesis.[75,76] However, clinical experience in humans has not substantiated that hypothesis.[77] Once breastfeeding has been established, the use of progestin-only contraceptives has not been shown to have an adverse effect on breast milk volume; in some studies, milk production has been enhanced. The quality of breast milk is not affected. Because of theoretical concerns over early neonatal exposure to exogenous steroids, several international organizations have urged that progestin-only methods not be initiated until at least 6 weeks postpartum.[60,78] Studies of DMPA initiated within 1 to 3 days postpartum,[77] 7 days postpartum,[79] or within 6 weeks postpartum[80] have found no adverse effects. In the U.S. MEC, family planning experts in the United States have endorsed the safety of administering DMPA immediately postpartum in women, classifying DMPA as category 2 immediately postpartum regardless of breastfeeding status.[74,81,82] Because DMPA does not carry the prothrombotic concern of estrogen-based contraceptives, it may be initiated immediately after delivery without increasing the risk of thromboembolism. (See Chapter 18 on Postpartum Contraception and Lactation.)

CANCER RISK AND DMPA

Breast cancer. There is no increase in the risk of breast cancer with DMPA use. In a pooled international study including 1,768 women with breast cancer and more than 13,000 controls, the overall relative risk associated with the use of DMPA was 1.1 (95% CI=0.97–1.4). There was no increased risk with longer use of DMPA; however, women who had used DMPA within the past 5 years had an increased risk of breast cancer (RR=2.0; 95% CI=1.5–2.8).[83] This increased risk may reflect either increased detection of breast cancer in DMPA users due to increased surveillance or accelerated growth of preexisting tumors. Two more recent studies have also shown no association between DMPA use and breast cancer, with no increased cancer risk with recent or current use.[84,85]

Reproductive tract cancers. There does not appear to be any association between invasive cervical cancer and DMPA use. A WHO Collaborative Study of 2,009 women with invasive cervical cancer and more than 9,000 controls failed to demonstrate a significantly increased risk (RR=1.1; 95% CI=1.0–1.3).[86] Another large case-control study similarly found no association between adenocarcinoma or adenosquamous carcinoma of the cervix and DMPA use.[87] Large WHO case-control studies have similarly demonstrated that DMPA use is not associated with ovarian cancer (RR=1.1; 95% CI=0.6, 1.8) and is associated with a significantly decreased risk of endometrial cancer (RR 0.2; 95% CI=0.1, 0.8).[47,48]

BONE DENSITY AND DMPA

The use of DMPA in contraceptive doses suppresses ovarian production of estradiol, a powerful inhibitor of bone resorption.[8] This has led to concern that DMPA may put women at risk of osteoporosis and resulting bone factures. Because minimal trauma bone fractures occur infrequently in reproductive-age women, the surrogate marker of skeletal health, bone mineral density (BMD), has been examined in many populations of current and previous DMPA users. DMPA is associated with a decrease in BMD[88–92] that is generally temporary and reversible.[93–95] Data suggest that the loss in BMD is rapid within the first 2 years of use, but after approximately 2 years of use, loss of BMD slows dramatically.[94–96] Although women have a decrease in BMD while using DMPA, studies have consistently demonstrated that BMD is regained back to baseline levels equivalent to that seen in non-DMPA users when DMPA is discontinued.[93–95] For women over 21 years, BMD values among women who had previously used DMPA 30 months or less are similar to those of never-users.[94] Other studies comparing past users of DMPA to never-users have similarly shown no difference in BMD.[97]

Although declines in BMD are concerning and recoveries reassuring, the most important question is whether DMPA use increases the risk of fracture, the clinically relevant outcome of interest. Our literature review identified only one case report of a low-trauma fracture in a long-term DMPA user.[98] A study of female military recruits evaluated risk factors for stress fractures during basic training and found that age, race, alcohol and tobacco use, weight-bearing exercise, lowest adult weight, corticosteroid use, and DMPA were associated with stress fractures.[99] However, this study was limited to women at high risk of fractures and may not be applicable to the general population. Another study, a cross-sectional study of developmentally delayed women suggests an increased risk of fractures in previous users of DMPA, a result that again may not be generalizable.[100] A recent case-control study utilized the United Kingdom General Practice Research Database to identify 17,527 women with any bone fracture and 70,130 controls in order to compare fracture rates between DMPA users and users of other hormonal contraceptives. The adjusted ORs for fracture in DMPA users were 1.17 to 1.54, with higher ORs noted in women with longer-term DMPA use. However, fracture rates were higher in DMPA users even before they received their first injection and fracture rate did not increase in these women after they started DMPA. Furthermore, while trauma-related fractures did occur at a higher rate in DMPA users, fragility fractures did not. All of this suggests the higher fracture rate observed in DMPA users in this study does not appear to be due to DMPA use.[140] A recent Cochrane Review found no randomized trials of DMPA and its effect on fracture risk.[101] A similar pattern of the decline in BMD followed by recovery that is seen in DMPA use is also observed with the hypoestrogenism that occurs with pregnancy and lactation.[102,103] Epidemiological evidence has not demonstrated any negative effect on fracture risk associated with pregnancy and lactation.[104]

The decreasing adolescent pregnancy rate in the United States has been paralleled by increased DMPA use in teenagers.[105,106] While this decreasing pregnancy rate likely has multiple contributing factors, the convenience of DMPA dosing for adolescents has likely played a role. Since the effects of contraceptives on bone mass may be particularly important for adolescents who have not yet reached peak bone mass, it is important to know if teenagers who have used DMPA regain bone mass after discontinuing DMPA.[107] A recent study suggests they do regain this bone mass, and that they regain it more quickly than older populations. One study of 170 adolescents (80 DMPA users and 90 controls) ages 14 to 18 years who underwent BMD testing every 6 months for 24 to 36 months, even after discontinuation of DMPA, found that use was associated with significant declines in BMD, but upon discontinuation, former users had a rapid and significant gain in BMD beyond the bone gain observed in control women.[95] This is reassuring and suggests that the bone loss associated with DMPA use is transient. Whether adolescents who use DMPA ultimately reach the same peak bone mass as they would have had they not used DMPA remains unknown. Similarly, we do not know the impact of prolonged DMPA use during adolescence on the risk of fracture later in life.

A separate, important question is whether prolonged DMPA use during the premenopausal years is associated with an increased risk of fracture during menopause. Limited data address this question. One study from New Zealand, where DMPA has been in use for a long time and many previous users are menopausal, did not demonstrate an association between prior DMPA use and postmenopausal fractures, although the study had limited statistical power to detect differences in fracture risk.[108] Another study found similar levels of BMD among women entering the menopause naturally (off hormones) and women with a history of prolonged DMPA use who continued use until they became menopausal. Those entering menopause naturally had a rapid decline in BMD, and those on DMPA had little additional loss with the transition to menopause, suggesting that they had already "lost the estrogen-sensitive component of bone."[109]

In November 2004 the FDA added a black box warning to the label of DMPA: "Women who use Depo-Provera Contraceptive Injection may lose significant bone mineral density. Bone loss is greater with increasing duration of use and may not be completely reversible. It is unknown if use of Depo-Provera Contraceptive Injection during adolescence or early adulthood, a critical period of bone accretion, will reduce peak bone mass and increase the risk for osteoporotic fracture in later life. Depo-Provera Contraceptive Injection should be used as a long-term birth control method (e.g., longer than 2 years) only if other birth control methods are inadequate."[110]

In June 2005, the World Health Organization reviewed the evidence on this subject. They concluded, "there should be no restriction on the use of DMPA, including no restriction on duration of use, among women aged 18 to 45 who are otherwise eligible to use the method." They further recommended that: "Among adolescents (menarche to < 18) and women over 45, the advantages of using DMPA usually outweigh the theoretical safety concerns regarding fracture risk. Since data are insufficient to determine if this is the case with long-term use among these age groups, the overall risks and benefits for continuing use of the method should be reconsidered over time with the individual user."[111] The Society for Adolescent Medicine has advocated for continued use of DMPA in teenage girls—"Continue prescribing DMPA to adolescent girls needing contraception with adequate explanation of benefits and potential risks"—and recommends adequate calcium and vitamin D intake, along with weight-bearing exercise for all adolescents on DMPA.[112] The American College of Obstetricians and Gynecologists states: "skeletal health concerns should not restrict use of DMPA in adult women. In adolescents, the advantages of DMPA likely outweigh the theoretical safety concerns regarding bone mineral density and factures. However, in the absence of long-term data in this population, consideration of long-term use should be individualized."[113]

Clinical management should be dictated by evidence that measures outcomes of interest (like fracture risk), not by surrogate markers of questionable clinical significance (such as bone densitometry in healthy premenopausal women).[114] Despite product labeling, BMD testing should play no role in the routine management of healthy DMPA users, because in premenopausal women there is no good correlation between bone densitometry results and fracture risk.[113,115,116] Similarly, using amenorrhea or serum estradiol levels to guide management is not helpful, because these factors have not consistently been associated with lower BMD or higher fracture risk among DMPA users.[92,96,117]

According to the WHO, "since the effect of DMPA on bone mineral density is largely reversible, any lifetime increase in fracture risk is likely to be small."[111] However, women with conditions that place them at high risk for osteoporosis and fracture, such as chronic corticosteroid use, disorders of bone metabolism, a strong family history of osteoporosis (that may represent a genetic mutation associated with fracture), or anorexia nervosa—may not be well suited for long-term DMPA use.

RISK OF SEXUALLY TRANSMITTED INFECTIONS AND DMPA

DMPA provides no protection against sexually transmitted infections (STIs), including HIV. Several observational studies have shown an association between DMPA use and acquisition of chlamydia,[46,118,119] though a recent systematic review suggests this association is weak.[120] In studies, DMPA use has been inconsistently associated with acquisition of gonorrhea.[46,119,120] While cervical ectopy may increase the presence or identification of chlamydia, ectopy is not an important mediator of the association between DMPA use and chlamydia infection.[46,119] It has been proposed that DMPA might increase the risk of chlamydia because progestins may enhance the growth of chlamydia or impact host immune factors that enable growth.[46,119] Alternatively, the observed relationship between DMPA use and chlamydia may be due to bias inherent in observational studies; women who choose DMPA may be at an increased risk of chlamydia because they are more likely to be a part of social-sexual circles where chlamydia has a higher prevalence.[121] No randomized controlled trial has addressed this question. Despite the association between DMPA use and chlamydia acquisition, DMPA use is associated with a decreased risk of pelvic inflammatory disease.[46,119] Presumably, the progestin-induced thickening of the cervical mucus inhibits ascent of bacteria to the upper genital tract.

Several studies in high-risk populations, including sex workers in Kenya and Thailand, have demonstrated an association between DMPA and HIV acquisition,[122–124] while studies in the general population have been mixed.[120,125,126] These differences may be due to study methodology, or they could be the result of variable levels of risk in different populations (i.e., sex workers with exposure to multiple strains of HIV versus family planning clients).[127] Whether DMPA use causes an increased risk of acquiring HIV in exposed women is unknown. WHO and the International Planned Parenthood Federation (IPPF) have not changed their practice guidelines on the use of DMPA. Nonetheless, all women at risk of acquiring an STI should be counseled to use condoms consistently and correctly.

PROVIDING DMPA

DMPA-IM is provided in either 1 cc vials or prefilled syringes containing 150 mg. The label states a 2-year shelf-life. Using a sterile needle and syringe, inject the DMPA deeply into the deltoid or the gluteus maximus muscle. Injections into the deltoid are less embarrassing but may be slightly more painful. The 21- to 23-gauge needle should be 2.5 to 4 cm long.[33] Immediately after injection do not massage the area over the injection, because it could lower the effectiveness of DMPA. DMPA-SC is available in prefilled, single-use syringes. Subcutaneous DMPA injections can be given in the anterior thigh or abdominal wall.

If a DMPA injection is given within 5 to 7 days of a normal last menstrual period or when switching from another effective contraceptive method, onset of contraceptive efficacy is within 24 hours and no back-up contraception is needed. The WHO states that DMPA can be given at any time in a menstrual cycle if the woman can be reasonably certain that she is not pregnant. If DMPA is given later than day 7 in the menstrual cycle, it is important that women use back-up contraception for 7 days and receive a follow-up pregnancy test several weeks later to diagnose pregnancy in a timely fashion. A recent study of immediate initiation of DMPA among 149 women who presented on cycle day 8 or later found that 47% of women continued to a second dose of DMPA, 92% returned for their follow up pregnancy test (half required many reminders) and 3 women were pregnant (2%).[128] Other studies have shown that the *Quick Start* (or *Depo Now*) method, of administering DMPA at any time that the patient presents to clinic, provided she and the provider are reasonably sure she is not pregnant, is safe, improves adherence, and results in fewer unwanted pregnancies in long-term follow-up.[129–131]

Schedule injections for every 3 months. After a single IM or SC DMPA injection, ovulation does not occur for at least 14 weeks (98 days).[2] Repeat DMPA IM or SC injections may be given as late as 14 to 17 weeks after a previous injection. For women who return more than 17 weeks after a previous injection, exclude pregnancy before re-injection, offer emergency contraception if they have had unprotected intercourse in the last 5 days, and have them use back-up contraception for 7 days after resuming DMPA. Giving DMPA injections in early pregnancy should be avoided if possible, because exposure has been associated with low-birthweight infants.[132] There is no increased risk of birth defects from pregnancies exposed to DMPA.[133,134] A prospective cohort study performed in Uganda, Zimbabwe, and Thailand examined 2,290 participants over 13,608 DMPA intervals and found that pregnancy rates were the same for repeat injections given at 13, 15, or 17 weeks from the last injection.[135] However, practice guidelines and manufacturer recommendations have not changed. The manufacturer recommends re-injection of DMPA-IM at 11 to 13 weeks after a previous injection, and re-injection of DMPA-SC at 12 to 14 weeks. The manufacturer recommends excluding pregnancy before proceeding with re-injection in women who return more than 13 weeks (91 days) after a previous DMPA-IM injection and more than 14 weeks (98 days) after a previous DMPA-SC injection.

At each re-injection visit, ask about any problems or concerns, the date of the last menstrual period, and any need for change in contraceptive or STI prevention. Record the patient's weight and blood pressure. If the client is not having any unacceptable symptoms or problems, she may continue getting DMPA injections. If she has had unprotected intercourse, offer her emergency contraception. Advise her that after 2 years of continuous use you will have to (1) discuss with her the impact of DMPA on BMD and the question of fracture risk, (2) reassess any underlying risk factors for bone fragility or fractures, and (3) re-evaluate whether DMPA continues to be the best contraceptive option for her. If DMPA remains her best contraceptive option, she may continue to get injections.

MANAGING DMPA PROBLEMS AND FOLLOW-UP

Menstrual changes. Inform women in advance that changes will occur in their menstrual cycles. Do not dismiss the impact of bleeding changes: they are the major reason that women discontinue this method. If bleeding occurs shortly after beginning DMPA, counsel patients that irregular bleeding decreases with use of DMPA. Spotting or breakthrough bleeding observed in prolonged use of DMPA may be managed by offering women one or more cycles of combined oral contraceptives, although the efficacy of this intervention has not been formally studied. Other options include short courses of exogenous estrogen[136] or a prostaglandin synthetase inhibitor such as mefenamic acid.[137] Each of these interventions has been shown to decrease bleeding in the short term; however, when these interventions are discontinued, irregular bleeding patterns resume.[136,137] A Cochrane Review of these interventions concluded there is not enough evidence of benefit to recommend the use of any one regimen in the treatment of menstrual irregularities experienced with DMPA.[138] Counseling helps continuation rates (see section on Effectiveness). Inform women that the irregular bleeding may return, but that over time the likelihood of amenorrhea will increase; in the context of DMPA use, amenorrhea is not harmful and does not require treatment.

Allergic reactions. Fortunately, severe anaphylactic reactions are rare. However, because DMPA is irretrievable once injected, have on hand emergency supportive measures such as epinephrine and diphenhydramine. Encourage patients to stay in the clinic/office area for 20 minutes following their first few injections. Those considering self-injection of DMPA-SC should receive their first one or two injections in a clinical setting, both to monitor for an allergic reaction and to learn safe self-injection technique.

Weight gain. DMPA is associated with weight gain in some women. In the one randomized study where DMPA was compared with a placebo injection, there was no difference in weight gain between the groups.[55] On average, the weight gain observed with DMPA use has been modest.[3,57,139] Women who gain a modest amount of weight should be encouraged to be careful about food intake and to exercise regularly. However, some women using DMPA have excessive weight gain. If the excessive weight gain is troublesome, cannot be controlled with diet and exercise, or has health consequences, these individual women should consider alternative methods of contraception.

U SER INSTRUCTIONS FOR DMPA

DMPA injections are very effective if you return on time for a repeat injection. Of 1,000 women who consistently get repeat injections on time, only 3 will become pregnant over a year's time.

1. DMPA injections have many *noncontraceptive benefits*. DMPA injections decrease—

- Menstrual blood flow

- Menstrual cramping

- Risk of anemia (low blood count)

- Risk of fibroids and bleeding from fibroids
- Risk of endometrial cancer
- Risk of pelvic infection
- Risk of ectopic pregnancy (a pregnancy outside of your uterus)
- Risk of a sickle cell crisis
- Frequency of grand mal seizures

2. **To use DMPA, you must be willing to accept unpredictable, frequent, or absent bleeding.** About 50% of women using DMPA will stop having any bleeding after a year of injections. This is to be expected and is not harmful to you.

3. **Have on hand a back-up contraceptive method** such as condoms, foam, spermicidal tablets or suppositories, or a diaphragm. You will need to use your back-up method for 1 week after your first injection. (This precaution may not be necessary if the first shot is given during the first 5 days after the beginning of your normal menstrual period.) Ask your clinician to give you a package or a prescription of an emergency contraceptive pill, such as ella, Plan B One-Step, or Next Choice, as a backup in case you have unprotected sex in the first week after your injection or if you are late for your next injection.

4. **Have latex or plastic condoms ready if you—**

- Are late for your injection
- May be at risk for a sexually transmitted infection, including infection with HIV, the virus that causes AIDS

5. Because of the rare possibility of an *allergic reaction*, you may be asked to remain in the vicinity of the clinic for 20 minutes after having your DMPA injection.

6. **Return to the clinic on time** for another injection. Mark your calendar for your next DMPA shot to be sure you will be on time. You may want to get your partner to mark his calendar too. Some programs are beginning to offer women (who have been using DMPA successfully) the opportunity to take home enough DMPA and syringes to last for a full year. If you would like to learn how to give yourself your DMPA injection, ask your clinician.

7. Depression and premenstrual symptoms may improve or become worse. If you become severely depressed, see your clinician immediately.

8. DMPA can decrease estrogen levels, which can cause a decrease in the density of your bones. In women who are in menopause

(usually 51 years old or older), decreased BMD can be associated with an increased risk of fractures. There is no evidence that DMPA use in pre-menopausal women increases the risk of fractures later in life. However, given the theoretical risk of fractures, let your clinician know if you frequently take corticosteroids or heparin, if you have fractured bones with minimal trauma, if you have a bone metabolism disease, if you have a strong family history of osteoporosis and fractures or if you have (or had) anorexia nervosa. Also, discuss bone health with your clinician if you plan to use DMPA for more than 2 years and are less than 18 years old or over 45 years old.[111]

9. Some DMPA users may gain weight. Be sure to eat a healthy balanced diet and exercise regularly. If you continue to gain weight excessively despite diet and exercise, discuss this with your clinician.

LATE FOR INJECTION

1. **If you realize after intercourse that you have missed your injection or are more than 4 weeks late for it,** use emergency contraception right away. If you do not have emergency contraception on hand, you can get emergency contraception from your pharmacy without a prescription if you are 17 years old or older. If you're younger than age 17, or want to use the prescription-only brand of EC called ella, visit the website www.not-2-late.com to find providers of emergency contraception nearest to you so you can get a prescription as soon as possible. In some states, you may be able to get emergency contraception from the pharmacist without a prescription, even if you're younger than 17. Visit www.EC-Help.org to find the closest pharmacy that can do this for you as soon as possible. Use another method until you are protected by another injection. If you realize you are late for your injection before you have intercourse, use another contraceptive method or abstain. Return as soon as possible for your shot.

2. If you are afraid you will forget your appointment for your next injection, the company that makes Depo Provera can email you reminders (www.depoprovera.com). Your doctor's office or clinic may also be able to call you or email you with reminders.

DMPA AND YOUR PERIODS

1. DMPA will make your periods less regular, and spotting between periods is fairly common. Eventually most women on

DMPA stop having periods completely. This is not harmful. Do *not* choose DMPA unless you do not mind having your periods change.

2. If your pattern of bleeding concerns you, contact your clinician. She may recommend that you return to the clinic for an evaluation to rule out the possibility of pregnancy or infection. If your bleeding is frequent or heavy, she may want to rule out anemia. She may recommend medications that you can use to decrease your bleeding.

3. If you discontinue taking DMPA, it may be a number of months before your periods return to normal after your last DMPA injection. However, there are medications, such as birth control pills, that can give you monthly withdrawal bleeding once you have stopped using DMPA.

DISCONTINUING DMPA

1. If you are more than 1 week late for your injection, use a back-up method of contraception as soon as you realize that you are going to be late. Use emergency contraception if you had unprotected intercourse. Visit your clinician as soon as possible for your injection. You will need to continue using a back-up method until you get your injection and for a week after that injection. Many clinicians will give you a pregnancy test to make sure you are not pregnant. If you are not sure if your intercourse was unprotected, use emergency contraception.

2. If you discontinue DMPA and do not want to become pregnant, start using a new contraceptive 13 weeks after your last shot. You may start birth control pills, have a contraceptive implant or intrauterine contraceptive placed, or use another contraceptive *before* it is time for your next injection.

3. If you are discontinuing DMPA because you want to become pregnant, remember that the contraceptive effect may take a number of months to go away. Start taking prenatal vitamins as soon as you decide to attempt pregnancy. Be patient.

DMPA AND PREGNANCY

1. DMPA injections may keep you from getting pregnant for more than 12 weeks (3 months) after your last shot. The average delay in return of fertility is about 10 months from the last injection. DMPA does not decrease your fertility in the long run.

2. If you are over age 35 and want to become pregnant in the near future, you may want to use an alternative contraceptive that has minimal or no delay in return of fertility after you stop using that method.

3. If you get pregnant while using DMPA, there is no increased risk of birth defects.[133,134]

DMPA WARNING SIGNALS

Serious health problems are very rare with DMPA use. Although DMPA is a highly effective contraceptive method, pregnancies do occur. If you feel pregnant, or think you might be pregnant, take a pregnancy test. See your clinician if you develop any of the following warning signals or if any other symptoms concern you:

- Repeated, very painful headaches
- Heavy bleeding
- Depression
- Severe, lower abdominal pain (may be a sign of pregnancy)
- Pus, prolonged pain, redness, itching or bleeding at injection site (may be a sign of infection).

> **Emergency Contraception:** Emergency contraceptive pills or insertion of a copper intrauterine contraceptive after unprotected intercourse substantially reduces the risk of pregnancy. (See Chapter 6 for more information.)

REFERENCES

1. Mishell DR, Jr. Pharmacokinetics of depot medroxyprogesterone acetate contraception. J Reprod Med. 1996;41(5 Suppl):381–390.
2. Jain J, Dutton C, Nicosia A, Wajszczuk C, Bode F, Mishell DR, Jr. Pharmacokinetics, ovulation suppression and return to ovulation follwoing a lower dose subcutaneous formulation of Depo-Provera. Contraception. 2004;70:11–18.
3. Jain J, Jakimiuk A, Bode F, Ross D, Kaunitz A. Contraceptive efficacy and safety of DMPA-SC. Contraception. 2004;70:269–275.
4. Petta CA, Faundes A, Dunson TR, et al. Timing of onset of contraceptive effectiveness in Depo-Provera users. II. Effects on ovarian function. Fertil Steril. 1998;70: 817–820.
5. Ismail AA, el-Faras A, Rocca M, el-Sibai FA, Toppozada M. Pituitary response to LHRH in long-term users of injectable contraceptives. Contraception. 1987;35: 487–495.
6. Paulen ME, Curtis KM. When can a woman have repeat progestogen-only injectables—depot medroxyprogesterone acetate or norethisterone enantate? Contraception. 2009;80:391–408.
7. Petta CA, Faundes A, Dunson TR, et al. Timing of onset of contraceptive effectiveness in Depo-Provera users: Part I. Changes in cervical mucus. Fertil Steril. 1998;69:252–257.

8. Croxatto HB. Mechanisms that explain the contraceptive action of progestin implants for women. Contraception. 2002;65:21–27.
9. Mishell DR, Jr. Long-acting contraceptive steroids. Postcoital contraceptives and anti-progestins. In: Mishell DR, Jr., Davajan V, Lobo R, eds. Infertility, contraception and reproductive endocrinology. Cambridge: Blackwell Scientific Publications; 1991.
10. Kaunitz AM, Darney PD, Ross D, Wolter KD, Speroff L. Subcutaneous DMPA vs. intramuscular DMPA: a 2-year randomized study of contraceptive efficacy and bone mineral density. Contraception. 2009;80:7–17.
11. Schwallie PC, Assenzo JR. Contraceptive use—efficacy study utilizing medroxyprogesterone acetate administered as an intramuscular injection once every 90 days. Fertil Steril. 1973;24:331–339.
12. Polaneczky M, Liblanc M. Long-term depot medroxyprogesterone acetate (Depo-Provera) use in inner-city adolescents. J Adolesc Health. 1998;23:81–88.
13. Moreau C, Cleland K, Trussell J. Contraceptive discontinuation attributed to method dissatisfaction in the United States. Contraception. 2007;76:267–272.
14. Paul C, Skegg DC, Williams S. Depot medroxyprogesterone acetate. Patterns of use and reasons for discontinuation. Contraception. 1997;56:209–214.
15. Potter LS, Dalberth BT, Canamar R, Betz M. Depot medroxyprogesterone acetate pioneers. A retrospective study at a North Carolina Health Department. Contraception. 1997;56:305–312.
16. Canto De Cetina TE, Canto P, Ordonez Luna M. Effect of counseling to improve compliance in Mexican women receiving depot-medroxyprogesterone acetate. Contraception. 2001;63:143–146.
17. Hubacher D, Goco N, Gonzalez B, Taylor D. Factors affecting continuation rates of DMPA. Contraception. 1999;60:345–351.
18. Davidson AR, Kalmuss D, Cushman LF, Romero D, Heartwell S, Rulin M. Injectable contraceptive discontinuation and subsequent unintended pregnancy among low-income women. Am J Public Health. 1997;87:1532–1534.
19. Goldberg AB, Cardenas LH, Hubbard AE, Darney PD. Post-abortion depot medroxyprogesterone acetate continuation rates: a randomized trial of cyclic estradiol. Contraception. 2002;66:215–220.
20. Lakha F, Henderson C, Glasier A. The acceptability of self-administration of subcutaneous Depo-Provera. Contraception. 2005;72:14–18.
21. McCann MF, Potter LS. Progestin-only oral contraception: a comprehensive review. Contraception. 1994;50 Suppl 1:S1–195.
22. Speroff L, Darney PD. A clinical guide for contraception. Third ed. Philadelphia: Lippincott Williams & Wilkins; 2001.
23. ACOG. Committee on Practice Guidelines. ACOG Practice Bulletin No. 73: Use of hormonal contraception in women with coexisting medical conditions. Obstet Gynecol. 2006;107:1453–1572.
24. Culwell KR, Curtis KM. Use of contraceptive methods by women with current venous thrombosis on anticoagulant therapy: a systematic review. Contraception. 2009;80:337–345.
25. Fu H, Darroch JE, Haas T, Ranjit N. Contraceptive failure rates: new estimates from the 1995 National Survey of Family Growth. Fam Plann Perspect. 1999;31:56–63.
26. Stevens-Simon C, Kelly L, Kulick R. A village would be nice but..it takes a long-acting contraceptive to prevent repeat adolescent pregnancies. Am J Prev Med. 2001;21:60–65.
27. Borgatta L, Murthy A, Chuang C, Beardsley L, Burnhill MS. Pregnancies diagnosed during Depo-Provera use. Contraception. 2002;66:169–172.
28. Belsey EM. Vaginal bleeding patterns among women using one natural and eight hormonal methods of contraception. Contraception. 1988;38:181–206.

29. Cromer BA, Smith RD, Blair JM, Dwyer J, Brown RT. A prospective study of adolescents who choose among levonorgestrel implant (Norplant), medroxyprogesterone acetate (Depo-Provera), or the combined oral contraceptive pill as contraception. Pediatrics. 1994;94:687–694.
30. Arias RD, Jain JK, Brucker C, Ross D, Ray A. Changes in bleeding patterns with depot medroxyprogesterone acetate subcutaneous injection 104 mg. Contraception. 2006;74:234–238.
31. Kaunitz AM. Injectable depot medroxyprogesterone acetate contraception: an update for U.S. clinicians. Int J Fertil Womens Med. 1998;43:73–83.
32. Dahan MH, Coffler MS, Patel KS. Oral contraceptives for inducing ovulation delay in orthodox Jewish women: a report of 2 cases. J Reprod Med. 2005;50:284–286.
33. Injectable contraceptives: their role in family planning. Geneva: World Health Organization; 1990.
34. Nanda K, Amaral E, Hays M, Viscola MA, Mehta N, Bahamondes L. Pharmacokinetic interactions between depot medroxyprogesterone acetate and combination antiretroviral therapy. Fertil Steril. 2008;90:965–971.
35. Hatcher RA, Schnare S. Ask the experts: progestin-only contraceptives. Contracept Technol Update. 1993;14:114–115.
36. Mattson RH, Cramer JA, Darney PD, Naftolin F. Use of oral contraceptives by women with epilepsy. JAMA. 11 1986;256:238–240.
37. Mattson RH, Rebar RW. Contraceptive methods for women with neurologic disorders. Am J Obstet Gynecol. 1993;168(6 Pt 2):2027–2032.
38. Rhodes ME, Frye CA. Actions at GABA(A) receptors in the hippocampus may mediate some antiseizure effects of progestins. Epilepsy Behav. 2005;6:320–327.
39. de Abood M, de Castillo Z, Guerrero F, Espino M, Austin KL. Effect of Depo-Provera or Microgynon on the painful crises of sickle cell anemia patients. Contraception. 1997;56:313–316.
40. Surrey ES. The role of progestins in treating the pain of endometriosis. J Minim Invasive Gynecol. 2006;13:528–534.
41. Walch K, Unfried G, Huber J, et al. Implanon versus medroxyprogesterone acetate: effects on pain scores in patients with symptomatic endometriosis—a pilot study. Contraception. 2009;79:29–34.
42. Crosignani PG, Luciano A, Ray A, Bergqvist A. Subcutaneous depot medroxyprogesterone acetate versus leuprolide acetate in the treatment of endometriosis-associated pain. Hum Reprod. 2005;21:248–56.
43. Johnson N, Fletcher H, Reid M. Depo medroxyprogesterone acetate (DMPA) therapy for uterine myomata prior to surgery. Int J Gynaecol Obstet. 2004;85:174–176.
44. Venkatachalam S, Bagratee JS, Moodley J. Medical management of uterine fibroids with medroxyprogesterone acetate (Depo Provera): a pilot study. J Obstet Gynaecol. 2004;24:798–800.
45. Lumbiganon P, Rugpao S, Phandhu-fung S, Laopaiboon M, Vudhikamraksa N, Werawatakul Y. Protective effect of depot-medroxyprogesterone acetate on surgically treated uterine leiomyomas: a multicentre case–control study. Br J Obstet Gynaecol. 1996;103:909–914.
46. Baeten J, Nyange P, Richardson B, et al. Hormonal contraception and risk of sexually transmitted disease acquisition: results from a prospective study. Am J Obstet Gynecol. 2001;185:380–385.
47. Depot-medroxyprogesterone acetate (DMPA) and risk of endometrial cancer. The WHO Collaborative Study of Neoplasia and Steroid Contraceptives. Int J Cancer. 9 1991;49:186–190.
48. Depot-medroxyprogesterone acetate (DMPA) and risk of epithelial ovarian cancer. The WHO Collaborative Study of Neoplasia and Steroid Contraceptives. Int J Cancer. 1991;49:191–195.
49. Prabhakaran S. Self-administration of injectable contraceptives. Contraception. 2008;77:315–317.

50. Gardner JM, Mishell DR, Jr. Analysis of bleeding patterns and resumption of fertility following discontinuation of a long acting injectable contraceptive. Fertil Steril. 1970;21:286–291.

51. Gray RH, Parker RA, Diethelm P. Vaginal bleeding disturbances associated with the discontinuation of long-acting injectable contraceptives. From the World Health Organization Special Programme for Research, Development, and Research Training in Human Reproduction; Task Force on Long-acting Systemic Agents for the Regulation of Fertility. Br J Obstet Gynaecol. 1981;88:317–321.

52. Hickey M, Dwarte D, Fraser IS. Superficial endometrial vascular fragility in Norplant users and in women with ovulatory dysfunctional uterine bleeding. Hum Reprod. 2000;15:1509–1514.

53. Bahamondes L, Del Castillo S, Tabares G, Arce XE, Perrotti M, Petta C. Comparison of weight increase in users of depot medroxyprogesterone acetate and copper IUD up to 5 years. Contraception. 2001;64:223–225.

54. Danli S, Qingxiang S, Guowei S. A multicentered clinical trial of the long-acting injectable contraceptive Depo Provera in Chinese women. Contraception. 2000;62:15–18.

55. Pelkman CL, Chow M, Heinbach RA, Rolls BJ. Short-term effects of a progestational contraceptive drug on food intake, resting energy expenditure, and body weight in young women. Am J Clin Nutr. 2001;73:19–26.

56. Curtis KM, Ravi A, Gaffield ML. Progestogen-only contraceptive use in obese women. Contraception. 2009;80:346–354.

57. Risser WL, Gefter LR, Barratt MS, Risser JM. Weight change in adolescents who used hormonal contraception. J Adolesc Health. 1999;24:433–436.

58. Bonny AE, Ziegler J, Harvey R, Debanne SM, Secic M, Cromer BA. Weight gain in obese and nonobese adolescent girls initiating depot medroxyprogesterone, oral contraceptive pills, or no hormonal contraceptive method. Arch Pediatr Adolesc Med. 2006;160:40–45.

59. Mangan SA, Larsen PG, Hudson S. Overweight teens at increased risk for weight gain while using depot medroxyprogesterone acetate. J Pediatr Adolesc Gynecol. 2002;15:79–82.

60. World Health Organization. Medical eligibility criteria for contraceptive use. 4th edition. Geneva: WHO, 2009.

61. Bonny A, Britto M, Huang B, Succop P, Slap G. Weight gain, adiposity, and eating behaviors among adolescent females on depot medroxyprogesterone acetate (DMPA). J Pediatr Adolesc Gynecol. 2004;17:109–115.

62. Pantoja M, Medeiros T, Baccarin MC, Morais SS, Bahamondes L, Fernandes AM. Variations in body mass index of users of depot-medroxyprogesterone acetate as a contraceptive. Contraception. 2010;81:107–111.

63. Westhoff C, Jain JK, Milsom I, Ray A. Changes in weight with depot medroxyprogesterone acetate subcutaneous injection 104 mg/0.65 mL. Contraception. 2007;75: 261–267.

64. Amatayakul K, Sivasomboon B, Thanangkul O. A study of the mechanism of weight gain in medroxyprogesterone acetate users. Contraception. 1980;22:605–622.

65. Civic D, Scholes D, Ichikawa L, et al. Depressive symptoms in users and non-users of depot medroxyprogesterone acetate. Contraception. 2000;61:385–390.

66. Gupta N, O'Brien R, Jacobsen LJ, et al. Mood changes in adolescents using depot-medroxyprogesterone acetate for contraception: a prospective study. J Pediatr Adolesc Gynecol. 2001;14:71–76.

67. Westhoff C, Truman C, Kalmuss D, et al. Depressive symptoms and Depo-Provera. Contraception. 1998;57:237–240.

68. Berenson AB, Odom SD, Breitkopf CR, Rahman M. Physiologic and psychologic symptoms associated with use of injectable contraception and 20 microg oral contraceptive pills. Am J Obstet Gynecol. 2008;199:351 e1–12.

69. Archer B, Irwin D, Jensen K, Johnson ME, Rorie J. Depot medroxyprogesterone. Management of side-effects commonly associated with its contraceptive use. J Nurse Midwifery. 1997;42:104–111.
70. Selo-Ojeme DO, Tillisi A, Welch CC. Anaphylaxis from medroxyprogesterone acetate. Obstet Gynecol. 2004;103(5 Pt 2):1045–1046.
71. Kongsayreepong R, Chutivongse S, George P, et al. A multicentre comparative study of serum lipids and apolipoproteins in long-term users of DMPA and a control group of IUD users. World Health Organization. Task Force on Long-Acting Systemic Agents for Fertility Regulation Special Programme of Research, Development and Research Training in Human Reproduction. Contraception. 1993;47:177–191.
72. Berenson AB, Rahman M, Wilkinson G. Effect of injectable and oral contraceptives on serum lipids. Obstet Gynecol. 2009;114:786–794.
73. Picardo C. Pharmacist-administered depot medroxyprogesterone acetate. Contraception. 2006;73:559–561.
74. Centers for Disease Control and Prevention. U.S. Medical Eligibility Criteria for Contraceptive Use, 2010. MMWR. 2010;59:(No. RR-4):1–85.
75. Kennedy KI, Short RV, Tully MR. Premature introduction of progestin-only contraceptive methods during lactation. Contraception. 1997;55:347–350.
76. Truitt ST, Fraser AB, Grimes DA, Gallo MF, Schulz KF. Combined hormonal versus nonhormonal versus progestin-only contraception in lactation. Cochrane Database Syst Rev. 2003:CD003988.
77. Halderman LD, Nelson AL. Impact of early postpartum administration of progestin-only hormonal contraceptives compared with nonhormonal contraceptives on short-term breast-feeding patterns. Am J Obstet Gynecol. 2002;186:1250–1256; discussion 1256–1258.
78. International Planned Parenthood Federation. IMAP statement on breast feeding, fertility and postpartum contraception. IPPF Med Bull. 1996;30:1–3.
79. McCann MF, Liskin LS, Piotrow PT, Rinehart W, Fox G. Breast-feeding, fertility, and family planning. Popul Rep J. 1981:J525–575.
80. Effects of hormonal contraceptives on breast milk composition and infant growth. World Health Organization (WHO) Task Force on Oral Contraceptives. Stud Fam Plann. 1988;19(6 Pt 1):361–369.
81. Rodriguez MI, Kaunitz AM. An evidence-based approach to postpartum use of depot medroxyprogesterone acetate in breastfeeding women. Contraception. 2009;80:4–6.
82. Speroff L, Mishell DR, Jr. The postpartum visit: it's time for a change in order to optimally initiate contraception. Contraception. 2008;78:90–98.
83. Skegg DC, Noonan EA, Paul C, Spears GF, Meirik O, Thomas DB. Depot medroxyprogesterone acetate and breast cancer. A pooled analysis of the World Health Organization and New Zealand studies. JAMA. 1995;273:799–804.
84. Shapiro S, Rosenberg L, Hoffman M, et al. Risk of breast cancer in relation to the use of injectable progestogen contraceptives and combined estrogen/progestogen contraceptives. Am J Epidemiol. 2000;151:396–403.
85. Strom BL, Berlin JA, Weber AL, et al. Absence of an effect of injectable and implantable progestin-only contraceptives on subsequent risk of breast cancer. Contraception. 2004;69:353–360.
86. Depot-medroxyprogesterone acetate (DMPA) and risk of invasive squamous cell cervical cancer. The WHO Collaborative Study of Neoplasia and Steroid Contraceptives. Contraception. 1992;45:299–312.
87. Thomas DB, Ray RM. Depot-medroxyprogesterone acetate (DMPA) and risk of invasive adenocarcinomas and adenosquamous carcinomas of the uterine cervix. WHO Collaborative Study of Neoplasia and Steroid Contraceptives. Contraception. 1995;52:307–312.

88. Berenson A, Breitkopf C, Grady J, Rickert V, Thomas A. Effects of hormonal contraception use on bone mineral density after 24 months of use. Obstet Gynecol. 2004;103:899–906.

89. Clark MK, Sowers M, Levy B, Nichols S. Bone mineral density loss and recovery during 48 months in first-time users of depot medroxyprogesterone acetate. Fertil Steril. 2006;86:1466–1474.

90. Cromer B, Stager M, Bonny A, et al. Depot medroxyprogesterone acetate, oral contraceptives and bone mineral density in a cohort of adolescent girls. J Adol Health. 2004;35:434–441.

91. Cundy T, Cornish J, Roberts H, Elder H, Reid I. Spinal bone density in women using depot medroxyprogesterone contraception. Obstet Gynecol. 1998;92:569–573.

92. Paiva L, Pinto-Neto A, Faundes A. Bone density among long-term users of medroxyprogesterone acetate as a contraceptive. Contraception. 1998;58:351–355.

93. Cundy T, Cornish J, Evans MC, Roberts H, Reid IR. Recovery of bone density in women who stop using medroxyprogesterone acetate. BMJ. 1994;308:247–248.

94. Scholes D, Lacroix A, Ichikawa L, Barlow W, Ott S. Injectable hormone contraception and bone density: results from a prospective study. Epidemiology. 2002;13:581–587.

95. Scholes D, Lacroix A, Ichikawa L, Barlow W, Ott S. Change in bone mineral density among adolescent women using and discontinuing depot medroxyprogesterone acetate contraception. Archives of Pediatric and Adolescent Medicine. 2005;159:139–144.

96. Clark M, Sowers M, Nichols S, Levy B. Bone mineral density changes over two years in first-time users of depot medroxyprogesterone acetate. Fertil Steril. 2004;82:1580–1586.

97. Petitti DB, Piaggio G, Mehta S, Cravioto MC, Meirik O. Steroid hormone contraception and bone mineral density: a cross-sectional study in an international population. The WHO Study of Hormonal Contraception and Bone Health. Obstet Gynecol. 2000;95:736–744.

98. Harkins GJ, Davis GD, Dettori J, Hibbert ML, Hoyt RA. Decline in bone mineral density with stress fractures in a woman on depot medroxyprogesterone acetate. A case report. J Reprod Med. 1999;44:309–312.

99. Lappe JM, Stegman MR, Recker RR. The impact of lifestyle factors on stress fractures in female Army recruits. Osteoporos Int. 2001;12:35–42.

100. Watson KC, Lentz MJ, Cain KC. Associations between fracture incidence and use of depot medroxyprogesterone acetate and anti-epileptic drugs in women with developmental disabilities. Womens Health Issues. 2006;16:346–352.

101. Lopez LM, Grimes DA, Schulz KF, Curtis KM. Steroidal contraceptives: effect on bone fractures in women. Cochrane Database Syst Rev. 2006:CD006033.

102. Chantry CJ, Auinger P, Byrd RS. Lactation among adolescent mothers and subsequent bone mineral density. Arch Pediatr Adolesc Med. 2004;158:650–656.

103. Sowers M, Corton G, Shapiro B, et al. Changes in bone density with lactation. JAMA. 23–30 1993;269:3130–3135.

104. Karlsson MK, Ahlborg HG, Karlsson C. Maternity and bone mineral density. Acta Orthop. 2005;76:2–13.

105. Santelli JS, Abma J, Ventura S, et al. Can changes in sexual behaviors among high school students explain the decline in teen pregnancy rates in the 1990s? J Adolesc Health. 2004;35:80–90.

106. Santelli JS, Lindberg LD, Finer LB, Singh S. Explaining recent declines in adolescent pregnancy in the United States: the contribution of abstinence and improved contraceptive use. Am J Public Health. 2007;97:150–156.

107. Curtis KM, Chrisman CE, Peterson HB. Contraception for women in selected circumstances. Obstet Gynecol. 2002;99:1100–1112.

108. Orr-Walker BJ, Evans MC, Ames RW, Clearwater JM, Cundy T, Reid IR. The effect of past use of the injectable contraceptive depot medroxyprogesterone acetate on bone mineral density in normal post-menopausal women. Clin Endocrinol (Oxf). 1998;49:615–618.

109. Cundy T, Cornish J, Roberts H, Reid I. Menopausal bone loss in long-term users of depot medroxyprogesterone acetate contraception. Am J Obstet Gynecol. 2002;186: 978–983.
110. Depo-Provera label. November 2004; http://www.accessdata.fda.gov/drugsatfda_docs/label/2004/20246s025lbl.pdf. Accessed April 8, 2010.
111. WHO statement on hormonal contraception and bone health. Wkly Epidemiol Rec. 2005;80:302–304.
112. Cromer BA, Scholes D, Berenson A, Cundy T, Clark MK, Kaunitz AM. Depot medroxyprogesterone acetate and bone mineral density in adolescents–the Black Box Warning: a Position Paper of the Society for Adolescent Medicine. J Adolesc Health. 2006;39:296–301.
113. ACOG Committee Opinion No. 415: Depot medroxyprogesterone acetate and bone effects. Obstet Gynecol. 2008;112:727–730.
114. Grimes DA, Schulz KF. Surrogate end points in clinical research: hazardous to your health. Obstet Gynecol. 2005;105(5 Pt 1):1114–1118.
115. Diagnosis of osteoporosis in men, premenopausal women, and children. J Clin Densitom. 2004;7:17–26.
116. Lewiecki EM. Premenopausal bone health assessment. Curr Rheumatol Rep. 2005;7:46–52.
117. Gbolade B, Ellis S, Murby B, Randall S, Kirkman R. Bone density in long term users of depot medroxyprogesterone acetate. Br J Obstet Gynaecol. 1998;105:790–794.
118. Jacobson D, Peralta L, Farmer M, Graham N, Gaydos C, Zenilman J. Relationship of hormonal contraception and cervical ectopy as measured by computerized planimetry to chlamydial infection in adolescents. STD. 1999;27:313–319.
119. Morrison C, Bright P, Wong E, et al. Hormonal contraceptive use, cervical ectopy, and the acquisition of cervical infections. STD. 2004;31:561–567.
120. Morrison CS, Turner AN, Jones LB. Highly effective contraception and acquisition of HIV and other sexually transmitted infections. Best Pract Res Clin Obstet Gynaecol. 2009;23:263–284.
121. Dayan L, Donovan B. Chlamydia, gonorrhoea, and injectable progesterone. Lancet. 16–22 2004;364:1387–1388.
122. Baeten JM, Benki S, Chohan V, et al. Hormonal contraceptive use, herpes simplex virus infection, and risk of HIV-1 acquisition among Kenyan women. AIDS. 20 2007;21:1771–1777.
123. Martin HL, Jr., Nyange PM, Richardson BA, et al. Hormonal contraception, sexually transmitted diseases, and risk of heterosexual transmission of human immunodeficiency virus type 1. J Infect Dis. 1998;178:1053–1059.
124. Ungchusak K, Rehle T, Thammapornpilap P, Spiegelman D, Brinkmann U, Siraprapasiri T. Determinants of HIV infection among female commercial sex workers in northeastern Thailand: results from a longitudinal study. J Acquir Immune Defic Syndr Hum Retrovirol. 15 1996;12:500–507.
125. Bulterys M, Chao A, Habimana P, Dushimimana A, Nawrocki P, Saah A. Incident HIV-1 infection in a cohort of young women in Butare, Rwanda. AIDS. 1994;8:1585–1591.
126. Morrison CS, Richardson BA, Mmiro F, et al. Hormonal contraception and the risk of HIV acquisition. AIDS. 2007;21:85–95.
127. Martin HL, Jr., Richardson BA, Mandaliya K, Achola JO, Overbaugh J, Kreiss JK. The early work on hormonal contraceptive use and HIV acquisition. J Acquir Immune Defic Syndr. 2005;38 Suppl 1:S12–14.
128. Sneed R, Westhoff C, Morroni C, Tiezzi L. A prospective study of immediate initiation of depo medroxyprogesterone acetate contraceptive injection. Contraception. 2005;71:99–103.
129. Lopez LM, Newmann SJ, Grimes DA, Nanda K, Schulz KF. Immediate start of hormonal contraceptives for contraception. Cochrane Database Syst Rev. 2008: CD006260.

130. Nelson AL, Katz T. Initiation and continuation rates seen in 2-year experience with Same Day injections of DMPA. Contraception. 2007;75:84–87.
131. Rickert VI, Tiezzi L, Lipshutz J, Leon J, Vaughan RD, Westhoff C. Depo Now: preventing unintended pregnancies among adolescents and young adults. J Adolesc Health. 2007;40:22–28.
132. Pardthaisong T, Gray RH. In utero exposure to steroid contraceptives and outcome of pregnancy. Am J Epidemiol. 15 1991;134:795–803.
133. Dahlberg K. Some effects of depo-medroxyprogesterone acetate (DMPA): observations in the nursing infant and in the long-term user. Int J Gynaecol Obstet. 1982;20:43–48.
134. Katz Z, Lancet M, Skornik J, Chemke J, Mogilner BM, Klinberg M. Teratogenicity of progestogens given during the first trimester of pregnancy. Obstet Gynecol. 1985;65:775–780.
135. Steiner MJ, Kwok C, Stanback J, et al. Injectable contraception: what should the longest interval be for reinjections? Contraception. 2008;77:410–414.
136. Said S, Sadek W, Rocca M, et al. Clinical evaluation of the therapeutic effectiveness of ethinyl oestradiol and oestrone sulphate on prolonged bleeding in women using depot medroxyprogesterone acetate for contraception. World Health Organization, Special Programme of Research, Development and Research Training in Human Reproduction, Task Force on Long-acting Systemic Agents for Fertility Regulation. Hum Reprod. 1996;11 Suppl 2:1–13.
137. Tantiwattanakul P, Taneepanichskul S. Effect of mefenamic acid on controlling irregular uterine bleeding in DMPA users. Contraception. 2004;70:277–279.
138. Abdel-Aleem H, d'Arcangues C, Vogelsong KM, Gulmezoglu AM. Treatment of vaginal bleeding irregularities induced by progestin only contraceptives. Cochrane Database Syst Rev. 2007:CD003449.
139. Mainwaring R, Hales HA, Stevenson K, et al. Metabolic parameter, bleeding, and weight changes in U.S. women using progestin only contraceptives. Contraception. 1995;51:149–153.

LATE REFERENCE

140. Meier C, Brauchli YB, Jick SS, Kraenzlin ME, Meier CR. Use of depot medroxyprogesterone acetate and fracture risk. J Clin Endocrinolo Metab 2010;95:4909-4916.

Progestin-Only Pills

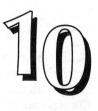

Elizabeth G. Raymond, MD, MPH

- Progestin-only pills contain a progestin hormone and no estrogen. A woman using progestin-only pills takes one tablet every day.

- Progestin-only pills are highly effective if taken as directed, although they are possibly less effective in typical use than are combined oral contraceptive pills.

- Progestin-only pills are safe for almost all women, including many women with contraindications to using combined oral contraceptive pills.

- The most common complaint of progestin-only pill users is irregular bleeding.

Progestin-only pills (POPs), sometimes called "minipills," contain a progestin hormone. One pill is taken every day with no hormone-free days. Only POPs containing norethindrone are currently available in the United States. POPs containing levonorgestrel, desogestrel, or other progestins are available in other countries. The amount of progestin in POPs is lower than the amount in combined oral contraceptive pills (COCs) containing the same compounds.

MECHANISM OF ACTION
POPs may prevent pregnancy by the following mechanisms:

- Ovulation is inhibited in a variable proportion of cycles.

- Cervical mucus is thickened and decreased in amount, which may prevent sperm penetration.

- The activity of the cilia in the fallopian tube is reduced, which may prevent the sperm and the egg from meeting.

- The endometrium is altered, which may inhibit implantation of a fertilized egg.

The specific mechanism active in a particular cycle may vary among women and, in any single woman, between cycles.[1] POPs containing desogestrel 75 mg inhibit ovulation more consistently than POPs containing levonorgestrel 30 mg.[2]

EFFECTIVENESS

POPs can be a highly effective contraceptive method when taken properly by motivated users. They are in the second tier of effectiveness, along with the patch and ring (see Figure 3–1 in Chapter 3 on Choosing a Contraceptive. In clinical studies, the proportion of women becoming pregnant in the first year of use was between 0% and 13%, and Pearl indices ranged up to 14 pregnancies per 100 woman-years (see Chapter 26, Contraceptive Efficacy).[1,3]

Scant data are available comparing efficacy of different POP products.[4] One randomized trial found no significant difference in efficacy between POPs containing norethindrone and POPs containing levonorgestrel.[5] Pregnancy rates in both POP groups in this trial were greater than 9% at one year, higher than in many other studies. Another randomized trial found substantially fewer pregnancies among women using POPs containing desogestrel (0.41 pregnancies/100 woman-years) than among women using POPs containing levonorgestrel (1.55 pregnancies/100 woman-years), although the difference did not reach statistical significance.[6] A third randomized trial conducted nearly 4 decades ago found similar and relatively low pregnancy rates in users of three POPs containing different hormones (2–4 pregnancies/100 woman-years), and a higher rate in users of POPs containing a fourth hormone. However, none of these four regimens is currently available.[7]

POPs are widely believed to be less effective than COCs. This belief may stem from the fact that the dose of hormone is lower in POPs than in COCs. However, data directly comparing actual pregnancy rates in users of the two methods are limited. One randomized trial comparing two COC and two POP preparations found that the pregnancy rate was significantly lower in one group of COC users than the rates in the other three groups. However, losses from the study for reasons other than pregnancy were very high in all the groups, which seriously compromised the comparisons.[5] Another small study comparing a POP to a COC (neither of which is currently marketed), found no pregnancies in either group, although the study contained only 43 women in each group who used the assigned method for only 6.7 and 9.2 cycles on average.[8]

In typical use, factors such as age, coital frequency, lactation, and compliance may influence pregnancy rates more than relatively minor differences in inherent method efficacy.[9,10]

Guidelines on use of POPs emphasize that for maximum efficacy, the pills must be taken within several hours of the same time every day. This recommendation is based primarily on data about serum progestin levels, which peak shortly after pill ingestion and then decline to nearly undetectable levels 24 hours later. In this respect, POPs differ from COCs, which produce higher and longer-lasting serum progestin levels. No clinical data are available that correlate pregnancy rates with timeliness in taking POPs.[1] One study suggests that POPs containing desogestrel 75 mg may inhibit ovulation reliably even when pills are occasionally taken 12 hours late.[11]

ADVANTAGES

POPs have many advantages for many women, as described below.

1. **Safety.** Because POPs contain lower doses of progestin than COCs and do not contain estrogen, they are presumably at least as safe as COCs and are quite likely safer. However, rigorous data on safety of POPs as distinct from or in comparison to COCs are relatively scant; therefore, it is not always possible to determine for certain which of the concerns related to COCs are not relevant to POP users. In general, data suggest that POPs containing norgestrel or norethindrone appear not to be associated with an overall clinically important increase in risk of hypertension,[12] cardiovascular disease,[13] breast cancer,[14] coagulation factors, or birth defects in women who accidentally take POPs during pregnancy.[1,15]

2. **Few contraindications.** According to the both the World Health Organization's Medical Eligibility Criteria for Contraceptive Use (WHO MEC)[16] and the corresponding United States document (U.S. *MEC*),[17] POPs can safely be used by almost all women (see section below on Providing the Method). These criteria list many fewer contraindications to POPs than to COCs (Chapter 4 on Medical Eligibility Criteria). This difference is partly rationalized by the absence of estrogen in POPs, which suggests that conditions that may be exacerbated by estrogen are not a contraindication to POP use. POPs are frequently recommended instead of COCs to breastfeeding women between 6 weeks and 6 months postpartum.

3. **Acceptable efficacy,** especially if the pills are taken as directed. See above.

4. **Improved menstrual symptoms for some women.** POPs cause menstrual cycle changes that are welcome to some women (see below under Disadvantages.) They may also reduce the severity of menstrual cramps and premenstrual tension symptoms.

5. **Simple, fixed daily regimen.** POP users take the same type of pill every day (same color and hormone content). In POP packages, every pill contains hormone; there is no pill-free week or hormone-free week.

6. **Immediate reversibility.** Limited data suggest that fertility is normal immediately after stopping use of POPs, regardless of the duration of POP use.[1]

7. **Non-contraceptive health benefits.** POPs may reduce the incidence of painful crises in women with sickle cell disease[18] and may be used to treat estrogen dermatitis related to the menstrual cycle.[19] Other non-contraceptive health benefits of POPs have not been rigorously studied. However, it seems reasonable to postulate that POPs might confer some of the same benefits as COCs, such as a reduced risk of uterine and ovarian cancers.

DISADVANTAGES AND CAUTIONS
POPs also have disadvantages, as described below.

1. **Menstrual cycle disturbances.** POPs cause bleeding changes in many or most users. The abnormal menstrual patterns are unpredictable and may include short cycles, irregular periods, intermenstrual bleeding and spotting, and less commonly, prolonged bleeding or amenorrhea. Analysis of bleeding patterns of women in six clinical trials studying various methods of contraception showed that POP users had less regular bleeding patterns and more total bleeding/spotting days over time than users of COCs. Whether or not bleeding patterns tend to become more regular with increased duration of POP use is unclear. Menstrual cycle disturbances are a common reason for discontinuing POPs, although some women consider the altered bleeding pattern, particularly if it constitutes less total bleeding than expected, to be a benefit of the method. One expert has suggested that POP users who have bleeding irregularities may be better protected from pregnancy than those who do not, because the irregularities indicate that the pills are disrupting the normal ovulatory hormonal cycles.[1,20-22]

2. **Other side effects.** Complaints by POP users include headaches, nausea, weight gain or loss, breast tenderness, depression, fatigue, decreased libido, androgenic symptoms such as hirsutism and acne, and other side effects. However, the precise extent to which these common symptoms are actually caused by the pills cannot be determined from available data.[1]

3. **Vulnerable efficacy.** To maximize contraceptive efficacy, POP users should be especially careful (more careful than users of

COCs) to take the pills at the same time each day and to use back-up methods such as condoms when taking drugs that may interact with the hormones in the pills or during periods of vomiting or diarrhea. This disadvantage may be less relevant to users of POPs containing desogestrel than to users of POPs containing norethindrone.

4. **Lower efficacy than some other methods in preventing ectopic pregnancy.** Rigorous data are not available about the effect of POPs on the absolute risk of ectopic pregnancy. One early report suggested that POP users may be at higher risk than users of no method or of other methods[23], but other data seem to refute that contention.[1] However, up to 10% of pregnancies that occur among POP users may be ectopic, a proportion higher than is seen in users of COCs or women who use no method at all. Thus, POPs appear not to prevent ectopic pregnancy as well as they prevent intrauterine pregnancy.[1]

5. **Possible increased risk of diabetes.** One study suggested that use of POPs during breastfeeding after a pregnancy complicated by gestational diabetes may increase the subsequent long-term risk of type II diabetes mellitus.[24] However, POPs are generally felt to be safe for use by diabetic women.

6. **Ovarian cysts.** Unlike COCs, which substantially inhibit ovarian activity and reduce the risk of functional ovarian cysts, POPs may be associated with an increased incidence of functional ovarian cysts or persistent follicles.[25] Most ovarian cysts cause minor or no symptoms and resolve without treatment.

7. **Lack of protection against sexually transmitted infections (STIs).** Progestin-only contraceptives provide no known substantial protection against STIs, including HIV.

8. **Possible increased risk of thromboembolic conditions in users of POPs containing desogestrel.** Controversy has existed about a possible increased risk of thrombosis in users of desogestrel-containing combined oral contraceptives (see Chapter 11, Combined Oral Contraceptives). Insufficient data exists on POPs containing this hormone to assess any possible association with clotting events. At this time (August, 2010), POPs containing desogestrel are not marketed in the United States.

9. **Limited availability.** In the United States, POPs are much less popular than COCs and may be more difficult for some women to obtain on short notice.

SPECIAL ISSUES

Breastfeeding: The physiologic effects of contraceptive steroids could, in theory, impair lactation. In addition, a small amount of the progestin in the pills passes into breast milk, which exposes a breastfeeding baby to the hormone.[26] A review of five randomized trials evaluating the use of hormonal contraceptives during breastfeeding found no clear evidence that POPs have a clinically important effect on milk volume or on infant growth and development. However, the quality of all the trials was poor, and the conclusions are therefore suspect.[27] Despite the paucity of evidence, the WHO *MEC* asserts that the risks of using POPs within the first 6 weeks postpartum generally outweigh the advantages. In contrast, the U.S. *MEC* indicates no restriction on use of POPs among breastfeeding women. One study conducted in Kenya found no evidence that the timing of initiation of POPs (6 weeks or 6 months postpartum) affected method continuation.[28]

Drug interactions: Interactions between POPs and other drugs have not been well studied. Because POPs produce relatively low progestin levels even in the absence of other drugs, POPs may not be an especially good hormonal contraceptive option for women who are taking certain drugs on a chronic basis. These drugs include rifampicin, certain anticonvulsants, some anti-retroviral drugs, and Saint John's Wort, which appear to affect metabolism of COCs. However, even for women on these drugs, POPs may be more effective than some other contraceptive methods, particularly barriers or natural family planning. Combined use of a barrier method and POPs might be the best choice for women taking potentially interacting drugs if they cannot use other highly effective contraceptive methods. Advise POP users to use a back-up method while temporarily taking a potentially interacting drug, and possibly for some period of time after stopping it.

PROVIDING THE METHOD

Almost all women can safely use POPs, including most women who are not eligible to take COCs. Neither the WHO *MEC* and U.S. *MEC* for POPs include any restriction based on age, smoking, hypertension, migraine without aura, uterine fibroids, diabetes, gall bladder disease, or sickle cell disease. No examination or laboratory test is needed to determine whether a woman is eligible to receive POPs.

The WHO and U.S. *MEC* list only a few Category 3 or 4 contraindications to POPs:

	WHO	US
Breastfeeding women less than 6 weeks postpartum	x	
Current deep venous thrombosis or pulmonary embolus	x	
History of bariatric surgery (malabsorptive procedures)		x
Systemic lupus erythematosus with positive or unknown antiphospholipid antibodies	x	x
Severe (decompensated) cirrhosis, benign or malignant liver tumors	x	x
Current or past breast cancer	x	x
Use of ritonavir-boosted protease inhibitors, certain anticonvulsants, (phenytoin, carbamazepine, barbiturates, primidone, topiramate, oxcarbazepine), rifampicin or rifabutin		

In addition, both the WHO and U.S. *MEC* note that POPs should be stopped if the user develops ischemic heart disease, stroke, or migraine with aura while using POPs.

POPs are not a good choice for women who cannot tolerate irregular bleeding or amenorrhea. Because they should be taken at close to the same hour each day, they may not be suitable for women whose schedules do not allow such consistency.

Counseling. Women considering POPs should be advised about their advantages and disadvantages, described above.

Timing of initiation. A woman may start taking POPs at any time (Quick Start) when it is reasonably certain that she is not pregnant. The WHO *Selected Practice Recommendations* indicate that no back-up method is needed if she starts POPs at any of the following times:

- During the first 5 days of her menstrual cycle

- Between 6 weeks and 6 months postpartum if she is fully or nearly fully breastfeeding and amenorrheic (Note: The U.S. *MEC* allows initiation without back-up between 0 and 6 weeks postpartum as well.)

- Within the first 21 days postpartum if she is not breastfeeding

- Immediately after an abortion

- The day after she stops another hormonal method (i.e., she is switching to POPs from another hormonal method with no break in between)

However, WHO recommends that if she starts POPs at any time other than these listed, she should use a back-up method such as male condoms for the first 2 days of taking POPs. Another, simpler, approach is to tell *all* POP users to use a back-up method (or abstain from vaginal sex) for the first 2 days after starting POPs.

Provide or prescribe as many packs of POPs as the patient wants.

M ANAGING PROBLEMS AND FOLLOW-UP

Abnormal bleeding in women using POPs can be managed by a number of approaches, including reassurance, prostaglandin inhibitors, estrogen supplementation, or a method switch.

If a woman becomes pregnant while using POPs, be vigilant for the possibility of ectopic pregnancy.

U SER INSTRUCTIONS FOR PROGESTIN-ONLY PILLS

To use POPs, follow these instructions:

1. Start taking the pills during the first 5 days of your normal menstrual period or on any day you are reasonably sure that you are not pregnant. If you are switching from estrogen-containing oral contraceptive pills (regular birth control pills), skip the 7 inactive pills at the end of the pack, and instead start the POPs the day after the last active pill.

2. **Use a back-up method** such as male condoms every time you have sex during the first 48 hours (2 days) after starting POPs. If you do not use a back-up method, abstain from vaginal sex for those first 2 days.

3. **Take 1 pill every day.** Choose a time and take the pill at that time or within 3 hours after that time.

4. Start the next pack the day after the last pack is finished. Do not take any break or days off between packs. Always have your next pack ready *before* you finish each pack.

5. **If you miss taking a pill** during the 3-hour window, take it as soon as you remember, even if that means you will take 2 pills in one day. Use a back-up method such as male condoms or abstain from vaginal sex during the next 48 hours. Take further pills at the usual time.

6. **If you vomit within 4 hours** after taking a pill, or if you have diarrhea, your body might not properly absorb the medicine in the POPs. Keep taking the pills on schedule, but use a back-up method such as male condoms every time you have sex, until 48 hours after the vomiting or diarrhea are over.

7. **Get a pregnancy test if—**

- Your menstrual period is late, and you have not taken all your pills on time, and you had sex without a condom or other back-up method

- You miss two periods in a row, even if you took all your POPs on time

- You are concerned about pregnancy for any reason.

  Keep taking the pills daily until you know the pregnancy test result. If the result is positive, then stop taking the pills and consult your clinician about your options. If the result is negative, then the late or missed periods are probably due to the pills and are not dangerous. Consult your clinician about other possible causes and your options.

8. Certain medicines and some over-the-counter preparations can reduce the effectiveness of POPs. If you take any other drug while using POPs, ask your clinician whether it might interact with POPs. If so, you should use a back-up method (such as male condoms) during the entire time you are taking the other drug and possibly for some time after you stop taking it. If you are planning to take the other drug for a long period of time, consult with your clinician about whether a contraceptive method other than POPs might be appropriate for you.

9. Changes in your menstrual periods (frequency and length and bleeding between periods) are common in women taking POPs. These changes are usually not dangerous. If you have unusual bleeding, keep taking the POPs. If the bleeding lasts for more than 8 days or is particularly heavy, or if you want to switch to another contraceptive method that is less likely to cause bleeding irregularities, consult your clinician.

10. If you have other problems or questions while taking POPs, keep taking the pills according to schedule while you figure out what to do.

11. If you stop taking POPs and do not want to become pregnant, start using another contraceptive immediately, or abstain from vaginal sex. Your ability to become pregnant returns right away after you stop POPs.

12. Consider using emergency contraception (emergency contraceptive pills or an intrauterine contraceptive) if you have had sex that was not properly protected by POPs or another contraceptive method (that is, if you did not follow the instructions above).

> **Emergency Contraception:** Emergency contraceptive pills or insertion of a copper intra-uterine contraceptive after unprotected intercourse substantially reduces the risk of preg-nancy. (See Chapter 6 for more information.)

REFERENCES

1. McCann MF, Potter LS. Progestin-only oral contraception: a comprehensive review. Contraception. 1994;50:S1–195.
2. Rice CF, Killick SR, Dieben T, Coelingh Bennink H. A comparison of the inhibition of ovulation achieved by desogestrel 75 micrograms and levonorgestrel 30 micrograms daily. Hum Reprod. 1999;14:982–5.
3. Lakha F, Ho PC, Van der Spuy ZM, et al. A novel estrogen-free oral contraceptive pill for women: multicentre, double-blind, randomized controlled trial of mifepris-tone and progestogen-only pill (levonorgestrel). Hum Reprod. 2007;22:2428–36.
4. Grimes DA, Lopez LM, O'Brien PA, Raymond EG. Progestin-only pills for contracep-tion. Cochrane Database Syst Rev. 2010;CD007541.
5. Sheth A, Jain U, Sharma S, et al. A randomized, double-blind study of two combined and two progestogen-only oral contraceptives. Contraception. 1982;25:243–52.
6. A double-blind study comparing the contraceptive efficacy, acceptability and safety of two progestogen-only pills containing desogestrel 75 micrograms/day or levonor-gestrel 30 micrograms/day. Collaborative Study Group on the Desogestrel-containing Progestogen-only Pill. Eur J Contracept Reprod Health Care. 1998;3:169–78.
7. Vessey M, Mears E, Andolsek L, Ogrinc-Oven M. Randomised double-blind trial of four oral progestagen-only contraceptives. Lancet. 1972;1:915–22.
8. Paulsen ML, Varaday A, Brown BW, Kalman SM. A andomized contraceptive trial comparing a daily progestogen with a combined oral contraceptive steroid. Contra-ception. 1974;9:497–506.
9. Vessey M, Lawless M, Yeates D, McPherson K. Progestogen-only oral contraception. Findings in a large prospective study with special reference to effectiveness. Br J Fam Plan. 1985;10:117–21.
10. Steiner M, Dominik R, Trussell J, Hertz-Picciott I. Measuring contraceptive effec-tiveness: a conceptual framework. Obstet Gynecol. 1996;88:24S-30S.
11. Korver T, Klipping C, Heger-Mahn D, Duijkers I, van Osta G, Dieben T. Maintenance of ovulation inhibition with the 75-microg desogestrel-only contraceptive pill (Cera-zette) after scheduled 12-h delays in tablet intake. Contraception. 2005;71:8–13.
12. Hussain SF. Progestogen-only pills and high blood pressure: is there an association? A literature review. Contraception. 2004;69:89–97.
13. Heinemann LA, Assmann A, DoMinh T, Garbe E. Oral progestogen-only contracep-tives and cardiovascular risk: results from the Transnational Study on Oral Contra-ceptives and the Health of Young Women. Eur J Contracept Reprod Health Care. 1999;4:67–73.
14. Skegg DC, Paul C, Spears GF, Williams SM. Progestogen-only oral contraceptives and risk of breast cancer in New Zealand. Cancer Causes Control. 1996;7:513–9.
15. Simpson JL, Phillips OP. Spermicides, hormonal contraception and congenital mal-formations. Adv Contracept. 1990;6:141–67.
16. World Health Organization. Medical Eligibility Criteria for Contraceptive Use. 4. Geneva: World Health Organization, 2009.
17. Centers for Disease Control and Prevention. U. S. Medical Eligibility Criteria for Contraceptive Use, 2010. MMWR. 2010;59 (No. RR-4):1–85.
18. de Abood M, de Castillo Z, Guerrero F, Espino M, Austin KL. Effect of Depo-Provera or Microgynon on the painful crises of sickle cell anemia patients. Contraception. 1997;56:313–6.

19. Randall K, Steele R. Estrogen dermatitis: treatment with progestin-only pill. Arch Dermatol. 2005;141:792–3.
20. Broome M, Fotherby K. Clinical experience with the progestogen-only pill. Contraception. 1990;42:489–95.
21. Belsey EM. Vaginal bleeding patterns among women using one natural and eight hormonal methods of contraception. Contraception. 1988;38:181–206.
22. Guillebaud J. Contraception—Your Questions Answered. 2nd. London: Churchill Livingstone, 1993.
23. Bergsjo P, Langengen H, Aas J. Tubal pregnancies in women using progestagen-only contraception. Acta Obstet Gynecol Scand. 1974;53:377–8.
24. Kjos SL, Peters RK, Xiang A, Thomas D, Schaefer U, Buchanan TA. Contraception and the risk of type 2 diabetes mellitus in Latina women with prior gestational diabetes mellitus. JAMA. 1998;280:533–8.
25. Tayob Y, Adams J, Jacobs HS, Guillebaud J. Ultrasound demonstration of increased frequency of functional ovarian cysts in women using progestogen-only oral contraception. Br J Obstet Gynaecol. 1985;92:1003–9.
26. Betrabet SS, Shikary ZK, Toddywalla VS, Toddywalla SP, Patel D, Saxena BN. ICMR Task Force Study on hormonal contraception. Transfer of norethisterone (NET) and levonorgestrel (LNg) from a single tablet into the infant's circulation through the mother's milk. Contraception. 1987;35:517–22.
27. Truitt ST, Fraser AB, Grimes DA, Gallo MF, Schulz KF. Hormonal contraception during lactation. systematic review of randomized controlled trials. Contraception. 2003;68:233–8.
28. Were EO, Kendall JZ, Nyongesa P. Randomised clinical trial to determine optimum initiation time of norgestrel-progestin only contraception in Eldoret Teaching Hospital, Kenya. East Afr Med J. 1997;74:103–7.

Combined Oral Contraceptives (COCs)

Anita L. Nelson, MD
Carrie Cwiak, MD, MPH

- For 50 years, combined oral contraceptives (COCs) have been the gold standard for birth control in the United States; up to 82% of U.S. women who have ever been sexually active have used COCs.[1]
- Due primarily to inconsistent use, each year 1 million U.S. COC users get pregnant.
- Women face many challenges to being successful pill users, but by changing our practice protocols to adopt Quick Start and simpler prescribing policies, we may reduce these barriers.
- Women may be reassured by pill safety messages and be more motivated by noncontraceptive benefits offered by COCs.

Combined oral contraceptives (COCs) have been almost synonymous with contraception in the United States for over half a century. As social and legal changes in the 1960s opened up opportunities for women to become more equal participants at home and in the workplace, the pill allowed women to take advantage of those opportunities. The pill gave couples (and women alone) greater ability to plan and prepare for childbearing (if they desired it). By unlinking coitus and childbearing, the pill enabled women to enjoy sexual activity without the fear of pregnancy. Beyond that, COCs made cyclic bleeding episodes predictable, so that women could plan their lives around their periods rather than having their lives unpredictably interrupted by their flows. Over the years, additional health benefits of pill use have become apparent. The pill's contributions to women's (and children's) health have been so enormous that the Centers for Disease Control and Prevention (CDC) recognized family planning (with oral contraceptives and condoms, in particular) as one of the 10 greatest public health achievements of the 20th century, on par with the vaccination and control of infectious disease.[2]

Unfortunately, 50 years later, these accomplishments are taken for granted, concerns about the safety of COCs are disproportionately magnified, and the noncontraceptive benefits of COCs are not appreciated by many women or by many clinicians. Even though 4 out of 5 sexually active women have used the pill, few women today have any idea what life for them would be like without the pill. In general, women underestimate their own fertility and they have little appreciation for the significant health risks posed by pregnancy. Women tend to view pregnancy as "natural," whereas pills are considered "artificial" and are thought by many COCs to be dangerous, but the facts paint a different picture (See Table 11–1).

Surveys show that the vast majority of women rank the pill as more hazardous to a woman's health than pregnancy.[3] In part, responsibility for this misperception rests with the informed consent process (and product labeling) that we have traditionally followed when offering pills to women: clinicians focus on the potential risks reported with pill use without comparing the magnitude of pill use risks to the magnitude of the risks associated with pregnancy. The only benefit that is listed for most pills is its low failure rate. This process assumes that without COCs, the woman would be abstinent and would not be at risk for pregnancy.

In the face of this one-sided information, it is not surprising that in the last 50 years, every hormonal birth control method has been the target of lawsuits. As a result, more restrictive wording and additional warnings have been added to product labeling. In the wake of negative publicity, women are reluctant to use these methods. These same forces drive up the cost of contraception. Companies stockpile profits to finance the litigation, which they see as inevitable, and need to recoup research costs and make profits in a much shorter time than ever before. Another unfortunate result of this boom-and-bust pattern[4] for contraceptive products is that many pharmaceutical companies have halted all research to develop new contraceptives.

Despite all the health benefits provided by contraception, the environment in which a woman lives does not always support contraception. Some in her family may desire her to become pregnant (to produce [grand]children). Others in her circle of friends may overtly oppose her use of contraception. Vocal and influential political groups might oppose a woman's right to control her own fertility.

Readers of this chapter will hopefully become more effective advocates for COCs if they understand more completely the evolution of the pill and the improvements that have been made to it over time and if they better appreciate the contraceptive and noncontraceptive health benefits offered by COCs. By understanding the challenges women face using pills correctly and consistently, and by adopting practices to over-

Table 11–1 Common myths that make women hesitate to use combined oral contraceptives (COCs)

Myths	Facts
Pregnancy is "natural" and therefore safe.	• Worldwide, over 340,000 women die each year from pregnancy and pregnancy-related causes. • Another 15 million women are severely disabled each year by pregnancy and delivery. • In the United States, a woman's lifetime risk of dying from pregnancy and pregnancy-related causes is 1 in 2,100. • The mortality rate associated with birth control pill use is 1 in 1,667,000.[86]
The pill reduces a woman's fertility even after she stops using it.	The pill is rapidly and completely reversible.
The pill causes cancer.	The pill protects against ovarian and endometrial cancer.
The pill causes depression.	The pill is no different than placebo for depression.
The pill causes weight gain.	Pill users have no greater weight gain than women taking placebo.
The pill causes acne.	Some pills are *treatment* for acne.
The pill causes abortion.	The pill reduces the need for abortion.
Monthly bleeding is needed with the pill.	Monthly bleeding with the pill offers no health benefits but can cause physical suffering.
The pill should not be used by women who— Smoke Have diabetes Are obese.	The pill can be used by— Smokers under 35 Most diabetics Heavy or obese women.
The pill should not be used by teens because it will disrupt their maturation.	Early use of the pill will not disturb development of the hypothalamic-pituitary-ovarian axis.

come those challenges, we can help women become more successful contraceptors. By providing pertinent patient information, we hope to make patient counseling messages more effective. However, information alone may not be enough. For contraception to achieve its full potential, we may need to assist women in incorporating contraception as an important part of their daily lives. For this we need to be culturally sensitive and chose our words more carefully, eliminating negative images associated with family planning.

HORMONES IN THE PILL

The history of the pill is one of remarkable evolution, reflecting increased knowledge about hormonal safety issues, changes in women's needs and demands, and enhancements designed to encourage more consistent pill use. The doses of the hormones in the pills have dramatically decreased. New hormone compounds have been introduced. Different formulations with different pill sequences have been developed. New health benefits have been documented. These technical changes paralleled legal and social changes that enabled women to gain access to COCs. Many people today are not aware of the fact that there was a time that it was illegal to prescribe or provide COCs. The last arrest made for prescribing COCs to a married woman was made in Connecticut in 1961—one year *after* the United States Food and Drug Administration (FDA) approved the first pill for contraception. FDA labeling did not discuss pill use for unmarried women until the 1970s.

The first pill approved by the FDA in May 1960 was Enovid-10. Enovid-10 had 21 active pills, which women took daily starting on the fifth day of menses. The 21 active pills were followed by 7 days off pills (hormone-free days), then the next cycle of 21 pills started. Each active pill contained 9.85 mg norethynodrel and 150 mcg mestranol—doses significantly higher than the doses in currently available COCs. To put it into context, if a woman today were to take all 21 active pills from a package of today's Ovcon-35 at once, she would still be taking a lower dose of progestin than women took every day with Enovid-10. Although the side effects of this first pill were impressive (nausea, vomiting, headaches, melasma, mastalgia), the women in the clinical trials took them with enthusiasm, because they were painfully familiar with their alternative—pregnancy.

PROGESTINS

Virtually all of the issues about COC safety relate to its estrogen component, but progestins provide the majority of the contraceptive actions of COCs. Progestins thicken the cervical mucus to block sperm entry into the upper genital tract and, depending upon progestin dose and potency, block LH surge and prevent ovulation. Therefore, with daily doses, therapeutic serum levels of progestins must be maintained for at least 24 hours, with an adequate margin to allow for variations in the ways individual women absorb and metabolize the hormone and to allow for some inconsistent pill use. The power of a particular progestin results not only from its intrinsic potency, but also from the dose that is used. Each compound has a different potency and different metabolic effects. In order to determine which formulation(s) might best match an individual woman's contraceptive and non-contraceptive needs, it is helpful to understand the properties of different progestins.

Progestins vary in their properties of bioavailability, dose needed for ovulation inhibition, and half-life. Much of a drug can be metabolized by the liver after it is first absorbed from the intestine and before it reaches the bloodstream. This first-pass metabolism is discussed in more detail in the Drug-Drug Interaction section. Individuals can differ significantly in their first-pass metabolisms. *Bioavailability* reflects the percentage of drug that is ultimately absorbed into the bloodstream. The higher the bioavailability, the lower the dose needed. A compound with greater bioavailability will also have less variation in absorption in a given individual or across a group of individuals. A clinical test of the potency of a progestin is *dose required for ovulation inhibition*.[5] Both bioavailability and dose required for ovulation inhibition are considered when the dose of a progestin is selected. The final property that can have significant clinical implications is the half-life of the progestin. *Half-life* is the time necessary for the blood level of a drug to fall to 50% of its maximum. The greater the serum half-life, the longer it stays in the patient's circulation. Longer half-lives of sex steroids in the pills are helpful in reducing the incidence of unscheduled spotting and bleeding. Longer half-lives also reduce the chance that missed pills will permit escape ovulation, and, therefore, may be more forgiving when pills are missed.

Natural progesterone is poorly absorbed from the gastrointestinal tract and is rapidly metabolized. At high doses, progesterone is sedating. For all these reasons, the original developers of the pill turned to more long-acting synthetic progestins derived from an androgen—19-nortestosterone. These progestins are rapidly absorbed; all progestins used in COCs reach maximum concentration within 1 to 3 hours after administration.[5,6]

Ten different progestins have been used in the COCs that have been sold in the United States. Several different classification systems for the progestins exist, but the one most commonly used system recapitulates the history of the pill in the United States by categorizing the progestins into the so-called "generations of progestins." The first three generations of progestins are derived from 19-nortestosterone. The fourth generation is drospirenone. Newer progestins are hybrids.

First-generation progestins. First-generation progestins include norethynodrel, norethindrone, norethindrone acetate, and ethynodiol diacetate. First-generation progestins are generally well-tolerated and have been extensively used for decades. Today they are found in many generic formulations and a few low-dose brand-name COCs. Because of its low progestational effect, one of these formulations (Ovcon) has proven very advantageous for use in women who have had gestational diabetes.[7] These compounds have the lowest potency and relatively short half-lives. The short half-life did not matter in the early, high-dose pills but as doses of progestin were decreased in the more modern pills, problems with unscheduled spotting and bleeding became more common.

Second-generation progestins. To solve the problem of unscheduled bleeding and spotting, the second-generation progestins (norgestrel and levonorgestrel) were designed to be significantly more potent and to have longer half-lives than the norethindrone-related progestins. *Levonorgestrel* is so potent that it has been the progestin used in most situations where a small amount of progestin needs to last for years—such as in the Norplant capsules and the Mirena Intrauterine System (LNg IUS). *Norgestrel* is a racemic mixture of the biologically active conformation of levonorgestrel and the inactive dextronorgestrel. To adjust for that difference, pills with norgestrel (Lo Ovral) have twice the amount of progestin as the equivalent pills with levonorgestrel (Nordette). The second-generation progestins have been associated with more androgen-related side effects such as adverse effect on lipids, oily skin, acne, and facial hair growth.

Third-generation progestins. Third-generation progestins (desogestrel, norgestimate and, elsewhere, gestodene) were introduced to maintain the potent progestational activity of the second-generation progestins, but to reduce androgenic side effects. Reduction in androgen impacts allows a fuller expression of the pill's estrogen impacts. This has some clinical benefits. One particular product (Ortho TriCyclen) with the third-generation progestin (norgestimate) was the first COC to earn approval from the FDA as an effective treatment for mild to moderate cystic acne. (see section on General Health Benefits). Another formulation (Mircette) has been shown to have no impact on glucose or insulin resistance.[287] On the other hand, concern arose that the increased expression of estrogen might increase the risk of venous thromboembolism (VTE). This concern introduced a pill scare in Europe until international studies were completed and correctly interpreted. (See the VTE Section in the Disadvantages and Health Issues.)

Fourth-generation progestins. Drospirenone is an analogue of spironolactone, a potassium-sparing diuretic used to treat hypertension. Drospirenone possesses antimineralocorticoid and anti-androgenic properties. These properties have led to new noncontraceptive applications, such as the treatment of premenstrual dysphoric disorder and acne, with a specific formulation containing this progestin. In the wake of concerns around possible increased VTE risk with the less androgenic third-generation formulations, those issues were also anticipated with drospirenone. They were clearly answered by large international studies (see VTE section in the Disadvantages and Health Issues.)

Next-generation progestins. More recently, newer progestins have been developed that have properties that are shared with different generations of progestins. They have more profound, diverse, and discreet effects on the endometrium than prior progestins. This class would include dienogestrel (United States) and nomegestrol (Europe).

A more functional categorization of the progestins is based on their metabolites. Under this system, there are three groups of progestins. See Table 11–2.

Another way to understand different progestins is to evaluate how each compares to the various properties of natural progesterone (see Table 11–3).

Table 11–2 Progestins used in oral contraceptives

Parent Component	Progesterone	10-Nortestosterone		17α Spironolactone
Class name	Pregnanes	Estranes	Gonanes	
Product Name	Medroxy-progesterone acetate*	Norethindrone	Norgestrel	Drospirenone
	Cyproterone acetate*	Norethindrone acetate	Levonorgestrel Desogestrel	
	Chormadinone acetate*	Ethynodiol diacetate	Norgestimate Gestodene*	

Dienogestrel
Nomegestrol*

*Not currently used in U.S. formulations

Table 11–3 Pharmacologic profile of progestins in animal models and half-lives in humans

	Progestogenic	Anti-androgenic	Anti-mineral-ocorticoid	Androgenic	Half life (hours) *
Progesterone	+	(+)	+	-	-
Norethindrone	+	-	-	(+)	5–13
Levonorgestrel	+	-	-	(+)	10
Desogestrel	+	-	-	(+)	12–24
Cyproterone acetate	+	+	-	-	
Drospirenone	+	+	+	-	31–33

+ Distinct effect

(+) Negligible effect

- No effect

* In humans

Sources: Krattenmacher R (2000),[8] Muhn P, et al. (1995),[9] Stanczyk FZ (2003),[5] Rapkin AJ, Winer SA (2007).[6]

ESTROGENS

Estrogen was added to birth control pills to provide better cycle control. Estradiol, the estrogen produced by the ovary, was not used in the first COCs because it was too weak to maintain endometrial support in the face of large doses of progestin. Instead, the early COCs used mestranol, a pro-drug that appeared as a contaminant in the first COC, Enovid. Mestranol is converted into the active form ethinyl estradiol (EE) when it is metabolized by the liver directly after absorption. Over time, the doses of mestranol used in COCs were reduced from 150 mcg to 100 mcg to 80 mcg and further to 50 mcg. Today mestranol is found in only a few 50 mcg pills. When the sub-50 mcg COCs were introduced, all of them contained bioactive EE. Today, most COCs in the United States contain 20, 25, 30, 35 or 50 mcg EE. One formulation contains only 10 mcg EE. Estradiol and estradiol esters have recently been introduced in pills that contain special progestins that have particularly strong endometrial activity.

COC FORMULATIONS

Over the decades, many different formulations of combined hormonal contraception have been introduced. This increased choice in COCs has enabled clinicians and patients to select formulations that would work for each individual woman. It also introduced a flexibility that allowed a woman who develops a problem with one formulation to switch to another formulation and not have to discontinue COC use. Formulations that provide monthly scheduled bleeding vary by the type of hormone, the amounts of the different hormones, and also the patterns of those hormones used in pills within the packet.

COCs with monthly cycling are available in either monophasic or multiphasic packages.

- Monophasic formulations have the same combination of estrogen and progestin in each active pill in the packet. Older formulations were available in 21 or 28 pill packs. The latter contains 7 placebo pills. Newer monophasic formulation packets contain 21 or 24 identical active pills and 4 or 7 placebo pills to total 28 pills. Reducing the number of placebo pills may improve the effectiveness of low-dose formulations.[288] One variation is a formulation with 21 identical active pills, 2 placebo pills, and 5 remaining pills that each contains 10 mcg EE.

- Multiphasic formulations have pills with different amounts of estrogen and progestin in the packet. Typically, biphasic formulations have 2 different combinations of estrogen and progestin in the active pills, and triphasic formulations have 3 different combinations of doses.

- Other pills offering more variable combinations of estrogen and progestin have recently been introduced to try to minimize hormonal exposure while providing reliable ovulation suppression and good cycle control.

Extended-cycle COCs (longer than 28-day cycles) represent an important step in the evolution of COCs. Physical and emotional suffering may be associated with scheduled monthly bleeding; women are more likely to complain of cramps, bloating, gastrointestinal upset, and headaches while taking the placebo pills than at any time when they are taking their active pills.[10] Limiting the number of bleeding episodes provides an additional noncontraceptive health benefit and motivates many women to be more consistent pill users.[11] The changes made to the original extended cycle pill formulations have mirrored the changes that were made in earlier years with monthly cycling pills. Extended cycle formulations are also diversified. Extended cycle pills have replaced placebo pills with tablets containing 10 mcg EE. One extended cycle formulation has reduced the estrogen dose in the active pill.[12] Multiphasic extended cycle formulations are in clinical trials.

In addition to the currently available FDA-approved products for extended-cycle pill use, the literature supports the safety and efficacy of using extended cycles of other formulations in reducing discomforts with monthly bleeding.[13,14] The challenge with use of other formulations for extended-cycle use is that it increases the cost of COC and introduces barriers for women who may not be able to get coverage for the extra packs of pills they will need to have to replace the placebo pills with active pills.

MECHANISM OF ACTION
COCs prevent fertilization and, therefore, qualify as contraceptives. There is no significant evidence that they work after fertilization. The progestins in all COCs provide most of the contraceptive effect by suppressing ovulation and thickening cervical mucus, although the estrogens also make a small contribution to ovulation suppression. Cycle control is enhanced by the estrogen.

Progestins inhibit ovulation by—

- Suppressing the release of gonadotropin releasing hormone (GnRH) from the hypothalamus
- Suppressing the surge of LH (luteinizing hormone) from the pituitary that induces ovulation

The progestin inhibits sperm activity by—

- Thickening the cervical mucus to prevent sperm entry into the upper genital tract

The estrogen decreases folliculogenesis by—

- Suppressing the release of FSH (follicle stimulating hormone) from the pituitary

The incidence of "escape ovulation" in COC users in earlier, higher dose pills was estimated to be around 2%. Breakthrough ovulation is probably higher in current lower-dose pills. In a study of 20 mcg pills, progesterone levels indicative of ovulation were found in 2 of 24 women (8.3%). In these situations, the impenetrability of the cervical mucus is the mechanism that prevents fertilization from occurring. Another study has documented that when 20 mcg EE pills were taken as directed, no escape ovulation was detected.[15]

EE and progestins have other effects on the reproductive system, but it has not been substantiated that any of these effects contributes significantly to the efficacy of COCs.

- Slowing of tubal motility and disruption of transport of the ova (may interfere with fertilization)

- Endometrial atrophy, changes in function of endometrial vessels, alterations in the matrix metalloproteinase content in the endometrium (progestin effects that might impede sperm motility and viability, or theoretically, could inhibit implantation)

- Localized edema of the endometrium (an estrogen effect that might affect implantation)

Because COCs so effectively suppress ovulation and block ascent of sperm into the upper genital tract, the potential impact on endometrial receptivity to implantation is almost academic. When the two primary mechanisms fail, the fact that pregnancy occurs despite the endometrial changes demonstrates that those endometrial changes do not significantly contribute to the pill's mechanism of action.

EFFECTIVENESS

COCs are in the second tier of contraceptive effectiveness because their first-year failure rate with typical use is 9% (see Figure 3–1 in the chapter on Choosing a Contraceptive). However, COCs have the potential to be in the top tier of efficacy, because with correct and consistent use, the first-year failure rate of most pills is less than 1%. The failure rates reported in clinical trials should not be confused with the *typical use* failure rate, because women in clinical trials are highly motivated, monitored closely, and reimbursed for the expenses they incur for study participation. Typical use failure rates, derived from real-world use in which some women use COCs correctly and others do not, are a better guide for patient counseling.

As hormone levels in pills have decreased dramatically over time, clinical pregnancy rates have increased due primarily to reasons unrelated to lower hormone doses. The most significant change has been that we can now diagnose pregnancy much earlier. When Enovid was in clinical trials, the only pregnancy test available was the "rabbit" test, which required that a woman have 6 weeks of amenorrhea before the test could detect the pregnancy. Today we can detect an implantation before the woman misses her menses. Given that many implantations are lost before 6 weeks, it is clear that it is difficult to compare the efficacy of different pills under these conditions. A second reason pregnancy rates appear to have increased is that the FDA changed the reporting criteria to include not only all the pregnancies that occur while the woman is using her COCs but also any pregnancies that are conceived within the first week or two after she stops using the method. Since pills are rapidly reversible, some pregnancies can occur immediately after their cessation.

Impact of behavior barriers to successful pill use. The gap that exists between *perfect use* failure rates and *typical use* failure rates is due to patient behaviors. Substantial barriers may prevent a patient from gaining timely access to her contraceptive supplies or to her consistent use of those methods. A study of how well women refilled their prescriptions for branded COCs showed that by 1 month, only 72% of women returned to the pharmacy on a timely basis to refill their prescriptions. Fewer than 30% of women returned to the pharmacy on time for 12 months of pills.[11] Requiring women to return each month for refills constitutes a major barrier to successful pill use. Studies have clearly demonstrated that women are much more likely to continue to use pills if they are given multiple packs at each visit.[11,16] Women who receive multiple packs have lower pregnancy rates.[289]

Possession of the COC pack does not guarantee correct daily use. One study, in which a computer chip was placed in the pill pack to record the date and time that a woman removed a pill from the pack, found that although most women thought that they took the pills on a daily basis, during the third cycle, 54% of women missed 3 or more pills.[17] It must be admitted that taking a pill each day for an asymptomatic condition is challenging. One way to motivate women to remember to take their pills is to link pill use to some other tangible benefit that they can appreciate—such as an improvement in acne or lighter or fewer bleeding episodes. Linking pill taking to some other daily activity (tooth brushing) has had mixed results. Programming cell phones to sound an alarm to remind the patient to take the pill may be more effective in younger women. Using formulations with fewer placebo pills might reduce the chance that a dominant follicle will form as a result of inconsistent pill use.[18]

Impact of attitudinal barriers to successful pill use. Contraceptive use requires ongoing commitment to be successful. Contraception is different from other preventive medications. People take insulin to prevent blindness, extremity amputations, and renal failure. No one ever wants any of those outcomes. However, with contraception, the picture is not so clear. Many women are ambivalent about wanting pregnancy.[19] Torn between two competing priorities, inconsistent pill use may be a way of letting a pregnancy happen, so that it can be accepted at some level as something "that was meant to be." Planning and preparing for pregnancy has not been adopted as a standard by women. Some women don't even understand the concept of "planning and preparing for pregnancy."[20]

Impact of discontinuation. Many pregnancies that are credited to the pill in typical use occur in the month when women discontinue COCs and do not adopt a new method of contraception. By 6 months, at least 28% of pill users have stopped the pill; by 1 year, that percentage approaches 33% to 50%.[21] Quite disturbingly, 42% of women who discontinued COC use did so *without* consulting their clinicians. Studies show that 11% of women discontinue their pills in the first month of use, and 19% of those who discontinue fail to adopt a new method.[22] Because of these concerns, **women starting the pill should also be given a second method** (such as condoms) that they can use in case they discontinue pill use before returning for follow-up. They should also be given a packet of or a prescription for emergency contraception (EC). At a minimum, inform women about the availability of EC.

IMPACT OF BODY WEIGHT ON COC EFFICACY

Given the growing number of reproductive-age women who are obese, the impact that patient weight might have on pill efficacy is important for public health as well as for personal health. Two early retrospective studies suggested that heavier women had higher pregnancy rates on COCs.[23,24] Interestingly, 75% of the women in the study weighed less than 154 lbs. Early follow-up studies also reported higher failure rates among obese women,[25] but causation could not be assigned. To investigate the issue in more detail, one pharmacokinetic study comparing obese to normal weight women using levonorgestrel pills noted significant differences in hormonal half-life, clearance, and time to reach steady state levels. However, escape ovulation measured by gonadotropin activity did not demonstrate any statistical difference between these two groups.[26] Another pharmacokinetic study, which compared hormone levels in normal weight women to hormone levels in obese women, found that peak hormone levels were lower in obese women, but follicular activity was not affected by the differences seen in hormone levels.[27] In a more direct study of potential efficacy, a prospective, double-blinded trial of two monophasic COCs found that the obese women and normal weight women who used their COCs correctly and consistently experienced substantial and comparable ovarian suppression as measured by progesterone levels.[28]

In clinical trials of various COC formulations in which weight, height, and COC type has been verified, there were *no* higher pregnancy rates in overweight/obese women than in slender women, whether using extended[29] or low-dose ($\leq$ 25 mcg EE) cyclic regimens.[30,31] Other analyses, including data from the National Surveys of Family Growth, found no increase in failure rates among obese women.[32] More conclusive data demonstrating no increase in failure rates in heavier women comes from the postmarketing surveillance studies in Europe, which showed that there was no trend of increasing pregnancy rates among women as weight increased.[33] Overall, the Society of Family Planning concluded that overweight and obese COC users appear to be at a similar or slightly higher risk of pregnancy compared with normal BMI women.[34]

ACOG has admonished clinicians to use any estrogen-containing contraceptive only "with caution in obese women (BMI >30) over age 35,"[35] reflecting the concern about an increased risk of venous thromboembolism (VTE) due to obesity. The medical eligibility criteria adapted by the United States (U.S. MEC) lists the use of COCs by obese women of any age as a category 2 condition.[36] (See Chapter 4.) Decreasing the pill-free interval or decreasing the number of pill-free intervals is clearly more acceptable than using higher-dose formulations in heavier women who are having unscheduled bleeding. Another option would be to switch to a vaginal ring, which could improve cycle control without increasing estrogen exposure.[37]

For recommendations regarding COC use following bariatric surgery, see section on Special Populations—Women with Medical Problems.

ADVANTAGES AND INDICATIONS

COCs provide women with safe, effective, and rapidly reversible control of their fertility; couples can plan and prepare for any pregnancies they may desire. In addition, COCs solve many menstrually related problems, not only by reducing medical problems associated with bleeding, but also by improving a woman's functionality, productivity and her quality of life. COCs also provide many other non-contraceptive health benefits.

General Advantages

1. **Effectiveness.** When women use COCs correctly and consistently, first-year pregnancy rates are below 1%. However, in typical use, these pregnancy rates are 9% (see Chapter 3.)

2. **Safety.** Despite widespread public perception that COCs are hazardous,[38] recent data about short- and long-term safety of pill use are very reassuring. Short-term safety is achieved by careful patient selection. Women are candidates for COCs when their health risks from COC use are less than the health risks they would face with pregnancy. (See U.S. MEC summarized in Chapter 4.) Since so many women get pregnant while they are "on the pill," we have extensive experience with fetal exposure to COCs; fetuses inadvertently exposed in utero to COCs are not at any greater risk for birth defects than are unexposed fetuses.[39,40]

   Long-term safety data about COCs have only recently become available. The Royal College of General Practitioners (RCGP) observed 46,112 women for up to 39 years, accumulating over 378,000 woman-years of observational data among never-users of COCs and 819,175 woman-years of experience among ever-users. Ever-users of COCs had a significant 12% *lower* rate of death from any cause than did never-users. The estimated absolute reduction in all causes of mortality for ever-users of COCs from that study was 52 per 100,000 woman-years.[41]

3. **An option throughout the reproductive years.** Healthy women can safely use COCs throughout their reproductive lives. Age itself is not a reason to avoid COCs. Moreover, the noncontraceptive impacts of the pill address specific issues for women in different age groups. Young women benefit from reduction in severe dysmenorrhea, primary menorrhagia, and acne. Perimenopausal women who are appropriate COC candidates often benefit from cycle control and hot flash reduction provided by this method.

4. **Rapid reversibility.** Return to fertility in women who stop COCs in order to conceive is comparable to that observed following discontinuation of other contraceptive methods.[42] Given the lower hormonal doses in modern COCs, there is no longer any post-pill amenorrhea. Baseline cycling will resume immediately. COC use neither hastens nor delays the onset of menopause.

Contraceptive Health Benefits

1. **Reduction of maternal deaths.** The maternal mortality rate in the United States is the highest it has been in 20 years[290] and now is 14.5 deaths per 100,000 live births in 2005.[291] Each year, an additional 34,000 women suffer such severe obstetrical complications that they almost die (called 'near misses').[292] Given that nearly half the pregnancies in this country are unintended, preventing those pregnancies could decrease maternal deaths.

2. **Reduction of ectopic pregnancies.** COCs reduce the risk of ectopic pregnancy by over 90%.[44,45] At least 1% of all US pregnancies are thought to be ectopic.

Menstrually Related Health Benefits

(See Chapter 20 for more details.)

1. **Decreased dysmenorrhea.** COCs significantly decrease menstrual cramps and pain. Although the original studies that demonstrated this benefit were based on high-dose formulations, low-dose formulations have also been shown to help even when given in the conventional cyclic fashion.[46] Overall, COC use reduces the incidence of dysmenorrhea by 60%.[47] The more severe the woman's pain is, the more effective COCs are in reducing her symptoms; severe dysmenorrhea is reduced by almost 90% with COC use.[48] In a randomized clinical trial for treatments of dysmenorrhea, low-dose COC users reported fewer absences from school and work and used less pain relief medicine than placebo users.[49] A recent review of existing literature concluded that for women who wish contraception, COCs are the preferred therapy for pain relief from dysmenorrhea; because COC use eliminates the risks associated with taking NSAIDs, it is a more suitable long-term option.[50] Continuous or extended-cycle COC use, which eliminates scheduled bleeding episodes for months at a time, provides even more significant relief from dysmenorrhea.

2. **Decreased menstrual blood loss.** COCs decrease the number of days of bleeding and the amount of blood women lose each cycle. In women with heavy menstrual bleeding, high-dose COC use reduced blood loss by 53%.[47] In studies of low-dose COCs (30 mcg EE), menstrual blood loss and duration of flow were also decreased.[51-53] In a newer study using a 20 mcg EE formulation, COCs reduced bleeding by 68%, as assessed by scores on a pictorial blood assessment chart (PBAC).[54] In that study, nearly 50% of women experienced a reduction in duration of menstrual

bleeding with COC use.[54] Women who use extended-cycle options reduce their numbers of scheduled bleeding episodes each year and further decrease their total menstrual blood loss.[55,56] The median number of days of bleeding after 84 days of pills is less than after 21 days of the same pills. These features are particularly important for women with idiopathic heavy menstrual bleeding, adenomyosis, and coagulation defects. Hormonal contraceptives, including COCs, are also first-line medical therapies for treatment of heavy menstrual bleeding due to fibroids.

3. **Regulation of bleeding.** Taken cyclically, COCs produce very predictable scheduled bleeding. This predictability allows women to plan their lives around their bleeding, rather than having to adapt their schedules to their flow whenever it starts. Women who use extended-cycle COCs gain even more control over their scheduled bleeding and, with time, over unscheduled spotting and bleeding.[55]

4. **Reduction in premenstrual syndrome (PMS) symptoms.** COCs can reduce physical PMS symptoms, such as mastalgia, cramping, and pain. Drospirenone-containing pills have also been shown to improve symptoms of water retention, bloating, negative affect, and increased appetite associated with menstruation.[57,58] In a comparative trial, drospirenone-containing pills reduced PMS symptoms more than did levonorgestrel-containing pills.[59] Extended-cycle low-dose levonorgestrel formulations may also be more effective than selective serotonin reuptake inhibitors (SSRIs) in reducing symptoms of PMS.[60]

5. **Reduction of premenstrual dysphoric disorder (PMDD).** As many as 18% of women of reproductive age may have PMDD, which, by definition, means that their symptoms are severe enough to cause distress.[61] In a randomized double-blind placebo-controlled study, one low-dose drospirenone-containing formulation with 24 active pills and 4 placebo pills reduced the severity and frequency of both the physical and behavioral symptoms of PMDD.[62] Women's ability to function and to interact socially during menses also improved. Based on these studies, it gained approval from the FDA as treatment for the symptoms of PMDD.

6. **Decreased anovulatory bleeding.** Low-dose COC use was associated with more than 80% improvement in anovulatory uterine bleeding in a randomized, double-blind, placebo-controlled study.[63] Anovulatory bleeding is a significant challenge for obese women, for women with polycystic ovarian syndrome (PCOS), and for women in the two extremes of their reproductive lives—menarche and perimenopause.

7. **Mittelschmerz relief.** By preventing ovulation, COCs can eliminate the midcycle pain (mittelschmerz) that some women experience with ovarian follicle swelling and oocyte extrusion.

8. **Reduced risk of post-ovulatory ovarian cysts.** Because COCs suppress ovulation, both monophasic and multiphasic COCs reduce a woman's risk of developing post-ovulatory (luteal) cysts,[64-68] including hemorrhagic corpus luteum cysts, which can pose a surgical emergency. However, low-dose pills taken cyclically (21/7) do not protect as well against follicular cyst formation, because they do not sufficiently suppress FSH levels.[67-70] Shortening the pill-free interval of a COC containing a progestin with a short half-life may not reduce the formation of ovarian follicles,[71] but there is evidence that shortening the pill-free interval of COCs containing progestins with a longer half-life is helpful at reducing follicular growth.[72] COCs are not a treatment for ovarian cysts because their use does not accelerate regression of existing cysts,[73] but COCs may prevent the formation of a new cyst, which might be mistaken for the original cyst on repeat exam. Extended cycle use of low-dose pills may more effectively reduce follicular ovarian cyst formation.

9. **Improvement in menstrual migraines.** Menstrual migraines are caused by estrogen withdrawal[74-76] and are mediated by prostaglandin release during menses. Cyclic COC use may worsen menstrual migraines because estrogen levels are higher with COC use; the end-of-cycle estrogen decline is more dramatic. On the other hand, menstrual migraine symptoms may be prevented for many months if a woman uses extended cycles and reduces her number of withdrawal bleeds.[77,78] (See the section on Headaches, in Managing Side Effects.)

General Health Benefits

1. **Ovarian cancer risk reduction.** Ovarian cancer is the most lethal gynecologic cancer. Most of the 21,550 cases diagnosed in 2010 in the United States were not detected until the women had advanced disease.[79] Women who use COCs are substantially less likely to develop epithelial ovarian cancer.[80] A collaborative reanalysis of data from 45 studies showed that ever-users of COCs had reduced risk of ovarian cancer that persisted for 30 years.[81] It is clear that the longer the duration of use, the greater the protection the pill provides against ovarian cancer. Monophasic formulations used for at least 10 years reduced a woman's risk of developing such cancers by 80%.[82,83] The Royal College of General Practitioners (RCGP) observational study with up to 39 years of follow-up found that ever-users were 47%

less likely to die from ovarian cancer than were never-users (RR 0.53 (0.38–0.72)).[41] This protective effect has also been seen with low-dose pills in most studies,[82–84] but some have reported less protection with a lower dose of progestin.[85]

Several mechanisms can explain the COCs' protection against epithelial ovarian carcinoma: increased apoptosis (programmed cell death) in the ovarian surface epithelium; decreased matrix metalloproteinase-2 activity (suggesting that COCs may work by inhibiting proteolytic activity)[86]; suppression of ovulation, which decreases the repeated epithelial damage that occurs each month with ovum extrusion; and reduction in gonadotropins (FSH and LH), which could help by reducing stimulation of steroid production and ovarian stimulation.[87]

A compelling argument can be made that COCs should be offered to otherwise healthy women who are at high risk for developing this carcinoma, even if they do not need contraception.[88,89] Women with a family history of ovarian cancer enjoy a greater reduction in ovarian cancer risk than do women with no such family history.[90] Women who used COCs for 4 years and had first degree relatives with ovarian cancer had a 90% reduction in their own ovarian cancer risk. Most studies have found that women with BRCA1 and BRCA2 mutations have similar protection from ovarian cancer with COC use.[83,91] For every 1,000 women with BRCA1 mutations, COC use could prevent 250 cases of ovarian cancer; for every 1,000 women with BRCA2 mutations, COC use would reduce 150 ovarian cancers.[92] One study did not support these findings. It reported that increased duration of use did not reduce the risk of ovarian cancer in multiparous BRCA1 or BRCA2 mutation carriers, but only a small segment (8.5%) of the study population had used COCs for 5 or more years.[93]

2. **Endometrial cancer risk reduction.** The incidence of endometrial cancer is increasing in the United States because women are living longer and are more likely to be obese. Women who are 50 pounds or more overweight have almost a 10-fold increased risk of developing endometrial cancer compared with normal weight controls. In 2009, the prevalence of obesity (BMI > 30) among adult U.S. women was 35.5%.[94] Over 40,000 U.S. women develop this cancer each year.[79] COC use for at least 12 months reduces a woman's risk of developing endometrial cancer by about 40%.[95] Women who use COCs for at least a decade reduce their risk of developing endometrial cancer by 80% compared with non-users.[95] This protection against endometrial cancer endures for up to 20 years after COC discontinuation.[96] For women who cur-

Table 11-4 COC use and cancer risk

Cancer Type	# of Cases in US— 2010	Impact of COC Use on Risk of Carcinoma				
		Significant Decrease	Some Decrease	Neutral	Some Increase	Significant Increase
Ovarian	21,880					
COC use < 5 yrs			X			
COC use ≥ 5 yrs		X				
Endometrial	43,470					
COC use < 1 yr			X			
COC use ≥ 1 yr		X				
Cervical	12,200					
COC use < 5 yrs				X		
COC use ≥ 5 yrs[1]					X	
Breast	207,090					
Age < 35					X	
Age ≥ 35				X		
Hepatic[2]	6,690			X		
Gallbladder	5,310			X		
Melanoma	9,010			X		

[1] No increased risk unless patient persistently infected with HR-HPV

[2] No increased risk, even in Hepatitis B virus carriers

Source: American Cancer Society Cancer Facts and Figures (2010).[79]

rently have endometrial hyperplasia (a precursor to endometrial carcinoma), COCs can be used as a treatment to reverse this condition and prevent endometrial carcinoma.

3. **Decreased risk of benign breast conditions.** COC users are less likely to develop fibrocystic breast changes, cysts, or fibroadenoma, and are less likely to experience progression of those breast conditions.[97] In one case-control study with over 500 women, the risk of benign breast conditions was lower in the COC users and markedly lower in women who started COC use before their first full-term pregnancy.[98] COC use does not reduce the risk of developing ductal hyperplasia with atypia, but it does not increase that risk.[99]

4. **Improvement of acne and hirsutism.** Dutch surveys reported that COC use reduced the prevalence of acne by over two thirds.[100] In prospective, randomized, placebo-controlled, double-blind trials, women who used selected COCs had a sig-

nificant reduction in the number and size of acne lesions.[101–103] Only three formulations have received formal FDA approval for treatment of mild to moderate acne (Ortho Tri-Cyclen, Estrostep, and YAZ), but other formulations may be somewhat effective.[104,105] A recent Cochrane review concluded that COCs in clinical trials are effective in reducing inflammatory and noninflammatory facial acne lesions. Few differences were found in acne effectiveness between the COC types that were included in the clinical trials.[106]

COCs reduce acne by suppressing ovarian production of testosterone and by inducing hepatic production of sex hormone binding globulin (SHBG). SHBG binds circulating testosterone and, thereby, reduces serum concentrations of free (biologically active) testosterone by up to 50%. Some formulations with drospirenone also block the testosterone receptors on the sebum glands and significantly reduce intracellular conversion of testosterone to dihydrotestosterone, which is the molecule that triggers the production of sebum. In addition, extended-cycle regimens and shortened pill-free intervals suppress endogenous androgen production more than 21/7 regimens.[107] COCs do not have an immediate impact on acne; women need to be advised that maximal effect may not be seen for up to 6 months.[101,102] SHBG levels may remain elevated for several months after discontinuation of COCs, leading a woman to conclude that her acne was cured, when it may not have been.[108]

Just as estrogen in COCs helps reduce androgen activation of sebum production, it also helps reduce that hormone's stimulation of androgen-sensitive (sexual) hair growth. With COC use, women with hirsutism have a reduction in the hair shaft diameter.[109,110] It generally takes 1 to 2 years to see the maximal beneficial effect of COCs on hirsutism. In these situations, the most appropriate formations will be those with progestins with low (or anti) androgen impact and high-dose estrogens. In addition, extended-cycle regimens and shortened hormone-free intervals suppress androgen production more than do cyclic 21/7 regimens.[107]

5. **Decreased risk of iron deficiency anemia.** By reducing menstrual blood loss, each cycle of COC use conserves a woman's hemoglobin and ferritin levels.[111] This benefit is especially important for women with sickle cell anemia or von Willebrand disease, women using anticoagulants (if they are MEC-eligible) or anticonvulsants, and women with fibroids, adenomyosis, or other causes of primary or secondary heavy menstrual bleeding

(see Chapter 20 on Menstrual Disorders). In the long run, this benefit is improved even further by extended-cycle COCs.

6. **Reducing symptoms of endometriosis.** Current or recent COC use is associated with a lower incidence of symptomatic endometriosis, especially among parous women.[112] The risk of developing endometriomas has also been found to be significantly lower in current COC users over the age of 25.[113] In addition, long-term cyclic and continuous use of COCs following laparoscopic excision of ovarian endometriomas has been found to significantly reduce and delay the recurrence of endometriomas.[114]

COCs decrease the menstrual pain suffered by women with endometriosis.[115] This benefit is enhanced by use of extended-cycle COCs, which reduce the number of painful episodes that women have. Also, with extended or continuous use of COCs, the progestins induce pseudodecidualization of the endometriotic implants, which makes them inactive and less likely to induce painful inflammation reactions during menses[116] or between menses. However, such treatment is not curative; the endometriotic implants undergo atrophy during treatment but remain ready for reactivation whenever COCs are stopped.[117]

7. **Treatment for hot flashes and other hormonal fluctuation symptoms in perimenopausal women.**[118,119] (See Chapter 25 on Perimenopause, Menopause and Postmenopause for more discussion)

8. **Fewer episodes of sickle cell crises and catamenial seizures, porphyria, and asthma.** Sickle cell crises are reduced by half by COC use.[120] Extended cycle and continuous use of COCs can significantly reduce menstrual exacerbations of seizure disorders, porphyria, and asthma (so called "catamenial" asthma).[121]

Other Potential Health Benefits

1. **Reduced risk of uterine fibroids.** COC users have fewer fibroids especially with long-term use,[122] but COC use early in life may increase risk of fibroid formation.[123] COCs are often prescribed to help women control the excess menstrual blood loss that leiomyomas can cause. In fact, many insurance carriers specify that women with small to moderate-sized fibroids must fail a trial of medical management (usually with COCs) for menorrhagia before they can be considered candidates for surgical therapies.

2. **Favorable impact on bone for high-risk women.** Women who have hypothalamic amenorrhea have low levels of circulating estrogens and are higher at risk for osteoporosis, and for fractures

later in life. COC use increases bone mineral density (BMD) in young women with hypothalamic amenorrhea[124] and in anorexic teenagers.[125] COC use by women with osteopenia due to anorexia nervosa is not sufficient to completely protect bone, but when added to anabolic agents such as insulin growth factor, COC use significantly improves that agent's effectiveness.[126] COC use also modulates the negative impact of smoking on BMD in young women and improves BMD in young women with irregular menses.[127]

For women with normal estrogen levels, the effect of low-dose (30 to 40 mcg EE) and ultra-low-dose (20 to 25 mcg EE) COCs on bone density is less clear. Studies of adolescent and premenopausal women typically measure bone mineral density and bone turnover markers because fracture is so rare in this population. A review of all randomized trials that compared different formulations of COCs found no negative effect on bone health overall, and slightly positive effects for some formulations over others.[128] Based on a systematic review, WHO concluded that adolescent COC users may gain less BMD than adolescent non-users while perimenopausal COC users generally have higher BMD compared with age-matched non-users.[129,130] Newer studies suggest a favorable impact on BMD later in life.[293]

3. **Influence on sexual enjoyment**. Controversy continues about the impact of COCs on sexual enjoyment. Because female sexuality is so complex, sexual appetite and enjoyment are affected by virtually everything in a woman's life. Reducing a woman's risk of pregnancy can permit her to enjoy the experience. The positive effect of COCs on endometriosis, dysmenorrhea, and unpredictable menses may improve sexual enjoyment for women with these problems. In reproductive-aged women, androgen levels do not strongly influence libido.[131] (See Libido discussion in section on Health Issues Incorrectly Attributed to Modern COC Use.)

4. **Source of folate or iron.** Some formulations have added extra minerals or vitamins to at least some of their active pills or their placebo pills. Iron is included in the placebo pills in some low-dose formulations. For women with heavy menstrual bleeding, this can be helpful in reducing their risk for anemia. Other formulations have a source of folate included in every pill to reduce the risk of neural tube defects in the fetuses conceived while the woman is on COCs (about 1 million pregnancies a year) or those conceived shortly after she stops the pill.

NONCONTRACEPTIVE APPLICATIONS FOR COCS

After underlying pathology has been ruled out, COCs are a first-line therapy off-label for otherwise healthy women who suffer from the following conditions, even if the women are not at risk for pregnancy:

- Heavy or prolonged menstrual bleeding
- Infrequent menses
- Painful menses
- Recurrent luteal phase ovarian cysts
- Family history of ovarian cancer
- Personal risk factors for endometrial cancer
- Acne or hirsutism
- Polycystic ovary syndrome (PCOS)

In addition, *extended use* of COC may be particularly helpful off-label for treatment for women with the following conditions:

- Painful menstruation
- Menstrually related PMS or PMDD symptoms
- Pain from endometriosis
- Anemia due to heavy or prolonged menstrual bleeding
- Developmentally delayed women whose monthly menstruations terrify them or those whose bleeding presents a hygiene challenge to their caregivers
- Hypothalamic amenorrhea, as seen in women with the athletic triad or isolated eating disorders
- Personal preference

COCs FOR EMERGENCY CONTRACEPTION

If emergency contraceptive products are not available, COCs with levonorgestrel or norgestrel may be used. One study suggests that COCs with norethindrone may be used for emergency contraception if norgestrel-related compounds are not available, but those formulations have slightly (but not significantly) higher failure rates (see Chapter 6 on Emergency Contraception).[132]

Societal Benefits

In addition to the health and quality of life benefits COCs have provided individual women and their children, COCs have had large societal impacts. Today, the biomass of our species exceeds the biomass of any other species on the face of the earth, which means that humans have a profound impact on the health of the planet. Since the introduction of COCs and IUDs, family size has dramatically diminished. In the United States the average birth rate in the 1950s was nearly 4; 50 years later it is barely at replacement levels at 2.1. As the world's human population has increased, major shortages of water and fuel have emerged, leading to social instability. COCs can slow population growth. When birth rates are lower, the resources available to each individual increases.

DISADVANTAGES AND CAUTIONS

Before a woman decides to use COCs, she should consider if she would be able to obtain COCs and to use them correctly and consistently. She should also balance the benefits she would get with COC use against the possible risks they pose for her in the context of her individual medical status.

GENERAL DISADVANTAGES

1. **Daily administration.** Inconsistent use of COCs reduces their potential for protection from pregnancy and increases the incidence of some side effects, especially unscheduled bleeding and spotting.[294] Studies demonstrate that most women miss several pills each month.[17]

2. **Expense and access challenges.** In most states, not all insurance plans are required to include contraception in a woman's benefit package. Many women must pay out of pocket for their COCs.[133] The cost of branded pills may easily exceed $80 per pack. Generic formulations are typically less expensive but often cost $30 or more per month. Pharmacies that have generic prescription programs (Wal-Mart, Target, and Walgreens) sell a limited number of generic COC formulations for $9 a pack. Even for systems that do provide contraceptive coverage, there may be a high copayment, especially for the more expensive formulations. Find out what a patient's coverage is and what her financial constraints may be when you help her choose a COC.

   Often, the number of packets dispensed at pharmacies is severely restricted, so women are required to return to pharmacies each month to purchase another package. The mismatch between calendar months with 30 to 31 days and pill packs with only 28 pills can present additional challenges in COC use. Women who desire to use extended cycles of pills are faced with even more difficulties in obtaining adequate pill supplies.

3. **Need for storage with ready access.** Adolescent women and adult women whose partners do not want them to use contraception may not have a secure place to store their pills. Practitioners need to confirm that the woman's plans for storage are realistic (school lockers are not an answer!) and to guide them to more private contraceptive methods, if needed. Homeless women and women who travel extensively may also have difficulty storing their pill packs.

4. **No protection against sexually transmitted infections (STIs).** Women at risk for STIs may use COCs, but they should be advised that COCs do not provide them protection from those infections. Advise them to reduce their risk for STIs by confining their sexual activity to mutually monogamous, uninfected partners, or by using condoms with every act of coitus.

Understanding Risk Estimates

Understanding the following fundamental statistical concepts will help in understanding the risks reported by studies and in interpreting those risks for our patients.

- *Relative risk,* generally represented as RR, represents the ratio of the probability that a complication will arise *with* pill use compared with the probability that the complication will arise *without* pill use. Mathematically, this is written—

$$RR = \frac{\text{Probability of developing condition X with pill use}}{\text{Probability of developing condition X without pill use}}$$

A relative risk of 1 means that pill use does not affect the risk one way (increase) or the other (decrease). Because pill use has no effect on eye color, the relative risk of having brown eyes with pill use would be 1.0. However, if some event happens more often in pill users, the relative risk will be greater than 1.0. If pill use reduces the risk of an event, the relative risk will be less than 1.0. For example, the relative risk of developing ovarian cancer after 10 years of COC use is 0.2, which means that long-term COC users have an 80% reduction in their risk of getting ovarian cancer ($1 - 0.2 = 0.8$). If there is only a slight increase in risk (RR=1.10, or a 10% increase), the clinical significance of the increase in risk is generally small unless the problem is very common or very serious. The "odds ratio" (OR) and the "hazard ratio" (HR) represent similar calculations and should be interpreted as a relative risk in clinical settings.

- *The absolute risk* of an event happening is especially important to know. Even if the relative risk is very high, the absolute risk of a complication may still be low, if the background risk in the population is low. For example the relative risk of developing liver tumors with COC use is 500. This risk appears to be enormous until you understand that this is such a rare tumor that the chance that a COC user will develop liver tumors (the absolute risk) is only 1 in 50,000. A large multiple of a rare event is still a rare event.

- The *attributable* risk reflects how much using pills changes a woman's risk from her background risk. Health problems (like headaches) happen to women whether or not they take COCs. The attributable risk is what a woman needs to know—how much more or less often she is apt to have headaches because she is using COCs.

- One final statistical principle is useful: the *confidence interval* (CI). Studies will report both a relative risk and the confidence interval. This is important because the relative risk calculated in a study is only an estimate. Studies are based on *samples* of women. No one study ever reflects the experience of every woman in the world. So when researchers calculate the relative risk for the women in their study, they also calculate (based on how many subjects were involved in the study and how similar the experiences of those women were) the limits in which the true answer could fall if all the women in the world were studied. The 95% confidence interval (95% CI) says that 95 times out of 100, the real answer lies between the 2 numbers quoted. For example, when a study of pills reports that RR = 1.5 (95% CI 1.2–1.7), the reader would know that the event occurred 50% more often with pill use than without it. However, the study also calculated with 95% confidence that the real risk lies somewhere between a 20% to 70% increase.

A crucial rule when interpreting the confidence interval is that a relative risk is statistically significant only if *both* confidence interval numbers reflect the same answer: either there is an increase or a decrease in risk. If the confidence interval includes the number 1, the relative risk is *not* statistically significant and should *not* change practice. For example, if a study reports RR = 2.5 (95% CI 0.7–4.8), the researchers are saying that the women in their study were 2.5 times more likely to have this complication when they used pills compared with women who did not use pills. However, they estimate that the real answer is that the complication risk could range widely, from 30% less often to 4.8 times more frequently. Obviously, because the study could not determine whether the complication risk increased or decreased with pill use, the outcome of the study should not alter anyone's clinical practice.

HEALTH ISSUES

1. **Pregnancy.** One of the most important health risks of COC use occurs when a woman becomes pregnant because the pill fails or because the she fails to take her COCs correctly and consistently. Even with excellent prenatal care, pregnancy carries with it significant health risks, including hemorrhage, infection, blood clots, stroke, heart attack, diabetes, hypertension, gallbladder disease, nausea, vomiting, kidney damage, liver dysfunction, choriocarcinoma, and even death. Delivery and postpartum periods pose significant health risks, both short-term (hemorrhage, infection, tissue damage, VTE, stroke, amniotic fluid embolism) and long-term (urinary and fecal incontinence). These are real risks the patient must understand when she selects the COC as her method, since there may be methods that could protect her even more effectively from pregnancy.

2. **Venous thromboembolism (VTE).** The best evidence supports the proposal that the increased risk of VTE in COC users is a class effect, dependent on estrogen dose and duration, and independent of the progestin used.[134] In recent years, a significant increase in the incidence of VTE has occurred in all clinical settings—in pregnancy, with estrogen-containing contraceptives, and among the general public. VTE can be a life-threatening condition; 200,000 new cases are diagnosed in the United States each year. Two-thirds of VTE cases are deep vein thromboses (DVTs); DVT carries a 6% mortality rate. The other third of VTE events involve pulmonary embolism, which has a 12% mortality rate. Only 40% of VTEs are idiopathic, with the rest attributable to an identified cause (surgery, trauma, etc.) or a risk factor. Risk factors for venous thrombosis include obesity, smoking, thrombophilia, and recent use of estrogen. VTE can develop in a variety of organs and present with different symptoms, as listed on Table 11–5.

Though the *relative risk* of thrombosis is increased with COC use, most COC users face a low *absolute risk* of thrombosis because VTE is a rare event in healthy young women. The incidence rate of VTE in reproductive-age women is half the rate reported for women of all ages.[135] The VTE risk during pregnancy is 98.5 per 100,000 women-years but rises to 511.2 per 100,000 women-years

Table 11–5 Thrombotic diseases attributable to COCs (See ACHES below)

ACHES	Diagnosis	Location of Pathology	Symptoms
A (Abdominal pain)	Mesenteric vein thrombosis	Intestines	Abdominal pain, vomiting, weakness
	Pelvic vein thrombosis	Pelvis	Lower abdominal pain, cramps
C (Chest pain)	Pulmonary embolism	Lung	Cough (including coughing up blood), chest pain, shortness of breath
	Myocardial infarction	Heart	Crushing chest pain, left arm and shoulder pain, shortness of breath, weakness
H (Headaches)	Stroke	Brain	Headache, weakness or numbness, visual problem, sudden intellectual impairment
E (Eye problems)	Retinal vein thrombosis	Eye	Headache, complete or partial loss of vision
S (Severe leg pain)	Thrombophlebitis	Leg	Swelling, heat or redness, tenderness in thigh or lower leg; calf pain

in the postpartum period.[136] The risk of pulmonary embolism during pregnancy is 10.6 per 100,000 women-years and during postpartum rises to 159.7 per 100,000 women-years.

Even though the doses of estrogen have significantly declined in pills since their introduction, the incidence of VTE events associated with COCs has increased over time. There are two reasons for this:

a. Risk factors for blood clots, such as obesity and age, have increased greatly in the last two decades. Estimates are that over one third of the adult women in the United States have a BMI greater than 30.[94] Today, many women are using COCs much later in life, as they postpone childbearing. More people have sedentary lifestyles with little physical activity.

b. Noninvasive, highly sensitive technologies, such as color flow Doppler ultrasounds, have replaced more invasive procedures, such as venograms, to diagnose DVTs. This has reduced the threshold for testing, so more VTEs are being diagnosed.

In addition to age and weight, some individual women may carry an increased genetic propensity to form clots. The increase in VTE risk seen with COC use is greatly magnified in the face of genetic thrombogenic mutation disorders, such as factor V Leiden mutation. The factor V Leiden mutation alone explains 30% of all cases of deep venous thromboses. In the United States, it is estimated that 5.3% of Caucasians, 2.2% of Hispanics, 1.2% of Blacks and Native Americans, and 0.5% of Asians carry this mutation. A WHO literature review reported that COC users with factor V Leiden mutations were 6.4 to 99.0 times more likely to form blood clots than were non-users without the mutation. Genetic mutations in prothrombin also increase VTE risks. When a carrier uses COCs, her VTE risk rises 100 times higher than noncarriers who do not use COCs.[137] For women with deficiencies in antithrombin, protein C, or protein S, the relative risks for VTE are 8 to 10, with an absolute risk of 120 to 150/100,000 a year. Despite the impact that these mutations may have on a woman's risk for thrombosis, routine laboratory screening for these mutations is not appropriate.[138] (For further discussion, see section on Patient Selection.)

The risk of VTE with COCs is greatest in the first 3 to 12 months of use and declines thereafter. It is for this reason that any study that compares VTE risk for different formulations must compare new start users. Obese COC users have as much as a 3-fold increased risk of VTE when compared with COC users of normal weight.[139] For this reason, it is imperative to control for patient weight in any study comparing different formulations. This is also why the American College of Obstetricians and Gynecologists (ACOG) recommends that women over age 35 with a BMI > 30 should use estrogen-containing contraception with caution,[35] although U.S. MEC rates obesity as a category 2 condition.

Tobacco smoking increases the risk of VTE, especially heavy smoking in young COC users. In one study (adjusted for age, BMI, and parity), smokers aged 18 to 39 who did not use COCs had double the risk of VTE compared with nonsmokers of the same age who did not use COCs. Smokers who did use COCs had a risk that was 8.8 times higher than nonsmokers who did not use COCs.[140] The risks showed a dose response among young smokers. Higher doses of estrogen are associated with greater risks of VTE. VTE risk with 50 mcg EE formulations is higher than that with 35 mcg EE formulations. Lower doses (≥35 mcg EE) have not demonstrated any increased safety.

Clinically significant VTE occurs when there is an imbalance between two sets of factors that control blood clot formation. Estrogen increases hepatic production of elements that promote clot formation by the extrinsic clotting system (Factor VII, Factor VIII, Factor X) and decreases the production of elements that promote clot lysis (tissue plasminogen activator, antiplasmin). COC users also develop an increased resistance to anticoagulant effect of activated protein C. The net result is a prothrombotic effect.

Progestins alone have virtually no impact on the clotting system, but when combined with estrogen, some progestins can modulate the strength of estrogen's production of extrinsic clotting factors, antithrombin,[141] fibrinolytics, and other steps in blood clot formation. In the mid-1990s, international studies indicated that pills containing the third-generation progestins desogestrel and gestodene (not available in the United States) were associated with higher rates of thrombosis (up to 2-fold increase) compared with formulations containing second-generation progestins levonorgestrel and norgestrel.[142-144] The hypothesis was that older, more androgenic progestins cancelled some of estrogen's impacts, so fewer prothrombotic factors would be produced. Because third-generation progestins were designed to reduce the androgenicity of progestin to allow fuller expression of the pill's estrogen component, such concerns about possible increased VTE risk were biologically plausible. Reassuringly, re-analyses of those early studies showed no increase in VTE risk with third-generation progestins, once corrections were made for biases related to recency of COC use and patient selection.[145] U.S. product labeling had been amended to include information about a potential increased risk, even though the risk was no longer apparent when the early studies were corrected and re-analyzed.

When the FDA approved the first drospirenone-containing COC, it required the manufacturer to conduct large-scale postmarketing surveillance studies to determine if there were any increased risk of this new anti-androgen progestin. As a result, two large studies found that, compared with other formulations, drospirenone-containing pills were *not* associated with higher risk of VTE; the absolute risks for all pills were about 180 to 190 VTE events per 100,000 women-years.[139,146] Two later studies reported that drospirenone had almost a 2-fold increased risk in VTE compared with levonorgestrel.[147,148] Although these studies included significant numbers of women, the FDA determined that one of the studies was significantly flawed (unreliable)[148] and the other study actually showed no increase in VTE risk.[147] There is no basis for concern that drospirenone-containing pills have higher rates of VTE risk compared with pills with other progestins.

Patients need to know the increase in VTE risk that they experience during COC use is a completely reversible risk. The risk of thrombosis usually disappears within 30 days after discontinuation.

3. **Myocardial Infarction (MI).** In healthy, nonsmoking U.S. women, the use of low-dose COCs (≤50 mcg EE) is not associated with any statistically significant risk of MI or stroke. One pooled analysis showed that the relative risk for MI was 1.0.[149] A meta-analysis of studies including high-dose COCs showed an overall relative risk of 2.48 for current users, but there was no increased risk for those women using 20 mcg formulations.[150] In a recent prospective study, use of low-dose COCs was not associated with an increased risk of MI.[151] Finally, the American College of Cardiology concluded that current COC formulations pose no increased myocardial infarction risk for current users.[152]

The risks for MI increase with age, but are greatly magnified by the combination of age, smoking, and hypertension.[150,153] In one meta-analysis of COC users, smoking, hypertension and dyslipidemia each were associated with a 9-fold increased risk for MI.[150] The absolute risk is low. Among nonsmoking women age 20–24, an estimated 4 per million who do not use COCs die from MI; that risk rises to 10 per million among smokers who use COCs.[154]

According to the U.S. MEC, women over 35 who smoke at least 15 cigarettes a day are not candidates for COC use[36]; however, because the increased risk of MI is reversible, once these women have stopped smoking or using nicotine-containing products for 3 to 12 months, they may become candidates for COC use. The older the woman and the more cigarettes she smokes, the longer the washout period must be.

International studies also demonstrate that COC use in women with uncontrolled hypertension increases the risk of MI. (See Table 11–6.) However, it is not as clear if well-controlled hypertension is equivalent to normotension. The U.S. MEC rates COC use by women with well-controlled or mildly elevated hypertension as a category "3" (the risks generally outweigh the benefits of use).[36] If you do prescribe COCs to a woman with treated hypertension, monitor her blood pressure carefully, because if she does not consistently take her prescribed medication, she may become ineligible for COC use.[155]

Early evidence suggested that second-generation progestins might be associated with a greater risk of MI.[150] However, those conclusions were based on limited numbers of cases. The more recent EURAS study that followed over 58,000 COC users found no difference in MI rates among users of various progestins.[139]

Several other findings about COC use and cardiovascular disease are reassuring. There is no increase in the risk of MI with increasing duration of use.[157] Past COC users have no increased risk due to their prior COC use.

Because the concerns for MI risks are related to arterial thrombosis (ATE) caused by *estrogen,* women who are not candidates for COCs because of concerns related to thrombosis may still be candidates for progestin-only methods.

4. **Stroke.** Cerebrovascular disease is rare in young reproductive-age women but becomes more common in women in their 40s. There are two types of stroke—ischemic and hemorrhagic. Each type has a different etiology and somewhat different risk factors to consider when prescribing COCs. Most evidence shows that healthy nonsmoking women using modern low-dose pills have no discernible increase in their risk for either ischemic or hemorrhagic stroke.[158]

Risk factors for stroke should be identified and women counseled to modify them, if possible. Risk factors for *ischemic* stroke include smoking, hypertension, diabetes, overweight or obesity, lower socioeconomic status, and migraine headaches with aura. Women with hypertension who use COCs have 3 times the risk of ischemic stroke as do COC users without hypertension.[159] Similarly, the risk of ischemic stroke is about 15 to 20 times higher in smokers compared with nonsmokers.[159] WHO studies also found a significant increase in the risk of ischemic stroke, but not hemorrhagic stroke, among COC users who experienced migraine with aura (odds ratio 3.0, 95% CI 1.3–11.3) and a nonsignificant increase in stroke among COC users who reported migraine without aura (OR 3.0, 95% CI 0.7–14.8)[160] (see Special Populations: Women with Headaches section, below). The WHO panel stated that migraineurs with aura have a higher risk of

Table 11–6 Age-specific estimates of attributable MI deaths due to low-dose COC use per 1 million users in international studies: the effect of smoking and hypertension

| | Risk of Myocardial Infarction/1,000,000 Users | | |
| | Age Range (years) | | |
Risk Category	20–24	30–34	40–44
Healthy nonsmokers	4	6	20
With smoking	10	20	200
With hypertension	100	120	450

Source: Farley TM, et al. (1998).[156]

stroke than those without aura, but no study had sufficient proof to examine risk of stroke by type of migraine.[161]

The risk factors for *hemorrhagic* stroke include age, hypertension, and smoking, but other factors, such as obesity and heavy alcohol use, are also important. The risk of hemorrhagic stroke increases 10-fold in COC users with hypertension compared with nonhypertensive users.[162] Current use of COCs raised the risk of hemorrhagic stroke only in developing countries, where blood pressure could not be monitored. The risk of hemorrhagic stroke in women who smoke is about double that of nonsmokers.[162] Smokers who use COCs may have up to triple the risk of stroke compared with nonsmoking non-users.

COC package inserts state, "The relative risk of hemorrhagic stroke is reported to be 1.2 for nonsmokers who used oral contraceptives, 2.6 for smokers who did not use oral contraceptives, 7.6 for smokers who used oral contraceptives, 1.8 for normotensive users, and 25.7 for users with severe hypertension. The attributable risk is also greater in older women.[163–165] There is no apparent increase in the risk of either type of stroke with increasing duration of COC use[166] or with past use of COCs.[161] Data are insufficient to make conclusions about how the type or dose of progestin might influence the risk of stroke,[167] but progestin-only methods do not increase the risk of stroke. COC use does not affect the risk of *subarachnoid* hemorrhage.[168]

5. **Hypertension.** The estrogen in COCs increases circulating levels of angiotensinogen. Some women are very sensitive to angiotensinogen metabolites (angiotensin) and experience increases in both their diastolic and systolic blood pressures with COCs. Estrogen, and to some extent progestins, enhance aldosterone activity, which results in fluid retention and, in turn, contributes to an increase in blood pressure. Most studies find no increase in clinically significant hypertension with low-dose COCs, although a 3 to 5 mmHg rise is not uncommon.[169,170] One study found that elevated blood pressure occurred in 41.5 cases per 10,000 COC users.[169] Women who experience hypertension attributable to COC use will normalize their blood pressures within 3 to 6 months of stopping estrogen-containing contraceptives.[152] The women whose readings do not return to normal should undergo a standard work-up; most will be found to have essential hypertension. **Women with significantly elevated blood pressure on COCs need to discontinue COCs immediately** and may need to be prescribed antihypertensive medication.

6. **Gallbladder disease.** Low-dose COCs have not been associated with the increased risk of cholelithiasis or cholecystitis that had been seen earlier with high-dose COCs. However, it may still be possible that low-dose COCs accelerate the development of symptomatic gallbladder disease in women with preexisting gallstones or sludge. COCs do not increase the risk of gallbladder cancer.[171]

7. **Cholestatic jaundice.** Active transport of bile can be impaired by high-dose COCs, resulting in cholestatic jaundice with pruritus. This condition reverses with discontinuation of hormones. The incidence in the general population using low-dose formulations is not known but is assumed to be very rare. Women who experience cholestatic jaundice with pregnancy should be offered estrogen-containing contraceptives with caution.

8. **Hepatic neoplasms.** Benign liver tumors have been associated with the use of high-dose COCs, especially with long-term use. Focal nodular hyperplasia may be increased nearly 3-fold in COC users, though its absolute risk is still small.[172] Preexisting hepatic lesions do not appear to be affected by COC use.

   Adenomas are the most clinically significant hepatic neoplasia, because they can cause rupture of the liver capsule, extensive intraperitoneal hemorrhage, and even death. Women may or may not have abdominal pain with adenomas; their liver function tests are usually normal. Palpate the liver edge as part of the annual physical exam. If the liver is enlarged or tender, discontinue COCs and evaluate with MRI or CT tests; ultrasound is not reliable. Tumor regression is expected after stopping COCs.

   Hepatocellular carcinoma risk is not increased with low-dose COC use.[173] Use of hormonal contraception by high-risk women (especially those with chronic hepatitis B infection) does not appear to increase the risk of hepatocellular carcinoma, but use may increase the risk in a low-risk population. (See Women with Medical Conditions, Liver Disease section, below.)

9. **Risks for acquiring STIs.** A systematic review of the literature concluded that women who use COCs are at increased risk for acquiring Chlamydia cervicitis, although the authors noted that nearly all the studies failed to adjust for confounders, had relatively small sample sizes, and were given a "poor" quality rating. The pooled odds ratio was 2.9 (95% CI 1.86–4.55).[174] A previous meta-analysis had concluded that women using COCs maybe more likely to have cervical ectopy and that women with cervical ectopy may be more likely to acquire chlamydial infec-

tion.[175] A prospective study found that cervical ectopy is a risk factor for cervicitis, but the presence of cervical ectopy did not change the association between COC use and cervicitis.[176] All this suggests that cervical ectopy may make the detection of chlamydial infection easier.[177] COC use does not increase a woman's risk for infection with gonorrhea, trichomoniasis, herpes, or syphilis.[174]

The data on HPV susceptibility with COC use are less certain. Review of cross-sectional studies found no evidence for a strong association between ever using COCs and having HPV infection.[178] Two subsequent prospective studies had conflicting results. One study of college students found a slight increase in HPV infection risk (HR = 1.4; 95% CI 1.01–1.8),[179] while a study of a broader age group (18 to 49 years) found no such association (OR = 0.7; 95% CI 0.2–2.0) after adjusting for risky sexual behavior.[180] Studies have not consistently shown any significantly higher risk for HPV acquisition among COC users.[178–180]

COCs influence transcription of natural antimicrobials in the human endometrium, which might increase a woman's vulnerability to upper-tract chlamydia or HIV infection.[181] The question of HIV susceptibility and COC use has now been answered by carefully designed clinical trials. HIV-uninfected women who used either COCs or injectable progestins for contraception were not at any significantly increased risk of acquiring HIV compared with women who used other non-barrier methods.[182] However, for young women and other subgroups, the association between hormonal contraception and HIV acquisition remains an unanswered question.[183] After reviewing the data, neither the U.S. MEC nor the International Planned Parenthood Federation (IPPF) has changed its current recommendations regarding hormonal contraceptive use.[36,184]

To reduce risks for STIs, women should choose to be sexually active with one uninfected, monogamous partner or, at minimum, use latex or polyurethane condoms with every act of vaginal or rectal intercourse and consider use of barriers with oral-genital contact too.

10. **Cervical dysplasia and cervical carcinoma.** Cervical dysplasia and cervical carcinoma are caused by the high-risk human papillomavirus (HPV), especially the high-risk subtypes HPV 16 and 18. In one study, women who used COCs for more than 5 years and who were infected with HPV had a 3- to 4-fold increased risk for in situ and invasive squamous cell cervical carcinoma compared to non-users.[185] A large meta-analysis of 28 studies including 12,531 women with cervical cancer found RR 1.1 after 5

years of COC use, RR 1.6 after 5 to 10 years, and RR 2.2 after more than 10 years.[186] However, this COC-associated risk is lower than the risk that is associated with high parity. For example, women with HPV infection who had 7 or more pregnancies had higher RR (8.29) for cervical cancer. Pregnancy before 18 years of age increases the relative risk for cervical cancer to 10.71.[187] Studies demonstrate that COC use may increase the risk of cervical adenocarcinoma (cancer of the glandular cells of the cervix).[188] COC use may also be associated with artifacts that mimic ASC-US (glycogen vacuoles create perinuclear halos in COC users) on liquid-based cytology tests. Reflex high-risk HPV testing will demonstrate that two thirds of those women have no virus.[189] Despite this slight increase in risk, even long-term COC users do not need to have cervical cytology testing performed more frequently or with more sensitive tests than required by their other risk factors.

11. **Melasma/Chloasma.** The estrogen in COCs stimulates melanocyte activity and can cause patchy brown discoloration on a woman's face, which can be very disturbing. Women with more melanocytes are more susceptible. Using the lowest dose of estrogen in pills, sunscreen, and hats can minimize this problem. Unfortunately, after pill discontinuation, the discoloration will generally only fade; it does not completely resolve.

HEALTH ISSUES INCORRECTLY ATTRIBUTED TO MODERN COC USE

In contrast to the issues discussed above where evidence may support concerns about risk, several other health risks have been inappropriately attributed to COC use. In part, this may be due to the increased safety of low-dose formulations compared with older, high-dose pills. In part, these myths arose from theoretical concerns that have lingered despite contrary results from clinical experience in the last 50 years. However, clinical experience and double-blind, prospective, placebo-controlled studies have shown that compared with placebo users, women using pills have no increased risks for having any of the problems listed as myths in the following section. It should be remembered that some women may be very sensitive to hormones and may experience side effects not generally encountered by other women.

1. **Myth: COCs adversely affect long-term fertility.** Return to fertility is very rapid following discontinuation of COCs. A comprehensive review of all studies published from 1960 to 2007 reveals that return of fertility in women who stop using COCs (either cyclic or extended-cycle regimens) in order to conceive is

comparable to that observed following cessation of other contraceptive methods. The 12-month conception rates ranged from 72% to 94%.[42] The return to fertility is so rapid and consistent that no more than a 2-week delay in menses is expected following discontinuation of COCs. There is no longer any significant "post-pill amenorrhea."

2. **Myth: In utero exposure to COCs will harm a pregnancy.** Women who become pregnant while using COCs have no higher rates of spontaneous abortion, preterm deliveries, birth defects or complications in the health of their offspring than do non-users.[190-194] The risks of significant congenital anomalies among infants of COC users is the same as that of the general population. No additional testing of fetal wellbeing is needed during the prenatal period for women who used COCs in the early months of pregnancy. Women who experience spontaneous losses following COC use should understand that their taking pills contributed nothing to that loss. Abortion should never be considered because of in utero exposure to COCs.

3. **Myth: Use of modern low-dose COCs increases the risk of breast cancer.** Older studies of early high-dose pills found a slight increase in the risk of breast cancer.[195] In a study that separated women who used pills before 1975 (when the estrogen dose was high) from those who used pills after 1975 (when sub-50 mcg EE formulations were in widespread use), earlier pill users were found to have an increased risk of subsequent breast cancer, while those using the low-dose formulations did not.[196] A convincing case-controlled study found no difference in pill use among women with breast cancer and those without that cancer.[197] Neither the duration of COC use nor age at starting COCs influenced the risk of breast cancer. A large Royal College study found no increase in the risk of breast cancer in ever-users of COCs compared with never-users (RR=0.98).[198] And the Royal College study that followed women for up to 39 years found that the relative risk for COC users was only 0.9 (95% CI 0.74–1.05).[41] Women who carry mutations for BRCA1 or BRCA2 and use COCs do not experience any increase in their already high risk of developing breast cancer.[92, 199] A later systematic review found that women with a family history of breast cancer do not increase their risk of disease by using COCs.[200]

4. **Myth: Pills reduce libido.** Postulating that women's sexual interest is driven by her circulating testosterone levels, some investigators have studied surrogate measures (such as SHBG levels) to estimate the impact of COCs on sexual health of women.[108] However, these studies fail to establish the validity of their sur-

rogate markers or to correct for compounding factors such as selection bias or length of relationships.[201] The impact of COC-induced changes in androgens was studied in a prospective investigation of the association between COC use and serum androgen levels (total testosterone, free testosterone and DHEA-S). Despite significant decreases in all androgens at 3 months, there was no evidence that these women experienced any reduction in enjoyment of sexual activity. The authors concluded that some women might be more sensitive to changes in the androgen than others.[108,202] A more recent study of DMPA vs. COCs showed marked differences on surrogate markers but no change in sexual function.[295] For reproductive-aged women, sexual desire and sexual activity are independent of serum testosterone levels.[296]

More direct information is available from clinical trials. In trials of a wide range and many different formulations of COCs, decreased libido has generally been reported by only 1% to 5% of users. Even in the clinical trial of the most estrogenic formulations with an antiandrogenic progestin, libido was one of the least frequent complaints.[165] The best evidence about the interactions between COCs and sexual desire comes from a study of using a pill with the anti-androgenic progestin drospirenone. Compared with their baselines, women using the drospirenone-containing COC had significant improvement in sexual enjoyment, sexual satisfaction, and frequency of orgasms, but no change in libido. Longer-term use was associated with significant increases in arousal and frequency of sexual activity.[203]

5. **Myth: COCs cause weight gain.** This has been difficult to assess because in clinical trials of contraceptive efficacy, all the weight that the women gained while on the COCs was attributed to the COC being tested. However, studies of COCs for noncontraceptive benefits that did include placebos do provide an opportunity to directly answer the question. Those studies found percent of women who gained excessive weight was the same among COC users as among placebo users.[204] A Cochrane review concluded that evidence supporting a causal association between COCs and weight gain has not been found.[205]

6. **Myth: COCs increase glucose intolerance and diabetes.** COCs currently available in the United States do not have any clinically significant adverse effect on carbohydrate metabolism[287] and do not produce an increase in diabetes.[206,207] Older COC formulations with high doses of sex steroids had a more profound impact on glucose tolerance and, in some instances, resulted in hyperglycemia with hyperinsulinemia. By contrast, in the

CARDIA study, current use of modern COCs was associated with *lower* glucose levels and with a lower odds ratio for diabetes.[208]

Concerns have been raised about COC use in women at risk for developing diabetes because progesterone is a competitive inhibitor of the insulin receptor, and estrogen influences the release of insulin from the pancreatic islet cells and decreases insulin sensitivity.[209] However, women with a history of gestational diabetes who used COCs with low progestin content had no higher risk of developing glucose intolerance or overt diabetes compared with controls who used nonhormonal methods when both groups were studied for up to 7 years.[210] Similarly, insulin resistance in women with polycystic ovarian syndrome does not predictably worsen with COC use.[211]

7. **Myth: COCs increase the risk of melanoma.** A pooled analysis of 10 case-control studies involving nearly 2,400 cases of melanoma revealed no correlation between COC use and the development of melanoma. Also, no effect of duration of use or current use was observed.[212] However, it is recommended that women with a history of melanoma refrain from getting pregnant and from using hormonal contraception for at least 2 years after their original therapy, because the risk of recurrence is highest during this time.[213]

8. **Myth: COCs should not be used by women with leiomyoma.** Leiomyoma (uterine fibroids) contain both estrogen and progesterone receptors. Because fibroids often shrink after menopause when estrogen levels decrease, it has been suggested that estrogen-containing contraceptives might increase the growth of these benign uterine tumors. However, clinical studies with low-dose COCs have found no impact on the risk of developing new fibroids or on increasing the size of pre-existing fibroids,[123,214,215] except in women who used COCs early in life.[123] In fact, COCs are often used to control excessive menstrual bleeding caused by fibroids, and long-term use may decrease the chances for fibroid development.

9. **Myth: Drospirenone-containing pills increase potassium levels in all women.** Drospirenone has antimineralocorticoid activity, which introduces the potential for hyperkalemia in high-risk patients; the 3 mg of drospirenone found in these formulations has the same impact on electrolytes as 25 mg of spironolactone. The EURAS multinational study noted no increase in arrhythmias in users of drospirenone-containing COCs compared with other COC formulations.[216] Use of these pills in combination with chronic daily use of ACE inhibitors,

angiotensin-II receptor antagonists, potassium-sparing diuretics, heparin, aldosterone antagonists, and NSAIDs may increase serum potassium. Note that *intermittent use* of NSAIDs does not pose any problems. If a woman is using other potassium-sparing drugs, test her potassium about 14 days after starting her first pack; if that value is normal, no further testing is needed for potassium.

PROVIDING COCs

Patient selection is the key to safe COC use. The benefits of COCs generally far outweigh the risks of COCs. However, some women have medical conditions or personal habits that increase their risk of developing serious complications with use of COCs. In addition to issues of medical safety, be aware that some women may not be good candidates for COCs because they are uncomfortable with COCs due to underlying beliefs about the nature of hormones in contraceptives, the desire for "natural" contraception, or a lack of belief in the importance of avoiding pregnancy.[217] Women seeking the most effective contraception may be better served by using intrauterine contraceptive (IUCs), implants, injections, or sterilization. Those who have difficulty with daily pill administration should consider all of the long lasting methods as well as the intermediate-acting combined hormonal methods, such as the transdermal patch or the vaginal ring.

Explore the patient's medical and reproductive health history and her family history to ensure that she has no conditions that would preclude her use of COCs. The U.S. Medical Eligibility Criteria for Contraceptive Use (U.S. MEC) provides a list of guidelines for practitioners to follow when assessing risks vs. benefits associated with the use of various contraceptive methods.[36] For a complete list of the Medical Eligibility Criteria for Contraceptive Use upon which to make your clinical decisions, see Chapter 4.

Discuss the potential noncontraceptive benefits and examine all the patient's lifestyle issues to ensure that she can realistically expect to take a pill each day. Anticipatory counseling about safety concerns can reduce later discontinuation. Determine if she wants to have monthly withdrawal bleeding or if she would prefer less frequent bleeding episodes. Ask if she has any other complaints that need to be addressed at this visit. In particular, find out if she needs STI testing or emergency contraception now or in the future. If she is at risk for STIs, advise her how to follow safer sex practices.

Measure the woman's blood pressure. Although the need for a breast and pelvic examination may be indicated by the patient's history or symptoms, neither is needed before initiating COCs in an asymptomatic woman.[218] A Pap smear is not needed prior to starting COCs.[218] STI testing, if needed for routine health care or because of her age or symptoms, can be serum or urine-based. No other screening tests are routinely needed unless the woman's history or blood pressure indicates a need for further assessment.[219] In particular, routine screening for thrombotic mutations is not recommended prior to prescribing estrogen-containing contraceptives.[220]

Once you have identified a woman as being a candidate for COCs, realize that despite the wide range of health *benefits*, attention in the public eye has been focused on possible health *risks* associated with COC use. Your patient probably has a distorted and inflated estimate of the health risks posed by COC use. Help her understand that her risks of not using protection (with pregnancy) are much greater than her risks of using COCs.

The FDA-approved prescribing information lists specific medical conditions that are not compatible with COC use. However, FDA package labeling for many drugs has been shown to be 20 to 30 years obsolete.[221] The U.S. MEC analysis represents an up-to-date evaluation of risks with COC use. Table 11–7 shows a list of medical conditions that preclude COC use from the FDA-approved prescribing information compared with the U.S. MEC Category 4 conditions. The latter represents the most up-to-date synthesis of available evidence for contraindications to COC use.

Prescribe or provide condoms and emergency contraception for all new start COC users. Many women discontinue pills without consulting their clinicians. Invest time teaching your patient how to use her condoms and emergency contraception (EC) so she knows how to use them as well as she knows how to use her COCs.

TIMING OF PILL INITIATION

Several different protocols can be helpful when starting a woman on a COC. Our goal in recommending ways to start COCs is to avoid creating any opportunity for accidental pregnancy. Therefore, the options listed in order of preference are as follows:

Quick Start

The preferred choice for pill initiation is the Quick Start or Same-Day Start method. Tell the woman to take the first pill in her pill pack on the day of her visit, as long as it is reasonably certain that she is not pregnant and is not in need of emergency contraception. If she needs emergency contraception, she should take her EC at once and start her COCs no later than the next day. Tell her to use a back-up method with her pills

Table 11–7 Medical conditions precluding COC use, as listed in COC prescribing information and compared with the U.S. Medical *Eligibility Criteria for Contraceptive Use*

Medical Conditions Precluding COC Use in Product Labeling	U.S. MEC Rating
Thrombophlebitis or thromboembolic disorder	4
Past history of deep vein thrombophlebitis or thromboembolic disorders	3/4
Cerebrovascular or coronary artery disease	4
Valvular heart disease with complications	4
Severe hypertension	4
Diabetes with vascular involvement	3/4
Headaches with focal neurological symptoms	4
Major surgery with prolonged immobilization	4
Breast cancer	4
Carcinoma of the endometrium	1
Other known or suspected estrogen-dependent neoplasia	Not discussed
Undiagnosed abnormal genital bleeding	2
Cholestatic jaundice of pregnancy	2
Jaundice with prior pill use	3
Hepatic adenomas	2
Known or suspected pregnancy	"Not applicable"
Hypersensitivity to any component of the product	Not discussed

Note: If two numbers appear, the first number represents the rating for COC initiation for pre-existing problems. The second number is the rating if the patient develops the problem while using COCs (continuation rating).

Source: Centers for Disease Control and Prevention (2010).[36]

for at least 7 days if she is not in the first 6 days of her cycle. If she has used ella for EC, advise that she use 14 days of a back-up method. With Quick Start, her next scheduled bleeding episode will be delayed until she completes the active pills in her pack and starts the placebo pills. If she has concern about an undetectable early pregnancy, she can start her pills and return for a urine pregnancy test if her scheduled bleeding does not occur when she is using the placebo pills. If she does not want to wait that long, advise her to be tested in 2 to 3 weeks. Reassure her that the hormones in the pills will not adversely affect an early pregnancy and the planned repeat pregnancy testing will detect the pregnancy early enough to begin the pregnancy care she chooses.

Quick Start is an off-label practice supported by good clinical research. Quick Start is preferred because other COC initial protocols generally leave a time gap between the time the patient is prescribed her pills and the time she is intended to start taking them. As many as 25% of young women given prescriptions for COCs that use one of the conventional start protocols (see below) fail to begin taking the pills as instructed because they conceive in the interim, forget the pill-taking instructions, fail to fill the prescription, or worry about taking the pill. [222,223] The Quick Start method improves continuation from the first pack of pills to the second pack when compared with conventional starts, although pill continuation rates are the same at 3 and 6 months.[224] No increase in pregnancy rates is shown with the Quick Start method and there is no increase in unscheduled spotting or bleeding.[225,226] The WHO endorses the Quick Start method.

First-Day Start

The First-Day start was introduced to gain early control of ovarian follicles during the first cycle. In this approach, a woman takes her first pill on the first day of her next period. It is important to have the woman determine that her period is normal—that it occurs at the predicted time and is preceded by symptoms that are usual for her. If there is any question that her period is not normal, she may want to rule out pregnancy, but she should start her first pill on the first day of bleeding while she is waiting for her pregnancy test results. No back-up contraception is needed when pills are started on the first day of menses.

Sunday Start

The Sunday Start used to be the most common method for starting pills. Women were told to start their first active pill on the first Sunday of their menses. For example, if a woman were to start bleeding on Friday, she should take her first pill two days later on Sunday. If her period were to start on Sunday, she should start on that day. Make sure the patient understands that she should not wait to start the first pill on the Sunday after her menses ends.

Today, the Sunday start is *not* generally recommended because it is often difficult for women to get refills when they need them on weekends. In addition, many women are working outside the home and prefer not to menstruate during their work week. However, some of the generic pill packages still direct a woman to use a Sunday start, so familiarity with this approach is still needed. If a woman starts her menses more than 5 days before starting her pills, she should use a back-up method for 7 days.

Switching from Other Methods

Women who switch from other methods can start COCs immediately, using the guidelines for the Quick Start initiation. For example, if a woman has her contraceptive implant or intrauterine contraceptive (IUC) removed, she should start her COCs that same day. Women who have had recent unprotected intercourse can be given emergency contraception (EC) immediately and told to start their COCs no later than the next day and to use a back-up method for at least the first 7-14 days of COC use. A urine pregnancy test in 2 to 3 weeks may be offered to detect any EC failures. Women using injectable methods generally start their COCs at the end of the effective period of their last injection. However, if a woman is more than 4 weeks late for reinjection, she can start the COCs on the visit day with a 7-day use of a back-up method. Add EC and follow-up pregnancy testing in 2 to 3 weeks if she has had recent (within last 5 days) unprotected sex after the date she was supposed to return for reinjections.

Cycling Patterns

The original pill formulations included hormone-free days to induce a monthly scheduled bleeding episode, which women would interpret as a normal (although generally lighter) menses.[227] Monthly bleeding was needed for acceptance of the pill because it reassured women that they were not pregnant and that their reproductive system was still functioning. Today it is recognized that monthly bleeding with COCs is not healthy. Monthly scheduled bleeding is not biologically necessary and does create health hazards, such as cramping and blood loss and other adverse impacts on quality of life.[10] Despite this, many women continue to prefer to bleed with COCs. Variations exist in the numbers of pills, content of active pills and the content of pills during the time when the woman has her scheduled bleeding episodes.

- *21/7 Formulations.* Most of the older cyclic formulations have 21 active pills and 7 placebo pills in a packet. This combination came from experience with the early high-dose pills. It often took 5 days without hormones for the progestins circulating in a woman's system to fall to levels that were low enough to permit endometrial sloughing. With today's lower-dose pills (20 to 35 mcg EE), women usually start bleeding about 2 days after their last active pill. Ovarian activity usually resumes even before a woman's bleeding starts. Many of the generic formulations today (and a few brand-name pills) still have 7 placebo pills. For women using these 21/7 formulations, it is very important that they do not have any delays in starting their next pill packs. Also ask about problems with unscheduled spotting and bleeding.

- *Shortened hormone-free interval.* Most of the newer pill formulations increased the number of active pills and decreased the number of placebo pills in a packet. Pregnancy rates are lower in the 24/4 formulations of low-dose pills (20 mcg EE) compared to 21/7 formulations.[288] Studies have demonstrated that having fewer hormone-free days also results in less ovarian stimulation to develop follicles and less ovarian production of estradiol to thicken the endometrium and cause unscheduled bleeding in the following cycle.[228,229] In a trial of 20 mcg EE pills, shortening the pill-free interval reduced the duration of scheduled bleeding.

  If a woman cannot get insurance coverage for formulations with shortened pill-free intervals, conventional pills can be used. The woman can start the first active pill in the next pack on the first day of her withdrawal bleeding (first day start each cycle). If she has no withdrawal bleeding by the 5th day of her placebos, she should start her next pack. Be aware that this approach results in more frequent bleeding episodes (every 25 days) and will cost the woman the price of at least an extra two packs of pills a year, unless the clinician can persuade the insurance company that there is a medical indication for this shortened pill interval.

- *Extended-cycle use.* Studies have documented that the majority of the pill's side effects (such as headache, cramping, breast tenderness, bloating or swelling) occur during the days women are taking their placebo pills, not when they are taking the active hormone-containing pills.[10] Because recent surveys have shown that many women would prefer to bleed less frequently than once a month,[230] it is time to re-educate pill users about the lack of need for monthly scheduled bleeding.[231] In one study of women who had no menstruation-related symptoms, 50% said they wanted to lessen the frequency of menstrual periods; half of these women wanted amenorrhea.[232]

  The purpose of menstruation is to end one cycle (in which no pregnancy began) and to prepare for the next cycle (which may result in pregnancy). Failure to menstruate without hormonal contraception may be an indication of pregnancy or significant illness. COC users are different; they are trying to avoid pregnancy. They have no biological need to endure artificial pill-induced scheduled bleeding on a monthly basis. Unless the patient wants to use bleeding as a reassurance that she is not pregnant, monthly cycling is not necessary; it is not healthy and may be avoided by extended COC use.

  In clinical studies, women with prolonged flow during spontaneous menses had fewer menstrually-related problems with extended-cycle COC use.[233] The majority of those women, in a clinical trial of extended cycle pills, continued to use them after the end of the study.[234] A Cochrane review reported that five out of six studies found that women's bleeding patterns were equivalent or improved with continuous-dosing regimens.[235] A regimen of extended pill use with extra packs of pills is cost-effective for women with heavy or prolonged menstrual bleeding.[236] Trials with extended cycles with COCs containing levonorgestrel, norethindrone, and drospirenone have all demonstrated safety and efficacy.[55] Other women for whom extended use would be particularly attractive are those with dysmenorrhea or menstrual migraines, and those on active military duty or other types of demanding jobs.

CHOOSING A FORMULATION

Clinicians in the United States have more than 70 COCs from which to choose. (See the color insert for photographs and formulations of pills available in the United States). Select a COC based on the hormonal dose and on the woman's clinical picture, her preferences, her past experiences with COCs, and cost. Both WHO and the FDA recommend using the lowest dose pill to reduce potential side effects, especially in women who have hormone sensitivity.[239] However, studies have shown that, compared with higher-dose formulations, several COCs containing 20 mcg EE (and generally 7 placebo pills) are associated with higher rates of unscheduled spotting and bleeding and, consequently, higher rates of discontinuation.[237] Figure 11–1 gives an algorithm to help clinicians and their patients select appropriate COCs.

PROVIDING ADEQUATE SUPPLIES

To facilitate access to contraception, WHO recommends providing up to 1 year's supply of COCs when a woman initiates pill use.[239] The practice of providing up to a 1-year supply can be continued at each annual visit. Studies have shown that women who are provided at least 3 cycles of pills are much more likely to continue to use the method for 3 months than are women who are required to return for monthly refills[16,297,298] and those given 13 cycles have lower pregnancy and abortion rates.[289]

Other Issues

Remember to instruct new COC users about condom use and provide them with condoms and EC in case they discontinue COC use or miss pills before returning.

Remind women that if they are scheduled for major surgery that will involve prolonged immobilization postoperatively, they should discon-

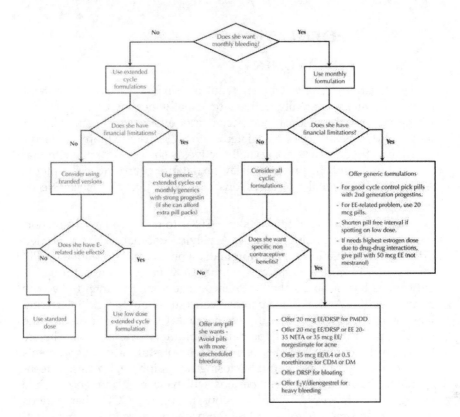

Figure 11-1 Helping a woman select a COC

tinue COCs 1 month prior to surgery. They should remind their clinicians about their COC use, so that they can be provided with appropriate antithrombosis therapy. COCs can be resumed after the patient has started to ambulate again.

FOLLOW-UP

Because side effects that may lead to pill discontinuation[238] generally appear in the first few months of COC use, a follow-up visit within 3 months may be beneficial, but dispensing policies should not be linked to follow-up visits.[239] Encourage women to return if problems develop or if they wish to change their method. Assess how well they are able to take their tablets each day. Recognize how difficult it may be for patients to remember to take pills daily,[240] and remind women that such daily pill-taking is critical for COC efficacy. As former Surgeon General C. Everett Koop said, "Drugs don't work in patients who don't take them." Responsiveness to patient concerns may increase patient continuation of COCs.

SPECIAL POPULATIONS
ADOLESCENT WOMEN

Menstruating teenage women who are sexually active or contemplating becoming sexually active are usually healthy. Therefore, for young women, the medical and social risks of pregnancy generally far outweigh the health risks associated with COC use. Explore the teen's decision to become (or stay) sexually active. Is she comfortable with that decision or would she prefer to delay sexual intercourse? (See Chapter 5, Abstinence, Noncoital Sex, and Nonsense: What Every Clinician Needs to Know.)

. Many teens can benefit from taking COCs to treat primary dysmenorrhea, anovulatory cycling, or acne. A pelvic examination is not needed prior to COC initiation for asymptomatic women (see the section on Pill Initiation). Reassure anxious parents that COC use for noncontraceptive indications has not been shown to encourage young women to become sexually active. Also assuage parents' concerns about the pill interfering with their daughter's physical development. COCs do not disrupt the orderly maturation of the hypothalamic-pituitary-ovarian axis. The estrogen in the current low-dose COCs does not stunt a young women's growth in height by prematurely closing her epiphyseal plates. A teenager who has had infrequent periods will have regular menses while taking COCs; however, when she stops taking her COCs, her periods will again become irregular, unless the primary cause of her menstrual disruption has been treated. Adolescent women using COCs do not accumulate increases in bone mineral density as rapidly as non-users; however, bone changes are rapidly reversed after COC cessation.[128,129]

Targeted counseling is important. Adolescent women may be more likely to abandon COCs because of minor side effects, such as nausea or spotting, so take all minor side effects in teenagers seriously.[238] Teens may find it more challenging to use COCs correctly and consistently than do older women. Provide concrete counseling to adolescents; studies show that adolescent women anticipate having side effects at much higher rates than actually occurs, and they expect to have no difficulty with consistent pill taking.[241] Instruct each teen who wants to use COCs about condom use, both for reducing her risk of acquiring STIs and for backup in case she discontinues taking the pill. Provide emergency contraception and detailed instructions on how to use it when she needs it.

Studies have shown that women of all ages more successfully use the once-a-week or once-a-month methods instead of taking a pill once a day, but teens benefit most from less frequent dosing.[242] For this reason, offer the vaginal ring and patch to teens who desire combined hormonal contraception.

The twelve color pages of pills are organized as follows:

Color photos of pills from lowest to highest estrogen dose

- Progestin-only pills with no estrogen: Micronor and NOR-QD

- Lowest estrogen pills with 20 micrograms of the estrogen,
  ethinyl estradiol: Alesse, Levlite, LoEstrin 1/20, and Mircette

- All of the 25-, 30- and 35-microgram pills (all ethinyl estradiol)

- All of the phasic pills

- Highest estrogen pills, with 50 micrograms of estrogen
  (ethinyl estradiol OR mestranol). Mestranol is converted in the body to
  ethinyl estradiol; 50 mcg of mestranol is equivalent to 35 mcg of ethinyl
  estradiol

*Pills which are pharmacologically exactly the same are grouped
within boxes. The color and packaging of pills dispensed in clinics
may differ from pills in pharmacies.*

Pills you can prescribe as emergency contraceptive pills

(A)

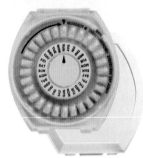

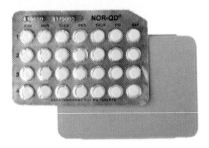

MICRONOR® TABLETS
28-DAY REGIMEN
(0.35 mg norethindrone)
(active pills lime green)
Ortho-McNeil

NOR-QD® TABLETS
(0.35 mg norethindrone)
(active pills yellow)
Watson

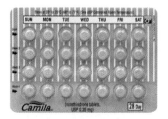

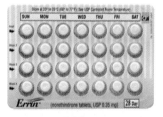

CAMILA®
(norethindrone tablets, USP 0.35 mg)
(active pills light pink)
Teva Pharmaceuticals USA

ERRIN®
(norethindrone tablets, USP 0.35 mg)
(active pills yellow)
Teva Pharmaceuticals USA

JOLIVETTE®
(0.35 mg norethindrone)
Watson

NORA-BE®
(0.35 mg norethindrone)
Watson

COMBINED PILLS - 20 microgram PILLS

LoSEASONIQUE®
(levonorgestrel/ethinyl estradiol/0.10mg/
20 mcg and ethinyl estridol 0.01 mg)
Teva Women's Health

(B)

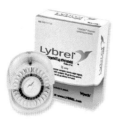

LYBREL™
(90 mcg levonorgestrel/20 mcg ethinyl estradiol)
(active pills pink)
Wyeth

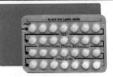

YAZ® 28 TABLETS
(3.0 mg drospirenone/20 mcg ethinyl estradiol)
(active pills pink)
Bayer

BEYAZ® 28 TABLETS
Beyaz = Yaz + 451mcg folic acid
Bayer

GIANVI® 28 TABLETS
(3.0 mg drospirenone/20 mcg ethinyl estradiol)
Teva Pharmaceuticals USA

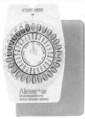

ALESSE® - 28 TABLETS
(0.1 mg levonorgestrel/20 mcg ethinyl estradiol)
(active pills pink)
Wyeth

SRONYX®
(0.1 mg levonorgestrel/
20mcg ethinyl estradiol)
Watson

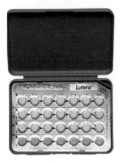

LUTERA™
(0.1 mg levonorgestrel/20 mcg ethinyl estradiol)
(active pills white)
Watson

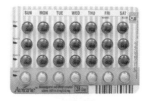

AVIANE®
(levonorgestrel/ethinyl estradiol tablets, USP 0.10 mg/20 mcg)
(active pills orange)
Teva Pharmaceuticals USA

LEVLITE™ - 28 TABLETS
(0.1 mg levonorgestrel/20 mcg ethinyl estradiol)
(active pills pink)
Bayer

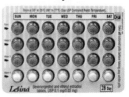

LESSINA®
(levonorgestrel/ethinyl estradiol tablets,
USP 0.1 mg/20 mcg)
(active pills pink)
Teva Pharmaceuticals USA

(c)

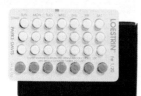

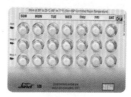

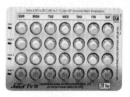

LOESTRIN® FE 1/20
(1 mg norethindrone acetate/
20 mcg ethinyl estradiol/
75 mg ferrous fumarate [7d])
(active pills white)
Teva Pharmaceuticals USA

JUNEL ™
(norethindrone acetate and
ethinyl estradiol tablets,
USP 1 mg/20 mcg)
(active pills light yellow)
Teva Pharmaceuticals USA

JUNEL ™ Fe
(norethindrone acetate and
ethinyl estradiol tablets, USP and
ferrous fumarate tablets 1 mg/20 mcg)
(active pills light yellow)
Teva Pharmaceuticals USA

MICROGESTIN® & MICROGESTIN FE®
(1mg norethindrone acetate/ 20 mcg ethinyl estradiol FE also contains /75 mg ferrous fumarate
Watson

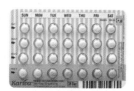

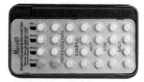

KARIVA®
(desogestrel/estradiol tablets 0.15 mg/
20 mcg and ethinyl estradiol tablets 0.01 mg)
(active pills white and light blue)
Teva Pharmaceuticals USA

MIRCETTE® - 28 TABLETS
(0.15 mg desogestrel/ 20 mcg ethinyl estradiol X
21 (white)/placebo X 2 (green)/
10 mcg ethinyl estradiol X 5 (yellow)
Teva Women's Health

MERCILON®
(0.15 mg desogestrel/20 mcg ethinyl
estradiol/10mcg ethinyl estradiol)
Schering-Plough

COMBINED PILLS - ESTRODIAL VALERATE

NATAZIA™

Natazia consists of 28 film-coated, unscored tablets in the following order:
- 2 dark yellow tablets each containing 3mg estradiol valerate
- 5 medium red tablets each containing 2mg estradiol valerate and 2mg dienogest
- 17 light yellow tablets each containing 2mg estradiol valerate and 3mg dienogest
- 2 dark red tablets each containing 1 mg estradiol valerate
- 2 white tablets (inert)

Bayer

(D)

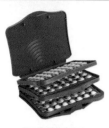
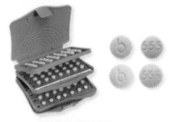

SEASONALE®
(0.15 mg levonorgestrel/
30 mcg ethinyl estradiol)
84 active pink pills
followed by 7 placebo pills
Teva Women's Health

SEASONIQUE®
(0.15 mg levonorgestrel/
30 mcg ethinyl estradiol)
84 active pink pills followed by
7 pills with 10 mcg ethinyl estradiol
Teva Women's Health

JOLESSA™
(0.15 mg levonorgestrel/
30 mcg ethinyl estradiol)
91 day regimen
Teva Women's Health

QUASENSE™
(0.15 mg levonorgestrel/
30 mcg ethinyl estradiol)
Watson Laboratories

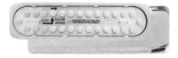

NORDETTE®-28 TABLETS
(0.15 mg levonorgestrel/30 mcg ethinyl estradiol)
(active pills light orange)
Teva Women's Health

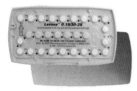
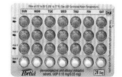
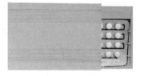

LEVORA TABLETS
(0.15 mg levonorgestrel/
30 mcg ethinyl estradiol)
(active pills white)
Watson

PORTIA®
(levonorgestrel and ethinyl estradiol
tablets, USP 0.15 mg/30 mcg)
(active pills pink)
Teva Pharmaceuticals USA

LEVLEN® 28 TABLETS
(0.15 mg levonorgestrel/
30 mcg ethinyl estradiol)
(active pills light orange)
Bayer

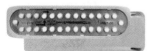
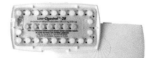
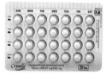

LO/OVRAL®-28 TABLETS
(0.3 mg norgestrel/
30 mcg ethinyl estradiol)
(active pills white)
Wyeth

LOW-OGESTREL® - 28
(0.3 mg norgestrel/
30 mcg ethinyl estradiol)
(active pills white)
Watson

CRYSELLE®
(0.3 mg norgestrel/
30 mcg ethinyl estradiol)
(active pills white)
Teva Pharmaceuticals USA

(E)

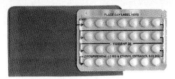

YASMIN® 28 TABLETS
(3.0 mg drospirenone/30 mcg ethinyl estradiol)
(active pills yellow)
Bayer

SAFYRAL™ 28 TABLETS
Safyral = Yasmin + 451mcg of folic acid
Bayer

OCELLA™ 28 TABLETS
(3.0 mg drospirenone/30 mcg ethinyl estradiol)
(active pills yellow)
Teva Pharmaceuticals USA

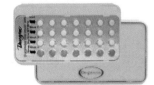
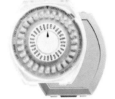
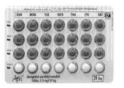

DESOGEN® 28 TABLETS
(0.15 mg desogestrel/
30 mcg ethinyl estradiol)
(active pills white)
Schering-Plough

SOLIA™
(0.15 mg desogestrel/30 mcg ethinyl estradiol)
Schering-Plough

**ORTHO-CEPT® TABLETS
28-DAY REGIMEN**
(0.15 mg desogestrel/
30 mcg ethinyl estradiol)
(active pills orange)
Ortho-McNeil

APRI®
(desogestrel/
ethinyl estradiol 0.15 mg/
0.03 mg tablets)
(active pills rose)
Teva Pharmaceuticals
USA

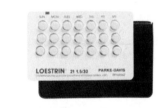
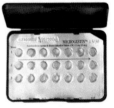

LOESTRIN® 21 1.5/30
(1.5 mg norethindrone acetate/30 mcg ethinyl estradiol)
(active pills green)
Teva Pharmaceuticals USA

MICROGESTIN® 1.5/30 with or without Fe
(1.5 mg norethindrone acetate/
30 mcg ethinyl estradiol)
Watson

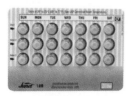
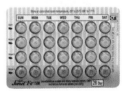

JUNEL ™
(norethindrone acetate and ethinyl estradiol
tablets, USP 1.5 mg./30 mcg.)
(active pills pink)
Teva Pharmaceuticals USA

JUNEL ™ Fe
(norethindrone acetate and ethinyl estradiol tablets,
USP and ferrous fumarate tablets 1.5 mg/30 mcg)
(active pills pink)
Teva Pharmaceuticals USA

(F)

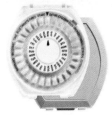

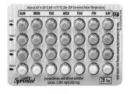

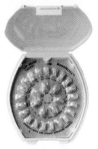

ORTHO-CYCLEN® 28 TABLETS
(0.25 mg norgestimate/
35 mcg ethinyl estradiol)
(active pills blue)
Ortho-McNeil

SPRINTEC®
(norgestimate and ethinyl estradiol tablets,
0.250 mg/35 mcg)
(active pills blue)
Teva Pharmaceuticals USA

MONONESESSA®
(norgestimate and
ethinyl estradiol tablets,
0.250 mg/35 mcg)
Watson

PREVIFEM™
(norgestimate and ethinyl estradiol tablets, 0.250 mg/35 mcg)
Teva Pharmaceuticals USA

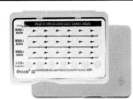

ZENCHENT®
(0.4 mg norethindrone/
35 mcg ethinyl estradiol)
Watson

FEMCON FE™
(0.4 mg norethindrone/
35 mcg ethinyl estradiol)
Warner-Chilcott

OVCON® 35 28-DAY
(0.4 mg norethindrone/
35 mcg ethinyl estradiol)
(active pills peach)
Warner-Chilcott
Now there is a chewable
Ovcon-35 pill!

**BALZIVA™ 1/35
21 OR 28 TABLETS**
(0.4 mg norethindrone/
35 mcg ethinyl estradiol)
Teva Pharmaceuticals USA

ZEOSA™
(0.4 mg norethindrone/
35 mcg ethinyl estradiol)
(chewable)
Teva Pharmaceuticals USA

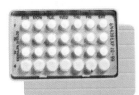

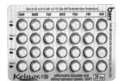

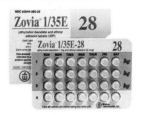

DEMULEN® 1/35-28
(1 mg ethynodiol diacetate/
35 mcg ethinyl estradiol)
(active pills white)
Pharmacia - A Division of Pfizer

KELNOR™
(ethynodiol diacetate 1 mg. and
ethinyl estradiol 35 mcg, USP)
(active pills light yellow)
Teva Pharmaceuticals USA

ZOVIA® 1/35E–28
(1 mg ethynodiol diacetate/
35 mcg ethinyl estradiol)
(active pills light pink)
Watson

(G)

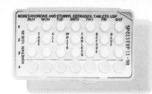

NORETHIN 1/35E–28
(1 mg norethindrone/35 mcg ethinyl estradiol)
(active pills white)
Shire

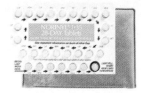

NORINYL® 1+35 28-DAY TABLETS
(1 mg norethindrone/35 mcg ethinyl estradiol)
(active pills yellow-green)
Watson

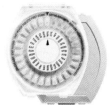

ORTHO-NOVUM® 1/35 28 TABLETS
(1 mg norethindrone/35 mcg ethinyl estradiol)
(active pills peach)
Ortho-McNeil

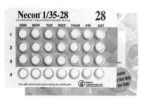

NECON® 1/35-28
(1 mg norethindrone/35 mcg ethinyl estradiol)
(active pills dark yellow)
Watson

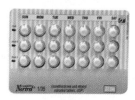

NORTREL®
(norethindrone and ethinyl estradiol tablets,
USP 1/35 mcg)
(active pills yellow)
Teva Pharmaceuticals USA

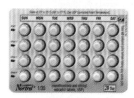

NORTREL®
(norethindrone and ethinyl estradiol tablets,
USP 1.0 mg/35 mcg 28-day regimen)
(active pills yellow)
Teva Pharmaceuticals USA

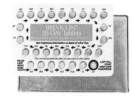

BREVICON® 28-DAY TABLETS
(0.5 mg norethindrone/35 mcg ethinyl estradiol)
(active pills blue)
Watson

NECON 0.5/35®
(0.5 mg norethindrone/35 mcg ethinyl estradiol)
Watson

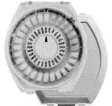

**MODICON® TABLETS
28-DAY REGIMEN**
(0.5 mg norethindrone/
35 mcg ethinyl estradiol)
(active pills white)
Ortho-McNeil

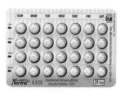

NORTREL®
(norethindrone and ethinyl estradiol
tablets, USP 0.5/35 mcg)
(active pills light yellow)
Teva Pharmaceuticals USA

(H)

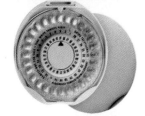

ORTHO TRI-CYCLEN® LO - 28 TABLETS
(norgestimate/ethinyl estradiol)
0.18 mg/25 mcg (7d) (white),
0.215 mg/25 mcg (7d) (light blue),
0.25 mg/25 mcg (7d) (dark blue)
remaining 7 placebo pills are green
Ortho-McNeil

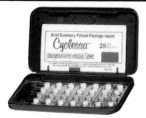

CYCLESSA®
(desogestrel/ethinyl estradiol - triphasic regimen)
0.1 mg/25 mcg (7d) (light yellow)
0.125 mg/25 mcg (7d) (orange)
0.150 mg/25 mcg (7d) (red)
Schering-Plough

VELIVET™
(desogestrel/ethinyl estradiol tablets - triphasic regimen)
(active pills beige, orange and pink)
Teva Pharmaceuticals USA

CESIA™
(desogestrel/ethinyl estradiol tablets - triphasic regimen)
Prasco

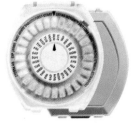

ORTHO-NOVUM® 10/11 - 28 TABLETS
(norethindrone/ethinyl estradiol)
0.5 mg/35 mcg (10d) (white),
1 mg/35 mcg (11d) (peach)
Ortho-McNeil

NECON® 10/11 - 28 TABLETS
(norethindrone/ethinyl estradiol)
0.5 mg/35 mcg (10d) (white),
1 mg/35 mcg (11d) (peach)
Watson

LEENA®
(norenthindrone/ethinyl estradiol) 0.5mg/35 mcg
(light blue), 1 mg/35 mcg (yellow-green)
Watson

ARANELLE™
(norenthindrone/ethinyl estradiol)
0.5mg/0.035mg (blue), 1 mg/35 mcg
Teva Pharmaceuticals USA

TRI-NORINYL®
(norenthindrone/ethinyl estradiol) 0.5mg/35 mcg
(blue), 1 mg/35 mcg (yellow-green)
Watson

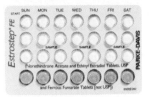

ESTROSTEP® FE - 28 TABLETS
(norethindrone acetate/ethinyl estradiol)
1 mg/20 mcg (5d) (white triangular),
1 mg/30 mcg (7d) (white square),
1 mg/35 mcg (9d), 75 mg ferrous
fumarate (7d) (white round)
Pfizer

TRI-LEGEST® FE
(norethindrone acetate/ethinyl estradiol)
1 mg/20 mcg (5d) , 1 mg/30 mcg (7d)
1 mg/35 mcg (9d), 75 mg ferrous fumarate (7d)
Teva Pharmaceuticals USA

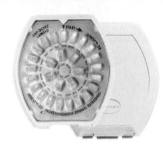

JENEST® 28 TABLETS
(norethindrone/ethinyl estradiol)
0.5 mg/35 mcg (7d) (white),
1 mg/35 mcg (14d) (peach)
Schering-Plough

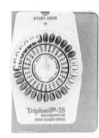

TRIPHASIL®- 28 TABLETS
(levonorgestrel/ethinyl estradiol–triphasic regimen)
0.050 mg/30 mcg (6d) (brown),
0.075 mg/40 mcg (5d) (white),
0.125 mg/30 mcg (10d) (light yellow)
Wyeth

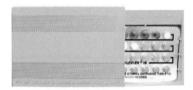

TRI-LEVLEN® 28 TABLETS
(levonorgestrel/ethinyl estradiol–triphasic regimen)
0.050 mg/30 mcg (6d) (brown),
0.075 mg/40 mcg (5d) (white),
0.125 mg/30 mcg (10d) (light yellow)
Bayer

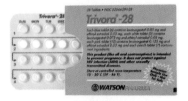

TRIVORA®
(levonorgestrel/ethinyl estradiol–triphasic regimen)
0.050 mg/30 mcg (6d), 0.075 mg/
40 mcg (5d), 0.125 mg/30 mcg (10d) (pink)
Watson

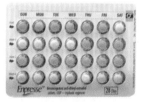

ENPRESSE®
(levonorgestrel and ethinyl estradiol tablets,
USP - triphasic regimen)
(active pills pink, white and orange)
Teva Pharmaceuticals USA

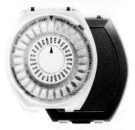

ORTHO TRI-CYCLEN® - 28 TABLETS
(norgestimate/ethinyl estradiol)
0.18 mg/35 mcg (7d) (white),
0.215 mg/35 mcg (7d) (light blue),
0.25 mg/35 mcg (7d) (blue)
Ortho-McNeil

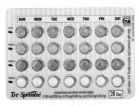

TRI-SPRINTEC®
(norgestimate and ethinyl estradiol tablets -
triphasic regimen)
(active pills gray, light blue and blue)
Teva Pharmaceuticals USA

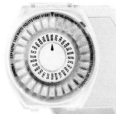

TRINESSA®
(norgestimate/ethinyl estradiol)
0.18 mg/35 mcg (7d) (white),
0.215 mg/35 mcg (7d) (light blue),
0.25 mg/35 mcg (7d) (dark blue)
remaining 7 placebo pills are green
Watson

TRI-PREVIFEM™ - 28 TABLETS
(norgestimate and
ethinyl estradiol tablets -
triphasic regimen)
Teva Pharmaceuticals USA

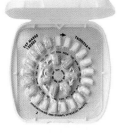

ORTHO-NOVUM® 7/7/7 - 28 TABLETS
(norethindrone/ethinyl estradiol)
0.5 mg/35 mcg (7d) (white),
0.75 mg/35 mcg (7d) (light peach),
1 mg/35 mcg (7d) (peach)
Ortho-McNeil

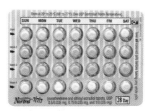

NORTREL® 7/7/7
(norethindrone and ethinyl estradiol tablets,
USP - triphasic regimen)
(active pills light yellow,
blue and peach)
Teva Pharmaceuticals USA

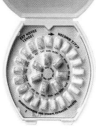

NECON® 7/7/7
0.5 mg/35 mcg (7d) (yellow),
0.75 mg/35 mcg (7d) (blue),
1 mg/35 mcg (7d) (peach)
Watson

(K)

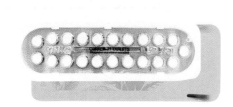

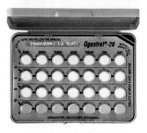

OVRAL® - 21 TABLETS
(0.5 mg norgestrel/50 mcg ethinyl estradiol)
(active pills white)
Wyeth

OGESTREL®
(0.5 mg norgestrel/50 mcg ethinyl estradiol)
(active pills white)
Watson

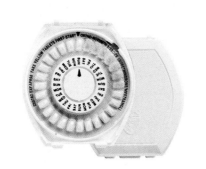

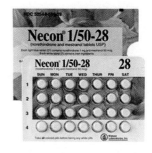

ORTHO-NOVUM® 1/50 - 28 TABLETS
(1 mg norethindrone/50 mcg mestranol)
(active pills yellow)
Ortho-McNeil

NECON® 1/50 - 28 TABLETS
(1 mg norethindrone/50 mcg mestranol)
Watson

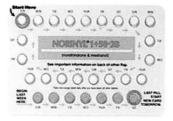

NORINYL® 1/50
(1 mg norethindrone/50 mcg mestranol)
Watson

(L)

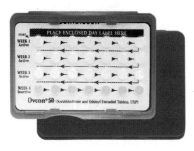

OVCON® 50 28-DAY
(1 mg norethindrone/50 mcg ethinyl estradiol)
(active pills yellow)
Warner-Chilcott

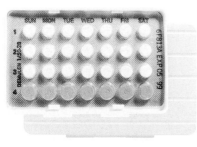

DEMULEN® 1/50-28
(1 mg ethynodiol diacetate/50 mcg ethinyl estradiol)
(active pills white)
Pharmacia - A Division of Pfizer

ZOVIA® 1/50
(1 mg ethynodiol diacetate/50 mcg ethinyl estradiol)
Watson

PILLS AS EMERGENCY CONTRACEPTIVES:
2 Different Approaches: Progestin-Only Pills OR Combined Pills

PROGESTIN-ONLY PILLS

Plan B

1 + 1 pill 12 hours apart OR
2 Plan B Pills *(white)* ASAP after unprotected sex

Plan B available without a prescription in pharmacies to women and men ≥ 18 years old. Plan B is NOT carried in all pharmacies. Check in advance. Ask your pharmacy to carry Plan B.

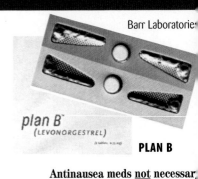

Barr Laboratories

plan B™
(LEVONORGESTREL)

PLAN B

Antinausea meds <u>not</u> necessary

COMBINED ORAL CONTRACEPTIVES

2 + 2 pills 12 hours apart
Ogestrel *(white pills)*
Ovral *(white pills)*

(Ogestrel and Ovral are NOT carried in all pharmacies. Check in advance.)

4 + 4 pills 12 hours apart
Cryselle *(white pills)*
Enpresse *(orange pills)*
Jolessa *(pink pills)*
Low-Ogestrel *(white pills)*
Lo-Ovral *(white pills)*
Levora *(white pills)*
Levlen *(light orange pills)*
Nordette *(light orange pills)*
Portia *(pink pills)*
Quasense *(white pills)*
Seasonale *(pink pills)*
Seasonique *(light blue pills)*
Triphasil *(yellow pills)*
Tri-Levlen *(yellow pills)*
Trivora *(pink pills)*

Have your patient take antinausea medication an hour before the first dose if using any of the combined oral contraceptives as emergency contraception. This is <u>not</u> necessary if using Plan B.

5 + 5 pills 12 hours apart
Alesse *(pink pills)*
Levlite *(pink pills)*
Aviane *(orange pills)*
Lessina *(pink pills)*
Lutera *(white pills)*

PERIMENOPAUSAL WOMEN

The balance between the benefits and the risks of COCs changes with women's age. As they get older, women's health risks of pregnancy increase (but their fertility diminishes) and they develop more severe medical problems. Healthy, non-obese, and nonsmoking women in their 40s are candidates for COCs. COCs can help reduce the risks of unscheduled bleeding and endometrial hyperplasia associated with anovulatory cycling during the perimenopausal years. Women in their 40s are at higher risk for heavy or prolonged menstrual bleeding and painful bleeding due to leiomyoma and adenomyosis. COCs can provide a medical alternative to surgical therapies, such as endometrial ablation or hysterectomy. Extended-cycle COC regimens help treat all these menstrual problems. COCs also help reduce the risk of ovarian and endometrial cancers later in life.

The American College of Obstetricians and Gynecologists (ACOG) cautions clinicians about using estrogen-containing contraceptives in obese women (BMI > 30 km/m²) over age 35.[35] ACOG's rationale is that both age and obesity are independent risk factors for venous thromboembolism; adding exogenous estrogen increases that risk. However, because pregnancy presents an even greater risk of deep venous thrombosis, COCs are not absolutely contraindicated when women cannot use other effective methods. The U.S. MEC rates obesity in woman at any age as a category 2 condition.[36]

No special testing is required prior to prescribing COCs for women in their 40s, except for blood pressure measurements. Screening measures such as clinical breast exams, serum lipids, and pelvic exam with cytology screens are important elements of well-woman care but do not need to be performed in apparently healthy asymptomatic women of any age prior to COC initiation.

COC users in their 40s or early 50s may not experience traditional symptoms of menopause while taking COCs. They generally do not experience menstrual irregularities or hot flashes, especially if the COCs are used on an extended basis. In this context, it may be difficult to detect when menopause occurs. (See Chapter 25 on Perimenopause, Menopause, and Postmenopause: Health Promotion Strategies.)

POSTPARTUM WOMEN

Pregnancy itself is a hypercoagulable state, the postpartum period is the time that the risk of venous thromboembolism (VTE) is greatest. As a result, it is generally recommended that postpartum women delay use of estrogen-containing contraception that could further increase VTE risk until at least 3 to 4 weeks after delivery, when those pregnancy-induced changes in the coagulation system start to resolve.

BREASTFEEDING WOMEN

High-dose estrogen used to be given to postpartum women to inhibit breast milk formation. From this outdated practice, theoretical concerns persisted for years that COCs would adversely affect the quality or quantity of breast milk production at any time while a woman breastfed. As reassuring evidence emerged, the American Academy of Pediatrics approved of estrogen-containing methods once some other source of nutrition (e.g., solid food) was added to the baby's diet. A thorough review of the world literature found that existing trials are insufficient to establish any effect of hormonal contraception on milk quality or its nutrients.[243] (See Chapter 18 on Postpartum Contraception and Lactation.) The U.S. MEC concluded that the benefits of COC use outweigh the risks in breastfeeding women after the first postpartum month, when hypercoagulability is decreased and the milk flow is established.[36]

WOMEN WITH MEDICAL PROBLEMS

Many medical conditions present no contraindications to use of COCs; for these conditions, COC use neither worsens disease progression nor increases risk of complications. These conditions are assigned categories "1" (use is not restricted) and "2" (benefits of use outweigh risks) in the U.S. MEC (see Chapter 4). These medical conditions include hypothyroidism and hyperthyroidism, rheumatoid arthritis, and sickle cell anemia, among others. Often COCs can help treat menstrual abnormalities associated with these medical problems. For example, the menstrual disturbances caused by thyroid disorders can be normalized by COC use. Women with sickle cell anemia benefit from less menstrual blood loss. In addition, medications used to treat conditions such as hyperthyroidism, rheumatoid arthritis, and convulsive disorders can be teratogenic, so unintended pregnancies that occur during treatment are at higher risk for birth defects. However, sometimes the medications used to treat medical conditions, such as depression and epilepsy, may interact with and decrease the efficacy of COCs (see Drug-Drug Interactions). Use of an additional method, or substitution of a nonhormonal or locally acting method, is therefore recommended in this situation. In the past, women who faced any significant health risks with COC use were prohibited from using COCs. This practice ignored the fact that pregnancy might pose the women even greater and more severe health threats. The risk of complications with COC use in women with medical problems must be weighed against the increased risks the woman would experience if she became pregnant. The appropriate yardstick to use to judge a woman's candidacy for COCs is whether COC use is safer for her current health than pregnancy would be.

Hypertension

Women with elevated blood pressure who use COCs have an increased risk of myocardial infarction and stroke.[244] Therefore, the U.S. MEC recommends that COC use is contraindicated in hypertensive women with uncontrolled blood pressure levels or advanced vascular disease, such as retinopathy or nephropathy (Category 4) and recommends against the use of COCs in women with well-controlled blood pressure, unless no other contraceptive method is available or acceptable (Category 3). In these cases, a progestin-only or nonhormonal method is still available. Women with a history of gestational hypertension or prehypertension (120–139 systolic or 80–89 diastolic) have no restrictions to COC use.

Diabetes

Diabetes increases a woman's risk for microvascular (retinopathy, nephropathy, neuropathy) and macrovascular (coronary artery disease, peripheral artery disease) complications. However, the use of low-dose COCs by women with diabetes mellitus does not appear to significantly alter glucose metabolism or increase risk of vascular complications.[245] Pills also provide a diabetic woman a chance to achieve a tight glucose control before conception to decrease maternal and fetal complications including serious malformations. Therefore, the U.S. MEC concluded that COCs may be used by women with diabetes who do not have vascular disease because the benefits outweigh the risks (Category 2). However, the U.S. MEC recommends against the initiation of COCs in women with diabetes who have co-existing vascular disease or who have had diabetes for over 20 years, unless no other contraceptive method is available or acceptable (Category 3). COC continuation is contraindicated in diabetic women who develop micro- or macrovascular complications during COC use (Category 4).[36] In each of these cases, the woman is still eligible for progestin-only or non-hormonal methods. Women with a history of gestational diabetes have no restrictions to COC use. In these women, more frequent screening may be needed because they are at higher risk of developing diabetes over time, but COC use does not appear to increase this risk.[246]

Headaches

Headache occurs commonly in reproductive-aged women. Before providing hormonal contraception to a woman with pre-existing headaches, characterize the type of headache she experiences. What a woman calls a "migraine" may actually be only a severe headache. The International Headache Society established guidelines for identifying headache type, including tension, cluster, and migraine headaches.[247] *Tension* headaches are the most common; they are bilateral in location, throbbing in nature, and mild to moderate in intensity. They may be associated with mild or no nausea, and either photo- or phonophobia. *Cluster* headaches are unilateral, severe in intensity, and occur in "clusters" over several days. They may be associated with sympathetic symptoms like eye tearing, nasal congestion, or a feeling of restlessness. There is no contraindication to the use of combined hormonal contraceptives in women with either tension or cluster headaches because there is no evidence to suggest that COCs cause any increased risk of complications.[248]

Migraine headaches are unilateral, throbbing in nature, moderate to severe in intensity, and are at least several hours in duration. They are exacerbated by physical activity, and associated with nausea and vomiting, photophobia and phonophobia. Migraines may be preceded by reversible, focal neurological symptoms that develop gradually, usually prior to onset of headache, and last no more than 60 minutes. Symptoms can include scotoma or flashing lights, loss of vision, numbness, tingling, or trouble speaking. A personal history of migraines is a risk factor for ischemic stroke, and the presence of aura further increases that risk. However, the absolute risk of stroke in young women is very low (5 to 10 per 100,000 women-years).[248] While COCs may be prescribed to young women with migraines without aura (Category 2), COCs are contraindicated in all migraineurs over age 35 years and in women of any age who experience migraines with aura (Category 4).[249]

Always ask *when* in a cycle a woman experiences her headaches or when in her cycle have they worsened on COCs. If the headaches occur during days of taking active pills, COCs should not be prescribed, although progestin-only methods would still be feasible. Headaches due to estrogen withdrawal are usually called *menstrual migraines*. These symptoms often improve with a shortened hormone-free interval or extended regimen of COCs. Although there is no evidence that a woman's stroke risk decreases if her migraines improve with extended COC use, the therapeutic relief in symptoms may provide enough benefit to outweigh the minimal risk.[248]

If a woman develops new headaches while on COCs or has worsening of her pre-existing headaches, she deserves prompt evaluation and probable discontinuation of estrogen-containing contraceptives. (See Managing Side Effects, Headaches.)

Tobacco Use

The first priority in caring for a woman who smokes tobacco is to encourage and help her to stop smoking entirely, or to reduce the number of cigarettes she smokes each day. Three to 12 months after stopping smoking, past smokers have the same COC-related cardiovascular risks as nonsmokers. Moderate and heavy smoking (i.e., at least 15 cigarettes a day) by women over age 35 precludes the use of COCs. Light smoking by women older than 35 merits caution (Category 3). Smoking increases a COC user's risk of heart attack nearly 13- to 14- fold.[250] Indeed, women who smoke as few as 1 to 4 cigarettes a day have a 2.5-fold increased risk of coronary heart disease.[251] The older the smoker, the more cigarettes she smokes, and the more comorbid cardiovascular risk factors she faces, the less likely she is to be a candidate for COCs. In otherwise healthy young women, the absolute risk of cardiovascular disease is low, so use of COCs by young women who smoke is still significantly safer than pregnancy.

In selecting a pill for smokers, the clinician is conflicted. On the one hand, the ideal pill would have the lowest estrogen content (to reduce arterial thrombosis) and the lowest androgenic activity (to minimize any adverse impacts on lipids). On the other hand, smokers tend to metabolize estrogen more rapidly and to increase SHBG levels more than nonsmokers do, so that a 20-mcg EE dose pill may not provide as much contraceptive efficacy for a smoker. There are no clinical trials to provide guidance. It may be prudent to start smokers and women who use a nicotine patch, gum, or other nicotine product on a 20-mcg EE formulation with a shortened hormone-free interval or other low-dose extended-cycle formulations. Vaginal contraceptive rings are another attractive option for smokers who want good cycle control.

HIV/AIDS

Worldwide, approximately 16 million adult women are infected with HIV,[252] 70% of whom are in their reproductive years. Millions more are at risk for acquiring the disease. With the increased use of antiretroviral therapy (ART), more HIV-infected women are surviving and are seeking reversible contraceptive methods. U.S. MEC recommendations are quite clear. COC use is rated Category 1 for HIV-infected women, whether or not they are diagnosed with AIDS.[36]

Several questions arise around the question of contraception and HIV infection:

- Will COC use increase the risk of transmission of HIV to an HIV-infected woman's uninfected partner? Correct and consistent use of male condoms remains the first-line recommendation to prevent partner-to-partner transmission. Only one study has directly investigated rates of female-to-male HIV transmission among couples using COCs. It found no increased transmission in those couples compared with controls who used no contraception.[253]

- Will COC use affect the efficacy of HIV treatments and will HIV therapies affect the efficacy of COCs? Some antiretroviral medications impact on COC metabolism. (See specific group of drug-drug interactions below.)

Systemic Lupus Erythematosus (SLE)

Four studies have shown that the incidence of disease flares does not increase in women with systemic lupus erythematosus (SLE) who use COCs, although women with severe disease were not studied. Antiphospholipid antibodies in SLE patients are a known risk factor for thromboembolism. Therefore, women with mild SLE manifestation may use COCs if they have no antiphospholipid antibodies.[254] Progestin-only methods are still a reasonable and safe alternative for all women with SLE.

Liver Disease

A systematic review found that COC use did not increase liver transaminase levels, hepatic inflammation, or fibrosis in women with chronic hepatitis, though studies were all limited by short duration of follow-up. Only one small trial investigated COC use in women with acute hepatitis and noted no increase in severity of disease with COC use. Women with chronic hepatitis or mild cirrhosis may use COCs. For women who are hepatitis carriers, COC use does not appear to precipitate liver failure or severe dysfunction. U.S. MEC rates COC use as Category 1 for both chronic viral hepatitis and carriers.[36] However, it is recommended that women with acute hepatitis or with a severe flare or cirrhosis avoid COC use.[255] Women with mild or compensated cirrhosis may use COCs, but those with severe disease should not (U.S. MEC Category 4). Women who have had pregnancy-related cholestasis might be at higher risk for cholestasis on COCs, so U.S. MEC rates their use as a Category 2. Women who have had cholestasis with prior COC use probably should not be given COCs unless other methods are not available.[36] In women who have focal nodular hyperplasia, a type of benign liver tumor, studies of COC use are limited, but nonetheless show no effect on tumor size. Use of COCs in women with hepatocellular adenoma or carcinoma is contraindicated.[256]

History of Bariatric Surgery

Fertility and ovulation rates increase in women after having bariatric surgery, so effective contraceptive use is important if women wish to avoid pregnancy at this time. No clinical trials have assessed the efficacy of COCs after bariatric surgery. A case series noted two COC failures in women after malabsorption surgery (biliopancreatic diversion, Roux-en-Y bypass). Nutritional deficiencies have been noted in patients after malabsorptive procedures, suggesting that COCs may also have been less well absorbed in these patients. An alternative method or use of a back-up method of contraception with the COCs is recommended. Transdermal or vaginal delivery may be more appropriate. On the other hand, women who have restrictive procedures (banding, gastrectomy) may use COCs.[257]

History of Organ Transplantation

Women with complications from organ transplants (graft failure, rejection, vasculopathy) or who are preparing for transplant surgery anticipating long immobilization should avoid COC use. The majority of anti-rejection medications show little or no interaction with hormonal levels of COCs. Following liver transplantation, COC users may need additional monitoring for signs of liver dysfunction or biliary stasis.[258]

DRUG-DRUG INTERACTIONS
GENERAL PRINCIPLES

One drug can alter the effectiveness of another drug in many ways. To evaluate possible drug-drug interactions with COCs, a clinician must first understand how the estrogen and progestin in COCs are absorbed, distributed, metabolized, and eliminated.

Absorption

Sex steroids in COCs are absorbed from the small intestine and shunted primarily through the liver (called *first-pass*). About 60% of the absorbed EE is conjugated by the intestinal mucosa and the liver to form glucuronic and sulfate conjugates. These conjugated estrogens are immediately excreted through the gallbladder back into the small intestines without entering into the bloodstream.[259] These conjugates cannot be reabsorbed from the small intestines. However, bacteria in the *large* intestine can enzymatically unconjugate the estrogen compounds. The newly freed estrogen is then absorbed from the colon and delivered to the liver via the enterohepatic circulation for additional hepatic passes for absorption into the bloodstream or for reconjugation and re-excretion back into the intestine, where it is ultimately eliminated in the feces. Sex steroids that do enter the woman's circulation are also ultimately conjugated hepatically and excreted in the urine.

Hepatic Effects

When EE is in contact with the liver, it induces profound changes in hepatic enzyme activity and protein synthesis. EE increases hepatic production of carrier proteins (e.g., sex hormone binding globulin, thyroxin binding globulin, and albumin). EE also activates cytochrome P-450 enzymes, increasing the rate at which many drugs are cleared by the liver from the bloodstream.

Effect of Other Drugs on COC Efficacy

Theoretically, interactions between COCs and other drugs could result from one or more of 3 actions:

1. Hepatic production of binding proteins

2. Influences on enterohepatic circulation

3. Changes in hepatic enzyme activity

Although COC-induced binding proteins are important for the treatment of acne or hirsutism, they do not affect the efficacy of any drugs. Other drugs do not induce binding globulins at rates that can affect COC efficacy. Therefore, there are no significant drug-drug interactions in this category.

The role that the enterohepatic circulation has on COC efficacy created considerable controversy. At the heart of the matter was the concern that use of broad-spectrum antibiotics, such as tetracycline and ampicillin, might destroy the bacteria needed in the colon to break down the estrogen conjugates and permit reabsorption (second pass) of the EE. Studies have shown that peak levels of serum EE are *not* altered when women take tetracycline,[260] doxycycline,[261] ampicillin, metronidazole[262] or quinolone antibiotics.[263] No enterohepatic recirculation of progestins occurs. Therefore, antibiotics that destroy colonic bacteria do not affect serum levels of progestin—the hormone that provides most of the contraceptive effects of the COC. Finally and most convincingly, women who have had an ileostomy and, therefore, have *no* enterohepatic recirculation, do not experience any reduction in the efficacy of COCs.[264]

The most important cause of drug-drug interaction with COCs is mediated through cytochrome P-450 enzyme activation. Increases in cytochrome P-450 start rapidly, but they are slow to normalize after COC cessation. Induction of P-450 will cause more rapid clearance of drugs that are metabolized by this pathway. One month after initiating COCs, patients using phenobarbital or other similar anticonvulsants should have levels of their anticonvulsants tested to ensure that those levels are still within the therapeutic range.

Similarly, drugs that affect the P-450 pathway may have an effect on the metabolic clearance of the hormones in COCs. Drugs that *increase* cytochrome P-450 activity can lower hormone levels while drugs that *decrease* cytochrome P-450 activity *raise* circulating levels of the hormones in COCs.

Other Drug Metabolism Issues

Complicating these recognized potential drug-drug interactions is the fact that there is great inter-individual variation in drug processing. Some women absorb fewer hormones from their intestines than others do. Some women's baseline cytochrome P-450 enzyme activity is greater than others. Some women's hepatic enzymes change in response to drugs more dramatically than others do. In addition, the drugs themselves may complicate the situation by requiring hepatic metabolism to transform them into their active forms. For example, mestranol must be metabolized in the liver to form the biologically active EE, and desogestrel is metabolized into the active etonogestrel. The extent of that transformation again varies from person to person. Beyond these biologic considerations is the concern that inconsistent use of COCs creates an opportunity for even higher failure rates.

SPECIFIC GROUPS OF DRUG-DRUG INTERACTIONS

Broad-spectrum Antibiotics

Hormone levels in women using COCs are not lowered by the use of ampicillin, amoxicillin, clarithromycin, metronidazole, quinolones (ciprofloxacin, ofloxacin), doxycycline, tetracycline or fluconazole. Virtually every COC user taking these antibiotics has hormone levels that remain well within the therapeutic range for contraceptive efficacy.[260–263,265,266] As a result, back-up methods should *not* be necessary unless the patient has problems taking her pills, e.g., if her underlying medical condition interferes with pill-taking or absorption. Long-term use of broad-spectrum antibiotics (such as erythromycin or tetracycline for acne) is also compatible with COC use; back-up methods are not routinely needed for pregnancy prevention.[266] The only antibiotics that profoundly affect COC potency are drugs that contain hepatic enzyme inducers: rifampin and rifapentine (Priftin), rifampin with INH, (Rifadin, Rimactane), Rifamate, Rifater (with INH and pyrazinamide) and griseofulvin (rarely used). Remember that rifampin is also widely used with other antibiotics to treat skin infections with methicillin-resistant Staphylococcus aureus (MRSA).

Table 11–8 Anticonvulsants that affect COCs' metabolism and clearance

Generic Name	Brand Name	Estrogen reduction	Progestin reduction	Other Uses of Drug
Carbamazepine	Tegretol Equetro	42%	58%	Trigeminal neuralgia, schizophrenia, bipolar disease
Felbamate	Felbatol	13%	42%	Neuropathic pain, migraines, bipolar disease
Lamotrigine	Lamictal	No change, but Lamotrigine levels drop	No change, but Lamotrigine levels drop	PTSD, Bipolar disease
Oxcarbazine	Trileptal	48%	32%	Bipolar disease, neuropathic pain
Phenobarbital	Generic	64–72%	0%	None
Phenytoin	Dilantin	49%	42%	None
Topiramate	Topamax	15–33%	0%	Migraines, bipolar disease, obesity

Provided courtesy of Michael Policar, MD, MPH

Anticonvulsants

Many drugs used today to control seizures are also used for other important applications, such as to reduce drug dependency and to treat depression. Some of these agents increase cytochrome P-450 clearance (see Table 11–8), while others do not (see Table 11-9). Because of their widespread applications, it is important to be familiar with each of their interactions with COCs. Lamotrigine (Lamictal) is a special case. Lamotrigine levels drop by 49% (41% to 64%) when COCs are started. Therefore, increase the woman's dose of lamotrigine during days of active COCs and then reduce the dose to her regular dose during the placebo pills. Extended cycle use of COCs greatly simplifies lamotrigine administration.

Antiretrovirals (ARVs)

The larger number of antiretroviral drugs now available, as well as their use in multiple-drug regimens, makes the issue of interaction with COCs all the more complex. Because many antiretrovirals (ARVs) are metabolized via the cytochrome P-450 pathway, their simultaneous use with COCs can either increase or decrease serum levels of estrogen or progestins. The Department of Health and Human Services published guidelines in 2009 that list all known interactions between currently used ARVs and COCs.[267] A review of the ARVs currently recommended for first-line treatment of newly infected persons might assist providers who work in settings in which high rates of new HIV infections occur. For women on alternative or advanced regimens, consulting the guidelines, package insert, and/or additional providers involved may be necessary.

Table 11–9. Anticonvulsants with no impact on COC metabolism

Generic Name	Brand Name
Clonazepam	Klonopin®
Ethosuximide	Zarontin®
Gabapentin	Neurontin®
Levetiracetam	Keppra®
Pregabalin	Lyrica®
Tiagabine	Gabitril®
Valproic acid	Depakene®, Depakote®
Vigabatrin	Sabril®
Zonisamide	Zonegran®

Classes of ARVs recommended for first-line treatment of newly infected persons include non-nucleoside reverse transcriptase inhibitors (NNRTI), nucleoside reverse transcriptase inhibitors (NRTI), protease inhibitors (PI) combined with ritonavir, and integrase inhibitors (INSTI).

- All NNRTIs interact with COCs via cytochrome P-450 metabolism. The most-recommended NNRTI, efavirenz, increases EE concentration levels by 37%, the clinical significance of which is unknown.
- NRTIs do not affect cytochrome P-450 metabolism, although some NRTIs are still metabolized through the liver; clinically significant interactions are not likely, but also not well studied.
- PIs interact with COCs via cytochrome P-450 metabolism, the most common of which, atazanavir and darunavir, both decrease EE levels when combined with ritonavir. Their effects on progestins appear to be minimal, but have not been well studied.
- INSTIs have no effect on cytochrome P-450 metabolism and do not interact with COCs.

Correct and consistent use of male condoms is recommended for all HIV-infected persons for prevention of partner-to-partner transmission of HIV and other STIs. In addition, women who use protease inhibitor-based regimens and rely on COCs for contraception should be counseled to either use a second method or to switch to a more effective contraceptive method based on these potential drug-drug interactions.

Other Prescription Drug Interactions

COCs may increase the effect of theophylline (used to treat asthma), tricyclic antidepressants, and the antipsychotic drugs diazepam (Valium) and chlordiazepoxide (Lithium). Doses of these drugs may need to be lowered with COC use.

Drospirenone acts as an antimineralocorticoid and can interact with other potassium-sparing drugs to cause hyperkalemia. Women using ACE inhibitors, angiotensin-II antagonists, potassium-sparing diuretics, heparin, aldosterone antagonists, and NSAIDS on a chronic daily basis to treat chronic conditions or diseases should have their serum potassium checked during the first cycle of drospirenone use (usually about 14 days after pill initiation). If those levels are normal, no future testing is necessary.

Over-The-Counter Drugs

St. John's Wort is taken by many women to treat mild depression. Because this botanical agent does not require a prescription, women sometimes neglect to tell their health care providers that they are using it. St. John's Wort greatly increases hepatic metabolism of exogenous estrogen and progestin. In one study of women using 35 mcg EE pills, St. John's Wort use was associated with a significant increase in the clearance of norethindrone and a significant reduction in the half-life of EE.[268] The FDA has alerted providers that St. John's Wort may decrease the therapeutic effect of COCs.[269] Women who use Orlistat to block fat absorption may also reduce intestinal absorption of COC hormones. This concern is magnified if the woman experiences diarrhea with Orlistat use.

M ANAGING MISSED PILLS

After having taken at least 7 pills at the correct time, women are at little risk for ovulation until they subsequently miss 7 consecutive pills. The conventional hormone-free interval provides these 7 days. Escape ovulation is much more likely to occur if pills are missed early in the packet and if the patient is using a lower-dose (20 mcg EE) pill. Therefore, the recommendations for coping with missed pills vary not only with the number of pills missed,[239] but also with the strength of the pill and the week in which the pills were missed. Management recommendations must include instructions about three items: when to take the missed (and subsequent) pills; when to use a back-up method; and when to use EC. The instructions for EC are covered in Chapter 6.

These recommendations are helpful for clinicians who are seeing patients when they miss pills. However, these recommendations are too complicated for many pill users, especially women with low literacy skills. Furthermore, the recommendations are based on the assumption that the women had taken all their earlier pills as directed. More than half of women miss 3 or more pills each cycle.[17] Finally, some of the recommendations may not be feasible in the United States. Women who are

Table 11–10 Instructions for missed pills, advice from Medicines and Healthcare Products Regulatory Agency (MHRA), 2011

If you forget to take a pill or start a pack late

Missing pills or starting the pack late may make your pill less effective. The chance of pregnancy after missing pills depends on *when* pills are missed and *how many* pills are missed. A pill is late when you have forgotten to take it at the usual time. A pill has been missed when it is more than 24 hours since the time you should have taken it.

- If you *miss 1 pill* anywhere in your pack, or start the new pack 1 day late, you will still have contraceptive cover. However, missing *2 or more pills* or starting the pack *2 or more days late* (more than 48 hours late) may affect your contraceptive cover. As soon as you realize you have missed any pills, take the last pill you missed immediately. In particular, during the 7-day pill-free break your ovaries are not getting any effects from the pill. If you make this pill-free break longer by forgetting 2 or more pills, your ovaries might release an egg and there is a real risk of becoming pregnant.

- Follow the advice below. If you are not sure what to do, continue to take your pill and use additional contraception, such as condoms, and seek advice as soon as possible.

If you have **missed 1 pill**, anywhere in the pack—
- Take the last pill you missed now, even if it means taking 2 pills in 1 day.
- Continue taking the rest of the pack as usual.
- No additional contraception needed.
- Take your 7-day break as usual.

If you have **missed 2 or more pills** *(more than 48 hours late)*, anywhere in the pack—
- Take the last pill you missed now, even if it means taking 2 pills in 1 day.
- Leave any earlier missed pills.
- Continue taking the rest of the pack as usual and use an extra method of contraception for the next 7 days.
- You may need emergency contraception—see below.
- You may need to start the next pack of pills without a break—see below.

Emergency contraception

If you have had unprotected sex in the previous 7 days and you have missed 2 or more pills (more than 48 hours late) **in the 1st week of a pack**, you may need emergency contraception. Get advice from your contraception clinic, family doctor, or a pharmacist about this.

Starting the next pack after missing 2 or more pills (more than 48 hours late)
- Finish the pack.
- Have the usual 7-day break.

If fewer than 7 pills are left in the pack after the missed pill—
- Finish the pack and begin a new one the next day (this means skipping the break).

told to skip the placebo pills and start the next packet may not be able to get another packet of pills until the usual refill time due to restrictive dispensing protocols required by third party payers. Therefore, a simplified protocol of missed pills is offered for advanced counseling of women (see below).

SIMPLIFIED MANAGEMENT OF MISSED PILLS

The rules about missed pills have been greatly simplified. However, they still do not account for any prior missed pills, the patient's confusion about the amount of hormones they are using, or any difficulties the woman may have in getting her next pill pack early. These issues have been addressed in the following simplified modifications of missed pill rules.

- If a woman remembers her pill within 12 hours of the time that she was to take it, she should take it immediately and take all the rest of the pills at the usual time.
  — No back-up method is needed.
  — No EC is needed.

- If a woman misses 1 pill for more than 12 hours, she should take today's pill now and use condoms or abstinence for the next 7 days.
  — No EC is needed.

- If a woman misses more than 1 pill, she should take today's pill and the last forgotten pill today (2 tablets in 1 day). The rest of the instructions depend upon which pills she missed:
  — If she has at least 7 active pills in the pack, she should use condoms for 7 days and use EC if she has had unprotected intercourse in the prior 7 days.
  — If she has 7 or fewer active pill in the pack, she has two options:

    1. Take the rest of the active pills. Skip the placebo pills and start the next pack of pills without interruption.
       — Use condoms or abstain for 7 days.
    2. Take the pills as in the pack.
       — Use condoms or abstinence until she has taken 7 of the pills in the next pack.
       — Use EC if she has had any unprotected intercourse in the prior 7 days.

These guidelines are still complicated for advanced counseling. *To simplify further,* consider telling a woman that—

- If she is late (<12 hours) in taking a pill, to take it immediately and continue with the other pills at the usual time.

- If she is later than 12 hours taking the pills, she should take the last missed pill right away and also take the pill she should take on time. She should use EC if she has had any unprotected intercourse in the past 7 days. She should use condoms or abstain until she has used 7 pills in a row.

Women who vomit within 2 hours of taking COCs or who have severe vomiting and diarrhea for 2 or more days should be treated as if they had missed pills.

Managing Side Effects

Management of side effects is crucial to successful use of COCs. In one study, 59% to 81% of women who discontinued COC use reported that they stopped due to side effects.[21] However, double-blind placebo-controlled trials have shown no difference in the incidence of any of the major side effects in COC users compared with placebo pill users; similar percentages of women in each group developed headaches, nausea, vomiting, mastalgia, excessive weight gain, etc.[270] In the original clinical trials in the 1950s, women who received placebos and were given counseling for COC's side effects reported side effects at almost precisely the same rates that the high-dose COC users reported.[271] However, some women may be more sensitive to exogenous hormones, so counsel all potential hormonal contraceptive users that side effects may be possible, but *not necessarily to be expected.*

Advise women that side effects are usually transient or responsive to changes in pill formulations. Familiarity with the hormones theoretically implicated in the different side effects can aid clinicians in selecting new formulations for patients (see Table 11–11). Some researchers have noted significant differences in rates of discontinuation among different groups of women. For example, discontinuation rates are higher among Bolivian women, who had lower endogenous hormone levels than did U.S. women.[272]

The side effects discussed are grouped by system: menstrually related side effects, symptomatic complaints, and metabolic effects.

Menstrually Related Side Effects

Absence of Scheduled Bleeding

Advise women that the amount of scheduled bleeding they will have with COCs may be significantly less than what they typically lose during their spontaneous cycling menses. Even scant bleeding or spotting on the placebo pills counts as a scheduled episode. The incidence of complete amenorrhea varies with different formulations and increases with dura-

Table 11–11 Estrogenic, progestogenic, and combined effects of COCs

Estrogen Related	Progesterone Related	Androgen Related
Weight gain in breast, hips, and thighs	Cyclic weight gain	Slow, steady weight gain
Cervical eversion or ectopy	Hypoglycemic headaches	Hirsutism
Increased blood pressure	Constipation, bloating	
Rise in gallbladder cholesterol	Fatigue	Elevated LDL-C
Melasma, telangiectasia	Depressive symptoms	Acne
Hepatocellular adenoma	Increased insulin resistance	Oily skin
Arterial thrombosis	Precipitation of gallbladder sludge or stones	
Venous thromboembolism		
Headaches	Nausea	
Increased HDL-C, and triglycerides	Mastalgia	
Nausea		
Mastalgia		

tion of use. Some women deliberately extend the number of active pills they use to achieve prolonged amenorrhea. For women using cyclic regimens of COCs who fail to have scheduled bleeding, obvious causes of amenorrhea (such as pregnancy and new medications) must be excluded. Other specific conditions, such as cervical stenosis, need to be evaluated, particularly if the patient has recently had cervical surgery (e.g., D&C, cone biopsy, LEEP, etc). When a woman uses COCs, it is far less likely that the usual causes of amenorrhea will be responsible for her lack of bleeding. Thyroid problems, prolactinoma, hypothalamic amenorrhea due to stress or excessive exercise, or anovulatory states (such as PCOS or obesity) are often masked by COCs. If a woman lacks the cyclic bleeding that she desires on COCs, switch her to a more estrogenic formulation or to a triphasic formulation with lower levels of progestin in the early pills. This will permit more endometrial proliferation.

Women who enjoy freedom from monthly scheduled bleeding with extended-cycle pills but just want to reassure themselves periodically that they are not pregnant may use home pregnancy tests or may want to monitor their basal body temperature (BBT). If a woman's BBT is lower than 98°F for 2 sequential days, the likelihood of pregnancy is very low.

Unscheduled Vaginal Spotting or Bleeding

Unscheduled spotting and bleeding occurs in 30% to 50% of women in the first few months of COC use. By the third pack of pills, 70% to 90% of women (depending upon the formulation) have no further unscheduled bleeding or spotting.

Before changing COC type, rule out more likely or more serious causes of unscheduled bleeding, such as pregnancy, infection (vaginitis and cervicitis), medications that block hormone absorption or increase their metabolism by the liver (anticonvulsants, cigarette smoking, St. John's Wort, rifampin), and gastrointestinal problems (vomiting and diarrhea) that may prevent adequate hormone absorption. *Remember that one of the most common causes of unscheduled spotting and bleeding is missed pills.*

Consider changing the woman's pill formulation if she has had persistent unscheduled spotting or bleeding after 2 to 3 months of COC use. Earlier changes are appropriate if a woman says she will discontinue COC use because of the bleeding. No research indicates that any specific COC is best at eliminating unscheduled spotting or bleeding. In part, such recommendations are not possible because the data reported on bleeding and spotting frequencies with different formulations are not comparable.[273,299] However, it may help to use the timing of the woman's unscheduled bleeding and spotting in her pill pack as a guide to decide which new formulation to recommend for her.

- Women who report spotting or bleeding *before they complete their active pills* probably need more endometrial support. Increase the progestin content of their pills, either by changing to a different monophasic formulation or by switching to a triphasic formulation that increases progestin levels in the last active pills.

- Women with continued spotting or bleeding *following their scheduled bleeding* may need more estrogen to proliferate the endometrium. Increase the estrogen in the first pills in the pack or decrease the progestin content of those first pills.

- The cause of *mid-cycle* spotting or bleeding is not clear. One approach to this relatively uncommon bleeding pattern is to use triphasic formulations that increase both estrogen and progestin in the middle pills.

- *Extended-cycle users* tend to experience unscheduled spotting and bleeding, especially after week 5 in the first cycle. Inform users that, as with all other pills, they will have more spotting when they begin taking pills. This unscheduled bleeding and spotting will decrease rapidly over time. However, if after having completed 21 days of pills a woman finds this bothersome, she can stop taking pills for 2 to 3 days to allow a withdrawal bleed to start. Then she should restart the active pills, taking at least 3 weeks of active pills before she stops again. As she takes pills in this flexible pattern, the length of time between unscheduled spotting and bleeding episodes will increase and she eventually will be able to take pills for 3 to 12 months at a time with little or no unscheduled spotting or bleeding.

SYSTEMIC SIDE EFFECTS

Weight Changes

Placebo-controlled, randomized clinical trials have demonstrated that, on average, women do *not* experience more weight gain with low-dose COCs than with placebo pills.[270] In a prospective trial of women using triphasic COCs with daily weight measurements for 4 months, no changes in mean weight fluctuations were noted during the cycle.[274] A 9-year study showed that COC use by adolescent women was *not* associated with either weight gain or increased body fat.[275] In clinical trials, women who use COCs do not typically gain more weight than they normally do in the same time interval without COCs. A Cochrane review confirmed that available evidence is insufficient to determine the effect of combination contraceptives on weight, but concluded that no large effect was evident.[276] However, it is important for clinicians to understand that what troubles a patient is her *perception* of weight changes and that often a woman's opinions about weight change in clinical trials may not correlate with measured changes on a scale.[277]

Any individual woman may respond robustly to any of the pill's hormones. Increases in the size of a woman's breasts, hips, and thighs reflect estrogen's influence on adipose cells (hypertrophy). Decreasing estrogen in the pill can reduce this impact. Weight gain similar to premenstrual fluid retention is due to increased aldosterone release and results from estrogen activity augmented by progesterone. In this situation, switch to a pill with both lower estrogen and lower progestin levels. Drospirenone-containing COCs, which have a mild diuretic effect, may also be an appropriate choice to deal with this problem. Steadily increasing weight may be attributed to the nitrogen retention and an increase in muscle mass stimulated by androgens. Although it is unlikely that the pill itself would be responsible for this type of weight gain, switching to a pill with low or no androgenic activity may address that patient's concerns. Every woman should be encouraged to adopt a healthy diet and to exercise routinely to achieve and maintain a healthy weight.

Headaches

Headaches occur commonly.[278] Randomized placebo-controlled trials have found that women using placebo pills experienced headaches as frequently as did COC users.[270] Nonetheless, new onset or worsening headaches in a COC user must be investigated, because those symptoms can indicate a serious medical problem, such as hypertension, transient ischemic attacks, or impending stroke. Approximately 4% of COC users discontinue pill use because of headaches.[279] Some women do appear to have higher risk of headache exacerbation or new onset headaches attributable to COC use. This risk is highest among women with a strong personal or family history of headache, especially migraines. The incidence increases with age, peaking in the late 40's.

Headache complaints decrease with continued use. Women experiencing headaches during the first cycle have only a 1 in 3 chance of having those headaches the second month of use. The risk drops to 1 in 10 by the third cycle. A systematic review of the literature found that there is no scientific evidence to support the common clinical practice of switching formulations to treat headache. However, the authors suggested that manipulation of the extent or duration of estrogen withdrawal might be beneficial, especially if headaches worsen during bleeding.[279] Stepwise evaluation of the headache is necessary. For discussion on headache classification, see section on Special Populations-Women with Medical Problems.

- **Confirm whether the headaches started or worsened in frequency or severity with the onset of COC use.** New or worsening symptoms prompt medical evaluation. Stop COCs during evaluation, especially if the headaches are severe or if the patient develops any aura with her headaches. Progestin-only pills may be used. If the headaches are not serious, consider lowering estrogen doses.

- **Rule out other causes.** Measure the patient's blood pressure. Obtain a personal history of medication use, caffeine intake, and other prescription, nonprescription, and recreational drug use. Inquire about recent trauma. Note if there are other associated problems with vision, sensation, or other functions. Evaluate for signs and symptoms of transient ischemic attacks, cerebrovascular accidents, temporal arteritis, sinusitis, viremia, sepsis, allergy, temporomandibular joint (TMJ) disorders, dental problems, drug use, alcohol or caffeine withdrawal, or central nervous system tumor. Treat appropriately.

- **Characterize the type of headache.** The consequences are different for different types of headaches. If a woman develops new-onset migraine or a worsening in the severity or frequency of her migraine headaches during her active pill days, she probably is no longer a candidate for COCs. *If she develops associated neurological auras, stop the COCs immediately* and provide contraception without estrogen. On the other hand, if her symptoms develop or worsen only on the days she takes placebo pills (when her estrogen levels drop), it may be possible to offer her extended use low-dose COCs to reduce her menstrual migraines, unless she experiences aura.

Mood Swings and Depression

Multiple studies have demonstrated that no increased risk of clinical depression occurs in women using COCs. Both estrogen and progestin in high-dose pills interact with tryptophans and serotonin; however, low-dose pills have not been implicated in any of these complaints.[280] Women on COCs remain solidly within normal ranges for all vitamins and do not require vitamin B supplementation to prevent depression because of COC use.[281]

Some women do report an increase in depressive symptoms, moodiness, and other emotional states when on COCs. This may represent an idiosyncratic response to hormones. They may respond to a decrease in hormone doses or pill cessation. However, it is also important to identify when in a woman's cycle these symptoms develop. If the symptoms appear just before the menses, then extended or continuous use of active pills may dampen her hormonal swings.[282] If the woman desires withdrawal bleeding, have her start her active pills from the next pack on the first day of her menses. The low-dose drospirenone-containing formulation that the FDA has approved for treatment of premenstrual dysphoric disorder (PMDD) may be helpful in this situation.[62]

If any concern exists about your patient suffering from an underlying depressive or anxiety disorder, these conditions deserve an explicit evaluation and treatment. Cessation of COCs is not adequate therapy and may not even be indicated. Suicidal women need emergency treatment by specialists.

Changes in Libido

During the reproductive years, a woman's libido is not associated with her circulating levels of testosterone.[63] Women's libido is much more likely to be affected by relationship issues, personal history, and coital techniques. When a patient complains of a decrease in libido, evaluate for depression and other life stresses. Ask about thyroid-related symptoms. In many women, COCs decrease vaginal secretions by reducing cervical secretions, which may be interpreted by the user as decreased arousal. In more extreme cases, the decrease in vaginal lubrication can make sexual intercourse painful. Consider using an estrogenic COC or the vaginal ring to increase lubrication. A link has been suggested between suppressed free testosterone with COC use and decreased libido.[283] However, randomized clinical trials have found that very few women complain of any change in libido except perhaps in women with pre-existing mood disorders. Despite this evidence, women who complain of decreased libido with COC use may benefit from an empiric trial with another pill (perhaps with a greater androgenic effect) if this change is not contraindicated and if it pleases the patient.

Skin Changes

Estrogen stimulates the production of melanocytes, which can cause darkening of pigmented areas (linea nigra) or dark patches on the face (*melasma* or *chloasma*). Women with darker skin pigment are more susceptible. After discontinuation of estrogen, the melasma fades slowly and often incompletely. Progestin-only methods may be preferable for at-risk women. Recommend consistent use of sunscreen and hats in at-risk COC users.

Estrogen can also stimulate the formation of telangiectasias, which are fine, dilated intracutaneous capillaries and small terminal arteries. Telangiectasias are not clinically significant, but may be cosmetically disturbing to a woman. Avoid the use of estrogen-containing hormonal methods in women troubled by telangiectasia.

Complaints that relate to the impact of androgens, such as worsening or new onset of *acne, oily skin,* or *hirsutism,* is reported in less than 5% of women in clinical trials. Consider other causes of androgen exposure (other medications, ovarian tumors, etc.) if her symptoms are severe. If it appears her COC may be contributing to her problem, switch to a COC formulation approved for treatment of acne. One clinical trial demonstrated that a drospirenone-containing COC was superior to the norgestimate formulation.[284] If these formulations are not available, use pills with low androgenicity and relatively high estrogen content.

Mastalgia

Both estrogen and progesterone affect the breast during the menstrual cycle. Ovulating women routinely experience a substantial increase in breast volume (up to 20%) during the luteal phase due to venous and lymphatic engorgement. Estrogen causes hypertrophy of the adipose cells in the breast and can increase breast size. In addition, both hormones stimulate the terminal ductal lobular tuft growth, especially in nulliparous women. Nearly 30% of women experience mastalgia or breast tenderness when they first start COCs. A proper-fitting bra is the first recommendation. Reduction of the doses of both steroids may be necessary if symptoms do not resolve rapidly enough to satisfy the patient. Lower-dose pills (20 mcg EE) produced less mastalgia than higher-dose (35 mcg EE) pills in one comparative trial.[280] Women using drospirenone-containing pills also report less mastalgia. If the symptoms develop just before menses, extended-cycle COC use can help.

Gastrointestinal Complaints

Working at the level of the central nervous system, estrogen can induce nausea or vomiting. Sex steroid hormones do not directly affect the gastric lining, although new research has demonstrated a hormonal impact on the intrinsic firing rate of the gastric pacemaker cells. Progesterone slows peristalsis and can increase constipation and sensations of bloating and distention. Most affected women acclimate to the hormones, and nausea resolves within 1 to 3 months of use. If a woman complains of nausea, she can try taking her pills with food or at night. Avoid double dosing by counseling the patient to catch up on any pills she forgets by taking pills at 12-hour intervals, rather than taking 2 pills at one time. In addition, advise more fluids and fresh fruits and vegetables. Women with recent onset of severe gastrointestinal symptoms should be evaluated promptly to rule out acute, serious problems that are unrelated to COC use, such as cholecystitis, appendicitis and diverticulitis, and reactivation of more chronic, intermittent problems, such as inflammatory bowel syndrome (IBS).

If vomiting or diarrhea is related to taking the pill, try the following approaches:

- Switch to a progestin-only formulation.

- Decrease hormone dose. A 20 mcg COC dramatically decreases nausea for many women. Add a back-up method until diarrhea resolves. A 10 mcg formulation may also be helpful.

If bloating and constipation are problems, a reduction in the progestin component in the pill may help. A progestin-only pill with its low dose may, paradoxically, be the best solution. Bloating associated with menses can be diminished by extended-cycle or continuous active pill use or use of a formulation with drospirenone.

Contact Lens Effects

Women who use contact lenses may note some visual changes or change in lens tolerance with COC use due to dry eyes. Normal saline eye drops often provide adequate treatment, but consultation with an ophthalmologist may be helpful.

Metabolic Effects (Hyperlipidemia)

Routine screening for lipids is not necessary before prescribing COCs unless a patient has pre-existing hyperlipidemia or a very strong family history of premature cardiovascular disease. Estrogen is known to decrease low-density lipoprotein cholesterol (LDL-C) and to increase high-density lipoprotein cholesterol (HDL-C), triglycerides, and total cholesterol levels. The androgen-derived progestins may be neutral or may reverse some of estrogen's stimulatory effects on HDL-C and triglycerides and may increase low-density lipoprotein cholesterol (LDL-C). The net effect depends upon the dose, potency, and estrogen/androgen balance of each formulation. If LDL levels rise or HDL levels drop significantly with COC use, change to a formulation with more estrogenic activity and less androgenic activity.

Hypertriglyceridemia is an independent risk factor for early cardiovascular disease in women. Although most modern COC formulations increase triglycerides by about 30%, these estrogen-induced triglyceride particles are different in size than endogenously produced triglycerides. COC-induced triglycerides do not appear to increase a woman's risk for atherosclerosis.[285] However, excessively high serum triglycerides (greater than 500 mg/dl) can cause pancreatitis. Therefore, women with triglycerides levels greater than 350 mg/dl should use COCs only with caution. Lower-dose pills (10 to 25 mcg EE) would be preferred to higher-dose ones. Progestin-only formulations may be a better choice.

USER INSTRUCTIONS FOR TAKING PILLS

Your health care provider has determined that you are a candidate for birth control pills. As you think about using birth control pills as your method of contraception, it is important that you know how pills work to protect you from pregnancy, how you should use your pills, and what to do if you have any problems while you are using them. This section provides information about those issues and answers questions women often ask about birth control pills.

HOW DO BIRTH CONTROL PILLS WORK?

Oral contraception pills prevent fertilization of a woman's egg by sperm. They do this first by stopping ovulation (release of an egg) and by making the mucus in the cervix so thick that sperm cannot enter into the uterus to fertilize the egg. Only about 1 woman in 100 will get pregnant during the first year of use of pills, if women take their pills every day on schedule. It is important that you use your method correctly and consistently to get the greatest pregnancy protection. If you ever decide to become pregnant, keep using your pill until you meet with your clinician and get checked out to see if you have any problems that should be resolved before you get pregnant.

WHAT ELSE DO BIRTH CONTROL PILLS DO FOR YOU?

In addition to preventing pregnancy, pills provide many other health benefits. They lower your risks of getting ovarian cancer, cancer of the lining of the uterus (endometrium), benign breast masses, and some other kinds of ovarian cysts. Pills decrease a woman's menstrual blood loss, her cramps, and the pain she has with menstruation. Pills tend to make acne and oily skin better. Pills also decrease your chance of having a dangerous ectopic pregnancy—a pregnancy outside of the uterus. Pills give women a chance to plan and prepare for any pregnancies they want to have so they will have safer pregnancies and healthier babies. In the 21st century, accidental pregnancy should be rare.

WHAT PILLS DO *NOT* DO FOR YOU

Remember: pills do not protect you from HIV/AIDS or other sexually transmitted infections (STIs). If you are at risk for an STI, use a male condom made of latex, isoprene, or polyurethane, or use a female condom, every time you have sexual intercourse.

GETTING STARTED

Your clinician will suggest one of three ways to begin taking pills:

- *Quick Start.* Take your first pill the day you visit your clinician. Unless you start your pills within 5 days of starting your period, use a back-up contraceptive method (such as condoms) for at least 7 days. Do not expect to get your period until you finish taking the active pills. You may also need to take emergency contraception (EC) right now if you have recently had unprotected intercourse in the last 5 days.

- *First-day Start.* Take your first pill on the first day of your next period. Be sure to use some other method, like condoms, every time you have sex until you start your pills.

- *Sunday Start.* Take your first pill on the first Sunday of your next period. Use a back-up method for 7 days. Be sure to use some other method, like condoms, every time you have sex until you start your pills.

Be sure to ask your clinician to give you a prescription for emergency contraceptives (EC). If you do not have a prescription, you can still purchase Plan B One-Step or Next Choice at the pharmacy, but your insurance probably will not pay for it. You will need government-approved identification. These ECs and other EC (ella) are all available by prescription. You should fill that prescription for EC and keep it on hand so that you will have it immediately available whenever you forget to take your pills on time before you have sex.

DAILY PILL ROUTINE

1. Take 1 pill from your pill pack daily. Combine your pill taking with a daily routine (brushing your teeth or taking off your earrings) or set the alarm on your cell phone to help you remember to take your pill each day.

2. Check your pack of pills each morning to make sure you took your pill the day before.

3. Use a back-up contraceptive method for 7 days if you—

    — Missed taking 2 or more pills in a row

    — Were late starting your new pill pack

    — Had severe vomiting or diarrhea

    — Start taking medication that lowers the ability of your body to absorb contraceptive hormones (see the instructions on Pills and Drug Interactions).

4. If you think you may have had sexual intercourse that was not adequately protected, consider using emergency contraception.

5. Use condoms every time you have intercourse if you suspect, even a little, that you or your partner may have a sexually transmitted infection. Remember, do not count on your partner to tell you that he has an infection. Most people who catch an infection get it from a partner who does not know he has it.

6. Every time you go to a health care provider, tell him that you are taking birth control pills.

7. If you want to bleed every month, your pills will be packed with pills for only one cycle in a packet. Usually there will be active pills and placebo pills in the packet with a total of 28 pills. Sometimes your packet will have fewer than 28 pills and you will be asked to take all the pills in the pack and wait until the end of 4 weeks to start another pack of pills.

8. If you are using pills to avoid having monthly bleeding, you will take an active pill each day at the same time for months at a time.

Figure 11–2 Simplified recommendations for missed pills

Did you have intercourse without extra protection in the 5 days before you missed your pill?

- If you are less than 12 hours late taking your pill, take it now and take your next pills at the time you usually would.
- If you are more than 12 hours late, take your missed pill now and any other pill you are supposed to take today. Finish taking all the other pills in your pack on time.
  — Use EC if in the last 5 days you had sex without protection.
  — Use abstinence or condoms with every act of sex until you have taken 7 active pills in a row.

9. Mark your calendar to remind yourself of the days you will begin a new pack of pills. Make sure you get your pill prescription refilled before you need to start your next pack. Some women mark their calendar each day as they take their pills.

10. You do *not* need to take a "rest" from taking pills. If you stop taking your pills, you could get pregnant.

11. What should you do if you miss any pills? Missing a pill means taking your pill late (more than 24 hours after the last one) or not taking it at all. To get the most correct answer about what to do, there are detailed instructions your clinician can provide you, depending upon what kind of pill you are taking, how many tablets you missed, and where in your packet you are. Otherwise, there are more simplified instructions found in Figure 11-2, which might over-treat you but will be easier to follow.

VOMITING OR DIARRHEA

Repeated vomiting or severe diarrhea can decrease your body's ability to absorb the pill's hormones. If you have vomiting or diarrhea, treat it as if you had missed pills. Use condoms as a back-up contraceptive for 7 days. Use emergency contraception, if you have had intercourse without using extra contraception while you were ill.

PILLS AND YOUR PERIODS

What changes can you expect in your bleeding?

1. *Short* and *scant bleeding.* When you use birth control pills, a drop of blood or a brown stain during the days you take the placebo pills counts as a "period."

2. *Spotting.* You may have very light bleeding, or spotting, between your periods for the first few months you are on the pills.

If you have bleeding between periods, be sure to take your pills at the same time every day and start each new package of pills on time. Spotting is generally not a sign of any serious problem. However, if you have bleeding between periods (especially after intercourse) and have not missed a pill or taken pills late, have your clinician check you for an infection or other problems. If the spotting between periods persists, it may be a sign that you may benefit from a different kind of pill. *Start each new package of pills on time.* Some clinicians recommend a back-up contraceptive method when you have spotting, especially if you are taking any medication that may make your birth control pill less effective.

3. *Missed period.* Many women miss their bleeding every now and then while they are using birth control pills. If you have not missed any pills and you miss one period without having any other signs of pregnancy, you are probably not pregnant. However, if you are worried, you may wish to get a pregnancy test. If you miss two periods, contact your clinician to get a pregnancy test or purchase a home pregnancy test.

PILLS AND PREGNANCY

If you decide that you want to become pregnant, see your health care provider for preconception counseling. If you are not already getting extra folic acid in your birth control pills, be sure to plan to take prenatal vitamins or extra folate for at least 30 days before you try to get pregnant. Once you stop taking the birth control pills, your fertility will return rapidly. The hormones in the pills do not linger in your system. Even if you accidently get pregnant while you are taking the pill, birth control pills will not adversely affect your pregnancy. You will not have any increase in risk of miscarriage, and your fetus will have no increased risk of having any birth defects.

PILL WARNING SIGNS

Pills have been studied extensively and are definitely safer than pregnancy. However, very rarely, pills can lead to serious problems. Here are the warning signals to watch out for while taking pills. These warning signs spell out the word ACHES. If you have any of these symptoms, it may or may not be related to pill use. Usually these warning signs have an explanation other than pills, but you need to get checked to be sure. *Do not ignore these problems or wait to see if they disappear on their own.* Stop your pill and check with your clinician as soon as possible—today if possible. (See Figure 11–3.) Be sure to use another birth control method until you find out if it is safe to use your birth control pills again.

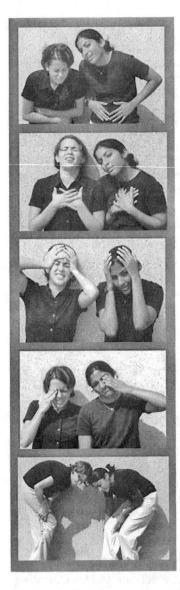

ABDOMINAL PAIN
- Blood clot in the pelvis or liver
- Benign liver tumor or gallbladder disease
- Pregnancy in your tubes

CHEST PAIN
- Blood clot in the lungs
- Heart attack
- Angina (heart pain)
- Breast lump

HEADACHES
- Stroke
- Migraine headache, blurred vision, spots, zigzag lines, weakness, difficulty speaking
- High blood pressure

EYE PROBLEMS
- Stroke
- Blurred vision, double vision, or loss of vision
- Migraine headache with blurred vision, spots, zigzag lines
- Blood clots in the eyes
- Change in shape of cornea (contacts don't fit)

SEVERE LEG PAIN
- Inflammation and blood clots of a vein in the leg

Figure 11–3 Pill warning signs—ACHES

You should also return to the office if you develop severe mood swings or depression, become jaundiced (yellow-colored skin), miss 2 periods or have signs of pregnancy.

Source: Hatcher RA, et al. (2003), with permission.

You should also stop your pills if you develop depression, jaundice (a yellowing of the skin), a breast lump, a fainting attack or collapse, a seizure (epilepsy), difficulty speaking, a blood pressure above 160/95 mm Hg, a severe allergic skin rash, or if you are immobilized (in a wheelchair or bedridden) after an accident or major surgery. If are planning to have major surgery, stop using your pills 4 weeks before your operation, and be sure to use another method to protect you from pregnancy. The risk of a blood clot in a vein is greatest if you have any of the following conditions: if you are overweight, immobile, have severe varicose veins, or if several members of your family have had a blood clot in a vein.

PILLS AND FUTURE FERTILITY

Pills are a good contraceptive choice for women who might want to become pregnant in the future. The birth control pill has no long-term effects on a woman's fertility. This means several things:

1. You are protected from pregnancy only when you are on the pill. You must use another method to protect yourself against pregnancy as soon as you stop the pill.

2. After you stop the pill, your fertility will be the same as it would have been at that age if you had never taken birth control pills.

   — The pill does not save your eggs. You will go through menopause at the same age you would have without using pills.

   — The pill does not use up your eggs.

3. If your periods were infrequent before you started the pill, they probably will be that way again after you stop the pill. The pill regulates your periods only when you use the pill.

4. By reducing the risk of some causes of infertility such as pelvic infections, uterine fibroids, ectopic pregnancies, ovarian cysts, ovarian cancer, endometrial cancer, and endometriosis, pills may protect your future ability to become pregnant after you stop using them.

PILLS AND SMOKING

If you smoke, do everything you can to stop smoking. This is the single most important thing you can do for your health. If you cannot stop, try to cut back on the number of cigarettes you smoke. If you smoke and use birth control pills, you need to watch carefully for the pill warning signals. If you smoke and you are over age 35 to 40, your clinician will probably not give you birth control pills with estrogen.

PILLS AND MOOD CHANGES

Usually, the pill has no effect on a woman's mood. However, if you notice mood changes—depression, irritability, or a change in sex drive—see your clinician. You may have another problem. If your clinician believes that your problem may be associated with the pills, switching brands may help you. Depression, premenstrual symptoms (PMS), and sexual pleasure can improve when women use birth control pills, but in some women, these problems may become worse. Newer ways of using pills have been found to help women deal with these problems.

PILLS AND DRUG INTERACTIONS

A few drugs you may need to take for medical conditions may interfere with the pill or the pill may interfere with how these drugs work. Be sure to tell *all* your clinicians that you are using birth control pills. Also, tell the clinician giving you your birth control pills about *all* of the other drugs (prescription, over-the-counter, and street drugs) that you are using. If you are using drugs such as rifampin, phenytoin, phenobarbital, topiramate, carbamazepine, or St. John's Wort, you may need to use different pills or another method of contraception. Do not worry about using antibiotics while you are on the pill. Women using HIV drugs may need lower- or higher-dose birth control pills.

PILLS AND THE MEDIA

Often there are stories in the news challenging the safety of the birth control pill. Sometimes ads run on television showcasing information about serious side effects with the pill. After hearing these stories, you might want to stop your pills. If you are doing well with your pills, keep using them. Do not stop your pills until you have a chance to talk to your clinician. Often these stories are wrong and do not apply to you at all.

REFERENCES

1. Mosher WD, Jones J. Use of Contraception in the United States: 1982–2008. National Center for Health Statistics. Vital Health Stat 23. 2010.
2. Centers for Disease Control and Prevention. Ten Great Public Health Achievements — United States, 1900–1999. Morbidity and Mortality Weekly Report. 1999;48: 241–64.
3. Bongaarts J, Bruce J. The Causes of Unmet Need for Contraception and the Social Content of Services. Studies in Family Planning. 1995;26:57–75.
4. Boonstra H, Duran V, Northington Gamble V, Blumenthal P, Dominguez L, Pies C. The 'boom and bust phenomenon': the hopes, dreams, and broken promises of the contraceptive revolution. Contraception. 2000;61:9–25.
5. Stanczyk FZ. All progestins are not created equal. Steroids. 2003;68:879–90.

6. Rapkin AJ, Winer SA. Drospirenone: a novel progestin. Expert Opin Pharmacother. 2007;8:989–99.
7. Kjos SL, Peters RK, Xiang A, Thomas D, Schaefer U, Buchanan TA. Contraception and the risk of type 2 diabetes mellitus in Latina women with prior gestational diabetes mellitus. JAMA. 1998;280:533–8.
8. Krattenmacher R. Drospirenone: pharmacology and pharmacokinetics of a unique progestogen. Contraception. 2000;62:29–38.
9. Muhn P, Fuhrmann U, Fritzemeier KH, Krattenmacher R, Schillinger E. Drospirenone: a novel progestogen with antimineralocorticoid and antiandrogenic activity. Ann N Y Acad Sci. 1995 Jun 12;761:311–35.
10. Sulak PJ, Scow RD, Preece C, Riggs MW, Kuehl TJ. Hormone withdrawal symptoms in oral contraceptive users. Obstet Gynecol. 2000;95:261–6.
11. Nelson AL, Westhoff C, Schnare SM. Real-world patterns of prescription refills for branded hormonal contraceptives: a reflection of contraceptive discontinuation. Obstet Gynecol. 2008;112:782–7.
12. Kroll R, Reape KZ, Margolis M. The efficacy and safety of a low-dose, 91-day, extended-regimen oral contraceptive with continuous ethinyl estradiol. Contraception. 2010;81:41–8.
13. Coffee AL, Sulak, PJ, Kuel TJ. Long-term assessment of symptomatology and satisfaction of an extended oral contraceptive regimen. Contraception. 2007;75:444–9
14. Machado RB, de Melo NR, Maia H Jr. Bleeding patterns and menstrual-related symptoms with the continuous use of a contraceptive combination of ethinylestradiol and drospirenone: a randomized study. Contraception. 2010;81:215
15. Spona J, Feichtinger W, Kindermann C, Wünsch C, Brill K. Inhibition of ovulation by an oral contraceptive containing 100 micrograms levonorgestrel in combination with 20 micrograms ethinylestradiol. Contraception. 1996;54:299–304.
16. Foster DG, Parvataneni R, de Bocanegra HT, Lewis C, Bradsberry M, Darney P. Number of oral contraceptive pill packages dispensed, method continuation, and costs. Obstet Gynecol. 2006;108:1107–14
17. Potter L, Oakley D, de Leon-Wong E, Cañamar R. Measuring compliance among oral contraceptive users. Fam Plann Perspect. 1996;28:154–8.
18. Tayob Y, Robinson G, Adams J, Nye M, Whitelaw N, Shaw RW, et al. Ultrasound appearance of the ovaries during the hormone-free interval. Br J Family Planning. 1990;16:94–6.
19. Nettleman MD, Chung H, Brewer J, Ayoola A, Reed PL. Reasons for unprotected intercourse: analysis of the PRAMS survey. Contraception. 2007;75:361–6. Erratum in: Contraception. 2007;76:413.
20. Moos MK, Petersen R, Meadows K, Melvin CL, Spitz AM. Pregnant women's perspectives on intendedness of pregnancy. Womens Health Issues. 1997;7:385–92.
21. Rosenberg MJ, Waugh MS. Oral contraceptive discontinuation: a prospective evaluation of frequency and reasons. Am J Obstet Gynecol. 1998;179:577–82.
22. Potter LS. Oral contraceptive compliance and its role in the effectiveness of the method. In Cramer JA, Spilker B, eds. Patient Compliance In Medical Practice And Clinical Trials. New York: Raven Press, 1991 pp 195–207.
23. Holt VL, Cushing-Haugen KL, Daling JR. Body weight and risk of oral contraceptive failure. Obstet Gynecol. 2002;99:820–7.
24. Holt VL, Scholes D, Wicklund KG, Cushing-Haugen KL, Daling JR. Body mass index, weight, and oral contraceptive failure risk. Obstet Gynecol. 2005;105:46–52.
25. Brunner Huber LR, Hogue CJ. The association between body weight, unintended pregnancy resulting in a livebirth, and contraception at the time of conception. Matern Child Health J. 2005;9:413–20.
26. Edelman AB, Carlson NE, Cherala G, Munar MY, Stouffer RL, Cameron JL, et al. Impact of obesity on oral contraceptive pharmacokinetics and hypothalamic-pituitary-ovarian activity. Contraception. 2009;80:119–27.

27. Westhoff CL, Torgal AH, Mayeda ER, Pike MC, Stanczyk FZ. Pharmacokinetics of a combined oral contraceptive in obese and normal-weight women. Contraception. 2010;81:474–80.

28. Westhoff CL, Torgal AH, Mayeda ER, Stanczyk FZ, Lerner JP, Benn EK, Paik M. Ovarian suppression in normal-weight and obese women during oral contraceptive use: a randomized controlled trial. Obstet Gynecol. 2010;116:275–83.

29. Anderson FD, Gibbons W, Portman D. Safety and efficacy of an extended-regimen oral contraceptive utilizing continuous low-dose ethinyl estradiol. Contraception. 2006;73:229–34.

30. Zhang H, LaGuardia KD, Creanga D. Higher body weight and body mass index are not associated with reduced efficacy in Ortho Tri-Cyclen Lo users (Abstract). Obstet Gynecol. 2006;50S:107.

31. Burkman RT, Fisher AC, Wan GJ, Barnowski CE, LaGuardia KD. Association between efficacy and body weight or body mass index for two low-dose oral contraceptives. Contraception. 2009;79:424–7.

32. Kaneshiro B, Edelman A, Carlson N, Nichols M, Jensen J. The relationship between body mass index and unintended pregnancy: results from the 2002 National Survey of Family Growth. Contraception. 2008;77:234–8.

33. Dinger JC, Cronin M, Möhner S, Schellschmidt I, Minh TD, Westhoff C. Oral contraceptive effectiveness according to body mass index, weight, age, and other factors. Am J Obstet Gynecol. 2009;201:263.e1–9.

34. Society of Family Planning, Higginbotham S. Contraceptive considerations in obese women: release date 1 September 2009, SFP Guideline 20091. Contraception. 2009;80:583–90.

35. ACOG Committee on Practice Bulletins-Gynecology. ACOG practice bulletin. No. 73: Use of hormonal contraception in women with coexisting medical conditions. Obstet Gynecol. 2006;107:1453–72.

36. Centers for Disease Control and Prevention. U. S. Medical Eligibility Criteria for Contraceptive Use, 2010. MMWR 2010;59:15–17.

37. Westhoff C, Osborne LM, Schafer JE, Morroni C. Bleeding patterns after immediate initiation of an oral compared with a vaginal hormonal contraceptive. Obstet Gynecol. 2005;106:89–96.

38. Tessler SL, Peipert JF. Perceptions of contraceptive effectiveness and health effects of oral contraception. Womens Health Issues. 1997;7:400–6.

39. Brent RL. Nongenital malformations following exposure to progestational drugs: the last chapter of an erroneous allegation. Birth Defects Res A Clin Mol Teratol. 2005;73:906–18.

40. Ahn HK, Poster presentation at annual meeting of Teratology Society, ObGyn News. 2005;40:7.

41. Hannaford PC, Iversen L, Macfarlane TV, Elliott AM, Angus V, Lee AJ. Mortality among contraceptive pill users: cohort evidence from Royal College of General Practitioners' Oral Contraception Study. BMJ. 2010;340:c927.

42. Barnhart KT, Schreiber CA. Return to fertility following discontinuation of oral contraceptives. Fertil Steril. 2009;91:659–63.

43. Centers for Disease Control and Prevention. Maternal Mortality and Related Concepts. Available from: www.cdc.gov/nchs/data/series/sr_03/sr03_033.pdf. Accessed 6/07/10.

44. Franks AL, Beral V, Cates W Jr, Hogue CJ. Contraception and ectopic pregnancy risk. Am J Obstet Gynecol. 1990;163(4 Pt 1):1120–3.

45. Marchbanks PA, Annegers JF, Coulam CB, Strathy JH, Kurland LT. Risk factors for ectopic pregnancy. A population-based study. JAMA. 1988;259:1823–7.

46. Milsom I, Sundell G, Andersch B. The influence of different combined oral contraceptives on the prevalence and severity of dysmenorrhea. Contraception. 1990;42:497–506.

47. Mishell DR Jr. Noncontraceptive health benefits of oral steroidal contraceptives. Am J Obstet Gynecol. 1982;142(6 Pt 2):809–16.
48. Robinson JC, Plichta S, Weisman CS, Nathanson CA, Ensminger M. Dysmenorrhea and use of oral contraceptives in adolescent women attending a family planning clinic. Am J Obstet Gynecol. 1992;166:578–83.
49. Davis AR, Westhoff C, O'Connell K, Gallagher N. Oral contraceptives for dysmenorrhea in adolescent girls: a randomized trial. Obstet Gynecol. 2005;106:97–104.
50. Zahradnik HP, Hanjalic-Beck A, Groth K. Nonsteroidal anti-inflammatory drugs and hormonal contraceptives for pain relief from dysmenorrhea: a review. Contraception. 2010;81:185–96.
51. Nilsson L, Rybo G. Treatment of menorrhagia. Am J Obstet Gynecol. 1971; 110:713–20.
52. Fraser IS, McCarron G. Randomized trial of 2 hormonal and 2 prostaglandin-inhibiting agents in women with a complaint of menorrhagia. Aust N Z J Obstet Gynaecol. 1991;31:66–70.
53. Farquhar C, Brown J. Oral contraceptive pill for heavy menstrual bleeding. Cochrane Database of Systematic Reviews. 2009, Issue 4. Art. No.: CD000154.
54. Endrikat J, Shapiro H, Lukkari-Lax E, Kunz M, Schmidt W, Fortier M. A Canadian, multicentre study comparing the efficacy of a levonorgestrel-releasing intrauterine system to an oral contraceptive in women with idiopathic menorrhagia. J Obstet Gynaecol Can. 2009;31:340–7.
55. Anderson FD, Hait H. A multicenter, randomized study of an extended cycle oral contraceptive. Contraception. 2003;68:89–96. Erratum in: Contraception. 2004;69:175.
56. Vandever MA, Kuehl TJ, Sulak PJ, Witt I, Coffee A, Wincek TJ, Reape KZ. Evaluation of pituitary-ovarian axis suppression with three oral contraceptive regimens. Contraception. 2008;77:162–70.
57. Parsey KS, Pong A. An open-label, multicenter study to evaluate Yasmin, a low-dose combination oral contraceptive containing drospirenone, a new progestogen. Contraception. 2000;61:105–11.
58. Borenstein J, Yu HT, Wade S, Chiou CF, Rapkin A. Effect of an oral contraceptive containing ethinyl estradiol and drospirenone on premenstrual symptomatology and health-related quality of life. J Reprod Med. 2003;48:79–85.
59. Sangthawan M, Taneepanichskul S. A comparative study of monophasic oral contraceptives containing either drospirenone 3 mg or levonorgestrel 150 microg on premenstrual symptoms. Contraception. 2005;71:1–7.
60. Freeman EW, Borisute H, Deal L, Smith L, Grubb GS, Constantine GD. A continuous-use regimen of levonorgestrelethinyl estradiol significantly alleviates cycle-related symptoms: results of a phase 3 study. Fertil Steril. 2005;84 (Suppl1):S25.
61. Halbreich U, Borenstein J, Pearlstein T, Kahn LS. The prevalence, impairment, impact, and burden of premenstrual dysphoric disorder (PMS/PMDD). Psychoneuroendocrinology. 2003;28 Suppl 3:1–23.
62. Yonkers KA, Brown C, Pearlstein TB, Foegh M, Sampson-Landers C, Rapkin A. Efficacy of a new low-dose oral contraceptive with drospirenone in premenstrual dysphoric disorder. Obstet Gynecol. 2005;106:492–501.
63. Davis A, Godwin A, Lippman J, Olson W, Kafrissen M. Triphasic norgestimate-ethinyl estradiol for treating dysfunctional uterine bleeding. Obstet Gynecol. 2000;96:913–20.
64. Lanes SF, Birmann B, Walker AM, Singer S. Oral contraceptive type and functional ovarian cysts. Am J Obstet Gynecol. 1992;166:956–61.
65. Vessey M, Metcalfe A, Wells C, McPherson K, et al. Ovarian neoplasms, functional ovarian cysts, and oral contraceptives. Br Med J (Clin Res Ed). 1987;294(6586): 1518–20.
66. Christensen JT, Boldsen JL, Westergaard JG. Functional ovarian cysts in premenopausal and gynecologically healthy women. Contraception. 2002;66:153–7.

67. Holt VL, Cushing-Haugen KL, Daling JR. Oral contraceptives, tubal sterilization, and functional ovarian cyst risk. Obstet Gynecol. 2003;102:252–8..

68. Young RL, Snabes MC, Frank ML, Reilly M. A randomized, double-blind, placebo-controlled comparison of the impact of low-dose and triphasic oral contraceptives on follicular development. Am J Obstet Gynecol. 1992;167:678–82.

69. Chiaffarino F, Parazzini F, La Vecchia C, Ricci E, Crosignani PG. Oral contraceptive use and benign gynecologic conditions. A review. Contraception. 1998;57:11–8.

70. Grimes DA, Godwin AJ, Rubin A, Smith JA, Lacarra M. Ovulation and follicular development associated with three low-dose oral contraceptives: a randomized controlled trial. Obstet Gynecol. 1994;83:29–34.

71. Rible RD, Taylor D, Wilson ML, Stanczyk FZ, Mishell DR Jr. Follicular development in a 7-day versus 4-day hormone-free interval with an oral contraceptive containing 20 mcg ethinyl estradiol and 1 mg norethindrone acetate. Contraception. 2009;79:182–8.

72. Willis SA, Kuehl TJ, Spiekerman AM, Sulak PJ. Greater inhibition of the pituitary—ovarianaxis in oral contraceptive regimens with a shortened hormone-free interval. Contraception 2006;74:100–3

73. MacKenna A, Fabres C, Alam V, Morales V. Clinical management of functional ovarian cysts: a prospective and randomized study. Hum Reprod. 2000;15:2567–9.

74. Loder EW. Menstrual migraine: pathophysiology, diagnosis, and impact. Headache. 2006;46 Suppl 2:S55–60.

75. Somerville BW. The role of estradiol withdrawal in the etiology of menstrual migraine. Neurology. 1972;22:355–65.

76. Somerville BW. The role of progesterone in menstrual migraine. Neurology. 1971;21:853–9.

77. Martin VT. Menstrual migraine: a review of prophylactic therapies. Curr Pain Headache Rep. 2004;8:229–37.

78. Harris M, Kaneshiro B. An evidence-based approach to hormonal contraception and headaches. Contraception. 2009;80:417–21.

79. American Cancer Society Cancer Facts & Figures 2010. Available at: http://www.cancer.org/docroot/stt/stt_0.asp?from=fast. Accessed 6/4/10.

80. Vessey MP, Painter R. Endometrial and ovarian cancer and oral contraceptives—findings in a large cohort study. Br J Cancer. 1995;71:1340–2.

81. Collaborative Group on Epidemiological Studies of Ovarian Cancer, Beral V, Doll R, Hermon C, Peto R, Reeves G. Ovarian cancer and oral contraceptives: collaborative reanalysis of data from 45 epidemiological studies including 23,257 women with ovarian cancer and 87,303 controls. Lancet. 2008;371:303–14.

82. Rosenberg L, Palmer JR, Zauber AG, Warshauer ME, et al. A case-control study of oral contraceptive use and invasive epithelial ovarian cancer. Am J Epidemiol. 1994;139:654–61.

83. Ness RB, Grisso JA, Klapper J, Schlesselman JJ, et al. Risk of ovarian cancer in relation to estrogen and progestin dose and use characteristics of oral contraceptives. SHARE Study Group. Steroid Hormones and Reproductions. Am J Epidemiol. 2000;152:233–41.

84. Royar J, Becher H, Chang-Claude J. Low-dose oral contraceptives: protective effect on ovarian cancer risk. Int J Cancer. 2001:5 370–4

85. Schildkraut JM, Calingaert B, Marchbanks PA, Moorman PG, Rodriguez GC. Impact of progestin and estrogen potency in oral contraceptives on ovarian cancer risk. J Natl Cancer Inst. 2002;94:32–8.

86. Romero IL, Gordon IO, Jagadeeswaran S, Mui KL, Lee WS, Dinulescu DM, et al. Effects of oral contraceptives or a gonadotropin-releasing hormone agonist on ovarian carcinogenesis in genetically engineered mice. Cancer Prev Res. 2009;2:792–9.

87. Lu KH, Yates MS, Mok SC. The monkey, the hen, and the mouse: models to advance ovarian cancer chemoprevention. Cancer Prev Res. 2009;2:773–5.

88. Jensen JT, Speroff L. Health benefits of oral contraceptives. Obstet Gynecol Clin North Am. 2000;27:705–21.

89. Gross TP, Schlesselman JJ. The estimated effect of oral contraceptive use on the cumulative risk of epithelial ovarian cancer. Obstet Gynecol. 1994;83:419–24.

90. Walker GR, Schlesselman JJ, Ness RB. Family history of cancer, oral contraceptive use, and ovarian cancer risk. Am J Obstet Gynecol. 2002;186:8–14.

91. Narod SA, Risch H, Moslehi R, Dorum A, et al. Oral contraceptives and the risk of hereditary ovarian cancer. Hereditary Ovarian Cancer Clinical Study Group. N Engl J Med. 1998;339:424–8.

92. Grenader T, Peretz T, Lifchitz M, Shavit L. BRCA1 and BRCA2 germ-line mutations and oral contraceptives: to use or not to use. Breast. 2005;14:264–8.

93. Modan B, Hartge P, Hirsh-Yechezkel G, Chetrit A, et al; National Israel Ovarian Cancer Study Group. Parity, oral contraceptives, and the risk of ovarian cancer among carriers and noncarriers of a BRCA1 or BRCA2 mutation. N Engl J Med. 2001;345:235–40.

94. Flegal KM, Carroll MD, Ogden CL, Curtin LR. Prevalence and trends in obesity among US adults, 1999–2008. JAMA. 2010;303:235–41.

95. Combination oral contraceptive use and the risk of endometrial cancer. The Cancer and Steroid Hormone Study of the Centers for Disease Control and the National Institute of Child Health and Human Development. JAMA. 1987;257:796–800.

96. Schlesselman JJ. Risk of endometrial cancer in relation to use of combined oral contraceptives. A practitioner's guide to meta-analysis. Hum Reprod. 1997;12:1851–63.

97. Brinton LA, Vessey MP, Flavel R, Yeates D. Risk factors for benign breast disease. Am J Epidemiol.1981;113:203–14.

98. Charreau I, Plu-Bureau G, Bachelot A, Contesso G, et al. Oral contraceptive use and risk of benign breast disease in a French case-control study of young women. Eur J Cancer Prev. 1993;2:147–54.

99. Rohan TE, Miller AB. A cohort study of oral contraceptive use and risk of benign breast disease. Int J Cancer. 1999;82:191–6.

100. Jemec GB, Linneberg A, Nielsen NH, Frolund L, et al. Have oral contraceptives reduced the prevalence of acne? A population-based study of acne vulgaris, tobacco smoking and oral contraceptives. Dermatology. 2002;204:179–84.

101. Redmond GP, Olson WH, Lippman JS, Kafrissen ME, et al. Norgestimate and ethinyl estradiol in the treatment of acne vulgaris: a randomized, placebo-controlled trial. Obstet Gynecol. 1997;89:615–22.

102. Lucky AW, Henderson TA, Olson WH, Robisch DM, et al. Effectiveness of norgestimate and ethinyl estradiol in treating moderate acne vulgaris. J Am Acad Dermatol. 1997;37(5 Pt 1):746–54.

103. Thorneycroft H, Gollnick H, Schellschmidt I. Superiority of a combined contraceptive containing drospirenone to a triphasic preparation containing norgestimate in acne treatment. Cutis. 2004;74:123–30.

104. Palatsi R, Hirvensalo E, Liukko P, Malmiharju T, Mattila L, Riihiluoma P, Ylostalo P. Serum total and unbound testosterone and sex hormone binding globulin (SHBG) in female acne patients treated with two different oral contraceptives. Acta Derm Venereol. 1984;64:517–23.

105. Wishart JM. An open study of Triphasil and Diane 50 in the treatment of acne. Australas J Dermatol. 1991;32:51–4.

106. Arowojolu AO, Gallo MF, Lopez LM, Grimes DA, Garner SE. Combined oral contraceptive pills for treatment of acne. Cochrane Database Syst Rev. 2009 Jul 8;:CD004425. Review.

107. Sullivan H, Furniss H, Spona J, Elstein M. Effect of 21-day and 24-day oral contraceptive regimens containing gestodene (60 microg) and ethinyl estradiol (15 microg) on ovarian activity. Fertil Steril. 1999; 72:115.

108. Panzer C, Wise S, Fantini G, Kang D, Munarriz R, Guay A, Goldstein I. Impact of oral contraceptives on sex hormone-binding globulin and androgen levels: a retrospective study in women with sexual dysfunction. J Sex Med. 2006;3:104–13.
109. Dewis P, Petsos P, Newman M, Anderson DC. The treatment of hirsutism with a combination of desogestrel and ethinyl oestradiol. Clin Endocrinol (Oxf). 1985;22: 29–36.
110. Lobo RA. The androgenicity of progestational agents. Int J Fertil. 1988;33 Suppl:6–12.
111. Task Force for Epidemiological Research on Reproductive Health, United Nations Development Programme/United Nations Population Fund/World Health Organization/World Bank Special Programme of Research, Development and Research Training in Human Reproduction, World Health Organization, Geneva, Switzerland. Effects of contraceptives on hemoglobin and ferritin. Contraception. 1998;58:262–73.
112. Sangi-Haghpeykar H, Poindexter AN 3rd. Epidemiology of endometriosis among parous women. Obstet Gynecol. 1995;85:983–92.
113. Westhoff C, Britton JA, Gammon MD, Wright T, Kelsey JL. Oral contraceptive and benign ovarian tumors. Am J Epidemiol. 2000;152:242–6.
114. Seracchioli R, Mabrouk M, Frascà C, Manuzzi L, Montanari G, Keramyda A, et al. Long-term cyclic and continuous oral contraceptive therapy and endometrioma recurrence: a randomized controlled trial. Fertil Steril. 2010;93:52–6.
115. Harada T, Momoeda M, Taketani Y, Hoshiai H, Terakawa N. Low-dose oral contraceptive pill for dysmenorrhea associated with endometriosis: a placebo-controlled, double-blind, randomized trial. Fertil Steril. 2008;90:1583–8.
116. Parazzini F, Ferraroni M, Bocciolone L, Tozzi L, Rubessa S, La Vecchia C. Contraceptive methods and risk of pelvic endometriosis. Contraception. 1994;49:47–55.
117. Nisolle-Pochet M, Casanas-Roux F, Donnez J. Histologic study of ovarian endometriosis after hormonal therapy. Fertil Steril. 1988;49:423–6. Erratum in: Fertil Steril 1988 Jul;50:184.
118. Shargil AA. Hormone replacement therapy in perimenopausal women with a triphasic contraceptive compound: a three-year prospective study. Int J Fertil. 1985;30:15, 18–28.
119. Casper RF, Dodin S, Reid RL, Study Investigators. The effect of 20 g ethinyl estradiol/1 mg norethindrone acetate (Minestrin_), a low-dose oral contraceptive, on vaginal bleeding patterns, hot flashes, and quality of life in symptomatic perimenopausal women. Menopause. 1997;4:139–47.
120. de Abood M, de Castillo Z, Guerrero F, Espino M, Austin KL. Effect of Depo-Provera or Microgynon on the painful crises of sickle cell anemia patients. Contraception. 1997;56:313–6.
121. Pinkerton JB, Guico-Pabie CJ, Taylor HS. Menstrual cycle-related exacerbation of disease. AJOG. 2010;202:221-231.
122. Chiaffarino F, Parazzini F, La Vecchia C, Marsico S, Surace M, Ricci E. Use of oral contraceptives and uterine fibroids: results from a case-control study. Br J Obstet Gynaecol. 1999;106:857–60.
123. Marshall LM, Spiegelman D, Goldman MB, Manson JE, Colditz GA, Barbieri R, et al. A prospective study of reproductive factors and oral contraceptive use in relation to the risk of uterine leiomyomata. Fertil Steril. 1998;70:432–9.
124. Hergenroeder AC, Smith EO, Shypailo R, Jones LA, Klish WJ, Ellis K. Bone mineral changes in young women with hypothalamic amenorrhea treated with oral contraceptives, medroxyprogesterone, or placebo over 12 months. Am J Obstet Gynecol. 1997;176:1017–25.
125. MacNeil JS. COC counters bone loss in anorexic teenagers. Ob.Gyn News. 2005 July 1.
126. Grinspoon S, Thomas L, Miller K, Herzog D, Klibanski A. Effects of recombinant human IGF-I and oral contraceptive administration on bone density in anorexia nervosa. J Clin Endocrinol Metab. 2002;87:2883–91.

127. Elgan C, Samsioe G, Dykes AK. Influence of smoking and oral contraceptives on bone mineral density and bone remodeling in young women: a 2-year study. Contraception. 2003;67:439–47.
128. Lopez LM, Grimes DA, Schulz KF, Curtis KM. Steroidal contraceptives: effect on bone fractures in women. Cochrane Database Syst Rev. 2009 Apr 15;:CD006033.
129. d'Arcangues C. WHO statement on hormonal contraception and bone health. Contraception. 2006;73:443–4.
130. Martins SL, Curtis KM, Glasier AF. Combined hormonal contraception and bone health: a systematic review. Contraception. 2006;73:445–69.
131. Davis AR, Castaño PM. Oral contraceptives and libido in women. Annu Rev Sex Res. 2004;15:297–320.
132. Ellertson C, Webb A, Blanchard K, Bigrigg A, Haskell S, Shochet T, Trussell J. Modifying the Yuzpe regimen of emergency contraception: a multicenter randomized controlled trial. Obstet Gynecol. 2003;101:1160–7.
133. Sonfield A, Gold RB, Frost JJ, Darroch JE. U.S. insurance coverage of contraceptives and the impact of contraceptive coverage mandates, 2002. Perspect Sex Reprod Health. 2004;36:72–9.
134. Shapiro S, Dinger J. Risk of venous thromboembolism among users of oral contraceptives: a review of two recently published studies. J Fam Plann Reprod Health Care. 2010;36:33–8.
135. Heinemann LA, Dinger JC. Range of published estimates of venous thromboembolism incidence in young women. Contraception. 2007;75:328–36.
136. Heit JA, Kobbervig CE, James AH, Petterson TM, Bailey KR, Melton LJ 3rd. Trends in the incidence of venous thromboembolism during pregnancy or postpartum: a 30-year population-based study. Ann Intern Med. 2005;143:697–706.
137. Vandenbroucke JP, Koster T, Briet E, Reitsma PH, Bertina RM, Rosendaal FR. Increased risk of venous thrombosis in oral-contraceptive users who are carriers of factor V Leiden mutation. Lancet. 1994;344:1453–7.
138. Vandenbroucke JP, van der Meer FJ, Helmerhorst FM, Rosendaal FR. Factor V Leiden: should we screen oral contraceptive users and pregnant women? BMJ. 1996;313:1127–30.
139. Dinger JC, Heinemann LAJ, Kuhl-Habich D. The safety of a drospirenone-containing oral contraceptive: final results from the European Active Surveillance study on Oral Contraceptives based on 142,475 women-years of observation. Contraception. 2007;75:344–54.
140. Pomp ER, Rosendaal FR, Doggen CJ. Smoking increases the risk of venous thrombosis and acts synergistically with oral contraceptive use. Am J Hematol. 2008;83: 97–102.
141. WHO Scientific Group. Cardiovascular disease and steroid hormone contraception. WHO Technical Report Series, No. 877. Geneva, World Health Organization, 1998.
142. Jick SS, Kaye JA, Russmann S, Jick H. Risk of nonfatal venous thromboembolism with oral contraceptives containing norgestimate or desogestrel compared with oral contraceptives containing levonorgestrel. Contraception. 2006;73:566–70.
143. Romero A, Alonso C, Rincón M, Medrano J, Santos JM, Calderón E, Marín I, González MA. Risk of venous thromboembolic disease in women A qualitative systematic review. Eur J Obstet Gynecol Reprod Biol. 2005;121:8–17.
144. World Health Organization Collaborative Study of Cardiovascular Disease and Steroid Hormone Contraception. Effect of different progestagens in low oestrogen oral contraceptives on venous thromboembolic disease. Lancet. 1995;346:1582–8.
145. Spitzer WO, Lewis MA, Heinemann LA, Thorogood M, MacRae KD. Third generation oral contraceptives and risk of venous thromboembolic disorders: an international case-control study. Transnational Research Group on Oral Contraceptives and the Health of Young Women. BMJ. 1996;312:83–8.
146. Seeger JD Laughlin L, Eng PM. Risk of thromboembolism in women taking ethinylestradiol/drospirenone and other oral contraceptives. Obstet Gynecol. 2007;110:587–93.

147. Lidegaard O.Hormonal contraception and risk of venous thromboembolism: national follow-up study. BMJ. 2009 Aug 13;339:b2890.

148. van Hylckama Vlieg A, Helmerhorst FM, Vandenbroucke JP, Doggen CJ, Rosendaal FR. The venous thrombotic risk of oral contraceptives, effects of oestrogen dose and progestogen type: results of the MEGA case-control study. BMJ. 2009;339:b2921.

149. Petitti DB. Combination estrogen-progestin oral contraceptives. N Engl J Med. 2003;349:1443–50.

150. Khader YS, Rice J, John L, Abueita O. Oral contraceptives use and the risk of myocardial infarction: a meta-analysis. Contraception. 2003;68:11–7.

151. Margolis KL, Adami HO, Luo J, Ye W, Weiderpass E. A prospective study of oral contraceptive use and risk of myocardial infarction among Swedish women. Fertil Steril. 2007;88:310–6.

152. Shufelt CL, Bairey Merz CN. Contraceptive hormone use and cardiovascular disease. J Am Coll Cardiol. 2009;53:221–31. Review. Erratum in: J Am Coll Cardiol. 2009;53:904.

153. Schwingl PJ, Ory HW, Visness CM. Estimates of the risk of cardiovascular death attributable to low-dose oral contraceptives in the United States. Am J Obstet Gynecol. 1999;180:241–9.

154. WHO Scientific Group. Cardiovascular disease and steroid hormone contraception. WHO Technical Report Series, No. 877. Geneva, World Health Organization, 1998.

155. Lubianca JN, Faccin CS, Fuchs FD. Oral contraceptives: a risk factor for uncontrolled blood pressure among hypertensive women. Contraception. 2003;67:19–24.

156. Farley TM, Collins J, Schlesselman JJ. Hormonal contraception and risk of cardiovascular disease. An international perspective. Contraception. 1998;57:211–30.

157. WHO Collaborative Study of Cardiovascular Disease and Steroid Hormone Contraception. Acute myocardial infarction and combined oral contraceptives: results of an international multicentre case-control study. Lancet. 1997;349:1202–9.

158. Petitti DB, Sidney S, Bernstein A, Wolf S, Quesenberry C, Ziel HK. Stroke in users of low-dose oral contraceptives. N Engl J Med. 1996;335:8–15.

159. WHO Collaborative Study of Cardiovascular Disease and Steroid Hormone Contraception. Ischaemic stroke and combined oral contraceptives: results of an international, multicentre, case-control study. Lancet. 1996;348:498–505.

160. Chang CL, Donaghy M, Poulter N. Migraine and stroke in young women: case-control study. The World Health Organisation Collaborative Study of Cardiovascular Disease and Steroid Hormone Contraception. BMJ. 1999;318:13–8.

161. Curtis KM, Chrisman CE, Peterson HB, WHO Programme for Mapping Best Practices in Reproductive Health. Contraception for women in selected circumstances. Obstet Gynecol. 2002;99:1100–12.

162. WHO Collaborative Study of Cardiovascular Disease and Steroid Hormone Contraception. Haemorrhagic stroke, overall stroke risk, and combined oral contraceptives: results of an international, multicentre, case-control study. Lancet. 1996;348:505–10.

163. Patient package insert for Alesse® (levonorgestrel and ethinyl estradiol tablets). Available at: www.accessdata.fda.gov/drugsatfda_docs/label/2008/020683s004s 006s007lbl.pdf. Accessed 6/8/10.

164. Patient package insert for Ortho Tri-Cyclen® (norgestimate/ethinyl estradiol). Available at: www.accessdata.fda.gov/drugsatfda_docs/label/2005/021690lbl.pdf. Accessed 6/8/10.

165. Patient package insert for YAZ® (drospirenone and ethinyl estradiol). Available at: www.accessdata.fda.gov/drugsatfda_docs/label/2010/021676s009lbl.pdf. Accessed 6/8/10.

166. Hannaford PC, Croft PR, Kay CR. Oral contraception and stroke. Evidence from the Royal College of General Practitioners' Oral Contraception Study. Stroke. 1994;25: 935–42.

167. Kemmeren JM, Tanis BC, van den Bosch MA, Bollen EL, Helmerhorst FM, van der Graaf Y, et al. Risk of Arterial Thrombosis in Relation to Oral Contraceptives (RATIO) study: oral contraceptives and the risk of ischemic stroke. Stroke, 2002;33:1202–1208.

168. Feigin VL, Rinkel GJ, Lawes CM, Algra A, Bennett DA, van Gijn J, Anderson CS. Risk factors for subarachnoid hemorrhage: an updated systematic review of epidemiological studies. Stroke. 2005;36:2773–2780.

169. Chasan-Taber L, Willett WC, Manson JE, Spiegelman D, Hunter DJ, Curhan G, Colditz GA, Stampfer MJ. Prospective study of oral contraceptives and hypertension among women in the United States. Circulation. 1996;94:483–9.

170. Darney P. Safety and efficacy of a triphasic oral contraceptive containing desogestrel: results of three multicenter trials. Contraception. 1993;48:323–37.

171. Milne R, Vessey M. The association of oral contraception with kidney cancer, colon cancer, gallbladder cancer (including extrahepatic bile duct cancer) and pituitary tumours. Contraception. 1991;43:667–93.

172. Scalori A, Tavani A, Gallus S, La Vecchia C, Colombo M. Oral contraceptives and the risk of focal nodular hyperplasia of the liver: a case-control study. Am J Obstet Gynecol. 2002;186:195–7.

173. The WHO Collaborative Study of Neoplasia and Steroid Contraceptives. Combined oral contraceptives and liver cancer. Int J Cancer. 1989;43:254–9.

174. Mohllajee AP, Curtis KM, Martins SL, Peterson HB. Hormonal contraceptive use and risk of sexually transmitted infections: a systematic review. Contraception. 2006;73:154–65.

175. Cottingham J, Hunter D. Chlamydia trachomatis and oral contraceptive use: a quantitative review. Genitourin Med. 1992;68:209–16.

176. Morrison CS, Bright P, Wong EL, Kwok C, Yacobson I, Gaydos CA, Tucker HT, Blumenthal PD. Hormonal contraceptive use, cervical ectopy, and the acquisition of cervical infections. Sex Transm Dis. 2004;31:561–7.

177. Rahm VA, Odlind V, Gnarpe H. Chlamydia trachomatis among sexually active teenage girls: influence of sampling location and clinical signs on the detection rate. Genitourin Med. 1990;66:66–9.

178. Green J, Berrington de Gonzalez A, Smith JS, Franceschi S, Appleby P, Plummer M, Beral V. Human papillomavirus infection and use of oral contraceptives. Br J Cancer. 2003;88:1713–20.

179. Winer RL, Lee SK, Hughes JP, Adam DE, Kiviat NB, Koutsky LA. Genital human papillomavirus infection: incidence and risk factors in a cohort of female university students. Am J Epidemiol. 2003;157:218–26. Erratum in: Am J Epidemiol. 2003;157:858.

180. Sellors JW, Karwalajtys TL, Kaczorowski J, Mahony JB, Lytwyn A, Chong S, et al. Survey of HPV in Ontario Women Group. Incidence, clearance and predictors of human papillomavirus infection in women. CMAJ. 2003;168:421–5.

181. Fleming DC, King AE, Williams AR, Critchley HO, Kelly RW. Hormonal contraception can suppress natural antimicrobial gene transcription in human endometrium. Fertil Steril. 2003;79:856–63.

182. Morrison CS, Richardson BA, Mmiro F, Chipato T, Celentano DD, Luoto J, et al. Hormonal Contraception and the Risk of HIV Acquisition (HC-HIV) Study Group. Hormonal contraception and the risk of HIV acquisition. AIDS. 2007;21:85–95.

183. Morrison CS, Chen PL, Kwok C, Richardson BA, Chipato T, Mugerwa R, Byamugisha J, Padian N, Celentano DD, Salata RA. Hormonal contraception and HIV acquisition: reanalysis using marginal structural modeling. AIDS. 2010;24:1778–81.

184. Terki F, Malhotra U. Medical and Service Delivery Guidelines for Sexual and Reproductive Health Services. Third edition. Powlson M, editor. London: International Planned Parenthood Federation; 2004.

185. Moreno V, Bosch FX, Munoz N, Meijer CJ, Shah KV, et al.; International Agency for Research on Cancer. Multicentric Cervical Cancer Study Group. Effect of oral contraceptives on risk of cervical cancer in women with human papillomavirus infection: the IARC multicentric case-control study. Lancet. 2002;359:1085–92.

186. Smith JS, Green J, Berrington de Gonzalez A, Appleby P, Peto J, Plummer M, et al. Cervical cancer and use of hormonal contraceptives: a systematic review. Lancet. 2003;361:1159–67.

187. Munoz N, Franceschi S, Bosetti C, Moreno V, et al.; International Agency for Research on Cancer. Multicentric Cervical Cancer Study Group. Role of parity and human papillomavirus in cervical cancer: the IARC multicentric case-control study. Lancet. 2002;359:1093–1101.

188. Ursin G, Peters RK, Henderson BE, d'Ablaing G 3rd, et al. Oral contraceptive use and adenocarcinoma of cervix. Lancet. 1994;344:1390–4.

189. Morrison C, Prokorym P, Piquero C, Wakely PE Jr, Nuovo GJ. Oral contraceptive pills are associated with artifacts in ThinPrep Pap smears that mimic low-grade squamous intraepithelial lesions. Cancer. 2003;99:75–82.

190. Raman-Wilms L, Tseng AL, Wighardt S, Einarson TR, Koren G. Fetal genital effects of first-trimester sex hormone exposure: a meta-analysis. Obstet Gynecol. 1995;85:141–9.

191. Lammer EJ, Cordero JF. Exogenous sex hormone exposure and the risk for major malformations. JAMA. 1986;255:3128–32.

192. Bracken MB. Oral contraception and congenital malformations in offspring: a review and meta-analysis of the prospective studies. Obstet Gynecol. 1990;76(3 Pt 2):552–57.

193. Cardy GC. Outcome of pregnancies after failed hormonal postcoital contraception an interim report. Br J Fam Plann. 1995;21:112–15.

194. Hemminki E, Gissler M, Merilainen J. Reproductive effects of in utero exposure to estrogen and progestin drugs. Fertil Steril. 1999;71:1092–8.

195. Collaborative Group on Hormonal Factors in Breast Cancer. Breast cancer and hormonal contraceptives: collaborative reanalysis of individual data on 53,297 women with breast cancer and 100,239 women without breast cancer from 54 epidemiological studies. Lancet. 1996;347:1713–27.

196. Grabrick DM, Hartmann LC, Cerhan JR, Vierkant RA, Therneau TM, Vachon CM, et al. Risk of breast cancer with oral contraceptive use in women with a family history of breast cancer. JAMA. 2000;284:1791–8.

197. Marchbanks PA, McDonald JA, Wilson HG, Folger SG, Mandel MG, Daling JR, et al. Oral contraceptives and the risk of breast cancer. N Engl J Med. 2002;346:2025–32.

198. Hannaford PC, Selvaraj S, Elliott AM, Angus V, Iversen L, Lee AJ. Cancer risk among users of oral contraceptives: cohort data from the Royal College of General Practitioner's oral contraception study. BMJ. 2007;335:651–4.

199. Figueiredo JC, Haile RW, Bernstein L, Malone KE, Largent J, Langholz B, et al. Oral contraceptives and postmenopausal hormones and risk of contralateral breast cancer among BRCA1 and BRCA2 mutation carriers and noncarriers: the WECARE Study. Breast Cancer Res Treat. 2010;120:175–83.

200. Gaffield ME, Culwell KR, Ravi A. Oral contraceptives and family history of breast cancer. Contraception. 2009;80:372–80.

201. Wallwiener CW, Wallwiener LM, Seeger H, Muck AO, Bitzer J, Wallwiner M. Prevalence of Sexual Dysfunction and Impact of Contraception in Female German Medical Students. J Sex Med. 2010 May 4 (Epub ahead of print)

202. Graham CA, Bancroft J, Doll HA, Greco T, Tanner A. Does oral contraceptive-induced reduction in free testosterone adversely affect the sexuality or mood of women? Psychoneuroendocrinology. 2007;32:246–55.

203. Caruso S, Agnello C, Intelisano G, Farina M, Di Mari L, Sparacino L, Cianci A. Prospective study on sexual behavior of women using 30 microg ethinylestradiol and 3 mg drospirenone oral contraceptive. Contraception. 2005;72:19–23.

204. Redmond G, Godwin AJ, Olson W, Lippman JS. Use of placebo controls in an oral contraceptive trial: methodological issues and adverse event incidence. Contraception. 1999;60:81–5.

205. Gallo MF, Lopez lM, Grimes Da, Schulz KF, Helmerhorst FM. Combination contraceptives: effects on weight. Cochrane Database Syst Rev. 2008; CD 003987 pub e

206. Chasan-Taber L, Willett WC, Stampfer MJ, Hunter DJ, Colditz GA, Spiegelman D, Manson JE. A prospective study of oral contraceptives and NIDDM among U.S. women. Diabetes Care. 1997;20:330–5.

207. Troisi RJ, Cowie CC, Harris MI. Oral contraceptive use and glucose metabolism in a national sample of women in the United States. Am J Obstet Gynecol 2000; 183:389–95.

208. Kim C, Siscovick DS, Sidney S, Lewis CE, Kiefe CI, Koepsell TD; CARDIA Study. Oral contraceptive use and association with glucose, insulin, and diabetes in young adult women: the CARDIA Study. Coronary Artery Risk Development in Young Adults. Diabetes Care. 2002;25:1027–32.

209. Kojima T, Lindheim SR, Duffy DM, Vijod MA, Stanczyk FZ, Lobo RA. Insulin sensitivity is decreased in normal women by doses of ethinyl estradiol used in oral contraceptives. Am J Obstet Gynecol. 1993;169:1540–4.

210. Kjos SL, Peters RK, Xiang A, Thomas D, Schaefer U, Buchanan TA. Contraception and the risk of type 2 diabetes mellitus in Latina women with prior gestational diabetes mellitus. JAMA. 1998;280:533–8.

211. Korytkowski MT, Mokan M, Horwitz MJ, Berga SL. Metabolic effects of oral contraceptives in women with polycystic ovary syndrome. J Clin Endocrinol Metab. 1995;80:3327.

212. Karagas MR, Stukel TA, Dykes J, Miglionico J, Greene MA, Carey M, et al. A pooled analysis of 10 case-control studies of melanoma and oral contraceptive use. Br J Cancer. 2002;86:1085–92.

213. Lens M, Bataille V. Melanoma in relation to reproductive and hormonal factors in women: current review on controversial issues. Cancer Causes Control. 2008;19: 437–42.

214. Ross RK, Pike MC, Vessey MP, Bull D, Yeates D, Casagrande JT. Risk factors for uterine fibroids: reduced risk associated with oral contraceptives. Br Med J (Clin Res Ed). 1986;293(6543):359–62. Erratum in: Br Med J (Clin Res Ed). 1986;293(6553):1027.

215. Parazzini F, Negri E, La Vecchia C, Fedele L, Rabaiotti M, Luchini L. Oral contraceptive use and risk of uterine fibroids. Obstet Gynecol .1992;79:430–3.

216. Loughlin J, Seeger JD, Eng PM, Foegh M, Clifford CR, Cutone J, Walker AM. Risk of hyperkalemia in women taking ethinylestradiol/drospirenone and other oral contraceptives. Contraception. 2008;78:377–83.

217. Cheung E, Free C. Factors influencing young women's decision making regarding hormonal contraceptives: a qualitative study. Contraception. 2005;71:426–31.

218. Stewart FH, Harper CC. Clinical breast and pelvic examination requirements for hormonal contraception: Current practice vs.evidence. JAMA. 2001;286:671–2.

219. Hannaford PC, Webb AM. Evidence-guided prescribing of combined oral contraceptives: consensus statement. An International Workshop at Mottram Hall, Wilmslow, U.K., March, 1996. Contraception. 1996;54:125–9.

220. Comp PC. Should coagulation tests be used to determine which oral contraceptive users have an increased risk of thrombophlebitis? Contraception. 2006;73:4–5.

221. Mullen WH, Anderson IB, Kim SY, Blanc PD, Olson KR. Incorrect overdose management advice in the Physicians' Desk Reference. Ann Emerg Med. 1997;29:255–61.

222. Oakley D, Sereika S, Bogue EL. Oral contraceptive pill use after an initial visit to a family planning clinic. Fam Plann Perspect. 1991;23:150–4.

223. Westhoff C, Kerns J, Morroni C, Cushman LF, Tiezzi L, Murphy PA. Quick start: novel oral contraceptive initiation method. Contraception. 2002;66:141–5.

224. Westhoff C, Heartwell S, Edwards S, Zieman M, Cushman L, Robilotto C, et al. Initiation of oral contraceptives using a quick start compared with a conventional start: a randomized controlled trial. Obstet Gynecol. 2007;109:1270–6.

225. Lara-Torre E, Schroeder B. Adolescent compliance and side effects with Quick Start initiation of oral contraceptive pills. Contraception. 2002;66:81–5.

226. Westhoff C, Morroni C, Kerns J, Murphy PA. Bleeding patterns after immediate vs. conventional oral contraceptive initiation: a randomized, controlled trial. Fertil Steril. 2003;79:322–9.

227. Gladwell M. John Rock's Error: What the co-inventor of the Pill didn't know about menstruation can endanger women's health. New Yorker Magazine. 2000 Mar 10:52–63.

228. Willis SA, Kuehl TJ, Spiekerman AM, Sulak PJ. Greater inhibition of the pituitary—ovarian axis in oral contraceptive regimens with a shortened hormone-free interval. Contraception. 2006;74:100–3.

229. Schlaff WD, Lynch AM, Hughes HD, Cedars MI, Smith DL. Manipulation of the hormone-free interval in oral contraceptive pill users: the effect on follicular suppression. Am J Obstet Gynecol. 2004;190:943–51.

230. Extended Regimen Contraception Clinical Proceedings. ARHP Clinical Proceedings. 2003 May 2. Available at: www.arhp.org/healthcareproviders/cme/onlinecme/extendedregimencp/index.cfm?ID=328.

231. Coutinho E, Segal S. Is menstruation obsolete? New York: Oxford University Press; 1999.

232. Ferrero S, Abbamonte LH, Giordano M, Alessandri F, Anserini P, Remorgida V, Ragni N. What is the desired menstrual frequency of women without menstruation-related symptoms? Contraception. 2006;73:537–41.

233. Miller L, Notter KM. Menstrual reduction with extended use of combination oral contraceptive pills: randomized controlled trial. Obstet Gynecol. 2001;98:771–8.

234. Sulak PJ, Kuehl TJ, Ortiz M, Shull BL. Acceptance of altering the standard 21-day/7-day oral contraceptive regimen to delay menses and reduce hormone withdrawal symptoms. Am J Obstet Gynecol. 2002;186:1142–9.

235. Edelman A, Gallo MF, Nichols MD, Jensen JT, Schulz KF, Grimes DA. Continuous versus cyclic use of combined oral contraceptives for contraception: systematic Cochrane review of randomized controlled trials. Hum Reprod. 2006;21:573–8.

236. Schwartz JL, Creinin MD, Pymar HC. The trimonthly combination oral contraceptive regimen: is it cost effective? Contraception 1999;60:263–267.

237. Gallo MF, Nanda K, Grimes DA, Lopez LM, Schulz KF. 20 microg versus >20 microg estrogen combined oral contraceptives for contraception. Cochrane Database Syst Rev. 2008 Oct 8;:CD003989. Review.

238. Westhoff CL, Heartwell S, Edwards S, Zieman M, Stuart G, Cwiak C, et al. Oral contraceptive discontinuation: do side effects matter? Am J Obstet Gynecol. 2007;196:412.e1–6.

239. World Health Organization. Selected practice recommendations for contraceptive use. Second ed. Geneva: World Health Organization;2004.

240. Osterberg L, Blaschke T. Adherence to medication. N Engl J Med. 2005;353:487–97.

241. Rosenthal SL, Cotton S, Ready JN, Potter LS, Succop PA. Adolescents' attitudes and experiences regarding levonorgestrel 100 mcg/ethinyl estradiol 20 mcg. J Pediatr Adolesc Gynecol. 2002;15:301–5.

242. Archer DF, Cullins V, Creasy GW, Fisher AC. The impact of improved compliance with a weekly contraceptive transdermal system (Ortho Evra) on contraceptive efficacy. Contraception. 2004;69:189–95.

243. Truitt ST, Fraser AB, Grimes DA, Gallo MF, Schulz KF. Combined hormonal versus nonhormonal versus progestin-only contraception in lactation. Cochrane Database Syst Rev. 2003;:CD003988.

244. Curtis KM, Mohllajee AP, Martins SL, Peterson HB. Combined oral contraceptive use among women with hypertension: a systematic review. Contraception 2006; 73:179–88.

245. Visser J, Snel M, Van Vliet HAAM. Hormonal versus non-hormonal contraceptives in women with diabetes mellitus type 1 and 2. Cochrane Database Syst Rev. 2006 Oct 18;:CD003990.

246. Nelson AL, Le MH, Musherraf Z, Vanberckelaer A. Intermediate-term glucose tolerance in women with a history of gestational diabetes: natural history and potential associations with breastfeeding and contraception. Am J Obstet Gynecol. 2008;198:699.e1–8.

247. International Headache Society. The international classification of headache disorders. 2nd edition. Cephalalgia. 2004;24:Suppl.

248. Harris M, Kaneshiro B. An evidence-based approach to hormonal contraception and headaches. Contraception. 2009;80:417–21.

249. Curtis KM, Mohllajee AP, Peterson HB. Use of combined oral contraceptives among women with migraine and nonmigrainous headaches: a systematic review. Contraception. 2006;73:189–94.

250. Chasan-Taber L, Stampfer M. Oral contraceptives and myocardial infarction—the search for the smoking gun. N Engl J Med. 2001;345:1841–2.

251. Willett WC, Green A, Stampfer MJ, Speizer FE, Colditz GA, Rosner B, et al. Relative and absolute excess risks of coronary heart disease among women who smoke cigarettes. N Engl J Med. 1987;317:1303–9.

252. Global HIV/AIDS estimates, end of 2008. Available from: http://www.avert.org/worldstats.htm Accessed 6/4/10.

253. Morrison CS, Turner AN, Jones LB. Highly effective contraception and acquisition of HIV and other sexually transmitted infections. Best Pract Res Clin Obstet Gynaecol. 2009;23:263–84.

254. Culwell KR, Curtis KM, del Carmen Cravioto M. Safety of contraceptive method use among women with systemic lupus erythematosus: a systematic review. Obstet Gynecol. 2009;114:341–53.

255. Kapp N, Tilley IB, Curtis KM. The effects of hormonal contraceptive use among women with viral hepatitis or cirrhosis of the liver: a systematic review. Contraception. 2009;80:381–6.

256. Kapp N, Curtis KM. Hormonal contraceptive use among women with liver tumors: a systematic review. Contraception. 2009;80:387–90.

257. Maggard MA, Yermilov I, Li Z, Maglione M, Newberry S, Suttorp M, et al. Pregnancy and fertility following bariatric surgery: a systematic review. JAMA. 2008;300:2286–96.

258. Estes CM, Westhoff C. Contraception for the transplant patient. Semin Perinatol. 2007;31:372–7.

259. Faculty of Family Planning and Reproductive Health Care Clinical Effectiveness Unit. FFPRHC Guidance (April 2005). Drug interactions with hormonal contraception. J Fam Plann Reprod Health Care 2005;31:139–51.

260. Murphy AA, Zacur HA, Charache P, Burkman RT. The effect of tetracycline on levels of oral contraceptives. Am J Obstet Gynecol. 1991;164:28–33.

261. Neely JL, Abate M, Swinker M, D'Angio R. The effect of doxycycline on serum levels of ethinyl estradiol, norethindrone, and endogenous progesterone. Obstet Gynecol.1991;77:416–20.

262. Joshi JV, Joshi UM, Sankholi GM, Krishna U, Mandlekar A, Chowdhury V, et al. A study of interaction of low-dose combination oral contraceptive with Ampicillin and Metronidazole. Contraception. 1980;22:643–52.

263. Maggiolo F, Puricelli G, Dottorini M, Caprioli S, Bianchi W, Suter F. The effect of ciprofloxacin on oral contraceptive steroid treatments. Drugs Exp Clin Res. 1991;17:451–4.

264. Grimmer SF, Back DJ, Orme ML, Cowie A, Gilmore I, Tjia J. The bioavailability of ethinyloestradiol and levonorgestrel in patients with an ileostomy. Contraception. 1986;33:51–9.

265. Friedman CI, Huneke AL, Kim MH, Powell J. The effect of ampicillin on oral contraceptive effectiveness. Obstet Gynecol. 1980;55:33–7.

266. Helms SE, Bredle DL, Zajic J, Jarjoura D, et al. Oral contraceptive failure rates and oral antibiotics. J Am Acad Dermatol. 1997;36:705–10.

267. Panel on Antiretroviral Guidelines for Adults and Adolescents. Guidelines for the use of antiretroviral agents in HIV-1-infected adults and adolescents. Department of Health and Human Services. December 1, 2009; 1–161. Available at http://www.aidsinfo.nih.gov/ContentFiles/AdultandAdolescentGL.pdf. Accessed April 2010.

268. Hall SD, Wang Z, Huang SM, Hamman MA, Vasavada N, Adigun AQ, et al. The interaction between St John's wort and an oral contraceptive. Clin Pharmacol Ther. 2003;74:525–35.

269. Henney JE. From the Food and Drug Administration. Risk of drug interactions with St. John's wort. JAMA. 2000;283:1679. (Also available at www.fda.gov/cder/drug/advisory/stjwort.htm).

270. Redmond G, Godwin AJ, Olson W, Lippman JS. Use of placebo controls in an oral contraceptive trial: methodological issues and adverse event incidence. Contraception. 1999;60:81–5.

271. Asbell B. The Pill: A biography of the drug that changed the world. New York: Random House 1995. p. 148.

272. Vitzthum VJ, Ringheim K. Hormonal contraception and physiology: a research-based theory of discontinuation due to side effects. Stud Fam Plann. 2005;36:13–32.

273. Thorneycroft IH. Cycle control with oral contraceptives: A review of the literature. Am J Obstet Gynecol. 1999;180:S280–7.

274. Rosenberg M. Weight change with oral contraceptive use and during the menstrual cycle. Results of daily measurements. Contraception. 1998;58:345–9.

275. Lloyd T, Lin HM, Matthews AE, Bentley CM, Legro RS. Oral contraceptive use by teenage women does not affect body composition. Obstet Gynecol. 2002;100:235–9.

276. Gallo MF, Lopez LM, Grimes DA, Schulz KF, Helmerhorst FM. Combination contraceptives: effects on weight. Cochrane Database Syst Rev. 2006;:CD003987.

277. O'Connell KJ, Osborne LM, Westhoff C. Measured and reported weight change for women using a vaginal contraceptive ring vs. a low-dose oral contraceptive. Contraception. 2005;72:323–7.

278. Scher AI, Stewart WF, Liberman J, Lipton RB. Prevalence of frequent headache in a population sample. Headache. 1998;38:497–506.

279. Loder EW, Buse DC, Golub JR. Headache as a side effect of combination estrogenprogestin oral contraceptives: a systematic review. Am J Obstet Gynecol. 2005;193:636–49.

280. Rosenberg MJ, Meyers A, Roy V. Efficacy, cycle control, and side effects of low- and lower-dose oral contraceptives: a randomized trial of 20 micrograms and 35 micrograms estrogen preparations. Contraception. 1999;60:321–9.

281. Mooij PN, Thomas CM, Doesburg WH, Eskes TK. Multivitamin supplementation in oral contraceptive users. Contraception. 1991;44:277–88.

282. Sulak PJ, Kuehl TJ, Ortiz M, Shull BL. Acceptance of altering the standard 21-day/7-day oral contraceptive regimen to delay menses and reduce hormone withdrawal symptoms. Am J Obstet Gynecol. 2002;186:1142–9.

283. Graham CA, Bancroft J, Doll HA, Greco T, Tanner A. Does oral contraceptive-induced reduction in free testosterone adversely affect the sexuality or mood of women? Psychoneuroendocrinology. 2007;32:246–55.

284. Thorneycroft H, Gollnick H, Schellschmidt I. Superiority of a combined contraceptive containing drospirenone to a triphasic preparation containing norgestimate in acne treatment. Cutis. 2004;74:123–30.

285. Walsh BW, Sacks FM. Effects of low dose oral contraceptives on very low density and low density lipoprotein metabolism. J Clin Invest. 1993;91:2126–32.

LATE REFERENCES

286. Trussell J, Jordan B. Reproductive health risks in perspective. Contraception. 2006;73:437–9.
287. Berenson AB, van den Berg P, Williams KJ, Rahman M. Effect of injectable and oral contraceptives on glucose and insulin levels. Obstet Gynecol. 2011;117:41–7.
288. Dinger J, Minh TD, Buttmann N, Bardenheuer K. Effectiveness of oral contraceptive pills in a large U.S. cohort comparing progestogen and regimen. Obstet Gynecol. 2011;117:33–40.
289. Foster DG, Hulett D, Bradsberry M, Darney P, Policar M. Number of oral contraceptive pill packages dispensed and subsequent unintended pregnancies. Obstet Gynecol. 2011;117:566–72.
290. Trends in maternal mortality: 1990 to 2008. Estimates developed by WHO, UNICEF, UNFPA, and The World Bank. Geneva, Switzerland: WHO Press, 2010.
291. Berg CJ, Callaghan WM, Syverson C, Henderson Z. Pregnancy-related mortality in the United States, 1998 to 2005. Obstet Gynecol. 2010;116:1302–9.
292. Kuklina EV, Meikle SF, Jamieson DJ, Whiteman MK, Barfield WD, Hillis SD, et al. Severe obstetrics morbidity in the United States: 1998-2005. Obstet Gynecol. 2009;113:293–9.
293. Wei S, Venn A, Ding C, Foley S, Laslett L, Jones G. The association between oral contraceptive use, bone mineral density and fractures in women aged 50–80 years. Contraception. 2011 (in press).
294. Thorneycroft IH: Cycle control with oral contraceptives: a review of the literature. Am J Obstet Gynecol. 1999;180:280–7.
295. Strufaldi R, Pompei LM, Steiner MI, Cunha EP, Ferreira JA, Peixoto S, Fernandes CE. Effects of two combined hormonal contraceptives with the same composition and different doses on female sexual function and plasma androgen levels. Contraception. 2010;82:147–54.
296. Davis AR, Castano PM. Oral contraceptives and libido in women. Ann Rev Sex Res. 2004;15:297–320.
297. Nelson AL, Pietersz D, Nelson LE, Aguilera L. Documented short-term continuation rates for combined hormonal contraceptives in an indigent population with ready access to contraceptive supplies. Am J Obstet Gynecol. 2007;196:599.e1–5.
298. Murphy PA, Brixner D. Hormonal contraceptive discontinuation patterns according to formulation: investigation of associations in an administrative claims database. Contraception. 2008;77:257–63.

Contraceptive Patch and Vaginal Contraceptive Ring

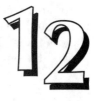

Kavita Nanda, MD, MHS

- Both the weekly contraceptive patch and the monthly vaginal contraceptive ring are highly effective in clinical trials: of 1,000 women using the patch or the ring, only 12 will become pregnant within a year.

- Neither the contraceptive patch nor the vaginal contraceptive ring requires daily use, which could facilitate consistent and correct use.

- Serum estrogen levels with the patch are higher than with COCs, while levels are lower with the vaginal ring. It is unclear whether the variation in levels leads to clinically significant differences in adverse outcomes.

- Reported side effects with the contraceptive patch and ring are similar to those with COCs, with the exception of skin reactions and breast tenderness with the patch and vaginal symptoms with the ring.

CONTRACEPTIVE PATCH

A transdermal contraceptive patch (Ortho Evra) was approved by the Food and Drug Administration (FDA) in 2002. It is a thin, flexible, 20 cm² patch with three layers: a beige outer protective polyester layer; a middle medicated adhesive layer; and a clear liner. Each patch contains 6 milligrams (mg) of norelgestromin (the primary active metabolite of norgestimate) and 0.75 mg of ethinyl estradiol (EE), and releases 150 micrograms (mcg) of norelgestromin and 20 mcg of EE daily. The patch can be applied to the buttocks, upper arm, lower abdomen, or upper torso (excluding the breasts). It is designed to mimic the 28-day dosing schedule of combined oral contraceptives (COCs), with 21 days of active hormones. Women use three 7-day patches for 1 week each, and then have a 7-day patch-free interval. Ortho Evra is dispensed in packages of three patches for the monthly cycle of use. Packages of a single replacement patch are also available.

Another weekly combined contraceptive patch, containing 1.9 mg gestodene and 0.9 mg EE, is under development and is currently in phase III clinical trials. The patch reviewed in this chapter is the Ortho Evra patch—the only contraceptive patch currently approved and marketed.

MECHANISM OF ACTION
The patch, like other combined hormonal contraceptives, works mainly by suppressing gonadotropins and preventing ovulation.[1] Other likely mechanisms of action include thickening of the cervical mucus to prevent sperm penetration and endometrial changes that could affect implantation.

EFFECTIVENESS
Patches belong in the second tier of contraceptive effectiveness (see Figure 3–1), with higher failure rates than those of IUDs and implants (see Chapter 26). In clinical trials and as reported in a Cochrane Review,[2] failure rates for patches were low and similar to those with COCs. Pearl indices for the patch range from 0.71 to 1.24 per 100 woman-years with overall use in trials, to 0.59 to 0.99 with perfect use.[3,4] In a pooled analysis of the three pivotal clinical trials, 15 pregnancies occurred in 22,160 treatment cycles, with an overall life-table failure rate of 0.8% (95% CI, 0.3%–1.3%) and overall Pearl index of 0.88 (95% CI, 0.44–1.33).[5] In this analysis, the contraceptive patch was less effective in obese women (see Special issues).

Although clinical trials showed higher correct and consistent use with the patch than with COCs,[4,6] pregnancy rates are similar to those with COCs.[2] In observational studies of typical use, patch users in the United Kingdom's General Practice Database had slightly higher pregnancy rates (0.34 per 100 women-years, 95% CI 0.13–0.69) compared with users of second- and third-generation COCs (0.16, 95% CI 0.14–0.17 and 0.12, 95% CI 0.10–0.15, respectively); however, women using the patch were younger than women using COCs.[7] In another observational study of new hormonal contraceptive users at high risk of unintended pregnancy, the Pearl index was 3.62 for COCs and 14.84 for the patch in 3,206 cycles.[8] Again, patch users in this study were dissimilar to COC users: they were less educated, had more prior pregnancies and abortions, and were more likely to be lost to follow-up immediately after receiving a prescription.

ADVANTAGES

1. **Convenience.** Some women find the weekly patch regimen more convenient than a daily pill regimen. In some studies, the weekly regimen appears to enhance consistent and correct use when compared with daily COC use, particularly among younger women.[3,4,6,9] Ease of use and no requirement for daily attention were among the main reported advantages.[9] However, the patch does not have higher continuation rates or lower failure rates than COCs.[7,8,10] Continuation rates with the patch in typical use populations were lower than with the vaginal ring (88% vs. 95% over 3 cycles, P=0.03)[11] or with COCs (67% vs. 89% over 3 cycles, P < .001; and 57% vs. 76% at 1 year, P=.004).[8]

2. **Forgiving.** Hormone levels remain therapeutic for at least 9 days after application of the second patch, suggesting that ovulation inhibition would be maintained even if a scheduled patch change was missed for as long as 2 days.[12] Additionally, missed patches (either forgetting to start a new patch or forgetting to change a patch) are less likely to lead to follicular growth or ovulation than missed COCs.[1] Hormone levels and ovulation are surrogate markers, however, and no studies have evaluated risk of pregnancy among patch wearers who miss patches.

3. **Adheres well under a variety of conditions.** In clinical trials, very few patches (< 5%) needed replacement because of complete or partial detachment. Heat, humidity, and exercise do not affect patch adhesion or pharmacokinetics.[12,13] In typical use, however, patch adhesion may be lower. In one three-cycle study, almost half of the women reported that the patch fell off at least once.[11]

4. **Verifiable.** The user can easily verify the presence of the patch. This reassurance about continued protection may reduce the anxiety some women report with COCs—questioning whether they remembered to take their daily pill and worrying that they might forget to take it.

5. **Cycle control comparable to COCs.** Although patch users may experience more breakthrough bleeding and spotting in the first 2 cycles, subsequent cycle control is comparable to that seen with COCs.[3,4] In a randomized cross-over trial comparing patch use to vaginal ring use, however, women switching to the patch were more likely than women switching

to the ring to experience longer periods (38% compared with 9%) and increased dysmenorrhea (29% compared with 16%).[11]

6. **No significant weight gain.** In a randomized placebo-controlled trial, the contraceptive patch was not associated with weight gain. In a pooled analysis of the clinical trials, the mean change in body weight from baseline to the end of treatment was an increase of 0.3 kg, and 79% of participants remained within 5% of their baseline weight.[14]

7. **Rapidly reversible.** Fertility returns rapidly in women discontinuing the patch; FSH and LH levels return to nearly baseline levels and 86% of women ovulate in the month following patch discontinuation.[1]

8. **No clinically significant metabolic effects.** Although the patch has not been studied in women with cardiovascular or other diseases, studies in healthy women have shown no clinically meaningful changes in hematology, blood chemistry, or bone turnover.[15-18] However, the impact of the patch on surrogate markers, such as cholesterol or coagulation tests, may not reflect the impact on outcomes of clinical interest such as myocardial infarction or stroke.[19]

9. **Noncontraceptive benefits.** Because the hormone levels and mechanisms of action are similar to those of COCs, the contraceptive patch may provide many of the same advantages and noncontraceptive health benefits (see Chapter 11 on Combined Oral Contraceptives). Data about long-term health benefits are not yet available.

10. **No need for oral administration.** Patches can be used by women who cannot take a pill orally or who have abnormal intestinal drug absorption.

11. **No effect on sexual function.** In one recent study, women switching from COCs to the patch had slightly higher sexual functioning scores.[20]

DISADVANTAGES AND CAUTIONS
POTENTIALLY SERIOUS HEALTH EFFECTS

1. **Risk of venous thromboembolism (VTE).** Media reports of deaths, allegedly from cardiovascular events, in healthy patch users have received great attention.[21] Serum ethinyl estradiol levels of patch users appear to be higher than those of women using a COC containing 35 mcg EE.[22] However, pharmacoki-

netic measures are surrogate markers and do not necessarily correlate with the magnitude of risk of rare estrogen-related complications such as VTE, stroke, or myocardial infarction. Epidemiologic data are conflicting. In the Cochrane review,[2] the risk of VTE with patch use was estimated to be 53 per 100,000 women (95% CI 1 to 294). A recent series of case-control studies found the risk of VTE diagnoses in women using the patch to be similar to that in women using COCs containing 35 mcg EE and norgestimate (overall OR 1.23 (0.86–1.77)).[23-25] VTE cases were identified by claims data review and were not confirmed by record review. Another series of studies, however, found the patch was associated with double the risk of VTE (OR 2.0; 95% CI 1.2–3.3) compared with COCs containing norgestimate.[26-27] In contrast to the previous series, VTEs were confirmed by medical record review. The authors included long-term pill users while including only new-start patch users, but a stratified analysis limited to new pill users showed similar findings.[27] Another study compared risk of VTE (diagnosed in two separate claims databases and combined with claims for anticoagulant use) of patch use compared with use of a COC containing 30 mcg EE and levonorgestrel. In this study, patch users in the PharMetrics database had a non-significant doubling of risk compared with users of levonorgestrel COCs (OR 2.0, 95% CI 0.9–4.1), while patch users in the MarketScan database had no increase in risk overall (OR 1.3, 95% CI 0.8–2.1). Results from both databases suggested that patch users aged over 40 were at increased risk of VTE compared with those who used levonorgestrel COCs, though confidence limits were wide.[28] Regardless, the risk of VTE with patch use is still far below the risk of VTE during pregnancy.

2. **Other health complications.** In clinical trials, other serious adverse events related to patch use included migraine, cholecystitis, parasthesia at the patch site, cervical adenocarcinoma in situ, and menorrhagia.[14] Although data are scarce, the contraceptive patch may also be associated with some of the rare but serious health complications associated with COCs, such as myocardial infarction, stroke, cholestatic jaundice, hepatic adenomas, or other conditions.

REPORTED SIDE EFFECTS

1. **Skin reactions.** One unique side effect, experienced by up to half of patch users, is a transient skin reaction, such as irritation, redness, pigment changes, or rash at the site of patch ap-

plication. These reactions lead to patch discontinuation less than 3% of the time, however. Most application-site reactions are mild to moderate, and the reactions do not appear more frequently over time.[14,29]

2. **Breast symptoms.** In a pooled analysis of the three pivotal clinical trials, 22.0% of patch users reported breast discomfort, engorgement, or pain, mainly in cycles 1 and 2. Breast symptoms were generally mild or moderate, decreased with continued use, and rarely led to patch discontinuation.[14] Compared with women using COCs and the vaginal ring, women using the patch are more likely to experience breast symptoms.[11,14]

3. **Headache.** In one study, 22% of women using either the patch or COCs reported headaches. Headaches led to discontinuation in 1.1% of patch users—a higher rate than in COC users.[14] Whether these symptoms are actually caused by the patch is unknown.

4. **Nausea.** Nausea is another frequent complaint, reported by approximately one fifth of both patch and COC users in a pooled study.[14] In the clinical trials, nausea led to patch discontinuation in 1.5% of women.[4] In the cross-over trial of patch vs. ring use, women switching to the patch were more likely than women switching to the ring to report frequent nausea (8% compared with 1%).[11]

SPECIAL ISSUES

OBESITY

Higher body weight is associated with lower serum levels of EE and norelgestromin in contraceptive patch users.[5] Furthermore, limited evidence suggests that women weighing more than 90 kg (198 lbs) may be at higher risk of pregnancy when using the contraceptive patch. In a pooled analysis of the three pivotal trials, 5 of the 15 pregnancies that occurred in patch users were in women weighing more than 90 kg, though such women comprised only 3% of the study population.[5] This decrease in effectiveness does not preclude use of the patch by heavier women, because such women are at risk for adverse outcomes from unplanned pregnancies. However, obese women may benefit from additional counseling regarding the importance of strict compliance with the patch regimen, use of a back-up method, and more effective alternative methods.

ADOLESCENTS

Adolescents using COCs are more likely than older women to experience problems with compliance and with unintended pregnancy. They are more likely than with COCs to use the contraceptive patch consistently and correctly.[6,30] However, they are more likely than older women to experience application site reactions and patch detachment, and should receive anticipatory counseling.[30,31] Ease of use, the lack of need for daily adherence, and the ease of concealment are among the main advantages reported by adolescents. However, in an observational study of teen mothers during the first year postpartum, repeat pregnancy rates were similar for patch users (32%) and COC users (30%) and higher than those of DMPA users (14%).[10] Although continuation rates for the patch were higher at 3 months than for the pill (71% vs. 51%), approximately half of both patch and COC users stopped the method by 1 year.[10] In a recent prospective cohort study of adolescent girls and women 15 to 24 years beginning a hormonal contraceptive method, continuation rates at 12 months were low for all methods, but were lowest for patch and DMPA initiators (10.9 and 12.1 per 100 person years, respectively). The pregnancy rate was highest for patch and ring initiators (30.1 and 30.5 per 100 person-years) compared with pill and DMPA initiators (16.5 and 16.1).[80]

POSTPARTUM WOMEN

Recommendations for timing of initiation of the contraceptive patch during the postpartum period, both, in breastfeeding and non-breastfeeding women, are the same as for COCs (see Chapters 4, 11 and 18).

PROVIDING THE METHOD

Explore the patient's medical, reproductive, and social history and conduct a review of systems to ensure that she does not have contraindications to the contraceptive patch. Generally, women who have medical or other contraindications to COC use (except for those related to intestinal absorption) also have contraindications to initiation and continuation of patch use. To identify such situations, please refer to Chapter 4 on Medical Eligibility Criteria, and Chapter 11 on COCs. Although not absolute contraindications, generalized skin conditions such as psoriasis, eczema, or sunburn, may prevent successful patch use.

Measure the woman's blood pressure, if possible. No other screening tests are routinely needed before starting the contraceptive patch unless her history, review of systems, or blood pressure reveal a contraindication or a need for further assessment.[32]

WHEN CAN A WOMAN START USING THE METHOD?

Time the initial placement of the patch to minimize the possibility that a woman is already pregnant or that she might become pregnant between initiation of the patch and onset of effectiveness of the patch. Serum levels of norelgestromin reach levels within the therapeutic range in 24 to 48 hours.[1,33] The contraceptive patch provides higher and more consistent estrogen levels than do COCs, and is associated with less breakthrough ovulation.[1,22] However, because the exact timing of onset of contraceptive effectiveness is unknown, recommendations for using a back-up method are conservative.

- *Menstruating women.* If a woman is menstruating and not using hormonal contraception, advise her of several options for initiating the patch:

  — On any day, if it is reasonably certain she is not pregnant (immediate start/Quick Start). A small randomized trial showed that immediate start of Ortho Evra on any cycle day was acceptable, although it did not lead to greater compliance or continuation rates compared with starting with menses.[34] Seven days of additional contraception and emergency contraceptive pills (if needed) are recommended with the immediate start approach.

  — On the first day of her menstrual period or on the Sunday following the first day of her menses. If she starts on the first day, she does not need additional contraceptive protection, but if she begins the patch after the first day of her period, the package insert recommends that she use an additional method of contraception for 7 days. She should also use emergency contraceptive pills (if needed). The calendar reminders that accompany the patches can accommodate either approach.

- *Switching from other methods.* Instruct a woman switching to the patch from COCs that she can start the first patch on the day her withdrawal bleeding starts; she does not need additional contraception. Alternatively, she can start on the Sunday following the start of her withdrawal bleed. If she begins the patch after the first day of her withdrawal bleed, the package insert recommends 7 days of additional contraception. She can also switch to the patch immediately and not wait until her next menstrual period; if she chooses this method she will not have a withdrawal bleed that month, and she will not need to use additional contraception. If a woman is switching from injectables, she should place the patch on the day she is due for her next injection. The Ortho Evra package insert does not provide instructions for women switching from other methods such as IUDs or implants; however, it is reasonable to follow the recommendations for COCs (see Chapter 11), because the hormonal mechanisms of action are similar.

- *After abortion or miscarriage.* After an abortion or miscarriage in the first or second trimester, women can start the patch immediately; additional contraception is not needed.[35] If the patch is not started within 5 days following a first-trimester abortion, the woman should follow the instructions for a woman who is menstruating.

- *After pregnancy.* Postpartum women who are not breastfeeding may start using the patch 3 weeks after delivery, if it is reasonably certain they are not pregnant; they should use additional contraception for 7 days. Breastfeeding women may begin the patch at or after 1 month postpartum if breastfeeding is well established.[35]

DOSING REGIMENS

Conventional use of the patch follows a 28-day cycle. A woman applies a new patch weekly for 3 weeks, leaves the patch off for a week to allow withdrawal bleeding, and then applies a new patch a week later. Extended use of combined hormonal contraceptives has been studied in healthy women who wish to avoid estrogen-withdrawal side effects during the hormone-free week or to avoid withdrawal bleeding.[36] Extended (84 days) use of the patch resulted in fewer days of bleeding and episodes of bleeding or spotting when compared with cyclic use.[37] Women in both groups reported more headache days during the patch-off weeks compared with patch-on weeks, but women in the extended group also reported more headache days per week while wearing the patch. Both regimens led to decreased headache frequency over time, and women in both groups were highly satisfied.[37] No published data evaluate long-term risks of extended patch use, however.

COUNSELING

Advise women of the advantages, potential risks, and side effects. Quality of counseling influences satisfaction with some contraceptive methods.[38] Women who have heard media reports about deaths associated with the patch may express concerns. Counsel them that the overall risk of death with patch use is extremely low and that to determine the exact risk will require many more years of use by many women.[21] Remind them that pregnancy carries higher risks of death due to thromboembolic complications than do hormonal contraceptive methods.

Advise women weighing more than 90 kg (198 lbs) that they should consider using a back up method of contraception or another more effective method.

Advise women to confirm periodically that the patch is firmly adherent, and to avoid using any creams, lotions, or oils near or at the patch site.

If multiple patches are given, advise women to store them at room temperature (25°C or 77°F) in their protective pouches, and not to put them in the refrigerator or freezer.

MANAGING PROBLEMS AND FOLLOW-UP

As with COCs, it is often preferable to prescribe or give a woman a full year's supply of patches at the very first visit and then encourage a revisit or two only if she has problems or side effects. Alternatively, prescribe 3 months supply with 5 refills, to allow ample time for a follow-up annual appointment.

Dislodged or detached patches. If the patch is partially or completely detached for less than 24 hours, instruct the woman to try to reapply it firmly, applying pressure for 10 seconds, and confirm that the edges are sticking well. If it does not stick well, tell her to remove the patch and apply a replacement. She should not use other adhesives or wraps to hold the patch in place. No additional contraception is needed, and the day she should change her patch will be the same. If the edges stick well, she can continue to use the patch for the full 7 days.

If the patch has been partially or completely detached for more than 24 hours or if the woman does not know how long it has been unstuck, instruct her to start a new patch cycle immediately and use additional contraceptive protection for 7 days. She will now have a new patch-change day. If she has had unprotected intercourse she may need emergency contraception.

Missed or forgotten patches. Missed or forgotten patches may mean that a woman has forgotten to place a patch at all in the first week of the cycle, or forgotten to remove and replace a patch during the 2nd or 3rd weeks. Management of forgotten patches depends upon which patch is missed and for how long (Table 12–1).

Application-site reactions. To decrease the risk of skin irritation, instruct women to rotate application sites when new patches are applied and not to apply the patch to areas of skin that are irritated or cut. If a woman experiences skin reactions at a patch application site, she can remove the patch and apply a new patch in a different location.

Other side effects. If a woman experiences breast symptoms, mild headaches, nausea, or breakthrough bleeding or spotting, advise her that

Table 12-1 Management of missed or forgotten patches

When patch forgotten/missed	Management
1st week	• If a patch is forgotten or is applied late during the first week, and the woman has had unprotected intercourse, provide emergency contraception.
	• Tell her to place a patch immediately.
	• She should use an additional contraceptive method or abstain for 7 days.
	• Remind her to change her patch each week, from now on; on the day of the week she started the new patch.
2nd–3rd week	• *1–2 days late:* If a woman forgets to remove and replace a patch, advise her to remove the old patch and replace it with a new patch immediately.
	• She needs no additional contraceptive method or emergency contraception.
	• *More than 2 days late:* Have her remove the old patch and place a new one immediately. Provide emergency contraception if she has had unprotected intercourse (especially if she is 4 days or more late in applying her patch). She should use additional contraception or abstain for 7 days.
	• Tell her to change the patch each week on the day of the week that she placed this new patch.
4th week	• If she forgets to remove her third patch, tell her to remove the patch.
	• She needs no additional contraceptive method or emergency contraception.
	• She should place a new one on the usual day.

these symptoms usually decrease over time; counsel her to try to continue using the patch.

Drug interactions. Although data are limited, the contraceptive effectiveness of the patch could be reduced by drugs that affect hepatic metabolism, similar to the effect on COCs (see Chapter 4 and Chapter 11). In one pharmacokinetic study, a short course of oral tetracycline did not significantly affect the pharmacokinetics of norelgestromin or EE.[12]

U SER INSTRUCTIONS FOR THE CONTRACEPTIVE PATCH

If multiple patches are given, store them at room temperature (25°C or 77°F) in their protective pouches, and do not put them in the refrigerator or freezer. Use 1 patch for 7 days. Apply a new patch once a week on the same day for 3 weeks in a row. During the fourth week, do not wear a patch. At the end of the week, start another cycle of patches.

Ask your clinician to provide you with a package of or a prescription for emergency contraceptive pills. If you forget you may also get these pills over-the-counter if you are 17 or older. You can use these pills if you have had sex that was not properly protected by the patch or by another contraceptive method (you forget to place a patch during the first week of the cycle, or you are more than 2 days late replacing a patch in the second or third week of the cycle).

Applying the Patch

1. Each patch is packaged in an individual foil packet. Open the pouch by tearing along the top edge and one side edge. Peel the foil pouch apart and open it. Using a fingernail to peel the unit off the foil pouch, lift out the patch along with its clear plastic cover—take care not to remove the clear liner as you remove the patch.

2. Fold the patch open. While holding onto one half, peel the plastic off the other half. Avoid touching the adhesive surface after you remove the liner.

3. Apply the sticky side of the opened patch to your skin, and then remove the other half of the clear liner. You can put the patch on your buttocks, abdomen, upper torso (except the breasts), or on the outside of your upper arm. Avoid placing patches in areas of friction, such as under bra straps or thongs. Only apply the patch to clean, dry skin, and never put it over skin that is irritated, sun-burned, red, or infected. Make sure there are no creams, oils, powder, sunscreen, or sweat on the skin—or the patch will not stick. Press firmly on the patch for 10 seconds. Run your finger around the edges of the patch to make sure that all parts of the patch are sticking properly.

Wearing the Patch

1. Keep the patch in the same place for 7 days; then remove it. Check the patch every day to make sure it is fully adherent. You can wear the patch while bathing, showering, swimming, and exercising.

2. After a week, apply a new patch in a different spot on your body. Every new patch should be applied on the same day of the week, called the patch change day. Because the hormone levels remain protective for up to 9 days, you do not need to apply a

new patch at exactly the same time of the day. Wear the new patch for 7 days. Repeat the procedure for a third week.

3. During the fourth week, do not wear a patch. You will begin your menstrual period.

4. After a week without wearing a patch, apply a new "first week" patch on the same day of the week you applied your other patches.

Removing the Patch

1. To remove the patch, grasp it by an edge and pull it off. Fold it closed on itself on the adhesive side to seal in the medication.

2. Discard the patch in the garbage; do not flush it into the toilet.

3. If any stickiness or adhesive remains on your skin, remove it by using baby oil or lotions.

VAGINAL CONTRACEPTIVE RING

A vaginal contraceptive ring (NuvaRing®) was approved by the FDA in 2001. NuvaRing is a soft, transparent, flexible ring of ethylene vinyl acetate copolymer, with an outer diameter of 54 mm and a cross-sectional diameter of 4 mm. The ring releases 120 mcg of etonogestrel (3-keto desogestrel), the major metabolite of desogestrel, and 15 mcg of EE daily. Each ring is designed to be placed vaginally once every 28 days; it is kept in place for 21 days and removed for a 7-day ring-free period to allow a withdrawal bleed.

Another hormonal contraceptive vaginal ring, releasing 150 mcg of the progestin nestorone and 15 mcg EE daily, is being developed by the Population Council, and is currently in clinical trials.[39] This ring is designed to be effective for 1 year; users keep the ring in place for 3 weeks, and then remove it for 1 week, reinserting the same ring a week later. A nestorone-only ring, available in Chile, Peru, Bolivia and Ecuador, is designed for use by breastfeeding women.[39]

The rest of this chapter will focus on the NuvaRing, because it is the only contraceptive vaginal ring currently approved by the FDA and marketed in the United States.

MECHANISM OF ACTION

The contraceptive mechanism of action of the combined vaginal ring is primarily ovulation suppression. Other likely mechanisms include effects on cervical mucus viscosity and endometrial thinning.[40]

EFFECTIVENESS

The vaginal contraceptive ring belongs in the second tier of contraceptive effectiveness; it has higher failure rates than IUDs and implants. Failure rates with the ring from clinical trials are low and similar to the patch and COCs (see Chapter 26).[41] Pearl indices range from 0.25 to 0.96 per 100 women-years with perfect use, to 0.65 to 1.23 overall.[41-44] In one study, more pregnancies occurred in North America sites than in European sites; the overall Pearl Index was 1.75 in North America and 0.65 in Europe; reasons for this difference are unclear.[42]

Theoretically, improved compliance associated with the ring's monthly regimen could lead to typical-use pregnancy rates lower than those with COCs, which require a daily regimen. Although a noncomparative trial showed rates of correct and consistent ring use (91%) higher than those of COC use in previous studies,[45] randomized comparative trials have demonstrated similar high compliance rates for both methods.[41,43] In typical use, pregnancy rates in ring users are low.[46,47] In a trial of young university students randomized to the ring or COCs, ring users were more compliant in the first 3 months than were COC users, but continuation rates were low in both groups at 6 months (26% for ring users and 29% for COCs users).[48]

ADVANTAGES

1. **Convenience.** Women in clinical trials report that the ring is easy to insert, comfortable to use, and easy to remove.[42,45,49] Women may easily verify that the device is in place. The ring's effectiveness does not depend on its position, because hormonal absorption occurs through the vaginal walls. The ring rests against the vaginal wall but does not exert pressure on the urethra; walking and movement do not lead to expulsion.[50] Although many women and their partners report feeling the ring during intercourse, this does not affect acceptability or continuation for most women.[45,51] Because the ring is left in place for 3 weeks at a time and is not coitally dependent, it is more convenient than other methods such as the diaphragm or COCs. In trials, 86% to 91% of ring users report perfect compliance,[42,43,45,51,52] but studies of typical use find lower compliance rates.[53] A randomized crossover study found higher 3-month continuation rates with the ring (94.6%) compared with the patch (88.2%).[11]

2. **Forgiving.** Hormone levels remain therapeutic for at least 35 days after application of the vaginal ring, suggesting that ovulation inhibition would be maintained even if a woman forgets

to remove the ring for up to 2 weeks beyond schedule. Additionally, ring use for as few as 3 days has been shown to suppress ovarian follicular growth (compared with 7 days for COCs).[54] Such removal is not recommended, however, and follicular size and ovulation are only surrogate markers; no studies have evaluated the risk of pregnancy due to dosing errors in ring use. The ring may be removed from the vagina for up to 3 hours without a decrease in effectiveness.

3. **Vaginal hormone delivery.** The vaginal route of delivery increases the bioavailability of hormones, thus enabling the use of a lower total hormone dose, potentially reducing side effects. The ring can be used by women who cannot swallow a pill and by women with abnormal intestinal absorption.

4. **Rapidly effective and rapidly reversible.** Hormone levels needed to suppress ovulation are achieved within the first day of vaginal ring use,[55] and as few as 3 consecutive days of vaginal ring use interferes with follicular growth. Return to ovulation after ring removal is rapid, occurring in a median of 17 to 19 days.[56]

5. **Excellent cycle control.** Compared with COCs, the ring is less likely to produce irregular bleeding, especially in the first few cycles. Most vaginal ring users experience withdrawal bleeding on schedule.[42,57-59]

6. **Does not cause weight gain.** In clinical studies, women are as likely to lose weight as to gain it when using the ring for a year.[41,60]

7. **No adverse effects on cervico-vaginal epithelium.** Ring use does not appear to have adverse effects on the cervico-vaginal epithelium or on cervical cytology.[42,61]

8. **No adverse endometrial effects.** Ring use for up to 2 years did not lead to endometrial hyperplasia or other adverse effects on endometrial histology.[62]

9. **Can be used concurrently with tampons.** Occasionally, a user may need to insert a ring while she is still having withdrawal bleeding. A pharmacokinetic study showed that tampons can be used concurrently with the ring without any effects on hormone absorption.[63] Ring users need to ensure that the ring is not inadvertently withdrawn at the time of tampon removal.

10. **Can be removed for up to 3 hours without compromising effectiveness.** Although most women and their partners do not report discomfort due to the ring during vaginal intercourse

the ring can be removed or left out for up to 3 hours in any 24-hour period without requiring a backup method.[64] The same ring can then be reinserted.

11. **Safe in women with latex allergies.**   Because the ring is made from vinyl acetate, women with latex allergies can use it safely.

12. **No clinically significant metabolic effects.**   In healthy women, the vaginal ring had no clinically important adverse effects on surrogate markers of disease such as heart rate, blood pressure, blood chemistries, lipids, adrenal and thyroid function, carbohydrate metabolism, or hematology.[42,45,65] In a study of women with type 1 diabetes, ring use did not adversely affect glycemic control or other metabolic measures.[66] These surrogate markers may not reflect the actual risk of adverse outcome, and no studies have examined long-term metabolic outcomes.

13. **Does not affect bone density.**   In one study, bone mineral density showed no change from baseline after as long as 24 months of contraceptive ring use.[67] The study did not include adolescents or perimenopausal women. No study has looked at risk of fractures.

14. **Noncontraceptive benefits.**   Because the hormonal levels and mechanisms of action are similar, the vaginal contraceptive ring may provide many of the same advantages and non-contraceptive health benefits that COCs do, although data about long-term health benefits are not yet available.

DISADVANTAGES AND CAUTIONS
POTENTIAL SERIOUS HEALTH RISKS

1. **Risk of venous thromboembolism.**   Although several cases of VTE have been reported with vaginal ring use,[68] no studies have been published evaluating this issue. In the Cochrane review,[2] the risk of VTE with ring use was estimated to be 149 per 100,000 women (95% CI 18–538). Etonogestrel, the progestin component of the ring, is a metabolite of desogestrel. Some studies have found that women using desogestrel-containing COCs at increased risk of VTE compared with women using COCs containing other progestins. Although ring users have progestin levels similar to those of COC users, their EE levels are 2-fold lower than those in women taking COCs with 35 mg EE and 3-fold lower than those in women

wearing the patch.[22] Pharmacokinetic measures are surrogate endpoints, however, and may not necessarily reflect a decreased risk of estrogen-related side effects or long-term risks.

2. **Other health complications.** Although data are scarce, the vaginal ring may be associated with other rare but serious health complications associated with COCs, such as myocardial infarction, stroke, cholestatic jaundice, gallbladder disease, hepatic adenomas, or other conditions.

3. **Toxic shock syndrome (TSS).** Very rare cases of TSS have been reported by ring users; some of these users were also using tampons.[64] Although causation has not been determined, any ring user with signs or symptoms of TSS should seek immediate medical evaluation and treatment.

REPORTED SIDE-EFFECTS

1. **Headache.** Headache is the most common reported hormonal side-effect of the ring, reported by 6% of users.[42,45]

2. **Vaginal symptoms.** In pivotal clinical trials, common reasons for discontinuation included vaginal symptoms such as foreign body sensation or coital problems, and 1% to 2.6% of ring users discontinued because of these symptoms or because of ring expulsion.[69] Other self-reported vaginal symptoms include vaginitis, leukorrhea, and vaginal discomfort. In a randomized comparative trial with COCs, however, the only vaginal symptom significantly associated with ring use was vaginal wetness; 63% of ring users reported vaginal wetness compared with 43% of COC users. Microbiological evaluation showed that ring use was associated with an increase only in hydrogen peroxide-producing Lactobacillus.[70]

3. **Other side effects.** Other reported side effects include decreased libido, nausea, and breast tenderness.[20,42,45,57] One study found that, in the first 3 months of use, fewer ring users called their providers about side effects than did patch or COC users.[71]

SPECIAL ISSUES

Adolescents

The vaginal contraceptive ring may be particularly appropriate for adolescents, because it offers both privacy and the convenience of monthly dosing. Improved consistent and correct use could ultimately lead to improved typical-use effectiveness. In the study of adolescent girls and young women,[80] ring continuation rates at 12 months were comparable to COC rates (29.4 and 32.7 per 100 person-years, respectively), but pregnancy rates were higher for patch and ring initiators (30.1 and 30.5 per 100 person-years) compared with pill and DMPA initiators (16.5 and 16.1). It is possible that adolescents may feel uncomfortable with a vaginal device; in one study of women aged 18 to 41, there was a trend towards increased sexual comfort with ring use with increasing age, for both the woman and her partner.[72]

Postpartum Women

Recommendations for timing of initiation of the vaginal ring postpartum during the postpartum period, both in breastfeeding and nonbreastfeeding women, are the same as for COCs (see Chapter 4 on Medical Eligibility Criteria, Chapter 11 on Combined Oral Contraceptives, and Chapter 18 on Postpartum Contraception and Lactation).

PROVIDING THE METHOD

Explore the patient's medical, reproductive, and social history and conduct a review of systems to ensure that she does not have contraindications to using the vaginal ring. Generally, women who have medical or other contraindications to COC use (except for those related to intestinal absorption) also have contraindications to the initiation and continuation of vaginal ring use.[35] To identify such situations, please refer to Chapter 4 on Medical Eligibility Criteria, and Chapter 11 on COCs. Additionally, women may not be suitable candidates for the vaginal ring if they have significant pelvic relaxation, vaginal stenosis or obstruction (if it prevents placement or retention of the ring), conditions that make the vagina more susceptible to irritation or ulceration, or an inability or unwillingness to touch their genitalia.

Measure the woman's blood pressure, if possible. No other screening tests are routinely needed before starting the contraceptive ring unless her history, review of systems, or blood pressure reveal a contraindication or a need for further assessment.[32]

WHEN CAN A WOMAN START USING THE METHOD?

Time initiation of the ring to minimize the possibility that a woman is already pregnant, and the risk that she might become pregnant between initiation of the ring and onset of effectiveness. The ring inhibits ovulation even when it is started on cycle day 5, and 3 days of ring use inhibited ovulation even with a follicle of up to 13 millimeters size. However, because the exact timing of contraceptive effectiveness is unknown, recommendations, based on the package insert, are conservative.

- *Menstruating women.* If a woman is menstruating and not using hormonal contraception, advise her that there are several options for initiating the ring:

  — On any day, if it is reasonably certain she is not pregnant (immediate start/Quick Start).[73] Seven days of additional contraception and emergency contraceptive pills (if needed) are recommended with the immediate start approach.

  — On the first day of her cycle (i.e., the first day of her menses). She needs no additional contraception.

  — On cycle days 2 to 5, even if she has not finished her menstrual bleeding. The manufacturer recommends that women inserting the ring between cycle days 2 to 5 should use an additional method of contraception (male or female condom or spermicide, but not diaphragm) for the first 7 days of ring use in the first cycle.

- *Switching from other methods.* Instruct a woman switching to the ring from COCs that she can insert the first ring on any day, but no later than the day following her usual hormone-free interval (the day she would start a new pack of pills). If she has used COCs consistently and correctly, no additional back-up contraceptive is needed. If she is switching from progestin-only pills, she may switch on any day, placing the first ring the day after she takes the last pill. Seven days of additional contraception is recommended. If a woman is switching from an implant or an IUD, she should place the first ring on the day that the implant or IUD is removed, and she should use additional contraception for 7 days. If she is switching from injectables, she should insert the ring the day she is due for her next injection.

- *After abortion or miscarriage.* If a woman has recently had a first or second trimester abortion or miscarriage, advise her that the ring may be inserted within 5 days; she needs no additional contraception. If she does not insert the ring within 5 days she will need to follow the recommendations for menstruating women not using hormonal contraception.

- *After pregnancy.* A postpartum woman who is not breastfeeding may start using the ring 3 weeks after delivery,[35] if it is reasonably certain she is not pregnant. She should use additional contraception for 7 days. Breastfeeding women may begin the patch at or after 1 month postpartum if breastfeeding is well established.[35]

DOSING REGIMENS

Conventional use of the ring follows a 28-day cycle. A woman inserts a new ring and keeps it in for 3 weeks, has a week when the ring is removed to allow withdrawal bleeding, and then inserts a new ring a week later. Extended use of combined hormonal contraceptives has been used to avoid estrogen-withdrawal side effects during the hormone-free week or to avoid bleeding in women who prefer amenorrhea. Extended ring cycles of 49, 91, or 364 days (with women changing the ring every 21 days) are well-tolerated and acceptable. Women experience few episodes of scheduled bleeding but may experience more unscheduled bleeding, which decreases over time.[74-76] Women with persistent or prolonged breakthrough bleeding or spotting may benefit from a short 4-day hormone-free interval.[77]

COUNSELING

Advise women considering the vaginal contraceptive ring about its advantages, potential risks, and side effects.

MANAGING PROBLEMS AND FOLLOW-UP

As for COCs and the patch, it is reasonable to prescribe a full year's supply of rings at the first visit. If a year's supply is dispensed at one time, advise the woman to refrigerate the rings at 2° to 8°C (36–46°F) to extend the shelf-life beyond 4 months. Rings may be stored for up to 4 months at 25°C (77°F).

EXPELLED RING

A woman may accidentally remove or expel her ring while removing a tampon, engaging in intercourse, or having a bowel movement. If the ring has been out of the vagina for less than 3 hours, no additional contraception is required. Instruct the woman to rinse the ring with lukewarm water and reinsert it as soon as possible. If a woman loses the ring, she should insert a new ring and continue the regimen without alteration.

During the first or second week, if the ring is removed or expelled and has been out of the vagina for more than 3 hours, it may still be reinserted. However, advise her that an additional contraceptive method should be used for the next 7 days, and offer her emergency contraception if she has had unprotected intercourse.

If a women in her third week of ring use reports that the ring has been out of her vagina for more than 3 hours, advise her to discard that ring. She can then choose one of two options:

- Insert a new ring immediately to begin a new 3-week cycle.
- Have a withdrawal bleed and insert a new ring no later than 7 days from when the last ring was removed/expelled. Advise the woman that this is an option only if the ring was used continuously for the preceding 7 days.

For either option, advise her to use an additional method of contraception until the new ring has been used continuously for 7 days.

PROLONGED USE

If a woman reports that the ring was left in the vagina for more than 3 weeks (but less than 4 weeks), advise her that it is still effective in preventing pregnancy. Counsel her to remove the ring and insert a new one after a 1-week interval. If the ring was left in place for more than 4 weeks, contraceptive effectiveness could be compromised. Consider pregnancy testing, and advise the woman to consider emergency contraception if indicated, and to use an additional contraceptive method until a new ring has been in place for at least 7 days.

DISCONNECTED (BROKEN) RING

If a woman calls to report that her ring has disconnected or broken, counsel her to discard the ring and replace it with a new ring. She does not need additional contraception.

VAGINAL SYMPTOMS

Advise women that they may perceive more vaginal discharge or wetness while using the ring, but that this does not signify infection. Counsel women that there is no increased risk of vaginal infection with ring use. However, if a woman complains of vulvovaginal itching or a foul odor, she should be evaluated and treated as needed.

OTHER SIDE EFFECTS

If a woman experiences headache, nausea, or breast tenderness, advise her that these symptoms usually decrease over time, and counsel her to try to continue using the ring.

DRUG INTERACTIONS

Although data are limited, drugs that affect hepatic metabolism could reduce the ring's effectiveness, just as they reduce the effectiveness of COCs (see Chapter 4 and Chapter 11). In a pharmacokinetic study, co-administration of three antimycotic formulations led to slight increases

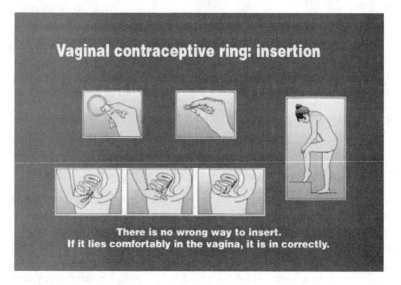

Source: Ballagh SA (2002), with permission courtesy of Organon USA.

Figure 12–1 Inserting the NuvaRing

in etonogestrel and EE levels, with suppositories having the greatest effect.[78] In another study, a single-dose of 100 mg nonoxynol-9 gel did not affect the serum concentrations of etonogestrel or EE.[79] Serum concentrations of etonogestrel and EE were also not affected by concomitant administration of 10 days of oral amoxicillin or doxycycline in standard dosages.[12]

USER INSTRUCTIONS FOR THE VAGINAL RING

1. Each ring comes in a reclosable foil pouch. After washing and drying your hands, remove the ring and keep the foil pouch for ring disposal.

2. Insert the ring into your vagina. Use any position you find most comfortable: standing with one leg up, squatting, or lying down. Squeeze the rim of the ring and put the leading edge into the opening of the vagina. If you feel the ring, just slide it farther into your vagina until it is comfortable; the muscles of your vagina should keep it in place. The exact position of the ring is not critical for its function.

3. Leave the ring in place for 3 weeks. You do not need to remove the ring for intercourse. If you do remove the ring for inter-

course, do not leave it out of the vagina for more than 3 hours in any 24-hour period.

4. After 3 weeks of use, remove the ring for 7 days. During this break, you will experience withdrawal bleeding. Remove the ring by hooking your index finger under the forward rim or by grasping the rim between your index and middle finger and pulling it out. Place the used ring in the foil pouch and throw it away in a trash container out of the reach of children and pets (do not flush it down the toilet).

5. After the 7-day break, insert a new vaginal ring to begin the cycle again. Insert the new ring on the same day of the week you inserted the previous ring, even if you have not finished your period.

6. If the ring is out of your vagina for more than 3 hours during the first 2 weeks, you might not be protected from pregnancy. Reinsert the ring as soon as possible and use an extra method of birth control (such as condoms or spermicide) until you have used the ring for 7 days in a row.

7. If the ring has been out for more than 3 hours during the third week, throw the ring away and choose 1 of the 2 options below:

   a. Insert a new ring immediately. This begins the next 3-week use period. You may not have a period but you may experience breakthrough spotting or bleeding.

   b. Have your period and insert a new ring no later than 7 days from the time the previous ring was removed or expelled. This option should be chosen only if the ring was used continuously for the preceding 7 days. In addition, you must use a barrier method (such as condoms or spermicide) until you have used the ring for 7 days in a row.

REFERENCES

1. Pierson RA, Archer DF, Moreau M, Shangold GA, Fisher AC, Creasy GW. Ortho Evra/Evra versus oral contraceptives: follicular development and ovulation in normal cycles and after an intentional dosing error. Fertil Steril. 2003;80:34–42.
2. Lopez LM, Grimes DA, Gallo MF, Schulz KF. Skin patch and vaginal ring versus combined oral contraceptives for contraception. Cochrane Database Syst Rev. 2008:CD003552.
3. Audet MC, Moreau M, Koltun WD, et al. Evaluation of contraceptive efficacy and cycle control of a transdermal contraceptive patch vs an oral contraceptive: a randomized controlled trial. JAMA. 2001;285:2347–54.
4. Urdl W, Apter D, Alperstein A, et al. Contraceptive efficacy, compliance and beyond: factors related to satisfaction with once-weekly transdermal compared with oral contraception. Eur J Obstet Gynecol Reprod Biol. 2005;121:202–10.

5. Zieman M, Guillebaud J, Weisberg E, Shangold GA, Fisher AC, Creasy GW. Contraceptive efficacy and cycle control with the Ortho Evra/Evra transdermal system: the analysis of pooled data. Fertil Steril. 2002;77:S13–8.

6. Archer DF, Bigrigg A, Smallwood GH, Shangold GA, Creasy GW, Fisher AC. Assessment of compliance with a weekly contraceptive patch (Ortho Evra/Evra) among North American women. Fertil Steril. 2002;77:S27–31.

7. Jick SS, Hagberg KW, Kaye JA, Jick H. The risk of unintended pregnancies in users of the contraceptive patch compared to users of oral contraceptives in the UK General Practice Research Database. Contraception. 2009;80:142–51.

8. Bakhru A, Stanwood N. Performance of contraceptive patch compared with oral contraceptive pill in a high-risk population. Obstet Gynecol. 2006;108:378–86.

9. Rubinstein ML, Halpern-Felsher BL, Irwin CEJ. An evaluation of the use of the transdermal contraceptive patch in adolescents. J Adolesc Health. 2004;34:395–401.

10. Thurman AR, Hammond N, Brown HE, Roddy ME. Preventing repeat teen pregnancy: postpartum depot medroxyprogesterone acetate, oral contraceptive pills, or the patch? J Pediatr Adolesc Gynecol. 2007;20:61–5.

11. Creinin MD, Meyn LA, Borgatta L, et al. Multicenter comparison of the contraceptive ring and patch: a randomized controlled trial. Obstet Gynecol. 2008;111:267–77.

12. Abrams LS, Skee D, Natarajan J, Wong FA. Pharmacokinetic overview of Ortho Evra/Evra. Fertil Steril. 2002;77:S3–12.

13. Zacur HA, Hedon B, Mansour D, Shangold GA, Fisher AC, Creasy GW. Integrated summary of Ortho Evra/Evra contraceptive patch adhesion in varied climates and conditions. Fertil Steril. 2002;77:S32–5.

14. Sibai BM, Odlind V, Meador ML, Shangold GA, Fisher AC, Creasy GW. A comparative and pooled analysis of the safety and tolerability of the contraceptive patch (Ortho Evra/Evra). Fertil Steril. 2002;77:S19–26.

15. Creasy GW, Fisher AC, Hall N, Shangold GA. Transdermal contraceptive patch delivering norelgestromin and ethinyl estradiol. Effects on the lipid profile. J Reprod Med. 2003;48:179–86.

16. Graziottin A. A review of transdermal hormonal contraception : focus on the ethinylestradiol/norelgestromin contraceptive patch. Treat Endocrinol. 2006;5:359–65.

17. Kiriwat O, Petyim S. The effects of transdermal contraception on lipid profiles, carbohydrate metabolism and coagulogram in Thai women. Gynecol Endocrinol. 2010;26:361–5.

18. Massaro M, Di Carlo C, Gargano V, Formisano C, Bifulco G, Nappi C. Effects of the contraceptive patch and the vaginal ring on bone metabolism and bone mineral density: a prospective, controlled, randomized study. Contraception. 2010;81:209–14.

19. Grimes DA, Schulz KF. Surrogate end points in clinical research: hazardous to your health. Obstet Gynecol. 2005;105:1114–8.

20. Gracia CR, Sammel MD, Charlesworth S, Lin H, Barnhart KT, Creinin MD. Sexual function in first-time contraceptive ring and contraceptive patch users. Fertil Steril. 2010;93:21–8.

21. Grimes DA, Mishell DR. Assessing Rare Event Reports: A Numerator in Search of a Denominator. Dialogues in Contraception. 2004;8:7.

22. van den Heuvel MW, van Bragt AJ, Alnabawy AK, Kaptein MC. Comparison of ethinylestradiol pharmacokinetics in three hormonal contraceptive formulations: the vaginal ring, the transdermal patch and an oral contraceptive. Contraception. 2005;72:168–74.

23. Jick SS, Kaye JA, Russmann S, Jick H. Risk of nonfatal venous thromboembolism in women using a contraceptive transdermal patch and oral contraceptives containing norgestimate and 35 microg of ethinyl estradiol. Contraception. 2006;73:223–8.

24. Jick S, Kaye JA, Li L, Jick H. Further results on the risk of nonfatal venous thromboembolism in users of the contraceptive transdermal patch compared to users of oral contraceptives containing norgestimate and 35 microg of ethinyl estradiol. Contraception. 2007;76:4–7.

25. Jick SS, Hagberg KW, Kaye JA. ORTHO EVRA and venous thromboembolism: an update. Contraception. 2010;81:452–3.
26. Cole JA, Norman H, Doherty M, Walker AM. Venous thromboembolism, myocardial infarction, and stroke among transdermal contraceptive system users. Obstet Gynecol. 2007;109:339–46.
27. Dore DD, Norman H, Loughlin J, Seeger JD. Extended case-control study results on thromboembolic outcomes among transdermal contraceptive users. Contraception. 81:408–13.
28. Jick SS, Hagberg KW, Hernandez RK, Kaye JA. Postmarketing study of ORTHO EVRA and levonorgestrel oral contraceptives containing hormonal contraceptives with 30 mcg of ethinyl estradiol in relation to nonfatal venous thromboembolism. Contraception. 2010;81:16–21.
29. Weisberg F, Bouchard C, Moreau M, et al. Preference for and satisfaction of Canadian women with the transdermal contraceptive patch versus previous contraceptive method: an open-label, multicentre study. J Obstet Gynaecol Can. 2005;27:350–9.
30. Rubinstein ML, Halpern-Felsher BL, Irwin CE, Jr. An evaluation of the use of the transdermal contraceptive patch in adolescents. J Adolesc Health. 2004;34:395–401.
31. Bodner K, Bodner-Adler B, Grunberger W. Evaluation of the contraceptive efficacy, compliance, and satisfaction with the transdermal contraceptive patch system Evra: a comparison between adolescent and adult users. Arch Gynecol Obstet. 2011;283:525–30.
32. Stewart FH, Harper CC, Ellertson CE, Grimes DA, Sawaya GF, Trussell J. Clinical breast and pelvic examination requirements for hormonal contraception: Current practice vs evidence. JAMA. 2001;285:2232–9.
33. Abrams LS, Skee DM, Natarajan J, Wong FA, Anderson GD. Pharmacokinetics of a contraceptive patch (Evra/Ortho Evra) containing norelgestromin and ethinyloestradiol at four application sites. Br J Clin Pharmacol. 2002;53:141–6.
34. Murthy AS, Creinin MD, Harwood B, Schreiber CA. Same-day initiation of the transdermal hormonal delivery system (contraceptive patch) versus traditional initiation methods. Contraception. 2005;72:333–6.
35. Centers for Disease Control and Prevention. U. S. Medical Eligibility Criteria for Contraceptive Use, 2010. MMWR 2010;59:(No. RR-4):1–85.
36. Miller L, Hughes JP. Continuous combination oral contraceptive pills to eliminate withdrawal bleeding: a randomized trial. Obstet Gynecol. 2003;101:653–61.
37. Stewart FH, Kaunitz AM, Laguardia KD, Karvois DL, Fisher AC, Friedman AJ. Extended use of transdermal norelgestromin/ethinyl estradiol: a randomized trial. Obstet Gynecol. 2005;105:1389–96.
38. Canto De Cetina TE, Canto P, Ordonez Luna M. Effect of counseling to improve compliance in Mexican women receiving depot-medroxyprogesterone acetate. Contraception. 2001;63:143–6.
39. Johansson ED, Sitruk-Ware R. New delivery systems in contraception: vaginal rings. Am J Obstet Gynecol. 2004;190:S54–9.
40. Duijkers IJ, Klipping C, Verhoeven CH, Dieben TO. Ovarian function with the contraceptive vaginal ring or an oral contraceptive: a randomized study. Hum Reprod. 2004;19:2668–73.
41. Oddsson K, Leifels-Fischer B, de Melo NR, et al. Efficacy and safety of a contraceptive vaginal ring (NuvaRing) compared with a combined oral contraceptive: a 1-year randomized trial. Contraception. 2005;71:176–82.
42. Dieben TO, Roumen FJ, Apter D. Efficacy, cycle control, and user acceptability of a novel combined contraceptive vaginal ring. Obstet Gynecol. 2002;100:585–93.
43. Ahrendt HJ, Nisand I, Bastianelli C, et al. Efficacy, acceptability and tolerability of the combined contraceptive ring, NuvaRing, compared with an oral contraceptive containing 30 microg of ethinyl estradiol and 3 mg of drospirenone. Contraception. 2006;74:451–7.

44. Mansour D, Inki P, Gemzell-Danielsson K. Efficacy of contraceptive methods: A review of the literature. Eur J Contracept Reprod Health Care. 2010;15:4–16.
45. Roumen F. Contraceptive efficacy and tolerability with a novel combined contraceptive vaginal ring, NuvaRing. Eur J Contracept Reprod Health Care. 2002;7 Suppl 2:19–24; discussion 37–9.
46. Merki-Feld GS, Hund M. Clinical experience with NuvaRing in daily practice in Switzerland: cycle control and acceptability among women of all reproductive ages. Eur J Contracept Reprod Health Care. 2007;12:240–7.
47. Brucker C, Karck U, Merkle E. Cycle control, tolerability, efficacy and acceptability of the vaginal contraceptive ring, NuvaRing: results of clinical experience in Germany. Eur J Contracept Reprod Health Care. 2008;13:31–8.
48. Gilliam ML, Neustadt A, Kozloski M, Mistretta S, Tilmon S, Godfrey E. Adherence and acceptability of the contraceptive ring compared with the pill among students: a randomized controlled trial. Obstet Gynecol. 2010;115:503–10.
49. Szarewski A. High acceptability and satisfaction with NuvaRing use. Eur J Contracept Reprod Health Care. 2002;7 Suppl 2:31–6; discussion 7–9.
50. Barnhart KT, Timbers K, Pretorius ES, Lin K, Shaunik A. In vivo assessment of NuvaRing(R) placement. Contraception. 2005;72:196–9.
51. Roumen FJ, op ten Berg MM, Hoomans EH. The combined contraceptive vaginal ring (NuvaRing): first experience in daily clinical practice in The Netherlands. Eur J Contracept Reprod Health Care. 2006;11:14–22.
52. Roumen FJ. Review of the combined contraceptive vaginal ring, NuvaRing. Ther Clin Risk Manag. 2008;4:441–51.
53. Lete I, Doval JL, Perez-Campos E, et al. Self-described impact of noncompliance among users of a combined hormonal contraceptive method. Contraception. 2008;77:276–82.
54. Killick S. Complete and robust ovulation inhibition with NuvaRing. Eur J Contracept Reprod Health Care. 2002;7 Suppl 2:13–8; discussion 37–9.
55. Timmer CJ, Mulders TM. Pharmacokinetics of etonogestrel and ethinylestradiol released from a combined contraceptive vaginal ring. Clin Pharmacokinet. 2000;39:233–42.
56. Mulders TM, Dieben TO, Bennink HJ. Ovarian function with a novel combined contraceptive vaginal ring. Hum Reprod. 2002;17:2594–9.
57. Bjarnadottir RI, Tuppurainen M, Killick SR. Comparison of cycle control with a combined contraceptive vaginal ring and oral levonorgestrel/ethinyl estradiol. Am J Obstet Gynecol. 2002;186:389–95.
58. Oddsson K, Leifels-Fischer B, Wiel-Masson D, et al. Superior cycle control with a contraceptive vaginal ring compared with an oral contraceptive containing 30 microg ethinylestradiol and 150 microg levonorgestrel: a randomized trial. Hum Reprod. 2005;20:557–62.
59. Milsom I, Lete I, Bjertnaes A, et al. Effects on cycle control and bodyweight of the combined contraceptive ring, NuvaRing, versus an oral contraceptive containing 30 microg ethinyl estradiol and 3 mg drospirenone. Hum Reprod. 2006;21:2304–11.
60. O'connell KJ, Osborne LM, Westhoff C. Measured and reported weight change for women using a vaginal contraceptive ring vs. a low-dose oral contraceptive. Contraception. 2005;72:323–7.
61. Roumen FJ, Boon ME, van Velzen D, Dieben TO, Coelingh Bennink HJ. The cervicovaginal epithelium during 20 cycles' use of a combined contraceptive vaginal ring. Hum Reprod. 1996;11:2443–8.
62. Bulten J, Grefte J, Siebers B, Dieben T. The combined contraceptive vaginal ring (NuvaRing) and endometrial histology. Contraception. 2005;72:362–5.
63. Verhoeven CH, Dieben TO. The combined contraceptive vaginal ring, NuvaRing, and tampon co-usage. Contraception. 2004;69:197–9.
64. Organon USA I, ed *NuvaRing prescribing information*. Roseland, NJ; 2005.

65. Tuppurainen M, Klimscheffskij R, Venhola M, Dieben TO. The combined contraceptive vaginal ring (NuvaRing) and lipid metabolism: a comparative study. Contraception. 2004;69:389–94.

66. Grigoryan OR, Grodnitskaya EE, Andreeva EN, Chebotnikova TV, Melnichenko GA. Use of the NuvaRing hormone-releasing system in late reproductive-age women with type 1 diabetes mellitus. Gynecol Endocrinol. 2008;24:99–104.

67. Massai R, Makarainen L, Kuukankorpi A, Klipping C, Duijkers I, Dieben T. The combined contraceptive vaginal ring and bone mineral density in healthy premenopausal women. Hum Reprod. 2005;20:2674–8.

68. Shum MK, Rajagopalan K, Lachant NA. Venous Thromboembolic Events in Women Using the NuvaRing(R). ASH Annual Meeting Abstracts. 2007;110:3994-.

69. Roumen FJ, Apter D, Mulders TM, Dieben TO. Efficacy, tolerability and acceptability of a novel contraceptive vaginal ring releasing etonogestrel and ethinyl oestradiol. Hum Reprod. 2001;16:469–75.

70. Veres S, Miller L, Burington B. A comparison between the vaginal ring and oral contraceptives. Obstet Gynecol. 2004;104:555–63.

71. Victor I, Fink RA. Comparing patient telephone callback rates for different hormonal birth control delivery systems. Am J Ther. 2006;13:507–12.

72. Novak A, de la Loge C, Abetz L, van der Meulen EA. The combined contraceptive vaginal ring, NuvaRing: an international study of user acceptability. Contraception. 2003;67:187–94.

73. Schafer JE, Osborne LM, Davis AR, Westhoff C. Acceptability and satisfaction using Quick Start with the contraceptive vaginal ring versus an oral contraceptive. Contraception. 2006;73:488–92.

74. Miller L, Verhoeven CH, Hout J. Extended regimens of the contraceptive vaginal ring: a randomized trial. Obstet Gynecol. 2005;106:473–82.

75. Guazzelli CA, Barreiros FA, Barbosa R, de Araujo FF, Moron AF. Extended regimens of the vaginal contraceptive ring: cycle control. Contraception. 2009;80:430–5.

76. Barreiros FA, Guazzelli CA, de Araujo FF, Barbosa R. Bleeding patterns of women using extended regimens of the contraceptive vaginal ring. Contraception. 2007; 75:204–8.

77. Sulak PJ, Smith V, Coffee A, Witt I, Kuehl AL, Kuehl TJ. Frequency and management of breakthrough bleeding with continuous use of the transvaginal contraceptive ring: a randomized controlled trial. Obstet Gynecol. 2008;112:563–71.

78. Verhoeven CH, van den Heuvel MW, Mulders TM, Dieben TO. The contraceptive vaginal ring, NuvaRing, and antimycotic co-medication. Contraception. 2004;69: 129–32.

79. Haring T, Mulders TM. The combined contraceptive ring NuvaRing and spermicide co-medication. Contraception. 2003;67:271–2.

LATE REFERENCE

80. Raine TR, Foster-Rosales A, Upadhyay UD, et al. One-year contraceptive continuation and pregnancy in adolescent girls and women initiating hormonal contraceptives. Obstet Gynecol. 2011;117:363–71.

Male Condoms

Lee Warner, PhD, MPH
Markus J. Steiner, PhD, MSPH

- When used consistently and correctly, male latex condoms can reduce the risk of pregnancy and many sexually transmitted infections (STIs), including human immunodeficiency virus (HIV).

- Condoms are inexpensive, available without a prescription, and easy to use.

- By preventing STIs and their long-term sequelae, condoms help protect future fertility.

- Clients at risk for STIs, particularly those in a new sexual relationship, should be encouraged to use condoms even if they already rely on more effective methods of contraception, because many infections are asymptomatic.

Male latex condoms remain the most widely available and commonly used barrier method to prevent sexually transmitted infections (STIs) in the United States. When used consistently and correctly, male condoms reduce the risk of pregnancy and most STIs, including human immunodeficiency virus (HIV), based on results from laboratory and clinical studies. Condom use has increased in recent years, according to national surveys of adolescents and adults,[1,2] largely in response to the HIV and STI epidemics. According to the National Youth Risk Behavior Surveys (YRBS), the prevalence of condom use at last intercourse increased by one-third among sexually active high school students between 1991 and 2007, from 46% to 61%.[2] Moreover, the most recent cycle of the National Survey of Family Growth (NSFG)[1] revealed that nearly 9 million reproductive-age women in the United States currently used condoms for contraception or protection from STIs, a figure comparable to that reported in the 2002 survey.[3] Among women using any contraceptive, 16% reported currently using male condoms for prevention of pregnancy, making it the third most popular method. Condom use thus continues to be an important part of public health efforts to prevent new cases of infection with HIV and other STIs.

MECHANISM OF ACTION

The male condom acts as a physical barrier by covering the penile glans and shaft. The condom prevents pregnancy by blocking the passage of semen; it prevents infections by covering the major portals of entry and exit for many STI pathogens. Because of their coitally-dependent nature, condoms must be used consistently and correctly with each act of intercourse to be effective. Among contraceptive methods that are physical barriers, condoms provide the most protection of the genital tract and effective protection against many STIs (see section on Special Issues).

A sheath worn over the penis can be traced as far back as 1350 B.C., when Egyptian men wore decorative covers for their penises. In 1564 A.D., Fallopius first described linen sheaths used to protect against syphilis.[4] Protective sheaths were made from dried animal intestines in the 18th century, when according to some sources, they were first given the name "condom," presumably after inventor Colonel Cundum.[5] The advent of vulcanized rubber in 1843 led to the mass production of condoms made from natural rubber latex.[5] In the past two decades, manufacturers also began to use synthetic materials (e.g., polyurethane) to develop new condom options for both men and women. (For more information on female condoms, see Chapter 14 on Vaginal Barriers and Spermicides.)

CONDOM OPTIONS

Male condoms are available in a variety of shapes, colors, and thicknesses, as well as with or without lubricants or spermicides, and with or without reservoir-tip or nipple-ends. Condoms can be straight-sided or tapered toward the closed end, textured (e.g., ribbed) or smooth, solid-colored or nearly transparent, and odorless or scented or flavored. Most condoms are about 7 inches (180 mm) long, 2 inches (52 mm) wide, and up to 0.003 inches (0.08 mm) thick.

Male condoms are made from three types of material—latex, natural membrane, and synthetic (Table 13–1). More than 80% of male condoms commercially available in the United States are manufactured from natural rubber latex ("rubber" condoms).[6] A small proportion (<5%) is made from the intestinal caecum of lambs ("natural skin," "natural membrane," or "lambskin" condoms). Unlike latex condoms, natural membrane condoms contain small pores that may permit the passage of viruses, including hepatitis B virus, herpes simplex virus, and HIV.[7,8] Because of this porosity, natural membrane condoms may not provide the

Table 13–1 Characteristics of latex, natural membrane, and synthetic condoms

Type	Latex	Natural Membrane	Synthetic
Material	Natural rubber	Lamb caecum	Polyurethane*
Lubricant use	Water-based only	Any	Any
Cost	Low	Moderate	Moderate/high
Recommended for prevention of pregnancy	Yes	Yes	Yes**
Recommended for prevention of STIs and HIV	Yes	No	Yes**

 * Most synthetic condoms currently available are made from polyurethane
** For latex sensitive or allergic persons

same level of protection against STIs as latex condoms.[9] No clinical data are available on the effectiveness of natural membrane condoms for STI prevention, however. The remaining 15% or so of male condoms are manufactured from polyurethane or other synthetic materials. Compared with latex condoms, synthetic condoms are generally more resistant to deterioration, have a longer shelf-life, and are compatible with use of both oil-based and water-based lubricants. For pregnancy prevention, synthetic male condoms have rates of failure similar to their latex counterparts.[10] The effectiveness of synthetic male condoms to prevent STIs has not been extensively studied, and FDA labeling restricts their recommended use to latex-sensitive or allergic persons; however, synthetic condoms are believed to provide STI protection similar to latex male condoms.

Spermicidal Condoms

Use of condoms lubricated with the spermicide nonoxynol-9 (N-9) is no longer recommended because of their higher cost, shorter shelf life, and lack of additive benefit as compared with other lubricated condoms.[11] Concerns have also been raised about genital ulceration and irritation resulting from high-frequency use of vaginal spermicidal N-9 products and the potential for facilitating transmission of STIs including HIV.[12] (See Chapter 14 on Vaginal Barriers and Spermicides.) Because the amount of N-9 contained in spermicidal condoms is much lower than that found in separately applied vaginal products,[13] spermicidal condoms are probably less likely to cause adverse effects; however, their use was associated with increased risk of urinary tract infections among young women in one study.[14]

In addition, other chemical products such as VivaGel have been proposed for coating condoms. No human data exist to support claims that adding chemicals to the outer coating of condoms provides any greater protection than uncoated condoms.

EFFECTIVENESS AGAINST PREGNANCY

Method failure of the male condom resulting in unintended pregnancy is uncommon. Of 100 couples using condoms, 2% are estimated to become pregnant during consistent and correct use during the first 12 months of use. (A summary of studies of contraceptive failure for the male condom, as well as a detailed discussion of the estimates used to derive these rates, can be found in Chapter 26 on Contraceptive Efficacy.)

Couples vary widely in their ability to use male condoms consistently and correctly. Among typical couples using condoms for contraception, about 18 of every 100 will become pregnant during the first year of typical use. The marked difference between the probabilities of pregnancy during typical use versus perfect use of condoms generally reflects errors in use, most notably the failure of couples to use condoms during every act of sexual intercourse. Several user behaviors, described later, likely contribute to the risk of unintended pregnancy and the transmission of infection despite condom use. Detailed instructions for condom use are provided at the end of this chapter.

CONDOM TESTING

Condoms are regulated as medical devices by the U.S. Food and Drug Administration (FDA), and manufacturing standards have become more stringent in recent years. Every condom is tested electronically for holes and weak spots before it is packaged and released for sale. Samples of condoms also undergo a series of additional laboratory tests for leakage, strength, dimensional requirements, and package integrity.[15] If the sample condoms fail any of these tests, the entire lot is rejected and destroyed to prevent access to the public. Imported condoms are required to comply with the same performance requirements as domestic condoms and should be equally safe. A 2009 Consumer Reports (CR) Survey showed that nearly all latex condoms tested met industry standards;[16] previous CR surveys have reported similar findings, while noting that test performance does not vary with price, thickness, or country of manufacture.[9]

ADVANTAGES AND INDICATIONS

Male condoms offer several noncontraceptive benefits to users.

1. **Protection against STIs.** When used consistently and correctly, condoms reduce the risk of many STIs, including HIV (see Spe-

cial Issues). By preventing STIs and their long-term sequelae, condoms also protect fertility

2. **Accessibility.** Usage does not require medical examination, prescription, or fitting.

3. **Low cost.** Condoms are among the most inexpensive and cost-effective contraceptives, especially considering the added protection against STIs. Condoms are available at low cost in both the private and public sectors and often for free from publicly funded programs.

4. **Delayed ejaculation.** For some men, condom use may help prolong intercourse and also prevent premature ejaculation.

5. **Portability.** Condoms can be easily and discretely carried by men or women, for example, in wallets or purses.

6. **Minimal side effects.** Because condoms are non-hormonal, they rarely cause medical problems among users. The most frequent side effect is most likely latex sensitivity; men or women with this condition can be directed to use synthetic condoms if STIs are of concern (see the section on Managing Problems and Follow-up in this chapter as well as chapter 4).

D ISADVANTAGES AND CAUTIONS
Male condoms also have disadvantages that may result in inconsistent or nonuse of the method.

1. **Reduced sensation.** Many men and their partners complain that condoms reduce sensitivity. Men should try different types of condoms to find ones that are most suitable for them.

2. **Lack of spontaneity.** Some men and their partners dislike interrupting foreplay to put on the condom and may find the coitally-dependent nature of condom use to be inconvenient.

3. **Problems with erection.** Some men cannot consistently maintain an erection during condom use, so condom use becomes unacceptable. In these cases, involving the partner in putting the condom on as part of foreplay may be helpful. Female condom use also may be appropriate (see Chapter 14 on Vaginal Barriers and Spermicides).

4. **Embarrassment and mistrust.** Some men and women may be embarrassed to obtain condoms or to suggest or initiate condom use because they perceive condom use implies a lack of trust or intimacy. Counsel clients (and partners, when possible) about their embarrassment and teach clients about condoms and how to negotiate their use. (See section on Providing Condoms—

Counseling). Encouraging clients to involve their partner in putting on the condom may help facilitate use.

5. **Lack of cooperation.** In some instances, men will not accept responsibility for contraception or prevention of infection, thus making male condom use impossible.

6. **Latex allergy.** Some men and women, especially health care workers repeatedly exposed to latex, may be allergic or sensitive to latex and thus unable to use latex condoms. Synthetic condoms are excellent alternatives.

SPECIAL ISSUES

Protection Against STIs and HIV

The primary noncontraceptive benefit of condom use is the protection conferred against STI. When placed on the penis before any genital contact and used throughout intercourse, condoms prevent direct contact with semen, genital lesions and subclinical viral shedding on the glans and shaft of the penis, and penile, vaginal, or anal discharges or infectious fluids. Condoms thus greatly reduce the risk of STIs that are transmitted primarily to or from the penile urethra (such as gonorrhea, chlamydia, trichomoniasis, hepatitis B infection, and HIV). Condoms also provide protection against STIs that are transmitted primarily through skin-to-skin contact or contact with mucosal surfaces (such as genital herpes, human papillomavirus [HPV], syphilis, and chancroid) to the extent that these areas are covered by the condom. Protection may be less when these STIs involve areas not covered by the condom.[13,17,18] In vitro laboratory studies indicate that latex condoms provide an effective physical barrier against passage of even the smallest sexually transmitted pathogen (hepatitis B). [7,8,19–25]

The level of protection for condoms is likely to vary for different STIs because STIs differ in their routes of transmission, as well as in their infectivity and prevalence.[26–28] Well-designed clinical studies of discordant couples (where one partner is infected and the other is not) have shown consistent use of latex condoms to be highly effective against heterosexual transmission of HIV infection, the most serious STI; thus, male condoms should be promoted to sexually active clients at risk for STI for this reason alone.[29] Two meta-analyses of these studies place the estimated effectiveness of consistent condom use between approximately 80% and 95%.[30,31]

Clinical studies of effectiveness against most other STIs suggest inconsistent protective effects for condoms.[17,19,28,32–35] Much of this inconsistency in estimates of the effectiveness of condom use can be attributed to limitations in study design, as the overall quality of clinical studies for these STIs is considerably weaker than for the HIV studies. Specifically, limitations in measurement of self-reported condom use and exposure to infected partners complicate interpretation of condom effectiveness estimates.[17,19,28,35-45] Recent studies and analyses[38,41,42,46-50] have empirically documented that effectiveness against many STIs is underestimated because of limitations in study design. Despite these limitations, studies and systematic reviews have found condom use to be associated with reduced risk of many STIs in addition to HIV, including gonorrhea, chlamydia, trichomoniasis, syphilis, genital herpes, HPV infection, and HPV-associated conditions.[28,32,33,34,35,45,51-68,109] We refer readers elsewhere for more extensive discussion of condom effectiveness for STI prevention.[17,28,35,37,67]

Condom Use During Anal and Oral Intercourse

Latex and synthetic condoms also can be used during anogenital and orogenital intercourse to reduce the risk of STI.[69] Latex sheets to be used for cunnilingus and anilingus have also been cleared by the FDA for over-the-counter sales, but no effectiveness data are available. Household plastic wrap (including the microwaveable variety) is another option for cunnilingus and anilingus, although it has not been manufactured or cleared by the FDA for medical applications, and no effectiveness data are available. Dental dams (or oral dams) and condoms adapted to form a barrier sheet have also been proposed as barriers for cunnilingus; however, their limited size may allow potentially infectious fluids to roll onto adjacent tissues, and these products also have not been evaluated or cleared by the FDA for this use.

CONDOM PROMOTION

Though general consensus holds that male condoms must play a central role in any STI/HIV prevention program,[70] the mix of condom promotion versus other prevention strategies (e.g., abstinence and mutual monogamy) remains controversial in many countries, including the United States. Condom promotion has been particularly controversial within specific settings and populations (e.g., adolescents).[71] Concerns also have been raised about the potential negative consequences of condom promotion,[72,73] because increased availability of condoms may not necessarily translate into sufficient use for effective STI prevention. For example, even among studies of heterosexual couples discordant for HIV or genital herpes simplex virus (HSV) for whom there is known risk for infection, fewer than half of couples report regular use of condoms.[30,31] Of increasing interest is whether interventions promoting condom use may result, paradoxically, in the onset or increased frequency of high-risk sexual activity, as hypothesized in some studies.[74,75]

No randomized controlled trials have evaluated whether such an effect exists or whether it outweighs the protective effects of condom use for persons at risk. However, a review of 174 condom-related prevention approaches concluded that interventions designed to reduce the risk of HIV infection do not increase unsafe sexual behavior.[76]

PROVIDING CONDOMS—COUNSELING

All clients should understand when to use condoms, how to use them most effectively, how to discuss condom use with their partner(s), and how to integrate condom use into intercourse:

Unintended pregnancy prevention. Advise men and women that condoms should be used with every act of intercourse regardless of cycle day because ovulation can occur on any cycle day.[77]

STI protection. Emphasize the need for condom use during all sexual activities that can transmit STIs and HIV. Recommend that clients use a new condom for each act of anal, vaginal, or oral intercourse when any risk of infection exists.[69] (See the section on Effectiveness against STIs and HIV.)

Dual method use. Encourage clients to use a condom plus another contraceptive. This could dramatically reduce the risk of both pregnancy and STI.[78] Use caution when recommending dual method use to clients, because simultaneous use of multiple methods can be overly cumbersome for some couples; instead they may opt to use no method of contraception at all. Follow the client's lead and perhaps suggest a brief trial period of dual method use. If this proves difficult for the client, consider recommending consistent and correct use of condoms alone to provide adequate protection against both pregnancy and infection. Emergency contraception can be used as a backup method against pregnancy in case a condom breaks, falls off, or is not used.

Tailored counseling. Adapt counseling messages on condom use to each client's needs. Clients may have formed their own attitudes about condom use and may have had varying experiences with condoms. Tailor the counseling session to each client's risk factors, abilities, needs, and readiness to change.[79]

Communication of pregnancy rates. Ensure clients choosing contraceptive methods (including condoms) understand the risks and benefits of the range of methods available. Although the ability to prevent pregnancy is often mentioned as the single most important criterion considered when choosing a method,[80-83] clients may have difficulty understanding typical use and perfect use pregnancy rates across methods.[82] Because clients may find it difficult to understand contraceptive failure rates, show them a scale of the relative effectiveness of contraceptives, as shown in Figure 3–1 (see Chapter 3 on Choosing a Contraceptive

Method). Consider using a similar approach when counseling clients about the ability of condoms to prevent STIs, including HIV (see the section on Protection Against STIs and HIV).

Personal benefits. Make sure clients understand how condom use benefits them personally. Explain that condoms protect future fertility by preventing long-term sequelae of STIs. (See Chapter 21 on Reproductive Tract Infections.) Strongly encourage pregnant women at high risk for STIs to use condoms to protect their fetus, their partner(s), and themselves.

Partner negotiation. Teach clients how to negotiate condom use with partners. Many clients may have contemplated using condoms but may be uncomfortable suggesting condom use to their partners. Teach clients how to negotiate condom use with their partner(s), and help them develop replies they can use when a partner objects to condoms. Assess the likelihood of a partner's negative reaction to the suggestion of condom use; some clients fear that they will be abused or abandoned if they insist on using condoms. Counsel or refer as appropriate if you detect battering or other forms of abuse. It is particularly important that a condom be available and its use agreed upon in advance by both partners.

Effective use. Make sure clients understand how to use condoms effectively. Emphasize that condoms are most effective when used correctly during every act of intercourse. Assessing condom use among clients is a two-tiered process. First ask clients how often they are using condoms (e.g., always, most of the time, sometimes, never). Then, to recognize potential misuse, ask clients to explain (and perhaps demonstrate on an appropriate model of a penis) how they use condoms. (See sections on Increasing Effective Use and Instructions for Condom Use.) Encourage clients to use condoms consistently and correctly with every act of anal, vaginal, and oral intercourse.

Suitability. Offer to help clients select a condom most suitable to their needs, which may include the female condom. Some clinics now provide a variety of condoms to clients, although one study[84] found that providing a choice of condoms increased acceptability but had no impact on levels of use or STI.

Practice. Encourage clients to practice using condoms. Many problems that occur during condom use can be attributed to inexperience[83] and can be overcome with practice. Users who have had negative experiences with condoms may be at risk of discontinuing condom use altogether[85]; encourage them to continue practicing with condoms. When providing instruction on how to use condoms, have the client unroll a condom onto a model of a penis or similarly shaped object (e.g., banana), both with eyes open and then again in the dark.

Provision of condoms. Provide each client a large number of condoms at low or no cost. Providing clients with a few condoms is only a short-term solution for clients who find the health care system inaccessible or who find it embarrassing to return repeatedly for condoms. Selling condoms, even at a low cost, dramatically reduces the number of condoms clients will obtain from a clinic compared with the number of free condoms they will take.

STRATEGIES FOR INCREASING EFFECTIVE CONDOM USE

Condom effectiveness depends heavily on the skill level and experience of the user.[17] Studies have documented relatively high levels of problems with condom use that may reduce their effectiveness, many of which can be minimized with appropriate counseling and practice. Interventions promoting condom use should address user-related behaviors that result in exposure to STIs and pregnancy, including the following:

1. **Failure to use condoms with every act of intercourse.** Nonuse of condoms, rather than poor condom quality or other condom-related problems, is the most common problem.[86,87] The highest single priority for any STI/HIV prevention program should be to address factors that lead to nonuse of condoms, including lack of device acceptability, poor skills for negotiating use with partners, and latex allergy or sensitivity. New strategies that emphasize condom use for contraception in addition to disease prevention[70] may help decrease nonuse. Persons at risk should be provided with an adequate supply of condoms at low or no cost.

2. **Failure to use condoms throughout intercourse.** Recent studies have documented that some men put condoms on after starting intercourse or remove condoms prior to ejaculation.[40,49,50,88–90] These behaviors represent product misuse and could expose partners to risk of pregnancy or STI despite condom use. Clients should be counseled to use condoms every time throughout intercourse, from beginning to end.

3. **Condom breakage and slippage.** Although users often fear that the condom will break or fall off during use, these events are rare with proper use and tend to be concentrated among a small proportion of users.[78] Most studies show that during vaginal sex, condoms break approximately 2 percent of the time during intercourse or withdrawal and a similar proportion slip off completely.[91–95] However, higher rates of breakage and slippage have been reported in a few studies.[96,97] Reviews of studies evaluating breakage and slippage during anal intercourse indicate that the rates may be slightly higher than during vaginal intercourse.[98–100] Advise users to have several condoms available in

Table 13–2 Examples of lubricant products that should and should not be used with natural rubber latex condoms[a]

Safe	Not safe
Egg whites	Baby oil
Glycerine	Cold creams
Saliva	Edible oils (olive, peanut, corn, sunflower)
Silicone	Hand and body lotions
Spermicides	Massage oil
Water	Petroleum jelly
Water-based lubricants (e.g., K-Y Jelly, Astroglide)	Rubbing alcohol
	Suntan oil and lotions
	Vegetable or mineral oil
	Vaginal infection medications in cream or suppository form

[a] All lubricants, including oil-based products, may generally be used with polyurethane condoms, although they may not be compatible with all synthetic condoms.

case a condom is torn or put on incorrectly, or repeated intercourse is desired.

4. **Improper lubricant use with latex condoms.** Unlike water-based lubricants (e.g., K-Y Jelly), oil-based lubricants (e.g., petroleum jelly, baby oil, and hand lotions) reduce latex condom integrity[101] and may facilitate breakage (see Table 13–2). People may use oil-based products as condom lubricants, mistaking them for water-based lubricants because they readily wash off with water. Because vaginal medications (e.g., for yeast infections) often contain oil-based ingredients that can damage latex condoms, advise clients to remain abstinent or use synthetic condoms until the medication is fully completed and the infection is cured. Note that oil-based products generally can be safely used as lubricants with polyurethane condoms, although they may not be compatible with all synthetic condoms.

MANAGING PROBLEMS AND FOLLOW-UP

Persons sensitive or allergic to natural rubber latex may experience irritation, allergic contact dermatitis, or systemic anaphylactic symptoms when exposed to latex-containing products.[102,103] While 1% to 6% of the U.S. population were previously estimated to be allergic to latex,[96] the prevalence of latex sensitivity is thought to be much higher among health care workers who have repeated exposure to latex-containing medical devices (e.g., surgical and examination gloves, catheters, intubation tubes, anesthesia masks, and dental dams).[102-104] Proteins in the latex appear to be the primary source of allergic reactions. All clients should be questioned for potential latex allergy.[103,104] Ask whether the client experiences itching, rash, or wheezing after wearing latex gloves or inflating a balloon.[104] If you suspect a client has generalized latex sensitivity, consider recommending synthetic condoms and refer the client for allergy skin testing.[105] While latex condom use is contraindicated for clients with general latex sensitivity, both synthetic and natural membrane condoms can be recommended for prevention of pregnancy, while only synthetic condoms should be recommended for prevention of STIs, including HIV.

Allergic reactions that occur only after exposure to latex condoms and not after exposure to other latex-containing products may be attributable to brand-specific condom attributes such as spermicides, lubricants, perfumes, local anesthetics, or other chemical agents added during the manufacturing process.[106] Advise clients to try different brands of latex and synthetic condoms. In any case, clients should immediately contact their health care provider for follow-up if they or their partner(s) experience a severe allergic reaction while using latex condoms or spermicides. Additional comprehensive information on latex allergy can also be obtained from the American Latex Allergy Association (see www.latexallergyresources.org). When counseling men and women about condom use, providers should bear in mind the possibility that client reports of latex sensitivity or allergy may in fact represent a simple dislike for condoms.

U SER INSTRUCTIONS FOR CONDOMS

Instructions for condom use are often overcomplicated and may have no scientific basis.[107] During a World Health Organization Experts Meeting (Geneva, June 22–24, 2005) to develop a Global Handbook for Family Planning Providers, consensus was reached on five key condom instructions.[17]

Five Key Instructions for Condom Use
1. Use a new condom for each act of intercourse if any risk of pregnancy or STI exists.
2. Before any genital contact, place the condom on the tip of the erect penis with the rolled side out.
3. Unroll the condom all the way to the base of the erect penis.
4. Immediately after ejaculation, hold the rim of the condom and withdraw the penis while it is still erect.
5. Throw away the used condom safely.

Updated, more detailed instructions for using condoms are included below:

Before Intercourse

1. Have on hand an adequate supply of latex or synthetic condoms and water-based lubricant if you think you may need to use a condom, even if you plan to use another contraceptive. Have extra condoms available in case the first is damaged, torn before use, or put on incorrectly. You will need a new condom if you have repeated intercourse.

2. Discuss condom use with your partner before you have intercourse.

At Time of Intercourse

1. Open the condom package carefully to avoid damaging it with fingernails, teeth, or other sharp objects.

2. Put on the condom before the penis comes in contact with the partner.

3. Unroll the condom a short distance to make sure the condom is being unrolled in the correct direction. Then hold the tip of the condom and unroll it down to the base of the erect penis. If the condom does not unroll easily, you probably put it on inside-out. Discard the condom and begin with a new one, because flipping it over and using it could expose your partner to infectious organisms contained in the pre-ejaculate.

4. Adequate lubrication is important. For latex condoms, use only water-based lubricants like water, lubricating jellies (e.g., K-Y Jelly), or spermicidal lubricants, jellies, foam, or suppositories. Avoid oil-based lubricants like cold cream, mineral oil, cooking oil, petroleum jelly, body lotions, massage oil, or baby oil, which can damage latex condoms (see Table 13–2).

5. Keep the condom on the penis until after intercourse. If the condom breaks or falls off during intercourse but before ejaculation, stop and put on a new condom. Use a new condom when you have prolonged intercourse, and when you have different types of intercourse within a single session (e.g., after anal sex, change the condom before having vaginal sex to decrease the risk of urinary tract infection).

After Intercourse

1. Soon after ejaculation, withdraw the penis while it is still erect. Hold the condom firmly against the base of the penis to prevent slippage and leakage of semen.

2. Check the condom for visible damage such as holes, then wrap it in tissue and discard. Do not flush condoms down the toilet.

3. If the condom breaks, falls off, leaks, is damaged, or is not used, the following may help:

   — Discuss the possibility of pregnancy or infection with your partner and contact your health care provider as soon as you can. Do not douche. Emergency contraception, now available without a prescription for persons aged 17 years and older, may be used to prevent pregnancy if it is started within 120 hours of having unprotected intercourse. Go to www.not-2-late.com to learn more about emergency contraception. (See Chapter 6 on Emergency Contraception.)

   — Gently wash the penis, vulva, anus, and adjacent areas with soap and water immediately after intercourse to help reduce the risk of acquiring an STI. Then insert an applicator full of spermicide into the vagina as soon as possible.

Repeated Intercourse

1. Use a new condom from "beginning to end" with each act of anal, vaginal, or oral intercourse. Do not reuse condoms.

Taking Care of Supplies

1. Store condoms in a cool and dry place out of direct sunlight (excessive heat will weaken latex). Latex condoms can probably be stored in a wallet for a short period of time (e.g., up to 1 month) when kept away from heat and sunlight.[108]

2. Check the expiration or manufacture date on the box or individual package of condoms. Expiration dates are marked as "Exp"; otherwise, the date is the manufacture date (MFG). Latex condoms should not be used beyond their expiration date or more than 5 years after the manufacturing date. Condoms in damaged packages or that show obvious signs of deterioration (e.g., brittleness, stickiness, or discoloration) should not be used regardless of their expiration date.

REFERENCES

1. Mosher WD, Jones J. Use of Contraception in the United States: 1982–2008. National Center for Health Statistics. Vital Health Stat. 2010;23(29). Available from http://www.cdc.gov/NCHS/data/series/sr_23/sr23_029.pdf [accessed October 4, 2010].

2. Centers for Disease Control and Prevention. Trends in HIV- and STD-related risk behaviors among high school students—United States, 1991–2007. MMWR. 2008;57: 817–22.

3. Mosher WD, Martinez GM, Chandra A, Abma JC, Willson SJ. Use of contraception and use of family planning services in the United States, 1982–2002. Advance data from vital and health statistics; no 350. Hyattsville, Maryland: National Center for Health Statistics. 2004.

4. Valdiserri RO. Cum hastis sic clypeatis: the turbulent history of the condom. Bull NY Acad Med. 1988;64:237–245.

5. Murphy JS. The condom industry in the United States, 1990. Jefferson NC: McFarland & Company, Inc., Publishers, 1990.

6. Global Industry Analysts, Inc. Condoms: A global business strategic report. San Jose, CA, March 2008, Publication # MCP-3209.

7. Carey RF, Lytle CD, Cyr WH. Implications of laboratory tests of condom integrity. Sex Transm Dis. 1999;26:216–220.

8. Lytle CD, Routson LB, Seaborn GB, et al. An in vitro evaluation of condoms as barriers to a small virus. Sex Transm Dis. 1997;24:161–164.

9. Consumer's Union: Condoms: Extra protection. Consumer Reports. 2005: February.

10. Gallo M, Grimes D, Lopez L, Schulz K. Non-latex versus latex male condoms for contraception. Cochrane Database Syst Rev. 2006; 1:CD003550.

11. Centers for Disease Control and Prevention. Nonoxynol-9 spermicide contraception use—United States 1999. MMWR. 2002;51:389–92.

12. Centers for Disease Control and Prevention. CDC statement on study results of products containing nonoxynol-9. MMWR. 2000;49:717–718.

13. Centers for Disease Control and Prevention. Sexually transmitted diseases treatment guidelines 2002. MMWR. 2002;51(No. RR-6).

14. Fihn SD, Boyko EJ, Normand EH, et al. Association between use of spermicide coated condoms and Escherichia coli urinary tract infection in young women. Am J Epidemiol. 1996;144:512–20.

15. ASTM (American Society for Testing Materials). Annual book of ASTM standards: Easton MD: ASTM: section 9, rubber. Volume 09.02 Rubber products; standard specifications for rubber contraceptives (male condoms-D3492). West Conshohocken, PA: American Society for Testing Materials, 1996.

16. Consumer Union: Seven of 20 condoms tested earn perfect score: Extra protection. Consumer Reports. 2009; December.

17. Steiner MJ, Warner L, Stone KM, Cates W Jr. Condoms and other barrier methods for prevention of STD/HIV infection, and pregnancy. In: Holmes KK, Sparling PF, Mardh P-A (editors). Sexually Transmitted Diseases, 4th ed. New York, NY: MacGraw-Hill, 2008.

18. Stone KM, Thomas E, Timyan J. Barrier methods for the prevention of sexually transmitted diseases. In: Holmes KK, Sparling FP, Mardh PA (editors). Sexually Transmitted Diseases, 3rd edition. New York: McGraw-Hill, 1998.

19. National Institute of Allergy and Infectious Diseases. Workshop summary: scientific evidence on condom effectiveness for sexually transmitted diseases prevention. July 20, 2001. www.niaid.nih.gov/dmid/stds/condomreport.pdf [Accessed October 27, 2010.]

20. Carey RF, Herman WA, Retta SM, et al. Effectiveness of latex condoms as a barrier to human immunodeficiency virus-sized particles under conditions of simulated use. Sex Transm Dis. 1992;19:230–4.

21. Conant MA, Spicer DW, Smith CD. Herpes simplex virus transmission: condom studies. Sex Transm Dis. 1984;11:94–5.

22. Katznelson S, Drew WL, Mintz L. Efficacy of the condom as a barrier to the transmission of cytomegalovirus. J Infect Dis. 1984;150:155–7.

23. Rietmeijer CA, Krebs JW, Feorina PM, et al. Condoms as physical and chemical barriers against human immunodeficiency virus. JAMA. 1988;259:1851–1853.

24. Van de Perre P, Jacobs D, Sprecher-Goldberger S. The latex condom, an efficient barrier against sexual transmission of AIDS-related viruses. AIDS. 1987;1:49–52

25. Judson FN, Ehret JM, Bodin GF, Levin MJ, Rietmeijer CA. In vitro evaluations of condoms with and without nonoxynol 9 as physical and chemical barriers against Chlamydia trachomatis, herpes simplex virus type 2, and human immunodeficiency virus. Sex Transm Dis. 1989; 16:51–6.

26. Cates W Jr. The condom forgiveness factor: the positive spin. Sex Transm Dis. 2002;29:350–2.

27. Mann JR, Stine CC, Vessey J. The role of disease-specific infectivity and number of disease exposures on long-term effectiveness of the latex condom. Sex Transm Dis. 2002;29:344–9.

28. Warner L, Stone KM, Macaluso M, Buehler J, Austin HD. A systematic review of design factors assessed in epidemiologic studies of condom effectiveness for preventing gonorrhea and chlamydia. Sex Transm Dis. 2006;33:36–51.

29. Cates W Jr. The NIH condom report: the glass is 90% full. Fam Plann Perspect. 2001;33:231–3.

30. Weller S, Davis K. Condom effectiveness in reducing heterosexual HIV transmission. Cochrane Database Syst Rev. 2001;(3):CD003255.

31. Pinkerton SD, Abramson PR. Effectiveness of condoms in preventing HIV transmission. Soc Sci Med. 1997;44:1303–1312

32. d'oro LC, Parazzini F, Naldi L, et al. Barrier methods of contraception, spermicides, and sexually transmitted diseases: A review. Genitourin Med. 1994;70:410.

33. Manhart LE, Koutsky LA. Do condoms prevent genital HPV infection, external genital warts, or cervical neoplasia? A meta-analysis. Sex Transm Dis. 2002; 29:725–35.

34. Centers for Disease Control and Prevention. Report to Congress: prevention of genital human papillomavirus infection, January 2004.

35. Holmes KK, Levine R, Weaver M. Effectiveness of condom in preventing sexually transmitted infections. Bull WHO. 2004; 84:454–461.

36. Aral SO, Peterman TA. Measuring outcomes of behavioural interventions for STD/HIV prevention. Int J STD AIDS. 1996;7 Suppl 2:30–8.

37. Crosby R, DiClemente RJ, Holtgrave DR, Wingood GM. Design, measurement, and analytical considerations for testing hypotheses relative to condom effectiveness against non-viral STIs. Sex Transm Inf. 2002;78:228–31.

38. Devine OJ, Aral SO. The impact of inaccurate reporting of condom use and imperfect diagnosis of sexually transmitted disease infection in studies of condom effectiveness: a simulation-based assessment. Sex Transm Dis. 2004;31:588–95.

39. Steiner MJ, Feldblum PJ, Padian N. Invited commentary: condom effectiveness—will prostate specific antigen shed new light on this perplexing problem: Am J Epidemiol. 2003;157:298–300.

40. Warner L, Clay-Warner J, Boles J, Williamson J. Assessing condom use practices. Implications for evaluating method and user effectiveness. Sex Transm Dis. 1998; 25:273–7.

41. Warner L, Macaluso M, Austin HD, et al. Application of the case-crossover design to reduce unmeasured confounding in studies of condom effectiveness. Am J Epidemiol. 2005;161:765–73.

42. Warner L, Newman DR, Austin HD, et al. Condom effectiveness for reducing transmission of gonorrhea and chlamydia: the importance of assessing partner infection.

43. Warner L, Macaluso M, Newman DR, et al. Re: Condom effectiveness for prevention of chlamydia trachomatis infection. Sex Transm Inf. 2006;82:265.

44. Zenilman JM, Weisman CS, Rompalo AM, et al. Condom use to prevent incident STDs: the validity of self-reported condom use. Sex Transm Dis. 1995;22:15–21.

45. Koss CA, Dunne EF. Warner L. A systematic review of epidemiologic studies assessing condom use and risk of syphilis. Sex Transm Dis. 2009;36:401–5.

46. Niccolai L, Rowhani-Rahbar A, Jenkins H, et al. Condom effectiveness for prevention of Chlamydia trachomatis infection. Sex Transm Inf. 2005;81:323–5.

47. Shlay JC, McClung MW, Patnaik JL, Douglas JM Jr. Comparison of sexually transmitted disease prevalence by reported condom use: errors among consistent condom users seen at an urban sexually transmitted disease clinic. Sex Transm Dis. 2004; 31:526–32.

48. Shlay JC, McClung MW, Patnaik JL, Douglas JM Jr. Comparison of sexually transmitted disease prevalence by reported level of condom use among patients attending an urban sexually transmitted disease clinic. Sex Transm Dis. 2004;31:154–160.

49. Paz-Bailey G, Koumans EH, Sternberg M, et al. The effect of correct and consistent condom use on chlamydial and gonococcal infection among urban adolescents. Arch Pediatr Adolesc Med. 2005;159:536–42

50. Warner L, Newman DR, Kamb ML, Fishbein M, Douglas JM Jr., Zenilman J, D'Anna L, Bolan G, Rogers J, Peterman TA, Project RESPECT Study Group. Problems with condom use among patients attending sexually transmitted disease clinics: prevalence, predictors, and relation to incident gonorrhea and chlamydia. Am J Epidemiol. 2008;167:341–49.

51. Winer RL, Hughes JP, Feng Q, et al. Condom use and the papillomavirus infection in young women. N Engl J Med. 2006;354:2645–2654.

52. Casper C, Wald A. Condom use and the prevention of genital herpes acquisition. Herpes. 2002;9:10–4.

53. Wald A, Langenberg AG, Krantz, et al. The relationship between condom use and herpes simplex virus acquisition. Ann Intern Med. 2005;143:707–713.

54. Wald A, Langenberg AG, Link K, et al. Effect of condoms on reducing the transmission of herpes simplex virus type 2 from men to women. JAMA. 2001;285:3100–6.

55. Barlow D. The condom and gonorrhoea. Lancet. 1977;222:811–812.

56. Ramstedt K, Forssman L, Giesecke J, Granath F. Risk factors for Chlamydia trachomatis in 6810 young women attending family planning clinics. Int J STD AIDS. 1992; 3:117–122.

57. Upchurch DM, Brady WE, Reichart CA, Hook EW III. Behavioral contributions to acquisition of gonorrhea in patients attending an inner-city sexually transmitted disease clinic. J Infect Dis. 1990;161:938–941.

58. Fennema JSA, van Ameijden EJC, Coutinho RA, van Den Hoek A. Clinical sexually transmitted diseases among human immunodeficiency virus-infected and noninfected drug-using prostitutes. Associated factors and interpretation of trends, 1986 to 1994. Sex Transm Dis. 1997;24:363–371.

59. Levine WC, Revollo R, Kaune V, et al. Decline in sexually transmitted disease prevalence in female Bolivian sex workers: impact of an HIV prevention project. AIDS. 1998;12:1899–1906.

60. Hooper RR, Reynolds GH, Jones OG, et al. Cohort study of venereal disease. I: the risk of gonorrhea transmission from infected women to men. Am J Epidemiol. 1978;108:136–144.

61. Baeten JM, Nyange PM, Richardson BA, et al. Hormonal contraception and risk of sexually transmitted disease acquisition: results from a prospective study. Am J Obstet Gynecol. 2001;185:380–5.

62. Cates W Jr., Holmes KK. Re: condom efficacy against gonorrhea and nongonococcal urethritis. Am J Epidemiol. 1996;143:843–844.

63. Sanchez J, Gutuzzo E, Escamilla J. Sexually transmitted infections in female sex workers: reduced by condom use but not by a limited periodic examination program. Sex Transm Dis. 1998;25:82–89.

64. Schwartz MA, Lafferty WE, Hughes JP, Handsfield HH. Risk factors for urethritis in heterosexual men. Sex Transm Dis .1997;24:449–455.

65. Hogewoning CJ, Bleeker MC, van den Brule AJ, et al. Condom use promotes regression of cervical intraepithelial neoplasia and clearance of human papillomavirus: a randomized clinical trial. Int J Cancer. 2003;107:811–6.

66. Bleeker MC, Hogewoning CJ, Voorhorst FJ, et al. Condom use promotes regression of human papillomavirus-associated penile lesions in male sexual partners of women with cervical intraepithelial neoplasia. Int J Cancer. 2003;107:804–10.
67. Alfonsi GA, Shlay J. The effectiveness of condoms for the prevention of sexually transmitted diseases. Current Women's Health Reviews. 2005;1:151–9.
68. Nielson CM, Harris RB, Nyitray AG, Dunne EF, Stone KM, Giuliano AR. Consistent condom use is associated with lower HPV prevalence in men. J Inf Dis., in press.
69. Centers for Disease Control and Prevention. Sexually transmitted diseases treatment guidelines 2010. MMWR 2010;59 (No. RR-12).
70. Halperin DT, Steiner MJ, Cassell MM, et al. The time has come for common ground on preventing sexual transmission of HIV. Lancet. 2004; 364:1913–5.
71. American Academy of Pediatrics, Committee on Adolescence. Condom use by adolescents. Pediatrics. 2001;107:1463–9.
72. Richens J, Imrie J, Copas A. Condoms and seat belts: the parallels and the lessons. Lancet. 2000;355:400–3.
73. Cassell MM, Halperin DT, Shelton JD, Stanton, D. Risk compensation: the Achilles' heel of innovations in HIV prevention? BMJ. 2006;332:605–7.
74. Kajubi P, Kamya MR, Kamya S, et al. Increasing condom use without reducing HIV risk: results of a controlled community trial in Uganda. J Acquir Immune Defic Syndr. 2005;40:77–82.
75. Imrie J, Stephenson JM, Cowan FM, et al. A cognitive behavioural intervention to reduce sexually transmitted infections among gay men: randomised trial. BMJ. 2001;322:1451–1456.
76. Smoak ND, Scott-Sheldon LA, Johnson BT, Cary MP. Sexual risk reduction interventions do not inadvertently increase the overall frequency of sexual behavior: A metaanalysis of 174 studies with 116,735 participants. J Acquir Immune Defic Syndro. 2006;41:374–384.
77. Wilcox AJ, Dunson DB, Weinberg CR, Trussell J, Baird DD. Likelihood of conception with a single act of intercourse: providing benchmark rates for assessment of postcoital contraceptives. Contraception. 2001;63:211–5.
78. Cates W Jr., Steiner MJ. Dual protection against unintended pregnancy and sexually transmitted infections: What is the best contraceptive approach? Sex Transm Dis. 2002;29:168–174.
79. Centers for Disease Control and Prevention. Revised guidelines for HIV counseling, testing and referral. MMWR. 2001;50:1–58.
80. Grady WR, Klepinger DH, Nelson-Wally A. Contraceptive characteristics: the perceptions and priorities of men and women. Fam Plann Perspect. 1999;31:168–75.
81. Edwards JE, Oldman A, Smith L, et al. Women's knowledge of, and attitudes to, contraceptive effectiveness and adverse health effects. Br J Fam Plann. 2000;26:73–80.
82. Steiner MJ, Dalebout S, Condon S, et al. Understanding risk: a randomized controlled trial of communicating contraceptive effectiveness. Obstet Gynecol. 2003;102:709–17.
83. Steiner M, Piedrahita C, Glover L, Joanis C. Can condom users likely to experience condom failure be identified? Fam Plann Perspect. 1993;25:220–223,226.
84. Steiner MJ, Hylton-Kong T, Figueroa JP, et al. Does a choice of condoms impact sexually transmitted infection incidence? A randomized, controlled trial. Sex Transm Dis. 2006;33:31–35.
85. Norris AE, Ford K. Associations between condom experiences and beliefs, intentions, and use in a sample of urban, low-income, African-American and Hispanic youth. AIDS Educ Prev. 1994;6:27–39.
86. Steiner MJ, Cates W Jr, Warner L. The real problem with male condoms is nonuse. Sex Transm Dis. 1999;26:459–62.
87. Warner L, Steiner MJ. Condom access does not ensure condom use: you've got to be putting me on. Sex Transm Inf. 2002;78:225.
88. Fishbein M, Pequegnat W. Evaluating AIDS prevention interventions using behavioral and biological outcome measures. Sex Transm Dis. 2000; 27:101–10.

89. Calzavara L, Burchell AN, Remis RS, et al. Delayed application of condoms is a risk factor for human immunodeficiency virus infection among homosexual and bisexual men. Am J Epidemiol. 2003;157:210–17.

90. Crosby RA, Sanders SA, Yarber WL, et al. Condom use errors and problems among college men. Sex Transm Dis. 2002;29:552–7.

91. Albert AE, Warner DL, Hatcher RA, Trussell J, Bennett C. Condom use among female commercial sex workers in Nevada's legal brothels. Am J Publ Health. 1995; 85:1514–1520.

92. Cook L, Nanda K, Taylor D. Randomized crossover trial comparing the eZ.on plastic condom and a latex condom. Contraception. 2001; 63:25–31.

93. Valappil T, Kelaghan J, Macaluso M, et al. Female condom and male condom failure among women at high risk of sexually transmitted diseases. Sex Transm Dis. 2005;32:35–43.

94. Macaluso M, Kelaghan J, Artz L, et al. Mechanical failure of the latex condom in a cohort of women at high STD risk. Sex Transm Dis. 1999;26:450–8.

95. Walsh TL, Frezieres RG, Peacock K, et al. Effectiveness of the male latex condom: combined results for three popular condom brands used as controls in randomized clinical trials. Contraception. 2004;70:407–13.

96. Mukenge-Tshibaka L, Alary M, Geraldo N, Lowndes CM. Incorrect condom use and frequent breakage among female sex workers and their clients. Int J STD AIDS. 2005;16:345–7.

97. Russell-Brown P, Piedrahita C, Foldesy R, et al. Comparison of condom breakage during human use with performance in laboratory testing. Contraception. 1992; 45:429–37.

98. Silverman BG, Gross TP. Use and effectiveness of condoms during anal intercourse. A review. Sex Transm Dis. 1997;24:11–7.

99. Richters J, Kippax S. Condoms for anal sex. In: Mindel A, editor. Condoms. First ed. London: BMJ Publishing Group, 2000, 132–146.

100. McBride KR, Fortenberry JD. Heterosexual anal sexuality and anal sex behaviors: a review. J Sex Research. 2010;47:123–35.

101. Voeller B, Coulson AH, Bernstein GS, Nakamura RM. Mineral oil lubricants cause rapid deterioration of latex condoms. Contraception .1989; 39:(1)95–102. 0010–7824.

102. Zaza S, Reeder JM, Charles LE, Jarvis WR. Latex sensitivity among perioperative nurses. AORN. 1994;60:806–812.

103. National Institute for Occupational Safety and Health. Preventing allergic reactions to natural rubber latex in the workplace [NIOSH alert]. National Institute for Occupational Safety and Health, June 1997 [DHHS (NIOSH) publication No. 97–135].

104. Food and Drug Administration. Allergic reactions to latex-containing medical devices [press release]. Rockville MD; Food and Drug Administration, March 29, 1991.

105. Yassin MS, Lierl MB, Fischer TJ, et al. Latex allergy in hospital employees. Ann Allergy. 1994;72:245–249.

106. Hamann CP, Kick SA. Update: immediate and delayed hypersensitivity to natural rubber latex. Cutis. 1993;52:307–311.

107. Spencer B, Gerofi J. Can we tell them how to do it? In: Mindel A, editor. Condoms. First ed. London: BMJ Publishing Group, 2000, 207–219.

108. Glasser G, Hatcher RA. The effect on condom integrity of carrying a condom in a wallet for three months [abstract]. Proceedings of the American College of Obstetricians and Gynecologists District IV Conference, November 1992. San Juan PR.

LATE REFERENCE

109. Martin ET, Krantz E, Gottlieb SC, et al. A pooled analysis of the effect of condoms in preventing HSV-2 acquisition. Arch Intern Med. 2009;169:1233–1240.

Vaginal Barriers and Spermicides

Willard Cates Jr., MD, MPH
Bryna Harwood, MD, MS

- Female condoms are a good alternative to male condoms and are a female-initiated contraceptive.

- Spermicides are a less effective method of contraception, but they avoid the use of hormones or the need for invasive procedures.

- Although these methods are relatively simple to use, they require more instruction and counseling from providers than do other methods.

- A variety of barrier methods and spermicide formulations are available, but they require ongoing motivation by the user to be effective.

- All of these methods can be initiated, inserted, and removed by the user, giving greater control in their use to women rather than to their providers or partners.

The use of vaginal barriers and spermicidal agents to prevent pregnancy dates back to antiquity, resulting in a diversity of products and formulations in the modern era. However despite development of several new products, the technology has changed little in recent decades. Most vaginal barriers are intended to be used with a spermicidal agent, and require a provider to fit and prescribe. The female condom is the exception. First approved by the U.S. Food and Drug Administration (FDA) in 1993 for over-the-counter sale in the United States, it does not require a spermicidal agent. Spermicidal products containing nonoxynol-9 (N-9) can also be purchased without prescription in pharmacies and supermarkets. They can be used alone, with a vaginal barrier method, or as an adjunct to any of the other contraceptive methods for added protection against pregnancy.

MECHANISM OF ACTION

All vaginal barriers and spermicides prevent fertilization by interfering with sperm transport into the female upper genital track.[1] Vaginal barriers work by mechanically blocking or killing sperm. The female condom provides a physical barrier that lines the vagina and partially shields the perineum without the use of any spermicidal agent. All other vaginal barriers combine both a physical barrier, to prevent sperm entry into the cervical canal, and a chemical, to kill sperm. The diaphragm and the cervical cap hold the spermicidal agent in place in front of the cervix.

Spermicidal preparations consist of two components: 1) a formulation (gel, foam, sponge, cream, film, suppository, or tablet), also called a carrier or base; and 2) a chemical that kills the sperm in different doses and concentrations. The sponge additionally absorbs and traps sperm in its spongy matrix that contains the spermicidal agent. For other products, the formulation helps disperse the spermicide in the vagina. In the case of viscous gel and foam, the formulation itself may provide both lubrication and an additional barrier effect. The active chemical agent in spermicide products available in the United States, nonoxynol-9 (N-9), is a surfactant that destroys the sperm cell membrane. Other surfactant products, including menfegol and benzalkonium chloride, are available in other parts of the world but are not licensed in the United States.

VAGINAL BARRIERS

The following products are currently available in the United States (Table 14–1).

Female Condoms. The Reality Female Condom (FC1) is a soft, loose-fitting polyurethane sheath, 7.8 cm in diameter and 17 cm long. It contains two flexible polyurethane rings. One smaller ring lies inside the vagina, at the closed end of the sheath, and serves as an insertion mechanism and internal anchor. The wider ring forms the external open end of the device and remains outside the vagina after insertion (Figure 14–1). The external portion of the device provides some barrier protection between the labia and the base of the penis during intercourse. The sheath is coated with a silicone-based lubricant; additional lubricant for the outside is provided with the device. The lubricant does not contain a spermicidal agent. Reality is approved for over-the-counter sale without prescription and is intended for single use. The expiration date is 5 years from the date of manufacture. The polyurethane used in the sheath is a thin (0.05 mm) but impermeable material with good heat transfer. It is stronger than latex and less likely to tear or break. It does not deteriorate with exposure to oil-based products and withstands storage better than latex does.

Table 14–1 Characteristics of vaginal barriers and spermicide contraceptives available in the United States

Method	Mechanism	Used with product	Prescription needed	Fitted by clinician	Single use or reusable	Material	Placement for use
Female condom	Mechanical barrier	Alone	No	One size	Single use	Polyurethane or nitrile sheath	Vagina and introitus
Diaphragm	Mechanical barrier	Spermicidal gel or cream	Yes	Yes	Reusable	Latex dome	Covers cervix and rests behind pubic arch
FemCap (cervical cap)	Mechanical barrier	Spermicidal gel or cream	Yes	Yes	Reusable	Silicone rubber bowl	Covers cervix and vaginal fornices
Spermicidal formulations	Spermicide	Alone or as above	No	No	Single use	Nonoxynol-9	Vagina

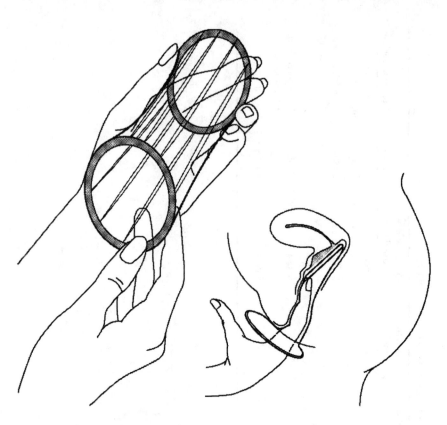

Figure 14–1 Reality Female Condom

Variations to the Reality design described above are available in some areas of the world.[2] The nitrile female condom, known as FC2, received FDA approval in 2009 and is available in about 100 countries. The FC2 makes less noise during intercourse than the Reality female condom and is less expensive than FC1. The PATH Woman's Condom (WC) is another new female condom currently in development.

Diaphragm.   This dome-shaped rubber cup has a flexible rim for ease with insertion. It is inserted into the vagina before intercourse so that the posterior rim rests in the posterior fornix and the anterior rim fits snugly behind the pubic bone. The dome of the diaphragm covers the cervix; spermicide is applied to the inside of the dome before insertion and is held in place near the surface of the cervix. Currently available diaphragms require a prescription, but new products for over-the-counter availability are being tested.

Once in position, the diaphragm may provide effective contraceptive protection for up to 6 hours. If a longer interval has elapsed, insertion of additional doses of spermicide into the vagina with an applicator (without removing the diaphragm) is recommended. After intercourse, the diaphragm should be left in place for at least 6 hours. Wearing it for longer than 24 hours is not recommended because of the rare risk of toxic shock syndrome (TSS). Diaphragms are available in sizes ranging from 50 mm to 95 mm (diameter) and in several styles. The styles differ in the inner construction of the circular rim.

Cervical Cap. FemCap is a bowl-shaped silicone rubber cap with a brim that flares outward. The concave side of the cap covers the cervix completely, while the rim fits against the vaginal fornices. The brim is taller on one end than the other; for proper positioning, the larger brim fits into the posterior vagina. Spermicide can be placed on the inside and the outside of the cap. The FemCap can be worn for up to 48 hours. A strap located on the convex side of the cap aids in removal. FemCap comes in three sizes and is available only by prescription.

SPERMICIDES

Spermicidal gels, creams, and foam are commonly marketed for use with a diaphragm, but they can also be used alone for contraception. One application delivers 52.5 mg to 150 mg of N-9, depending on the product: the spermicide concentration ranges from 8% to 12.5% in foam, and from 2% to 4% in gels and creams.

Spermicidal suppositories can be used alone for contraception or with a condom. Suppositories have a spermicide concentration of 3% to 5% and provide 100 mg to 125 mg of N-9. Adequate time between insertion and intercourse (10 to 15 minutes depending on the product) is essential for the spermicide to dissolve and disperse. Incomplete dissolution of the suppository may reduce its contraceptive efficacy and may cause an uncomfortable gritty sensation or friction for either partner.

Spermicidal film containing N-9 can be used alone for contraception or with condoms, diaphragms or cervical caps. Each paper-thin sheet of film has a spermicide concentration of 28% and contains 72 mg to 100 mg of N-9. The sheet must be inserted on or near the cervix at least 15 minutes before intercourse to allow time for the sheet to melt and disperse. Placing film on the tip of the penis for insertion is not recommended; the film will not have adequate time to dissolve, and it may not be properly placed so as to cover the cervical os.

The *contraceptive sponge* is a single-use vaginal spermicide. This small, pillow-shaped polyurethane sponge contains 1 gram of N-9 spermicide. The concave dimple on one side is designed to fit over the cervix and decrease the chance of dislodgement during intercourse (Figure 14–2). The other side of the sponge incorporates a woven polyester loop to facilitate removal. The sponge, made in one size, is available over-the-counter. It is moistened with tap water prior to use and inserted deep into the vagina. The sponge protects for up to 24 hours, no matter how

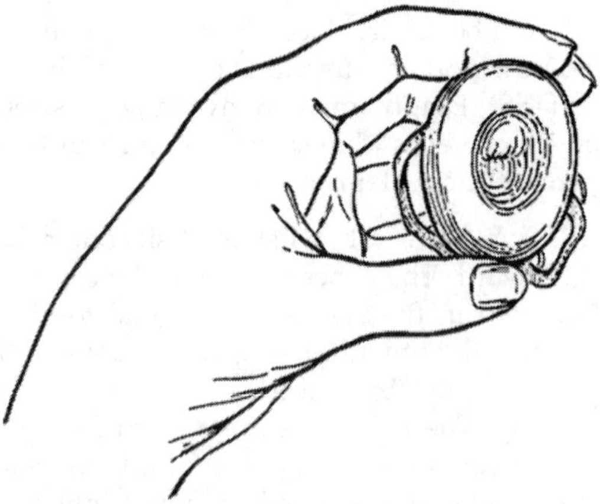

Figure 14–2 Contraceptive sponge

many times intercourse occurs. After intercourse, the sponge must be left in place for at least 6 hours before it is removed and discarded. Wearing the sponge for longer than 24 to 30 hours is not recommended because of the rare risk of TSS.

EFFECTIVENESS

The effectiveness of all of these barrier/spermicidal methods depends on anticipatory motivation at the time of each coital act. Thus the difference between "perfect use" and "typical use" is greater than those methods that don't require coital attention. While pregnancy rates vary across studies, these methods of contraception overall are less effective than hormonal or long-acting methods and more similar to withdrawal and fertility awareness methods in both perfect use and typical use rates. Thus, pregnancy rates associated with perfect use in the first year are approximately 5% for vaginal barriers and approximately 20% for spermicides.[1-5] The rates for typical use range between 10% to 30% for these barrier methods.[1-5] Most published clinical trials of spermicide used alone for contraception do not meet current standards for study design and analysis; thus, we must be cautious when comparing the contraceptive effectiveness of spermicides to other contraceptive methods across studies. However, the dose of spermicide is directly associated with the efficacy of spermicidal methods; a gel containing a low dose of spermicide (52.5 mg of nonoxynol-9) was less effective than gels containing 100 or 150 mg. No difference was found between a gel, a film, and a suppository each containing 100 mg of nonoxynol-9.[6]

> **Emergency Contraception:** Emergency contraceptive pills or insertion of a copper intrauterine contraceptive after unprotected intercourse substantially reduces the risk of pregnancy. (See Chapter 6 for more information.)

Other factors related to the user are associated with decreased efficacy with some of these methods. Parity has been associated with decreased effectiveness of cervical caps and vaginal sponges. For nulliparous women, all vaginal barrier devices provide similar levels of contraceptive effectiveness with typical use. For parous women who use the cap consistently, the pregnancy rate at one year was 20.5%, more than twice the 9.5% pregnancy rate among nulliparous women.[7] Similar results were seen with the contraceptive sponge: the one-year pregnancy rate among parous women with consistent use was 27.0%, almost three times higher than that of nulliparous women (9.9%).[7] In studies of the diaphragm, the almost twice higher pregnancy rate associated with consistent use among parous women compared with nulliparous women did not reach statistical significance.

The different failure rates reported in studies for these methods are not entirely accounted for by consistently correct use or parity. The wide range reflects the profound effect of differences among study populations in fertility characteristics such as age and coital frequency. For example, women who used the diaphragm consistently and had intercourse 3 or more times weekly were almost 3 times as likely to experience a pregnancy compared with women who had intercourse less than three times weekly (9.7% vs. 3.4%).[7] In studies of spermicidal formulations, the measured efficacy of the method also differs between studies but so does the age and sexual behavior of the populations studied. In a study of spermicidal formulations with younger participants who on average had more frequent coitus, the 6-month pregnancy rates were $\geq 25\%$ compared with $< 15\%$ in a study with older participants who had coitus less frequently.[5,6]

Furthermore, a woman is most likely to succeed with a method that is compatible with her sexual routines. For example, her comfort with using an applicator or vaginal placement, the degree of lubricating effect, the proper fit of a device, or any required delay for a suppository or film to melt may influence a woman's ability to use any of these methods effectively.

The addition of a spermicide to a diaphragm or cervical cap may improve the efficacy of both methods. Several studies suggest that spermicide may be helpful in improving contraceptive effectiveness with some of these devices. Women using the diaphragm without spermicide had a pregnancy rate of 29 pregnancies per 100 women within 12 months, while those using a diaphragm with spermicide had a rate of 21 per 100 women.[3] In contrast, in a 6-month study, women using a type of cervical cap without spermicide experienced almost twice as many pregnancies as those who used it in combination with spermicide (9.3 vs. 5.6 pregnancies per 100 women).[8]

ADVANTAGES

CONTRACEPTIVE ADVANTAGES

Vaginal barriers and spermicides have certain advantages over other contraceptive methods that make them a useful option in certain contexts for both short-term and long-term contraception. They are non-hormonal, user-controlled, and immediately effective. They avoid the rare but serious medical risks associated with hormonal methods or those that require a medical procedure. In addition, they avoid certain discomforts of other methods. They do not cause systemic side effects, nor do they alter a woman's endogenous hormone patterns. Vaginal barrier methods and spermicides do not generally require partner involvement in the decision to insert them. For women who need contraception only intermittently, these methods can be available for immediate protection whenever needed, no matter how long the interval between uses. The female condom and all spermicide formulations, including the contraceptive sponge, can be purchased over-the-counter and do not require the user to seek medical consultation to obtain the method, and none require a clinician visit to discontinue use. Finally, because these are user controlled, immediately effective methods, they offer a simple option for a woman who needs back-up contraception, for instance when using the quickstart method of hormonal contraception initiation, when oral contraceptives are forgotten, or when prescription contraceptives are refilled late.

SEXUALLY TRANSMITTED INFECTION (STI) PROTECTION

If vaginal barriers were to protect against transmission or acquisition of STIs, it could be the most important noncontraceptive benefit.[9,10] However, only the female condom has been shown to prevent STIs in rigorous studies. The female condom lines the vagina completely, preventing direct contact between the penis and vagina. The condom traps semen and is then discarded. The female condoms are strong and impermeable to organisms as small as HIV. Unless the female condom slips out of place or is torn, or the penis gets misrouted between the female condom and vaginal wall, the protection against STI exposure should be equivalent to that provided by male condoms. Consistent, correct use of female condoms appears effective in preventing reinfection with trichomonas.[11] In addition, giving sex workers female condoms to use when male condoms were refused led to slightly lower STI rates in Thai brothels than only providing male condoms.[12]

Studies of women who use a diaphragm or contraceptive sponge differ in their reported reduction of gonorrhea, chlamydia, and trichomoniasis.[13–15] The presence of a mechanical barrier with a spermicide, to reduce exposure of the fragile cervical epithelium to semen and microbes, could theoretically reduce infection risk. Unfortunately, studies to date have failed to demonstrate a reduction in infection risk with the diaphragm and male condoms compared with male condom use alone.[16]

Currently available spermicides containing nonoxynol-9 are ineffective as microbicides, in particular as HIV-preventive measures.[17] Thus, spermicides used alone are not recommended to prevent HIV or other STIs. Furthermore, frequent use (more than 2 times per day) of spermicides causes more vulvovaginal epithelial disruption,[18] which theoretically could increase susceptibility to HIV. In a high-risk population using a vaginal gel with nonoxynol-9 more than three applications per day on average, the risk of HIV acquisition was *increased* compared with placebo.[19]

We have a critical need for female-initiated topical methods to prevent STIs, including infection with HIV. However, the most promising topical products currently in development are based on antiretroviral (ARV) agents and do not have contraceptive properties. For example, tenofovir gel, an ARV, used before and after sex was found to protect against both HIV and HSV.[20] No effect on pregnancy was noted.

CERVICAL NEOPLASIA PROTECTION

Several observational studies show a lower risk of cervical dysplasia and cancer among women using the diaphragm. Because cervical infection with certain strains of human papillomavirus virus (HPV) plays an etiologic part in cervical neoplasia, diaphragm use may reduce the risk of HPV. However, in a randomized trial use of the diaphragm and lubricant gel did not demonstrate a protective effect against HPV acquisition and clearance superior to male condom use.[21] It may be that women who choose to use the diaphragm may be at lower risk for HPV for reasons unrelated to effects of the diaphragm itself.

DISADVANTAGES AND CAUTIONS

Few serious medical problems are associated with use of vaginal barriers. The vast majority of women are medically appropriate candidates for their use. Toxic shock syndrome is a potentially life threatening but rare complication of use of vaginal barriers and the contraceptive sponge.

Local Irritation. Temporary skin irritation involving the vulva, vagina, or penis caused by either local toxicity or allergy to the formulation is the most common problem associated with spermicide use. When you suspect an allergy, suggest the client try another contraceptive method. Although vaginal epithelial disruption has been associated with frequent use (twice a day or more) of spermicides containing N-9, this is usually asymptomatic. In a low-risk population, long-term use of N-9 containing methods was not associated with epithelial disruption.[22] Similarly, barrier methods may irritate the vaginal epithelium. If any signs of irritation or inflammation are noted, or if symptoms of irritation are reported, review the frequency of use (for spermicides) and duration of use (for barrier methods). If the reported use is appropriate, consider recommending another method of contraception.

Vaginal and urinary tract infections. Use of a diaphragm with spermicide during sexual intercourse is associated with increased vaginal colonization with Escherichia coli and may lead to an increase in urinary tract infections.[23] As noted above, frequent use of spermicides with N-9 in a high risk population is associated with an increased risk of HIV acquisition, and a dose dependent relationship between N-9 formulations and alterations in vaginal flora in a low risk population has been demonstrated.[24]

Toxic shock syndrome (TSS). TSS is a rare but serious disorder caused by the systemic release of toxin(s) by certain strains of Staphylococcus aureus. Most TSS occurs in association with prolonged tampon use during menses; nonmenstrual TSS risk is increased for women who use a diaphragm or a contraceptive sponge. However, the risk attributable to the use of these contraceptives is low.[25] Nevertheless, patients using vaginal barriers and the contraceptive sponge need to be aware of the danger signs and symptoms of TSS and receive instructions consistent with recommended TSS precautions.

Systemic effects and pregnancy exposure. No serious systemic side effects have been reported in association with human use of spermicides in conjunction with vaginal barriers. Safety concerns have centered on the issue of fetal exposure related to their accidental use during early pregnancy. However, composite data show no true association exists between spermicide use and fetal defects.[26]

Removal. Problems with removal of some vaginal barriers are fairly common. Foul odor and vaginal discharge are likely to occur if a diaphragm or sponge is inadvertently left in the vagina for more than a few days. Symptoms abate promptly when the device is removed.

Common dislikes. Many aspects of these methods may be unpleasant to women depending upon their experiences and preferences. For instance, all of these methods involve inserting something vaginally, which may be uncomfortable or unpleasant for some. Others dislike the noise of female condoms during intercourse. The main complaints reported with spermicides are the messiness, experiencing leakage of spermicides, and excessive lubrication. Some couples find the taste of spermicide unpleasant when they engage in oral-genital sex. Occasionally, women find the effervescence of foaming vaginal suppositories unpleasant.

CAUTIONS

The following conditions may make use of one or more of the vaginal barrier methods or spermicides inadvisable:

1. Allergy to spermicide, rubber, latex, polyurethane, the spermicidal agent, or ingredients in the base

2. Abnormalities in vaginal anatomy that interfere with a satisfactory fit, stable placement, or retention of a vaginal barrier device or spermicide

3. Inability to learn or difficulty with correct insertion technique

4. History of TSS (except female condom and spermicides other than the contraceptive sponge)

5. Repeated UTIs (except female condom)

6. Lack of trained personnel to fit the device or lack of clinical time to provide instruction (for the diaphragm and FemCap)

7. Full-term delivery within the past 6 weeks, recent spontaneous or induced abortion, or vaginal bleeding from any cause, including menstrual flow (for FemCap and sponges)

8. (*For N-9 spermicides*) If STI/HIV exposure is likely, situations that would involve frequent use, defined as 2 times or more a day

In addition, certain precautions should be noted which affect the efficacy of these methods.

1. Female and male condoms should not be used together; they can adhere to each other, causing slippage or displacement of one or both devices.

2. Douching is not a method of contraception, even when a spermicide is in the douching solution. While douching is not recommended generally because of the association with vaginal infections, douching may also decrease the efficacy of spermicides. A woman who has used a vaginal spermicide for contraception should not douche until at least 6 hours after sexual intercourse to avoid washing away the spermicide prematurely.

PROVIDING VAGINAL BARRIER AND SPERMICIDES

Vaginal barriers and spermicides vary by how they are obtained and how they are fitted, inserted, and used by women. In addition, ongoing motivation for correct and consistent use is essential for the efficacy of all of these methods. Therefore, clinicians can assist women in choosing a method with which is she is most likely to be successful (Table 14–2):

1. Counsel women individually on their own risk of unintended pregnancy. The higher the risk of pregnancy, the less effective any of these methods will be. Individual characteristics that may increase the risk of unintended pregnancy include:

   — Frequent intercourse (3 times or more per week on average)

   — Age less than 30 years

   — Parity (cervical cap, sponge)

   — Circumstances that make consistent use difficult

   — Previous contraceptive failure with vaginal barriers or spermicides

   — Chaotic situations such as known abuse of alcohol or other illicit drugs

   If the woman is at high risk for method failure, encourage her to consider using either a more effective contraceptive method or a combination of methods

2. Advise women that these methods should be used with every act of intercourse *regardless of cycle day,* because ovulation (and therefore pregnancy) can occur on ANY CYCLE DAY.[27]

3. Inform women about emergency contraception (postcoital contraception), offer to provide it to all women in advance of need, and provide information on how to obtain EC if needed and how to use it (See Chapter 6 on Emergency Contraception).

4. Counsel women on their individual risk of STI acquisition or transmission. For women at increased risk of STI, male or female condoms are recommended. Male and female condoms should not be used simultaneously.

5. Advise women to avoid lubricants such as mineral oil, baby oil, suntan oil, vegetable oil, and butter; and vaginal medications such as Femstat cream, Monistat cream, estrogen cream, and Vagisil when using a barrier made of latex (diaphragm). These products have a rapid, deleterious effect on the integrity of the latex. They will not affect silicon (the FemCap) or polyurethane (the Reality Female Condom). If additional lubrication is needed, a vaginal spermicide or a product intended for use with latex condoms would be reasonable options.

6. Personalize the choice of the vaginal barrier or spermicide for the individual woman. The differences in efficacy and instruc-

tions for use may make one option easier or more appealing for an individual woman.

GUIDELINES FOR INDIVIDUAL METHODS:

Female condom. The Reality Condom is available over the internet or counter and does not require a clinician's visit for initiation or use. However, if you perform a routine pelvic examination, you can confirm that the pelvic anatomy would permit the use of the female condom, or advise the woman if her pelvic anatomy—such as a septate vagina or severe uterine prolapse—may interfere with the method.

Diaphragm. Diaphragms are available only by prescription and require a pelvic examination and fitting to ensure proper size and placement of the device. During a pelvic examination, the correct diaphragm size can be estimated by measuring the distance from the posterior vaginal vault to the pubic arch. Insert your index and middle fingers into the vagina until your middle finger reaches the posterior vault of the vagina. Then using your thumb, mark the point at which your index finger touches the pubic bone. Place the diaphragm rim on the tip of your middle finger. The opposite rim should lie just in front of your thumb.

Now that you have selected the diaphragm size, fold the rim of the diaphragm so that it is collapsed and insert the diaphragm into the patient's vagina with the convex side facing the cervix. The device should rest snugly in the vagina, but without tension against the vaginal walls. Its rim should be in contact with the lateral walls and posterior fornix, and there should be just enough space to insert one fingertip comfortably between the inside of the pubic arch and the anterior edge of the diaphragm rim.

Choose the largest size that is comfortable for the patient. You will often need to try more than one rim size to ensure a proper fit. If the diaphragm is too small, it may not remain in position during intercourse. Vaginal depth increases during sexual arousal (3 cm to 5 cm in nulliparous women). A diaphragm that is too large, however, may cause vaginal pressure, discomfort, vaginal ulceration, and recurrent UTI. One approach to assessing fit is to have the patient bear down while the diaphragm is in place. The largest size that does not dislodge or expel is a proper fit. Allow the woman to practice insertion and removal. After she inserts the diaphragm, check to see if she is experiencing any discomfort and examine her to confirm proper placement. Have the woman attempt to void with the diaphragm in place to make certain that the urethra is not obstructed by the diaphragm.

Cervical Cap. FemCap is available only by prescription and a pelvic examination is required for fitting. The three sizes of FemCap are intended to correspond to a woman's obstetric history. Women who have never been pregnant should use the smallest size (internal rim diameter 22 mm); women who have miscarried or had a cesarean section should use the middle size (26 mm); and women who have vaginally delivered a full-term baby should use the largest size (30 mm). To confirm the fit, insert the FemCap into the vagina by squeezing it and pushing it deep into the vagina with the convex bowl facing upward toward the cervix and the long rim entering first. When the device is released in place over the cervix, the unfolding dome should create suction between the rim of the cap and the cervix. Check with your finger to make sure that the cervix is completely covered. To remove the Femcap, rotate the device in any direction. Push the tip of your finger against the dome of the device to dimple it. This will break the suction and allow room for your finger to fit between the dome and the removal strap. Hook the strap with your finger and gently pull the device down and out. Allow the woman to practice insertion and removal. After she inserts the device, check to see if the cervix is covered, the cervical cap is properly placed, and the woman is comfortable.

Spermicides. All spermicidal methods (spermicidal foam, gel, cream, film or suppository, and contraceptive sponge) are currently available over the counter without the need for a prescription or a clinician visit.

MANAGING PROBLEMS AND FOLLOW-UP

None of these methods require specific or special follow-up. Women using a fitted device should have that fit checked annually, or after significant weight change (gain or loss of 10 or more pounds) or pregnancy. However, with the exception of vaginal delivery, women rarely need to change the size of a diaphragm after any of those events. Routine well-woman visits are an opportunity to assess contraceptive needs and plans for all women at risk of unintended pregnancy, regardless of current contraceptive method. Take the opportunity to ask, in an open-ended fashion, how the method is working, and in particular if she is having any difficulty or discomfort, or if she desires a different method. Vaginal barriers (excepting female condoms) should be replaced annually or sooner if they are not water-tight.

Problems caused by vaginal barrier methods may require clinical intervention. Recurrent vaginal or vulvar irritation, without evidence of infection, may indicate an allergy or sensitivity to the product (i.e., spermicide or latex). If symptoms persist for more than one or two days after discontinuation of the method, evaluate the patient for another etiology, such as STI exposure, yeast vaginitis, or bacterial vaginosis. Changing to an alternative product with a different formulation or changing to a less concentrated product may help.

Recurrent urinary tract infection (UTI), recurrent yeast infection, and bacterial vaginosis may be associated with contraceptive sponges or diaphragms. If a diaphragm user experiences recurring UTIs, consider refitting her with a smaller diaphragm size or an alternative rim style. If her UTI problems persist despite these measures, changing to an alternative method of contraception that avoids the use spermicide may reduce the risk of UTI.

A vaginal barrier user who develops signs or symptoms of TSS requires urgent and intensive evaluation and treatment with antibiotics and supportive care. If her symptoms are severe, she will need hospitalization. A woman who has had TSS in the past has an increased risk for repeat TSS, so she should avoid using vaginal barriers.

U SER INSTRUCTIONS FOR VAGINAL BARRIER METHODS AND SPERMICIDES

1. Use your method every time you have vaginal intercourse. Be sure your vaginal barrier or spermicide is in place before your partner's penis enters your vagina.

2. If you feel unsure about the proper fit or placement of your diaphragm, FemCap, or sponge, use spermicides and/or male condoms until you see your clinician to be sure your insertion technique is correct.

3. If you have problems with recurring bladder infections or vaginal yeast infections, discuss these with your clinician.

4. You can use male condoms along with your diaphragm, sponge, FemCap, or spermicide if you wish. Using this combination, you will have effective protection against both pregnancy and sexually transmitted infection.

5. Do not use a male condom along with a female condom; the two may stick to each other and increase the chance your female condom will dislodge or the male condom will slip off.

6. No conclusive studies show just how long a spermicide is fully active or exactly how long the diaphragm or sponge must be left in place after intercourse. The most important thing is consistent and correct use.

7. Douching after intercourse is not recommended. If you are using a diaphragm or sponge, and choose to douche, wait at least 6 hours after intercourse to avoid washing away spermicide.

8. If you are using a diaphragm or sponge, learn the danger signs for toxic shock syndrome and watch for them. These signs include sudden high fever, chills, vomiting, diarrhea, muscle aches and sunburn-like rash. If you have a high fever and one or more of the other danger signs, you may have early toxic shock syndrome. Remove the sponge or diaphragm and contact your clinician immediately, or go to a hospital emergency room.

TAKING CARE OF YOUR VAGINAL BARRIER METHOD

1. Store your supplies in a convenient location that is clean, cool, and out of direct sunlight.

2. Wash your spermicide inserter, diaphragm, or cap after each use. Plain soap is best; avoid deodorant soap or perfumed soap. **Do not use talcum powder** on your diaphragm or cap, or in the case.

3. Check your vaginal barrier before each use to make sure there are no holes or tears and that the device is not damaged in any way.

4. Contact with oil-based products can deteriorate a diaphragm. Do not use oil-based vaginal medications or lubricants when you are using a diaphragm. Some examples include petroleum jelly (Vaseline), mineral oil, hand lotion, vegetable oil, cold cream, and cocoa butter as well as common vaginal yeast creams and vaginal hormone creams. If you need extra lubrication for intercourse, contraceptive jelly is a good choice, or you can try a water-soluble lubricant specifically intended for use with condoms.

Emergency Contraception: Emergency contraceptive pills or insertion of a copper intrauterine contraceptive after unprotected intercourse substantially reduces the risk of pregnancy.

REFERENCES

1. Trussell J, Sturgen K, Strickler J, Dominik R. Comparative contraceptive efficacy of the female condom and other barrier methods. Fam Plann Perspect. 1994;26:66–72.
2. Hoke TH, Stone KM, Steiner MJ, Warner L, Cates W, Jr. Female Condoms. In: UpToDate. Waltham, MA: UpToDate; 2010.
3. Cook L, Nanda K, Grimes D. Diaphragm versus diaphragm with spermicides for contraception. Cochrane Database Syst Rev. 2001:CD002031.
4. Grimes DA, Lopez L, Raymond EG, Halpern V, Nanda K, Schulz KF. Spermicide used alone for contraception. Cochrane Database Syst Rev. 2005:CD005218.

5. Raymond E, Dominik R. Contraceptive effectiveness of two spermicides: a randomized trial. Obstet Gynecol. 1999;93:896–903.
6. Raymond EG, Chen PL, Luoto J. Contraceptive effectiveness and safety of five nonoxynol-9 spermicides: a randomized trial. Obstet Gynecol. 2004;103:430–439.
7. Trussell J, Strickler J, Vaughan B. Contraceptive efficacy of the diaphragm, the sponge and the cervical cap. Fam Plann Perspect. 1993;25:100–105, 135.
8. Mauck C, Glover LH, Miller E, et al. Lea's Shield: a study of the safety and efficacy of a new vaginal barrier contraceptive used with and without spermicide. Contraception. 1996;53:329–335.
9. Moench TR, Chipato T, Padian NS. Preventing disease by protecting the cervix: the unexplored promise of internal vaginal barrier devices. AIDS. 2001;15:1595–1602.
10. Minnis AM, Padian NS. Effectiveness of female controlled barrier methods in preventing sexually transmitted infections and HIV: current evidence and future research directions. Sex Transm Infect. 2005;81:193–200.
11. Soper DE, Shoupe D, Shangold GA, Shangold MM, Gutmann J, Mercer L. Prevention of vaginal trichomoniasis by compliant use of the female condom. Sex Transm Dis. 1993;20:137–139.
12. Fontanet AL, Saba J, Chandelying V, et al. Protection against sexually transmitted diseases by granting sex workers in Thailand the choice of using the male or female condom: results from a randomized controlled trial. AIDS. 1998;12:1851–1859.
13. Cates W, Jr., Stone KM. Family planning, sexually transmitted diseases and contraceptive choice: a literature update–Part I. Fam Plann Perspect. 1992;24:75–84.
14. d'Oro LC, Parazzini F, Naldi L, La Vecchia C. Barrier methods of contraception, spermicides, and sexually transmitted diseases: a review. Genitourin Med. 1994;70:410–417.
15. Ramjee G, van der Straten A, Chipato T, et al. The diaphragm and lubricant gel for prevention of cervical sexually transmitted infections: results of a randomized controlled trial. PLoS One. 2008;3:e3488.
16. Padian NS, van der Straten A, Ramjee G, et al. Diaphragm and lubricant gel for prevention of HIV acquisition in southern African women: a randomised controlled trial. Lancet. 2007;370:251–261.
17. McCormack S, Hayes R, Lacey CJ, Johnson AM. Microbicides in HIV prevention. BMJ. 2001;322:410–413.
18. Roddy RE, Cordero M, Cordero C, Fortney JA. A dosing study of nonoxynol-9 and genital irritation. Int J STD AIDS. 1993;4:165–170.
19. Van Damme L, Ramjee G, Alary M, et al. Effectiveness of COL-1492, a nonoxynol-9 vaginal gel, on HIV-1 transmission in female sex workers: a randomised controlled trial. Lancet. 2002;360:971–977.
20. Karim QA, Karim SSA, Frohlich JA, Grobler AC, Baxter C, Mansoor LE, et al. Effectiveness and safety of tenofovir gel, an antiretroviral microbicide, for the prevention of HIV infection in women. Science. 2010;329:1168–1174.
21. Sawaya GF, Chirenje MZ, Magure MT, et al. Effect of diaphragm and lubricant gel provision on human papillomavirus infection among women provided with condoms: a randomized controlled trial. Obstet Gynecol. 2008;112:990–997.
22. Harwood B, Meyn LA, Ballagh SA, Raymond EG, Archer DF, Creinin MD. Cervicovaginal colposcopic lesions associated with 5 nonoxynol-9 vaginal spermicide formulations. Am J Obstet Gynecol. 2008;198:32 e31–37.
23. Hooton TM, Roberts PL, Stamm WE. Effects of recent sexual activity and use of a diaphragm on the vaginal microflora. Clin Infect Dis. 1994;19:274–278.
24. Schreiber CA, Meyn LA, Creinin MD, Barnhart KT, Hillier SL. Effects of long-term use of nonoxynol-9 on vaginal flora. Obstet Gynecol. 2006;107:136–143.
25. Schwartz B, Gaventa S, Broome CV, et al. Nonmenstrual toxic shock syndrome associated with barrier contraceptives: report of a case-control study. Rev Infect Dis. 1989;11 Suppl 1:S43–48; discussion S48–49.

26. Gallaway MS, Waller DK, Canfield MA, Scheuerle A. The association between use of spermicides or male condoms and major structural birth defects. Contraception. 2009;80:422–429.
27. Wilcox AJ, Dunson DB, Weinberg CR, Trussell J, Baird DD. Likelihood of conception with a single act of intercourse: providing benchmark rates for assessment of post-coital contraceptives. Contraception. 2001;63:211–215.

Coitus Interruptus (Withdrawal)

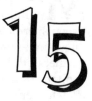

Deborah Kowal, MA, PA

- Coitus interruptus does not eliminate the risk of sexually transmitted infections (STIs): the pre-ejaculate can contain HIV-infected cells, and lesions or ulcers on the genitals can transmit pathogens.

- Spermatozoa appear in the pre-ejaculatory fluid of some men and could cause pregnancy even if the man withdraws prior to ejaculation.

- Half of all sexually active women report having relied on coitus interruptus at some point in their lives.

Coitus interruptus is simply the practice of withdrawing the penis from the vagina and away from external genital organs of the woman before ejaculation, with the intention of avoiding pregnancy. Coitus interruptus, or the withdrawal method, was a natural response to the discovery that ejaculation into the vagina caused pregnancy.[1] The method was probably widely practiced throughout history, playing a role in fertility declines occurring prior to the advent of the pill. Although the 2006-2008 National Survey of Family Growth (NSFG) reports that the prevalence of women using a contraceptive who currently rely on coitus interruptus is only 5.2%,[2] this figure probably belies more widespread practice. In a re-examination of 2002 NSFG data that included women who reported currently using withdrawal *and* another method, the percentage increased from 4% to 11%.[3]

In recent years, couples have increasingly relied on coitus interruptus. When sexually active women were asked if they had *ever* practiced withdrawal, more than half (58.8%) answered affirmatively in 2006-2008, compared with 25% in 1992 and 41% in 1995.[2] Only pills and condoms were more often reported as methods "ever used" by the respondents. Withdrawal is also widely practiced among adolescent women aged 15 to 19. Although less than 1% reported using withdrawal as their current method, more than half (55%) reported ever having used the method.[4]

MECHANISM OF ACTION

Withdrawal prevents fertilization by preventing the contact between spermatozoa and the ovum. The couple may have penile-vaginal intercourse until ejaculation is impending, at which time the male partner withdraws his penis from the vagina and away from the external genitalia of the female partner. The man must rely on his own sensations to determine when he is about to ejaculate. The pre-ejaculate, which is usually released just prior to full ejaculation, generally goes unnoticed by both the man and the woman during their course of sexual activity and so cannot be relied upon as a sign that ejaculation is about to occur.

EFFECTIVENESS

Withdrawal is in the bottom tier of contraceptive effectiveness (see Table 3–1). For typical users, our best guess based on the 1995 and 2002 National Survey of Family Growth (NSFG) has been that the probability of pregnancy among typical users would be about 22% during the first year of use. Among couples practicing withdrawal perfectly, the probability of pregnancy among perfect users might be about 4% in the initial year of use (Table 3–1). The immense difference between the 22% failure rate in typical users and the 4% rate if used perfectly attests to the difficulty couples have in using withdrawal consistently and correctly.

In itself, the pre-ejaculate, a lubricating secretion produced by the Littre or Cowper's glands, presumably contains no sperm. Although two studies examining the pre-ejaculate for the presence of spermatozoa found none,[5,6] two other studies found spermatozoa, though in small numbers. In one of these studies,[7] 8 of 23 samples contained clumps of a few hundred sperm, which could theoretically have posed a risk of fertilization. In a recent study designed specifically to determine whether pre-ejaculate contained sperm potentially capable of fertilizing an egg, researchers examined the samples within 2 hours of production.[8] The pre-ejaculate of 37% of men contained motile sperm, though the number of sperm in each sample was low. Because the number of sperm in each pre-ejaculate was low, the risk of pregnancy would be low, though not zero. Each man in the study was consistent in either leaking or not leaking sperm in with the pre-ejaculate fluid.

As with other methods, withdrawal's efficacy in preventing pregnancy probably may depend not only on characteristics of the method (whether the man's pre-ejaculate contains sperm), but also on characteristics of the user. Men who are less experienced with using the method or who have difficulty in foretelling when ejaculation will occur could have a greater risk of failure. It may be that certain cultural factors influence how successful a couple may be in using withdrawal. A recent study found that Hispanic women relying on withdrawal were less likely to experience accidental pregnancy than were black or white women.[9]

A DVANTAGES AND INDICATIONS

As a method of contraception, withdrawal has several distinct advantages. It costs nothing, requires no devices, involves no chemicals, and is available in any situation. Some couples may select withdrawal as their method because it requires no physical examination or contact with a clinic or pharmacy.[10] Practicing coitus interruptus causes no medical side effects. It also enables men to take a responsible and active role in fertility regulation and may foster a dialogue on contraception and sexuality between the partners.[11,12] Couples who cannot or do not wish to use other contraceptive methods and who can accept the potential for unintended pregnancy may find withdrawal an acceptable alternative. It is also a back-up contraceptive that is always available.

D ISADVANTAGES AND CAUTIONS

Some men produce pre-ejaculate fluid that contains spermatozoa and theoretically could fertilize an egg.[8]

The method is unforgiving of incorrect or inconsistent use, leading to a probability of pregnancy in typical users that is substantially higher than the rates for hormonal methods or intrauterine contraceptives (IUCs). One reason for contraceptive failure may be a man's fear that he lacks the self-control demanded by the method.[13] The man may feel the urge to achieve deeper penetration at the time of impending orgasm and may not withdraw in sufficient time to avoid depositing semen in his partner's vagina or on her external genitalia. The woman may be close to an orgasm when the man is close to ejaculation and starts to withdraw his penis from her vagina; her response may be to grip her legs around her partner to hold him inside her, thus preventing him from withdrawing before he ejaculates. For some couples, interruption of the excitement or plateau phase of the sexual response cycle may diminish pleasure.

In addition, some men have difficulty foretelling when they will ejaculate. Some women may feel anxiety in relinquishing control over contraceptive behavior to men.

SPECIAL ISSUES

Because not all pathogens are limited to seminal fluid, withdrawal does not completely protect couples from exposure to STIs presenting with actively infective surface lesions such as those from herpes genitalis or human papilloma virus.[15]

The seminal fluid that emerges from the penis prior to ejaculation may contain some human immunodeficiency virus (HIV).[7,15] However, coitus interruptus may decrease HIV exposure by reducing the amount of semen that enters the woman's vagina. In stable discordant couples (the man was infected with HIV and the woman was not), coitus interruptus cut the HIV conversion rate of women by half in one study,[16] and by a larger percentage in another study.[17] Because these studies examined only stable heterosexual couples, the findings may not hold true for women with several HIV-infected partners.

Although coitus interruptus may be less likely than intercourse with ejaculation to transmit HIV, women have become infected while their partners consistently practiced withdrawal. Coitus interruptus has not been studied as a way to reduce HIV transmission from woman to man.

USE PATTERNS

Withdrawal can be used in a variety of different patterns. It can be combined with other methods—such as pills, condoms, or fertility awareness methods—to increase contraceptive efficacy, as long as the two methods are used concurrently. Among women reporting current use of withdrawal, 31% reported current condom use and 5% reported current use of rhythm or natural family planning.[3] Therefore, giving couples information on the fertile period can lower their risk of pregnancy when they use coitus interruptus. Some couples rely on coitus interruptus interchangeably with fertility awareness methods or condoms, presumably to increase convenience. In one study of college males, 43% reported using withdrawal during the initial phases of intercourse and then applying a condom for intravaginal ejaculation.[18] Some couples may share contraceptive responsibility; for example, the woman may use a modern contraceptive for a while and then the man may use withdrawal.[11]

The popular misperception is that adolescents use withdrawal only as a back-up method during spontaneous, unanticipated sexual activity.[19] However, adolescents often choose to rely on withdrawal; these teens may view condoms and withdrawal as categorically similar, as the only male methods of contraception and as methods that do not require a visit to a clinician.[20] In addition, factors involving the individual, the relationship, and the adolescent's family appear to influence withdrawal use.

COUNSELING ABOUT COITUS INTERRUPTUS

Most users can learn to use withdrawal on their own and become skillful users.[11] Therefore, the majority of men and women who rely on withdrawal may not bring up the topic of withdrawal with their health care provider. According to one study, men and women often did not believe withdrawal was a legitimate contraceptive method and therefore did not talk with their health care providers about using withdrawal, even when discussing contraception.[21]

Consequently, you need to discuss withdrawal in the clinical setting, especially given that a large proportion of the at-risk population will at one time or another rely on this method.[3] Some users or potential users may have questions related to the fertile period, emergency contraception, and the risk of any negative health effects, including exposure to STIs. When counseling adolescents, consider their withdrawal use within the context of other contraceptive behaviors, sexual behaviors and attitudes, and relationships.[20]

Finally, inform the couple about emergency contraception, including intrauterine contraception, and provide a supply of emergency contraceptive pills and instruct them on their use to help decrease the risk of pregnancy.

USER INSTRUCTIONS FOR WITHDRAWAL

1. To practice withdrawal, the man should withdraw his penis from his partner's vagina when he feels he is about to ejaculate, making sure that ejaculation occurs away from his partner's genitalia.

2. Withdrawal is not a good contraceptive method if the man cannot predictably withdraw prior to ejaculation.

3. A man may release pre-ejaculate fluid as soon as the penis becomes erect to as late as just before ejaculation. In some men, this pre-ejaculate fluid may contain small numbers of sperm, which could possibly cause a pregnancy. A man may not be aware that he has released pre-ejaculate fluid.

4. If more than one intercourse takes place within a relatively short period of time, the man should urinate and wipe off the tip of his penis before intercourse to remove any sperm remaining from a previous ejaculation.

5. Withdrawal does not effectively protect against sexually transmitted infections (STIs), including infection with the human immunodeficiency virus (HIV). Abstinence or use of latex or plastic condoms provide better protection.

6. Learn what options are available for postcoital protection should any ejaculate come in contact with the vagina. If you think you may have been exposed to a risk of pregnancy, contact your clinician about emergency contraception. (You can also go to www.not-2-late.com.)

Emergency Contraception: Emergency contraceptive pills or insertion of a copper intrauterine contraceptive after unprotected intercourse substantially reduces the risk of pregnancy. (See Chapter 6 for more information.)

REFERENCES

1. Robertson W. An illustrated history of contraception. Park Ridge NJ: Parthenon Publishing Group, 1990.
2. Mosher WD, Jones J. Use of Contraception in the United States: 1982–2008. National Center for Health Statistics. Vital Health Stat. 2010;23(29). Available from http://www.cdc.gov/NCHS/data/series/sr_23/sr23_029.pdf
3. Jones RK, Fennell J, Higgins JA, Blanchard K. Better than nothing or savvy risk-reduction practice? The importance of withdrawal. Contraception. 2009;79:407–410.
4. Abma JC, Martinez GM, Mosher WD, Dawson, BS. Teenagers in the United States: sexual activity, contraceptive use, and childbearing, 2002. National Center for Health Statistics. Vital Health Stat. 2004;23(24).
5. Ilaria G, Jacobs JL, Polsky B, Koll B, Baron P, MacLow C, Armstrong D, Schlegel PN. Detection of HIV-1 DNA sequences in pre-ejaculatory fluid [Letter]. Lancet. 1992;340:1469.
6. Zukerman Z, Weiss DB, Orvieto R. Does preejaculatory penile secretion originating from Cowper's gland contain sperm? J Assist Reprod Genet. 2003;20:157–159.
7. Pudney J, Oneta M, Mayer K, Seage G, Anderson D. Pre-ejaculatory fluid as potential vector for sexual transmission of HIV-1 [Letter]. Lancet. 1992;340:1470.
8. Killick SR, Leary C, Trussell J, Guthrie KA. Sperm content of pre-ejaculatory fluid. Hum Fertil., doi:10.3109/14647273.2010.520798.
9. Ranjit N, Bankole A, Darroch J, Singh, S. Contraceptive failure in the first two years of use: differences across socioeconomic subgroups. Fam Plann Perspect. 2001;33: 19–27.
10. Rogow D, Horowitz S. Withdrawal: a review of the literature and an agenda for research. Stud Fam Plann. 1995;26:140–153.
11. Ortayli N, Bulut A, Ozugurlu M, Cokar M. Why withdrawal? Why not withdrawal? Reprod Health Matters. 2005;13:164–173.
12. Schneider J, Schneider P. Sex and responsibility in an age of fertility decline: a Sicilian case study. Soc Sci Med. 1991;33:885–95.
13. De Visser, R, Delayed application of condoms, withdrawal and negotiation of safer sex among heterosexual young adults, AIDS Care. 2004;16:315–322.
14. Whittaker PG, Merkh RD, Henry-Moss D, Hock-Long L. Withdrawal attitudes and experiences: a qualitative perspective among young urban adults. Perspect Sex Repro H. 2010;42:102–9.
15. Howe JE, Minkoff HL, Duerr AC. Contraceptives and HIV. AIDS. 1994;8:861–871.
16. Musicco M, Nicolosi A, Saracco A, Lazzarin A (for the Italian Study Group on HIV Heterosexual Transmission). The role of contraceptive practices in HIV sexual transmission from man to woman. In: Nicolosi A (ed). HIV epidemiology: models and methods. New York: Raven Press, Ltd., 1994:121–135.

17. DiVincenzi I (for the European Study Group). A longitudinal study of human immunodeficiency virus transmission by heterosexual partners. N Engl J Med. 1994;331:341–346.
18. Crosby RA, Sanders SA, Yarber WL, et al. Condom use errors and problems among college men. Sex Transm Dis. 2002;29:552–557.
19. Woods JL. Hensel DJ, Fortenberry JD. Contraceptive withdrawal in adolescents: a complex picture of usage. Adolesc Gynecol. 2009;22:233–237.
20. Horner JR, Salazar LF, Romer D, Vanable PA, DiClemente R, Carey MP, Valois RF, Stanton BF, Brown LK. Withdrawal (coitus interruptus) as a sexual risk reduction strategy: perspectives from African-American adolescents. Arch Sex Behav. 2009;38:779–787.
21. Sznitman SR, Romer D, Brown LK, DiClemente RJ, Valois RF, Vanable PA, Carey MP, Stanton B. Prevalence, correlates, and sexually transmitted infection risk related to coitus interruptus among African-American adolescents. Sex Transm Dis. 2009;36:218–220.

Fertility Awareness-Based Methods

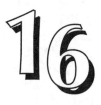

Victoria H. Jennings, PhD
Anne E. Burke, MD, MPH

- Fertility awareness helps couples understand how to avoid pregnancy or how to become pregnant.

- Regardless of whether they use family planning, or which method they use, most women and men can find value in learning fertility awareness.

Fertility Awareness-Based (FAB) methods of family planning depend on identifying the "fertile window," or the days in each menstrual cycle when intercourse is most likely to result in a pregnancy. Some FAB methods may simply involve keeping track of cycle days to understand on which days of her cycle a woman is most likely to be fertile. Other FAB methods involve observing, recording, and interpreting the body's fertility signs.[1]

FAB methods rely on five biological facts:[2]

- The periodicity of fertility and infertility

- A single ovulation each cycle

- The limited lifespan of the ovum (which can be fertilized only in the short time span of 12–24 hours after release)

- The limited lifetime of sperm in cervical mucus and the upper genital tract (3 to 5 days)

- A woman's ability to monitor cycle length or cycle-related symptoms and signs

To avoid pregnancy, couples either use another method or do not have intercourse during the fertile time. Couples who use a barrier method on fertile days are using a fertility awareness-combined method, while those who abstain are using natural family planning.[3]

MECHANISM OF ACTION

FAB methods of family planning use one or more indicators to identify the beginning and end of the fertile time during the menstrual cycle. FAB methods discussed throughout this chapter include the Standard Days Method, the TwoDay Method, the Billings Ovulation Method, Symptothermal Method, and the Calendar Rhythm Method. FAB methods are effective when they are used correctly. However, with incorrect use, unprotected intercourse takes place precisely when the woman is potentially fertile.

In most cycles, ovulation occurs on or very near the middle of the cycle.[4] The fertile window of the menstrual cycle lasts for only about 6 days (the 5 days preceding ovulation and the day of ovulation), related to the lifespan of the gametes.[5,6] Even though ovulation does not occur on the same day each cycle, in cycles that range between 26 and 32 days long (approximately 78% of cycles) the fertile window is highly likely to fall within cycle days 8 to 19.[7] In shorter or longer cycles, the fertile window shifts accordingly.

Two FAB methods, the Standard Days Method and the Calendar Rhythm Method, involve counting the days in the menstrual cycle to identify the fertile days. The Standard Days Method requires only that the woman know the day of her menstrual cycle in order to consider herself potentially fertile on days 8 through 19. Prior to starting the Calendar Rhythm Method, the woman must have recorded the length of her previous 6 to 12 menstrual cycles in order to identify the longest and shortest of these cycles. Once these are collected, calculations are performed to identify the probable days of fertility during the current cycle. While survey results show that, in many countries, a significant number of couples state that they are using the "rhythm" or "calendar rhythm" method,[8] most have little understanding of its proper use and simply abstain from intercourse on a few days of the woman's cycle when they believe, often erroneously, that the woman is most likely to become pregnant. It appears that "calendar rhythm" has become a generic term for "occasional abstinence."

Other FAB methods, such as the TwoDay Method, the Billings Ovulation Method (and variants such as the Creighton Model),[9] and the Symptothermal Method, involve actual observation of fertility signs such as presence or absence of secretions, changes in characteristics of cervical secretions, or changes in basal body temperature. Changes in these signs are caused by fluctuations in circulating hormone levels during the cycle. Women who use these methods identify the start of the fertile time by observing cervical secretions. To identify the end of the fertile time, women can observe their cervical secretions as well as monitor the change in their basal body temperature.

EFFECTIVENESS

Successful use of FAB methods depends on (1) the accuracy of the method in identifying the woman's actual fertile window, (2) the ability to correctly identify the fertile time, and (3) the ability to follow the instructions of the method—that is, to use a barrier method or to avoid intercourse on the days the method identifies as fertile.

There are no recent randomized controlled trials of FAB methods.[10] Efficacy studies of individual FAB methods show that among perfect users (i.e., those who correctly and consistently use a barrier method or avoid intercourse during the fertile time), the percentage of women experiencing an unintended pregnancy during the first year of use ranges from 0.4% to 5%, depending on the method used during the fertile days.[11] In typical use (i.e., correct and consistent use during some cycles, but incorrect or inconsistent use during others), pregnancy rates are higher, about 12% to 24%. Success rates for FAB methods may also vary from country to country.[12] (See Chapter 26 on Contraceptive Efficacy.) *Family Planning: A Global Handbook for Providers*, one of the World Health Organization's cornerstone family planning documents, places what they call fertility awareness methods in the third tier of contraceptive effectiveness along with male and female condoms and diaphragms.[1]

Standard Days Method. The first-year probability of pregnancy for women using the Standard Days Method is about 5% if the method is used correctly. When including correct and incorrect use in efficacy trials, as well as data from other field studies, the probability of pregnancy has been estimated at about 12%.[13] Providers who taught the women participating in the efficacy study how to use the Standard Days Method received 1 to 2 days of training in the method and had no prior experience with it. When the Standard Days Method is offered by experienced providers, efficacy may improve.

Calendar Rhythm Method. Estimates of pregnancy rates for the Calendar Rhythm Method vary widely, partially because the estimates come from flawed studies. One meta-analysis reported a first-year pregnancy rate of 5% with correct use, although the studies included did not consistently identify the parameters of the method.[14] The probability of pregnancy during the first year of typical use of the Calendar Rhythm Method is estimated to be about 13%, based on a meta-analysis of published studies,[15] but no well-designed prospective studies have been conducted, and no data are available from national surveys.

TwoDay Method. The first-year probability of pregnancy is 3.5% for women who use the method correctly. Adding correct use and incorrect use, the probability of pregnancy, based on the results of clinical trials, is just under 14% in the first year of use. Providers who taught the women participating in the efficacy study how to use the TwoDay Method had no prior experience with any FAB method and received 1 to 2 days of training in the TwoDay Method.[12] Thus, similar to the Standard Days Method, it is possible that failure rates will decrease as provider experience increases.

Billings Ovulation Method. The first-year probability of pregnancy for methods based on using only changes in characteristics of cervical secretions detected at the opening of the woman's vagina to identify the beginning and end of the fertile time is about 3% among perfect users and up to 22% among all users in studies.[16-18] Most efficacy studies of the Billings Ovulation Method did not enroll women until they had completed 3 cycles of use, and most study providers had extensive training and experience with the method.

Symptothermal Method. The first-year probability of pregnancy among couples who use two or more fertility indicators (usually cervical secretions and basal body temperature, but others such as cervix position or a calendar calculation may also be used as a "double check" to identify the start and end of the fertile time) is about 0.4% among perfect users and as high as 13% to 20% among all users in clinical trials.[19,20] Several efficacy studies of the Symptothermal Method include women who already had used the method for at least 3 cycles and who had learned the method from experienced providers.

ADVANTAGES AND INDICATIONS

Studies in several countries have shown that characteristics of FAB methods that are perceived by some to be advantages may be perceived by others as disadvantages. For example, the importance of the male partner's participation in method use is positive for some couples[21,22] but difficult to achieve for others. Some women choose FAB methods precisely because of the need for daily awareness of fertility signs or cycle day, while others find this burdensome. For many women, the lack of side effects of FAB methods offsets their higher failure rates.[20,21] Indeed, studies have shown that most women who choose FAB methods either began practicing family planning for the first time or stopped using another method several months before initiating FAB method use—mostly because of their concerns about side effects with other methods.[20]

Fertility awareness is important for all women and men, regardless of which family planning method they use or whether they choose to use family planning at all. Fertility awareness increases the users' knowledge of their reproductive potential and enhances self-reliance. Fertility awareness information can be used for a number of purposes:

To avoid pregnancy. For maximum effectiveness, couples should abstain from intercourse or use a barrier method during the entire fertile time of the woman's menstrual cycle.

To become pregnant. Couples have intercourse on days the woman is potentially fertile. Depending on the method used, these may include days 8 to 19 of the cycle, or the days she observes cervical secretions. Women are most likely to become pregnant if they have intercourse within 1 to 2 days of ovulation.[4]

To detect pregnancy. A postovulatory temperature rise (see the section on Basal Body Temperature Charting) sustained for 18 or more days is an excellent early indicator that pregnancy is underway.

To detect impaired fertility. Charting fertility signs costs relatively little and can aid in diagnosing and treating fertility problems due to infrequent or absent ovulation. Women who do not ovulate tend to have a meandering basal body temperature pattern throughout the cycle, rather than the typical pattern (lower in the first part of the cycle and higher in the second). Cervical secretions similarly may be absent or not conform to the typical pattern.

To detect a need for medical attention. Changes in cervical and vaginal secretions, abdominal pain, and other signs or symptoms may indicate the need for medical attention. (See Chapter 21 on Reproductive Tract Infections.)

DISADVANTAGES AND CAUTIONS

FAB methods produce no physical side effects. Like many other methods, however, they offer no protection against sexually transmitted infections (STIs), including infection with the human immunodeficiency virus (HIV). Also, lack of the male partner's cooperation will be a distinct obstacle for women who wish to practice abstinence or use an alternative method during the fertile time. Certain conditions that increase the likelihood of irregular cycles may make FAB more difficult to use, and women with these conditions require more extensive counseling and follow-up:

- Recent childbirth
- Current breastfeeding
- Recent menarche
- Anovulatory cycling as with polycystic ovarian syndrome (PCOS) or obesity-related infrequent cycles
- Recent discontinuation of hormonal contraceptive methods

- Approaching menopause

FAB methods are not recommended for women with the following difficulties:

- Inability to abstain or use other contraceptive methods during the fertile days

- Irregular cycles, including postpartum until cycle regularity has returned (Standard Days Method)

- Inability to interpret their fertility signs correctly (Billings Ovulation Method, Symptothermal Method) or to recognize the presence of secretions (TwoDay Method)

- Persistent reproductive tract infections or vaginitis that affect the signs of fertility (Billings Ovulation Method, TwoDay Method, Symptothermal Method)

- Intermenstrual bleeding not distinguishable from menstruation or that masks secretions

- Reluctance to access vaginal secretions (Billings Ovulation, Symptothermal, TwoDay Method)

Postpartum/breastfeeding women will require additional counseling to use Billings Ovulation Method, Symptothermal Method, or TwoDay Method.

SPECIAL ISSUES

Acceptability

Studies have shown that relatively few family planning providers routinely include information about FAB methods in their discussions with patients. A survey of approximately 500 physicians in the United States found that one-third did not mention FAB methods to their patients at all, while 40% mentioned it to selected women. When asked by a patient for information about a FAB method, most physicians described either calendar rhythm or basal body temperature.[23] In another study, nurse-midwives similarly offered little information on FAB methods, based on their perception that these methods are not effective or are inappropriate for their patients,[24] suggesting the potential for provider bias. However, one study suggests that as many as 20% of women seeking family planning services would be interested in a FAB method if it were explained to them appropriately.[22] Recent data from the U.S. National Survey of Family Growth reports that about 25% of American couples have used periodic abstinence or natural family planning at least once.[25]

Recent development of FAB methods that are easy to use may increase interest and availability. This could benefit many women, including those who prefer nonmedical methods, those who are dissatisfied with other methods, the almost 25% of women in the United States between ages 15 and 44 who ever have used periodic abstinence, and the 59% who have used withdrawal.[26] In addition, it is relatively easy to incorporate a discussion of the simpler methods into the context of regular clinical services, thus making the methods more widely available. Ongoing operations research at clinics in California and Massachusetts has demonstrated that it is feasible to integrate the Standard Days Method (SDM) and that clients are interested in the method. One community-based health center in California reported that nearly 120 women adopted SDM in the first year the method was offered.[21]

Some providers and program managers worry that using a FAB method will hamper a couple's sexual life, making the method less acceptable and leading to discontinuation of use. Recent statistical analysis of intercourse patterns of users of the Standard Days Method and of the TwoDay Method show that users of these methods have intercourse almost as frequently as users of other modern methods (5.6 and 5.5 coital acts per month, respectively). The pattern differs, however, as the couples who use these two FAB methods tend to have sex more frequently during the infertile days before and after the fertile window, and avoid sex during their fertile days.[27]

Safety

Because unintended pregnancies among couples who use FAB methods usually result from having intercourse at the beginning or end of the fertile time, concerns have been raised about the risk of birth defects or poor pregnancy outcomes due to aged ovum or sperm. Research has shown that no such increased risks exist.[28,29] An exception is that, in one prospective study, women with a history of spontaneous abortion had a greater chance of having another spontaneous abortion when conception occurred very early or late in the fertile time (23% compared with 10% to 15%).[26] Reassure your clients that FAB methods do not pose a threat to the health of mothers and their children.

Sex Selection

A study of about 1,000 births showed no association between the timing of conception and the sex ratio at birth.[30] These results do not substantiate claims that couples can select the sex of their child by timing intercourse.

PROVIDING FERTILITY AWARENESS-BASED METHODS

To use FAB methods, couples must adjust their sexual behavior according to their fertility intentions. Users of FAB methods will need to avoid unprotected intercourse for about 10 to 17 days of the woman's menstrual cycle, depending on her cycle length and the method used. Successful use of these methods therefore requires that a couple be able to communicate effectively with each other about sexual matters.

Studies conducted by the Institute for Reproductive Health at Georgetown University have shown that it takes less than 20 minutes for a woman to learn that she should consider herself fertile on days 8 to 19 of her cycle and to keep track of her cycle days (to use the Standard Days Method) or to learn how to notice the presence or absence of secretions (to use the TwoDay Method).[25] Counseling may be needed to help her use the methods correctly. Couples using other FAB methods need an instructor's teaching to observe, record, and interpret the woman's fertility signs and patterns. The National Health Service in Great Britain estimates that it takes 4 to 6 hours over two to three cycles to teach a woman fertility awareness skills, including charting fertility signs (cervical secretions and basal body temperature) and identifying the fertile time.[31]

A critical component of providing FAB methods is helping women/couples decide how they want to handle their fertile days (i.e. by abstaining or using another method) to avoid pregnancy. Those who choose to use a barrier method (a fertility awareness-combined method) on those days should be instructed on correct use of the method and counseled accordingly.

> **Emergency Contraception:** Emergency contraceptive pills or insertion of a copper intrauterine contraceptive after unprotected intercourse substantially reduces the risk of pregnancy. (See Chapter 6 for more information.)

USER INSTRUCTIONS FOR FERTILITY AWARENESS-BASED METHODS

STANDARD DAYS METHOD

The Standard Days Method is most appropriate for women who usually have cycles between 26 and 32 days long. Approximately 78% of women can expect to meet this requirement at any time. A woman's cycle length should be reassessed as she ages. To use the Standard Days Method, you will need to track the days of your menstrual cycle, starting with the day your menstrual bleeding begins.

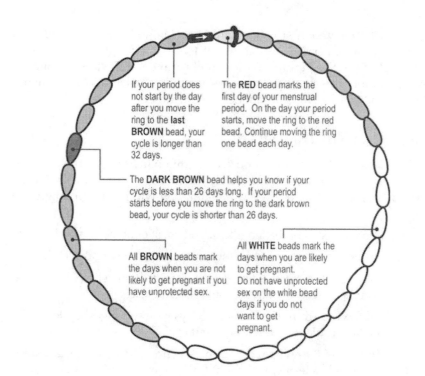

If your period does not start by the day after you move the ring to the **last** **BROWN** bead, your cycle is longer than 32 days.

The **RED** bead marks the first day of your menstrual period. On the day your period starts, move the ring to the red bead. Continue moving the ring one bead each day.

The **DARK BROWN** bead helps you know if your cycle is less than 26 days long. If your period starts before you move the ring to the dark brown bead, your cycle is shorter than 26 days.

All **BROWN** beads mark the days when you are not likely to get pregnant if you have unprotected sex.

All **WHITE** beads mark the days when you are likely to get pregnant. Do not have unprotected sex on the white bead days if you do not want to get pregnant.

Figure 16–1 CycleBeads for Standard Days method

1. Count the first day of your menstrual bleeding as day 1.

2. Continue counting every day.

3. On days 1 to 7, you can have unprotected intercourse. (You may be bleeding on these days.)

4. On days 8 to 19, you should use a barrier method or avoid intercourse if you do not want to become pregnant.

5. From day 20 through the end of your cycle, you can have unprotected intercourse.

6. The Standard Days Method works best for women who usually have cycles between 26 and 32 days long. If you have more than 1 cycle in 1 year that is shorter than 26 days or longer than 32 days, you should contact your provider to discuss the possibility of using another method.

7. **To prevent pregnancy.** Unprotected intercourse is permitted on days 1 to 7 and from day 20 until the end of your cycle. On days 8 to 19, use a barrier method or avoid intercourse.

8. **To become pregnant.** Unprotected intercourse is suggested every other day between days 8 and 19 of your cycle.

Most women who use the Standard Days Method use CycleBeads or a software program based on this visual tool to help them keep track of their cycle days. See Figure 16–1 for an illustration of CycleBeads and instructions for use. Software versions include iCycleBeads for iPhones and CycleBeads for Android phones, among others.

CALENDAR RHYTHM METHOD

The Calendar Rhythm Method was traditionally taught to women in preparation for marriage, but is rarely taught today, and thus is not described here in detail. To use this method, you will need to follow these steps:

1. Keep a record of the lengths of your past 6 menstrual cycles.

2. Find the longest and shortest of your past menstrual cycles.

3. Subtract 18 from the number of days in your shortest cycle to find the first fertile day in your current cycle.

4. Subtract 11 from the number of days in your longest cycle to find the last fertile day in your current cycle.

5. **To prevent pregnancy.** From the first through the last days identified as fertile, you should use a barrier method or avoid intercourse if you do not want to become pregnant.

6. **To become pregnant.** Intercourse is suggested every other day on the days identified as fertile.

7. Update the calculation every cycle to determine your fertile days.

Example: If the lengths of the past six cycles were 29, 27, 30, 28, 29 and 26 days,

Shortest cycle was 27 days long → 27–18 = 9 (first fertile day)

Longest cycle was 30 days long → 30–11= 19 (last fertile day)

Thus, for the current cycle, probable fertile days are 9 through 19.

Women who have very irregular cycles can use the Calendar-Rhythm method, but would have many days identified as potentially fertile, with many of those being false positives.

TWODAY METHOD

The TwoDay Method is based on the presence or absence of cervical secretions. If a woman notices cervical secretions of any type TODAY or YESTERDAY, she considers herself fertile TODAY. If she did not notice any secretions TODAY or YESTERDAY she considers herself not fertile TODAY.[32] This algorithm is illustrated in Figure 16–2.

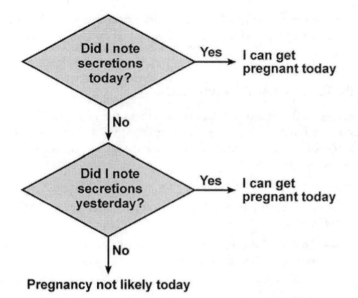

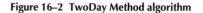

Pregnancy not likely today

Figure 16–2 TwoDay Method algorithm

To use the TwoDay Method:

1. Check for secretions every day before you urinate, in the afternoon and in the evening. You can:

   —Look at the secretions in your underwear or in toilet paper,

   —Touch the secretions in your vulva, or

   —Feel the sensation of wetness at your vulva.

2. Determine whether you are fertile or not TODAY based on the presence or absence of secretions. You can ask yourself these two questions:

   —Did I notice ANY secretions of any type TODAY?

   —Did I notice ANY secretions of any type YESTERDAY?

   If you noticed ANY secretions TODAY or YESTERDAY, you can become pregnant if you have sex today. If you did not notice secretions of any type today or yesterday, you are not likely to get pregnant if you have sex today.

3. **To prevent pregnancy.** Avoid unprotected intercourse if you noticed any secretions of any type either today or yesterday.

4. **To become pregnant.** Unprotected intercourse is suggested every other day on days with secretions.

5. If you have continuous secretions for more than two weeks, or if your secretions are malodorous or irritating, you may have an

infection that requires medical attention and should contact your healthcare provider. (See Chapter 21 on Reproductive Tract Infections.)

BILLINGS OVULATION METHOD

Changes in the characteristics of cervical mucus signal the beginning and end of the fertile time, even among those who have irregular cycles. Assistance of a trained instructor is necessary for correct use of the Billings Ovulation Method.

To use the Billings Ovulation Method:

- Observe your cervical secretions by 'the look, the touch, and the feel':

  — *Look* at the secretions on your underwear, fingers, or toilet paper to determine color and consistency.

  — *Touch* the secretions to determine their stretch and slipperiness.

  — *Feel* how wet the sensation is at your vulva.

When they first appear, the secretions may be scant but sticky and thick, with a cloudy or whitish color. Highly fertile secretions are abundant, clear, stretchy, wet, and slippery. Ovulation most likely occurs within 1 day before, during, or 1 day after the last day of abundant, clear, stretchy, slippery cervical secretions (peak day). If your secretions do not follow this pattern, you may have an infection that requires medical attention and should contact your healthcare provider. (See Chapter 21 on Reproductive Tract Infections.) When you are observing your cervical secretions, do not douche. Douching can wash out the secretions, making it very difficult to notice changes.

Use your cervical secretions to identify the beginning and end of the fertile time:

1. Observe your cervical secretions every day, beginning the day after your menstrual bleeding has stopped, and record them daily on a special chart (Figure 16–3). To help you avoid confusing cervical secretions with semen and normal sexual lubrication, some counselors advise complete sexual abstinence throughout the first cycle. Alternatively, you can use a condom every time you have sex during that cycle. Remember, your own lubrication can increase the secretions you find when you check after sex.

2. Check secretions each time before and after you urinate by wiping (front to back) with tissue paper. Note and record the color and appearance (yellow, white, clear, or cloudy) and feel

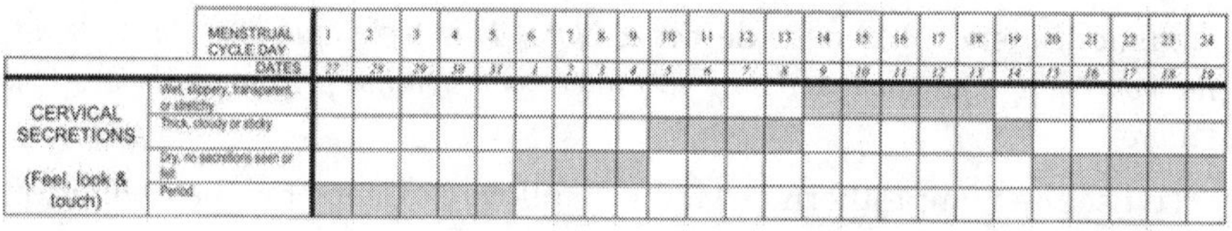

		MENSTRUAL CYCLE DAY DATES	1	2	3	4	5	6	7	8	9	10	11	12	13	14	15	16	17	18	19	20	21	22	23	24
CERVICAL SECRETIONS (Feel, look & touch)			27	28	29	30	31	1	2	3	4	5	6	7	8	9	10	11	12	13	14	15	16	17	18	19
	Wet, slippery, transparent, or stretchy																									
	Thick, cloudy or sticky																									
	Dry, no secretions seen or felt																									
	Period																									

Figure 16–3 Cervical secretion variations during a model menstrual cycle

(dry, wet, or slippery), and consistency (thick, sticky, or stretchy) of the secretions by pulling it between your thumb and index finger. Also, note and chart the sensations of dryness, moistness, or wetness at your vulva. Always record the 'most fertile' observations you see during the day. (Reminder: *Most fertile* means abundant, clear, stretchy, and slippery.)

3. **To prevent pregnancy.** Check for secretions as soon as your menses ends. (Some counselors recommend avoiding intercourse or using a barrier method during menses because it is difficult to detect secretions when they are mixed with menstrual blood.) You can have sexual intercourse on preovulatory days if no secretions are present. (Some counselors recommend abstaining the next day and night following intercourse to allow time for bodily fluids to drain out of your body so you will not confuse semen and arousal fluids with cervical secretions. The following day, check your cervical secretions.) The fertile time begins when cervical secretions are first observed and ends on the 4th day after the *peak day* (see above).

4. **To become pregnant.** Intercourse is suggested every other day when cervical secretions are present. The probability of pregnancy is greatest when the secretions are abundant, clear, stretchy, and slippery. Most women need help in the first few cycles to interpret their cervical secretion patterns and charts to determine the fertile time.

SYMPTOTHERMAL METHOD

Some couples prefer to observe more than one indicator of the woman's fertility. Most couples who use a combined, or symptothermal, approach use both cervical secretions and basal body temperature (BBT) to identify the fertile time.

The BBT is the temperature of the body at rest. It is lower in the first part of the cycle, rises to a higher level beginning around the time of ovulation, and remains at the higher level for the rest of the cycle. By taking her temperature when she first wakes in the morning and recording her temperature on a chart each day of her menstrual cycle, a woman can retrospectively identify whether she has ovulated and, thus, calculate the end of her fertile time. *Note: This technique by itself will not give you enough advance warning to protect you against pregnancy before you ovulate.*

To use the Symptothermal Method, follow the steps for the Ovulation Method. In addition, take and record your BBT as follows to determine the postovulatory infertile time:

1. Take your BBT every morning at the same time before getting out of bed (after at least 3 hours of sleep). A special calibrated thermometer makes temperature reading easier. Take the BBT orally, rectally, or vaginally, but take it at the same site each day so changes in temperature can be detected accurately.

2. Record your BBT readings daily on a chart (Figure 16–4). Connect the dots for each day to make a line between successive days (day 2 to day 3, and so on).

3. Your temperature will probably rise at least 0.4 degrees F° around the time of ovulation and remain elevated until the next menses begins. Your actual temperature and maximum temperature are not important, just the rise over the baseline (preovulatory) temperatures.

4. If you have 3 continuous days of higher temperatures (above the baseline) following 6 days of lower temperatures, you have probably ovulated and your postovulatory infertile time has

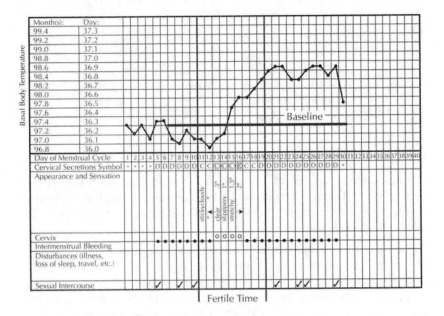

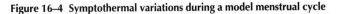

Figure 16–4 Symptothermal variations during a model menstrual cycle

begun. To see the baseline and rise clearly on the chart, highlight the chart at the 0.1 degree line just above the lower (preovulatory) temperatures. When you record 3 continuous temperatures above this line, and the last temperature is 0.4 degrees higher than this line, your postovulatory infertile time has begun.

5. If you cannot detect a sustained rise in BBT, you may not have ovulated in that cycle. A true postovulatory BBT rise usually persists 10 days or longer.

6. Some women notice a temperature drop about 12 to 24 hours before it begins to rise after ovulation, whereas others have no drop in temperature at all. A drop in your BBT probably means ovulation will occur the next day.

7. **To prevent pregnancy.** Rely on your cervical secretions to identify the beginning of your fertile time. Your BBT can help you identify the end of your fertile time. You should use another method or not have intercourse during the fertile time if you do not want to become pregnant.

8. **To become pregnant.** It is often difficult to predict fertile days using BBT. By the time the rise is detected, you are probably in the infertile phase of your menstrual cycle and have missed the opportunity to become pregnant. To become pregnant, you should rely on your cervical secretions.

FAB METHOD COMPARISON

FAB methods differ from each other in terms of the protocol for determining the fertile time and identifying which days to avoid unprotected intercourse, the amount of time typically needed to learn the method, and the materials needed to use it. Table 16–1 compares FAB method protocols and requirements.

FAB METHODS IN DEVELOPMENT

Home Test Kits for Ovulation Prediction and Detection

There are many products available that can help women identify their fertile days. Unfortunately, many of these do not provide enough advance warning of impending ovulation to be useful for pregnancy prevention, given that sperm can survive for up to 5 to 7 days in the vagina. These products include mini microscopes to see ferning of saliva or of cervical mucus (PG53, PC2000, Maybe Baby) as well as handheld computers that measure and correlate day of the cycle with BBT (Babycomp, Ladycomp, Bioself 2000, Cyclotest 2 Plus). Research to evaluate potential effectiveness of some of these devices to prevent pregnancy suggests that

Table 16–1 FAB method protocols

Method	Observations	Days to avoid unprotected intercourse
Standard Days Method	• Track cycle days beginning with first day of menses • Note days 8–19 of cycle	• Days 8–19 of cycle Total: 12 days per cycle
Calendar Method	• Record cycle lengths for 6–12 cycles • Identify shortest and longest cycles • Shortest minus 18: beginning of fertile window • Longest minus 11: end of fertile window	• Days identified as fertile by calculations (repeat calculations every cycle) Total: Depends on cycle-length variability
TwoDay Method	• Note presence or absence of cervical secretions • Record on chart	• All days with secretions • One day following days with secretions Total: Approximately 10–14
Ovulation Method	• Monitor cervical secretions daily • Assess quality and quantity of secretions • Record observations on chart	• Menses • Preovulatory days following days with intercourse • All days with fertile-type secretions • Until 4 days past "peak" day Total: Approximately 14–17 days each cycle
Symptothermal Method	• Monitor cervical secretions daily • Assess quantity and quality of secretions • Take basal temperature daily • Record observations on chart	• Menses • Preovulatory days following days with intercourse • All days with secretions • Until 3 days of higher temperatures following 6 lower temperatures, or 4 days past peak Total: Approximately 12–17 days each cycle

mini microscope-type devices would have high failure rates.[2] Studies to assess the potential contraceptive efficacy of devices with computing capability are mixed.[33,34,35] Persona is a device that measures urinary hormone metabolites to identify the fertile days and combines that information with the length of the woman's previous menstrual cycles. It was shown in a European study to have a failure rate of 6% with correct use.[36] A new version of this device is in development. ClearPlan, a device similar to Persona, is currently being tested by researchers at Marquette University for use in conjunction with monitoring cervical secretions.[37]

Some of these devices are more user-friendly than others. Some require that the user enter more information or are more difficult to operate. Likewise, the information some of them provide is easier to interpret than others. Cost can be an issue, as some of the devices cost several hundred dollars plus the cost of supplies. Additional research (including efficacy trials) is needed before currently available kits and devices can be confidently recommended for pregnancy prevention.

REFERENCES

1. World Health Organization. Family Planning: A Global Handbook for Family Providers. Geneva: World Health Organization, 2007. Available at http://info.k4health.org/globalhandbook/#msword. Last accessed September 26, 2010.
2. Freundl G, Godehardt E, Kern PA, Frank-Hermann P, Koubenec HJ, Gnoth C. Estimated maximum failure rates of cycle monitors using daily conception probabilities in the menstrual cycle. Hum Reprod. 2003;18:2628–2633.
3. World Health Organization. Natural family planning: a guide to provision of services. Geneva: WHO, 1988.
4. Lamprecht VM, Grummer-Strawn L. Development of new formulas to identify the fertile time of the menstrual cycle. Contraception. 1996;54:339–343.
5. Wilcox AJ, Weinberg CR, Baird DD. Timing of sexual intercourse in relation to ovulation. N Engl J Med. 1995;333:1517–1521.
6. Wilcox AJ. Dunson D, Baird DB. The timing of the "fertile window" in the menstrual cycle: day specific estimates from a prospective study. BMJ. 2000;321:1259–1262.
7. Arévalo M, Sinai I, Jennings V. A fixed formula to define the fertile window of the menstrual cycle as the basis of a simple method of natural family planning. Contraception. 2000;60:357–360.
8. Che Y, Cleland JG, Ali MM. Periodic abstinence in developing countries: an assessment of failure rates and consequences. Contraception. 2004;69:15–21.
9. Fehring RJ, Lawrence D, and Philpot C: Use Effectiveness of the Creighton Model Ovulation Method of Natural Family Planning. J Obstet Gynecol, and Neonat Nurs. 23:303–309, 1994.
10. Grimes D, Gallo M, Grigorieva V, Nanda K, Schultz K. Fertility awareness-based methods for contraception: systematic review of randomized controlled trials. Contraception. 2005;72:85–90.
11. Mansour D, Inki P, Gemzell-Danielsson K. Efficacy of contraceptive methods: a review of the literature. Eur J Contracep Repr. 2010;15:14–16.
12. Freundl G, Sivin I, Batár I. State of the art of non-hormonal methods of contraception: IV. Natural family planning. Eur J Contracept Reprod Health Care. 2010;15:113–23.
13. Arévalo M, Jennings V, Sinai I. Efficacy of the Standard Days Method of family planning. Contraception. 2002;65:333–338.
14. Dicker D, Wachsman T, Feldbergt D. The vaginal contraception diaphragm and the condom: an evaluation and comparison of two barrier methods with the rhythm method. Contraception. 1989; 40:497–503.
15. Kambic RT, Lamprecht V. Calendar rhythm efficacy: a review. Adv Contracept. 1996;12:123–128.
16. Trussell J, Grummer-Strawn L. Contraceptive failure of the ovulation method of periodic abstinence. Fam Plann Perspect. 1990;22:65–75.

17. World Health Organization. A prospective multicentre trial of the ovulation method of natural family planning. II. The effectiveness phase. Fertil Steril. 1981; 36:591–598.

18. Bhargava H, Bhatia JC, Ramachandran L, Rohatgi P, Sinha A. Field trial of Billings ovulation method of natural family planning. Contraception. 1996;53:69–74.

19. Frank-Herrmann P, Freundl G, Baur S, Bremme M, Doring GK, Godehardt EAJ, Sottong U. Effectiveness and acceptability of the symptothermal method of natural family planning in Germany. Am J Obstet Gynecol .1991;165:2052–2054.

20. Frank-Herrmann P, Heil J, Gnoth C, Toledo E, Baur S, Pyper C, Jenetzky E, Strowitzki T, Freundl G. The effectiveness of a fertility awareness based method to avoid pregnancy in relation to a couple's sexual behaviour during the fertile time: a prospective longitudinal study. Hum Reprod.. 2007;22:1310–9.

21. Gribble, JN, Lundgren RI, Velasquez C, Anastasi EE . Being strategic about contraceptive introduction: the experience of the Standard Days Method®. Contraception. 2008;77: 147–154.

22. Lavoie, K. Improving family planning services for women and their partners: a couple-focused approach. Institute for Reproductive Health, Georgetown University. 2009.

23. Stanford JB, Thurman PB, Lemaire JC. Physicians' knowledge and practices regarding natural family planning. Obstet Gynecol. 1999;94:672–678.

24. Mikolajczyk RT, Stanford JB, Rauchfuss M. Factors influencing the choice to use modern natural family planning. Contraception. 2003;67:253–258.

25. Mosher WD, Jones J. Use of Contraception in the United States: 1982–2008. National Center for Health Statistics. Vital Health Stat. 2010;23.(29). Available from http://www.cdc.gov/NCHS/data/series/sr_23/sr23_029.pdf [Accessed September 25, 2010].

26. Stanford JB, Lemaire JC, Fox A. Interest in natural family planning among female family practice patients. Fam Pract Res J. 1994; 14:237–49.

27. Sinai I, Arevalo M. It's all in the timing: coital frequency and fertility awareness-based methods of family planning. J Biosoc Sci. 2006;38:763–77.

28. Gray RH, Simpson JL, Kambic RT, Queenan JT, Mena P, Perez A, Barbato M. Timing of conception and the risk of spontaneous abortion among pregnancies occurring during use of natural family planning. Am J Obstet Gynecol. 1995;172:1567–1572.

29. Simpson JL, Gray R, Perez A, Mena P, Queenan JT, Barbato M, Pardo F, Kambic R, Jennings V. Fertilization involving aging gametes, major birth defects and Down's syndrome. Lancet. 2002; 359:1670–1671.

30. Gray RH, Simpson JL, Bitto AC, Queenan JT, Chuanjun L. Sex Ratio associated in timing of insemination and length of the follicular phase in planned and unplanned pregnancies during use of NFP. Hum Reprod. 1998;13:1397–1400.

31. Clubb EM, Pyper CM, Knight J. A pilot study on teaching natural family planning in general practice. Natural family planning: current knowledge and new strategies for the 1990s, Part II 1992:130–132.

32. Sinai I, Arevalo M, Jennings V. The TwoDay algorithm: a new algorithm to identify the fertile time of the menstrual cycle. Contraception. 1999;60:65–70.

33. Fehring R, Raviele K, Schneider M. A comparison of the fertile phase as determined by the Clearplan Easy Fertility Monitor and self-assessment of cervical mucus. Contraception. 2003;69:9–14.

34. Bonnar J, Flynn A, Freundl G, Kirkman R, Royston R, Snowden R. Personal hormone monitoring for contraception. Br J Fam Plan. 2000; 26:178–9.

35. Guida M, Bramante S, Acunzo G, Pellicano M, Cirillo D, Nappi C. Diagnosis of fertility with a personal hormonal evaluation test. Minerva Ginecol. 2003; 55:167–73.

36. Bonnar J, Flynn A, Freundl G, Kirkman R, Royston R, Snowden R. Personal hormone monitoring for contraception. Br J Fam Plann. 1999;24:128–34.

37. Fehring RJ, Schneider M, Barron ML, Raviele K. Cohort comparison of two fertility-awareness based methods of family planning. J Reprod Med. 2009;54:165–70.

Female and Male Sterilization

Danielle Roncari, MD
Melody Y. Hou, MD, MPH, FACOG

- Sterilization is one of the safest, most effective, and most cost-effective contraceptive methods.

- Contraceptive sterilization (female and male) is the most widely used method of family planning in the world in both developed and developing countries.

- Current female methods of sterilization include transabdominal and transcervical approaches.

- Achieving pregnancy after sterilization is expensive, requires either costly assisted reproductive technology (such as in vitro fertilization, or IVF) or highly technical surgery, and results cannot be guaranteed.

- Patients should be advised that sterilization procedures should be considered permanent and do not provide any protection against sexually transmitted infections, including HIV infection.

Tubal sterilization and vasectomy are safe and effective permanent methods of contraception. Sterilization continues to be the most commonly used contraceptive method in the United States, with 15 million U.S. women relying on either female or male sterilization.[1] Approximately 700,000 tubal sterilizations and 500,000 vasectomies[2] are performed in the United States annually.[2,3] Of all women using a contraceptive method in 2006–2008, 16.7% relied on female sterilization and 6.1% relied on male sterilization.[4]

Worldwide, 220 million couples use tubal sterilization or vasectomy as their contraceptive method of choice.[5]

A couple should consider both vasectomy and tubal sterilization as options for permanent contraception. They are comparable in effectiveness, although vasectomy is simpler, safer, and less expensive.

There is no medical condition that would absolutely prohibit sterilization, although some conditions and circumstances may require certain precautions with the procedure. (See Chapter 4 on Medical Eligibility Criteria.)

FEMALE STERILIZATION

The most common methods of female sterilization in the United States are interval tubal sterilization using a laparoscopic approach under general anesthesia and postpartum tubal sterilization using a subumbilical minilaparotomy approach. Recently, the U.S. Food and Drug Administration (FDA) approved the female sterilization systems Essure and Adiana, which use a transcervical approach. Long-term data on these systems are limited. This and transcervical sterilization's unique mechanism of action and technique should be considered during counseling and procedure planning for sterilization.

MECHANISM OF ACTION

Sterilization for women blocks fertilization by cutting or occluding the fallopian tubes to prevent the sperm and egg from uniting. (See Figure 17–1.)

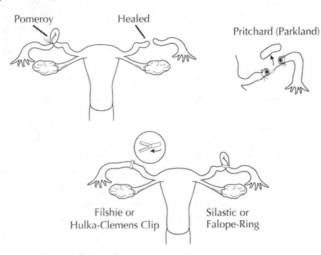

Figure 17–1 Tubal sterilization techniques

EFFECTIVENESS

Following completion of childbearing, women spend approximately 20 years using contraception. Tubal sterilization is far more effective than reversible contraceptive methods that are short-term and user-dependent, such as oral contraceptives, condoms, and injectable methods. The World Health Organization places both female and male sterilization in the top tier of contraceptive effectiveness. The overall first-year typical use failure rate of tubal sterilization is 0.5%, and 0.15% for vasectomy. (See Table 26–1.)

Failure rates of tubal sterilization are roughly comparable with those of long-acting reversible methods of contraception, the contraceptive implant and the intrauterine contraception (IUC). The copper T 380A IUC has a 5-year cumulative failure rate of 14 per 1,000 procedures, and levonorgestrel-releasing IUCs range from 5 to 11 failures per 1,000 procedures.[6–9] The rate of failure with Implanon is estimated at 0.05% within the first year of use (see Table 26–1). The Centers for Disease Control and Prevention in 1996 conducted the Collaborative Review of Sterilization (CREST), a large, prospective, multicenter observational study of over 10,000 women undergoing transabdominal sterilization who were followed up to 14 years. They concluded that transabdominal tubal sterilization is highly effective.[10] Analysis of CREST data found a 5-year cumulative probability of failure of aggregated sterilization methods of 13 per 1,000 procedures.[10] The risk of sterilization failure persists for years after the procedure and varies by several factors, including method and age. The younger a woman was at the time of sterilization, the more likely she was to have had a sterilization failure. Postpartum partial salpingectomy had the lowest 5-year and 10-year cumulative pregnancy rates: 6.3 per 1,000 and 7.5 per 1,000 procedures, respectively. The highest 10-year cumulative pregnancy rate was for women under 28 who had sterilization with bipolar coagulation, 54 pregnancies per 1,000 women.[10] It should be noted that the CREST study on transabdominal sterilizations evaluated certain methods early in their clinical use, so the long-term failure rates with these methods do not necessarily reflect those with current use. The CREST study was also completed prior to the introduction of the popular Filshie clip in the United States in 1996. The United Kingdom, however, has experience with the Filshie clip since 1975, and The Royal College Working Party on Sterilization in 1999 estimated that Filshie clip efficacy compares favorably to other methods with a crude failure rate of 2 to 3 per 1,000 women.[11]

At the time of writing, two transcervical sterilization systems are available in the United States, Essure and Adiana. In the two clinical trials on which FDA approval for Essure was primarily based, no pregnancies were reported in the more than 600 patients using the device up to 5 years, and the method was found to be highly acceptable.[12,13] However, even in clinical trials in which candidates were carefully screened to rule out tubal disease or adhesions which could complicate placement of the Essure micro inserts, the bilateral placement success rate was 81% to 98% (with 2 separate attempts). By 6 months, all women with successful placement had tubal occlusion demonstrated on HSG, but at 3 months, 3.5% did not.[14] There are case reports of pregnancies occurring among women who were not part of any clinical trial, but none have occurred in women in whom successful occlusion has been confirmed via hysterosalpingogram (HSG). Instead, most of these pregnancies have been attributed to patient or clinician noncompliance with manufacturer's instructions or clinician error in interpreting the postprocedure HSG.[15] In a prospective trial of Adiana, there was a 1.1% rate of failure in the first year and a 1.8% rate of failure by the third year. Data collection is still ongoing, but there have been further confirmed pregnancies in the fourth and fifth years, even after successful occlusion was confirmed.[16] The rates for Adiana are higher than the failure rates seen in the CREST study with other forms of female sterilization methods except for the Hulka-Clemens spring clip.[10] Longer-term efficacy has not been fully assessed for either system.

Ectopic Pregnancy

Because spontaneous pregnancy after sterilization is rare, the overall risk of ectopic pregnancy is lower than that of the general population. However, if a pregnancy does occur after sterilization, the chance that it will be ectopic is considerable, although the risk varies with the method of sterilization. An analysis of CREST data found that roughly 30% of post-sterilization pregnancies were ectopic.[17] The 10-year cumulative probability of ectopic pregnancy after transabdominal tubal sterilization by all methods was 7.3 per 1,000 procedures. For Filshie clip applicators and Falope rings the 10-year cumulative probability was 8.5 and 7.3 per 1,000 procedures respectively. Postpartum salpingectomy has the lowest risk of ectopic pregnancy at 1.5 per 1,000 procedures. The risk of ectopic pregnancy did not diminish with the length of time since the tubal sterilization but did vary inversely with the age of the women. For all methods except postpartum partial salpingectomy, the probability of ectopic pregnancy was greater for women sterilized before age 30 years than for women sterilized at age 30 years or older. Furthermore, young women sterilized by bipolar tubal coagulation had a 10-year cumulative probability of ectopic pregnancy of 31.9 per 1,000 procedures.[17] To date, equivalent data on ectopic risk for transcervical sterilization are unavailable, although there have been 2 ectopic pregnancies reported in the first 2 years of the Adiana trial and no reported or published postmarketing cases of an ectopic pregnancy after Essure placement.[12,16]

Intrauterine Pregnancy

When intrauterine pregnancy occurs after transabdominal tubal sterilization, there is no known added risk to the woman or her fetus. Pregnancy outcomes are unclear with Essure left in-situ, since a portion of the coils trail into the uterine cavity. However, the effect of these trailing coils on pregnancy may not be as detrimental as previously thought, since on follow-up hysteroscopy, the trailing coils appear to shorten and become completely encapsulated in tissue.[18] Unintended intrauterine pregnancies have been reported following transcervical sterilization but all were conceived prior to complete tubal occlusion and ended with either successful delivery or elective termination, with complication rates not higher than that of the general population.[15,19] Because these outcome data are from case reports and series, more generalizable statements about transcervical sterilization and safety in pregnancy cannot be made.

ADVANTAGES AND INDICATIONS

Female sterilization is ideal for those women who are certain they wish no further children and need a reliable contraceptive method. Advantages include the following:

- Permanence
- High effectiveness
- High acceptability
- Safety
- Quick recovery
- Lack of significant long-term side effects
- Cost effectiveness
- No need to buy anything
- No need for partner compliance
- No need to interrupt lovemaking
- Privacy of choice

DISADVANTAGES AND CAUTIONS

Female sterilization is not recommended for anyone who is unsure of her desire regarding future fertility. Disadvantages include the following:

- Permanence: Restoring fertility after sterilization is difficult though possible. It is expensive, requires either costly assisted reproductive technology (such as IVF) or highly technical major surgery, and results cannot be guaranteed.

- All surgical procedures carry some risk specific to the nature of the surgery and anesthetic used.
- Regret for decision is high among some groups of women.
- Procedures require surgeon, procedure room (aseptic conditions), trained assistants, medications, and surgical equipment.
- Expense is high at the time of the procedure.
- Probability of pregnancy being ectopic is higher if method fails.
- Sterilization provides no protection against sexually transmitted infections (STIs), including infection with the human immunodeficiency virus (HIV).

Women with medical conditions or other special characteristics may have precautions for sterilization that differ from those of healthy women or women without these medical conditions or characteristics. To identify situations in which this is the case, please refer to the table on sterilization in Chapter 4, Medical Eligibility Criteria.

SAFETY

Tubal sterilization is a safe method of contraception. Death from transabdominal tubal sterilization is extremely rare, and overall complication rates are low. Mortality rates in the United States have been estimated at 1 to 4 deaths per 100,000 procedures.[20–23] Most deaths in the United States have been associated with anesthetic complications.[24] In the CREST study, no deaths were reported among 9,475 women who underwent interval laparoscopic tubal ligation.[25]

Major complications from transabdominal tubal sterilization are also uncommon. The complication rates for tubal sterilization, which includes conversion to laparotomy, blood transfusion, febrile morbidity, and rehospitalization, are estimated to be 0.9 to 1.6 per 100 procedures.[25] The types of complications vary by the type of surgical procedure and anesthesia, as well as if energy is used for tubal occlusion. Intraoperative complications include damage to bowel, bladder, or major vessels. Rarely, laparotomy and/or blood transfusion may be required to manage these events. Postoperative complications include wound infection and possible prolonged pelvic or abdominal pain. Risk factors for complications during transabdominal tubal sterilization include previous abdominal or pelvic surgery and obesity.[25]

Based on published literature, major complications other than pregnancy from transcervical sterilization have not been reported. Tubal perforation was reported in 1% to 3% of Essure cases. Micro inserts were found in the intraperitoneal cavity in 0.5% to 3% of women, and other incorrect placements were found in 0.5% of them. No perforations were reported during the Adiana trial.[13,16] In addition to infection, bleeding, and injury to surrounding organs, potential complications might include hypervolemia from hysteroscopy in less than 1% of cases. Fluid absorbance may be of particular interest during Adiana placement, since the procedure requires nonionic solution during hysteroscopy.[13,16] There are case reports of pelvic pain following Essure placement, with relief following laparoscopic or hysteroscopic removal even 11 months postoperatively, but there are no randomized trials that compare transcervical sterilization safety or postprocedure patient pain with that of transabdominal sterilization.[26,27]

Anesthetic risks include idiosyncratic reaction to local anesthesia, or airway control and ventilation complications associated with the use of general anesthesia.

SPECIAL ISSUES

Cancer Prevention

Case control and cohort studies have consistently shown a reduced risk of ovarian cancer following transabdominal tubal sterilization.[28–30] The protective effect of transabdominal tubal sterilization on ovarian cancer persists over many years. A large case-control study showed tubal sterilization was associated with a 39% reduction in the risk of ovarian cancer. The risk remained low up to 25 years after surgery and was irrespective of sterilization technique.[28] Results of a cohort study of more than 65,000 Danish women not only showed an overall decrease in the risk of ovarian cancer, but also a reduced rate of endometrial cancer, although the association was not as strong.[29]

The protective effect of transabdominal tubal sterilization on ovarian cancer risk also extends to carriers of the BRCA1 mutation, according to one study.[31,32] The risk reduction does not appear to include carriers of BRCA2, although this may be due to the small sample size.[32] Combined oral contraceptive (COC) use, especially long term use, confers more protection in BRCA1 carriers, but the combination of COCs and tubal ligation offered greater protection than either method alone, conferring a risk reduction of 72%.[32]

The biological mechanism for ovarian cancer reduction in women who have undergone transabdominal tubal sterilization is unknown. Possible theories include routine screening for occult ovarian pathology at the time of pelvic surgery, blockage of the ascent of potentially carcinogenic agents such as talc or an immeasurable effect on ovarian function or hormone levels.

Studies examining the relationship between tubal sterilization and breast cancer are mixed. One prospective cohort study of 619,199 women suggests an inverse association between tubal sterilization and breast cancer mortality, with a stronger protective benefit related to younger age at time of sterilization.[33] However, data from the Nurses' Health Study and Cancer and Steroid Hormone Study yielded no association with breast cancer risk.[34,35] Unmeasured confounding related to differences in screening practices may explain inconsistent study outcomes.

The impact of transcervical sterilization on these cancers has not been studied.

Menstrual Abnormalities

The long-term health effects of tubal sterilization on menstrual pattern appear to be negligible. Early studies of menstrual disturbances (post-tubal ligation syndrome) after sterilization failed to account for confounding variables, such as presterilization use of hormonal contraceptives that can mask underlying menstrual dysfunction.[36-38] The fact that women who have postpartum sterilization may have inaccurate memories of their menses or the impact that weight gain during pregnancy has on the menses is not understood by many women. Most recent studies that account for these factors have found little or no difference in menstrual patterns between women before and after transabdominal sterilization.[38-45] Although 2 to 4% of women in the Essure and Adiana trials reported a disturbance in their menstrual patterns, the relationship of the menstrual abnormalities to transcervical sterilization is unclear, and the same concerns about confounding by discontinuation of hormonal contraception apply.[13,16]

Ovarian Function, Vascular Changes and Potential Effects

A decrease in ovarian blood supply has been postulated as a mechanism by which tubal ligation might protect against ovarian cancer. Several studies have recently evaluated the vascular effects of tubal ligation and subsequent ovarian function as well as possible long-term outcomes such as menopausal symptoms and osteoporosis. A prospective matched cohort evaluation of ovarian reserve and function in women undergoing laparoscopic tubal sterilization using bipolar coagulation showed no functional impact after 5 years.[46] Another prospective study of minilaparotomy and laparoscopic tubal ligation found no difference in uterine or ovarian blood flow or ovarian hormone secretion after 6 months.[47]

Despite relatively strong evidence that ovarian function and vascular resistance are not affected by tubal ligation,[46-48] there are conflicting reports on the association of tubal sterilization and menopausal symptoms.[49,50] Prospective randomized controlled trials are warranted before making definitive conclusions.

Hysterectomy

Although there is no known biologic mechanism to support a causal relationship between tubal sterilization and hysterectomy, there is a strong reported association between transabdominal sterilization and hysterectomy (RR, 1.6–4.4).[43,51–55] Women who undergo tubal sterilization appear to be 4 to 5 times more likely to undergo hysterectomy than those whose partners underwent vasectomy. Increased risk was associated with a presterilization history of menstrual or other benign gynecologic disorders.[51] This association suggests a tendency of surgeons to move to hysterectomy rather than to use medical therapy or conservative surgery when a woman no longer wishes to preserve her fertility. There are no data yet on the rate of hysterectomy following transcervical sterilization.

Sexuality

A study of female marital sexuality found no detrimental long-term effects from female or male sterilization. Conversely, the study found an increase in coital frequency after 1 year among women who had undergone transabdominal tubal sterilization as compared with women not planning sterilization.[56]

A CREST study to determine if interval tubal sterilization leads to a change in female sexual interest or pleasure found that interval tubal sterilization is unlikely to result in changed sexual interest or pleasure. Among those women with changes, the majority experienced positive sexual effects.[56,57]

Endometrial Ablation and Tubal Sterilization

Endometrial ablation has become an increasingly popular treatment for heavy or prolonged uterine bleeding. Women are advised not to undergo ablation unless they have completed childbearing due to the increased risk of abnormal placentation (e.g., placenta accreta), spontaneous abortion and preterm delivery in a subsequent pregnancy.[58] Sterilization is thus an appealing contraceptive option for these women. However, after ablation, endometrial tissue can persist or regenerate in the cornual regions of the uterine cavity, even when the remaining cavity may be reduced in size or completely obliterated by the procedure.[59] For patients undergoing tubal sterilization in addition to an ablation, retrograde bleeding from persistent endometrial tissue in the cornua and in the isolated areas in the myometrium into the proximal tubal segment can cause painful distention known as post-ablation tubal sterilization syndrome.[60] The frequency of post-ablation tubal sterilization syndrome is unknown.

Transcervical sterilization may have a lower risk of post-ablation tubal sterilization syndrome because the occlusion occurs in the tubocornual junction, but this has not been studied. Performing transcervical sterilization concurrent with ablation is not advisable, due to the difficulty in reading the HSG to determine whether the tubes have been occluded, but successful concomitant procedures have been reported.[175] Manufacturer instructions for both Essure and Adiana recommend confirming that the tubes are occluded prior to performing any planned ablations.[13,16] Global radiofrequency ablation, such as the NovaSure system, is not recommended with Essure microinserts in-situ due to the potential risk of energy conduction along the stainless steel core and damage to surrounding organs, but there are case reports of successful combined NovaSure and Essure procedures. Studies have, however, demonstrated the safety of global thermal methods, such as ThermaChoice, and endometrial resection with careful avoidance of the microinserts in the cornua.[15,61,62]

RISK OF REGRET

Most women who choose sterilization as a contraceptive method never regret their decision; however, because of relationship changes and other life events, regret is always possible. Women who undergo sterilization before the age of 30 are at greater risk for regret.[63–65] The cumulative probability of regret over 14 years of follow-up in the CREST study was 12.7%.[61] However, the probability was 20.3% for women aged 30 years or younger at the time of sterilization, compared with 5.9% for women older than 30 years at the time of sterilization. The CREST data also showed similar high levels of regret for interval sterilization within 1 year of delivery (22.3%) as for postpartum sterilization after vaginal delivery (23.7%) and cesarean delivery (20.7%). The cumulative probability of regret diminished steadily with the interval between delivery and sterilization.[61] Post-abortion sterilization was not associated with increased regret when compared with interval sterilization.[63,66–68]

Analysis of the data from the CREST study showed the 14-year cumulative probability of requesting reversal information was 14.3%, but in women under the age of 24 who underwent sterilization, the request for reversal information was as high as 40.4%.[65] The number of women who requested information about IVF was undocumented.

Risk factors for increased regret include having received less information about the procedure, having had less access to information or support for other contraceptive method use, and having made the decision under pressure from a spouse or because of medical indications.[65,69,70]

Younger women are at greater risk for regret given the longevity of their future fertility and the opportunity for life changes such as divorce and remarriage or the death of a child.

Thorough and effective counseling is crucial in reducing regret in women undergoing sterilization. Counseling should be in a language the patient can easily understand. Both the patient and her partner (when appropriate) should be counseled, and risk factors for regret should be addressed.[71] The presence of strong risk factors for regret (such as age) should not be used to uniformly restrict sterilization. Instead, these risk factors should be indicators for more extensive counseling before undergoing sterilization. The availability of the highly effective IUCs and implants will result in fewer young women choosing sterilization prematurely.

Desire for Pregnancy Following Tubal Sterilization

Sterilization should be considered permanent, but even with careful counseling some women will have a change in personal circumstance and later desire more children. In-vitro fertilization (IVF) or microsurgical tubal reversal can be considered if attempting pregnancy following transabdominal sterilization. Success is not guaranteed with either approach.

The choice between IVF and tubal surgery to achieve pregnancy following surgical tubal sterilization is dependent on multiple factors, including the age of the woman at the time of treatment, severity of the tubal damage and remaining tubal length, as well as other fertility factors. With careful case selection and meticulous surgical technique, reasonable pregnancy rates can be achieved following microsurgical reversal of tubal sterilization.[72]

Surgery, especially major abdominal surgery, carries operative risks as well as risks due to anesthesia. Ectopic pregnancy is more common among pregnancies occurring after surgical reversal of female sterilization. Ectopic pregnancy rates range from 1% to 7%—higher rates can be observed in specific anatomical situations.[72] Nonetheless, sterilization reversal may be appealing for younger women, couples who desire more than a single additional pregnancy, or those who are not comfortable with IVF. Both IVF and reversal surgery are costly and are often not covered by health insurance. Finally, those couples utilizing tubal reversal surgery may have the need for future contraception. A large Canadian study showed that 23% of women obtaining tubal reversal following sterilization went on to obtain a subsequent sterilization.[73]

There are limited data on the likelihood that women can become pregnant after reversal of transcervical sterilization, or on what the outcomes may be for any pregnancies that occur. One of the issues with transcervical sterilization is the location of the implants within the tubocornual junction rather than the tube itself, and the tissue ingrowth into the implants. There are anecdotal reports of Essure reversals via removal of the implants and reimplantation of the tubes, with one subsequent spontaneous pregnancy and birth at the time of this writing, but none yet published in the literature.[74] IVF implantation and pregnancy outcomes are unknown with Essure left in-situ, since a portion of the coils trail into the uterine cavity. However, there are case reports of successful IVF pregnancies following transcervical sterilization, especially several years after coil placement.[75]

PROVIDING FEMALE STERILIZATION
COUNSELING GUIDELINES FOR FEMALE STERILIZATION

The goal of counseling is to help clients select a contraceptive method that they will use, that will be effective, that is most consistent with their reproductive intentions, and that will not have adverse effects. The permanence of sterilization methods is a significant consideration with respect to counseling.

The factors contributing to an individual's decision about female sterilization vary. Each woman needs to weigh the risks, benefits, effectiveness, and side effects of the various contraceptive options available to her, as well as her personal need to use a barrier method for protection against sexually transmitted infections, especially HIV/AIDS.

Counseling should address the following:

1. **Provide choices.** Present highly effective, long-acting, temporary methods as options, such as the contraceptive implant or IUC, as well as male sterilization.

2. **Assess the client's understanding of the procedure.** Although awareness of female sterilization is widespread in the United States, review the procedure with your clients so that she correctly understands each sterilization procedure, its effectiveness, and risks and has no misconceptions.

3. **Facilitate the decision-making process.** Give the client sufficient time to make a thoughtful, informed decision about a permanent method of contraception, especially women having immediate postpartum or post-abortion (spontaneous or induced) sterilization. The woman should have decided she wants a permanent method well before delivery or a pregnancy-related event or procedure.

4. **Provide information about possible failure.** Inform clients that sterilization is not 100% successful and that failure can

occur, even years after the procedure was performed. Additionally, there is a significant risk of ectopic pregnancy if the method fails.

5. **Discuss STI prevention.** Tubal sterilization will not provide protection against sexually transmitted infections, including HIV. Thoroughly explain the risk to the client or her partner(s). Condom use will be necessary if the client is at risk of such infections.

Components of Presterilization Counseling [76]

- Permanent nature of the procedure
- Alternative methods of contraception available (reversible methods as well as vasectomy)
- Reasons for choosing sterilization
- Screening for risk indicators for regret
- Details of the procedure, including risks and benefits of anesthesia
- The possibility of failure and risk of ectopic pregnancy
- The need to use condoms for protection against sexually transmitted diseases, including HIV
- Need for post-procedure confirmation following transcervical sterilization methods
- Federal and state Medicaid regulations regarding informed consent, including age of the client, circumstances in which consent is obtained, and interval from time of consent to procedure

Informed Consent

Informed consent is a voluntary decision made by a person who is able to give consent and is fully informed regarding a particular surgical procedure and its consequences. Provide information on tubal sterilization in a language that the client can understand. The client must always sign or mark an informed consent form indicating that she understands the type of operation and intended permanence, possibility of failure, and risks and benefits, including the option to decline sterilization without loss of medical or financial benefits. The surgeon or authorized representative must also sign the form. Written informed consent should document, but not substitute for, the provider's active involvement in the client's informed decision to have tubal sterilization. Ensure that she has knowingly and freely requested the procedure. Understand that the initial consent for sterilization often represents only a consent to obtain surgical consent later for the actual procedure. The state's consents do not replace the surgical consent, which must be obtained at the time of the procedure.

Policy and Legal Issues

Knowledge of state and local guidelines is important in the counseling and consent process. Some states have requirements about the consent process, forms and the requirements, which must be adhered to, even if private funding is used.

- Strict adherence to informed choice and consent procedures is mandatory prior to sterilization.[77]

- Partner or spousal consent in the United States is not legally required.[78]

- Clients using federal or state funds for sterilization must be age 21 or older and mentally competent; they must wait 30 days after signing consent before receiving a sterilization procedure. There may be exceptions in cases of premature delivery,[78] where women must sign their informed consent 30 days prior to either estimated date of delivery or actual delivery date.

Arbitrary decisions by health professionals to restrict access to sterilization have been judged by courts in the United States to violate a woman's basic rights. The policy and legal status of providing sterilization for mentally challenged individuals remains a problem. Health care providers, policy makers, and the public should be aware of the ethical and legal issues involved in providing voluntary sterilization to those who may not be able to give informed consent.[79]

TIMING

Tubal sterilization can be performed at the time of cesarean delivery, postpartum, after spontaneous or therapeutic abortion, or as an interval procedure (unrelated in time to a pregnancy). The timing of the procedure influences both the surgical approach and the method of tubal occlusion. For patients relying on federal or state funding, Medicaid regulations require that the abortion consent and the sterilization consent be obtained on separate occasions.

Postpartum Sterilization

Postpartum sterilization is performed after 10% of all hospital deliveries in the United States.[76] Approximately half of all sterilization procedures are performed in this period.[3] Sterilization may be done at the time of cesarean delivery or via minilaparotomy following vaginal delivery and should not extend the patient's hospital stay. Postpartum minilaparotomy should be done in a medically stable patient prior to the onset of significant uterine involution (within 1 to 2 days following delivery). Fully assess maternal and neonatal well-being prior to sterilization. Consider postponing sterilization in the presence of medical or obstetric complications.[74] Individualize the choice of anesthetic technique based on obstetrical outcomes and maternal risk factors. However, regional anesthesia is usually preferred over general anesthesia.[80] Local anesthesia with sedation has been used but little data exist on its effectiveness.[81]

Postpartum sterilization requires counseling and informed consent before labor and delivery.[82,83] Obtain the woman's consent during prenatal care, when the patient can make an informed decision, review the risks and benefits of the procedure, and consider alternative methods of contraception. For patients without private insurance who rely on federally funded insurance programs, consider the regulations that address the timing of consent.[79]

Interval Tubal Sterilization

In the United States, approximately one half of all tubal sterilizations are performed as interval procedures.[3] Although *transabdominal* tubal sterilization can be done at any time during the menstrual cycle, performing the procedure during the patient's follicular phase reduces the likelihood of concurrent (luteal phase) pregnancy, as does the patient's use of an effective method of contraception before sterilization. Same-day, highly sensitive urine pregnancy tests will detect pregnancies as early as 1 week after conception.[84] The introduction of *transcervical* devices, Essure and Adiana, has expanded women's sterilization options. For these procedures, performing them in the early follicular phase not only reduces the chance of pregnancy but may also provide technical advantages.

Postabortion sterilization

Approximately 3.5% of all sterilizations are performed after an elective or spontaneous abortion.[85] Sterilization, either laparoscopically or via minilaparotomy, following uncomplicated first and second trimester abortions, can be provided without added risk over interval sterilization.[86] To avoid additional risk, use a single anesthetic for both the abortion and the sterilization. Transcervical sterilization should not be performed immediately after an abortion procedure due to poor visualization via hysteroscopic methods.[13,16]

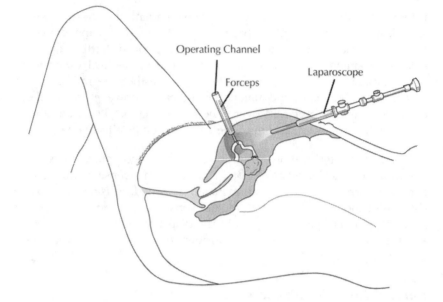

Figure 17–2 Laparoscopy

Options For Approach

There are 2 basic approaches to female sterilization—transabdominal, via minilaparotomy or laparoscopy, and transcervical. The transvaginal approach is rarely used and is associated with an increased rate of postoperative infections and other potential complications. Hysterectomy, whether performed through a vaginal or abdominal approach, carries a much higher risk of morbidity and mortality than other sterilization procedures. Hysterectomy should not be performed for contraceptive purposes alone.

The transabdominal approach is currently the most common approach to tubal sterilization in the United States.[3] *Laparoscopy* is most commonly used for interval sterilization and is usually performed as an outpatient procedure. The advantage of laparoscopy over other surgical approaches includes the opportunity to inspect under direct visualization the abdominal and pelvic organs. Laparoscopy results in barely visible incision scars and a rapid return to full activity for the patient. The disadvantages of laparoscopy include the special training required, possible difficulty accessing the fallopian tubes due to prior surgery or adhesions, and the risk of bowel, bladder, or major vessel injuries following insertion of laparoscopic instruments. (See Figures 17–2 and 17–3.)

In the United States, *minilaparotomy* is most commonly used for postpartum procedures prior to involution of the uterus. A small 2 to 3 cm

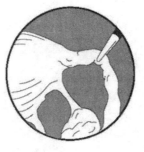

Figure 17–3 A laparoscopy instrument grasps one tube in preparation for electrocoagulation or application of a ring or clip

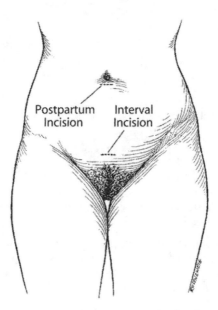

Figure 17–4 Minilaparotomy incision site and size

incision is made below the umbilicus, allowing easy access to the fallopian tubes. (See Figure 17–4.) Minilaparotomy requires only basic surgical instruments and training, although there is still a small risk of injury to the bowel, bladder, and other adjacent structures. In developing countries where laparoscopy is not available, suprapubic or minilaparotomy is frequently used for interval or first trimester post-abortion tubal sterilization.

Transcervical approaches to tubal sterilization involve gaining access to the fallopian tubes via the cervix. There are currently two FDA-approved methods in the United States. The Essure device, introduced in 2002, is a soft, flexible, micro-insert that is placed, by hysteroscopic guid-

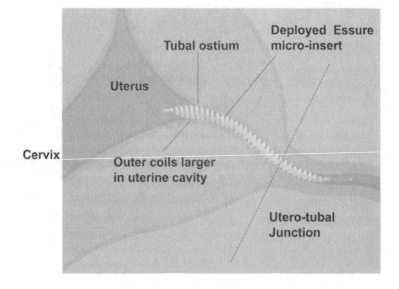

Figure 17–5 Hysteroscopic placement of Essure micro-insert within the tubal lumen

ance, in the proximal section of each fallopian tube (Figure 17–5).[13] Adiana was approved by the FDA in 2009. A specially designed catheter-electrode is introduced, by hysteroscopic guidance, into each tubal ostium to create a tubal lesion via radiofrequency energy. A silicone matrix is then deployed into the thermal lesion site (Figure 17–6).[16]

Clinicians require special training to perform either hysteroscopic method, which can be done only as interval procedures. In less than 30 minutes, either method can be provided under local anesthesia, with or without sedation, in a properly equipped physician's office with appropriately dedicated resources for post-procedure recovery.

Successful placement is not guaranteed, and either procedure may be abandoned due to abnormal findings at the time of hysteroscopy or from failed attempts to place one or both devices. Data from the original prospective multicenter trials of Essure reported successful bilateral placement rates of 86% after 1 procedure.[87] A study published in 2004 reported 98% success in single-attempt bilateral placement using an improved catheter design, which is now widely available.[88] A systematic review published in 2010 reported bilateral placement success rate of 81% to 98% (with up to two attempts).[14] The initial trials of Adiana showed a 94% successful placement with one procedure. Rates increased to 95% after a second procedure.[87]

Placement of transcervical devices may be difficult because of anatomical features such as tubal or uterine scarring.[87] Effectiveness with either method is dependent on growth and formation of tubal scar tissue.

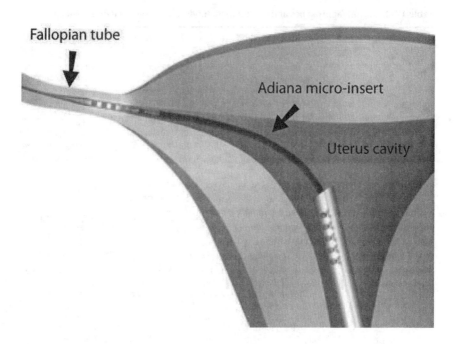

Fallopian tube

Adiana micro-insert

Uterus cavity

Figure 17–6 Adiana transcervical micro-insert. Courtesy of Hologic, Inc. and affiliates

Therefore, the woman must use an alternate method of reliable contraception for at least 3 months following either procedure, until a HSG demonstrates that both tubes are occluded.[13,16]

CHOICE OF OCCLUSION METHOD

The choice of occlusion method depends on the provider's training, personal experience, the patient's medical history including prior abdominal or uterine surgery, availability of supplies, and ultimately, the approach. The transabdominal minilaparotomy approach allows for ligation and transection of the fallopian tubes, whereas laparoscopic procedures use special instruments to apply clips, bands, or electrocoagulation for complete occlusion. There are currently two devices for transcervical tubal occlusion as described in the previous section.

Laparoscopic Occlusion Methods

It is possible to do a Pomeroy sterilization procedure with an endoscopy loop. Electrocoagulation for tubal occlusion is used exclusively with laparoscopic sterilization. Bipolar electrocoagulation is the most common laparoscopic occlusion method in the United States.[89] Unipolar

Table 17–1 Various approaches and occlusion methods (advantages and disadvantages)

Approach	Occlusion Method	Advantages	Disadvantages
Laparoscopy	1. Silastic bands or Falope-rings 2. Filshie or Hulka clips 3. Bipolar electrocoagulation 4. Unipolar electrocoagulation	1. Single incision with either single-punch or double-punch technique 2. Less pain than from minilaparotomy 3. Low complication rate 4. Short recovery time	1. Need for specialist with method-specific training 2. Necessary equipment is often difficult to obtain and maintain 3. Need a fully equipped operating and recovery room with trained staff
Transcervical	1. Essure 2. Adiana	1. May be performed under local anesthesia 2. No incisions or scars 3. Can be safely performed in an outpatient setting	1. Long-term effectiveness not known 2. Requires initial 3 months of back-up contraception and confirmatory HSG
Suprapubic Minilaparotomy	1. Pomeroy and Pritchard (Parkland) technique 2. Silastic bands or Falope-rings 3. Filshie or Hulka clips	1. Local or general anesthesia 2. Incision site usually not visible (below pubic hairline)	1. Difficult technique if the woman is obese, the uterus immobile or the tubes have adhesions 2. Recovery can be more painful than with laparoscopy
Postpartum Sterilization			
Subumbilical Minilaparotomy	1. Pomeroy or Pritchard (Parkland) technique 2. Filshie clip	1. Convenience 2. Lower costs 3. Ease of surgery 4. Does not necessarily extend hospital stay beyond that for a normal delivery	1. Electrocoagulation not indicated 2. Filshie clip requires special postpartum applicator 3. Counseling must be prior to labor to reduce risk of regret
Cesarean Section	1. Pomeroy or Pritchard (Parkland) technique 2. Filshie clip	1. Convenience 2. Lower costs 3. Anatomy fully visible	1. Cesareans should not be performed solely to occlude the tubes 2. Other disadvantages from subumbilical minilaparotomy apply
Postabortion Sterilization			
Laparoscopy	1. Silastic bands or Falope-rings 2. Filshie or Hulka clips 3. Bipolar electrocoagulation 4. Unipolar electrocoagulation	1. Convenience 2. Client motivation	1. Need for careful counseling with consideration of risk of regret 2. If using general anesthesia, may increase the amount of blood loss with abortion procedure
Suprapubic Minilaparotomy	Pomeroy and Pritchard (Parkland) techniques	Same as above	Same as above

electrocoagulation is not commonly used because of an association with thermal bowel injury. At least 3 cm of the isthmic portion of the tube must be coagulated using sufficient energy to achieve maximum efficacy.[89] Use of a current meter rather than visualizing tissue blanching during bipolar coagulation more accurately indicates complete coagulation and is associated with improved efficacy rates[90,91] Ectopic pregnancy rates are higher with electrocoagulation methods than with other occlusion methods. In the CREST study, the risk of ectopic pregnancy for women who underwent sterilization by bipolar coagulation before the age of 30 was 27 times higher than for those women who had a postpartum partial salpingectomy (31.9 vs. 1.2 ectopic pregnancies per 1,000 procedures).[17]

Mechanical occlusion devices commonly used with laparoscopic sterilization in the United States include the silastic band (Falope Ring), the Filshie clip, and the Hulka-Clemens clip. All require special applicators and are most effective when used to occlude normal-appearing tubes. None of these methods involve risk of electrical burn.[92,93] While sterilization should always be considered a permanent method, these devices typically destroy less of the fallopian tube than electrocoagulation methods, making future reversal efforts more likely to succeed.[89]

The silastic band was first developed in the 1970s in pursuit of a safer, non-thermal method. Two centimeters of tube is contained in a constricted loop following application. With this method, it is possible to lacerate the tube or surrounding vessels, and application may be more difficult when tubal abnormalities are present, such as adhesions or edema. The silastic band is one of the most commonly used tubal sterilization devices worldwide.

The Hulka-Clemens clip was developed in the same time period as the silastic band, and was introduced in the United States in 1972. The hinged spring-loaded plastic clip with interlocking teeth is loaded in a special applicator and applied perpendicular to the tube across the isthmus. A popular method since it destroys less than 1 cm of tissue, the Hulka clip's popularity decreased once its relatively high failure rate was recognized. The cumulative 10-year failure rate in the CREST study for the Hulka-Clemens clip was 3.65%.[10]

In September 1996, the FDA approved the Filshie clip for use as a new contraceptive device in the United States. The hinged Filshie clip is made of titanium with a silicone rubber lining, which expands to keep the tube compressed as it flattens. It is easier to use than other occlusion devices, destroys a minimal amount of the fallopian tube (5 mm), and has a high efficacy.[94] It requires a special applicator for interval laparoscopic sterilization and for postpartum sterilization.[94,95] The Filshie clip has a similar safety and efficacy profile as other occlusion devices with data from the

UK demonstrating a crude failure rate of 2 to 3 in 1,000 women.[11] Studies do not support routine application of multiple clips per tube.

Transcervical Occlusion Methods

Essure and Adiana are transcervical mechanical occlusion devices. Both methods are considered irreversible and require an alternate method of reliable contraception be used until an HSG documents a successful occlusion. Both microinserts are placed through a hysteroscope. Essure consists of two concentric metal coils. The nickel titanium outer coil anchors the device in the tubal lumen; the inner stainless steel coil anchors synthetic polyester fibers and causes a benign inflammatory response. The inflammation stimulates growth of fibrous tissue, which occludes the tubes over the subsequent few weeks. During the Adiana procedure, bipolar radiofrequency energy is used to first create a superficial 5 mm tubal lesion. A 3.5 mm silicone matrix is then placed into the tube at the site of this lesion. Over the next few weeks, fibroblast tissue grows into the porous matrix architecture.[87]

Transcervical devices have relatively few contraindications and are acceptable alternatives in patients with significant medical problems who require permanent contraception. However, these methods rely on inflammation and scar tissue formation to cause tubal occlusion. Therefore, caution women who are immunocompromised from HIV infection, immunosuppression medications, or chemotherapy that while data are lacking, success rates may be lower in immunocompromised women.[13,16] Nickel allergy is a contraindication specifically for Essure, as the effects from the small amount of nickel in the microinserts have not been examined in these women. Women who have a possible nickel allergy should pursue formal allergy testing before undergoing sterilization via Essure.[13] In addition, because transcervical sterilization requires the use of a HSG to confirm successful occlusion, allergy to contrast dye is a contraindication for the procedure. While the presence and position of Essure devices can be confirmed using ultrasound and other imaging modalities such as CT and MRI, these modalities are off-label in the United States and are not considered sufficient to prove successful occlusion.[96,97]

Transabdominal Ligation Methods

Tubal occlusion at the time of Cesarean delivery, and postpartum or interval minilaparotomy and traditional laparotomy is usually performed by ligation and resection of a portion of both fallopian tubes. A variety of techniques have been described, including the Pomeroy and Parkland methods (Figure 17–1).[83] The most common variation of the Pomeroy method is the substitution of plain catgut, which degrades more rapidly, replacing the original chromic suture type. The Irving and Uchida methods involve ligating and excising a segment of the tube and burying the proximal end either in the myometrium (Irving) or in the mesosalpinx (Uchida). Occasionally the distal end is also buried in the mesosalpinx, although it is more frequently left exposed. The Irving and Uchida methods are seldom used in the United States, although failures with these two methods are exceedingly rare.[83]

ANESTHESIA AND PAIN MANAGEMENT

Short-acting general anesthesia or regional anesthesia is most frequently used for female transabdominal sterilization procedures in the United States. The current trend today is toward out-patient-based surgery. Transcervical devices may be provided using local anesthesia or minimal intravenous sedation. The use of a nonsteroidal anti-inflammatory is recommended 1 to 2 hours prior to transcervical procedures to both control pain and reduce risk of tubal spasm that can prevent placement of the microinserts.

Advantages of local anesthesia include lower complication rates, lower cost of the procedure, quicker recovery, better postoperative course with fewer or milder side effects, and high acceptance by most patients. By not compromising the normal physiological control of vital functions, a high level of safety can be maintained. *All* anesthetic methods, however, need the attention of a trained professional who carefully monitors the patient and the drugs used. Avoid high doses of opioid (narcotic) analgesics and benzodiazepine (tranquilizer) sedatives that can compromise ventilation, sometimes dramatically, and may cause cardiovascular depression.[83] For complete information on anesthetic techniques and regimens, go to www.engenderhealth.org (Mini-laparotomy for Female Sterilization: An illustrated guide for providers, 2003: pg 27–31.)[98]

MANAGING PROBLEMS AND FOLLOW-UP

Major complications from tubal sterilizations are uncommon and vary by study definition, occurring at levels that range from 1 to 3.5%.[25,92,93] The types of complications vary by the type of surgical procedure and anesthesia. Among the risks are hemorrhage, infection, and the risk of death from anesthesia. The risk of these complications can be reduced by careful screening, use of local anesthesia with light sedation, close monitoring of vital signs, good asepsis, and careful surgical technique. The seriousness of complications can often be minimized by early recognition and aggressive management.

Intraoperative complications recognized during surgery can be avoided or attended to by an experienced surgeon and by adherence to standard protocols. Although complications from laparoscopy are NOT more common than that from minilaparotomy, some are more severe. Because of the blind entry into the abdomen and the proximity of major blood vessels, bowel and other organs, prompt recognition of injury to these structures is paramount. No patient should leave the recovery room without both verbal and clear written instructions for follow-up, including 24 hour contact information for concerns or emergencies, immediate self care, and a follow-up visit.

Women who undergo transcervical sterilization must return for a HSG for occlusion confirmation 3 months after the procedure. In a successful placement, the HSG will demonstrate that the device is placed in both fallopian tubes and that there is no peritoneal spillage. The tubes may fail to occlude for idiopathic reasons or because the insert has been placed incorrectly, with possible myometrial perforation or loss of the insert intra-abdominally or externally. If perforation is suspected, obtain an ultrasound (for Essure or Adiana) or a flat abdominal plain film (for Essure) to assess the position of the inserts.[87] If occlusion has not been achieved and the inserts are in the correct location, a repeat HSG may be performed 6 months postoperatively, with the woman continuing her method of contraception.[16] If correct placement is assured and occlusion is not achieved at 6 months, tell the client that she cannot rely on her transcervical procedure and must use another method.[13,16] She may consider transabdominal sterilization at this point as well as reversible methods, including long-acting methods such as IUCs or implants.

USER INSTRUCTIONS FOR FEMALE STERILIZATION

PREOPERATIVE INSTRUCTIONS

1. Be completely sure of your decision to have a sterilization procedure. You must be certain that you understand and desire the permanence of sterilization. You can change your mind at any time before the operation.

2. If you intend on having sedation or general anesthesia, do not eat or drink anything 6 hours prior to your procedure, and bring someone who can accompany you home after the procedure.

POSTOPERATIVE INSTRUCTIONS

1. **Avoid intercourse** for 1 to 2 weeks. When you resume having intercourse, stop if it is uncomfortable.

2. Return to the clinic or contact the clinic or provider promptly if you develop:

Condition:	Action:
Temperature: > 100.4 degrees Fahrenheit	Contact your provider immediately
Fainting: Fainting spells	Contact your provider immediately
Pain: Abdominal pain that is persistent, severe and/or increasing after 12 hours	Contact your provider immediately
Incision site issues: (if transabdominal) Bleeding or spotting from incision sites	Put pressure and tape x 12 hours. If condition continues or worsens, contact provider
Pus or discharge from incision sites	Clean with povidone-iodine or peroxide 2 times a day. If condition continues or worsens, contact provider
Stitch in wound	It will eventually fall out (unless a permanent suture was put in place, which will need to be removed by your provider)

3. Take one or two analgesic tablets at 4- to 6-hour intervals if you need them for pain (Note to provider: name and dose should be specified.). Do not use aspirin since it may promote bleeding.

4. If you think you are pregnant at any time in the future, return to the clinic immediately. Although pregnancy after female sterilization is rare, when it does occur, chances are increased that it will be outside the uterus (an ectopic pregnancy). This is a dangerous, life-threatening condition and must be treated immediately.

5. You should know this method of birth control is permanent. Reversal surgery is possible under certain conditions, but it is expensive and requires highly technical and major surgery. Both reversal surgery and IVF results cannot be guaranteed.

Further instructions for **transabdominal** procedures:

6. **Return to the clinic** 1 to 2 weeks after the procedure to make sure the healing process is normal.

7. **Avoid strenuous lifting** for 1 week to allow the incisions to heal.

8. You may bathe 48 hours after surgery but avoid putting tension on the incision and do not rub or irritate the incision for 1 week. Dry the incision site after bathing.

9. Stitches will dissolve and do not require removal. (Note to provider: this instruction must be modified if nonabsorbable sutures such as silk are used).

Further instructions for **transcervical** procedures:

6. **Please return to your clinician for the confirmatory test** (known as a hysterosalpingogram or HSG) in 3 months so the success of the procedure can be assessed.

7. **Continue with your contraceptive method** until success of the sterilization procedure has been confirmed (with an HSG). Until success is confirmed, you cannot rely on this method for contraception.

MALE STERILIZATION

Male sterilization or vasectomy is one of the safest and most effective family planning methods. It is also one of the few contraceptive options available to men. Nearly all vasectomies are performed using local anesthesia. The no-scalpel approach to the vas, developed in China in the mid-1970s, has become common throughout the world. It takes 5 to 10 minutes for preoperative preparation and administration of local anesthesia and then an additional 5 to 15 minutes to perform. Recent research on surgical techniques and postoperative care has led to changes in clinical guidelines and practice in many settings.

MECHANISM OF ACTION
Sterilization for men blocks fertilization by cutting or occluding both vas deferens so that sperm can no longer pass out of the body in the ejaculate.

EFFECTIVENESS
Vasectomy is highly effective and is one of the most reliable contraceptive methods.[99–103] The first-year failure rate in the United States is estimated to be 0.15% (see Table 26–1), with a range of 0% to 0.5%. In general, vasectomy failure rates are believed to be similar to those for female sterilization and lower than those for reversible methods.

It is very difficult to interpret the published literature on vasectomy efficacy because follow-up is usually short-term; many studies are retrospective, anecdotal and of low quality; a wide variety of occlusion methods are used; and there is no standard definition of what constitutes failure.[104] Few studies present failure rates based on pregnancies after vasectomy; most report failures as failure to reach azoospermia (i.e., no sperm in the ejaculate). The relationship between sperm counts after vasectomy and the risk of pregnancy is not well understood, nor can it be readily measured. When pregnancy rates are reported, there are two complicating factors. Since vasectomy is not immediately effective, pregnancies may be related to failure to use another contraceptive until sperm are cleared from the reproductive tract. One quarter to one half of pregnancies after vasectomy may occur during this time.[101,102,105] In addition, pregnancies may not always be attributable to the men who underwent the vasectomy. True failure of the technique can result from spontaneous recanalization of the vas, division or occlusion of the wrong structure during surgery, and rarely a congenital duplication of the vas that went unnoticed during the procedure. It is clear, nevertheless, that pregnancy can occur long after the vasectomy procedure.

ADVANTAGES

Vasectomy is safer, less expensive, and as effective as female sterilization. It is ideal for men and couples who need a reliable contraceptive method and are certain that they desire no further children. When both female and male sterilization are acceptable to a couple, vasectomy would be the preferred surgical contraceptive method due to its safety, although individuals and couples need to make their own informed decision. The main advantages of vasectomy are as follows:

- Permanence
- High effectiveness
- High acceptability
- Safety
- Quick recovery
- Lack of significant long-term side effects
- Cost-effectiveness (most cost-effective of all contraceptive methods)
- No need to buy anything
- No need for partner compliance
- No need to interrupt lovemaking
- Privacy of choice
- Removal of contraceptive burden from the woman
- Successful reversal rates are higher than those following tubal sterilization

DISADVANTAGES AND CAUTIONS

Male sterilization is not recommended for anyone who is not sure of his desire to end future fertility. One caution that must be kept in mind is that vasectomy is not effective until all sperm in the reproductive tract are cleared. As a contraceptive method, vasectomy provides indirect protection from pregnancy for women—a woman has to rely on the man being truthful about having had a vasectomy and about knowing that his semen is free of sperm.

The major disadvantages of vasectomy are as follows:

- Permanence: Pregnancy after male sterilization is difficult, though possible. It is expensive, requires either costly assisted reproductive technology (such as IVF with intracytoplasmic sperm injection (ICSI)) or highly technical surgery, and results cannot be guaranteed.

- **All surgical procedures carry some risk specific to the nature of the surgery and anesthetic used.**

- Regret for decision: regret can be high among some groups of men

- Need for trained surgeon or other health professional, procedure room (aseptic conditions), trained assistants, medications, surgical equipment

- Expense at the time of the procedure

- Lack of protection against sexually transmitted infections (STIs), including infection with HIV

Men with medical conditions or other special characteristics may have precautions for sterilization that differ from those for men without these conditions or characteristics. These men will need further counseling before they can give informed consent for male sterilization.[106]

SAFETY

Vasectomy appears to be largely safe, with risks no greater than those found with any of the contraceptive options for women. Mortality due to vasectomy is extremely rare.[107-109] Although there are a few reports of vasectomy-related mortality, the most comprehensive study, based on over 400,000 vasectomies worldwide, found a procedure-related mortality rate of 0.5 deaths per 100,000 vasectomized men.[109]

Extensive research has been conducted on the potential physiological effects and long-term sequelae of vasectomy. No significant long-term physical or mental health effects have been found. Numerous well-designed studies have consistently shown no adverse effects of vasectomy in terms of heart disease, prostate or testicular cancer, immune complex disorders, and a variety of other conditions.[99,110,111] Sexual function remains unaffected, and vasectomy does not lead to impotence or other sexual difficulties, or to any reduction in the amount of semen ejaculated. Vasectomy has been reported to have no negative effects on sexuality, with some studies demonstrating a positive effect, perhaps because of the reduced worry about unintended pregnancy.[57,112–114]

SPECIAL ISSUES

Antisperm Antibodies

Antisperm antibodies appear in 50% to 80% of men following vasectomy, compared to only 8% to 21% of men in the general population.[115,116] The theoretical concern that these antibodies may have adverse health consequences has led to numerous studies, which have shown no evidence of any immunologic or other diseases related to the formation of antisperm antibodies after vasectomy.[112,117,118] Antisperm antibodies may play a role in decreased fertility after vasectomy reversal, although results are conflicting.[119–122] Current consensus is that fertility following vasectomy reversal is only inhibited by high levels of antisperm antibodies.[123] However, there remains much debate regarding the interpretation and clinical relevancy of different types of antisperm antibody tests.[124,125] In addition, the class of antibody may have more clinical significance than titer level, with IgA antibodies leading to greater fertility impairment than IgG antibodies.[125]

Prostate Cancer

The incidence of prostate cancer is rising, and is the most commonly diagnosed cancer among men in the United States.[126] Little is known about the etiology and pathogenesis of prostate cancer, and few risk factors have been identified.[127] Since the mid-1980s, there have been over a dozen epidemiological studies of the risk of prostate cancer after vasectomy reported in the literature. Results have been difficult to interpret because of conflicting study findings, lack of a convincing biological mechanism for vasectomy causing prostate cancer, and generally weak associations when they have been found.[128,129] In addition, the potential for bias in some studies was high and likely led to an overestimation of any effect.[128–130] A panel of experts gathered by the U.S. National Institutes of Health in 1993 concluded that no change in the current practice of vasectomy was necessary nor should vasectomy reversal be done as a prostate cancer prevention measure.[131] More recent studies continue to find no relation between vasectomy and risk of prostate cancer.[131–136]

Chronic Testicular Pain (also referred to as postvasectomy pain syndrome)

Some men report severe chronic testicular pain or discomfort after vasectomy. While up to one-third to one-half of men have reported occasional testicular discomfort following vasectomy, only a small percentage of all vasectomized men (no more than 2% to 3%) said the pain had a negative impact on their lives or that they regretted having had the vasectomy because of chronic pain.[137-139] There are limited data on chronic testicular pain in the general population and only one study of postvasectomy pain included a control group. In that study, 47% of vasectomized men reported having occasional testicular discomfort compared to 23% of the controls, with 6% and 2%, respectively, seeking medical advice.[140] None of the men reported they regretted having had a vasectomy because of the pain. The cause of chronic testicular pain after vasectomy is poorly understood but may be related to epididymal or vas congestion, back pressure-induced epididymal tubule rupture, sperm granuloma formation, or nerve entrapment.[141,142] Conservative therapy such as nonsteroidal anti-inflammatory drugs, sitz baths, antibiotics, or spermatic cord blocks is sufficient treatment in most cases. When this fails, there is some evidence that vasectomy reversal, epididymectomy or denervation of the spermatic cord may be helpful.[141,142] During counseling it is important to mention that a small percentage of men experience chronic testicular pain following vasectomy.

RISK OF REGRET

The vast majority of men who have a vasectomy do not regret their decision. Regret among men after vasectomy, most often reported as less than 5%, is lower than the reported regret among women after female sterilization.[143,144] Regret among women whose husbands had a vasectomy has been reported to be slightly higher than men's regret at 6% to 8% but is similar to regret in women who had a tubal ligation.[64,145] Regret following a vasectomy is more common among men who, at the time of the vasectomy, were less than 30 years old, were in an unstable marriage, had no or very young children, or made the decision to have a vasectomy during a time of financial crisis or for reasons related to a pregnancy.[99,144,146] The need for good counseling prior to vasectomy is underscored by the fact that some men who express regret have had a complication following the procedure or a problem that they perceived to be caused by the vasectomy. Men with risk factors for regret should receive more in-depth counseling to make sure that vasectomy is the right contraceptive choice. Men should not be denied the procedure if they decide they want it.

Desire for Pregnancy Following Vasectomy

Vasectomy should be considered permanent, but even with careful counseling, some men will request reversal. The most common reason that men request vasectomy reversal is that they want another child because they have changed partners, changed their mind, or lost a child.[99, 147] Vasectomy reversal or assisted reproductive technologies can be used; however, success cannot be guaranteed. In addition, these techniques are technically complex, require special skills and are costly.

Both macroscopic and microsurgical techniques have been used for vasectomy reversal. The current consensus is that the microsurgical techniques are more successful.[148] The percentage of men with sperm in the ejaculate ranges from 75% to 100% after microsurgical reversal.[147,149] However, presence of sperm should not be presented to men as the measure of success, since pregnancy is the desired outcome. Reported pregnancy rates are lower, ranging from 38% to 89%.[147,149–151]

The time elapsed between vasectomy and reversal is a major factor in the success of reversal; the longer the interval between vasectomy and reversal, the less likely the man is to be fertile after the reversal. Reversal is usually more successful when done within 10 years after vasectomy. Pregnancy rates drop to less than 50% when reversal is performed more than 10 to 15 years after vasectomy.[147,150,151] Other factors that affect the success of vasectomy reversal include the skill of the surgeon, the type of vasectomy procedure originally performed, levels of antisperm antibodies, the age of the female partner, and partial obstruction of the vas after the reversal surgery that prevents movement of sperm through the vas.[152]

Assisted reproduction technologies have been successful in vasectomized men who want children but do not want a vasectomy reversal or have had one or more unsuccessful reversal surgeries. Sperm can be retrieved from the epididymis or the testis and then used for intracytoplasmic sperm injection (ICSI). Pregnancy rates per attempt following ICSI with IVF using epididymal and testicular sperm are reported to be 25% to 36% and 17% to 36%, respectively.[153] Several studies have found that similar to the case with vasectomy reversal, a negative correlation appears to exist between pregnancy rates and time elapsed from the vasectomy until ICSI.[154–156] However, there are also two reports that found no association between the time since vasectomy and the outcome of ICSI.[157,158]

Vasectomy reversal has been shown to be equally or more successful and less costly than ICSI following epididymal sperm aspiration.[151,155,156,159] Surgical reversal appears to be a better first choice for vasectomized men who wish to have children.[160,161] This is the case even in men who are undergoing repeat vasectomy reversal surgery due to a previously failed reversal attempt.[162] However, factors in deciding whether to have a reversal or ICSI with IVF should not only include cost but should also take into consideration the age and fertility of the partner and the number of children desired.

PROVIDING MALE STERILIZATION

Vasectomy is a surgical method of permanent sterilization for men that involves cutting or tying the vas deferens. It is one of the most effective, safe, and inexpensive forms of contraception. In the United States, it is one of the three least expensive forms of contraception. Failure rates range from 0% to 2%, with most studies reporting failure as less than 1%.[10] Some conditions and circumstances may indicate that certain precautions should be taken or that the procedure should be delayed. These include localized problems that make vasectomy more difficult to perform (such as inguinal hernia, large hydrocele or varicocele, and cryptorchidism) or conditions that may increase the likelihood of complications (such as diabetes, coagulation disorders, anticoagulation medications or AIDS).[104]

COUNSELING GUIDELINES FOR VASECTOMY

The goal of counseling is to help clients select a contraceptive method that they will use, that will be effective, that is most consistent with their reproductive intentions, and that will not have adverse effects. The permanence of vasectomy is a significant consideration with respect to counseling.

The factors contributing to an individual's decision about vasectomy vary. Each man needs to weigh the risks, benefits, effectiveness, and side effects of the various contraceptive options available to him and his partner, as well as his personal need to use a barrier method for protection against sexually transmitted infections, especially HIV/AIDS.

Counseling for men interested in vasectomy should address the following:

1. **Provide choices.** Present highly effective, long-acting, reversible methods such as the contraceptive implant or IUCs as options available to the man's partner.

2. **Assess the client's understanding of the procedure.** Awareness of vasectomy is fairly widespread in the United States, but there are often misconceptions about the procedure. Review the procedure with the client so that he correctly understands the procedure and has no misconceptions. Men should be informed that chronic testicular pain can occur after vasectomy, but occurrence is rare.

3. **Facilitate the decision-making process.** Give the client sufficient time to make a thoughtful, informed decision about vasectomy, especially when a man's partner has just given birth or had an abortion, or when there are financial, marital, or sexual problems.

4. **Provide information about possible failure.** Inform the client that vasectomy, although highly effective, is not 100% successful and that failure can occur, even years after the procedure was performed.

5. **Discuss STI prevention.** Vasectomy will not provide protection against sexually transmitted infections, including HIV. This should be thoroughly explained to the client or his partner(s). Condom use will be necessary if the client is at risk of such infections.

6. **Emphasize the need for effectiveness confirmation.** Men should be advised that vasectomy is not immediately effective, that success should be confirmed by semen analysis if possible, and that another contraceptive should be used until their provider says they can rely on the vasectomy alone.

Components of Pre-vasectomy Counseling

- Permanent nature of the procedure
- Alternative methods of contraception available (including permanent and reversible methods for partners)
- Reasons for choosing sterilization
- Screening for risk indicators for regret
- Details of the procedure, including risks and benefits of anesthesia
- The possibility of failure
- The need to use condoms for protection against sexually transmitted diseases, including HIV
- Need for post-procedure confirmation
- Federal and State Medicaid regulations regarding informed consent, including age of the client, circumstances in which consent is obtained, and interval from time of consent to procedure

Informed Consent

Informed consent is a voluntary decision made by a person who has been fully informed regarding a procedure and its consequences. Provide the information on vasectomy in a language the client can understand. The client must always sign or mark an informed consent form indicating that they understand the vasectomy procedure, its intended permanence, the possibility of failure, the risks and benefits, and the option to change his mind about having a vasectomy at any time prior to the procedure without loss of medical or financial benefits. The surgeon or authorized representative must also sign the form. Written informed consent should document, but not substitute for, the provider's active involvement in the client's informed decision making process to have a vasectomy, in order to ensure that he has knowingly and freely requested the procedure.

Policy/Legal Issues

See female sterilization section.

Preoperative Screening

Take a preoperative history and evaluate the general health condition of the client with particular attention to assessing the inguinal area, scrotum, and testicles to see if there are factors that might affect the procedure. Laboratory examinations are not routinely performed, but should be available in case the history or physical suggest they might be indicated (e.g., liver function, bleeding and clotting time, etc.). Clip the hair from around the scrotum and penis, if this was not already done at home. Shaving the scrotum is no longer recommended, as this significantly increases the chance of surgical-site infection. Strict adherence to good infection prevention practices and aseptic technique is crucial for the safety of the procedure and essential to prevent both immediate and long-term infectious morbidity and mortality. Both conventional and no-scalpel vasectomies are performed almost exclusively under local anesthesia alone, using 1% lidocaine. Pre-medication, sedation, or regional or general anesthesia is rarely needed and unnecessarily increases the risk and the costs associated with the procedure.

APPROACHES TO THE VAS

The first step in a vasectomy is to identify and immobilize the vas through the skin of the scrotum, and then to deliver the vas. There are two approaches to delivering the vas: conventional vasectomy and no-scalpel vasectomy.

For conventional vasectomy, the skin and muscle overlying the vas are incised with a scalpel. Generally only the area around the skin entry site is anesthetized. Some surgeons use a single midline incision, and others make two lateral incisions in the scrotal skin, one overlying each vas deferens (Figure 17–7). The incision(s) are typically closed with absorbable suture after the vasectomy is completed.

An alternative approach, no-scalpel vasectomy, is used in many family planning programs around the world, including many in the United States. No-scalpel vasectomy (also known as NSV) was developed in 1974 in China. The anesthetic technique used with NSV includes

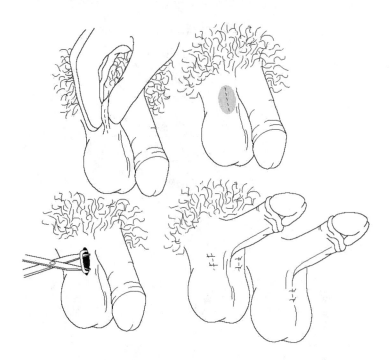

Figure 17–7 Sites of vasectomy incisions

a deep injection of anesthesia alongside each vas to create a perivasal block, as well as anesthetizing the skin. In addition, two specialized instruments, a ringed clamp and a dissecting forceps, are used in the NSV procedure. Both vasa are reached through the same small midline puncture in the scrotum rather than through a scalpel incision, and sutures are not needed (Figure 17–8). A detailed description can be found at www.engenderhealth.org (No-Scalpel Vasectomy: An Illustrated Guide For Surgeons).[163]

The NSV approach has a number of advantages over the conventional scalpel method: fewer complications, including infection and hematoma, less pain during the procedure and immediate follow-up period, and earlier resumption of sexual activity after surgery.[164] Several modifications to the NSV approach have also been reported in the literature.[165–167]

OCCLUSION METHODS

Once the vas has been delivered through the skin, it is then occluded. A variety of methods are used, including ligation with sutures, chemical occlusion, thermal or electrocautery, application of clips, excision of a segment of the vas, fascial interposition, or some combination of these.

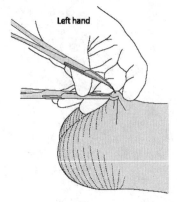

A. Inserting both tips of the dissecting forceps into the puncture site

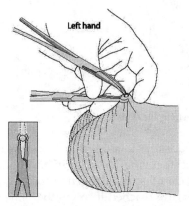

B. Spreading the tissues to make a skin opening twice the diameter of the vas

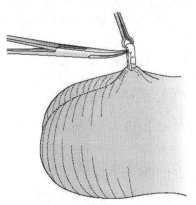

C. Grasping a partial thickness of the elevated vas

Source: Engenderhealth (2007)[163] with permission.

Figure 17–8 No-scalpel vasectomy

The same techniques are used to occlude the vas whether using conventional or no-scalpel vasectomy.

Ligation and excision of a section of the vas is the most common technique worldwide. Another popular occlusion technique is cautery—electrosurgical or thermal. This is done by inserting a needle electrode or a cautery device into the vas lumen and desiccating the luminal mucosa of the vas to create a firm scar that will occlude the vas. Sometimes a segment of the vas is removed as well. Clips can be applied to the vas to compress a narrow segment and block the passage of sperm. With this method, after division of the vas, a clip is applied to both of the cut ends. Sometimes a segment of the vas is removed.

Fascial interposition is widely used to reduce the risk of recanalization. It can be used with any of the occlusion methods described above. This technique involves placing a tissue barrier between the cut end of the vas by suturing or securing with a clip the thin layer of tissue that surrounds the vas over one of the cut ends. A controversial and less widespread modification performed by some surgeons is to occlude the proximal end of the vas but leave the testicular end of the vas open, called open-ended vasectomy. Theoretically, this method is thought to allow sperm to flow out of the vas, which may minimize pressure and damage on the epididymis. Success rates for vasectomy reversal may be higher with open-ended vasectomy; however, no studies have been reported in the literature. Some surgeons irrigate the distal vas deferens with sterile water or a spermicidal solution to hasten sperm clearance. There have not been any well-designed randomized trials validating this practice.[168] Finally, a randomized trial showed fewer adverse events but also decreased effectiveness of an intra-vas device of urethane filled with nylon thread when compared with the no-scalpel method.[169]

Choice of occlusion method depends on the provider's training and personal experience, but there are some differences in effectiveness among different occlusion techniques. Trials comparing vasectomy using clips versus more traditional techniques of ligation have not shown a difference in failure.[168] Results of a randomized controlled trial demonstrated that use of fascial interposition with ligation and excision significantly improved the effectiveness of vasectomy, so ligation and excision without fascial interposition should no longer be recommended.[170] Cautery has been shown to be highly effective and was found to significantly reduce failures compared to ligation and excision with fascial interposition.[104,171,172] Data are lacking on use of fascial interposition with cautery, chemical occlusion methods, differences in the effectiveness of thermal and electrocautery, and the importance of removing a segment of the vas.[168]

MANAGING PROBLEMS AND FOLLOW-UP

Vasectomy is a minor surgical procedure. Fewer than 3% of cases require medical attention.[168] Intraoperative complications such as vasovagal reaction, lidocaine toxicity, and excessive bleeding are unusual and can generally be prevented if appropriate guidelines and procedures are followed. Postoperative complications such as bleeding or infection as well as failure, although infrequent, do occur. Most postoperative complications are minor and subside within one or two weeks. The most frequent complaints after surgery are swelling of the scrotum, bruising, pain, and minor bleeding under the skin. A scrotal support, mild pain medication, and local application of ice are usually sufficient for treatment. More significant complications such as heavy bleeding, hematoma, or infection are quite rare. Careful surgical technique, aseptic technique, early recognition of a problem, and proper postoperative care and follow-up greatly reduce the risks of both minor and major complications after vasectomy.

The standard accepted endpoint of vasectomy has traditionally been achievement of azoospermia, although some have suggested that men with low numbers of nonmotile sperm after vasectomy are at low risk of causing pregnancy and can rely on their vasectomy for contraception.[99] It is generally recommended that men have a semen analysis to confirm vasectomy success, although recommendations on when men should return in terms of time or number of ejaculations after vasectomy vary widely. In resource-poor settings, semen analysis may not be available or practical. To reduce the risk of pregnancy, men in resource-poor settings should use another form of contraception until 12 weeks after vasectomy.[170,173,174]

USER INSTRUCTIONS FOR VASECTOMY

Preoperative Instructions

1. Be completely sure of your decision to have a vasectomy. You must be certain you understand and desire the permanence of vasectomy. You can change your mind at any time before the operation.

2. Before surgery while you are home, use scissors to cut all hair from around the penis and scrotum to about 1/4-inch in length. Do not shave.

3. Shower or bathe, washing the penis and scrotum thoroughly to remove all loose hairs.

4. If possible, bring someone who can accompany you home after the procedure. Do not ride a bicycle; avoid walking long distances or using other transportation that may rub or put pressure on the scrotum.

5. Bring a pair of tight-fitting underwear or athletic supporter to support the scrotum and minimize swelling.

6. Plan to remain quiet for about 48 hours following the vasectomy. A 48-hour rest and limited mobility is important to decrease the risk of complications.

Postoperative Instructions

1. **Rest for 2 days** following surgery. You will probably be able to resume your normal activities after 2 or 3 days as you gradually become more comfortable.

2. **Wear a scrotal support for 2 days** (e.g., brief-style underwear). If possible, keep an ice pack on the scrotum for at least 4 hours to reduce the chances of swelling, bleeding, and discomfort.

3. **Avoid intercourse for 2 to 3 days.** You may resume sexual intercourse after 2 or 3 days if you feel it would be comfortable; but remember, you are not sterile immediately.

4. **Avoid strenuous physical exercise for 1 week.** Strenuous exercise means hard physical exertion, lifting or straining that could bring pressure to the groin or scrotum.

5. If you have pain or discomfort, simple analgesics taken at intervals of 4 to 6 hours usually give adequate relief. (Note to provider: name and dose should be specified.)

6. Do not shower or bathe for the first 24 hours after the vasectomy.

7. The stitches will dissolve and do not have to be removed. (Note to provider: this instruction must be modified if nonabsorbable skin sutures, such as silk, are used or if no skin sutures are used.)

8. It is important for you to know what is normal and what is not normal following your surgery. You will probably have some pain and swelling in the scrotal region; the scrotum may be somewhat discolored. These conditions are normal and should not worry you. Occasionally, blood from a tiny blood vessel may escape into the scrotum at the time of surgery, and bleeding may continue. Notify the provider who performed your vasectomy if you have any of the following danger signs or if you notice any other unusual body changes:

Condition:	Action:
Temperature > 100.4 degrees Fahrenheit	Contact your provider immediately
Pain preventing sleep or work	If unrelieved by analgesic, contact your provider
Incision site Redness, discharge or inflammation at the incision site	Clean with povidone-iodine or peroxide twice a day. If redness in skin increases or the pus or discharge persist, contact your provider
Bleeding from the incision site	Place pressure on the area for 10 minutes. If bleeding continues, contact your provider
Swelling greater than twice normal size	Contact your provider
Nodules larger than a nickel, painful and tender	Contact your provider
Stitches causing extreme pulling sensation	Contact your provider

9. **Use condoms or other contraceptive method** until you know that you're sterile. For many men, sperm will not be cleared from the body until after a minimum of 3 months. Until then, use condoms or another contraceptive method to prevent pregnancy. The best way of finding out if you are sterile is to have your semen looked at under a microscope about 3 months after the vasectomy.

10. Remember, vasectomy is permanent. Reversal surgery or assisted reproductive technologies are possible under certain conditions, but are expensive and require highly technical procedures. Results are not guaranteed.

REFERENCES

1. Mosher WD, Martinez GM, Chandra A, Abma JC, Willson SJ. Use of contraception and use of family planning services in the United States: 1982–2002. Adv Data. 2004:1–36.
2. Magnani RJ, Haws JM, Morgan GT, Gargiullo PM, Pollack AE, Koonin LM. Vasectomy in the United States, 1991 and 1995. Am J Public Health. 1999;89:92–4.
3. MacKay AP, Kieke BA, Jr., Koonin LM, Beattie K. Tubal sterilization in the United States, 1994–1996. Fam Plann Perspect. 2001;33:161–5.
4. Mosher WD, Jones J. Use of Contraception in the United States: 1982–2008. National Center for Health Statistics. Vital Health Stat. 2010;23(29). Available from http://www.cdc.gov/NCHS/data/series/sr_23/sr23_029.pdf. Accessed: 3 August 2010).
5. EngenderHealth. Contraceptive Sterilization: global issues and trends. New York; 2002.
6. Fortney JA, Feldblum PJ, Raymond EG. Intrauterine devices. The optimal long-term contraceptive method? J Reprod Med. 1999;44:269–74.
7. Andersson K, Odlind V, Rybo G. Levonorgestrel-releasing and copper-releasing (Nova T) IUCs during five years of use: a randomized comparative trial. Contraception. 1994;49:56–72.

8. Sivin I, el Mahgoub S, McCarthy T, Mishell DR, Shoupe D, Alvarez F, et al. Long-term contraception with the levonorgestrel 20 mcg/day (LNg 20) and the copper T 380Ag intrauterine devices: a five-year randomized study. Contraception. 1990;42:361–78.

9. Luukkainen T, Allonen H, Haukkamaa M, Lahteenmaki P, Nilsson CG, Toivonen J. Five years' experience with levonorgestrel-releasing IUDs. Contraception. 1986;33:139–48.

10. Peterson HB, Xia Z, Hughes JM, Wilcox LS, Tylor LR, Trussell J. The risk of pregnancy after tubal sterilization: findings from the U.S. Collaborative Review of Sterilization. Am J Obstet Gynecol. 1996;174:1161–8; discussion 8–70.

11. Shaw RR, I., Settatree, R., Templeton, A., Filschie, G.M., Argent, V.P. Male and Female Sterilization. Evidence Based Guidelines No. 4. In. London: Royal College of Obstetricians and Gynaecologists; 1999.

12. FDA approves new female sterilization device. FDA Talk Paper 2002;T02–41:1–2.

13. Essure Permanent Birth Control System. Instructions for Use. Conceptus, Inc.; 2009.

14. Hurskainen R, Hovi S, Gissler M, Grahn R, Kukkonen-Harjula K, Nord-Saari M, Makela M. Hysteroscopic tubal sterilization: a systematic review of the Essure system. Fertil Steril. 2010. 94:16–19.

15. Smith RD. Contemporary hysteroscopic methods for female sterilization. Int J Gynaecol Obstet. 2010;108:79–84.

16. Adiana Permanent Contraception. Instructions for use. Hologic, Inc.; 2009.

17. Peterson HB, Xia Z, Hughes JM, Wilcox LS, Tylor LR, Trussell J. The risk of ectopic pregnancy after tubal sterilization. U.S. Collaborative Review of Sterilization Working Group. N Engl J Med. 1997;336:762–7.

18. Kerin JF, Munday D, Ritossa M, Rosen D. Tissue encapsulation of the proximal Essure micro-insert from the uterine cavity following hysteroscopic sterilization. J Minim Invasive Gynecol. 2007;14:202–4.

19. Moses AW, Burgis JT, Bacon JL, Risinger J. Pregnancy after Essure placement: report of two cases. Fertil Steril. 2008;89:724 e9–11.

20. Escobedo LG, Peterson HB, Grubb GS, Franks AL. Case-fatality rates for tubal sterilization in U.S. hospitals, 1979 to 1980. Am J Obstet Gynecol. 1989;160:147–50.

21. Hulka JF, Phillips JM, Peterson HB, Surrey MW. Laparoscopic sterilization: American Association of Gynecologic Laparoscopists' 1993 membership survey. J Am Assoc Gynecol Laparosc. 1995;2:137–8.

22. Peterson HB, Ory HW, Greenspan JR, Tyler CW, Jr. Deaths associated with laparoscopic sterilization by unipolar electrocoagulating devices, 1978 and 1979. Am J Obstet Gynecol. 1981;139:141–3.

23. Peterson HB, Hulka JF, Phillips JM, Surrey MW. Laparoscopic sterilization. American Association of Gynecologic Laparoscopists 1991 membership survey. J Reprod Med. 1993;38:574–6.

24. Peterson HB, DeStefano F, Rubin GL, Greenspan JR, Lee NC, Ory HW. Deaths attributable to tubal sterilization in the United States, 1977 to 1981. Am J Obstet Gynecol. 1983;146:131–6.

25. Jamieson DJ, Hillis SD, Duerr A, Marchbanks PA, Costello C, Peterson HB. Complications of interval laparoscopic tubal sterilization: findings from the United States Collaborative Review of Sterilization. Obstet Gynecol. 2000;96:997–1002.

26. Hur HC, Mansuria SM, Chen BA, Lee TT. Laparoscopic management of hysteroscopic Essure sterilization complications: report of 3 cases. J Minim Invasive Gynecol. 2008;15:362–5.

27. Lannon BM, Lee SY. Techniques for removal of the Essure hysteroscopic tubal occlusion device. Fertil Steril 2007;88:497 e13–4.

28. Green A, Purdie D, Bain C, Siskind V, Russell P, Quinn M, et al. Tubal sterilisation, hysterectomy and decreased risk of ovarian cancer. Survey of Women's Health Study Group. Int J Cancer. 1997;71:948–51.

29. Kjaer SK, Mellemkjaer L, Brinton LA, Johansen C, Gridley G, Olsen JH. Tubal sterilization and risk of ovarian, endometrial and cervical cancer. A Danish population-based follow-up study of more than 65 000 sterilized women. Int J Epidemiol. 2004;33:596–602.
30. Irwin KL, Weiss NS, Lee NC, Peterson HB. Tubal sterilization, hysterectomy, and the subsequent occurrence of epithelial ovarian cancer. Am J Epidemiol. 1991;134:362–9.
31. McGuire V, Felberg A, Mills M, Ostrow KL, DiCioccio R, John EM, et al. Relation of contraceptive and reproductive history to ovarian cancer risk in carriers and noncarriers of BRCA1 gene mutations. Am J Epidemiol. 2004;160:613–8.
32. Narod SA, Sun P, Ghadirian P, Lynch H, Isaacs C, Garberg J, et al. Tubal ligation and risk of ovarian cancer in carriers of BRCA1 or BRCA2 mutations: a case-control study. Lancet. 2001;357:1467–70.
33. Calle EE, Rodriguez C, Walker KA, Wingo PA, Petrelli JM, Thun MJ. Tubal sterilization and risk of breast cancer mortality in US women. Cancer Causes Control. 2001;12:127–35.
34. Eliassen AH, Colditz GA, Rosner B, Hankinson SE. Tubal sterilization in relation to breast cancer risk. Int J Cancer. 2006;118:2026–30.
35. Irwin KL, Lee NC, Peterson HB, Rubin GL, Wingo PA, Mandel MG. Hysterectomy, tubal sterilization, and the risk of breast cancer. Am J Epidemiol. 1988;127:1192–201.
36. Poma PA. Tubal sterilization and later hospitalizations. J Reprod Med 1980;25:272–8.
37. Alder E, Cook A, Gray J, Tyrer G, Warner P, Bancroft J, et al. The effects of sterilisation: a comparison of sterilised women with the wives of vasectomised men. Contraception. 1981;23:45–54.
38. Gentile GP, Kaufman SC, Helbig DW. Is there any evidence for a post-tubal sterilization syndrome? Fertil Steril. 1998;69:179–86.
39. Bhiwandiwala PP, Mumford SD, Feldblum PJ. Menstrual pattern changes following laparoscopic sterilization with different occlusion techniques: a review of 10,004 cases. Am J Obstet Gynecol. 1983;145:684–94.
40. DeStefano F, Perlman JA, Peterson HB, Diamond EL. Long-term risk of menstrual disturbances after tubal sterilization. Am J Obstet Gynecol. 1985;152:835–41.
41. Foulkes J, Chamberlain G. Effects of sterilization on menstruation. South Med J. 1985;78:544–7.
42. Rivera R, Gaitan JR, Ruiz R, Hurley DP, Arenas M, Flores C, et al. Menstrual patterns and progesterone circulating levels following different procedures of tubal occlusion. Contraception. 1989;40:157–69.
43. Rulin MC, Davidson AR, Philliber SG, Graves WL, Cushman LF. Long-term effect of tubal sterilization on menstrual indices and pelvic pain. Obstet Gynecol. 1993;82:118–21.
44. Sahwi S, Toppozada M, Kamel M, Anwar MY, Ismail AA. Changes in menstrual blood loss after four methods of female tubal sterilization. Contraception. 1989;40:387–98.
45. Thranov I, Hertz JB, Kjer JJ, Andressen A, Micic S, Nielsen J, et al. Hormonal and menstrual changes after laparoscopic sterilization by Falope-rings or Filshie-clips. Fertil Steril. 1992;57:751–5.
46. Carmona F, Cristobal P, Casamitjana R, Balasch J. Effect of tubal sterilization on ovarian follicular reserve and function. Am J Obstet Gynecol. 2003;189:447–52.
47. Cevrioglu AS, Degirmenci B, Acar M, Yilmazer M, Erol D, Kahraman A, et al. Examination of changes caused by tubal sterilization in ovarian hormone secretion and uterine and ovarian artery blood flow rates. Contraception. 2004;70:467–73.
48. Yazici G, Arslan M, Pata O, Oz U, Aban M. Ovarian function and vascular resistance after tubal sterilization. J Reprod Med. 2004;49:379–83.
49. Whiteman MK, Miller KP, Tomic D, Langenberg P, Flaws JA. Tubal sterilization and hot flashes. Fertil Steril. 2004;82:502–4.
50. Wyshak G. Menopausal symptoms and psychological distress in women with and without tubal sterilization. Psychosomatics. 2004;45:403–13.

51. Hillis SD, Marchbanks PA, Tylor LR, Peterson HB. Higher hysterectomy risk for sterilized than nonsterilized women: findings from the U.S. Collaborative Review of Sterilization. The U.S. Collaborative Review of Sterilization Working Group. Obstet Gynecol. 1998;91:241–6.
52. Cohen MM. Long-term risk of hysterectomy after tubal sterilization. Am J Epidemiol. 1987;125:410–9.
53. Goldhaber MK, Armstrong MA, Golditch IM, Sheehe PR, Petitti DB, Friedman GD. Long-term risk of hysterectomy among 80,007 sterilized and comparison women at Kaiser Permanente, 1971–1987. Am J Epidemiol. 1993;138:508–21.
54. Kendrick JS, Rubin GL, Lee NC, Schulz KF, Peterson HB, Nolan TF. Hysterectomy performed within 1 year after tubal sterilization. Fertil Steril. 1985;44:606–10.
55. Stergachis A, Shy KK, Grothaus LC, Wagner EH, Hecht JA, Anderson G, et al. Tubal sterilization and the long-term risk of hysterectomy. JAMA 1990;264:2893–8.
56. Costello C, Hillis SD, Marchbanks PA, Jamieson DJ, Peterson HB. The effect of interval tubal sterilization on sexual interest and pleasure. Obstet Gynecol. 2002;100: 511–7.
57. Shain RN, Miller WB, Holden AE, Rosenthal M. Impact of tubal sterilization and vasectomy on female marital sexuality: results of a controlled longitudinal study. Am J Obstet Gynecol. 1991;164:763–71.
58. Lo JS, Pickersgill A. Pregnancy after endometrial ablation: English literature review and case report. J Minim Invasive Gynecol. 2006;13:88–91.
59. McCausland AM, McCausland VM. Frequency of symptomatic cornual hematometra and postablation tubal sterilization syndrome after total rollerball endometrial ablation: a 10-year follow-up. Am J Obstet Gynecol. 2002;186:1274–80; discussion 80–3.
60. Webb JC, Bush MR, Wood MD, Park GS. Hematosalpinx with pelvic pain after endometrial ablation confirms the postablation-tubal sterilization syndrome. J Am Assoc Gynecol Laparosc. 1996;3:419–21.
61. Valle RF, Valdez J, Wright TC, Kenney M. Concomitant Essure tubal sterilization and Thermachoice endometrial ablation: feasibility and safety. Fertil Steril. 2006;86:152–8.
62. Donnadieu AC, Fernandez H. The role of Essure sterilization performed simultaneously with endometrial ablation. Curr Opin Obstet Gynecol. 2008;20:359–63.
63. Hillis SD, Marchbanks PA, Tylor LR, Peterson HB. Poststerilization regret: findings from the United States Collaborative Review of Sterilization. Obstet Gynecol. 1999;93:889–95.
64. Jamieson DJ, Kaufman SC, Costello C, Hillis SD, Marchbanks PA, Peterson HB. A comparison of women's regret after vasectomy versus tubal sterilization. Obstet Gynecol. 2002;99:1073–9.
65. Schmidt JE, Hillis SD, Marchbanks PA, Jeng G, Peterson HB. Requesting information about and obtaining reversal after tubal sterilization: findings from the U.S. Collaborative Review of Sterilization. Fertil Steril. 2000;74:892–8.
66. Wilcox LS, Chu SY, Eaker ED, Zeger SL, Peterson HB. Risk factors for regret after tubal sterilization: 5 years of follow-up in a prospective study. Fertil Steril. 1991;55:927–33.
67. Cheng MC, Cheong J, Ratnam SS, Belsey MA, Edstrom KE, Pinol A, et al. Psychosocial sequelae of abortion and sterilization: a controlled study of 200 women randomly allocated to either a concurrent or interval abortion and sterilization. Asia Oceania J Obstet Gynaecol. 1986;12:193–200.
68. Wilcox LS, Chu SY, Peterson HB. Characteristics of women who considered or obtained tubal reanastomosis: results from a prospective study of tubal sterilization. Obstet Gynecol. 1990;75:661–5.
69. Boring CC, Rochat RW, Becerra J. Sterilization regret among Puerto Rican women. Fertil Steril. 1988;49:973–81.
70. Neuhaus W, Bolte A. Prognostic factors for preoperative consultation of women desiring sterilization: findings of a retrospective analysis. J Psychosom Obstet Gynaecol. 1995;16:45–50.

71. Ledger WL. Implications of an irreversible procedure. Fertil Steril. 2004;82:1473; author reply 4.
72. Lee DM, Patton PE. Tubal Surgery and Treatment of Infertility. In: Sciarra JJ, editor. Gynecology & Obstetrics. Philadelphia: Lippincott Williams & Wilkins; 2004.
73. Trussell J, Guilbert E, Hedley A. Sterilization failure, sterilization reversal, and pregnancy after sterilization reversal in Quebec. Obstet Gynecol. 2003;101:677–84.
74. Lakeshore Tubal Reversal Center [Internet]. Gainsville CA: Lakeshore Tubal Reversal Center; c2010 [cited 2010 May 5], Essure and Adiana Tubal Occlusions. Available from:
http://www.pregnantagain.com/tubal_reversal/Essure_Tubal_Occlusion.php.
75. Kerin JF, Cattanach S. Successful pregnancy outcome with the use of in vitro fertilization after Essure hysteroscopic sterilization. Fertil Steril. 2007;87:1212 e1–4.
76. Pollack AE, Soderstrom RM. Female Tubal Sterilization. In: Corson SL, Derman RJ, Tyrer LB, editors. Fertility Control. 2nd ed. London, Ontario: Goldin Publishers; 1994:293–317.
77. Soderstrom R. Clinical challenges: share warning information, court case teaches. Contraceptive Technology Update 1981;2:8–9.
78. Sterilization of persons in federally assisted family planning projects. 42 CFR 50 Subpart B (2004).
79. American College of Obstetricians and Gynecologists. Sterilization of women, including those with mental disabilities. ACOG Committee Opinion 371. Washington, D.C.: American College of Obstetricians and Gynecologists; July 2007.
80. Practice guidelines for obstetric anesthesia: an updated report by the American Society of Anesthesiologists Task Force on Obstetric Anesthesia. Anesthesiology 2007;106:843–63.
81. Bucklin BA, Smith CV. Postpartum tubal ligation: safety, timing, and other implications for anesthesia. Anesth Analg. 1999;89:1269–74.
82. American College of Obstetricians and Gynecologists. Tubal ligation with cesarean delivery. ACOG Committee Opinion 205. Washington, D.C.: American College of Obstetricians and Gynecologists; August 1998.
83. Peterson HB, Pollack AE, Warshaw JS. Tubal Sterilization. In: Rock JA, Jones HW, editors. Te Linde's Operative Gynecology. 10th ed. Philadelphia: Lippincott Williams & Wilkins; 2008:609–28.
84. Kasliwal A, Farquharson RG. Pregnancy testing prior to sterilisation. BJOG. 2000;107:1407–9.
85. Centers for Disease Control and Prevention. Surgical sterilization surveillance 1976–1978. In. Atlanta: Centers for Disease Control; 1981.
86. Akhter HH, Flock ML, Rubin GL. Safety of abortion and tubal sterilization performed separately versus concurrently. Am J Obstet Gynecol. 1985;152:619–23.
87. Palmer SN, Greenberg JA. Transcervical sterilization: a comparison of Essure® permanent birth control system and Adiana® permanent contraception system. Rev Obstet Gynecol. 2009;2:84–92.
88. Kerin JF, Munday DN, Ritossa MG, Pesce A, Rosen D. Essure hysteroscopic sterilization: results based on utilizing a new coil catheter delivery system. J Am Assoc Gynecol Laparosc. 2004;11:388–93.
89. American College of Obstetricians and Gynecologists. Benefits and risks of sterilization. ACOG Practice Bulletin No. 46. Washington, D.C.: American College of Obstetricians and Gynecologists; Sept 2003.
90. Peterson HB, Xia Z, Wilcox LS, Tylor LR, Trussell J. Pregnancy after tubal sterilization with bipolar electrocoagulation. U.S. Collaborative Review of Sterilization Working Group. Obstet Gynecol. 1999;94:163–7.
91. Soderstrom RM, Levy BS, Engel T. Reducing bipolar sterilization failures. Obstet Gynecol. 1989;74:60–3.

92. Sokal D, Gates D, Amatya R, Dominik R. Two randomized controlled trials comparing the tubal ring and Filshie clip for tubal sterilization. Fertil Steril. 2000;74:525–33.
93. Dominik R, Gates D, Sokal D, Cordero M, Lasso de la Vega J, Remes Ruiz A, et al. Two randomized controlled trials comparing the Hulka and Filshie Clips for tubal sterilization. Contraception. 2000;62:169–75.
94. Sterilization device to offer ease of use. Contracept Technol Update. 1996;17:53–64.
95. Update on female sterilization. The Contraception Report. 1996;7:13–4.
96. Wittmer MH, Brown DL, Hartman RP, Famuyide AO, Kawashima A, King BF. Sonography, CT, and MRI appearance of the Essure microinsert permanent birth control device. AJR Am J Roentgenol. 2006;187:959–64.
97. Teoh M, Meagher S, Kovacs G. Ultrasound detection of the Essure permanent birth control device: a case series. Aust N Z J Obstet Gynaecol. 2003;43:378–80.
98. EngenderHealth. Minilaparotomy for Female Sterilization: An illustrated guide for providers. New York: EngenderHealth; 2003.
99. EngenderHealth. Male Sterilization. In: Contraceptive Sterilization: Global Issues and Trends. New York: EngenderHealth; 2002:161–77.
100. Wang D. Contraceptive failure in China. Contraception. 2002;66:173–8.
101. Nazerali H, Thapa S, Hays M, Pathak LR, Pandey KR, Sokal DC. Vasectomy effectiveness in Nepal: a retrospective study. Contraception. 2003;67:397–401.
102. Jamieson DJ, Costello C, Trussell J, Hillis SD, Marchbanks PA, Peterson HB. The risk of pregnancy after vasectomy. Obstet Gynecol. 2004;103:848–50.
103. Hieu DT, Luong TT, Anh PT, Ngoc DH, Duong LQ. The acceptability, efficacy and safety of quinacrine non-surgical sterilization (QS), tubectomy and vasectomy in 5 provinces in the Red River Delta, Vietnam: a follow-up of 15,190 cases. Int J Gynaecol Obstet. 2003;83 Suppl 2:S77–85.
104. Labrecque M, Dufresne C, Barone MA, St-Hilaire K. Vasectomy surgical techniques: a systematic review. BMC Med. 2004;2:21.
105. Deneux-Tharaux C, Kahn E, Nazerali H, Sokal DC. Pregnancy rates after vasectomy: a survey of US urologists. Contraception. 2004;69:401–6.
106. World Health Organization. Medical Eligibility Criteria for Contraceptive Use. 4th ed. Geneva: World Health Organization; 2009.
107. Grimes DA, Satterthwaite AP, Rochat RW, Akhter N. Deaths from contraceptive sterilization in Bangladesh: rates, causes, and prevention. Obstet Gynecol. 1982;60:635–40.
108. Grimes DA, Peterson HB, Rosenberg MJ, Fishburne JI, Jr, Rochat RW, et al. Sterilization-attributable deaths in Bangladesh. Int J Gynaecol Obstet. 1982;20:149–54.
109. Khairullah Z, Huber DH, Gonzales B. Declining mortality in international sterilization services. Int J Gynaecol Obstet. 1992;39:41–50.
110. Manson JE, Ridker PM, Spelsberg A, Ajani U, Lotufo PA, Hennekens CH. Vasectomy and subsequent cardiovascular disease in US physicians. Contraception. 1999;59:181–6.
111. Coady SA, Sharrett AR, Zheng ZJ, Evans GW, Heiss G. Vasectomy, inflammation, atherosclerosis and long-term followup for cardiovascular diseases: no associations in the atherosclerosis risk in communities study. J Urol. 2002;167:204–7.
112. Petitti DB, Klein R, Kipp H, Kahn W, Siegelaub AB, Friedman GD. A survey of personal habits, symptoms of illness, and histories of disease in man with and without vasectomies. Am J Public Health. 1982;72:476–80.
113. Hofmeyr DG, Greeff AP. The influence of a vasectomy on the marital relationship and sexual satisfaction of the married man. J Sex Marital Ther. 2002;28:339–51.
114. Miller WB, Shain RN, Pasta DJ. The pre- and poststerilization predictors of poststerilization regret in husbands and wives. J Nerv Ment Dis. 1991;179:602–8.
115. Ghazeeri GS, Kutteh WH. Autoimmune factors in reproductive failure. Curr Opin Obstet Gynecol. 2001;13:287–91.

116. Gubin DA, Dmochowski R, Kutteh WH. Multivariant analysis of men from infertile couples with and without antisperm antibodies. Am J Reprod Immunol. 1998;39: 157–60.
117. Giovannucci E, Tosteson TD, Speizer FE, Vessey MP, Colditz GA. A long-term study of mortality in men who have undergone vasectomy. N Engl J Med. 1992;326:1392–8.
118. Massey FJ, Jr., Bernstein GS, O'Fallon WM, Schuman LM, Coulson AH, Crozier R, et al. Vasectomy and health. Results from a large cohort study. JAMA. 1984;252:1023–9.
119. Huang MK, Wu X, Fu C, Zou P, Gao X, Huang Q. Multiple factors affecting human repregnancy after microsurgical vasovasostomy. Reprod Contracept. 1997;8:92–100.
120. Meinertz H, Linnet L, Fogh-Andersen P, Hjort T. Antisperm antibodies and fertility after vasovasostomy: a follow-up study of 216 men. Fertil Steril. 1990;54:315–21.
121. Newton RA. IgG antisperm antibodies attached to sperm do not correlate with infertility following vasovasostomy. Microsurgery. 1988;9:278–80.
122. Carbone DJ, Jr., Shah A, Thomas AJ, Jr., Agarwal A. Partial obstruction, not antisperm antibodies, causing infertility after vasovasostomy. J Urol. 1998;159:827–30.
123. Lea IA, Adoyo P, O'Rand MG. Autoimmunogenicity of the human sperm protein Sp17 in vasectomized men and identification of linear B cell epitopes. Fertil Steril. 1997;67:355–61.
124. Helmerhorst FM, Finken MJ, Erwich JJ. Antisperm antibodies: detection assays for antisperm antibodies: what do they test? Hum Reprod. 1999;14:1669–71.
125. Hjort T. Antisperm antibodies. Antisperm antibodies and infertility: an unsolvable question? Hum Reprod. 1999;14:2423–6.
126. Chan JM, Jou RM, Carroll PR. The relative impact and future burden of prostate cancer in the United States. J Urol. 2004;172:S13–6; discussion S7.
127. Bostwick DG, Burke HB, Djakiew D, Euling S, Ho SM, Landolph J, et al. Human prostate cancer risk factors. Cancer. 2004;101:2371–490.
128. Bernal-Delgado E, Latour-Perez J, Pradas-Arnal F, Gomez-Lopez LI. The association between vasectomy and prostate cancer: a systematic review of the literature. Fertil Steril. 1998;70:191–200.
129. Dennis LK, Dawson DV, Resnick MI. Vasectomy and the risk of prostate cancer: a meta-analysis examining vasectomy status, age at vasectomy, and time since vasectomy. Prostate Cancer Prostatic Dis. 2002;5:193–203.
130. Millard PS. Review: bias may contribute to association of vasectomy with prostate cancer. West J Med. 1999;171:91.
131. Healy B. From the National Institutes of Health: does vasectomy cause prostate cancer? JAMA. 1993;269:2620.
132. Lynge E. Prostate cancer is not increased in men with vasectomy in Denmark. J Urol. 2002;168:488–90.
133. Peterson HB, Howards SS. Vasectomy and prostate cancer: the evidence to date. Fertil Steril. 1998;70:201–3.
134. Holt SK, Salinas CA, Stanford JL. Vasectomy and the risk of prostate cancer. J Urol. 2008;180:2565–7; discussion 7–8.
135. Cox B, Sneyd MJ, Paul C, Delahunt B, Skegg DC. Vasectomy and risk of prostate cancer. JAMA. 2002;287:3110–5.
136. Schwingl PJ, Meirik O, Kapp N, Farley TM. Prostate cancer and vasectomy: a hospital-based case-control study in China, Nepal and the Republic of Korea. Contraception. 2009;79:363–8.
137. Choe JM, Kirkemo AK. Questionnaire-based outcomes study of nononcological postvasectomy complications. J Urol. 1996;155:1284–6.
138. Ehn BE, Liljestrand J. A long-term follow-up of 108 vasectomized men. Good counselling routines are important. Scand J Urol Nephrol. 1995;29:477–81.
139. Manikandan R, Srirangam SJ, Pearson E, Collins GN. Early and late morbidity after vasectomy: a comparison of chronic scrotal pain at 1 and 10 years. BJU Int. 2004;93:571–4.

140. Morris C, Mishra K, Kirkman RJ. A study to assess the prevalence of chronic testicular pain in post-vasectomy men compared to non-vasectomised men. J Fam Plann Reprod Health Care. 2002;28:142–4.
141. Christiansen CG, Sandlow JI. Testicular pain following vasectomy: a review of post-vasectomy pain syndrome. J Androl. 2003;24:293–8.
142. Granitsiotis P, Kirk D. Chronic testicular pain: an overview. Eur Urol. 2004;45:430–6.
143. Shain RN. Psychosocial consequences of vasectomy in developed and developing countries. In: Goldsmith A, Spieler JM, Sciearra J, Zatuchni GI, editors. Male contraception: Advances and future prospects. Philadelphia: Harper and Row; 1986:34–53.
144. Holman CD, Wisniewski ZS, Semmens JB, Rouse IL, Bass AJ. Population-based outcomes after 28,246 in-hospital vasectomies and 1,902 vasovasostomies in Western Australia. BJU Int. 2000;86:1043–9.
145. Pitaktepsombati P, Janowitz B. Sterilization acceptance and regret in Thailand. Contraception. 1991;44:623–37.
146. Potts JM, Pasqualotto FF, Nelson D, Thomas AJ, Jr., Agarwal A. Patient characteristics associated with vasectomy reversal. J Urol. 1999;161:1835–9.
147. Belker AM, Thomas AJ, Jr., Fuchs EF, Konnak JW, Sharlip ID. Results of 1,469 microsurgical vasectomy reversals by the Vasovasostomy Study Group. J Urol. 1991;145:505–11.
148. Vasectomy reversal. Fertil Steril. 2004;82 Suppl 1:S194–8.
149. Lee HY. A 20-year experience with vasovasostomy. J Urol 1986;136:413–5.
150. Takihara H. The treatment of obstructive azoospermia in male infertility—past, present, and future. Urology. 1998;51:150–5.
151. Boorjian S, Lipkin M, Goldstein M. The impact of obstructive interval and sperm granuloma on outcome of vasectomy reversal. J Urol. 2004;171:304–6.
152. Nagler HM, Jung H. Factors predicting successful microsurgical vasectomy reversal. Urol Clin North Am. 2009;36:383–90.
153. Pollack AP, Barone MA. Reversing vasectomy. In: Sciarra JJ, editor. Gynecology & Obstetrics, Vol 6. Philadelphia: Lippincot Williams & Wilkins; 2000.
154. Borges EJ, Rossi-Ferragut LM, Pasqualoto FF, Rocha CC, Iaconelli AJ. Different intervals between vasectomy and sperm retrieval interfere in the reproductive capacity from vasectomized men. J Assist Reprod Genet. 2003;20:33–7.
155. Kolettis PN, Sabanegh ES, D'Amico A M, Box L, Sebesta M, Burns JR. Outcomes for vasectomy reversal performed after obstructive intervals of at least 10 years. Urology. 2002;60:885–8.
156. Fuchs EF, Burt RA. Vasectomy reversal performed 15 years or more after vasectomy: correlation of pregnancy outcome with partner age and with pregnancy results of in vitro fertilization with intracytoplasmic sperm injection. Fertil Steril. 2002;77:516–9.
157. Sukcharoen N, Sithipravej T, Promviengchai S, Chinpilas V, Boonkasemsanti W. No differences in outcome of surgical sperm retrieval with intracytoplasmic sperm injection at different intervals after vasectomy. Fertil Steril. 2000;74:174–5.
158. Nicopoullos JD, Gilling-Smith C, Almeida PA, Ramsay JW. Effect of time since vasectomy and maternal age on intracytoplasmic sperm injection success in men with obstructive azoospermia after vasectomy. Fertil Steril. 2004;82:367–73.
159. Robb P, Sandlow JI. Cost-effectiveness of vasectomy reversal. Urol Clin North Am. 2009;36:391–6.
160. Kolettis PN, Thomas AJ, Jr. Vasoepididymostomy for vasectomy reversal: a critical assessment in the era of intracytoplasmic sperm injection. J Urol. 1997;158:467–70.
161. Pasqualotto FF, Lucon AM, Sobreiro BP, Pasqualotto EB, Arap S. The best infertility treatment for vasectomized men: assisted reproduction or vasectomy reversal? Rev Hosp Clin Fac Med Sao Paulo. 2004;59:312–5.
162. Donovan JF, Jr., DiBaise M, Sparks AE, Kessler J, Sandlow JI. Comparison of microscopic epididymal sperm aspiration and intracytoplasmic sperm injection/in-vitro fertilization with repeat microscopic reconstruction following vasectomy: is second attempt vas reversal worth the effort? Hum Reprod. 1998;13:387–93.

163. EngenderHealth. No-scalpel vasectomy curriculum: A training course for vasectomy providers and assistants: Trainer's manual. New York:EngenderHealth, 2007.
164. Cook LA, Pun A, van Vliet H, Gallo MF, Lopez LM. Scalpel versus no-scalpel incision for vasectomy. Cochrane Database Syst Rev. 2007:CD004112.
165. Black T, Francome C. Comparison of Marie Stopes scalpel and electrocautery no-scalpel vasectomy techniques. J Fam Plann Reprod Health Care. 2003;29:32–4.
166. Chen KC. A novel instrument-independent no-scalpel vasectomy - a comparative study against the standard instrument-dependent no-scalpel vasectomy. Int J Androl. 2004;27:222–7.
167. Jones JS. Percutaneous vasectomy: a simple modification eliminates the steep learning curve of no-scalpel vasectomy. J Urol. 2003;169:1434–6.
168. Cook LA, Van Vliet H, Lopez LM, Pun A, Gallo MF. Vasectomy occlusion techniques for male sterilization. Cochrane Database Syst Rev. 2007:CD003991.
169. Song L, Gu Y, Lu W, Liang X, Chen Z. A phase II randomized controlled trial of a novel male contraception, an intra-vas device. Int J Androl. 2006;29:489–95.
170. Sokal D, Irsula B, Hays M, Chen-Mok M, Barone MA. Vasectomy by ligation and excision, with or without fascial interposition: a randomized controlled trial [ISRCTN77781689]. BMC Med. 2004;2:6.
171. Barone MA, Irsula B, Chen-Mok M, Sokal DC. Effectiveness of vasectomy using cautery. BMC Urol. 2004;4:10.
172. Sokal D, Irsula B, Chen-Mok M, Labrecque M, Barone MA. A comparison of vas occlusion techniques: cautery more effective than ligation and excision with fascial interposition. BMC Urol. 2004;4:12.
173. Barone MA, Nazerali H, Cortes M, Chen-Mok M, Pollack AE, Sokal D. A prospective study of time and number of ejaculations to azoospermia after vasectomy by ligation and excision. J Urol. 2003;170:892–6.
174. World Health Organization. Selected Practice Recommendations for Contraceptive Use. 2nd ed. Geneva: World Health Organization; 2004.

LATE REFERENCE

175. Donnadieu AC, Deffieux X, Gervaise A, Faivre E, Frydman R, Fernandez H. Essure sterilization associated with endometrial ablation. Int J Gynaecol Obstet. 2007;97:139–142.

Postpartum Contraception and Lactation

Kathy I. Kennedy, DrPH, MA
James Trussell, PhD

- Breast milk is the ideal source of nutrition for infants and confers immunological protection against many infections. It reduces the risk of some chronic diseases and includes factors that support growth. Family planning clinicians can play an important role in promoting breastfeeding.

- The Lactational Amenorrhea Method (LAM) is a highly effective, *temporary* method of contraception. To maintain effective protection against pregnancy, another method of contraception must be used as soon as menstruation resumes, the frequency or duration of breastfeeds is reduced, bottle feeds or regular food supplements are introduced, or the baby reaches 6 months of age.

- Other good contraceptive options for lactating women are (1) barrier methods, such as the male or female condom, which also confer protection against sexually transmitted infections; (2) the Copper T 380A intrauterine contraceptive (IUC) (3) *progestin-only* methods such as the progestin-only pill, Implanon or Depo-Provera, or the levonorgestrel intrauterine contraceptive (LNg IUC); and (4) the permanent methods, male or female sterilization for women or couples who want no more children.

- The *combined hormonal methods* administered in pills, patches, injectables, or vaginal rings are not good contraceptive options for lactating women; substitutes can usually be found until breastfeeding is finished.

- HIV can be transmitted through breastmilk. Therefore, in the United States, where safe alternatives to breastmilk are available, HIV-infected mothers are advised to avoid breastfeeding.

After childbirth, the recommended period before attempting the next pregnancy is at least 24 months.[1] However, especially if she is not fully breastfeeding, a woman soon becomes capable of becoming pregnant again since the postpartum period of infertility may be brief. Although the breastfeeding woman will have a longer period of infertility than will the nonbreastfeeding woman, her fertility usually returns during weaning, as the frequency of breastfeeds decreases. During weaning, the breastfeeding woman should use a contraceptive method so that she may breastfeed for as long as she chooses before becoming pregnant again. Fortunately, most family planning methods are compatible with breastfeeding, and the provider can play an important role in promoting both contraception and breastfeeding. In addition to helping to devise a postpartum plan for contraception, the provider can ensure that the new mother has several essential breastfeeding experiences and lessons while still in the hospital, prior to discharge after delivery (see Figure 18–1[2]). Human milk is the ideal source of nutrition for infants and confers immunological protection against many infections. Health experts around the globe have declared that all women should be enabled to breastfeed exclusively for 6 months,[3–11] to continue to breastfeed for 1 year[4,5,8,11] or 2 years or beyond,[3,9] and to have access to family planning information and services that allow them to sustain breastfeeding.[12]

POSTPARTUM INFERTILITY

During pregnancy, cyclic ovarian function is suspended. The corpus luteum, which arises from the ovulated follicle, secretes steroids, including estrogen and progesterone, that are essential in maintaining the early weeks of pregnancy. Later, steroids secreted by the placenta emerge to play a more dominant role in hormonal support of the pregnancy. Luteal and placental steroids suppress the mother's circulating levels of follicle stimulating hormone (FSH) and luteinizing hormone (LH) but more importantly disrupt their pulsatile release from her pituitary.[13] When the placenta is delivered, the inhibiting effects of estrogen and progesterone are removed so that levels of FSH and LH gradually rise and the pituitary resumes the pulsatile release of FSH and LH.[14]

Most nonlactating women resume menses within 4 to 6 weeks of delivery, but about one third of first cycles are anovulatory, and a high proportion of first ovulatory cycles have a deficient corpus luteum that secretes subnormal amounts of steroids. In the second and third menstrual cycles, 15% are anovulatory and 25% of ovulatory cycles have luteal-phase defects. On average, the first ovulation occurs 45 days postpartum, although few first ovulations are followed by normal luteal phases.[15] The duration of postpartum infertility is variable and unpredictable.

Figure 18–1 Clinical guidelines for the establishment of exclusive breastfeeding

1. Facilitate breastfeeding within the first hour after birth and provide for continuous skin-to-skin contact between mother and infant until after the first feeding.
2. Assist the mother and infant in achieving a comfortable position and effective latch (attachment).
3. Keep the mother and infant together during the entire postpartum stay.
4. Teach mothers to recognize and respond to early infant feeding cues and confirm that the baby is being fed at least 8 times in each 24 hours.
5. Confirm that mothers understand the physiology of milk production, especially the role of milk removal.
6. Confirm that mothers know how to wake a sleepy infant.
7. Avoid using pacifiers, artificial nipples, and supplements, unless medically indicated.
8. Observe and document at least one breastfeeding in each 8-hour period during the immediate postpartum period.
9. Assess the mother and infant for signs of effective breastfeeding and intervene if transfer of milk is inadequate.
10. Identify maternal and infant risk factors that may impact the mother's or infant's ability to breastfeed effectively and provide appropriate assistance and follow-up.
11. Identify any maternal and infant contraindications to breastfeeding.
12. If medically indicated, provide additional nutrition using a method of supplementation that is least likely to compromise the transition to exclusive breastfeeding.
13. Confirm that the infant has a scheduled appointment with a primary care provider or health worker within 5 to 7 days after birth.
14. Provide appropriate breastfeeding education materials.
15. Support exclusive breastfeeding during any illness or hospitalization of the mother or infant.
16. Comply with the *International Code of Marketing of Breast-milk Substitutes* and subsequent WHA resolutions, and avoid distribution of infant feeding product samples and advertisements for such products.
17. Include family members or significant others in breastfeeding education.
18. Provide anticipatory guidance for common problems that can interfere with exclusive breastfeeding.
19. Confirm that mothers understand normal breastfed infant behaviors and have realistic expectations regarding infant care and breastfeeding.
20. Discuss contraceptive options and their possible effect on milk production.

Source: International Lactation Consultant Association (2005).[2] Reprinted with permission.

LACTATIONAL INFERTILITY

Breastfeeding further extends the period of infertility and depresses ovarian function.[16] Plasma levels of FSH return to normal follicular phase values by 4 to 8 weeks postpartum in breastfeeding women.[17] In contrast, LH pulsation is disorganized in terms of the frequency or the amplitude of the LH pulse in the majority of lactating women throughout most of the period of lactational amenorrhea.[18]

Nipple and areola sensitivity increases at birth.[19] Infant suckling stimulates the nerve endings in the nipple and areola. Nerve impulses are passed to the hypothalamus, stimulating the release of various hormones, including prolactin. Prolactin controls the rate of milk production but is not believed to play a major role in suppressing ovarian function.[20]

Instead, suckling appears to disrupt the pulsatile release of gonadotropin releasing hormone (GnRH) by the hypothalamus,[17] perhaps by increasing hypothalamic β-endorphin production.[21] The interference with GnRH in turn averts the normal pulsatility of LH, which is required for follicle stimulation in the ovary. Small amounts of secreted estrogen at this time are insufficient to trigger an LH surge necessary to induce ovulation.[17,22]

Ovulation can occur even though the breastfeeding mother has not yet resumed menstruation. Only about 60% of ovulations preceding first menses have an adequate luteal phase.[23] Lactational amenorrhea becomes increasingly unreliable as an indicator of infertility beyond 6 months postpartum. The probability that ovulation will precede the first menses increases over time:[23,24]

- 33% to 45% during the first 3 months postpartum
- 64% to 71% during months 4 through 12
- 87% to 100% after 12 months.

Full or nearly full (unsupplemented) breastfeeding is associated with longer periods of lactational amenorrhea and infertility than is supplemented breastfeeding. Frequent stimulation of the breast by suckling day and night helps maintain the cascade of neuroendocrine events that produces the contraceptive effect.[25] The breastfeeding characteristics that contribute significantly to delay the return of ovulation include a high frequency of breastfeeds, a long total duration of feedings, a short interval between breastfeeds, and the presence of night feeds.[24,26] Milk production appears to be reduced far more by supplementary bottle feeds than by supplementary cup and spoon feeds.[24]

CONTRACEPTIVE BENEFITS OF LACTATION

In both traditional societies and developing countries, lactation plays a major role in prolonging birth intervals and thereby reducing fertility.[27] In developed countries, however, breastfeeding has a much smaller contraceptive impact because proportionately fewer infants are breastfed, and those who are breastfed are completely weaned at earlier ages. For example, in Indonesia, 96% of infants are breastfed, and those who are breastfed are not completely weaned until they are 2 years old on average.[28] In contrast, in the United States, only 74% of infants are ever breastfed with only 21% still breastfeeding at 1 year.[29] Work outside the home is a major barrier to breastfeeding in the United States and around the world. The International Lactation Consultants Association and the International Labor Organization and others endorse the right of women to be supported to breastfeed in the context of their paid and unpaid work.[30]

THE LACTATIONAL AMENORRHEA METHOD (LAM) OF CONTRACEPTION

Women who breastfeed can learn to make use of breastfeeding's natural contraceptive effect. If the woman feeds her infant only from her breast (or gives supplemental non-breastmilk feeds only to a minor extent) and has not experienced her first postpartum menses (defined as any bleeding occurring after 56 days postpartum), then breastfeeding provides more than 98% protection from pregnancy in the first 6 months following a birth.[25,31,32] See Figures 18–2 and 18–3. The Lactational Amenorrhea Method (LAM) is the proactive application of exclusive breastfeeding during lactational amenorrhea for the first 6 months after delivery. Four prospective clinical studies of the contraceptive effect of LAM demonstrated cumulative 6-month life-table perfect-use probability of pregnancy ranging from 0.5% to 1.5% among women who relied solely on LAM.[33–36] While pregnancy rates during the use of LAM compare favorably with those for many other methods of contraception (see Chapter 26 on Contraceptive Efficacy), even greater efficacy could be achieved by a combination of breastfeeding and use of an additional method of contraception.

LAM requires "full or nearly full" breastfeeding because the infant who obtains nearly all nutritional requirements through breastfeeding is providing maximal suckling stimulation at the breast. As long as additional foods do not decrease this optimal amount of suckling, small amounts of supplementation should have little or no effect on the return of fertility. Thus, if LAM is to be used, supplements should be given only infrequently, in small amounts, and not by bottle. The only real challenge concerning the correct use of LAM is determining the allowable extent of supplementation to the infant's diet, if the mother wishes to supplement. Figure 18–2 defines different infant feeding patterns and can be helpful in determining whether the woman is fully or nearly fully breastfeeding.[31,37] *Milk expression, such as by hand or pump, is not a substitute for breastfeeding in terms of its fertility-inhibiting effect.* A study of LAM used by working women reported an elevated 6-month probability of pregnancy (5.2%) indicating that frequent suckling, despite adequate milk production and full breastfeeding, is necessary to acquire the benefits of LAM.[38]

Experience with LAM in the United States is limited, and it is unknown whether more women would breastfeed if they appreciated the contraceptive effect of breastfeeding (or the other benefits of breastfeeding). Some U.S. women are already highly motivated to breastfeed, and they would be good candidates to use LAM as a temporary contraceptive option.[39] Women who choose to use LAM are basically choosing to fully or nearly fully breastfeed for at least some period (up to 6

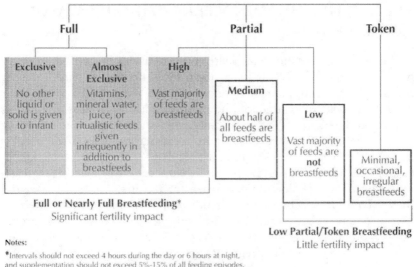

Full			Partial		Token

Exclusive

No other liquid or solid is given to infant

Almost Exclusive

Vitamins, mineral water, juice, or ritualistic feeds given infrequently in addition to breastfeeds

High

Vast majority of feeds are breastfeeds

Medium

About half of all feeds are breastfeeds

Low

Vast majority of feeds are **not** breastfeeds

Minimal, occasional, irregular breastfeeds

Full or Nearly Full Breastfeeding*
Significant fertility impact

Low Partial/Token Breastfeeding
Little fertility impact

Notes:

*Intervals should not exceed 4 hours during the day or 6 hours at night, and supplementation should not exceed 5%-15% of all feeding episodes, preferably fewer. While the high-partial pattern is adequate for fertility suppression, the woman should be counseled that any supplementation or disruption of the breastfeeding pattern can increase the risk of fertility return.

Source: Labbok et al. (1994).[31]

Figure 18–2 Schema for breastfeeding definition

months), so the choice to use LAM should be associated with the motivation to maintain good breastfeeding practices. In the United States, LAM may be best promoted in the context of breastfeeding support (from the healthcare system, friends, employers), which facilitates full/nearly full breastfeeding and maximizes the duration of amenorrhea[40] and the duration for which women can use LAM.

If a woman wishes to avoid becoming pregnant when LAM protection expires, then she must begin to use another contraceptive method at that time.[41,42]

POSTPARTUM SEXUALITY

Most American couples resume sexual intercourse within several weeks of delivery. Among U.S. lactating women, 66% are sexually active in the first month postpartum and 88% are sexually active in the second month postpartum.[43] In small samples of breastfeeding Western women, monthly coital frequency in the second month postpartum averaged 2.4, increasing to 3.2 to 4.9 in the third postpartum month.[44]

Contraception is only one counseling issue for postpartum women. Women—and men—may experience reduced sexual feelings associated with bodily changes caused by pregnancy and delivery. Discussion of these bodily changes may help to alleviate a couple's anxiety:

Ask the mother, or advise her to ask herself, these three questions:

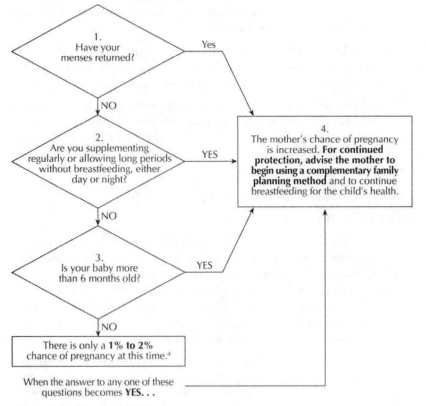

Source: Labbok et al. (1994).[31]

Figure 18–3 LAM: Lactational Amenorrhea Method

- Tenderness in the perineum may make intercourse painful, especially if there has been an episiotomy.

- Reduced postpartum estrogen secretion may result in diminished vaginal lubrication.

- Most women experience a heavy and bloody lochial discharge for a couple of weeks postpartum. This may interfere with a woman's sexual feeling.

- Couples may find that the exhaustion caused by the around-the-clock responsibilities of being a new parent temporarily decreases sexual drive.

- Lactation may diminish the erotic significance of the breasts. Couples need to communicate feelings about whether sucking or touching the breasts is acceptable.

- Bonding between mother and child creates skills and commitment in the mother and trust and security in the infant but may interfere with the mother's emotional availability to her partner.

- Conversely, a birth (especially if planned) can be an exceedingly joyous experience that can enhance sexual intimacy. To some men and women, the shape or fullness of the lactating breast is particularly arousing.

INITIATING CONTRACEPTIVE USE POSTPARTUM

Counseling for postpartum contraception should begin in the prenatal period because many methods can be provided at the time of delivery or during the hospital stay, such as intrauterine contraception (IUC) and female sterilization. For these methods provided immediately upon delivery, it is important to plan in advance, preferably in the prenatal period, so informed choice is valid and method choice and initiation is uncomplicated, convenient, and cost-effective.

Traditionally, a postpartum follow-up consultation occurred at 6 weeks because the uterus had mostly involuted and healed by this time. However, a physical exam can reasonably occur at any time between 3 and 8 weeks postpartum. In terms of contraceptive service delivery, routine adherence to the 6-week convention does not seem appropriate.[45] Therefore an individual approach to timing postpartum follow-up and contraceptive initiation is indicated. Although nearly all contraceptive methods can be used postpartum, the methods vary in terms of when in the postpartum period they should be initiated:[46-48]

- 6 weeks is too late to begin contraception for nonbreastfeeding mothers who wish to start using oral contraceptives, the patch, the vaginal ring, Implanon, or Depo-Provera.[49]

- 3 weeks is too soon for inserting an IUC (if not inserted immediately postpartum) or fitting a diaphragm.

- If the couple has been unable to select a contraceptive method by the time of hospital discharge, they should plan a postpartum visit for 3 weeks.[50]

When the couple's method of choice cannot be initiated during the hospital stay after delivery, they can choose temporary methods such as LAM or the brief use of condoms and plan to initiate a longer-term method later. Schedule the first postpartum visit for the most logical time based on the longer-term method choice. For example, if a breast-feeding woman will be using the Copper 380A IUC (and did not receive one within 10 minutes of the delivery of the placenta), schedule her follow-up visit for 4 weeks postpartum, with the plan for her to use condoms or LAM until that time. To help ensure success, provide a package of lubricated condoms at hospital discharge, and instruct her about the need for and use of LAM and the condoms. Perhaps most important, contact the woman 2 to 4 weeks after delivery to check on her postpartum recovery and breastfeeding success, and to confirm and support her personal contraception plan.

A systematic review of the research on the effectiveness of postpartum counseling for contraception found that postpartum education results in more family planning use and fewer unplanned pregnancies.[51] As mentioned above, antenatal counseling is essential for informed choice for the immediate postpartum use of long acting and permanent methods. Women appear to be open and interested in family planning information at a variety of times, and their individual circumstances and opinions undoubtedly change over time as well. Thus, strategies for counseling before and after delivery and during the hospital stay all have their place. A recent U.S. study found that mothers are comfortable talking with their infant's health care provider about contraception.[52] Accordingly, we should not be limited to conventional approaches when considering the best time and place to reach women regarding their needs for contraception.

The following considerations may prove useful when counseling and providing contraceptives to the postpartum woman, whether or not she is breastfeeding:

- *Withdrawal* may be a good method for couples in the postpartum period. Withdrawal is effective if used correctly and consistently. (See Chapter 26.)

- *Condoms* are an attractive option. Postpartum endometritis is a serious complication. The risk of introducing bacteria into the uterus is elevated before cervical closure is complete, i.e., for about 6 to 8 weeks.

- *Barrier method* use may need to be delayed:

  — Episiotomies may still be tender. Fitting a woman for a diaphragm may cause discomfort.

  — Avoid the diaphragm and contraceptive sponge until 6 weeks after delivery. The diaphragm cannot be (re)fitted properly until that time. Moreover, the risk of toxic shock syndrome is increased when blood, including the postpartum lochia, is present.[53] (See Chapter 14.)

— The sponge (though not the diaphragm) has much higher failure rates among women who have delivered a child than among women who have not, *even during perfect use*. (See Chapter 26.) Inform women about this substantial decrease in efficacy for parous women so they can make an informed choice of a contraceptive method.

- *Postpartum abstinence*, if practiced properly, is 100% effective in preventing pregnancy. It can, however, be notoriously difficult to maintain. Counsel women about other contraceptive methods should they desire to resume intercourse.

- *Copper intrauterine contraceptives (IUCs)* are best inserted postpartum, either (1) immediately (within 10 minutes) after the expulsion of the placenta, or (2) after 4 weeks postpartum. (It is less desirable to insert an IUC in the period between because of the high expulsion rate that occurs during uterine involution.) An IUC can be inserted immediately after a cesarean delivery through the uterine incision.[54] Avoid IUC insertion when premature rupture of the membranes, prolonged labor, or fever has occurred, because of the elevated risk of infection.[55,56] Immediate postpartum insertion has not been associated with excessive bleeding or endometritis.[57] Expulsion rates following postpartum insertion are higher than those following interval insertion, but they are lower for immediate than for delayed postpartum insertion.[58] A small study compared the expulsion of Copper T380A IUCs inserted within the first 10 minutes after placental delivery (using a ring forceps inserted through the uterine cervix) with the same type of IUC placed through the hysterotomy site transoperatively in women who delivered by cesarean section. Expulsion was detected by ultrasound and not just clinical examination. In women who delivered vaginally, 50% of the IUCs had been expelled, while none were missing among those who delivered surgically.[59]

- *Sterilization* presents excellent options for appropriate candidates:

— Vasectomy is an appropriate postpartum choice for couples who want a permanent method. As soon as the health of the mother and infant is determined to be sound, the vasectomy can be performed. If the woman is breastfeeding, a back-up method may not be needed while waiting for confirmation that the vasectomy has taken effect.[18,46] As with tubal ligation, vasectomy requires counseling and reflection under nonstressful circumstances, preferably before delivery.[46,47]

— Tubal ligation performed during the immediate postpartum period can be a more cost-effective and simpler technique than interval sterilization. While tubal ligation is a highly effective method of contraception, a small risk of sterilization failure persists for at least a decade. However, partial salpingectomy performed postpartum carries the lowest known 10-year pregnancy risk of any female sterilization procedure.[60] Discuss immediate postpartum sterilization well before the delivery to help ensure that consent is fully informed.[61] Take great care that the woman is confident of this choice,[62] since the performance of tubal sterilization during the postpartum period is a risk factor for regret.[60,63] (See Chapter 17 on Female and Male Sterilization.) After a vaginal delivery, sterilization should be performed by minilaparotomy within 48 hours or else delayed for 4 to 6 weeks. After 48 hours, access to the tubes is reduced and the risk of infection increased.[61] Tubal ligation can be performed through the abdominal incision after a cesarean delivery. As with minilaparotomy after vaginal delivery, cesarean sterilization may need to be delayed in the case of complications, such as severe pre-eclampsia, eclampsia, premature rupture of the membranes, sepsis, fever, severe hemorrhage, uterine rupture or perforation.[47,64]

POSTPARTUM CONTRACEPTION FOR THE NONBREASTFEEDING WOMAN

If she wishes to avoid becoming pregnant, the nonbreastfeeding woman should begin using a contraceptive method immediately postpartum or at least by the beginning of the fourth postpartum week.[49] Most nonbreastfeeding mothers have few restrictions placed on which method of contraceptive they can choose. Nonetheless, a few guidelines—in addition to those given above—are warranted:

- Combined oral contraceptives (COCs) and the combined patch, injectable, and vaginal ring may be *prescribed* immediately postpartum. However, caution women not to use them until at least 3 full weeks after delivery.[46–48,54] The risk of postpartum thrombophlebitis and thromboembolism in the postpartum period is 5 times the risk during pregnancy, and remains elevated through at least the 6th postpartum week.[65] Some leaders in the field advise the postponement of COCs until 4[66] to 6.5 weeks,[45] since COCs may increase the risk of venous thromboembolic disease 2 to 4 fold.[67] Product labeling cautions the deferral of COCs until 4–6 weeks postpartum in non-breastfeeding women.[66]

- Caution women that it is difficult to practice fertility awareness before their cycles are reestablished and cyclic signs of fertility return.

- Suggest that lubricated condoms are a good option at least for the short period before the woman becomes better suited to her preferred method.

- Implanon can be inserted and Depo-Provera can be safely injected immediately postpartum. Discuss these options before delivery to ensure that consent is fully informed.

POSTPARTUM CONTRACEPTION FOR THE BREASTFEEDING WOMAN

NONHORMONAL METHODS

General comments regarding contraceptive use among postpartum women are given above. In addition, the following considerations are relevant for women who are breastfeeding. Breastfeeding is a condition for which there is no restriction on the use of nonhormonal methods.[47,54]

Tubal ligation can be performed immediately postpartum, although it can disrupt lactation if it requires general anesthesia or separation of mother and infant. Both problems can be minimized by performing the procedure with only regional or local anesthetic.[68] If tubal ligation does not occur while the mother is on the delivery table, breastfeeding should occur just before she receives anesthesia, and be delayed immediately after, to reduce the transfer of the anesthetic agent to the infant.[69,70] As soon as the mother is awake enough to hold her baby, it is safe for her to breastfeed.

Copper T 380A IUCs are also a good choice for breastfeeding women. The copper on the Copper T does not affect the quantity or quality of breastmilk.[71] (See the following section on Hormonal Methods for information on the IUCs containing a progestin.) Some women experience mild uterine cramping when they breastfeed with an IUC in place, but the cramping does not usually interfere with lactation or with the effectiveness of the IUC. IUC insertion is less painful, and pain and bleeding removal rates are lower, for the lactating mother.[72,73] Although case reports and small studies suggested that the risk of uterine perforation is higher among breastfeeding women, larger studies find low rates of perforation in both breastfeeding and nonbreastfeeding women.[56,74]

Spermicides and barrier methods have no effect on the ability to breastfeed. The lubricated condom is especially useful in the postpartum period because of increased vaginal dryness. Spermicides also may help offset dryness due to estrogen deficiency. In the United States, barrier methods are the most widely used contraceptive among lactating mothers in the first 6 months postpartum.[43] In animal studies, nonoxynol-9 is absorbed through the skin and secreted in breastmilk.[75] The question of whether nonoxynol-9 is secreted in breastmilk has not been completely evaluated in humans. (See Chapter 14 on Vaginal Barriers and Spermicides.)

Lactational Amenorrhea Method (LAM) provides effective protection against pregnancy for up to 6 months postpartum. If continued protection is desired, another method of contraception must be introduced when the LAM criteria indicate a return to the risk of pregnancy. It is useful and acceptable to many women to have a back-up method in hand to begin when any of the LAM criteria no longer apply. (See the detailed description of LAM earlier in this chapter.)

Fertility awareness methods can be difficult to use during the return of fertility, which can extend for many cycles during lactation.[76] The couple needs to abstain for 2 weeks in order to establish a "basic infertile pattern" of cervical mucus (and other) symptoms. Intercourse can then occur every other night unless/until there is some change in the basic infertile pattern, in which case more abstinence is necessary.[77] The changing fertility symptoms after the first postpartum menses may be especially difficult for new users to identify, and may lead to an increased risk for unplanned pregnancy.[78]

Basal body temperature cannot be ascertained unless a woman has at least 6 hours of uninterrupted sleep. Thus, the woman who gets up in the night to care for her infant is precluded from using the temperature symptom to help determine her fertility status.

The rules for using the symptothermal method during breastfeeding have been found to detect the onset of true fertility extremely well. However, these same rules often necessitate many days of abstinence when there is virtually no risk of pregnancy.[79] However, if they use the proposed new "TwoDay Method," breastfeeding women who want to use a fertility awareness method may need to abstain for fewer days.[80] Recommend LAM to users of fertility awareness methods who are breastfeeding. LAM can eliminate the requirements for abstinence for up to 6 months with no apparent additional risk of unplanned pregnancy.[81] The transition from LAM use to the use of a fertility awareness method begins with the establishment of a basic infertile pattern.[77,79]

HORMONAL METHODS

The use of hormonal contraception by breastfeeding women is an area of dispute among experts.[82] Since all steroids pass through the breastmilk to the infant, the WHO, the International Planned Parenthood Federation (IPPF), and the Academy for Breastfeeding Medicine do not consider hormonal methods of contraception to be the category of first choice for breastfeeding women.[46-48,83,84]

The WHO finds COCs during breastfeeding to pose an unacceptable health risk in the first 6 months postpartum, and thereafter the advantages generally outweigh the risks. They find that progestin-only methods (except LNg IUCs) are not usually recommended for breastfeeding women earlier than 6 weeks postpartum, and thereafter there is no restriction.[47,48] These recommendations, recently reiterated by WHO, are based on the admittedly theoretical concern that early neonatal exposure to exogenous steroids, which have passed from the contraceptive into the milk, should be avoided when alternative methods are available.[85] The binding capacity of plasma is low, the neonatal liver is not well able to conjugate and oxidize drugs, and the immature kidneys are inefficient in excretion.[18,88] Unable to be cleared from the infant's circulation, exogenous steroids or their metabolites may "compete with natural hormones for receptor sites in sex organs, brain or other tissues."[86] Experts issue their caution because animal literature has indicated long-term effects from inappropriate hormone exposure at critical postpartum periods.[85,86]

In the absence of definitive human research to support or refute this concern, the U.S. Centers for Disease Control and Prevention (CDC) and the U.K. Faculty of Sexual and Reproductive Health Care offer less restrictive guidance. They do not find that COCs pose "an unacceptable health risk," and, while not indicating that they are completely without restriction, they advise that most progestin-only methods have advantages that generally outweigh the risks during breastfeeding, even from the time of delivery.[54,87]

Progestin-only contraceptives such as Implanon, the LNg IUC, Depo-Provera, and progestin-only pills do not (with a possible caveat explained below) have adverse effects on lactation, and some studies suggest they may even increase milk volume. They do not appear to have adverse effects on infant growth and development.[88] In addition, their contraceptive efficacy is high (see Chapter 26), and they are simple to use. Therefore, these methods are good options for lactating women who wish to postpone a subsequent pregnancy. The U.S. CDC advises that progestin-only methods can be used in the first month postpartum as the advantages generally outweigh the risks during breastfeeding.[54]

Although progestin-only contraceptives probably have no adverse effects on lactation or infant health, little research has been conducted on their immediate postpartum use, since initiation prior to 6 weeks has been discouraged. The precipitous withdrawal of natural progesterone, usually 30 to 40 hours after birth, triggers the production of copious amounts of mature milk (although the mother may not perceive breast fullness for 50 to 73 hours), and the related changes in milk composition are largely completed by 72 hours.[89]

The receipt of a high-dose of exogenous progestin (as with a Depo-Provera injection or in the first week after the insertion of an implant) before this process is complete may interfere with the successful or optimal establishment of milk synthesis. This reasoning argues for a delay in commencing progestin-only contraception, especially injectable formulas, until the mature milk has come in.[90] If a breastfeeding woman's informed choice is to use Depo-Provera (or another high dose of exogenous progestin) as soon as possible after delivery, and no other appropriate methods are available or acceptable, then her care providers should facilitate her receipt of the injection immediately after her mature milk comes in. Among other approaches, this can be accomplished (a) by delaying hospital discharge (during which period breastfeeding support can be provided), or (b) by scheduling a nurse home visit after the 7th postpartum day, during which visit the injection can be given and continued breastfeeding support can be provided. (In some cases, particularly among diabetic or obese women, mature milk may not come in for 5 to 7 days.) Many clinicians are deeply concerned about preventing early subsequent pregnancies in women described to be at high risk for not initiating a contraceptive method early enough. Either of the innovative approaches suggested above (and undoubtedly others) may reach women who are simultaneously at high risk for early breastfeeding cessation and early unplanned pregnancy, and we may be able to serve more than one of her needs by modifying the way we think about and deliver postpartum care. The aforementioned review of studies of postpartum family planning education concluded that "Health care providers can test in their own environment the programs that appear to be appropriate for their population, location and resources".[51] The authors found that structured home visiting programs resulted in better contraceptive use, and programs with multiple contacts do not always cost more than standard care.[51]

Some studies of Depo-Provera and progestin-only pills have found no overall deleterious effect of progestin on milk volume when begun as early as the first week postpartum,[91,92] suggesting that very early exposure to progestin-only contraceptives is not always detrimental to lactogenesis. However, in these studies, progestin might have been initiated after the withdrawal of natural progesterone. Similarly, a study of progestin-only methods saw no effect of progestin method use on breastfeeding duration or child growth, but the average time to administration of the method was more than 2 days postpartum. Also, women were not randomized into the treatment groups, and breastfeeding duration was short for all women.[93]

Studies in China and Bolivia showed that breastfeeding women tolerate Depo-Provera's disruption of menstrual cyclicity better than nonbreastfeeding women, and their method continuation rates are higher.[94,95] A progesterone-releasing vaginal ring is effective during lactation and is associated with prolonged lactational amenorrhea, which represents a health benefit for the woman.[96] Studies of other progestin-only contraceptives initiated after 6 weeks postpartum show that lactational amenorrhea is prolonged.[97]

As with the Copper T 380A IUC, the CDC advises that the LNg IUC can be inserted at any time, including on the delivery table and during uterine involution, although for breastfeeding women they do not classify LNg IUC use as a condition with no restriction. In the absence of evidence that compares risks of different insertion times, they find that the advantages of the method generally outweigh the risks. However, in a recent study, 97 breastfeeding women were randomized to receive an LNg IUC within 10 minutes of delivery versus at 6 to 8 weeks postpartum. The percent breastfeeding was the same at 6 to 8 weeks postpartum, but became significantly and increasingly lower at 3 and 6 months in the group with immediate progesterone IUC insertion.[98]

Until there are better studies of the effects of neonatal exposure to steroid hormones in the first 6 weeks postpartum, and until there are better studies of the effect of exogenous progestins on the critical period of lactogenesis in the first 2 to 7 days postpartum, informed choice will remain important. South African investigators provided women with appropriate information about immediate versus delayed progestin injection, and women were able to make their own decisions about the timing of initiation.[99]

Combined hormonal contraceptives (the combined pill, patch, injectable, and vaginal ring) have been the subject of a systematic review, in which 3 of 4 randomized controlled studies of the effects of COCs on breastfeeding showed decreased durations of breastfeeding.[100] WHO considers this and other evidence to absolutely contraindicate the use of COCs in the first 6 weeks of breastfeeding and to relatively contraindicate it in the period from 6 weeks to 6 months.[47] The CDC interprets the evidence as less restrictive, advising that the risks outweigh the advantages in the first month, but that advantages outweigh the risks thereafter.[54]

As described in the section on COCs for nonbreastfeeding women, it is prudent for all women to avoid methods containing estrogen for at least 3 and up to 6 weeks postpartum. In the United States, progestin-only methods are as widely available as methods containing estrogen, and since breastfeeding women are at a reduced risk of pregnancy (especially during amenorrhea and full breastfeeding), it may be possible to avoid COC use altogether during breastfeeding. There is no need for breastfeeding women using progestin-only pills to switch to COCs during lactation. However, if it is the woman's informed choice to make this switch, it is best to do so after 6 months postpartum.[101]

EFFECTS OF HORMONAL CONTRACEPTION ON THE BREASTFED INFANT

Contraceptive steroids taken by the mother can be transferred to the nursing infant through breastmilk. The amounts, however, are small. Nevertheless, it is prudent to avoid exposing the neonate to exogenous steroids, which are not easily bound in plasma, conjugated by the liver, or excreted; additionally, the exogenous steroids may compete with natural hormones for receptor sites. While concern about the possible effects on the liver, sex organs, and other tissues of the neonate or premature infant is theoretical, exposure should be avoided wherever possible. Although studies are few and numbers are small, it appears that:

- The dose of contraceptive ethinyl estradiol reaching the infant of a mother taking combined pills is typically 1% or less of the maternal dose.[85]

- The quantity of progestin transferred to mother's milk varies with the type of progestin. The 17-hydroxy compounds (such as medroxyprogesterone acetate) enter the milk at approximately the same level as is found in the mother's blood, whereas the 19-nor compounds (such as norgestrel and norethindrone) enter the milk at only one-tenth the level in the blood.[102]

Hormonal contraceptive use during lactation is not the only possible source of estrogen and progestin exposure for the infant. When a mother becomes pregnant and continues to breastfeed a prior infant, that child is exposed to estrogen and progesterone in the mother's milk. Dairy cattle may also be pregnant at the time that they are milked, so that cow's milk and infant formula made from it may have relatively high levels of estrogen and progesterone.

Drug absorption, distribution, metabolism, and elimination are poorly understood in neonates. Although early studies of high-dose oral contraceptives did demonstrate some effect of hormones on nursing babies,[103] most of those reports were anecdotal and have not been corroborated in women using low-dose pills. One study of the male offspring of women who had used Depo-Provera found no effect on infant hormone regulation associated with breastfeeding exposure.[104]

EMERGENCY CONTRACEPTION AND THE BREASTFEEDING WOMAN

There is little if any published experience with emergency contraception during breastfeeding. Given what is known in general about both breastfeeding and contraception, the U. K. Faculty of Family Planning and Reproductive Health Care Clinical Effectiveness Unit advises breastfeeding women that a contraceptive failure or unprotected sex before postpartum day 21 does not require the use of an emergency method, and that an IUC can be inserted as emergency contraception beginning in the fourth week.[105] The WHO and the CDC indicate that progestin-only pills can be used for emergency contraception with no restriction on use by breastfeeding women.[47,54] Although researchers have cautioned women to discontinue nursing for 8 to 24 hours after using progesterone-only emergency contraception,[106] once a breastfeeding woman starts a hormonal method, she can follow the emergency contraception guidance that corresponds to that method.[105]

B REASTFEEDING: ADVANTAGES TO THE INFANT

The practice of breastfeeding facilitates attachment—the psychological bond between mother and infant. Mother's milk has both nutritional and anti-infective advantages for the infant. The infant ingests host-protecting, humoral, and allergy prophylaxis factors. These are particularly concentrated in the colostrum, the high-protein, high-anti-oxidant fluid secreted in the first few days postpartum. The particular mixtures of protein, fat, carbohydrate, and trace elements change to meet the infant's evolving needs as breastfeeding proceeds from month to month.[107,108] There are both short-term and long-term health benefits of breastfeeding to the infant, and few, if any, liabilities. Even in developed country settings, breastfeeding reduces the risk of acute otitis media, nonspecific diarrheal disease, respiratory tract infections, atopic dermatitis, asthma, type 1 diabetes, childhood leukemia, sudden infant death syndrome, and necrotizing enterocolitis.[109] Later in life, significant positive effects of having been breastfed are seen in blood pressure, serum cholesterol, overweight and obesity, and type 2 diabetes.[110]

Most medications taken by the breastfeeding mother are safe for the infant, and excellent references are available that distinguish those medications which may require an interruption of breastfeeding.[111,112] In the United States there are few contraindications to breastfeeding,[112] with illicit drug use and maternal human immunodeficiency virus (HIV) infection as notable exceptions.[113]

BREASTFEEDING AND HIV

HIV, which causes acquired immune deficiency syndrome (AIDS), can be transmitted by an infected mother to her infant in utero, during childbirth, and through breastmilk. That HIV can be transmitted by breastfeeding has been conclusively demonstrated by case reports, laboratory data, and epidemiologic studies. Rates of vertical transmission during pregnancy and delivery are about 15% to 25%, and an additional 5% to 20% can become infected through breastfeeding.[114] Thus, the majority of infants who are infected with HIV acquire the infection in utero or during childbirth, and the majority of infants who are breastfed by HIV-positive mothers do not become infected.

HIV transmission via breastmilk is greatest when the mother's viral load is high and HIV immune status is poor. The risk of transmission is probably also affected by inflammatory breast conditions (such as mastitis), the mother's nutritional status, mode of feeding (exclusive breastfeeding is associated with less risk), and possibly HIV-specific anti-infective activities of the milk, (such as inhibiting the binding of HIV glycoproteins to CD4 molecules.[114-117]) The duration of breastfeeding is associated with the risk of transmission, and the rate is a relatively constant 1% per month from about 4 to 6 months postpartum to about 18 months.[114]

It is clear that breastfeeding can be a route for HIV transmission. It is also clear that breastmilk is normally protective (albeit to an unknown degree) against enveloped viruses such as HIV. Since antiretroviral therapy and exclusive breastfeeding can profoundly reduce the risk of breastfeeding transmission, and since many HIV-infected infants live in environments with extraordinary competing risks of infant mortality, the WHO recommends, "... that national authorities in each country decide which infant feeding practice, i.e., breastfeeding with an antiretroviral intervention to reduce transmission or avoidance of all breastfeeding..." to advocate in their jurisdictions.[118] According to U.S. authorities, HIV-infected mothers *in the United States* should be counseled not to breastfeed or provide their milk to other infants.[112,113,119] Mother to child transmission of HIV during pregnancy and delivery also is reduced profoundly through antiretroviral prophylaxis (and in some places also by cesarean delivery).[120]

BREASTFEEDING: EFFECTS ON THE MOTHER

Breastfeeding has a major protective effect against premenopausal cancers of the ovary, endometrium, and breast and protects against type 2 diabetes.[4,5,109,121-123] Mother's milk is free and is always available at the right temperature, in contrast to infant formula. Breastfeeding also promotes emotional bonding between mother and infant. Finally, the breastfeeding mother experiences a rapid return of uterine tone. Oxytocin, which induces uterine contraction, is released from the posterior pituitary when the nipple is stimulated by suckling.

During lactation, the body's estrogen levels are very low, and vaginal lubrication may be less than usual and begin later during sexual intercourse. Vaginal lubrication improves when cycling resumes or when the frequency of breastfeeding declines. Nursing mothers have added requirements for calories, protein, calcium, and iron, as well as several vitamins and other micronutrients. The increased needs for specific nutrients can be provided by a well-balanced diet, although U.S. women are often encouraged to continue their prenatal vitamins during breastfeeding. Supplements are generally unnecessary unless the diet is deficient in one or more of these nutrients.[124,125]

INSTRUCTIONS FOR AND INFORMATION ABOUT BREASTFEEDING

1. Congratulations! Enjoy your baby, rest, and keep in touch with your clinician.

2. Health experts concur that all women should be enabled to breastfeed, to breastfeed exclusively for 6 months, and to continue supplemented breastfeeding for 12 to 24 months or longer.

3. **If you are not breastfeeding, begin using a contraceptive method before or at your first sexual encounter.** You can become pregnant before your first menstrual period after childbirth because ovulation can begin before menstruation.

4. **If you are breastfeeding and providing bottle supplements, begin using a contraceptive method as soon as your clinician advises based on the method you have chosen.**

5. **If you are breastfeeding and using the Lactational Amenorrhea Method (LAM) as a temporary method of contraception, breastfeed your baby on demand, avoid any bottle feeds, and provide any minimal supplements by cup or spoon.** Begin using another method of contraception when you resume menstruation (defined as any bleeding after 56 days postpartum), when you reduce the frequency or duration of breastfeeds, when you introduce bottle feeds or regular food supplements, or when your baby turns 6 months old. (See Figures 18–2 and 18–3.)

6. **You can become pregnant while breastfeeding your baby,** although the risk is greatly reduced before your first menstrual

period; in the first 6 months of amenorrhea when you feed your baby on demand, avoid any bottle feeds, and provide minimal supplements by cup or spoon, your risk of pregnancy will be about 2%, equivalent to or lower than the risk associated with many other contraceptive methods. Most U.S. women do not follow breastfeeding patterns that confer maximum protection against pregnancy. However, women who choose LAM may adopt breastfeeding behaviors that maximize both milk production and the duration of amenorrhea.

7. **Breastfeeding is a convenient, inexpensive, and nutritious way to feed your baby and it helps to protect the baby against infection, diarrhea, allergy, and sudden infant death syndrome. It also offers you protection against cancer of the breast, ovary, and uterus.**

8. **Neither intercourse nor menstruation affects the quality or quantity of your breastmilk. You do not need to stop breastfeeding because you start having intercourse again or start your period.** You can continue breastfeeding when you start using another contraceptive method.

9. **Lubricants, such as K-Y Jelly, spermicides, or saliva, may make intercourse easier after childbirth** because decreased estrogen production during breastfeeding diminishes vaginal lubrication.

10. **When you are nursing your child, your own nutrition is important.** Women can usually obtain all the calories and nutrients they need to breastfeed through their usual diet. There is no need to buy any special foods. Just eat a sensible, well-balanced diet, which is always a good idea.

11. **Avoid smoking.** Nursing women who smoke may transfer nicotine to their infant through their breastmilk. Nicotine is a poison that can harm the child. Inhaling smoke, as well as second-hand smoke, is also harmful to the baby. Smoking may also influence your ability to produce milk and decrease your supply.

12. **Alcohol that you drink will be passed to your baby through breastmilk.** Your baby will have more difficulty metabolizing alcohol than you do, especially in the first few weeks after delivery. No good studies have been conducted to assess what level of alcohol consumption is safe. Thus it seems prudent to drink only modest amounts of alcohol and wait several hours after you have had a drink to nurse your baby, if possible.

13. **If you are using any medications while breastfeeding, be sure to tell your physician.** You can breastfeed while using virtually all common drugs. However, for some medications you may need advice concerning the best timing for ingestion to decrease infant exposure.

14. **If you are infected with HIV, be sure to get antiretroviral treatment. HIV, the virus that causes AIDS, can be transmitted to your baby through breastmilk.** For this reason, most experts recommend that you not breastfeed your baby if you live in a country where replacement feedings are acceptable, feasible, affordable, sustainable and safe, as in the United States.

15. **It is indeed possible to combine work and breastfeeding successfully,** yet any separation of mother from infant for more than a few hours can create challenges to breastfeeding. Working women (or any breastfeeding woman!) should be sure to locate, preferably before delivery, a certified lactation consultant who can help in the event of any difficulty, from engorgement to declining milk supply. Lactation consultants are highly trained to give advice on a broad spectrum of breastfeeding issues, including the storage and transport of expressed milk, and can often help you rent an electric breast pump if you need one. The headquarters of the International Lactation Consultant Association can help you locate a certified lactation consultant near you (Website: http://www.ilca.org).

RESOURCE MATERIALS

Academy of Breastfeeding Medicine: Clinical Protocols. (Guidelines for the care of breastfeeding mothers and infants.) Available from: www.bfmed.org/Resources/Protocols.aspx [cited 2010 July 18].

International Lactation Consultant Association (ILCA): Clinical Guidelines for the Establishment of Exclusive Breastfeeding. Raleigh: ILCA; June 2005. Available from: www.ilca.org/files/resources/ilca_publications/ClinicalGuidelines2005.pdf [cited 2010 July 18]. Other ILCA resources to support breastfeeding are available at www.ilca.org. [cited 2010 July 18].

REFERENCES

1. World Health Organization: Report of a WHO technical consultation on birth spacing. 2007 WHO Press, WHO/RHR/07.1 World Health Organization, Geneva, Switzerland. [cited 2010 July 18]. Available from: http://www.who.int/making_pregnancy_safer/documents/birth_spacing05/en/index.html

2. International Lactation Consultant Association (ILCA). Clinical guidelines for the establishment of exclusive breastfeeding. Raleigh (NC): ILCA; 2005 June. [cited 2010 July 18]. Available from: http://www.ilca.org/files/resources/ilca_publications/ClinicalGuidelines2005.pdf

3. World Health Assembly. Infant and young child nutrition. Fifty-fourth World Health Assembly Resolution WHA54.2. Geneva (Switzerland):WHO, 2001 May 18. [updated 2001 May 18;cited 2010 Jun 7]; [about 4 pages]. Available from: http://apps.who.int/gb/archive/pdf_files/WHA54/ea54r2.pdf

4. American Academy of Pediatrics. Breastfeeding and the use of human milk. Pediatrics. 2005 [cited 2010 Jun 7];115:496–506. Available from: http://www.pediatrics.org/cgi/content/full/115/2/496

5. U.S. Department of Health and Human Services, Office of Women's Health. Breastfeeding—HHS blueprint for action on breastfeeding. Washington (DC): The Department; 2000 [cited 2010 Jun 7]. Available from: http://www.womenshealth.gov/archive/breastfeeding/programs/blueprints/bluprntbk2.pdf

6. World Health Organization. The optimal duration of exclusive breastfeeding: report of an expert consultation. Geneva (Switzerland): 2001 March 28–30. Geneva (Switzerland): WHO; 2002 [cited 2010 Jun 7]. Available from: http://whqlibdoc.who.int/hq/2001/WHO_NHD_01.09.pdf

7. Kramer MS, Kakuma R. The optimal duration of exclusive breastfeeding: a systematic review. Geneva (Switzerland): WHO; 2002: WHO/FCH/CAH/01.23. [cited 2010 Jun 7]. Available from: http://www.who.int/nutrition/topics/optimal_duration_of_exc_bfeeding_review_eng.pdf

8. American Dietetic Association. Position of the American Dietetic Association: promoting and supporting breastfeeding. J Am Diet Assoc. 2009;109:1926–42.

9. Academy for Breastfeeding Medicine. ABM Statements Position on breastfeeding. Breastfeeding Medicine 2008;3:267–270.

10. American College of Obstetrics and Gynecology. Breastfeeding: maternal and infant aspects. ACOG Committee Opinion Number 361. Obstet Gynecol 2007;109:479–80.

11. American Academy of Family Physicians. Breastfeeding (Policy Statement) 2007. [cited 2010 July 18]. Available from: http://www.aafp.org/online/en/home/policy/policies/b/breastfeedingpolicy.html

12. UNICEF. Innocenti declaration on the protection, promotion and support of breastfeeding. New York: UNICEF; 1990.

13. Hodgen GD, Itskovitz J. Recognition and maintenance of pregnancy. In: Knobil E, Neill JD, Ewing LL, Greenwald GS, Markert CL, Pfaff DW, (eds). The physiology of reproduction. New York: Raven Press; 1988:1995–2021.

14. Willson JR. The puerperium. In: Willson JR, Carrington ER, Ledger WJ, Laros RK, Mattox JH, (eds). Obstetrics and gynecology. 8th ed. St. Louis (MO): CV Mosby Company; 1987:598–607.

15. Gray RH, Campbell OM, Zacur H, Labbok MH, MacRae SL. Postpartum return of ovarian activity in non-breastfeeding women monitored by urinary assays. J Clin Endocrinol Metab. 1987;64:645–50.

16. McNeilly AS. Lactational control of reproduction. Reprod Fertil Dev. 2001;13:583–90.

17. McNeilly AS. Neuroendocrine changes and fertility in breastfeeding women. Prog Brain Res. 2001;133:207–14.

18. Díaz S, Croxatto HB. Contraception in lactating women. Curr Opin Obstet Gynecol. 1993;5:815–22.

19. Robinson JE, Short RV. Changes in breast sensitivity at puberty, during the menstrual cycle, and at parturition. Br Med J. 1977;1:1188–91.

20. Díaz S, Seron-Ferre M, Croxatto HB, Veldhuis J. Neuroendocrine mechanisms of lactational infertility in women. Biol Res. 1995;28:155–63.

21. Gordon K, Renfree MB, Short RV, Clarke IJ. Hypothalamo-pituitary portal blood concentrations of β-endorphin during suckling in the ewe. J Reprod Fertil. 1987;79: 397–408.

22. McNeilly AS, Tay CCK, Glasier A. Physiological mechanisms underlying lactational amenorrhea. In: Campbell KL, Wood JW, (eds). Human reproductive ecology: interactions of environment, fertility and behavior. New York: Academy of Sciences; 1994. p. 145–55.

23. Lewis PR, Brown JB, Renfree MB, Short RV. The resumption of ovulation and menstruation in a well-nourished population of women breastfeeding for an extended period of time. Fertil Steril. 1991;55:529–36.

24. Campbell OMR, Gray RH. Characteristics and determinants of postpartum ovarian function in women in the United States. Am J Obstet Gynecol. 1993;169:55–60.

25. Kennedy KI, Rivera R, McNeilly AS. Consensus statement on the use of breastfeeding as a family planning method. Contraception. 1989;39:477–96.

26. Gray RH, Campbell OM, Apelo R, Eslami SS, Zacur H, Ramos RM, Gehret JC, Labbok MH. Risk of ovulation during lactation. Lancet. 1990;335:25–9.

27. Becker S, Rutstein S, Labbok MH. Estimation of births averted due to breast-feeding and increases in levels of contraception needed to substitute for breast-feeding. J Bios Sci. 2003;35:559–74.

28. Demographic and Health Surveys. Indonesia demographic and health survey 1997. Calverton: Macro International Inc., 1998.

29. Centers for Disease Control and Prevention. Breastfeeding trends and updated national health objectives for exclusive breastfeeding – United States, birth years 2000–2004. MMWR. 2007;56:760–763.

30. International Lactation Consultant Association. Position paper on breastfeeding and work. Raleigh (NC): ILCA; 2007 December. [cited 2010 July 18]. Available from: http://www.ilca.org/files/resources/ilca_publications/ BreasfeedingandWorkPP.pdf

31. Labbok M, Cooney K, Coly S. Guidelines: breastfeeding, family planning, and the Lactational Amenorrhea Method—LAM. Washington (DC): Institute for Reproductive Health, Georgetown University, 1994.

32. World Health Organization. The WHO multinational study of breastfeeding and lactational amenorrhea: III. Pregnancy during breastfeeding. Fertil Steril. 1999;72: 431–40.

33. Kazi A, Kennedy KI, Visness CM, Khan T. Effectiveness of the Lactational Amenorrhea Method in Pakistan. Fertil Steril. 1995;64:717–23.

34. Labbok MH, Hight-Laukaran V, Peterson AE, Fletcher V, von Hertzen H, Van Look PFA. Multicenter study of the Lactational Amenorrhea Method (LAM): I. Efficacy, duration, and implications for clinical application. Contraception.1997;55:327–36.

35. Pérez A, Labbok MH, Queenan JT. Clinical study of the Lactational Amenorrhoea Method for family planning. Lancet. 1992;339:968–70.

36. Ramos R, Kennedy KI, Visness CM. Effectiveness of lactational amenorrhea in prevention of pregnancy in Manila, the Philippines: non-comparative prospective trial. BMJ. 1996;313:909–12.

37. Labbok M, Krasovec K. Toward consistency in breastfeeding definitions. Stud Fam Plann. 1990;21:226–30.

38. Valdés V, Labbok MH, Pugin E, Pérez A. The efficacy of the lactational amernorrhea method (LAM) among working women. Contraception. 2000;62:217–19.

39. Hight-Laukaran V, Labbok MH, Peterson AE, Fletcher V, von Hertzen H, Van Look PFA. Multicenter study of the Lactational Amenorrhea Method (LAM): II. Acceptability, utility, and policy implications. Contraception. 1997;55:337–46.

40. Valdés V, Pérez A, Labbok M, Pugin E, Zambrano I, Catalan S. The impact of a hospital and clinic-based breastfeeding promotion programme in a middle class urban environment. J Trop Pediatr. 1993;39:142–51.

41. Kennedy KI, Labbok MH, Van Look PFA. Consensus statement—Lactational Amenorrhea Method for family planning. Int J Gynaecol Obstet. 1996;54:55–7.

42. Van Look PFA. Lactational Amenorrhoea Method for family planning. BMJ. 996;313:893–4.

43. Ford K, Labbok M. Contraceptive usage during lactation in the United States: an update. Am J Public Health. 1987;77:79–81.
44. Visness CM, Kennedy KI. The frequency of coitus during breastfeeding. Birth. 1997;24:253–7.
45. Speroff L and Mishell DR: The postpartum visit: it's time for a change in order to optimally initiate contraception. Contraception 2008; 78:90–98.
46. International Planned Parenthood Federation (IPPF). IMAP Statement on postpartum contraception and breast feeding. IPPF Med Bull. 2008;42:1–5.
47. World Health Organization. Medical eligibility criteria for contraceptive use, 4th ed. Geneva (Switzerland): World Health Organization; 2009, Department of Reproductive Health [cited 2010 July 18]. Available from: http://www.who.int/reproductive-health/publications/family_planning/9789241563888/en/index.html .
48. World Health Organization. Selected practice recommendations for contraceptive use. 2nd ed. Geneva (Switzerland): World Health Organization; Reproductive Health and Research Division; 2004 [updated 2008;cited 2010 Jun 7]. Available from: http://www.who.int/reproductivehealth/publications/family_planning/9241562846index/en/.
49. Guillebaud J. Postpartum contraception unnecessary before three weeks. BMJ. 1993;307:1560–1.
50. Speroff L, Darney PD. A clinical guide for contraception. 2nd ed. Baltimore (MD): Williams and Wilkins; 1996.
51. Lopez LM, Hiller JE, Grimes DA. Education for contraceptive use by women after childbirth. Cochrane Database of Systematic Reviews 2010, Issue 1. Art. No.: CD001863. DOI: 10.1002/14651858.CD001863.pub2.
52. Fagan EB, Rodman E, Sorensen EA, Landis S, and Colvin GF: A survey of mothers' comfort discussing contraception with infant providers at well-child visits. South Med J. 2009;102:260–4.
53. Faich G, Pearson K, Fleming D, Sobel S, Anello C. Toxic shock syndrome and the vaginal contraceptive sponge. JAMA. 1986;255:216–8.
54. Centers for Disease Control and Prevention. U S. Medical Eligibility Criteria for Contraceptive Use, 2010. MMWR 2010;59:1–85.
55. O'Hanley K, Huber DH. Postpartum IUDs: keys for success. Contraception. 1992;45:351–61.
56. Treiman K, Liskin L, Kols A, Rinehart W. IUDs—An Update. Popul Rep. 1995 [cited 2010 Jun 7];B(6). Available from: http://info.k4health.org/pr/b6/b6.pdf
57. Welkovic S, Costa LOBF, Faúndes A, Ximenes RA, Costa CFF. Postpartum bleeding and infection after post-placental IUD insertion. Contraception. 2009;80:327–36.
58. Kapp N and Curtis K: Intrauterine device insertion during the postpartum period: a systematic review. Contraception. 2009;80:327–336.
59. Letti Müller AL, Lopes Ramos JG, Martins-Costa SH, Palma Dias RS, Valério EG, Hammes LS, Glitz CL, Zucatto AE, Vettori DV, Magalhães JA. Transvaginal ultrasonographic assessment of the expulsion rate of intrauterine devices inserted in the immediate postpartum period: a pilot study. Contraception. 2005;72:192–5.
60. Peterson HB: Sterilization. Obstet Gynecol. 2008;111:189–203.
61. Association for Voluntary Surgical Contraception. Safe and voluntary surgical contraception. New York: AVSC International; 1995.
62. American College of Obstetricians and Gynecologists. Benefits and Risks of sterilization. Obstet Gynecol. 2003;102:647–58.
63. Wilcox LS, Chu SY, Eaker ED, Zeger SL, Peterson HB. Risk factors for regret after tubal sterilization: 5 years of follow-up in a prospective study. Fertil Steril. 1991;55:927–33.
64. Chi IC, Thapa S. Postpartum tubal sterilization: an international perspective on some programmatic issues. J Biosoc Sci. 1993;25:51–61.

65. Heit JA, Kobbervig CE, James AH, Petterson TM, Bailey KR and MeltonLJ: Trends in the incidence of venous thromboembolism during pregnancy or postpartum: a 30-year population-based study.Ann Intern Med. 2005;143:697–706.
66. American College of Obstetricians and Gynecologists. Use of hormonal contraception in women with coexisting medical conditions. Obstet Gynecol. 2006:107:1453–72.
67. Sidney S, Petitti DB, Soff GA, Cundiff DL,Tolan KK and Qusenberry CP: Venous thromboembolic disease in users of low-estrogen combined estrogen-progestin oral contraceptives. Contraception. 2004;70:3–10.
68. Labbok MH. Contraception during lactation: considerations in advising the individual and in formulating programme guidelines. J Biosoc Sci. 1985;9 Suppl:S55–66.
69. American Academy of Pediatrics Committee on Drugs. The transfer of drugs and other chemicals into human milk. Pediatrics. 1994;93:137–50.
70. Burkman RT. Puerperium and breast-feeding. Curr Opin Obstet Gynecol. 1993;5:683–7.
71. Wenof M, Aubert JM, Reyniak JV. Serum prolactin levels in short-term and long-term use of inert plastic and copper intrauterine devices. Contraception. 1979;19:21–7.
72. Chi I, Potts M, Wilkens LR, Champion CB. Performance of the copper T-380A intrauterine device in breastfeeding women. Contraception. 1989;39:603–18.
73. Farr G, Rivera R. Interactions between intrauterine contraceptive device use and breast-feeding status at time of intrauterine contraceptive device insertion: analysis of TCu-380A acceptors in developing countries. Am J Obstet Gynecol. 1992;167:144–51.
74. Andersson K, Ryde-Blomquist E, Lindell K, Odlind V, Milson I. Perforations with intrauterine devices: report from a Swedish survey. Contraception. 1998;57:251–5.
75. Chvapil M, Eskelson CD, Stiffel V, Owen JA, Droegemueller W. Studies on nonoxynol-9. II. Intravaginal absorption, distribution, metabolism and excretion in rats and rabbits. Contraception. 1980;22:325–39.
76. Howie PW. Natural regulation of fertility. Br Med Bull. 1993;49:182–99.
77. Parenteau-Carreau S, Cooney KA. Breastfeeding, Lactational Amenorrhea Method, and natural family planning interface: teaching guide. Washington (DC): Institute for Reproductive Health, Georgetown University; 1994.
78. Labbok MH, Stallings RY, Shah F, Pérez A, Klaus H, Jacobson M, Muruthi T. Ovulation method use during breastfeeding: is there increased risk of unplanned pregnancy? Am J Obstet Gynecol. 1991;165:2031–6.
79. Kennedy KI, Gross BA, Parenteau-Carreau S, Flynn AM, Brown JB, Visness CM. Breastfeeding and the symptothermal method. Stud Fam Plann. 1995;26:107–15.
80. Arevalo M, Jennings V and Sinai I. Application of simple fertility awareness–based methods of family planning to breastfeeding women. Fertil Steril. 2003;80:1241–8.
81. Kennedy KI, Parenteau-Carreau S, Flynn A, Gross B, Brown JB, Visness C. The natural family planning - Lactational Amenorrhea Method interface: observations from a prospective study of breastfeeding users of natural family planning. Am J Obstet Gynecol. 1991;165:2020–6.
82. Johansson E, Odlind V. The passage of exogenous hormones into breast milk—possible effects. Int J Gynaecol Obstet. 1987;25 Suppl:S111–4.
83. International Planned Parenthood Federation. IMAP statement on hormonal methods of contraception. IPPF Med Bull. 2002;36:1–8.
84. Academy for Breastfeeding Medicine. Clinical Protocol #13 Contraception during breastfeeding. Breastfeeding Medicine. 2006;1:43–51.
85. World Health Organization. Technical consultation on hormonal contraceptive use during lactation and effects on the newborn Summary report. WHO/RHR/10.05 Geneva (Switzerland): World Health Organization; Reproductive Health and Research Division; 2010 [cited 2010 July 18]. Available from: http://whqlibdoc.who.int/hq/2010/WHO_RHR_10.05_eng.pdf.

86. Harlap S. Exposure to contraceptive hormones through breast milk—are there long-term health and behavioral consequences? Int J Gynaecol Obstet. 1987;(25 Suppl):S47–55.
87. Faculty of Sexual and Reproductive Healthcare:UK medical eligibility criteria for contraceptive use (2009). Faculty of Sexual and Reproductive Healthcare Aberdene, United Kingdom. [cited 2010 July 18]. Available from: http://www.fsrh.org/admin/uploads/UKMEC2009.pdf.
88. Kapp N, Curtis K and Nanda K: Progestogen-only contraceptive use among breast-feeding women: a systematic review. Contraception. 2010;82:17–37.
89. Jones E and Spencer SA: The physiology of lactation. Pediatrics and Child Health. 2007;17:244–8.
90. Kennedy KI, Short RV, Tully MR. Premature introduction of progestin-only contraceptive methods during lactation. Contraception. 1997;55:347–50.
91. McCann MF, Moggia AV, Higgins JE, Potts M, Becker C. The effects of a progestin-only oral contraceptive (Levonorgestrel 0.03 mg) on breast-feeding. Contraception. 1989;40:635–48.
92. Moggia AV, Harris GS, Dunson TR, Diaz R, Moggia MS, Ferrer MA, McMullen SL. A comparative study of a progestin-only oral contraceptive versus non-hormonal methods in lactating women in Buenos Aires, Argentina. Contraception. 1991;44: 31–43.
93. Halderman LD and Nelson AL. Impact of early postpartum administration of progestin-only hormonal contraceptives compared with nonhormonal contraceptives on short-term breast-feeding patterns. Am J Obstet Gynecol. 2002;186:1250–8.
94. Danli S, Qingxiang S, Guowei S. A multicentered clinical trial of the long-acting injectable contraceptive Depo Provera in Chinese women. Contraception. 2000;62:15–8.
95. Hubacher D, Goco N, Gonzalez B, Taylor D. Factors affecting continuation rates of DMPA. Contraception. 1999;60:345–51.
96. Nath A and Sitruk-Ware R: Progesterone vaginal ring for contraceptive use during lactation. Contraception. 2010;82:428–34.
97. Díaz S, Zepeda A, Maturana X, Reyes MV, Miranda P, Casado ME, Peralta O, Croxatto HB. Fertility regulation in nursing women. IX. Contraceptive performance, duration of lactation, infant growth, and bleeding patterns during use of progesterone vaginal rings, progestin-only pills, Norplant® implants, and Copper T 380-A intrauterine devices. Contraception. 1997;56:223–32.
98. Chen BA, Creinin M, Reeves MS and Schwarz EB: Breastfeeding continuation among women using the levonorgestrel-releasing intrauterine device after vaginal delivery. Contraception. 2009;80:204–5.
99. Hani A, Moss M, Cooper D, Morroni C, Hoffman M. Informed choice–the timing of postpartum contraceptive initiation. S Afr Med J. 2003;93:862–4.
100. Kapp N and Curtis K: Combined oral contraceptive use among breastfeeding women: a systematic review. Contraception. 2010;82:10–16.
101. Visness CM, Rivera R. Progestin-only pill use and pill switching during breast-feeding. Contraception. 1995;51:279–81.
102. Toddywalla VS, Mehta S, Virkar KD, Saxena BN. Release of 19-nor-testosterone type of contraceptive steroids through different drug delivery systems into serum and breast milk of lactating women. Contraception. 1980;21:217–23.
103. Curtis EM. Oral-contraceptive feminization of a normal male infant. Obstet Gynecol. 1964;23:295–96.
104. Virutamasen P, Leepipatpaiboon S, Kriengsinyot R, Vichaidith P, Muia PN, Sekadde-Kigondu CB, Mati JKG, Forest MG, Dikkeschei LD, Wolthers BG, d'Arcangues C. Pharmacodynamic effects of depot-medroxyprogesterone acetate (DMPA) administered to lactating women on their male infants. Contraception. 1996;54:153–7.
105. Faculty of Family Planning and Reproductive Health Care Clinical Effectiveness Unit. Contraceptive choices for breastfeeding women. J Fam Plann Reprod Health Care. 2004;30:181–9.

106. Gainer E, Massai R, Lillo S, Reyes V, Forcelledo ML, Caviedes R et al: Levonorgestrel pharmacokinetics in plasma and milk of lactating women who take 1.5 mg for emergency contraception. Human Reproduction. 2007;22(6):1578–1584.
107. Heinig MJ, Dewey KG. Health Advantages of breastfeeding for infants: a critical review. Nutrition Research Reviews. 1996;9:89–110.
108. Riordan J and Wambach K (eds): Breastfeeding and Human Lactation (4th ed). Sudbury, MA: Jones and Bartlett, 2010.
109. Ip S, Chung M, Raman G, Chew P, Magula N, DeVine D, et al. Breastfeeding and Maternal and Infant Health Outcomes in Developed Countries. Evidence Report/Technology Assessment No. 153 (Prepared by Tufts-New England Medical Center Evidence-based Practice Center, under Contract No. 290–02–0022). AHRQ Publication No. 07-E007. Rockville, MD: Agency for Healthcare Research and Quality. April 2007. [cited 2010 July 18]. Available from: http://www.ahrq.gov/downloads/pub/evidence/pdf/brfout/brfout.pdf.
110. World Health Organization. Horta BL, Bahl R, Martines JC, Victora CG. Evidence on the long-term effects of breastfeeding. Systematic reviews and meta-analyses. 2007 WHO Press, World Health Organization, Geneva, Switzerland, [cited 2010 July 18]. Available from: http://whqlibdoc.who.int/publications/2007/9789241595230_eng.pdf.
111. American Academy of Pediatrics. The transfer of drugs and other chemicals into human milk. Pediatrics. 2001;108:776–89.
112. Lawrence RA. A review of the medical benefits and contraindications to breastfeeding in the United States. (Maternal and Child Health Technical Information Bulletin). Arlington (VA): National Center for Education in Maternal and Child Health; 1997. [cited 2010 Jun 7] Available from: http://www.mchlibrary.info/pubs/PDFs/BreastfeedingTIB.pdf
113. American Academy of Pediatrics. Human milk, breastfeeding and the transmission of Human Immunodeficiency Virus in the United States. Pediatrics. 1995;96:977–9.
114. World Health Organization: HIV transmission through breastfeeding: a review of available evidence : 2007 update. Geneva (Switzerland): World Health Organization; 2008, [cited 2010 July 18]. Available from: http://whqlibdoc.who.int/publications/2008/9789241596596_eng.pdf.
115. Bélec L, Bouquety JC, Georges AJ, Siopathis MR, Martin PMV. Antibodies to human immunodeficiency virus in the breast milk of healthy seropositive women. Pediatrics. 1990;85:1022–6.
116. Newburg DS, Viscidi RP, Ruff A, Yolken RH. A human milk factor inhibits binding of human immunodeficiency virus to the CD4 receptor. Pediatr Res. 1992;31:22–8.
117. Van de Perre P, Simonon A, Hitimana DG, Dabis F, Msellati P, Mukamabano B, Butera JB, Van Goethem C, Karita E, Lepage P. Infective and anti-infective properties of breastmilk from HIV-1-infected women. Lancet. 1993;341:914–8.
118. World Health Organization: Guidelines on HIV and infant feeding. 2010. Principles and recommendations for infant feeding in the context of HIV and a summary of evidence. Geneva (Switzerland): World Health Organization; 2010, [cited 2010 July 18]. Available from: http://whqlibdoc.who.int/publications/2010/9789241599535_eng.pdf.
119. Centers for Disease Control. Recommendations for assisting in the prevention of perinatal transmission of human T-lymphotropic virus type III/lymphadenopathy-associated virus and acquired immunodeficiency syndrome. Morb Mortal Wkly Rep. 1985;34:721–6, 731–2.
120. Newell M.Current issues in the prevention of mother-to-child transmission of HIV-1 infection. Trans R Soc Trop Med Hyg. 2006;100:1–5.
121. Eaton SB, Pike MC, Short RV, Lee NC, Trussell J, Hatcher RA, Wood JW, Worthman CM, Blurton-Jones NG, Konner MJ, Hill KR, Bailey R, Hurtado AM. Women's reproductive cancers in evolutionary context. Q Rev Biol. 1994;69:353–67.

122. Rosenblatt KA, Thomas DB. Prolonged lactation and endometrial cancer: WHO Collaborative Study of Neoplasia and Steroid Contraceptives. Int J Epidemiol. 1995;24:499–503.
123. Speroff L, Glass RH, Kase NG. Clinical gynecologic endocrinology and infertility. 5th ed. Baltimore (MD): Williams & Wilkins; 1994.
124. Institute of Medicine. Nutrition during lactation. Washington (DC): National Academy Press; 1991.
125. Worthington-Roberts BS, Williams SR. Nutrition in pregnancy and lactation. 5th ed. St. Louis (MO): Mosby-Year Book; 1993:340.

Contraceptive Research and Development

19

Jill Schwartz, MD
Henry L. Gabelnick, PhD

- New discoveries in biotechnology, genetics, immunology, and molecular biology have the potential to accelerate innovation; we urgently need multipurpose technologies that provide both pregnancy and STI, HIV/AIDS prevention.

- Research to develop systemic methods for men is ongoing, but the introduction of new options for men is not likely to occur in the near future.

- Although entirely new and innovative options are not likely to occur in the near future, modifications of existing methods such as a contraceptive ring that will last for a year and a generic levonorgestrel intrauterine contraceptive (IUC) that would last for 7 years may be available in the short term.

- Contraceptive research has the potential to stimulate new thinking about regimens and requirements for service delivery. Methods with simpler rules for use and fewer obstacles to initiating the method could improve a user's ability to use contraceptives more effectively.

- Increased resources are needed for both public and private sectors in the field of contraception.

CONTRACEPTIVE RESEARCH OVERVIEW
WHY IS CONTRACEPTIVE RESEARCH NEEDED?

In addition to the intuitive appeal of assuring the latest, best medications and technologies in all medical fields, the need for improvement in the field of contraception is clear from public health statistics. First, data from the 2006–2008 National Survey of Family Growth (NSFG) indicate that the percentage of all U.S. women ages 15 to 44 who were at risk for unintended pregnancy but using no method increased from 7.5% in 1995 to 10.7% in 2002 and decreased only slightly to 10.6 in 2006–2008.[1] In the developing world, 200 million women seek to delay or avoid having a birth but are not using contraception.[2] The United Nations estimates that by 2050 this so-called unmet need will grow by 40 percent as record numbers of women enter the reproductive years.[3] Second, the impact of the HIV epidemic on reproductive-age women has created an urgent need for methods that provide dual protection—against both unintended pregnancy and sexually transmitted infections (STIs) including HIV/AIDS. Worldwide, this is an imperative problem, but it is also important for many couples in the United States.

Disappointingly, because no improvement in contraceptive effectiveness occurred between 1995 and 2002, the Healthy People 2010 goal of reducing overall probability of contraceptive failure to 7% is likely out of reach, although some encouraging trends in the NSFG show increased uptake of effective methods such as intrauterine contraception.[1,4] Although couples have a range of contraceptive methods available now, almost half of all pregnancies in the United States are unintended.[5] Many unintended pregnancies occur because the couple was not using a method at the time, but some 1.5 million annually in the United States occur among contraceptive users.[6] A small proportion of unintended pregnancies among contraceptive users are attributable to method failure, but most failures instead reflect inconsistent or incorrect use of a method, or interruptions in use. Improved education on correct method use is critically important to successful use, but highly effective, long-acting reversible contraception, often called *forgettable contraception*, can significantly reduce failures due to nonadherence and method discontinuation—behavioral aspects associated with combined oral contraceptives (COCs) and barrier methods.[7]

Contraceptive research in the past focused on finding highly effective methods and on improving method safety. Contraceptive research that aims to improve affordability and access may provide the potential to help reduce unintended pregnancy by reducing obstacles to initiating and continuing a method. In addition to making existing methods accessible, ongoing contraceptive research to improve methods also plays an important role in addressing unmet need and unintended pregnancies. Much effort and research priority have concentrated on the improvement of existing methods so that they have fewer side effects and are easier and more appealing to use. For example, research has sought methods that have non-contraceptive benefits such as clearer skin or increased libido. The developments of new delivery systems, extended dosing and research to reduce typical delays in initiation of contraception have sought to improve adherence and acceptability.

While COCs were revolutionary when introduced in 1960, 2010 marks their 50th anniversary in the United States. Over that half of a century, women's lifestyles have changed and modern contraceptive needs continue to evolve as women enter different reproductive life phases, accentuating the need for a wide variety of methods. Women with serious chronic diseases that make use of hormonal products inadvisable have limited alternative options, as do women who experience unacceptable side effects when using hormonal products. Continued efforts to develop entirely new categories of contraceptives would help both of these groups and might have important advantages for other women as well. Existing methods do not meet the needs of all; we need to revitalize interest in the development of new and innovative contraceptive methods that will meet the needs of today's and tomorrow's couples.

The widening HIV pandemic and the role that STIs play in accelerating HIV spread make it an urgent priority to find methods that can prevent pregnancy *and* reduce infection. Some evidence exists that hormonal contraception alters immune function in the genital tract.[8,9] Depot-medroxyprogesterone acetate (DMPA) was associated with increased acquisition of cervical chlamydial and gonococcal infections in a prospective cohort study.[10] Concern about a possible association between hormonal contraceptive use and increased risk of HIV infection has triggered research into this question.[11] Prospective analyses of hormonal contraceptive use and HIV acquisition found that high-risk groups of women, HSV-2 negative women and women younger than 25 who used DMPA or COCs may be at increased risk of HIV acquisition.[12-13] Further research is needed, but if current hormonal methods do turn out to increase HIV acquisition, then new methods based on other mechanisms of action will be desperately needed for women who are at high individual risk for acquiring HIV.

This chapter provides information practitioners can use in supporting or advocating for adequate research funding, and for educational presentations about the future of contraception. It also describes new methods available elsewhere, which are ready for imminent introduction or reintroduction in the United States, and which may become available in the near future, especially new microbicide and barrier options. The chapter also reviews the status of male methods, although the time horizon for these possibilities may be longer.

A BRIEF HISTORY OF CONTRACEPTIVE RESEARCH

Modern private-sector contraceptive research began in the 1950s and led to the first oral contraceptive pill (Enovid), approved by the Food and Drug Administration (FDA) in 1960, and the marketing of the Lippes Loop and the Saf-T-Coil intrauterine contraceptives (IUCs), in the early 1960s (see Table 19–1). At its peak in the late 1970s, sizable invest-

Table 19–1 Method timeline: date of introduction and/or FDA approval[a]

1839	Condoms mass-produced by Goodyear (vulcanized rubber)
1925	Diaphragms manufactured in United States
1960	Estrogen plus progestin oral contraceptive pill—Enovid
1962	Lippes Loop licensed
1982	Contraceptive sponge (withdrawn in 1994)
1984	Cu T 380A copper-releasing intrauterine device
1988	Prentif cavity-rim cervical cap
1990	Levonorgestrel 6-rod implant device (subsequently withdrawn from sale)—Norplant
1992	3-month progestin injectable—medroxyprogesterone acetate—Depo-Provera
1994	Female condom—Reality (currently named FC1)
1996	Levonorgestrel 2-rod implant device (not marketed)—Jadelle
1998	Estrogen plus progestin emergency contraceptive—dedicated product (Preven)
1999	Progestin emergency contraceptive—(Plan B)
2000	Estradiol cypionate and medroxyprogesterone acetate monthly injectable (subsequently withdrawn from sale)—Lunelle
2000	Mifepristone antiprogestin for early abortion
2000	Levonorgestrel-releasing intrauterine system—Mirena
2001	Etonogestrel/ethinyl estradiol vaginal ring—NuvaRing (approved 2001, marketed in US 2002)
2002	Contraceptive patch—Ortho Evra
2002	Lea's Shield barrier device (not currently available)
2003	FemCap barrier device
2003	Transcervical permanent sterilization device—Essure
2004	Etonogestrel single-rod implant—Implanon
2005	Contraceptive sponge reintroduced—Today
2005	Depo-Subq Provera 104—FDA Approval
2006	Etonogestrel single-rod implant—Implanon
2009	Ulipristal acetate (approved in Europe for EC)—ellaOne
2009	Latex female condom (FDA approved)—FC2
2009	Transcervical permanent sterilization device—Adiana
2010	Ulipristal acetate—ella (FDA approved)

[a] Note: This table does not include the many oral contraceptive pill products introduced following the 1960 approval for Enovid, the first "pill." Pill development has provided major improvements, especially with gradual reduction in the hormone dose for both the estrogen and progestin components, and development and introduction of improved progestins and extended use. Intrauterine devices introduced after the Lippes Loop but no longer available also are not listed.

ments in contraceptive research were being made by at least six large U.S. companies.[14]

Support for basic research prior to 1950, and continuing through the 1980s, was provided principally by three visionary foundations—Rockefeller, Mellon, and Ford—and was critical in establishing the basis for most of the methods available today. Public research funding began when the National Institute of Child Health and Human Development (NICHD) was established at the National Institutes of Health (NIH) in 1963. Soon after, the U.S. Agency for International Development (USAID) allocated additional research funding.

Private-sector involvement after 1970 declined, however, and focused on improvements in hormonal formulations. The level of public and foundation funding for research, after significant growth in the 1960s and early 1970s, also slowed in the 1980s.[15] By 1990, an Institute of Medicine report concluded that declining and sporadic funding from foundations and public sources and the decreased interest of most pharmaceutical companies threatened to reduce the pool of scientific personnel and resources for the field.[14] The committee noted that resource limitations would be likely to delay the application of new biotechnology, genetic engineering, and molecular biology discoveries that otherwise might provide significant advances in contraception.

During the 1980s and 1990s, the increasing complexity of regulatory review for new drugs and devices along with concerns about product liability and public controversy in the field of contraception also had a detrimental effect on the development of new methods, especially in the United States.[16] Damaging litigation following the Dalkon Shield scandal led to withdrawal of other IUCs from the market in the 1970s, and attacks against Norplant beginning in 1994 were followed by a dramatic decline in its sales. Large companies were logically more reluctant to assume the financial risks involved in development of innovative approaches, and smaller companies lacked sufficient resources to do so. Initial development of new approaches, therefore, became increasingly dependent on public sector resources and research organizations.

Development of a new drug or device is a long and costly process (see Table 19–2). Drug discovery and device invention typically involve many discarded possibilities before an option promising enough to warrant human studies is identified. Human studies require IND (Investigational New Drug) or IDE (Investigational Device Exemption) approval by the FDA, and applications must include a review of laboratory and toxicology testing in animals. For drugs, human studies are conducted in phases to assess safety (Phase I), effectiveness (Phase II), and extended safety and effectiveness in clinical use (Phase III). Research data from these studies provide the basis for a New Drug Application (NDA) to the FDA. If the product is approved, the data are the basis for product labeling, including dosing, instructions, and indications. When the NDA is approved, the company is entitled to sell and market the drug for the approved indications. FDA processes for reviewing applications for device approval (called PMA—Premarket Approval applications) are similar, although somewhat more complex.[14]

Reviewing available information in 2004, the Institute of Medicine Committee on New Frontiers in Contraceptive Development concluded that development of a new drug takes 10 to 14 years and involves an investment of $400 million to $800 million.[17] The investment in contraceptive research and development from all sectors is insufficient to develop more than just a handful of new possibilities. Although private sector companies are investing in research on drugs for conditions that primarily affect women, contraception is not a high priority.

However, the tide may be turning in favor of funding for contraceptive research. Federal funding for women's health research saw large increases in their base funding in FY 2009.[18] The Bill and Melinda Gates Institute for Population and Reproductive Health, along with other international and national partners, organized an international conference on family planning research and best practices in Kampala, Uganda, in 2009. Plans were made to invest in the next 5 to 10 years in contraceptive technologies suitable for use in developing country settings. The public and private total, however, is modest in relation to the estimated development cost for even a single new product.

The urgent need for methods that women can use to protect against HIV/AIDS and STIs as well as pregnancy has infused the contraceptive development field with new vitality and some new resources. Although the primary sources of funding for this effort have been public sector and foundation grants, private sector organizations have begun to work in this area. The steady increase in contraceptive use in developing countries—a vast potential market for products estimated to include 2.5 billion women by the year 2025—along with the successful introduction of new products (including the hormone-releasing vaginal ring, the patch, the levonorgestrel intrauterine system, and dedicated extended-use oral contraceptives) has helped create renewed interest in contraceptive development at major pharmaceutical companies.

WHAT IS NEEDED?

More public funding. Along with all women's health issues, resources for contraceptive development research continue to lag behind research in other areas. Governments and foundations need to help reverse this trend. Inadequate resources means the opportunity to apply major advances in immunology, genetics, and molecular biology is delayed or lost. These shortcomings are tragic because the human need is

Table 19–2 The drug development process

Preclinical Development	
Concept and synthesis	
Production of sufficient drug quantity for research	
Formulation to provide suitable dose and administration route	
Preclinical Research	
Toxicology, safety and effectiveness (animals)	1–3 years
Investigational New Drug Application (IND) Filed	
Reviewed by FDA	30 days for FDA staff review but questions can prolong
FDA Acceptance permits research use for human subjects	
Clinical Research (human subjects)	
Phase 1 Fewer than 100 subjects to establish safety	6 mo–1 year
Phase 2 100 + human subjects to establish effectiveness	6 mo–2 years
Phase 3 Sufficient subject number (1000 +) to confirm safety, effectiveness and dosage	1–4 years
New Drug Application (NDA) Filed	
Reviewed by FDA	2 mo–7 years for FDA review*
FDA Approval for Marketing	
Postmarketing Surveillance	
Adverse event reporting	
Additional studies as required in FDA Approval Decision	

Source: adapted from Mastroianni, 1990.[7]

* Review and decision by FDA staff, with recommendations to FDA from Advisory Committee.

great. Contraceptive options that could make a dent in the rate of unintended pregnancy would have a huge health impact—certainly comparable to that of a major heart disease or cancer breakthrough. Not everyone will develop these important diseases, but almost everyone does need effective contraception, and unintended pregnancy involves serious health risks for young people that translate to high losses in years of productive life.

Support for increased participation of private-sector companies. Biotechnology companies that work in this field should be applauded, and they will be assisted by efforts to increase public awareness of the importance of this research area and to diminish the controversy about family planning and reproductive health in national public policy. Commitment to providing adequate public funding of family planning services and supplies for low income couples in the United States, and as part of international aid, can also fortify the private sector involvement in the field.

Development of innovative approaches. In addition to methods that protect against both infection and pregnancy, investment is needed to pursue entirely new approaches as well as improvements in existing hormonal methods.

CURRENT CONTRACEPTIVE RESEARCH
CHEMICAL BARRIERS AND MICROBICIDES

Chemical barriers have been used for contraception in conjunction with cervical caps and diaphragms, and also alone as foams, suppositories, tablets, creams, and gels. Although nonoxynol-9 (N-9)-containing vaginal spermicides have been available over-the-counter for more than 50 years, a paucity of information exists regarding the effectiveness of these products. A multi-center trial evaluating the effectiveness of five N-9 products (52.5 mg gel, 100 mg gel, 150 mg gel, 100 mg suppository, and 100 mg film) found that the 6-month failure rates with typical use (14%–22%) were in the range previously accepted for spermicide and barrier method users (except in the lowest dose, the 52.5 mg gel).[19]

The Today contraceptive sponge, previously marketed for more than a decade in the United States but not available since 1994, returned to the U.S. market in 2005 and was re-introduced in 2009 in more than 13,000 drug stores across the United States and online. Other contraceptive sponge options (Protectaid, containing a lower concentration of N-9 along with benzalkonium chloride, and Pharmatex, containing benzalkonium chloride) are available outside the United States, but are not approved by the FDA.

In addition to their spermicidal effect, currently marketed products— N-9 in the United States and similar detergents in other countries—also kill bacteria and viruses when tested in the laboratory. This microbicidal effect led to the initial hope that existing products might also reduce infection risk in actual use. Contrary to the hope, however, research on the effect of N-9 spermicide use by women in a high-risk group found higher HIV incidence with spermicide use than with use of a placebo.[20–22] Vaginal irritation caused by the N-9 may have compromised normal vaginal defenses against infection, leaving women more vulnerable.[23] (See Chapter 14 on Vaginal Barriers and Spermicides.) Other available spermicide detergents also may cause irritation. Because of the potential harm, N-9 use is no longer recommended for women at high risk for HIV/AIDS, and it also should not be used as a lubricant for rectal intercourse. Efforts to find methods to prevent infection have therefore turned to the task of finding entirely new microbicide options.[24]

The challenge in microbicide development is to find an option that is effective in stopping bacterial or viral infection but does not cause irritation. Ideally, a product might even enhance natural infection defenses and protect against irritation. The potential for protecting users against HIV infection or other pathogens is based on the microbicide's ability to kill or inactivate HIV or pathogens. Alternatively, a microbicide could act by interfering with essential steps in the infection process, such as cell attachment or entry, or replication of the pathogen. Demonstrating safety during conception and through pregnancy, however, would be a formidable research challenge. Agents that were once hoped to have dual protection against HIV and pregnancy, such as cellulose sulfate and C31G, have demonstrated no effect against HIV transmission in clinical trials.[25] Second-generation microbicides such as tenofovir, dapivirine, and UC781 are antiretrovirals being developed as gel formulations and intravaginal rings (IVRs). Efforts are ongoing to develop dual protection systems that combine antiretroviral microbicides with hormonal contraceptives for release from an IVR and offer promise as multipurpose prevention technologies. CONRAD is developing a vaginal ring containing tenofovir with levonorgestrel (LNg) to provide both HIV prevention and contraception in the same product. Combining dapivirine and LNg in a vaginal ring, the International Partnership for Microbicides is collaborating with the Population Council to also develop a multipurpose ring. Research related to microbicide development may also prove to have unanticipated long-term benefits. The microbicide effort has required a major investment in basic research on vaginal physiology and on the pathophysiology of HIV/AIDS and STI transmission. Advances are likely to be helpful in combating common problems such as bacterial vaginosis, and have already produced some important findings. The complex vaginal ecosystem was previously little understood. It is a delicate system that can easily be disrupted by trauma or by chemical alteration. "Mildly" toxic exposures to compounds such as N-9 or a solution that is too acid or too alkaline can disrupt normal vaginal bacteria and impair the normal defenses against infection. Use of "hygiene" products including douching solutions seems to create much more significant problems than previously recognized.

MECHANICAL BARRIER METHODS

Renewed attention has been directed to development of new mechanical barriers in parallel with the emphasis on microbicide development. A mechanical barrier may be helpful for use in conjunction with a new microbicide, and some hope exists that a barrier may itself provide some protection against transmission of infection. Providing a physical shield for the cervix is a plausible strategy since the cervical epithelium is an important infection target: it is the primary site for chlamydial infection and contains a rich supply of immune system cells that are the target for the initial uptake of HIV.[26]

Research is also ongoing to develop new, improved cervical barrier devices that are appropriate for use along with a microbicide. A device under development, the SILCS diaphragm, is an intravaginal single size cervical barrier device that has performed well in postcoital testing and is undergoing a contraceptive effectiveness study in the United States.[27] The BufferGel Duet is a disposable, one-size-fits-all, clear diaphragm made of dipped polyurethane that is being studied prefilled with BufferGel, a candidate contraceptive microbicide. A contraceptive study conducted by the NICHD showed that BufferGel used with an Ortho All-Flex diaphragm worked about as well as N-9 used with a diaphragm but whether or not BufferGel will be marketed as a contraceptive gel is unclear.[28] Evaluating a method that does not require provider fitting is of interest. A method that is available over-the counter would have the potential to be adopted more widely if the combination of a vaginal barrier and microbicide proves to be effective in helping reduce HIV/AIDS and STI transmission.

New female condom prototypes are under development. The FC2 Female Condom is a second-generation female condom with the same design and instructions for use as the FC Female Condom (formerly Reality). It is made of synthetic latex instead of polyurethane, to improve affordability, and was approved by the FDA in 2009. The Reddy female condom, also known as the VA feminine condom and as V-Amour, is held in place inside the vagina by a soft sponge inside the condom, rather than a ring as used in the FC Female Condom, and has received CE Marking. PATH has a new female condom in development with a dissolving capsule intended to make insertion easier, a polyurethane condom pouch with foam dots to allow gentle cling to the vaginal walls, and a soft outer ring. A clinical trial assessing the contraceptive efficacy of the Woman's Condom is expected to begin in 2010. In addition, panty condoms such as the Silk Parasol Panty Condom and the Natural Sensation Female Panty Condom have been developed but are not available in the United States.

New male condom models have been developed with alternative materials other than latex and with design modifications. Synthetic nonlatex materials can be used by people who have latex allergies, can be used with oil-based lubricants, may transmit heat better than latex, and may have longer shelf-lives. Despite male preference for synthetic nonlatex condoms such as Avanti and eZ-on, nonlatex condoms broke or slipped more often than latex condoms; however, most were as effective as latex condoms in preventing pregnancy.[29] Innovative condom designs that are spiral shaped and loose fitting to increase friction and sexual pleasure have been developed and successfully marketed by large companies.

HORMONAL AND SYSTEMIC METHODS FOR WOMEN

Hormonal methods have been the mainstay of reversible contraception because of their safety and effectiveness. New developments have provided methods with a lower hormone dose, improved progestin options, and a drug delivery mechanism that simplifies use. Several options used in other countries, however, are not available in the United States, including implants and injectables that have already received FDA approval and initial marketing here.

Progestin implants gained a small but appreciative user group because of their extremely high efficacy and simplicity of use. Their average continuation rate is higher than that with other reversible methods.[30] The original 6-rod progestin-releasing implant—Norplant—was approved by the FDA in 1990. Complications of insertion and removal limited its appeal. Sales of the product were stopped in 2000, and the company announced in 2002 that it did not plan to reintroduce the device.

An improved, 2-rod version of this method—Jadelle—is currently marketed in Europe by Schering Oy. Jadelle received FDA approval in 1996 but has not yet been sold in the United States. Sino-Implant (II) is a generic 2-rod-system equivalent to Jadelle. It contains 75 mg of LNg per rod and can be manufactured at lower cost than other contraceptive implants. Sino-Implant has been widely distributed in China and Indonesia and is being introduced in resource-constrained settings.[31] The only implant currently available in the United States is Implanon, which has been marketed in Europe and Australia for several years and received FDA approval in July 2006. A new generation Depo Provera injectable, the lower-dose 3-month Depo-Sub Q Provera 104 is available in the United States and several European countries.[32] An additional innovation now being studied is the provision of Depo Provera in a prefilled single-use syringe, Uniject, that could be self-administered subcutaneously thereby increasing user access. Levonorgestrel Butanoate (LB), a long-acting intramuscular progestin formulation intended to provide highly effective contraception with potentially fewer side effects, was initially tested by the WHO more than two decades ago. Formulation stability problems led to a hiatus in further clinical testing, but a new formulation has been developed with the support of CONRAD and NICHD and is scheduled to begin Phase I testing shortly.

The combination estrogen and progestin injectable, Lunelle, had a history similar to that of Norplant. Although this method is marketed in many other countries, it was available only briefly in the United States, then voluntarily recalled by Pharmacia in 2002. The Concept Foundation is seeking FDA approval of Cyclofem, a monthly injectable contraceptive with the same composition as Lunelle, with the ultimate goal to manufacture and market Cyclofem in India. Approval of Cyclofem by the FDA would also allow reintroduction to the U.S. market.

Nestorone, a nonandrogenic progestin, might provide incidental "side benefits" related to the characteristics of the progestin or a method with fewer undesirable side effects. The Population Council has developed a hormonal contraceptive vaginal ring containing nestorone and ethinyl estradiol (EE) that may be used for one year. This was found to be safe and effective in a Phase 3 clinical trial with the use of the ring for 3 weeks and then removal for one week for 13 cycles.[33] The NDA is currently being prepared for submission to the FDA.

The contraceptive patch provides another way to administer hormonal methods; however, recent studies have shown that women using the norelgestromin/EE patch are exposed to more estrogen and are at a higher risk for venous thromboembolism. Newer patches with lower levels of hormones are in development.

The development of approaches to block hormone receptors might also provide new contraceptive options. The anti-progestin mifepristone has been studied for use as an emergency contraceptive after unprotected intercourse, for low-dose, daily use and for use as a once-a-month regimen. Such regimens can provide contraceptive protection, but they have caused menstrual disruption. Further basic research is ongoing to identify and evaluate other members of the anti-progestin family.[34] One such progesterone receptor modulator candidate with many of the same antagonistic activities as mifepristone is ulipristal acetate, which has been shown to be effective as an emergency contraception for up to 5 days after unprotected sex in Phase III trials and is available in Europe.[35,36] Ulipristal acetate was approved by the FDA in August 2010 and is now sold by prescription under the name ella.

In the future, systemic methods may be developed that do not disrupt normal hormone cycles. For example, a narrowly targeted method with effect only on zona pellucida binding of sperm, or factors essential for ovulation or implantation, might provide effective contraception without the side effects related to hormone disruption. These approaches may lead to the development of methods that could be used monthly. The ability of nonsteroidal anti-inflammatory drugs to interfere with follicular rupture has been known for some time, and, as such, cyclooxygenase-2 (COX-2) inhibitors have great potential as an alternative to hormonal methods to block ovulation and at the same time maintain ovarian cyclicity. Studies in women have shown that oral COX-2 inhibitors administered around the time of the ovulatory LH surge can prevent or delay follicle rupture, as assessed by ultrasound, without alteration of hormone levels or menstrual cycle length.[37] Studies in macaques have shown that oral COX-2 administration resulted in oocytes trapped within luteinized follicles.[38] These data support further investigation of COX-2 inhibitors as possible monthly contraceptives.

In the preclinical discovery phase, when developing a new contraceptive lead, it is necessary to identify a target specific for the reproductive tract that can be inhibited. Initial preclinical research has identified several such targets, and among those, leukemia inhibitory factor (LIF) and pro-protein convertase 6 (PC6) might be feasible targets for inhibition, as they play essential roles in implantation. Development of such options will require more basic research and a better understanding of the molecular biology and biochemistry involved, making it unlikely that these options would be put into clinical use in the near future.

SYSTEMIC METHODS FOR MEN

Although the percentage of the world's couples that rely on male methods (condoms, withdrawal, and vasectomy) has increased, the development of systemic methods for men has been slow. Part of the reason is that the physiology of male fertility is a difficult challenge: sperm are continuously produced, with maturation and development over an interval of weeks. Issues like adverse reactions, side effects, acceptability, and affordability are more powerful constraints now than they were in the 1950s when female systemic methods were devised, because a high standard has been set. Three possible approaches include (1) blocking hormonal support for testicular cell function by stopping pituitary LH and FSH, (2) interfering with seminiferous tubule function to stop sperm production, and (3) disrupting maturation, functioning, and/or transport of sperm after they are produced. Targeting the second or third approach would have significant advantages, but except for gossypol, no method has yet been developed sufficiently for clinical studies.[39] Current research has focused on the first option.

Two proof of concept studies have been conducted using large doses of testosterone enanthate as a male contraceptive; however, the frequent injections were not well accepted.[40,41] Suppression of testicular cells responsible for sperm development has the incidental effect of stopping testosterone production and, along with it, libido and potency. Too much testosterone has unfavorable effects on lipids, acne, weight gain, and possibly mood. Hormonal methods for men, therefore, must provide an ideal amount of testosterone to avoid these effects, but at the same time ensure effective hormonal suppression of sperm production. Regimens most likely to become available first involve an androgen administered along with a progestin sufficient to suppress LH, the normal pituitary stimulus for testicular cell hormone and sperm production.

The combination of the etonorgestrel implant (good for a year) and intramuscular testosterone undeconoate (TU) administered bimonthly was studied as a possible method of male contraception. While this was well tolerated and effective, two methods of delivery were not ideal, and this combination is not being pursued further.[42] Longer-acting preparations such as TU coupled with norethisterone enanthate also permit longer dosing intervals.[43] TU (1000 mg) and NET-EN (200mg) is being administered bi-monthly in an ongoing trial under the auspices of CONRAD and WHO.

Non-hormonal possibilities have been evaluated as systemic contraceptives for men. Large studies with Gossypol, derived from cottonseed oil, have found that it can provide effective sperm suppression without changing testosterone production or libido.[44] Other non-hormonal options being considered for development are anti-cancer drugs such as lonidamine. These agents are known to reduce normal sperm production, and it may be possible to find a compound that has a high effectiveness in reducing sperm but an acceptable toxicity profile in other respects.

Glyceraldehyde-3-phosphate dehydrogenase is a glycolytic enzyme that is encoded by the GAPDHS gene (known as GAPDH-2 in the human) expressed only during spermatogenesis and is tightly bound to the sperm flagellum.[45] Since it is required for sperm motility and male fertility, GAPDH-2 may be a useful target for contraception in men.

INTRAUTERINE CONTRACEPTIVES (IUC)

Currently two IUCs are marketed in the United States: a copper releasing device marketed as ParaGard T380A and a levonorgestrel releasing system marketed under the brand name Mirena. Several improvements for existing intrauterine contraceptives are being investigated with the hope of reducing cost and reducing the discomfort and cramping that some women experience, and of providing an intrauterine option for women whose uterine depths are too small to accommodate the currently available devices.

A lower-dose Mirena with LNg delivery of 12 mcg and 16 mcg is in clinical trials. The LNg20, manufactured by Leiras Pharmaceuticals in Finland, is currently being studied in the United States by Medicines360 with the hopes of extending the use from 5 to 7 years and to gain FDA approval of a lower cost option. Other IUCs available outside the United States include both the frameless GyneFix and the frameless FibroPlant LNg IUC, which both possess unique features but require the technical skill of correct anchoring of the devices. GyneFix carries copper tubes on a suture embedded in the endometrium and provides efficacy similar to that provided by the copper T.[46–48] The FibroPlant-LNg is also anchored in the myometrium but instead of using copper tubes, releases LNg from a fibrous delivery system and has recently been shown to decrease menstrual blood loss in women with menorrhagia.[49,50] A T-shaped LNg-releasing IUC, called Femilis, with a small version for nulliparous women, called Femilis Slim, is in development. These aim to simplify insertion procedures with a push-in technique that does not require highly skilled providers. Innovative copper-containing IUCs that release an NSAID are being developed in China.

METHODS FOR STERILIZATION

In the United States and worldwide, sterilization surgery is one of the most widely used of all contraceptive options. Research to improve sterilization approaches therefore aims to increase both safety and effectiveness of the procedures, as well as lower the cost and simplify the technologies to avoid the need for surgical facilities and general anesthesia.

Minimally invasive transcervical sterilization methods for women are currently available, and others are being studied. The transcervical sterilization device Essure was approved by the FDA in 2002, and Adiana was approved by the FDA in 2009. Ovabloc is an outpatient alternative to laparoscopic sterilization, available in the Netherlands, whereby liquid silicone elastomer is inserted into both uterine tubes, with the aid of hysteroscopy vision, and sets to form plugs in the tubal openings.[51]

Low-technology methods of female transcervical nonsurgical sterilization that will not require hysteroscopy have been studied since the 1960s by a wide variety of researchers and organizations. The goal is to develop a product that employs a simple method to deliver an active chemical or device to produce permanent tubal occlusion leading to female infertility.

Of the possible chemical agents evaluated in animal and clinical trials, quinacrine has been the most widely studied for female nonsurgical sterilization. The use of quinacrine for nonsurgical sterilization has been halted in several countries due to safety, efficacy, and ethical concerns. A study of a cancer cluster among women in Chile concluded that the cluster was unrelated to quinacrine, but a single suspicious uterine cancer remained as a provocative finding.[52] In a 10-year follow up of patients sterilized with quinacrine, risks to health were felt to be minimal but effectiveness was less than for other forms of sterilization.[53,54] A further follow-up of Chilean women concluded that rates of cancer among quinacrine-treated women are similar to population-based rates.[55] Nevertheless, findings from small animal toxicology studies still pose concerns.[56] A Phase I safety study of quinacrine was conducted in the United States with the FDA concurrence.[57]

In 1999, erythromycin was offered as an alternative agent with the potential to cause sufficient sclerosis in animals to occlude the fallopian tubes.[58] As animal studies continued, a Phase I study of crushed erythromycin tablets concluded that the failure rate of intrauterine insertion of erythromycin was unacceptably high.[59] More carefully designed studies using an improved erythromycin delivery method and formulation may be warranted.

Both conventional and no-scalpel vasectomies are safe and effective procedures performed almost exclusively under local anesthesia. Investigators have explored alternatives to surgical sterilization for men, including chemical injections and formed in-place plugs, but questions over the safety of these chemicals and material have slowed down this research.[60] One intra-vas device known as the "SHUG" has been in development for many years and is now known as the Intra Vas Device (IVD).[61] The IVD consists of two hollow silicone plugs joined by a thread. The plugs are placed in the vas and the thread left outside the vas to facilitate removal. While this is a promising approach, research on this method has lost momentum. Another potential approach, Reversible Inhibition of Sperm under Guidance (RISUG), consists of styrene maleic anhydride (SMA) powder dissolved in dimethyl sulfoxide (DMSO), which is injected into the vas to partially block it. Not only does the SMA block the vas, but it also actively kills sperm.[62] A Phase III trial in India sponsored by the Indian Council of Medical Research is ongoing.

IMPROVING USE-EFFECTIVENESS

Since hormonal methods are effective and widely used, recent research has focused on new delivery systems and extended dosing to increase choice and to make methods easier for women to use correctly and consistently. With the knowledge that poor communication between healthcare providers and consumers, including inadequate education regarding emergency contraception, may contribute to the occurrence of unintended pregnancies,[63–64] research into better communication strategies is warranted. Such research suggests that the presentation of pregnancy risk categories rather than standard numeric risk for available methods best conveys pregnancy risks.[65] In addition, active interventions, such as electronic mail reminders, may improve oral contraceptive compliance.[66] Continued research into simple ways of improving regimens, such as the development of novel initiation methods,[67] remove obstacles to use and may improve successful use.

THE 21ST CENTURY

Compared with the extraordinary advances in pharmaceuticals in other fields, progress in development of contraceptives has been modest. With the 50th anniversary of COCs in the United States, most of the options now in wide use are variations of half-century-old hormonal suppression technology. Major innovations in contraception technologies will only occur if a sustained commitment from both public and private funders is assured. This is a time for renewed effort and fortified resources to develop new methods not only for couples in developed countries, but also for those in less affluent nations whose lives would be so greatly improved.

REFERENCES

1. Mosher WD, Jones J. Use of contraception in the United States: 1982–2002. Vital and Health Statistics. 2010; Series 23, Number 29;1–44.
2. Singh S, Darroch JE, Vlassof M, Nadeau J. Adding it up: the benefits of investing in sexual and reproductive health care. New York: Alan Guttmacher Institue; 2003. Available online at www.guttmacher.org/pubs/addingitup.pdf
3. UNAIDS, AIDS Epidemic Update. December 2005.
4. Kost K, Vaughan SB, Trussell J, Bankole A. Estimates of contraceptive failure from the 2002 National Survey of Family Growth. Contraception. 2008;77:10–21
5. Finer LB, Henshaw SK. Disparities in rates of unintended pregnancy in the United States, 1994 and 2001. Perspect Sex Reprod Health. 2006;38:90–6.
6. Frost JJ, Darroch JF. Factors associated with contraceptive choice and inconsistent method use, United States, 2004. Perspectives on Sexual and Reproductive Health. 2008;40:94–104.
7. Grimes DA. Forgettable contraception. Contraception. 2009;80:497–9.
8. Mostad SB, Overbaugh J, DeVange DM, et al. Hormonal contraception, vitamin A deficiency, and other risk factors for shedding of HIV-1 infected cells from the cervix and vagina. Lancet. 1997;350:922–927.
9. Prakash M, Patterson S and Kapembwa MS. Hormonal upregulation of CCR5 expression on T lymphocytes as a possible mechanism for increased HIV-1 risk J Acquir Immune Defic Syndr. 2005;38 (Suppl 1):S14–6.
10. Morrison CS, Bright P, Wong EL, Kwok C, Yacobson I, Gaydos CA, Tucker HT, Blumenthal PD. Hormonal contraceptive use, cervical ectopy, and the acquisition of cervical infections. Sex Transm Dis. 2004;31:561–7
11. Morrison CS, Richardson BA, Celentano DD, Chipato T, Mmiro F, Mugerwa R, Padian NS, Rugpao S, Salata RA. Prospective clinical trials designed to assess the use of hormonal contraceptives and risk of HIV acquisition. J Acquir Immune Defic Syndr. 2005;38 (Suppl 1):S17–8.
12. Morrison CS, Richardson BA, Mmiro F, Chipato T, Celentano DD, Luoto J, Mugerwa R, Padian NS, Rugpao S, Van Der Pol B, Brown JM, Cornelisse, P, Salata RA. Hormonal contraception and the risk of HIV acquisition. AIDS. 2007; 21;85–95.
13. Morrison CS, Chen PL, Kwok C, Richardson BA, Chipato T, Mugerwa R, Byamugisha J, Padian N, Celentano DD, Salata RA. Hormonal contraception and HIV acquisition: reanalysis using marginal structural modeling. AIDS. 2010;24:1778–81.
14. Mastroianni LJ, Donaldson PJ, Kane FJ, Jr., editors. Developing new contraceptives: obstacles and opportunities. Washington, D.C.: National Academy Press;1990.
15. Harrison PF, Rosenfield A, editors. Contraceptive research and development: looking to the future. Washington, D.C.: National Academy Press;1996.
16. Harrison PF, Rosenfield A. Research, introduction, and use: advancing from Norplant. Contraception. 1998;58:323–334.
17. Nass SJ, Strauss JF III, Editors. New Frontiers in contraceptive research: a blueprint for action. Washington, D.C.: National Academics Press, 2004.
18. Society for Women's Health Research. Issue: Federal Funding for Women's Health Research. www.womenshealthresearch.org http://www.womenshealthresearch.org/site/PageServer?pagename=policy_issues_funding

19. Raymond EG, Chen PL, Luoto J. Contraceptive effectiveness and safety of five nonoxynol-9 spermicides: a randomized trial. Obstet Gynecol. 2004;103: 430–439.
20. Roddy RE, Zekeng L, Ryan KA, Tamoufe U, Weir SS, Wong EL. A controlled trial of nonoxynol-9 film to reduce male-to-female transmission of sexually transmitted diseases. N Engl J Med. 1998;339:504–510.
21. Roddy RE, Zekeng L, Ryan KA, Tamoufe U, Tweedy KG. Effect of nonoxynol-9 gel on urogenital gonorrhea and chlamydial infection: a randomized controlled trial. JAMA. 2002;287:1117–1122.
22. Van Damme L, Ramjee G, Alary M, et al. Effectiveness of COL-1492, a nonoxynol-9 vaginal gel, on HIV-1 transmission in female sex workers: a randomised controlled trial. Lancet. 2002;360:971–977.
23. Roddy RE, Cordero M, Cordero C, Fortney JA. A dosing study of nonoxynol-9 and genital irritation. Int J STD AIDS. 1993;4:165–170.
24. Richardson BA. Nonoxynol-9 as a vaginal microbicide for prevention of sexually transmitted infections: it's time to move on. JAMA. 2002;287:1171–1172.
25. van de Wijgert J, Shattock RJ. Vaginal microbicides: moving ahead after an unexpected setback. AIDS. 2007;21:2369–2376
26. Moench TR, Chipato T, Padian NS. Preventing disease by protecting the cervix: the unexplored promise of internal vaginal barrier devices. AIDS. 2001;15:1595–1602.
27. Schwartz JL, Ballagh S, Creinin M, Rountree R, Kilbourne-Brook M, Mauck CK, Callahan M. SILCS diaphragm: postcoital testing of a new single size contraceptive device. Contraception. 2008;78:237–244
28. Barnhart KT, Rosenberg MJ, MacKay HT, Blithe DL, Higgins J, Walsh T, Wan L, Thomas M, Creinin MD, Westhoff C, Schlaff W, Archer DF, Ayers C, Kaunitz A, Das S, Moench TR. Contraceptive efficacy of a novel spermicidal microbicide used with a diaphragm: a randomized controlled trial. Obstet Gynecol. 2007;110:577–86.
29. Gallo, MF, Grimes, DA, Schulz, KF. Non-latex versus latex male condoms for contraception. Cochrane Database of Systematic Reviews 2003;CD003550. Review
30. Meirik O. Implantable contraceptives for women. Contraception. 2002;65:1–2.
31. Steiner MJ, Luo D, Cancel AM, Jenkins K, Asante D, Vahdat H, Meng H. Increasing Access by Introducing a Low-Cost Contraceptive Implant in Resource Constrained Countries. International Conference on Family Planning: Research and Best Practices E04:3 Kampala, Uganda; 2009.
32. Kaunitz AM et al. Subcutaneous DMPA vs. intramuscular DMPA: a 2-year randomized study of contraceptive efficacy and bone mineral density. Contraception. 2009; 80:7–17.
33. Merkatz R, Sitruk-Ware R, Sivin I.Mensch B, Hewett P, Coone M, Hoskin E. Development and acceptability of the NES/EE CVR: A Year-Long, User Controlled Contraceptive Method. International Conference on Family Planning: Research and Best Practices E01:Kampala, Uganda; 2009.
34. Van Look PF, von Hertzen H. Clinical uses of antiprogestogens. Hum Reprod Update. 1995;1:19–34.
35. Creinin MD, Schlaff W, Archer DF, Wan L, Frezieres R, Thomas M, Rosenberg M, Higgins J. Progesterone receptor modulator for emergency contraception: a randomized controlled trial. Obstet Gynecol. 2006;108:1089–1097.
36. Glasier AF, Cameron ST, Fine PM, Logan SJS, Casale W, Van Horn J, Sogor L, Blithe DL, Scherrer B, Mathe H, Jaspart A, Ulmann A, Gainer E. Ulipristal acetate versus levonorgestrel for emergency contraception: a randomised non-inferiority trial and meta-analysis Lancet. 2010;375:555–62.
37. Jesam C, Salvatierra AM, Schwartz JL, Croxatto HB. Suppression of follicular rupture with meloxicam, a cyclooxygenase-2 inhibitor: potential for emergency contraception. Hum Reprod. 2010; 25:368–373.
38. Hester KE, Harper MJ, Duffy DM. Oral administration of the cyclooxygenase-2 (COX-2) inhibitor meloxicam blocks ovulation in nonhuman primates when administered to simulate emergency contraception. Hum Reprod. 2010;25:360–7.

39. Brady BM, Anderson RA. Advances in male contraception. Expert Opin Investig Drugs. 2002;11:333–344.
40. World Health Organization Task Force on Methods for the Regulation of Male Fertility. Contraceptive efficacy of testosterone-induced azoospermia in normal men. Lancet. 1990;336:955–959.
41. World Health Organization Task Force on Methods for the Regulation of Male Fertility. Contraceptive efficacy of testosterone-induced azoospermia and oligospermia in normal men. Fertil Steril. 1996;65:821–829.
42. Mommers E, Kersemaekers WM, Elliesen J, Kepers M, Apter D, Behre HM, Beynon J, Bouloux PM, Constantino A, Gerbershagen HP, Grønlund L, Heger-Mahn D, Huhtaniemi I, Koldewijn EL, Lange C, Lindenberg S, Meriggiola MC, Meuleman E, Mulders PF, Nieschlag E, Perheentupa A, Solomon A, Väisälä L, Wu FC, Zitzmann M. Male hormonal contraception: a double-blind, placebo-controlled study. J Clin Endocrinol Metab. 2008;93:2572–2580.
43. Meriggiola MC, Constantino A, Saad F, D'Emidio L, Morselli Labate AM, Bertaccini A, Bremner WJ, Rudolph I, Ernst M, Kirsch B, Martorana G, Pelusi G. Norethisterone enanthate plus testosterone undecanoate for male contraception: effects of various injection intervals on spermatogenesis, reproductive hormones, testis, and prostate. J Clin Endocrinol Metab. 1990;90:2005–14.
44. Coutinho EM. Gossypol: a contraceptive for men. Contraception. 2002;65: 259–263.
45. Welch JE, Brown PL, O'Brien DA, Magyar PL, Bunch DO, Mori C, Eddy EM. Human glyceraldehyde 3-phosphate dehydrogenase-2 gene is expressed specifically in spermatogenic cells. J Androl. 2000;21 (2): 328–38.
46. Wu S, Hu J, Wildemeersch D. Performance of the frameless GyneFix and the TCu380A IUDs in a 3-year multicenter, randomized, comparative trial in parous women. Contraception. 2000;61:91–98.
47. Wildemeersch D, Cao X, Zhang W, et al. Efficacy of a mini version of the frameless GyneFix intrauterine system (IUS) with effective copper surface area of 200 mm2. Contraception. 2002;66:237–241.
48. Wildemeersch D, Batar I, Affandi B, et al. The 'frameless' intrauterine system for long-term, reversible contraception: a review of 15 years of clinical experience. J Obstet Gynaecol Res. 2003;29:164–173.
49. Wildemeersch D, Schacht E, Wildemeersch P. Contraception and treatment in the perimenopause with a novel "frameless" intrauterine levonorgestrel-releasing drug delivery system: an extended pilot study. Contraception. 2002;66:93–99.
50. Andrade A, Wildemeersch D. Menstrual blood loss in women using the frameless FibroPlant LNG-IUS. Contraception. 2009;79:134–8.
51. Ligt-Veneman NG, Tinga DJ, Kragt H, Brandsma G, van der Leij G The efficacy of intratubal silicone in the Ovabloc hysteroscopic method of sterilization. Acta Obstet Gynecol Scand. 1999;78:824–825
52. Sokal, D. C., A. Dabancens, R. Guzman-Serani, and J. Zipper.. 2000. Cancer risk among women sterilized with transcervical quinacrine in Chile: an update through 1996. Fertil Steril 74:169–71.
53. Sokal DC, Hieu do T, Loan ND, Hubacher D, Nanda K, Weiner DH, Vach TH. Safety of quinacrine contraceptive pellets: results from 10-year follow-up in Vietnam. Contraception. 2008;78:66–72.
54. Sokal DC, Hieu do T, Loan ND, Hubacher D, Nanda K, Weiner DH, Vach TH. Contraceptive effectiveness of two insertions of quinacrine: results from 10-year follow-up in Vietnam. Contraception. 2008; 78:61–65.
55. Sokal DC, Trujillo V, Guzmán SC, Guzman-Serani R, Wheeless A, Hubacher D. Cancer risk after sterilization with transcervical quinacrine: updated findings from a Chilean cohort. Contraception. 2010; 81:75–78.
56. Cancel AM, Smith T, Rehkemper U, Dillberger J, Sokal D and McClain RM. A one-year neonatal mouse carcinogenesis study of quinacrine dihydrochloride. Int J Toxicol. 2006;25:109–18.

57. Lippes J, Brar M, Gerbracht K, Neff P, Kokkinakis S. An FDA phase I clinical trial of quinacrine sterilization (QS). Int J Gynaecol Obstet. 2003;83 Suppl 2:S45–9.
58. Fail PA, Martin P, Sokal D. Comparative effects of quinacrine and erythomycin in adult female rats: a nonsurgical sterilization study. Fertil Steril. 2000;73:387–94.
59. Bairagy NR and Mullick BC. Use of erythromycin for nonsurgical female sterilization in West Bengal, India: a study of 790 cases. Contraception. 2004;69:47–9.
60. Engender Health, Contraceptive Sterilization: Global Issues and Trends, 2002.
61. Zaneveld LJD, De Castro MP, Faria G, et al. The soft hollow plug ("SHUG"): a potentially reversible vas deferens blocking device. In Griffin PD, Rajalakshmi M (eds) Male Contraception: Present and Future. New Delhi: New Age International, pp.293
62. Guha SK, Singh G, Ansari S, Kumar S, Srivastava A, Koul V, Das HC, Malhotra RL, Das SK Phase II clinical trial of a vas deferens injectable contraceptive for the male. Contraception. 1997; 56:245–250.
63. Jones R, Darroch JE, Henshaw SK. Contraceptive use among U.S. women having abortions in 2000–2001. Perspect Sex Reprod Health. 2002;34:294–93.
64. Isaacs JN, Creinin MD. Miscommunication between healthcare providers and patients may result in unplanned pregnancies. Contraception. 2003;68:373–76.
65. Steiner MJ, Dalebout S, Condon S, Dominik R, Trusell J. Understanding risk: A randomized controlled trial of communicating contraceptive effectiveness. Obstet Gynecol. 2003;102:709–17.
66. Fox MC, Creinin MD, Murthy AS, Harwood B, Reid LM. Feasibility study of the use of a daily electronic mail reminder to improve oral contraceptive compliance. Contraception. 2003;68:365–71.
67. Westhoff C, Kerns J, Morroni C, et al. Quick Start: a novel oral contraceptive initiation method. Contraception. 2002;66:141–45.

Menstrual Disorders

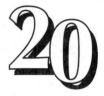

Anita L. Nelson, MD
Susie B. Baldwin MD, MPH

- A new terminology has been developed to describe abnormalities in menstrual cycling.

- Infrequent menses due to lack of progesterone increase the risk for endometrial cancer, while infrequent or absent menses due to lack of estrogen increase the risk for osteoporosis.

- Definitions and treatments for polycystic ovarian syndrome (PCOS) have changed. Insulin-sensitizing drugs are rarely indicated.

- Menstrual bleeding is heavy when a woman says it is heavy.

- New therapies have gained approval from the Food and Drug Administration (FDA) for the treatment of heavy menstrual bleeding.

- Many medical problems flare with menstruation and can be controlled by menstrual suppression.

Menstrual disorders cause considerable morbidity among reproductive-aged women. This chapter will discuss the diagnosis and treatment of a variety of disorders in menstrual bleeding patterns and the additional problems that are caused by menstruation and the hormonal shifts that occur during the menstrual cycle.

In order to understand and describe abnormal bleeding, it is necessary to understand the normal menstrual cycle. (See Chapter 2.) A new terminology has been introduced to describe the major dimension of menses and to more accurately describe different menstrual abnormalities.[1] This new vocabulary for menstruation is needed because the existing one is imprecise. For example, what does *irregular bleeding* mean? Does *menorrhagia* mean prolonged bleeding or excessive blood loss or both? The term *dysfunctional uterine bleeding* is used so loosely today that it may refer to virtually any abnormal bleeding pattern. The new terminology specifically describes disorders that can occur in four different aspects of menses:

Table 20–1   Characterization of menstrual patterns: new terminology

Clinical dimensions of menstruation and menstrual cycle	Descriptive terms	Normal limits (5th to 95th percentiles)
Frequency of menses	Frequent	<24 days
	Normal	24–38 days
	Infrequent	>38 days
Regularity of menses (cycle to cycle variation over 12 months)	Absent	-
	Regular	Variation ±2 to 20 days
	Irregular	Variation > 20 days
Duration of flow	Prolonged	>8.0 days
	Normal	4.5–8.0 days
	Shortened	<4.5 days
Volume of monthly blood loss	Heavy	>80 mL
	Normal	5–80 mL
	Light	<5 mL

Fraser IS, et al. (2007),[2] with permission.

- Frequency of bleeding
- Regularity of cycles (cycle to cycle variation over 12 months)
- Duration of flow
- Amount of blood lost

The normal values for these variables are listed in Table 20–1. The terms to use when describing abnormalities in any of the variables are also provided there. Although this level of detail may seem cumbersome, the new terminology provides a comprehensive description of bleeding and can lead more directly to appropriate testing and diagnosis. For example, a woman who menstruates every 20 days, flows for 4 days, and loses 90 ml of blood would be described as having regular, frequent cycles of normal duration with heavy bleeding. On the other hand, a woman whose flow lasts 9 days with a blood loss of 75 ml would be described as having prolonged, regular cyclic bleeding. A woman whose cycle varies in length from 23 to 45 days would have cycles with irregular variability. A woman whose menses occurred only 3 to 4 times a year would be described as having infrequent menses. This chapter will utilize this new terminology.

MENSTRUAL BLEEDING DISORDERS
AMENORRHEA

The most common causes of amenorrhea are pregnancy, lactation, menopause, and contraceptives. However, in about 3% to 4% of reproductive-aged women with amenorrhea, the absence of bleeding is due to other causes.[3] The majority of those women have premature ovarian insufficiency or an extreme version of one of three other conditions: polycystic ovarian syndrome, hyperprolactinemia, or hypothalamic amenorrhea. An exhaustive list of uncommon genetic, anatomic, and enzymatic abnormalities accounts for the remaining cases. Women who never experience menstruation are more likely to have one of these uncommon abnormalities than are women who stop bleeding after menarche, but the etiologies for both primary and secondary amenorrhea are often similar.

Reproductive endocrinologists have persuasively argued that the distinction between primary amenorrhea (no menarche) or secondary amenorrhea (cessation of bleeding after menarche) should be eliminated. To evaluate women for any type of amenorrhea, they recommend a comprehensive set of laboratory tests—including thyroid-stimulating hormone (TSH), prolactin, follicle stimulating hormone (FSH), luteinizing hormone (LH), and estradiol.[3] These results can be used to identify groups of disorders as shown in Figure 20–1. However, most family planning clinics and primary care providers have limited resources and limited expertise to care for the more unusual pathologies associated with primary amenorrhea, while secondary amenorrhea is comfortably within their scope of practice. Therefore, the distinction between primary amenorrhea and secondary amenorrhea is maintained in this text.

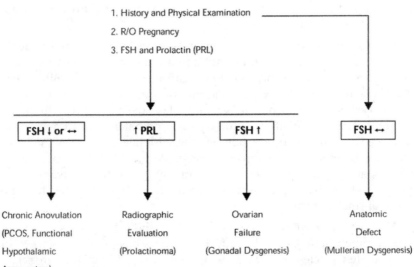

Practice Committee of American Society for Reproductive Medicine. Fertil Steril (2008),[3] with permission.

Figure 20–1 Suggested flow diagram aiding in the evaluation of women with amenorrhea

FAILURE OF MENARCHE (PRIMARY AMENORRHEA)

The mean age of menarche (first menstrual bleeding episode) is 12.5 years in the United States, and the mean age of menopause (the last menstrual bleeding episode) is 51.3 years. The first manifestation of puberty is either breast budding (thelarche) or axillary/pubic hair growth (adrenarche). These changes should start between the ages of 8 and 13 years. Girls go through a normal progression of Tanner stages of breast and pubic hair development, followed by a growth spurt and weight gain just prior to menarche. The usual time interval from thelarche to menarche is 2 years. A work-up is needed for girls who have no thelarche or adrenarche by age 13, for those who have no menses by age 15, and for those who enter puberty on time but have no menses within the following 5 years.[3]

The differential diagnosis for a lack of menarche is wide-ranging. It includes anatomical, genetic, enzymatic and psychologic causes. Anatomical defects, such as an imperforate hymen or a transverse vaginal septum, may mask the onset of menses. These obstructions can usually be treated with surgical excision. Most other cases of primary amenorrhea should be referred to reproductive endocrinologists, but preliminary evaluation can often be initiated by generalists.

A thorough personal history, a physical exam, and a family history can suggest specific etiologies. The work-up of primary amenorrhea can be organized into four different pathways based on the presence or absence of breasts and a uterus.

Uterus, no breasts. Women who have no breasts but have a uterus can be assumed to lack ovarian estrogen production. This can represent premature ovarian insufficiency due to chromosomal abnormalities (e.g., Turner syndrome [45, X], mosaicism, or pure gonadal dysgenesis), ovarian enzyme deficiency (17α-hydroxylase deficiency), or childhood chemotherapy or radiation. Pituitary or hypothalamic dysfunction can also prevent estrogen production by otherwise healthy ovaries. A classic example of this is Kallmann syndrome. Women with Kallmann syndrome lack gonadotropin releasing hormone (GnRH) and retain an infantile body with no secondary sexual characteristics. They also have no sense of smell (anosmia).

No breasts, no uterus. Women who lack both breasts and a uterus are extremely rare. Generally, affected women have one of a variety of enzyme deficiencies (17, 20 desmolase deficiency; 17 alpha-hydroxylase deficiency in a 46, XY) or lack any gonads after birth (but in utero had testicular tissue to prevent the formation of a uterus).

Breasts, no uterus. For women who have no uterus but have normal breast development demonstrating estrogen exposure, there are only a few major possible etiologies. One possible cause of this phenotype is a

46, XY karyotype with androgen insensitivity. Patients with complete androgen insensitivity lack all secondary sexual hair and may be found to have bilateral inguinal masses (testes). The other possible etiology of normal breast development with congenital absence of a uterus is Müllerian agenesis. Ten percent of cases of primary amenorrhea are due to complete uterine agenesis, making it the second most common cause of this condition. Müllerian agenesis is associated with other urogenital malformations, especially in the urinary tract (kidney and ureteral abnormalities). A testosterone level can distinguish between androgen insensitivity and Müllerian agenesis. If testosterone levels are elevated into the male range, karyotyping is helpful to confirm the diagnosis of androgen insensitivity. These patients are genetically male; their estrogen comes from peripheral conversion of testosterone. These women should retain their sexual identity (since they are phenotypically female), but require removal of their gonads to prevent the development of gonadoblastoma, which occurs in more than 20% of cases. If they desire children, women with congenital absence of the uterus must adopt or utilize egg donation and surrogates to carry their pregnancies.

Breasts, uterus. Most women with primary amenorrhea have both a uterus and breasts. As discussed above, congenital obstruction of menstrual flow (by vaginal septa, imperforate hymen, etc.) can be ruled out by examination or imaging studies. The remaining evaluations are virtually the same as the evaluations needed for secondary amenorrhea, with the exception that galactorrhea and pituitary adenomas tend to be much more frequent in this population; up to 25% of women in this category will have elevated prolactin levels and evidence of tumor on magnetic resonance imaging (MRI).

SECONDARY AMENORRHEA

When women who have previously menstruated unexpectedly stop menstruating, the first test that needs to be performed is a pregnancy test, except for patients who consistently use hormonal contraceptives that are known to reduce episodes of bleeding, such as the levonorgestrel (LNg) intrauterine contraceptive, depot medroxyprogesterone acetate (DMPA), or extended cycle combined hormonal methods. Pregnancy testing in these cases is not needed unless the patient is experiencing other signs or symptoms of pregnancy. It should be noted that with modern low-dose pills, it is no longer appropriate to attribute any delay in return of menses to "post-pill amenorrhea;" cyclic bleeding should return within 2 weeks of stopping all combined hormonal methods. If the onset of amenorrhea follows a combined uterine procedure (such as a dilation and curettage to treat a septic abortion or postpartum hemorrhage), evaluate the endometrial cavity for adhesions (Asherman's syndrome). For amenorrhea following a cervical LEEP or cone biopsy, rule out cervical stenosis.

The question is: how long must a woman go without bleeding to be diagnosed with secondary amenorrhea? Today the diagnosis is most often made when a woman lacks any spotting or bleeding for a period of time that is *3 times her normal cycle length*. Prior to that, her diagnosis is formally termed *delayed menses*. For a woman with monthly cycles, the interval needed to declare amenorrhea would be 3 months. A woman who usually had menses every other month would have to wait 6 months (2 months x 3) to be given this diagnosis. However, that patient would warrant earlier evaluation for her infrequent menses (see below).

The lack of uterine bleeding can reflect one of two different endocrine states: a lack of *estrogen* to stimulate growth of the endometrium or a lack of *progesterone* to offset unopposed estrogen stimulation. Lack of estrogen carries with it the risks of menopause, such as osteoporosis, early cardiovascular disease, and atrophic vaginitis. On the other hand, unopposed estrogen stimulation significantly increases the risk for developing endometrial hyperplasia and endometrial cancer. Rarely, in the presence of both estrogen and progesterone, other local factors can affect the endometrium. A classic example of this is relatively high levels of testosterone that block the ability of endogenous estrogen to stimulate endometrial cells.

Secondary amenorrhea in reproductive-aged women not using hormonal contraception can indicate either a problem confined to the reproductive system or a systemic medical problem. Even if a woman with secondary amenorrhea does not desire fertility, she must be evaluated, because the medical problem underlying her amenorrhea may require treatment.

History and physical examination. The evaluation of amenorrhea begins with a thorough history and physical examination. Take a detailed menstrual history and inquire about vasomotor symptoms. Question the patient about recent changes in her weight, dietary habits, acne, hair growth, and cold or heat intolerance. Ask about galactorrhea, recent pregnancy, recent breastfeeding, recent genital tract procedures, prior chemotherapy or irradiation, stress, and exercise patterns. Medical problems, such as uncontrolled juvenile diabetes, end-stage renal disease, AIDS, malabsorption, hepatic failure, Cushing syndrome, sarcoidosis, acromegaly, and craniopharyngiomas, can cause amenorrhea. Also obtain a personal and family history of medical problems, especially endocrine problems that might influence menstrual cycling.

Obtain a complete drug history, because all classes of medications (prescription, over-the-counter, and street recreational drugs) include some drugs that can induce amenorrhea or infrequent bleeding. Of course, long-acting progestin birth control methods, such as DMPA and LNg intrauterine contraception and extended cycle use of combined oral contraceptives (COCs) or vaginal rings, induce amenorrhea. However, many other prescription drugs also affect cycling. Phenothiazine derivatives, phenothiazine-like compounds, haloperidol, selective serotonin reuptake inhibitors (SSRIs), reserpine derivatives, metoclopramide, sulpiride, promazine, cimetidine, verapamil, opiates, diazepams, tricyclic antidepressants, methyldopa, amphetamines and marijuana can cause amenorrhea. The high levels of prolactin can cause amenorrhea; less dramatic elevations in prolactin are associated with infrequent menses (see below). Note that androgenic drugs, sometimes used to improve athletic performance or libido, may be compounded or obtained by patients in unconventional ways.

On examination, pay close attention to signs of androgen excess (hirsutism, balding, acne, voice changes, and clitoromegaly), insulin resistance (acanthosis nigricans), hypoestrogenism (dry, flattened vaginal mucosa), prolactin excess (galactorrhea), thyroid dysfunction (skin, pulse, and reflex changes), or changes indicating other systemic diseases. Check the patient's index and middle fingers for any signs of calluses on the dorsal surface, and look for yellow staining on the inner surfaces of her teeth, which might suggest induced vomiting associated with eating disorders.[4]

Laboratory tests. Order laboratory tests that are appropriate for the woman's history, physical exam, immediate fertility desires, and personal and family history. Once pregnancy is ruled out, the most common tests are TSH and prolactin, although total testosterone or FSH can also be very helpful. However, not all tests are needed in every case, particularly in a resource-restricted clinical setting. For example, consider tests that may be appropriate for the following women who have secondary amenorrhea:

- A 25-year-old woman with increasing weight and decreased energy may be best served by first testing her TSH.

- A 23-year-old woman who complains of hot flashes and a dry vagina should be first tested for FSH.

- A 19-year-old woman with progressively worsening hirsutism would need 17-α hydroxyprogesterone, total testosterone, and possibly, DHEAS levels to rule out adult-onset congenital adrenal hyperplasia and androgen-producing tumors.

- A 24-year-old nulliparous, hirsute woman who desires pregnancy would most likely benefit from having all these tests done.

More extensive testing may be needed after the results of the first round of tests suggest a specific problem. For example, a woman with elevated TSH needs additional testing to determine the cause of her thyroid deficiency. A woman with elevated prolactin (especially if >70 ng/dL) without a history of medication or drug use to explain that elevation needs to have imaging studies (usually MRI) of her pituitary gland and adjacent areas to rule out pituitary prolactinoma, empty-sella syndrome, craniopharyngioma, and other obstructive lesions.

The 23-year-old with no bleeding for 8 months, whose FSH is in the postmenopausal range, should have that diagnosis confirmed by repeating her FSH and testing her LH and estradiol. If both gonadotropins are elevated and her estradiol is low, she has premature ovarian insufficiency and is menopausal. Because she is under 30, it would be prudent to check her karyotype to identify chromosomal abnormalities, such as Turner syndrome, the presence of Y chromosome, or other abnormalities that might also impact other family members. Nearly 40% of women who experience ovarian insufficiency between ages 30 and 40 have anti-ovarian antibodies. Women with antibodies to their ovarian tissue are also likely to later develop other auto-antibodies to their thyroid or parathyroid or adrenal glands. Therefore, periodic screening for failure of those organs is indicated.

A woman whose prolactin is normal, but whose gonadotropin and estrogen levels are low or low normal, probably has hypothalamic amenorrhea. This condition can result from excessive exercise, eating disorders, or other significant stress. The athletic triad (amenorrhea, eating disorder, and osteoporosis) represents a classic presentation of this condition.[4,6,7] Eating disorders are generally chronic conditions that require long-term therapy and monitoring.[5]

While blood tests are being analyzed, it is quite reasonable to give women with secondary amenorrhea a short course of progestin therapy (MPA 10 mg or norethindrone acetate 5 mg once daily for 10 days) to offset possible endometrial stimulation from unopposed estrogen. In the past, the results of this so-called *progestin challenge test* were used as part of the work-up of amenorrhea. Today the progestin is considered therapeutic, not diagnostic. This is because the results do not reliably support any diagnosis. The presence of withdrawal bleeding after progestin challenge does not necessarily demonstrate ovarian estradiol production. Peripheral aromatization of androgens can produce weaker estrogens that can stimulate the endometrium; some postmenopausal woman can even be induced to bleed following short-term treatment with progestin. On the other hand, the absence of bleeding after MPA does not absolutely verify the absence of ovarian estrogen production. High circulating levels of androgen can block estrogen's proliferative impact on endometrial cells.

Treatments for Secondary Amenorrhea

If a specific etiology is identified by the work-up, therapy can be targeted:

- Prolactinomas are generally treated medically with bromocriptine or cabergoline.
- Hypothyroidism can be treated with thyroxin.
- Testosterone-producing tumors must be surgically removed.
- Women with Kallmann's syndrome need pulsatile GnRH to help them develop secondary sexual characteristics, after which time they require supportive hormonal therapies, as do other women with estrogen deficiency.

Progestin therapy. Women with secondary amenorrhea due to anovulation require progestin therapy to mitigate the harmful effect of unopposed estrogen on the endometrium. Progestin can be administered cyclically, following a variety of protocols. Medroxyprogesterone acetate (MPA) or norethindrone acetate (NETA) is often given for the first 10 days of each month. Alternatively, women may prefer to have some degree of endometrial suppression with progestin-only methods, such as the LNg intrauterine contraceptive, the implant, or progestin-only pills. Of course, anovulatory women may be able to use combined hormonal contraceptive methods either cyclically or continuously if they do not have contraindications to estrogen.

Estrogen therapy. Reproductive-aged women whose amenorrhea is caused by estrogen deficiency may reduce their risk for osteoporosis by taking estrogen. If they have a uterus, add progestin.[6] Many younger women feel a stigma in using postmenopausal products and prefer to use estrogen-containing contraceptive products; they may also derive greater bone mineral density benefits from those products.[7,142] Of note, many women with amenorrhea appreciate freedom from menstrual bleeding and are excellent candidates for extended cycle use of oral contraceptives or vaginal rings (see Chapters 11 and 12).

INFREQUENT MENSES

Infrequent menstruation is a very common problem that can be associated with heavy or prolonged bleeding episodes. The conditions that cause secondary amenorrhea—hypothyroidism, androgen-excess conditions, and obesity-induced anovulatory cycling—also commonly cause infrequent menses. Once pregnancy is ruled out, most cases are found to be associated with estrogen production but with a lack of progesterone. Occasionally, women may experience intermittent estrogen deficiency, which is generally associated with intermittent strenuous exercise, seasonal sports, periodic extreme stress, or severe depression, all of which affect the hypothalamus. The history and physical exam needed for women presenting with infrequent menses are virtually the same as for secondary amenorrhea, except that a more detailed history of recent menstrual trends is appropriate. Ask about symptoms of ovulation (Mittelschmerz) and moliminal complaints (bloating, cramping, or breast tenderness that typically herald the onset of menses). Ask about bleeding patterns over time, and examine these in the context of life events, activities, and changes in weight.

Polycystic Ovarian Syndrome (PCOS)

Polycystic ovarian syndrome (PCOS) is a common cause of infrequent bleeding and is the most common endocrinopathy of reproductive-aged women. Depending upon the definition used, 7% to 10% of women meet all the criteria for PCOS, but up to 20% of women have some manifestation of androgen excess. With increasing prevalence of obesity, these estimates may increase.[8]

The 1990 NIH definition of PCOS requires that the women have chronic anovulation, i.e., fewer than 8 menses per year. In addition to infrequent bleeding, this classic definition specifies that the woman have either hyperandrogenemia (high normal or slightly elevated levels of circulating testosterone) or hyperandrogenism (hirsutism, acne, male-balding pattern). Hirsutism must be distinguished from virilization. The latter is characterized by irreversible changes, such as voice deepening and clitoromegaly.

PCOS is really a diagnosis of exclusion; other conditions that could explain these signs and symptoms must be excluded before the woman can be diagnosed with PCOS. Most importantly, pregnancy, thyroid dysfunction, prolactinoma, pituitary or hypothalamic suppression, and medication-induced infrequent menses must be ruled out first.

After adoption of the 1990 NIH definition, reproductive endocrinologists pressed for the definition to be expanded to include the relatively rare cases of hirsute women who have monthly menses.[9] This expansion was sought because ovarian function in these hirsute women was found to be very similar to that seen in women with classic PCOS; these women also face challenges with infertility that are identical to those faced by women with PCOS. To include these cycling hirsute women, a new definition of PCOS was advanced in 2003 called the Rotterdam definition of PCOS.[10] The Rotterdam definition requires that in the absence of other causes, women can be diagnosed with PCOS when they meet at least two of the following three criteria:

- Infrequent menses (<8 per year)
- Hyperandrogenism or hyperandrogenemia
- Polycystic-appearing ovaries on ultrasound

From this definition, it is clear that the old 1990 NIH Consensus definition is still valid; it is met when the patient meets the first two criteria. A polycystic-appearing ovary is defined on ultrasound imaging when at least 13 preantral follicles (2 to 9 mm) peripherally oriented can be seen in any one plane. This appearance of the ovary is used to demonstrate anovulation when combined with one of the other two criteria. It is important to note that the presence of a polycystic-appearing ovary does *not* by *itself* make the diagnosis of PCOS.[11] Anovulation associated with *any* condition can induce polycystic-appearing ovaries.

The laboratory tests needed to confirm the diagnosis of PCOS using the Rotterdam definition are generally intended to rule out other etiologies, just as they were under the older NIH Consensus criteria. Here again, selection of initial tests is driven by the patient's clinical presentation and her immediate fertility desires.

Women with PCOS have an increased risk of developing diabetes at a younger age.[12] Therefore, glucose tolerance testing may be very important to their health, even if it is not part of diagnosing PCOS. The best test is a 2-hour glucose tolerance test with a 75 g glucose load; this test can clearly identify prediabetes (100–125 fasting blood sugar, or a 2-hour-glucose level between 140 to 200) as well as overt diabetes ($\geq$126 fasting blood sugar, or a 2-hour glucose >200). Other tests, such as FBS or hemoglobin A1C, can be used, but they are less sensitive in diagnosing diabetes and often miss the diagnosis of prediabetes. Almost half of women with PCOS (both lean and obese) also have metabolic syndrome, which may also put them at increased risk for future cardiovascular problems.[13] Therefore, obese women and those with elevated blood pressure may benefit from receiving a lipid profile as part of their well-woman care, even though this testing is not needed to diagnose PCOS. Also screen women with PCOS carefully for depression.

It is also important to know which tests are *not* indicated to make the diagnosis of PCOS. Because tests that can accurately diagnose insulin resistance are not commercially available, and since knowing that women have insulin resistance does *not* affect the choice of treatment, routine testing for insulin resistance with fasting insulin levels is *not* indicated.[14] Older tests, such as the LH/FSH ratio, are also not relevant.[15] Finally, in the absence of a pelvic mass, it is generally *not* necessary to order a pelvic ultrasound for patients who meet the other two criteria for PCOS.[10,14,16]

Other Causes of Infrequent Menses

Infrequent menses usually result from anovulation, which can have other etiologies, as noted in the work-up for PCOS. Clinical symptoms such as fatigue, weight gain, constipation, and depressive moods can suggest hypothyroidism; an elevated TSH can confirm the diagnosis and distinguish it from depression. Prolactinomas more often cause infrequent menses than lack of menses, especially when those pituitary tumors produce lower levels of prolactin. Similarly, centrally acting medications, such as lithium and others that interfere with dopamine, raise prolactin levels and commonly cause infrequent bleeding in their users.

An increasingly common cause of infrequent bleeding during reproductive years is obesity-related anovulation; obese women often have polycystic-appearing ovaries reflecting their chronic anovulation. Technically, criteria 1 and 3 of the Rotterdam definition, would qualify them for the diagnosis of PCOS. However, since they have no androgen excess, most experts have objected to labeling these ladies as having PCOS.[16] This issue should be clarified in subsequent refinements of the definition of PCOS that are expected in the near future.

Women with intermittent challenges from eating disorders, excessive exercise, or stress may present with infrequent menses due to estrogen deficiency. Bulimia can present in women who have normal weight or are overweight; the stress of the disease itself causes hypothalamic amenorrhea. The diagnosis of hypothalamic amenorrhea can be verified by a normal prolactin and TSH but low gonadotropins (FSH with or without LH) with low estradiol.

Treatment for Women with Infrequent Menses

Treatment of women with infrequent menses depends upon their diagnoses, their immediate fertility desires, and other health challenges. Women with underlying problems such as hyperprolactinemia and hypothyroidism should receive targeted therapies for those issues, but they should also be provided progestin until their menses normalize. Contraception during this time is also important, because thyroid abnormalities can adversely affect pregnancy outcomes. Prolactinomas can grow during pregnancy. Women with eating disorders need specific psychological and other professional help to deal with those long-term problems, but they will need estrogen and progestin to protect their bones while they are recovering.

Weight loss. Women not seeking pregnancy who have chronic anovulation caused by either PCOS or obesity can be treated with similar therapies. The first and most effective intervention for overweight women with or without PCOS focuses on lifestyle changes, with particular emphasis on weight loss and exercise. It is important to emphasize to patients that a combination of long-term healthy eating, including a diet rich in fruit, vegetables, fiber, and lean proteins, *and* consistent engagement in physical activity, are the keys to losing weight and maintaining a healthy weight. Despite the fact that various diets make often outrageous claims about their efficacies, research has shown that there are few differences in outcomes among them overall.[17] Recent research has suggested that important genetic differences may make some people more resistant to weight loss with diets that work for other people. This is an exciting development that may allow clinicians to individualize diet recommendations in the future. For now, encouraging women to find a safe diet they can follow over the long term is the goal.[17] To lose weight, women with PCOS must maintain low-calorie diets for prolonged periods of time. Reducing their intake to 500 to 600 kcal a day below subsistence level can mean that they are allowed to consume only 1000 calories kcal a day. In order to be successful on such stringent diets, women need significant support and understanding from their providers and from their loved ones.

Providers should encourage women to find a form of physical activity they enjoy, and to make a lifetime commitment to engaging in exercise. Exercise is critically important to every weight loss program, and to the maintenance of a healthy weight, because to lose weight, calories consumed need to be lower than the calories being expended. Exercise helps consume calories and promotes cardiovascular health, balance, and quality sleep. Sleep disorders contribute to insulin resistance, increase cardiovascular disease risk, and are associated with obesity. Therefore, sleep, diet, and exercise comprise an inter-related triad of key health promotion messages for women of all ages.

Therapeutic agents. Some medical agents have been shown to help women with PCOS enhance their weight loss. The most successful of these is Orlistat, taken 60 mg orally before each meal. Orlistat works by blocking absorption of fats out of the intestine. When patients on Orlistat consume foods high in fat, they experience very unpleasant flatus and diarrhea. In a comparative clinical trial, the Orlistat-treated group of PCOS women had over 4 times as much weight loss than women treated without Orlistat.[18]

Routine use of insulin-sensitizing agents for women with PCOS is now discouraged by the American College of Obstetricians and Gynecologists (ACOG), the American Society for Reproductive Medicine (ASRM), and other authorities.[14,15] Metformin may be appropriate in the treatment of women with PCOS who also have metabolic syndrome and prediabetes, but its use in this context is still controversial.

Women with anovulatory infrequent menses need a progestin to protect their endometrial linings from the long-term effects of unopposed estrogen: endometrial hyperplasia and endometrial carcinoma. Women who are at least 50 pounds overweight have a 10-fold increased risk of endometrial carcinoma. Because obese women do occasionally ovulate, they also need contraception if they are sexually active. Progestin-only methods such as DMPA, the LNg intrauterine contraceptive, and progestin-only pills provide substantial endometrial protection and good contraceptive efficacy without inducing periodic bleeding. Many women with PCOS appreciate their freedom from bleeding and are excellent candidates for long-acting methods; however, some women with PCOS or other women with infrequent bleeding desire monthly bleeding. Combined hormonal methods may be more appropriate for them, unless obesity will reduce efficacy (contraceptive patch) or will increase the risk of thrombosis (as in women over 35 years of age). (See Chapters 11 and 12.)[19]

Infertility treatment. The treatment of infertility in women with PCOS has changed dramatically in recent years. In women who are overweight, the first step has always been to encourage weight loss. For overweight and obese women with PCOS, a loss of only 10% to 15% of baseline weight can restore ovulation. First-line medical therapy for ovulation induction is clomiphene citrate (it is no longer insulin-sensitizing agents, such as metformin). Randomized comparative clinical trials have clearly demonstrated that clomiphene citrate is superior to extended-release metformin in producing higher rates of ovulation, pregnancy, and live births.[20] Second-line therapies include ovulation induction, laparoscopic ovarian drilling and, perhaps, aromatase inhibitors. ACOG recommendations include clomiphen citrate with metformin as a second-line option.[14] The 2008 Consensus on Infertility Treatment stated that metformin use for infertility treatment in women with PCOS should be restricted to those with glucose intolerance.[15]

For long-term health promotion, women who have PCOS complicated by obesity, cigarette smoking, dyslipidemia, hypertension, impaired glucose tolerance, and subclinical vascular disease need to be recognized as being at risk for cardiovascular disease. Women with PCOS and metabolic syndrome or type 2 diabetes are at high risk. For this reason, the Androgen Excess and Polycystic Ovary Syndrome Society recommended in 2010 that all women with PCOS be assessed for body mass index (BMI), waist circumference, serum lipids, serum glucose, and blood pressure measurement. Additional targeted testing was also recommended. Oral glucose tolerance testing was recommended for PCOS women with obesity, advanced reproductive age, personal history of gestational diabetes, and family history of diabetes. Mood disorder assessment is recommended for all PCOS women. The Society also recommended lifestyle management for primary prevention of cardiovascular disease, targeting low-density and non-high density lipoprotein cholesterol. Insulin-sensitizing agents should be recommended for glucose intolerance.[21]

It is interesting to note that these recommendations would generally apply to women with those complications even in the absence of PCOS. This suggests that rather than having PCOS be the focus of the woman's medical conditions, it may be possible that PCOS may be better viewed as a modifier. For example, the woman's diagnosis should focus on her major problem, such as obesity with PCOS or infertility due to PCOS.

HEAVY OR PROLONGED MENSTRUAL BLEEDING

Heavy menstrual bleeding (HMB) is a common gynecologic problem affecting 9% to 14% of healthy women, although one survey found that 30% of women consider their bleeding to be excessive.[22] Women with HMB are 45% more likely to use health services and 27% less likely to work. If they do work, it has been estimated that their annual income is $1,692 less than women with normal menses.[23] Studies have shown that one third of uteri that were removed to control HMB were normal on pathological examination.[24]

The prevalence of heavy menstrual bleeding depends upon how it is defined. The classic definition is the loss of greater than 80 mL of blood per cycle. However, in daily life, the amount of blood loss is very difficult to quantify. Pad counts are not a reliable measure because of difference in product absorbancy and in women's fastidiousness. Interpretation of hemoglobin levels can be complicated by variations in dietary intake of iron. Losses as great as 800 to 1000 mL per cycle can occur without anemia in women with iron rich diets and supplements.[25] By the time a woman does decrease her hemoglobin, she has lost a considerable amount of blood.

A practical new definition of HMB advances the idea that a woman's blood loss is excessive *when she says it is excessive*. This definition illustrates that the key factor in making a diagnosis of HMB is not the *amount of blood* that a woman loses, which is difficult to ascertain, but how a woman's HMB *disrupts her life*. A woman whose total blood loss is only 60 mL/month, but whose flow is so heavy for 2 hours each cycle that she must remain restroom-bound, clearly has excessive bleeding. Of course a woman with blood loss so excessive that she becomes anemic must be diagnosed even if she does not complain. Another important consideration is that women lose a lot more than just blood with menstruation. Only about half of the menstrual fluid is blood; the rest of the material comes from the cervical and uterine secretions.[26] When we estimate that the woman's blood loss is 150 mL/cycle, we need to recognize that she has to contain over 300 mL of fluid onto the surface area of sanitary protection products, which can be a very challenging task that often results in staining episodes.

Etiologies. The differential diagnoses of excessive blood loss are extensive. Pregnancy complications must always be ruled out. Gynecologic causes include benign neoplasia such as uterine leiomyoma (fibroids), adenomyosis, and endometrial and endocervical polyps, along with serious pathology such as uterine hyperplasia, cervical and endometrial cancers.

Very commonly overlooked causes of HMB are the inherited and acquired disorders of hemostasis. In one study of over 100 women with physician-diagnosed HMB, 47% had a hemostatic abnormality including von Willebrand disease, idiopathic thrombocytopenia purpura, aplastic anemia, and platelet dysfunction. The most common abnormality was a platelet aggregation defect.[27] Although classic teaching reports that women with coagulation defects generally have other symptoms, such as easy bruising or bleeding gums, HMB often is the only symptom in woman with a bleeding diathesis.[28] Women with von Willebrand disease have lifelong histories of prolonged and heavy menstrual bleeding patterns. On the other hand, women with acquired disorders often have histories of having lighter menses earlier in their lives. Bleeding disorders should be ruled out in collaboration with a hematologist.[29,30]

Excessive blood loss can also result from systemic diseases or medication use. Hepatic disease, such as cirrhosis of the liver and active hepatitis, can disrupt production of clotting factors and vitamin K synthesis, resulting in HMB. Heavy menstrual bleeding is also found in early renal failure, adrenal hyperplasia, and some hematologic cancers, as well as with thyroid dysfunction. Anticoagulants will usually cause heavy menstrual bleeding, as will some anticonvulsants (phenytoin, phenobarbital), digitalis, nonhormonal intrauterine contraception, and chronic use of aspirin or nonsteroidal anti-inflammatory drugs (NSAIDs).

Cervical and endometrial biopsies are needed to rule out endometrial hyperplasia and cervical or uterine carcinoma in women with intermenstrual or postcoital bleeding and in high-risk women with unexplained heavy or prolonged menstrual bleeding. A dilation and curettage may be needed if the patient is hemodynamically unstable and if her acute heavy bleeding does not respond to the recommended hormonal therapies. Ultrasound studies can identify uterine leiomyoma that may contribute to heavy bleeding. Saline infusion sonography or hysteroscopy can better visualize endometrial polyps and other intracavity lesions that cause heavy menstrual bleeding. Saline infusion studies are better tolerated by women than office hysteroscopy.[31]

More frequently, women with HMB have *functional* problems with excessive endometrial fibrinolysis, a prostaglandin imbalance, vessel instability, or inhibition of matrix metalloproteinase activity. Only about half of women with heavy menstrual bleeding have an anatomical pathology identified at the time of hysterectomy.[32]

Treatments of Heavy Menstrual Bleeding

There are increasing numbers of treatments for women with HMB. Choice depends upon the age of the patient, the severity of her symptoms, the presence of other pelvic pathology, and her plans for childbearing. Many of the therapies are used off-label but are based on substantial clinical experience.

Acute bleeding. To arrest acute, heavy menstrual bleeding, various hormonal regimens are available. The classic treatment was with intravenous estrogen (conjugated equine estrogen 20 to 25 mg every 3 to 4 hours) for 24 hours.[33] Oral estrogen (conjugated equine estrogen 2.5 mg every 6 hours) has generally replaced the use of intravenous estrogen because oral preparations are often more available, require less frequent dosing and achieve efficacy similar to intravenous therapy. With either of these treatments, bleeding should slow in 12 to 24 hours at which time a progestin (MPA 5–10 mg daily) should be added. Reduce the doses of the estrogen in 3 to 5 days and maintain treatment for about 1 month, to allow the patient's hemoglobin to normalize. Taper the doses to reduce the risk of thrombosis but maintain amenorrhea. Treatment with high-dose combined oral contraceptive (COC) pills (50 mcg ethinyl estradiol [EE]/0.5 mg norgestrel 2 times daily or 35 mcg EE/1 mg norethindrone acetate 3 times a day) for 5 days, then once daily for up to 30 days, is slightly less effective than the earlier sequential hormonal regimens, but compliance has been reported to be better. Most recently, a regimen of high-dose progestin therapy (MPA 20 mg 3 times daily for 7 days, followed by MPA 20 mg once daily for 21 days) has been reported to be as effective as COC pills.[34] Because this regimen does not expose patients to any estrogen-related adverse events, it is gaining in popularity.

Chronic bleeding. Chronic heavy menstrual bleeding can be caused by an imbalance of prostaglandins favoring those that cause vasodilation (prostaglandin E) over those that cause vasoconstriction (prostaglandin $F_{2\alpha}$).[35] Higher levels of prostaglandins have been found in the menstrual fluid of women with HMB compared with controls. PGE receptors are found in higher concentrations in women with HMB. High-dose NSAIDs increase the ratio of prostaglandin $F_{2\alpha}$/prostaglandin E_2, and when taken from onset of menses until the end of the heavy flow days can reduce total menstrual blood loss by 20% to 45%. See Table 20–2 for appropriate doses. A Cochrane Database Review demonstrated that blood loss reduction was not affected by the particular NSAID used, but that low-dose NSAIDs were far less effective than high-dose regimens.[36] Women with gastric ulcers should avoid NSAIDs, or at least consider concomitant use of proton pump inhibitors (PPIs).

Antifibrinolytic therapy, as reported in a Cochrane review,[39] resulted in a 40% to 50% reduction in mean blood loss. Some women with chronic

Table 20–2 NSAID regimens for treatment of chronic heavy menstrual bleeding

Mefenamic acid

- 500 mg TID first 4–5 days of menses
- 500 mg TID from 4–5 days prior to menses to cessation
- 500 mg initially; 200 mg QID for 3–5 days

Naproxen

- 500 mg at onset and 3–5 hours later; 500 mg BID for 5 days
- 500 mg in AM and 250 in PM for two days; 250 mg BID for 7 days
- 500 mg; 250 mg QID for 4 days
- 550 mg; 275 mg QID for 5 days

Ibuprofen

- 600 mg daily or 1200 mg daily—not as effective
- 800 mg TID for 5 days (Norplant trial)

Lethaby A, et al. (2007).[36]

heavy and prolonged bleeding have increased endometrial plasminogen activity that promotes fibrinolysis;[37,38] when normal blood clots form in the vessels of these women, those clots are lysed, and the women's bleeding persists. The antifibrinolytic agent tranexamic acid has been used in Europe for treatment of HMB for more than 3 decades. It has been judged to be so safe that in Sweden, tranexamic acid has been available over-the-counter for more than a decade. There is now a version of tranexamic acid available by prescription in the United States (Lysteda). In clinical trials, women who took this tranexamic acid 650 mg 2 tabs orally 3 times a day for up to the first 5 days of menses experienced a 39% reduction in menstrual blood loss.[40] Reflecting previous theoretical concerns about the possibility that drugs that block lysis of fibrin clots might create a hypercoagulable state, the FDA labeling for Lysteda advises caution in prescribing this product for women who use estrogen-containing contraceptives.

Hormonal therapies are even more effective in treating HMB. Progesterone can be effectively used to help control chronic excessive menstrual blood loss. Cyclic progestin (MPA 10 mg or norethindrone acetate 5 mg daily for 10 days a month) is most useful for women with chronic anovulation but may even increase blood loss in ovulating women.[41] (See prior section.) For women with monthly cycling, progestin-only pills, progestin injections, and progestin-containing intrauterine contraceptives offer variable control of bleeding as well as pregnancy protection. The progestin-only pill (POP) decreases estrogen-stimulated endometrial proliferation to reduce blood loss. DMPA initially increases unscheduled spotting and bleeding but, over the longer term, usually results in cessation of spotting and bleeding by reducing ovarian estrogen production and by directly suppressing the endometrium.[42] Both POPs and DMPA are commonly used to treat heavy or prolonged menstrual bleeding, even though their use for this indication is off-label. Similarly, COC pills are routinely used off-label to reduce cyclic bleeding. COCs act both by thinning the endometrium and by altering plasminogen-activating enzymes. Most of the studies demonstrating clinical efficacy of pills in the treatment of HMB are based on higher-dose formulations, but there is one clinical trial using low-dose pills to treat heavy menstrual bleeding. That study showed that low-dose pills reduced menstrual blood loss by 68%.[43] Use of extended-cycle COCs and vaginal rings also reduces total blood loss in women with HMB.[44,45]

The LNg intrauterine contraceptive is the most effective medical therapy for HMB. It has the U.S. FDA approval as well as the approval of regulatory authorities in over 100 other countries to be used for the treatment of HMB. In clinical trials of women with HMB documented by eluting hematin from sanitary pads, women who randomized to the LNg intrauterine contraceptive had a median reduction in blood loss of 62% by 3 months and a 71% reduction by 6 months, 85% of women both normalized their blood loss and reduced their flow by more than 50%.[46] In an early comparative trial of LNg intrauterine contraceptive, NSAIDs, and tranexamic acid, LNg intrauterine contraceptive was significantly better than an antifibrolytic agent, which in turn was better than NSAIDs.[47]

Outpatient endometrial ablation has been increasingly popular for the treatment of heavy menstrual bleeding. Over 500,000 procedures are done in the United States each year. Women who are treated with endometrial ablation must have finished their childbearing and be committed to using effective contraception until menopause. Pregnancies that occur after the destruction of the endometrium are associated with increased risk of spontaneous abortion and with very serious problems with placentation, including placenta accreta and placenta percreta.[48–50] Early studies had found that there was no difference between ablation and LNg intrauterine contraceptive therapy after 1 year.[51] A recent meta-analysis shows even earlier equivalence. Starting at about 3 months, the efficacy of the LNg intrauterine contraceptive was comparable to that of all the different (first and second generation) ablation techniques.[52] A newer study comparing the LNg intrauterine contraceptive to thermal balloon ablation reported that menstrual bleeding was less in the LNg intrauterine contraceptive group at 6 and 12 months. However, intermenstrual bleeding and spotting was lower in the ablation group at those time points. By 12 months, there was no difference between the treatment groups.[53] Cost, safety, and reversibility make the LNg intrauterine contraceptive first-line therapy compared with endometrial ablation. Endometrial ablation is more expensive, requires more analgesia/ anesthesia, must be coupled with an effective method of contraception, and is less effective in treating adenomyosis.

Studies have also demonstrated the cost-effectiveness of the LNg intrauterine contraceptive compared with hysterectomy as first-line therapy for women with HMB without other pelvic pathology. One randomized 5-year study comparing LNg intrauterine contraceptive use to hysterectomy found that 58% of women who randomized to LNg intrauterine contraceptive avoided surgery.[54] Reserving hysterectomy for use only in women with pelvic pathology and to those who do not respond to LNg intrauterine contraceptive therapy would significantly reduce health care costs associated with treatment of HMB.

OTHER ABNORMAL BLEEDING PATTERNS IN PREMENOPAUSAL WOMEN

Postcoital bleeding or increased or renewed bleeding after removal of tampons may raise concerns about cervical or vaginal pathology. In younger women, the most common cause is chlamydia cervicitis. In older women, benign lesions such as cervical polyps and more serious problems, such as cervical carcinoma, present with these types of bleeding patterns.

Intermenstrual bleeding is often associated with significant endometrial pathology, such as endometrial hyperplasia or carcinoma. Rarely, reproductive-aged women may have midcycle spotting associated with ovulation. Women who miss birth control pills have unscheduled spotting and bleeding, which could be considered under this category.

PAINFUL MENSES (DYSMENORRHEA)

Dysmenorrhea, Greek for painful menstruation, is classified as *primary dysmenorrhea* (intrinsic and usually of early onset) or *secondary dysmenorrhea* (due to some other physical cause and usually of later onset). Even though the word to describe this problem comes from ancient Greek roots, dysmenorrhea has only recently been recognized as a medical problem. Before the 1970s, there were virtually no scientific articles studying any aspect of the problem, despite the fact that women have suffered from dysmenorrhea throughout time. In a study of young women attending a family planning clinic, 72% of those surveyed reported having experienced dysmenorrhea; for 15%, the symptoms were severe enough to interfere with their normal activities.[55] Among adult menstruating women, dysmenorrhea was reported by 40%; over 10% reported severe limitations of their activities for 1 to 3 days per cycle.[56] Many women with dysmenorrhea also experience nausea, vomiting, diarrhea, headaches, or lightheadedness. Symptoms often vary in severity from cycle to cycle but generally are present each month throughout the reproductive years. Younger women lose days at school, and older women are hampered at home and in the workplace.

PRIMARY DYSMENORRHEA

Primary dysmenorrhea has physiologic, not psychological, causes. While early investigators believed that dysmenorrhea occurred in "maladjusted women who were intensely rejecting their feminine role and who suffered from deep hostility,"[57] today we understand that the problem is not in the woman's head, but in her uterus. Measurements with intrauterine pressure catheters demonstrate that women with primary dysmenorrhea generate intrauterine pressures similar to pressures seen during the second stage of labor.[58,59]

Women with primary dysmenorrhea are generally ovulatory and produce progesterone in the luteal phase. Progesterone stimulates the production of prostaglandins in the base of the endometrium. These prostaglandins are released when the endometrium sloughs. Women with primary dysmenorrhea produce excessive amounts of prostaglandin $F_{2\alpha}$.[60] Prostaglandin $F_{2\alpha}$ increases the force of uterine contractions; uterine contractions reduce uterine blood flow, causing ischemia. This ischemia directly causes pain and sensitizes afferent nerve fibers in the uterus to other painful stimuli, which augments the patient's perception of pain. When these same prostaglandins are injected into the general circulation by uterine contractions, they can induce headache, nausea, vomiting, and diarrhea. Other etiologies of primary dysmenorrhea, such as structural abnormalities of the uterus (blind horns), cervix (stenotic os), or vagina (transverse septa), can usually be ruled out by a careful pelvic examination and radiographic studies.

Symptomatic therapies include rest, applying a heating pad, or using teas or over-the-counter medications to treat the discomfort. A vitamin E 200 unit given twice a day for 2 days before menses and for 3 days after onset reduces both pain severity and duration.[61] Usually, however, women seeking medical care have already tried many of these measures without success and require therapies targeting the underlying causes of their complaints. Several therapeutic interventions are effective for dysmenorrhea, including direct prostaglandin inhibitors and hormonal contraceptives. These therapies can be used individually or in combination.

Prostaglandin synthetase inhibitors such as NSAIDs and COX-2 inhibitors are more effective than placebo in treating dysmenorrhea: approximately 80% of women with dysmenorrhea feel relief with these agents. The drugs improve cramping pain and also reduce backache, headaches, and blood loss. In some women, NSAIDs may cause gastrointestinal symptoms. A recent comprehensive review concluded that NSAIDs are first-line therapy for dysmenorrhea in women who do not want to use contraception.[62] In contrast, aspirin is no more effective than placebo for dysmenorrhea and can increase menstrual blood loss. While COX-2 inhibitors reduce dysmenorrhea, they have been linked to cardiovascular risk and, therefore, are generally not prescribed for this indication.

Hormonal contraceptives have been used extensively off-label to reduce menstrual cramping. Older studies showed that within 3 to 4 months of beginning combined oral contraceptive (COC) therapy, 90% of women experience marked decreases in the severity of pain.[63,64] A review of studies using lower-dose formulations concluded that COCs were the preferred therapy for dysmenorrhea for women who wish to use contraception, because the additional benefit of such relief was not linked to any other risks and eliminated the risks of NSAID use.[62]

Women can achieve additional relief from dysmenorrhea by using extended cycle COCs[65] or extended cycles with contraceptive vaginal rings. The ring has not been tested for dysmenorrhea, but extended ring use does significantly reduce the days of bleeding[66] and, therefore, may be expected to reduce the pain related to menstruation.

DMPA is also helpful in treating dysmenorrhea. After their third injection, nearly half of DMPA users become amenorrheic and avoid dysmenorrhea altogether. The LNg intrauterine contraceptive is also an excellent choice for women with dysmenorrhea, because menstrual blood loss and duration of bleeding are significantly reduced. By 12 months of use, 20% of women have amenorrhea. Newer therapies are under investigation to treat dysmenorrhea by blocking the hormone vasopressin, which causes the uterus to contract.

A recent systematic review of acupuncture for primary dysmenorrhea concluded that there is promising evidence in the form of randomized clinical trials for the use of acupuncture in the treatment of primary dysmenorrhea compared with pharmacologic treatment or herbal medication. However, the results are limited by flaws in study design. Compared with sham acupuncture, the effectiveness of acupuncture is not convincing.[67]

SECONDARY DYSMENORRHEA

Women with secondary dysmenorrhea also complain of painful uterine cramping with menses but may have other accompanying complaints, such as dyspareunia or non-menstrual pelvic pain. The pain that women with secondary dysmenorrhea experience is, by definition, due to uterine or pelvic pathology.

The most common causes of secondary dysmenorrhea are adenomyosis, endometriosis, pelvic adhesions, and neoplasia. *Adenomyosis* is the presence of endometrial glands and stroma in the myometrium; in *endometriosis*, the endometrial glands and stoma implant outside the uterus. Monthly hormonal cycling causes cyclic sloughing of endometrial cells into the surrounding tissue, which causes intense, usually painful, local inflammation.

The treatment of secondary dysmenorrhea should be targeted to the underlying problems and should reflect the patient's desire for fertility. In the absence of problems requiring surgical intervention, the treatments helpful for primary dysmenorrhea (especially those that eliminate menses) often successfully reduce symptoms of secondary dysmenorrhea. In particular, Depo-subQ provera 104 is an FDA-approved therapy for the treatment of dysmenorrhea associated with endometriosis. The magnitude of pain reduction seen in the clinical trials with Depo-subQ provera 104 matched the pain score reductions seen with gonadotropin releasing hormone (GnRH) agonists.[68,69] In clinical trials, the LNg intrauterine contraceptive has been effective in the treatment of dysmenorrhea caused by endometriosis, and also has shrunk the size of endometriotic implants, particularly those that are located near the uterus.[70]

Other medications are available to treat dysmenorrhea by inducing amenorrhea, but their use is limited due to side effects and cost. Danazol, an androgen used to treat endometriosis, effectively induces amenorrhea but can be used for only 4 to 6 months due to androgenic side effects such as acne, hirsutism, oily skin, clitoral enlargement, and voice deepening. GnRH agonists also induce amenorrhea and, thereby, eliminate dysmenorrhea. However, GnRH use is also limited to 4 to 6 months because it causes hypoestrogenic side effects such as vasomotor symptoms (hot flashes), vaginal dryness, and loss of bone mineralization. GnRH agonists have been combined with estrogen/progestin add-back therapy for long-term treatment of endometriosis.[71] Aromatase inhibitors have also been found to reduce pain (generally dysmenorrhea) induced by endometriosis.[72]

If these interventions are not sufficiently effective, or if the patient seeks fertility, more definitive surgical approaches may be needed. For example, secondary dysmenorrhea caused by pelvic scarring may benefit from surgical lysis of adhesions. Hysterectomy is reserved for treatment of incapacitating dysmenorrhea unresponsive to more conservative measures and only in women who do not desire future childbearing.

PREMENSTRUAL SYNDROME (PMS) AND PREMENSTRUAL DYSPHORIC DISORDER (PMDD)

Nearly 90% of women experience some discomfort with their menses. With ovulation, problems with fluid retention, bloating, mood disorders, and breast tenderness are common. For many women, these symptoms are not significant, but in 20% to 30%, they affect a woman's activities,[73] and in 3% to 8%, the problem rises to the level of qualifying for a psychiatrically defined disorder.

Premenstrual syndrome (PMS) is a heterogeneous collection of signs and symptoms that share one common characteristic: a temporal relationship to the menstrual cycle. PMS is the cyclic appearance of at least one symptom during the luteal phase, followed by an entirely symptom-free interval beginning a few days after the onset of menses. ACOG diagnostic criteria for PMS include over 150 symptoms including physical symptoms of abdominal bloating, breast tenderness, headaches, extremity edema, and psychological and behavioral symptoms of anxiety, depression, confusion, social withdrawal, angry outbursts, and irritability.[74] Other commonly reported manifestations of PMS include fatigue, thirst, appetite changes, and crying spells. To be considered clinically significant, PMS symptoms must interfere with a woman's work, lifestyle, or interpersonal relationships. PMS can increase relationship strain, sexual dysfunction, social isolation, work absenteeism, and risk for suicide. Studies have demonstrated that PMS results in poorer self-reported mental and physical health, increased use of health services, and higher health care costs for sufferers.[75,76]

Premenstrual dysphoric disorder (PMDD) is a more severe form of PMS with a very specific definition. The American Psychiatric Association requires the manifestation of at least 5 symptoms during the 10 premenstrual days, with relief by the fourth day of menses.[77] (See Table 20-3.) By definition, at least one of the five required symptoms must represent a change in mood that is severe enough to interfere with the woman's occupational or social functions for at least 2 consecutive cycles.

Etiologies. What causes PMS/PMDD? Multiple factors likely play a role in the etiology. Early investigators suggested that PMS may be due to a lack of progesterone,[78] but subsequent research failed to find a difference between PMS sufferers and controls in levels of progesterone or any other major hormones including estradiol, FSH, LH, prolactin, SHBG, or testosterone.[79,80] However, women with PMS may be more biologically vulnerable to normal fluctuations in hormone levels than are women without the syndrome.[81]

Table 20–3 DSM IV-TM criteria for premenstrual dysphoric disorder

Symptoms

Core Symptoms

- Markedly depressed mood, feelings of hopelessness, self deprecation
- Suddenly feeling sad or tearful, with increased sensitivity to personal rejection
- Marked anxiety, tension, feelings of being "keyed up" or "on edge"
- Persistent and marked irritability, anger, or increased interpersonal conflicts

Other Symptoms

- Fatigue, lethargy, or marked lack of energy
- Insomnia or hypersomnia
- Marked change in appetite or cravings for certain foods
- Decreased interest in usual activities
- Subjective sense of having difficulty in concentrating
- Feeling out of control or overwhelmed
- Other physical symptoms, such as breast tenderness, joint or muscle pain, a sensation of "bloating" or weight gain, pain, etc.

Criteria

- 5 emotional and physical symptoms, including at least 1 core symptom
- Must occur during last week of luteal phase and remit soon after onset of menses
- Must markedly interfere with work, school or with social activities and relationships with others
- Must not be an exacerbation of symptoms of another disorder although it may be superimposed on one
- Confirmed by prospective daily rating during at least 2 consecutive menstrual cycles

American Psychiatric Association. DSM-IV-TR (2000),[77] with permission.

Other investigators have hypothesized that PMS may be caused by low beta-endorphin levels,[82,83] low adrenocorticotropin levels,[84] abnormal prostaglandin production, or endogenous hormone allergies, but research has not consistently supported any of these hypotheses. Studies of PMS sufferers have failed to identify deficiencies of magnesium, zinc, vitamin A, vitamin E, thiamine, or vitamin B6.[85] At least one epidemiologic investigation has revealed an association between post-traumatic stress disorder (PTSD) or trauma and PMS/PMDD.[86]

Scientists now believe that PMS/PMDD likely results from a complex interaction between ovarian hormones, central nervous system neurotransmitters such as serotonin and gamma-aminobutyric acid (GABA), and neurohormonal systems like the renin-angiotensin-aldosterone system.[87,88] Evidence suggests that serotonin dysregulation, in particular, plays a role in the pathogenesis of many of the psychological elements in PMS, including tension, irritability, and dysphoria.[89]

Diagnosis. The differential diagnosis of PMS/PMDD includes other dysthymic and depressive disorders, generalized anxiety disorder, and hypothyroidism. Take a detailed history to begin differentiating between these conditions. For many women, clinical depression and other serious problems worsen premenstrually but never completely abate; women who do not experience a symptom-free interval do not have PMS or PMDD.[90] As many as half the women with self-diagnosed PMS have other problems, which require careful evaluation and therapies different from those for PMS.[91] Some women may have PMDD symptoms as well as an underlying or concomitant psychiatric problem; in one study, 59% of women diagnosed with PMDD also had clinical depression or an anxiety disorder.[92]

In general, laboratory tests are not needed to diagnose PMS. In some cases, however, the clinician must rule out hypothyroidism, because a patient with low levels of thyroid hormone may present with fatigue, bloating, depression, and irritability. Laboratory testing to measure sex steroid hormone levels is unnecessary in the evaluation of PMS.

The key to diagnosing PMS/PMDD is prospective charting of symptoms by the patient, for at least 2 to 3 menstrual cycles. Research studies have validated a few assessment tools for this purpose, including the Premenstrual Symptoms Screening Tool, the Calendar of Premenstrual Experiences, and the Daily Record of Severity of Problems.[93–95] A woman generally can successfully document her symptoms by taking notes on a regular calendar, writing down the symptoms she experiences each day, along with their severity, and recording the dates of her menses. A woman who is overwhelmed by a series of complaints can chart only the 3 to 5 complaints that most profoundly bother her. Ideally, this chart should also include her weight and, if possible, a record of her basal body temperature or home ovulation test results. Have the patient document any medications she uses during this time.

Have the patient return in 2 to 3 months. Carefully study the pattern of her symptoms. Symptoms do not need to recur with equal intensity in each cycle; different symptoms may occur during different cycles. Again, the key to diagnosing PMS/PMDD is the timing of symptoms—they must appear in the luteal phase and disappear soon after the onset of menses.

TREATMENT OF PMS/PMDD

Treatment of Premenstrual Syndrome

PMS treatment is strongly influenced by a placebo effect. In a wide range of studies, researchers report that 40% to 94% of patients will improve in the short term regardless of the treatment used. This reinforces the need to rely on placebo-controlled studies rather than on case reports or personal testimonials to determine the true efficacy of a particular drug or treatment for PMS.

Treatment requires a comprehensive, individualized approach. For women with physiologic menstrual changes, provide reassurance, emotional support, and education. Both the patient and her family may benefit from a discussion of the hormonal changes associated with PMS. Charting the symptoms helps validate the diagnosis, but may also help the patient gain more insight into her problem and give her a greater sense of control. If therapy is initiated, have her continue her charting so that she can identify which interventions improve her symptoms.

For women with mild to moderate PMS, consider directing treatment toward their specific symptoms. Breast tenderness can be eased with a fitted support or sports bra. Abdominal pain and backache respond well to the therapies outlined under the discussion of dysmenorrhea, including NSAIDs (to reduce prostaglandin production) and extended-cycle COCs or vaginal rings, LNg intrauterine contraception, and DMPA.

Increasing evidence underscores the importance of exercise in maintaining physical and mental health. Clinicians should encourage women with PMS to engage in regular physical activity. Vigorous exercise may improve mood as well as reduce stress and physical complaints in PMS.[96,97] Results from one investigation demonstrated that aerobic exercise helped more than bodybuilding exercise in reducing PMS symptoms.[98] Smoking cessation, limiting of alcohol intake, and regular sleep have all been found to be helpful.[99]

For years, dietary manipulations have been recommended in the treatment of PMS, but for the most part, randomized controlled trials have not demonstrated any efficacy for this approach. Clinicians have traditionally advised patients with PMS to avoid caffeine, chocolate, alcohol, and salt, but no data exist to demonstrate the efficacy of these dietary modifications. The commonly-held belief that coffee worsens PMS, for example, stems from two studies in the 1980s that demonstrated an association between caffeinated beverages and PMS.[100] These studies, however, were cross-sectional in design, so it is not possible to conclude that caffeine intake among these women *caused* PMS; it is equally likely that women with PMS-related fatigue may self-medicate with caffeinated drinks. Carbohydrate-rich food and beverages may reduce food cravings and other symptoms; a small double-blind, randomized controlled trial found that a high-carbohydrate beverage consumed during the late luteal phase reduced not only carbohydrate cravings, but also reduced symptoms of depression, anger, and confusion reported by women with PMS.[101]

Vitamins and minerals have also been recommended to reduce PMS symptoms. Pyridoxine (vitamin B6) is important in the biosynthesis of neurotransmitters and may help with PMS symptoms, especially breast pain and depression. Most placebo-controlled studies have reported improvement among women with PMS, but an evidence-based review of pyridoxine found "insufficient evidence" to conclusively support its efficacy.[102–104] Peripheral neuropathy can occur when pyridoxine is taken at daily doses as low as 100 mg to 200 mg, so caution patients that if they use this vitamin, they must do so in moderation.

Limited but conflicting evidence suggests that supplementation with vitamin E or magnesium may reduce PMS symptoms, along with dysmenorrhea, perhaps by reducing prostaglandin levels.[105–107] Again, advise patients that more is not always better with supplements, and that their dose of vitamin E should not exceed 400 IU per day.[108]

Strong evidence does exist for the use of calcium supplementation in PMS. In the Nurses Health Study II, a large longitudinal cohort, women who consumed the most vitamin D and calcium were the least likely to develop PMS during 10 years of follow-up.[109] In addition, randomized controlled trials have demonstrated a reduction of PMS symptoms among women taking 1,200 to 1,600 mg of calcium carbonate daily.[110,111] Calcium may affect PMS symptomatology through its interaction with estrogen and parathyroid hormone. Higher doses of calcium should be avoided in women with histories of renal stones.

Herbal agents have grown in popularity in the United States and are used frequently by women for PMS. Chasteberry tree extract (Vitex agnus-castus in Latin) is used commonly in Europe for PMS and clinical breast pain; it is approved by the German Commission E for these indications. Small, randomized controlled trials support its use.[112] Evening primrose oil is also popularly used in Europe for PMS and breast tenderness (mastalgia), but randomized controlled studies have not validated the efficacy of this herb in the treatment of PMS.[113]

Progesterone supplementation, often with hormonal products marketed as natural or bio-identical, remains popular among women as a treatment for any degree of PMS despite scientific evidence of its lack of effectiveness.[80] A recent, comprehensive review of progesterone as a treatment for PMS failed to find evidence that this remedy is effective, *or that it is ineffective.*[114]

Ovulation suppressants may also be helpful in the treatment of PMS. COCs sometimes benefit women with mild to moderate symptoms of bloating and breast pain. However, for some COC users, depression, breast tenderness, and bloating increase with pill use, especially during the placebo pill days. Randomized, controlled trials of cyclic COC use for treatment of PMS have generated mixed results. Extended-cycle dosing of COCs, vaginal contraceptive rings and DMPA may aid PMS sufferers not only by suppressing ovulation, but also by reducing the number of withdrawal bleeding episodes (and associated symptoms) they experience.

Trials of cognitive therapy, group therapy, and relaxation therapy have shown that these modalities may improve physical or psychological symptoms of PMS, although few studies have randomized patients.[115] Stress management, anger management, self-help, biofeedback, acupuncture, reflexology, or light therapy may help some women.[115-118]

Treatment for Premenstrual Dysphoric Disorder

PMDD requires a different medical approach to deal with its severe symptoms and mood disorders. There are two classes of FDA-approved medications to treat the physical and emotional symptoms of PMDD. The first is a class of anti-depressant drugs known as selective serotonin reuptake inhibitors (SSRIs). Many randomized, placebo-controlled trials have demonstrated that SSRIs reduce both physical and psychological PMDD symptoms.[119-121] The FDA has specifically approved three drugs for PMDD (fluoxetine, sertraline, and paroxetine), which can be given at low doses continuously (every day) or intermittently (only during the luteal phase). Research has found that other agents related to SSRIs are equally effective, including citalopram and venlafaxine.[122] If one agent is not successful, try another one before abandoning SSRIs as a class, because an individual's response may vary from drug to drug. Recommend that the woman use effective contraception when she is using SSRIs.

Most women tolerate SSRIs without incident, but these medications can cause side effects, including nausea, decreased libido, and insomnia. Clinicians should counsel patients about these potential side effects and inquire about them at follow-up visits. The risk for side effects is related to dose; the use of low-dose SSRIs often suffices in treating both PMS and PMDD, and may minimize side effects;[123] monthly dosing during the luteal phase has also proven effective in PMDD, with rapid improvement of symptoms noted within a day or two of the first dose each cycle.[124]

The other FDA-approved therapy for PMDD is the monophasic oral contraceptive with active pills containing 20 mcg EE and 3 mg drospirenone in a 24/4 formulation. Randomized placebo-controlled, double-blinded clinical prospective studies found that both mood disorders and physical complaints of PMDD were reduced by about 50% with this COC, which was significantly superior to the placebo effect.[125] Interestingly, this is the same order of magnitude seen in response to SSRIs.

Clinical experience supports off-label use of other medications to treat PMDD. For women who cannot tolerate SSRIs but who would benefit from psychotropic medication, buspirone and anxiolytic medications provide an alternative.[126] Alprazolam has demonstrated efficacy in PMDD, but the most effective pattern of use has not been defined. Some studies have found therapeutic response with intermittent use of alprazolam (e.g., 4 to 5 days preceding menses), while other studies have found such protocols no better than placebo. The clinician must individualize therapy. To avoid withdrawal symptoms, taper the alprazolam each time it is discontinued. Be careful when prescribing anxiolytic medicines because they are habit-forming and have potential for abuse. Women with histories of alcoholism or other substance abuse are not appropriate candidates. Caution women that the drug may make them feel drowsy; the first dose should be taken at home, before bedtime, to gauge its effect.

Counseling may be very beneficial for women with PMDD and their families. Stress management, anger management, self–help support groups, individual and couple therapy, cognitive behavioral therapy, and light therapy all have been reported to provide relief.[117] Selection depends upon an individual woman's symptoms and her ability to access resources.

MENSTRUAL EXACERBATION OF OTHER MEDICAL CONDITIONS

Worsening of medical conditions is very common during the luteal phase and during menses.[127] This may reflect the complex, often poorly understood interplay of hormones with other physiologic processes throughout the body. A classic example is menstrual migraines; about 50% of migraine headaches in women are menstrually related.[128] About 7% to 9% of women with migraines have them only with menses, while 35% to 40% of migraine sufferers experience worsening of headaches with menses.[129-132] One approach to menstrual migraine has been to treat prophylactically during at-risk times with standard migraine treatments. Some have recommended home fertility monitors to predict menses more accurately, to better time therapy.[133] However, because headaches have been definitely linked to a decline in estrogen levels,[134,135] another approach has been to suppress menses with extended cycle hormones or to provide estrogen supplementation during bleeding days. The use of estrogen is appropriate only for women who do not suffer neurologic auras preceding the onset of their migraines or suffer worsening of their headaches with estrogen exposure (see Chapter 11).

Women with seizure disorders frequently experience acute exacerbations of their convulsive activity with menstruation; 10% to 70% of women with epilepsy are affected by catamenial (menses-related) epilepsy.[136,137] Premenstrual increases in asthma attacks have been reported in up to 40% of women with this problem.[138] Virtually every woman knows that acne lesions tend to blossom around the time of menses. Less common medical conditions that flare around the time of menses include acute intermittent porphyria, diabetes, erythema multiforme, glaucoma, hereditary angioedema, rheumatoid arthritis, and multiple sclerosis.[127]

Mental health problems tend to become more symptomatic at the time of menses. Women with anxiety disorders and pain disorders tend to experience more anxiety and panic attacks during menses. Symptoms of obsessive-compulsive disorders have been found to increase before menstruation, and women with psychotic disorders also tend to suffer more intense symptoms during menses.[139] Worsening of symptoms of schizophrenia during the luteal phase has been reported.[139,140] There is some evidence that women with bulimia may experience increased food cravings premenstrually.[141]

Suppressing ovulation alone (ENG implant) or eliminating menses by controlling the endometrium alone (LNg intrauterine contraceptive) may not suffice as adequate therapy for women whose medical conditions fluctuate in response to hormonal cycling. However, it is possible to prevent hormonal fluctuations with DMPA or extended cycle use of combined hormonal methods. Selection of the appropriate method depends upon the woman's health, as well as her personal preferences.

REFERENCES

1. Fraser IS, Critchley HO, Munro MG, Broder M; Writing Group for this Menstrual Agreement Process. A process designed to lead to international agreement on terminologies and definitions used to describe abnormalities of menstrual bleeding. *Fertil Steril.* 2007;87:466–76.
2. Fraser IS, Critchley HO, Munro MG. Abnormal uterine bleeding: getting our terminology straight. Curr Opin Obstet Gynecol. 2007;19:591–5.
3. Practice Committee of American Society for Reproductive Medicine. Current evaluation of amenorrhea. Fertil Steril. 2008;90(5 Suppl):S219–25.
4. Drinkwater BL, Bruemner B, Chesnut CH 3rd. Menstrual history as a determinant of current bone density in young athletes. JAMA. 1990;263:545–8.
5. Garner DM, Rosen LW, Barry D. Eating disorders among athletes. Research and recommendations. Child Adolesc Psychiatr Clin N Am. 1998;7:839–57.
6. Shangold M, Rebar RW, Wentz AC, Schiff I. Evaluation and management of menstrual dysfunction in athletes. JAMA. 1990;263:1665–9.

7. Hergenroeder AC, Smith EO, Shypailo R, Jones LA, Klish WJ, Ellis K. Bone mineral changes in young women with hypothalamic amenorrhea treated with oral contraceptives, medroxyprogesterone or placebo over 12 months. Am J Obstet Gynecol. 1997;176:1017–25.
8. Yildiz BO, Knochenhauer ES, Azziz R. Impact of obesity on the risk for polycystic ovary syndrome. J Clin Endocrinol Metab. 2008;93:162–8.
9. Carmina E, Lobo RA. Polycystic ovaries in Hirsute women with normal menses. Am J Med. 2001;111:602–6.
10. Rotterdam ESHRE/ASRM-Sponsored PCOS Consensus Workshop Group. Revised 2003 consensus on diagnostic criteria and long-term health risks related to polycystic ovary syndrome. Fertil Steril. 2004;81:19–25.
11. Legro RS, Chiu P, Kunselman AR, Bentley CM, Dodson WC, Dunaif A. Polycystic ovaries are common in women with hyperandrogenic chronic anovulation but do not predict metabolic or reproductive phenotype. J Clin Endocrinol Metab. 2005;90:2571–9.
12. Apridonidze T, Essah PA, Iuorno MJ, Nestler JE. Prevalence and characteristics of the metabolic syndrome in women with polycystic ovary syndrome. J Clin Endocrinol Metab. 2005;90:1929–35.
13. Graf MJ, Richards CJ, Brown V, Meissner L, Dunaif A. The independent effects of hyperandrogenaemia, hyperinsulinaemia, and obesity on lipid and lipoprotein profiles in women. Clin Endocrinol. 1990;33:119–31.
14. ACOG Committee on Practice Bulletins–Gynecology. ACOG Practice Bulletin No. 108: Polycystic ovary syndrome. Obstet Gynecol. 2009;114:936–49.
15. Thessaloniki ESHRE/ASRM-Sponsored PCOS Consensus Workshop Group. Consensus on infertility treatment related to polycystic ovary syndrome. Fertil Steril. 2008;89:505–22.
16. Azziz R. Diagnostic criteria for polycystic ovary syndrome: a reappraisal. Fertil Steril. 2005;83:1343–6.
17. Pereira MA, Swain J, Goldfine AB, Rifai N, Ludwig DS. Effects of a low-glycemic load diet on resting energy expenditure and heart disease risk factors during weight loss. JAMA. 2004;292:2482–90.
18. Jayagopal V, Kilpatrick ES, Holding S, Jennings PE, Atkin SL. Orlistat is as beneficial as metformin in the treatment of polycystic ovarian syndrome. J Clin Endocrinol Metab. 2005;90:729–33.
19. Dragoman M, Davis A, Banks E. Contraceptive options for women with preexisting medical conditions. J Womens Health (Larchmt). 2010;19:575–80.
20. Legro RS, Barnhart HX, Schlaff WD, Carr BR, Diamond MP, Carson SA, et al. Cooperative Multicenter Reproductive Medicine Network. Clomiphene, metformin, or both for infertility in the polycystic ovary syndrome. N Engl J Med. 2007;356:551–66.
21. Wild RA, Carmina E, Diamanti-Kandarakis E, Dokras A, Escobar-Morreale HF, Futterweit W, et al. Assessment of cardiovascular risk and prevention of cardiovascular disease in women with the polycystic ovary syndrome: a consensus statement by the Androgen Excess and Polycystic Ovary Syndrome (AE-PCOS) Society. J Clin Endocrinol Metab. 2010;95:2038–49.
22. Prentice A. Fortnightly review. Medical management of menorrhagia. BMJ. 1999;319:1343–5.
23. Côté I, Jacobs P, Cumming D. Work loss associated with increased menstrual loss in the United States. Obstet Gynecol. 2002;100:683–7.
24. Gath D, Cooper P, Day A. Hysterectomy and psychiatric disorder: I. Levels of psychiatric morbidity before and after hysterectomy. Br J Psychiatry. 1982;140:335–42.
25. Chimbira TH, Anderson AB, Turnbull A. Relation between measured menstrual blood loss and patient's subjective assessment of loss, duration of bleeding, number of sanitary towels used, uterine weight and endometrial surface area. Br J Obstet Gynaecol. 1980;87:603–9.

26. Fraser IS, McCarron G, Markham R, Resta T. Blood and total fluid content of menstrual discharge. Obstet Gynecol. 1985;65:194–8.
27. Philipp CS, Faiz A, Dowling N, Dilley A, Michaels LA, Ayers C, et al. Age and the prevalence of bleeding disorders in women with menorrhagia. Obstet Gynecol. 2005;105:61–6.
28. Kadir RA, Economides DL, Sabin CA, Owens D, Lee CA. Frequency of inherited bleeding disorders in women with menorrhagia. Lancet. 1998;351:485–9.
29. Claessens EA, Cowell CA. Dysfunctional uterine bleeding in the adolescent. Pediatr Clin North Am. 1981;28:369–71.
30. Munro MG, Lukes AS. Abnormal Uterine Bleeding and Underlying Hemostatic Disorders Consensus Group. Abnormal uterine bleeding and underlying hemostatic disorders: report of a consensus process. Fertil Steril. 2005;84:1335–7.
31. Widrich T, Bradley LD, Mitchinson AR, Collins RL. Comparison of saline infusion sonography with office hysteroscopy for the evaluation of the endometrium. Am J Obstet Gynecol. 1996;174:1327–34.
32. Clarke A, Black N, Rowe P, Mott S, Howle K. Indications for and outcome of total abdominal hysterectomy for benign disease: a prospective cohort study. Br J Obstet Gynaecol. 1995;102:611–20.
33. DeVore GR, Owens O, Kase N. Use of intravenous Premarin in the treatment of dysfunctional uterine bleeding–a double-blind randomized control study. Obstet Gynecol. 1982;59:285–91.
34. Munro MG, Mainor N, Basu R, Brisinger M, Barreda L. Oral medroxyprogesterone acetate and combination oral contraceptives for acute uterine bleeding: a randomized controlled trial. Obstet Gynecol. 2006;108:924–9.
35. Rees MC, Anderson AB, Demers LM, Turnbull AC. Prostaglandins in menstrual fluid in menorrhagia and dysmenorrhoea. Br J Obstet Gynaecol. 1984;91:673–80.
36. Lethaby A, Augood C, Duckitt K, Farquhar C. Nonsteroidal anti-inflammatory drugs for heavy menstrual bleeding. Cochrane Database Syst Rev. 2007 Oct 17:CD000400.
37. Edlund M, Blombäck M, He S. On the correlation between local fibrinolytic activity in menstrual fluid and total blood loss during menstruation and effects of desmopressin. Blood Coagul Fibrinolysis. 2003;14:593–8.
38. Gleeson N, Devitt M, Sheppard BL, Bonnar J. Endometrial fibrinolytic enzymes in women with normal menstruation and dysfunctional uterine bleeding. Br J Obstet Gynaecol. 1993;100:768–71.
39. Lethaby A, Farquhar C, Cooke I. Antifibrinolytics for heavy menstrual bleeding. Cochrane Database Syst Rev. 2000:CD000249.
40. FDA Approves Lysteda to Treat Heavy Menstrual Bleeding. Found at: www.fda. gov/NewsEvents/Newsroom/PressAnnouncements/2009/ucm190551.htm (accessed 04–27–10)
41. Preston JT, Cameron IT, Adams EJ, Smith SK. Comparative study of tranexamic acid and norethisterone in the treatment of ovulatory menorrhagia. Br J Obstet Gynaecol. 1995;102:401–6.
42. Schwallie PC, Assenzo JR. Contraceptive use–efficacy study utilizing medroxyprogesterone acetate administered as an intramuscular injection once every 90 days. Fertil Steril. 1973;24:331–9.
43. Endrikat J, Shapiro H, Lukkari-Lax E, Kunz M, Schmidt W, Fortier M. A Canadian, multicentre study comparing the efficacy of a levonorgestrel-releasing intrauterine system to an oral contraceptive in women with idiopathic menorrhagia. J Obstet Gynaecol Can. 2009;31:340–7.
44. Anderson FD, Hait H. A multicenter, randomized study of an extended cycle oral contraceptive. Contraception. 2003;68:89–96. Erratum in: Contraception 2004;69:175.
45. Miller L, Verhoeven CH, Hout J. Extended regimens of the contraceptive vaginal ring: a randomized trial. Obstet Gynecol. 2005;106:473–82.

46. Nelson AL. The LNG-IUS in Heavy Menstrual Bleeding: First-line treatment based on comprehensive clinical data. Presented at XIX FIGO World Congress of Gynecology and Obstetrics, Cape Town, South Africa 10/4–10/9/09.

47. Milsom I, Andersson K, Andersch B, Rybo G. A comparison of flurbiprofen, tranexamic acid, and a levonorgestrel-releasing intrauterine contraceptive device in the treatment of idiopathic menorrhagia. Am J Obstet Gynecol. 1991;164:879–83.

48. Cook JR, Seman EI. Pregnancy following endometrial ablation: case history and literature review. Obstet Gynecol Surv. 2003;58:551–6.

49. Hare AA, Olah KS. Pregnancy following endometrial ablation: a review article. J Obstet Gynaecol. 2005;25:108–14.

50. Lo JS, Pickersgill A. Pregnancy after endometrial ablation: English literature review and case report. J Minim Invasive Gynecol. 2006;13:88–91.

51. Marjoribanks J, Lethaby A, Farquhar C. Surgery versus medical therapy for heavy menstrual bleeding. Cochrane Database Syst Rev. 2006 Apr 19:CD003855.

52. Kaunitz AM, Meredith S, Inki P, Kubba A, Sanchez-Ramos L. Levonorgestrel-releasing intrauterine system and endometrial ablation in heavy menstrual bleeding: a systematic review and meta-analysis. Obstet Gynecol. 2009;113:1104–16.

53. de Souza SS, Camargos AF, de Rezende CP, Pereira FA, Araújo CA, Silva Filho AL. A randomized prospective trial comparing the levonorgestrel-releasing intrauterine system with thermal balloon ablation for the treatment of heavy menstrual bleeding. Contraception. 2010;81:226–31.

54. Hurskainen R, Teperi J, Rissanen P, Aalto AM, Grenman S, Kivelä A, et al. Clinical outcomes and costs with the levonorgestrel-releasing intrauterine system or hysterectomy for treatment of menorrhagia: randomized trial 5-year follow-up. JAMA. 2004;291:1456–63.

55. Andersch B, Milsom I. An epidemiologic study of young women with dysmenorrhea. Am J Obstet Gynecol. 1982;144:655–60.

56. Avant RF. Dysmenorrhea. Prim Care. 1988;15:549–59.

57. Berry C, McGuire FL. Menstrual distress and acceptance of sexual role. Am J Obstet Gynecol. 1972;114:83–7.

58. Smith RP. Cyclic pelvic pain and dysmenorrhea. Obstet Gynecol Clin North Am. 1993;20:753–64.

59. Wilson L, Kurzrok R. Uterine contractility in functional dysmenorrhea. Endocrinology. 1940;27:23–8.

60. Pickles VR, Hall WJ, Best FA, Smith GN. Prostaglandins in endometrium and menstrual fluid from normal and dysmenorrhoic subjects. J Obstet Gynaecol Br Commonw. 1965;72:185–92.

61. Ziaei S, Zakeri M, Kazemnejad A. A randomised controlled trial of vitamin E in the treatment of primary dysmenorrhoea. BJOG. 2005;112:466–9.

62. Zahradnik HP, Hanjalic-Beck A, Groth K. Nonsteroidal anti-inflammatory drugs and hormonal contraceptives for pain relief from dysmenorrhea: a review. Contraception. 2010;81:185–96.

63. Milsom I, Sundell G, Andersch B. The influence of different combined oral contraceptives on the prevalence and severity of dysmenorrhea. Contraception 1990; 42:497–506.

64. Robinson JC, Plichta S, Weisman CS, Nathanson CA, Ensminger M. Dysmenorrhea and use of oral contraceptives in adolescent women attending a family planning clinic. Am J Obstet Gynecol. 1992;166:578–83.

65. Coffee AL, Sulak PJ, Kuehl TJ. Long-term assessment of symptomatology and satisfaction of an extended oral contraceptive regimen. Contraception. 2007;75:444–9.

66. Miller L, Verhoeven CH, Hout J. Extended regimens of the contraceptive vaginal ring: a randomized trial. Obstet Gynecol. 2005;106:473–82.

67. Cho SH, Hwang EW. Acupuncture for primary dysmenorrhoea: a systematic review. BJOG. 2010;117:509–21.

68. Crosignani PG, Luciano A, Ray A, Bergqvist A. Subcutaneous depot medroxy-progesterone acetate versus leuprolide acetate in the treatment of endometriosis-associated pain. Hum Reprod. 2006;21:248–56.
69. Schlaff WD, Carson SA, Luciano A, Ross D, Bergqvist A. Subcutaneous injection of depot medroxyprogesterone acetate compared with leuprolide acetate in the treatment of endometriosis-associated pain. Fertil Steril. 2006;85:314–25.
70. Fedele L, Bianchi S, Raffaelli R, Portuese A, Dorta M. Treatment of adenomyosis-associated menorrhagia with a levonorgestrel-releasing intrauterine device. Fertil Steril. 1997;68:426–9.
71. Zupi E, Marconi D, Sbracia M, Zullo F, De Vivo B, Exacustos C, et al. Add-back therapy in the treatment of endometriosis-associated pain. Fertil Steril. 2004;82:1303–8.
72. Nawathe A, Patwardhan S, Yates D, Harrison GR, Khan KS. Systematic review of the effects of aromatase inhibitors on pain associated with endometriosis. BJOG. 2008;115:818–22. Review. Erratum in: BJOG. 2008;115:1069.
73. Arias RD. Premenstrual syndrome. In: Mishell DR Jr, Goodwin TM, Brener PF (eds). Management of common problems in obstetrics and gynecology, 4th ed. Boston: Blackwell Publishers, 2001.
74. ACOG Committee on Practice Bulletins. Premenstrual syndrome. ACOG Practice Bulletin 15. Washington DC: American College of Obstetricians and Gynecologists, 2000.
75. Borenstein JE, Dean BB, Endicott J, et al. Health and economic impact of the premenstrual syndrome. J Reprod Med. 2003;48:515–24.
76. Borenstein J, Chiou CF, Dean B, Wong J, Wade S. Estimating direct and indirect costs of premenstrual syndrome. J Occup Environ Med. 2005;47:26–33.
77. American Psychiatric Association. Diagnostic and statistical manual of mental disorders, fourth edition text revision (DSM-IV-TR). Washington DC: American Psychiatric Association, 2000:771–774.
78. Dalton K. The premenstrual syndrome and progesterone therapy, 2nd ed. Chicago: Mosby-Year Book Medical Publisher, 1984.
79. Rubinow DR, Hoban MC, Grover GN, Galloway DS, Roy-Byrne P, Andersen R, et al. Changes in plasma hormones across the menstrual cycle in patients with menstrually related mood disorder and in control subjects. Am J Obstet Gynecol. 1988;158:5–11.
80. Freeman EW, Rickels K, Sondheimer SJ, Polansky M. A double-blind trial of oral progesterone, alprazolam, and placebo in treatment of severe premenstrual syndrome. JAMA. 1995;274:51–7.
81. Schmidt PJ, Nieman LK, Danaceau MA, Adams LF, Rubinow DR. Differential behavioral effects of gonadal steroids in women with and those without premenstrual syndrome. New Engl J Med. 1998;338:209–16.
82. Chuong CJ, Coulam CB, Kao PC, Bergstralh EJ, Go VL. Neuropeptide levels in premenstrual syndrome. Fertil Steril. 1985;44:760–5.
83. Straneva PA, Maixner W, Light KC, Pedersen CA, Costello NL, Girdler SS. Menstrual cycle, beta-endorphins, and pain sensitivity in premenstrual dysphoric disorder. Health Psychol. 2002;4:358–67.
84. Redei E, Freeman EW. Preliminary evidence for plasma adrenocorticotropin levels as biological correlates of premenstrual symptoms. Acta Endocrinol. (Copenh) 1993; 128:536–42.
85. Mira M, Stewart PM, Abraham SF. Vitamin and trace element status in premenstrual syndrome. Am J Clin Nutr. 1988;47:636–641.
86. Perkonigg A, Yonkers KA, Pfister H., Lieb R, Wittchen HU. Risk factors for premenstrual dysphoric disorder in a community sample of young women: the role of traumatic events and posttraumatic stress disorder. J Clin Psychiatry. 2004;65:1314–22.
87. Mortola JF. Premenstrual syndrome-pathophysiologic considerations. New Engl J Med. 1998;338:256–7.

88. Halbreich U, Monacelli E. Some clues to the etiology of premenstrual syndrome/premenstrual dysphoric disorder. Prim Psychiatry. 2004;11:33–40.
89. Rapkin AJ. The role of serotonin in premenstrual syndrome. Clin Obstet Gynecol. 1992;35:629–36.
90. Rubinow DR, Roy-Bryne P, Hoban MC, et al. Prospective assessment of menstrually related mood disorders. Am J Psychiatry. 1984;141:684–6.
91. Harrison WM, Rabkin JG, Endicott J. Psychiatric evaluation of premenstrual changes. Psychosomatics. 1985;26:789–92,795,798–9.
92. Fava M, Pedrazzi F, Guaraldi GP, Romano G, Genazzani AR, Facchinetti F. Comorbid anxiety and depression among patients with late luteal phase dysphoric disorder. J Anxiety Disorders. 1992;6:325–35.
93. Steiner M, Macdougall M, Brown E. The premenstrual symptoms screening tool (PSST) for clinicians. Arch Women Ment Health. 2003;6:203–9.
94. Feuerstein M, Shaw WS. Measurement properties of the calendar of premenstrual experience in patients with premenstrual syndrome. J Reprod Med. 2002;47:279–89.
95. Endicott J, Nee J, Harrison W. Daily record of severity of problems (DRSP): reliability and validity. Arch Women Ment Health. 2006;9:41–9.
96. Choi PY, Salmon P. Symptom changes across the menstrual cycle in competitive sportswomen, exercisers, and sedentary women. Br J Clin Psychol. 1995;34:447–60.
97. Prior JC, Vigna Y, Sciarretta D, Alojado N Schulzer M. Conditioning exercise decreases premenstrual symptoms: a prospective controlled 6 month trial. Fertil Steril. 1987;47:402–8.
98. Steege JF, Blumenthal JA. The effects of aerobic exercise on premenstrual symptoms in middle-aged women: a preliminary study. J Psychosom Res. 1993;37:127–33.
99. Johnson WG, Carr-Nangle RE, Bergeron KC. Macronutrient intake, eating habits, and exercise as moderators of menstrual distress in healthy women. Psychosom Med. 1995;57:324–30.
100. Rossignol AM. Caffeine-containing beverages and premenstrual syndrome in young women. Am J Public Health. 1985;75:1335–7.
101. Sayegh R, Schiff I, Wurtman J, et al. The effect of a carbohydrate- beverage on mood, appetite, and cognitive function in women with premenstrual syndrome. Obstet Gynecol. 1995;86:520–528.
102. Stevinson C, Ernst E. Complementary and alternative therapies for premenstrual syndrome: a systematic review of randomized controlled trials. Am J Obstet Gynecol. 2001;185:227–35.
103. Wyatt KM, Dimmock PW, Jones PW, Shaughn O'Brien PM. Efficacy of vitamin B-6 in the treatment of premenstrual syndrome: systematic review. BMJ. 1999;318:1375–81.
104. London RS, Bradley L, Chiamori NY. Effect of a nutritional supplement on premenstrual symptomatology in women with premenstrual syndrome: a doubleblind longitudinal study. J Am Coll Nutr. 1991;10:494.
105. Facchinetti F, Borella P, Sances G, et al. Oral magnesium successfully relieves premenstrual mood changes. Obstet Gynecol. 1991;78:177–81.
106. Girman A, Lee R, Kligler B. An integrative medicine approach to premenstrual syndrome. Am J Obstet Gynecol. 2003;188:S56–65.
107. Walker AF, De Souza MC, Vickers MF, Abeyasekera S, Collins ML, Trinca LA. Magnesium supplementation alleviates premenstrual symptoms of fluid retention. J Womens Health. 1998;7:1157–65.
108. Miller ER, Pastor-Barriuso R, Dalal D, et al. Meta-analysis: high-dosage vitamin E supplementation may increase all-cause mortality. Ann Intern Med. 2005;142:37–46.
109. Bertone-Johnson ER, Hankinson SE, Bendich A, et al. Calcium and vitamin D intake and risk of incident premenstrual syndrome. Arch Intern Med. 2005;165:1246–52.
110. Thys-Jacobs S, Ceccarelli S, Bierman A, Weisman H, Cohen M, Alvir J. Calcium supplementation in premenstrual syndrome: a randomized crossover trial. J Gen Intern Med. 1989;4:183–9.

111. Thys-Jacobs S, Starkey P, Bernstein D, Tian J. Calcium carbonate and the premenstrual syndrome: effects on premenstrual and menstrual symptoms. Premenstrual Syndrome Study Group. Am J Obstet Gynecol. 1998;179:444–52.

112. Blumenthal M. German Federal Institute for Drugs and Medical Devices. Commission E. Herbal Medicine: expanded Commission E monographs. 1st ed. Newton, MA: Integrative Medicine Communications, 2000.

113. Budeiri D, Li Wan Po A, Dornan JC. Is evening primrose oil of value in the treatment of premenstrual syndrome? Control Clin Trials. 1996;17:60–8.

114. Ford O, Lethaby A, Roberts H, Mol BW. Progesterone for premenstrual syndrome. Cochrane Database Syst Rev. 2009; CD003415.

115. Goodale IL, Domar AD, Benson H. Alleviation of premenstrual syndrome with the relaxation response. Obstet Gynecol. 1990;75:649–655.

116. Oleson T, Flocco W. Randomized controlled study of premenstrual symptoms treated with ear, hand and foot reflexology. Obstet Gynecol.1993;82:906–911.

117. Van Zak DB. Biofeedback treatments for premenstrual and premenstrual affective syndromes. Int J Psychosom. 1994;41:53–60.

118. Lam RW, Carter D, Misri S, et al. A controlled study of light therapy in women with late luteal phase disorder. Psychiatry Res.1999;86:185–92.

119. Steiner M, Steinberg S, Stewart D, Carter D, Berger C, Reid R, et al. Fluoxetine in the treatment of premenstrual dysphoria. N Engl J Med. 1995; 332:1529–1534.

120. Yonkers KA, Halbreich U, Freeman E, et al. Symptomatic improvement of premenstrual dysphoric disorder with sertraline treatment. A randomized controlled trial. Sertraline Premenstrual Dysphoric Collaborative Study Group. JAMA. 1997;278: 983–8.

121. Steiner M, Hirschberg AL, Bergeron R, et al. Luteal phase dosing with paroxetine controlled release (CR) in the treatment of premenstrual dysphoric disorder. Am J Obstet Gynecol. 2005;193:352–60.

122. Freeman EW, Rickels K, Yonkers KA, et al. Venlafaxine in the treatment of premenstrual dysphoric disorder. Obstet Gynecol. 2001;98:737–44.

123. Steiner M, Steinberg S, Stewart D, Carter D, Berger C, Reid R, et al. Fluoxetine in the treatment of premenstrual dysphoria. N Engl J Med. 1995;332:1529–1534.

124. Halbreich U and Smoller JW. Intermittent luteal phase sertraline treatment of dysphoric premenstrual syndrome. J Clin Psychiatry. 1997;58:399–402.

125. Yonkers KA, Brown C, Pearlstein TB, Foegh M, Sampson-Landers C, Rapkin A. Efficacy of a new low-dose oral contraceptive with drospirenone in premenstrual dysphoric disorder. Obstet Gynecol. 2005;106:492–501.

126. Rapkin AJ, Winer SA. The pharmacologic management of premenstrual dysphoric disorder. Expert Opin Pharmacother. 2008;9:429–45.

127. Pinkerton JV, Guico-Pabia CJ, Taylor HS. Menstrual cycle-related exacerbation of disease. Am J Obstet Gynecol. 2010;202:221–31.

128. Brandes JL. The influence of estrogen on migraine: a systematic review. JAMA. 2006;295:1824–30.

129. Martin V, Brandes JL. IMED Communications. Strategies for optimizing management of menstrual migraine. J Fam Pract. 2005;54:S1–7;quiz S8.

130. Cupini LM, Matteis M, Troisi E, et al. Sex-hormone-related events in migrainous females. A clinical comparative study between migraine with aura and migraine without aura. Cephalalgia. 1995;15:140–4.

131. Granella F, Sances G, Allais G, et al. Characteristics of menstrual and nonmenstrual attacks in women with menstrually related migraine referred to headache centres. Cephalalgia. 2004;24:707–16.

132. Martin VT. Menstrual migraine: a review of prophylactic therapies. Curr Pain Headache Rep. 2004;8:229–37.

133. MacGregor EA, Frith A, Ellis J, Aspinall L. Predicting menstrual migraine with a home-use fertility monitor. Neurology. 2005;64:561–3.

134. Somerville BW. The role of estradiol withdrawal in the etiology of menstrual migraine. Neurology. 1972;22:355–365.
135. Somerville BW. The role of progesterone in menstrual migraine. Neurology. 1971; 21:853–9.
136. Reddy DS. Pharmacology of catamenial epilepsy. Methods Find Exp Clin Pharmacol. 2004;26:547–61.
137. Foldvary-Schaefer N, Falcone T. Catamenial epilepsy: pathophysiology, diagnosis, and management. Neurology. 2003;61:S2–15.
138. Tan KS. Premenstrual asthma: epidemiology, pathogenesis and treatment. Drugs. 2001;61:2079–86.
139. Hsiao MC, Hsiao CC, Liu CY. Premenstrual symptoms and premenstrual exacerbation in patients with psychiatric disorders. Psychiatry Clin Neurosci. 2004;58:186–90.
140. Dennerstein L, Judd F, Davies B. Psychosis and the menstrual cycle. Med J Aust. 1983;1:524–6.
141. Gladis MM, Walsh BT. Premenstrual exacerbation of binge eating in bulimia. Am J Psychiatry. 1987;144:1592–5.

LATE REFERENCE

142. Wei S, Venn A, Dig C, Foley S, Laslett L, Jones G. The association between oral contraceptive use, bone mineral density and fractures in women aged 50–80 years. Contraception. 2011 (in press).

Reproductive Tract Infections, Including HIV and Other Sexually Transmitted Infections

Jeanne M. Marrazzo, MD, MPH
Willard Cates, Jr., MD, MPH

- Reproductive tract infections (RTI) are frequently encountered by reproductive health professionals.

- RTI include both sexually transmitted infections and also other common infections of the genital tract, such as bacterial vaginosis and vulvovaginal candidiasis.

- RTI can have four serious health consequences:

  — Tubal occlusion leading to infertility and ectopic pregnancy

  — Pregnancy loss and neonatal morbidity caused by transmission of the infection to the infant during pregnancy and childbirth

  — Genital cancers

  — Enhanced transmission of the human immunodeficiency virus (HIV)

- Assessing a client's risks for RTI can help the client better select appropriate contraceptive methods and help the clinician provide better care. Ask each patient, "What do you do to protect yourself from infection with HIV and other sexually transmitted infections?"

- Preventing RTI and their consequences requires sexually active persons to adopt safer sexual behaviors and clinicians to diagnose and treat existing infections effectively.

- Because reproductive-age women constitute a major segment of the HIV epidemic in the United States, reproductive health care settings are a critical conduit to HIV testing. Offer counseling and voluntary HIV testing to each patient.

- Routine HIV testing for all pregnant women is the standard of care for prenatal services. Be certain that HIV-infected pregnant women have access to antiretroviral drug regimens that can improve health status, reduce viral load, and reduce the likelihood of perinatal transmission.

In *Contraceptive Technology*, the generic term RTI covers three types of infections: (1) sexually transmitted infections (STI), (2) vaginal infections including bacterial vaginosis and candidiasis, and (3) iatrogenic infections associated with the insertion of intrauterine contraception (IUC) or induced abortion. While prevention of infection through risk reduction and screening/treatment are the most effective ways to reduce the adverse consequences of RTI, recognition and correct management of RTI that do occur can prevent complications in the individual and interrupt transmission in the community. This chapter provides general background about RTI management in the reproductive health care setting.

MAGNITUDE AND RISKS OF RTI

The number of people infected with RTI or affected by their consequences is a major problem for society.[1] For example, in 2008, the highest number of sexually transmitted *Chlamydia trachomatis* cases (well over one million: 1,210,523) were reported to the Centers for Disease Control and Prevention (CDC).[2] This is the largest number of infections ever reported to CDC for any condition. STI are the most common cause of pelvic inflammatory diseases (PID). Infertility caused by PID accounts for billions of healthcare costs, as well as major emotional cost. Although deaths due to some RTI (primarily syphilis and PID) have declined over the past four decades, bacterial RTI still cause almost one third of the reproductive mortality in the United States, and HIV-related mortality has become a leading cause of death in reproductive-age persons—particularly women—worldwide.

While the prevalence of RTI by individual pathogen and across different geographic regions varies considerably, some general trends are consistently observed. For example, individuals under 25 years of age account for a majority of RTI cases, with two-thirds of cases of gonorrhea and chlamydia reported in persons less than 25 years of age. Rates of chlamydia, gonorrhea, and PID are highest in adolescents and decline steadily with increasing age. RTI are also concentrated in socio-geographic clusters, so-called "core populations," that generally reflect sexual networks, regional variation in disease prevalence and, possibly, access to care.

Finally, most RTI exhibit a "biological sexism." Compared with men, women suffer more severe long-term consequences, including PID, infertility, ectopic pregnancy, chronic pelvic pain, and cervical cancer. Women may also be less likely to seek health care for assessment of RTI-related symptoms, because a higher proportion of their RTI are asymptomatic or unrecognized as being serious. Due to the transmission dynamics of vaginal intercourse, women are more likely than men to acquire RTI from any single heterosexual encounter. The risk of acquisition increases when trauma occurs to the genital mucosa, as may be the case in sexual assault, but it decreases in the absence of penile-vaginal intercourse, as is the case with sex between women.

TRANSMISSION OF RTI

The probability that unprotected sexual intercourse will lead to RTI or its consequences differs from the probability of unintended pregnancy (Table 21–1). The risk of pregnancy varies according to the menstrual cycle. In contrast, while numerous complex factors probably modulate susceptibility to RTI, the risk of acquisition depends on (1) having sex with an infected person, (2) the gender of the infected person, (3) transmissibility of the particular RTI, and (4) use of barrier or other protective measures.[3] For example, the risk of acquiring gonorrhea from a single act of vaginal intercourse (where one partner is infectious) is approximately 25% for men and 50% for women. The probability of suffering consequences from an RTI depends on whether or not proper diagnosis and treatment occur. In the case of HIV, the quantity of serum (and presumably genital) HIV viral load directly influences risk of transmitting HIV

Table 21–1 Comparative risk of adverse consequences from coitus: RTI and unintended pregnancy

Unintended pregnancy/coital act[a]	• 17%–30% midcycle • < 1% during menses
Gonococcal transmission/coital act[b]	• 50% infected male, uninfected female • 25% infected female, uninfected male
PID per woman infected with cervical gonorrhea[c]	• 40% if not treated • 0% if promptly and adequately treated
Tubal infertility per PID episode[d]	• 8% after first episode • 20% after second episode • 40% after third or more episodes

[a] Trussell J, Kost K. Contraceptive failure in the United States: a critical review of the literature. Stud Fam Plann 1987;18:237–83.

[b] Anderson RM. Transmission dynamics of sexually transmitted infections. In: Holmes KK, et al., ed. Sexually Transmitted Diseases. 3rd ed. New York: McGraw Hill; 1999:25–37.

[c] Platt R, Rice PA, McCormack WM. Risk of acquiring gonorrhea and prevalence of abnormal adnexal findings among women recently exposed to gonorrhea. JAMA. 1983;250:3205-9.

[d] Westrom L, Joesoef R, Reynolds G, Hagdu A, Thompson SE. Pelvic inflammatory disease and fertility. A cohort study of 1,844 women with laparoscopically verified disease and 657 control women with normal laparoscopic results. Sex Transm Dis. 1992;19:195–9.

to vulnerable partners. HIV viral load is extremely high in the context of early infection (the first several months after a person acquires the virus). Because sexual transmission of HIV frequently occurs during this early infection interval,[4] persons at risk need to consider HIV protection at all times.

Research related to preventing sexual transmission of HIV is ongoing. Most recently, studies in Africa indicate that circumcision of male partners can significantly reduce the risk of these men acquiring HIV and other RTI from their female partners.[5] Topical microbicides containing antiretroviral agents, like tenofovir, also appear to hold promise for protecting women against infection with HIV.[13]

R TI RISK ASSESSMENT, PREVENTION AND RISK BEHAVIORS

Different individuals accept different levels of risk. Not everyone will follow every safer sex recommendation but, with the proper knowledge, each person can make his or her own informed choices about reducing risk. While some prevention messages are universal and should be reinforced (for example, barrier methods when appropriate), the use of client-centered counseling highlights the need to individualize risk assessment and tailor risk reduction plans. The latter may include a discussion on selecting sex partners and building skills for negotiating safer sex.

Preventive measures for avoiding RTI transmission are generally consistent with guidelines for reducing risk of HIV infection. Risk-free options include having a mutually faithful relationship with an uninfected partner or completely abstaining from sexual activities that involve semen, blood, or other body fluids, or that allow for skin-to-skin contact. Examining a partner for lesions, discussing each new partner's previous sexual history, and avoiding partners who have had many previous sex partners, or known high-risk partners, can augment other measures to prevent RTI transmission. Educating people about their bodies and teaching them to be active participants in their health care gives them more control over their reproductive health.

Contraceptive Choice

Choice of contraception directly affects the risk of RTI (Table 21–2). Condoms reduce the risks of both bacterial and viral RTI; the evidence is strongest for condom effectiveness against HIV, trichomoniasis, genital herpes, and gonorrhea.[3] No recent data support spermicides' ability to prevent bacterial or viral infections, including HIV.[3] Diaphragms provide a barrier against cervical infection, but recent data have not demonstrated protection against HIV and most other RTI.[6] In addition, diaphragms have been associated with changes in vaginal flora and urinary tract infections. Although oral contraceptives are usually associated with an increase in chlamydia detected in the cervix, they protect against symptomatic PID, but not asymptomatic endometritis.[7] Depot medroxy-progesterone acetate (DMPA) use has been associated with an increased risk of HIV acquisition and of chlamydial RTI infection in some studies.[8,9] Intrauterine contraception (IUC) is associated with a transient increased risk of PID in the first month after insertion, but after this, the RTI risk declines to levels seen in women without IUC. IUC has a strong record of safety, even for HIV-infected women.[11] At present, the data are insufficient to state whether the progesterone-releasing method of IUC has a differential effect on RTI acquisition or natural history.

Microbicides, defined as substances used topically that interrupt the ability of infectious agents to establish infection, hold promise for prevention of both HIV and other STI. (See Chapter 14 on Vaginal Barriers and Spermicides and Chapter 19 on Contraceptive Research and Development.) The search for a nonspecific microbicide that offers protection against a wide variety of STI, including HIV, has yielded disappointing results, and no available microbicide offers protection against RTI. In one study, frequent use of nonoxynol-9 gel was associated with an increased risk of HIV acquisition.[12] However, vaginal delivery of drugs such as tenofovir, with specific antiretroviral activity against HIV, appears more promising. Use of tenofovir gel applied vaginally before and after sexual intercourse significantly reduced the rate of HIV acquisition (by 39%) in

Table 21–2 Effects of contraceptives on bacterial and viral RTI

Contraceptive Methods	Bacterial RTI	Viral RTI
Condoms	Protective	Protective
Spermicides	No evidence of protection	Not protective
Diaphragms	Protective against cervical infection	Protective against cervical neoplasia
Hormonal Contraceptives	Associated with increased cervical chlamydia Protective against symptomatic PID, but not unrecognized endometritis Effect may depend on estrogen vs. progesterone effects	Not protective
IUD	Associated with PID in first month after insertion	Not protective
Fertility Awareness	Not protective	Not protective

Source: Adapted from Cates and Padian (2000).[10]
See chapters on specific contraceptive methods for details.

a study of South African women.[13] Additional dosing regimens (e.g., daily use) are under study.

Other Risk Behaviors

In addition to sexual behaviors, other practices have been linked to RTI risk. Routine douching for hygiene has been associated with an increased risk of PID and ectopic pregnancy. Douching is a risk factor for bacterial vaginosis because it eradicates commensal hydrogen peroxide-producing vaginal *Lactobacillus* species.[14] Genital washing or urinating postcoitally have been poorly studied but appear to have little effect, if any, on reducing the risk of acquiring an RTI. In some studies, these practices have been associated with an increased risk of HIV acquisition. Finally, post-exposure prophylaxis (for example, after an unprotected sexual encounter in which RTI is suspected in one partner) has not been well studied for RTI prevention; it is currently recommended only in managing sexual assault.

Drug use influences the transmission of RTI. Although not sexually transmitted, blood-borne transmission through needle sharing occurs for hepatitis C, hepatitis B, and HIV. While hepatitis C is not typically considered an RTI, this virus has been identified in genital secretions (particularly in HIV-infected persons,[15] and the risk of sexual transmission, while probably low in the absence of exposure to blood, is not zero. Use of drugs such as methamphetamine and cocaine—whether through intravenous, intranasal, or other routes—has been associated with risky sexual behaviors. Outbreaks of syphilis, antibiotic-resistant gonorrhea, and chancroid have been linked to drug-related sexual behaviors and to sexual networks of drug users. Crystal methamphetamine has figured prominently in national outbreaks of syphilis in men who have sex with men, and the drug is especially harmful for its disinhibitory effects on sexual behavior. Abuse of alcohol, particularly binge drinking, has also been associated with risky sexual practices, including not using condoms;[16] alcohol abuse is a notable concern for adolescents.

ASSESSMENT, DIAGNOSIS, AND TREATMENT OF RTI

Comprehensive RTI-related care begins with routine risk assessment. Risk assessment should not be discarded due to common assumptions based on prior experience either with the individual patient (for example, a married patient) or with "representative" types of patients (for example, patients who identify as "lesbian"). At a minimum, ask clients about recent numbers of sex partners, anatomic sites exposed during sex (vagina, rectum, oropharynx), and personal protective measures (e.g.,

Table 21–3 Recommendations for annual screening of women for genital infection with *Chlamydia trachomatis*

- All asymptomatic sexually active women < 25 years old
- Women of any age at risk for infection, defined as
  - Inconsistent condom use
  - New sex partner in preceding 3 months
  - Multiple sex partners in preceding 3 months
- Presence of cervicitis

Ref: U.S. Preventive Services Task Force.[18]

condoms). Risk assessment also helps clinicians provide better contraceptive counseling and more cost-efficient RTI management. Balance the variety of demographic, behavioral, and clinical information (other than laboratory test results) to assess the likelihood that clients are infected with an RTI or are at high risk of future infection and to counsel clients in selecting appropriate contraceptive methods. For example, an RTI risk assessment scale can help identify women who may be good candidates for barrier methods or inappropriate candidates for IUC.[17]

Laboratory diagnosis of most RTI can be performed in nearly every reproductive health care setting. For example, over the past decade, routine screening for chlamydia has been associated with a decreased prevalence of the infection among clients attending family planning clinics in several regions of the country, and with concomitant declines in PID and ectopic pregnancy.[18] In addition, some family planning clinics have extended their range of services to male clients, including RTI diagnosis, treatment, and counseling. Many clinics provide *expedited partner management*, defined as provision of medications or a prescription for the partner of the index woman being treated, without a requirement for examination.

Routine screening for RTI. Because most RTI are asymptomatic and do not cause clinical signs such as cervicitis or PID, routine screening can provide early detection and prompt treatment, thus interrupting the progression to the sequelae of untreated disease. Chlamydial infections are the prototype, since up to 90% of these infections cause neither symptoms nor clinical signs (namely, cervicitis) in women. The U.S. Preventive Services Task Force recommends routine annual screening for target groups of women, as delineated in Table 21–3.[18] Indications for gonorrhea screening are less clear, but take into account the patient's recent history of STI, her high-risk exposures (for example, sex with a partner having chlamydia or gonorrhea, or with a symptomatic partner), and the local prevalence.[19] Adults in the United States should be screened for HIV at least once, and more frequently if at ongoing risk of acquisition.[19] Patients should be counseled about the asymptomatic nature of most RTI and that transmission typically occurs in the absence of symptoms.[20]

COUNSELING PATIENTS ABOUT RTI DIAGNOSIS AND TREATMENT

Counseling patients with RTI requires an approach different than that generally used in family planning settings. For couples trying to prevent unplanned pregnancies, counseling is typically nondirective to allow maximal opportunity for them to make an informed choice of the best contraceptive method. However, for patients who have RTI, *directive* counseling is important to prevent new infections, increase adherence to treatment and follow-up, and offer guidance on talking to partners about their RTI exposure. Patients must be made aware of both the potential serious consequences of RTI and the behaviors that increase the likelihood of reinfection.

Education about infection and treatment. Make sure patients understand what RTI they have, how it is transmitted, why it must be treated, and exactly when and how to take prescribed medication. Because unpleasant side effects from some medications may discourage patients from continuing treatment, discuss what to expect and ways to minimize side effects. For example, doxycycline taken on an empty stomach may cause nausea that prompts the patient to stop taking the medication. Advise taking the medication with food.

Completion of treatment. Urge patients to finish their entire supply of medication even though symptoms, if present, may diminish or disappear in a few days. Discontinuing antibiotics before the infection is completely cured can lead to recurrent infection and increase the likelihood that hard-to-cure strains of the pathogen may flourish.

Abstinence during treatment. Advise patients to avoid sex until they complete the full course of therapy (or, for single-dose therapy like azithromycin, for the week following treatment).

Partner management. Failure to treat the partners of women with RTI is the most important risk factor influencing the high rates of chlamydia and gonorrhea recurrence in the months after initial treatment. An increasing number of family planning professionals are being trained in partner management skills. Confidentiality is crucial, just as it is in all aspects of family planning and RTI care. Sex partner(s) should be notified and treated to prevent both reinfection of the patient and spread of disease through the community. Assist patients in notifying their partners by coaching them in partner notification techniques (patient referral) and using local sexually transmitted disease program staff (provider referral) to help evaluate and treat partners. Increasingly, the approach of *expedited partner management*, in which the patient is given either drugs or a prescription to give to partners without requiring that the partner be examined, has been recognized as a highly effective way to increase the likelihood that partners are treated. Legal regulations about the provision of expedited partner management vary by state; the CDC maintains updated information on its website at www.cdc.gov/std/ept

Comfort and support. Be attentive to patients' physical and psychosocial comfort to enhance adherence with treatment. Treat nausea, pain, itching, or other physiologic discomforts symptomatically, if possible. This is especially critical for women who may be experiencing a first episode of symptomatic genital herpes, for example, or for women with highly symptomatic vulvovaginal candidiasis. Overcoming the psychosocial component of genital discomfort is exceedingly important in RTI treatment. Patients may be afraid or ashamed to ask a partner to seek treatment, embarrassed to admit their sexual practices, or concerned about confidentiality. Reinforcing that most STI are relatively common, and often transmitted when people are experiencing no symptoms can help to minimize the stigma associated with these infections.

Concurrent infections. Managing RTI requires that clinicians have a high index of suspicion for other infections. A patient may have two or more RTI concurrently. Be alert for symptoms that differ from those normally associated with the primary RTI infection.

STI reporting. All states require that certain STIs, including chlamydia, gonorrhea, syphilis, and chancroid, be reported to public health officials; many states have instituted reporting systems for others, such as genital herpes. Nearly all states require that HIV infection and AIDS be reported. Reporting is not a breach of confidentiality; in fact, statutory protection of clients' names is a crucial part of control strategies. Accurate reporting helps identify trends in disease, gain resources for high prevalence communities, and evaluate RTI control efforts. Resources to assist with this process can be found online at state STD program websites, which are listed at the National Coalition of STD Directors website at www.ncsddc.org/programsites.htm.

RTI DURING PREGNANCY

Question pregnant women and their sex partners about their risk of RTI; counsel them about the possibility of transmitting an infection to their infant. Because of the severe effects RTI may have on both the pregnancy and the developing fetus, assess whether the pregnant woman should be screened for infections with HIV, syphilis, hepatitis B, chlamydia, and gonorrhea, and trichomoniasis (Tables 21–4 and 21–5). Encourage screening for HIV to detect infected women who could benefit

Table 21-4 Risks of sexually transmitted bacteria and related syndromes in pregnancy and childbirth

Organism/Syndrome	Maternal Infection Rate (%)[a]	Infant Effects	Transmission Risk from Infected Mother	Prevention	Treatment of Mother, Neonate
Neisseria gonorrhoeae	1–30	Conjunctivitis, sepsis, meningitis	Approximately 30%	Screening; test mother; apply ocular prophylaxis	Ceftriaxone
Chlamydia trachomatis	2–25	Conjunctivitis, pneumonia, bronchiolitis, otitis media	25%–50% conjunctivitis, 5%–15% pneumonia	Screening in third trimester: test mother, apply ocular prophylaxis	Azithromycin Amoxicillin Erythromycin
Treponema pallidum	0.01–15	Congenital syphilis, neonatal death	50%	Serologic screening in early and late pregnancy	Penicillin
Trichomonas vaginalis	3–35	Low birth-weight, preterm delivery	N/A	Screening	Metronidazole
Bacterial vaginosis	10–35	Low birth-weight, preterm delivery	N/A	Screening	Metronidazole Clindamycin

Source: Adapted from Cates (1995).[3]

[a] Percentage of pregnant women with evidence of infection

Table 21-5 Risks of sexually transmitted viruses and related syndromes in pregnancy and childbirth

Organism/Syndrome	Maternal Infection Rate (%)[a]	Infant Effects	Transmission Risk from Infected Mother	Prevention	Treatment of Mother, Neonate
Hepatitis B Virus	1–10	Hepatitis, cirrhosis	10%–90%	Active HBV immunization	Post-exposure passive HBV immunization
Herpes Simplex Virus	1–30	Disseminated, central nervous system, localized lesions	Recurrent: 3% at delivery; primary: 30% at delivery	Cesarean delivery if lesions present at delivery	Acyclovir
Human Papillomavirus	10–60	Laryngeal papillomatosis	Rare	None	Surgical
Human Immunodeficiency Virus	0.01–40	Pediatric AIDS	27% without ART < 5% with ART	Pregnancy prevention; ART during pregnancy	Antiretrovirals (ART)

Source: Adapted from Cates (1995).[3]

[a] Percentage of pregnant women with evidence of infection

from prophylactic antiretroviral therapy to reduce maternal-to-infant transmission. Routine screening for human papillomavirus (HPV) is not recommended. Screening for herpes simplex virus type-2 (HSV-2) infection is not routinely recommended. Depending on the individual woman's concerns, HSV screening can be considered on a case-by-case basis. If serologic testing is obtained, it is critical to use a glycoprotein-G-based test, because this is the only type of assay that can reliably distinguish between antibody formed in response to HSV-2 infection from that formed in response to HSV-1 infection (a common cause of oral infection), and an increasing cause of genital herpes.

The management of specific RTI is discussed in the Alphabetical Catalog of RTI at the end of this chapter. For more complete information on RTI in pregnant women, refer to Guidelines for Perinatal Care, jointly published by the American College of Obstetricians and Gynecologists and the American Academy of Pediatrics.[21]

RTI AND SEXUAL ASSAULT

In cases of sexual assault and abuse, clinicians must attend not only to physical and psychological trauma, but also to the possibility of pregnancy or RTI. Any of the sexually transmissible infections, including HIV, can be acquired during a sexual assault. Some RTI, such as gonorrhea or syphilis, are almost exclusively sexually transmitted and are therefore useful markers of assault in persons who have not been sexually active. To reduce the risk of pregnancy, offer emergency contraception (see Chapter 6 on Emergency Contraception). To reduce risk of RTI, the CDC recommends the following approach:[22]

Adult evaluation. If possible, evaluate the victim within 24 hours of the assault and take specimens for culture of N. gonorrhoeae and C. trachomatis. Examine vaginal fluid microscopically for trichomoniasis and bacterial vaginosis (BV). Perform a pregnancy test, and keep a frozen serum sample for possible testing in the future. If treatment is not administered, schedule a repeat evaluation for 2 weeks later. Presumptive treatment may be provided at the victim's request. Advise clients to use condoms until the test results are reported. While no regimen provides coverage against all potential pathogens, the following should be effective against the most frequent RTI:

- Cefixime 400 milligrams (mg) given orally in a single dose OR Ceftriaxone 250 mg given intramuscularly (IM)
- Metronidazole 2 grams (g) given orally
- Azithromycin 1 g given orally
- Hepatitis B vaccination, first dose

- Post-exposure prophylaxis against HIV, depending on risk assessment

Child evaluation. In general, the presence of an RTI in a child beyond the neonatal period suggests sexual abuse. However, unlike gonorrhea or syphilis, specific infections such as bacterial vaginosis (BV), genital mycoplasmas, and genital warts are not conclusive evidence of sexual abuse. Evaluation is essentially the same as described for adult victims, except culture specimens should be collected from the pharynx and rectum as well as from the vagina or urethra because the child's report of assault may not be complete. Presumptive treatment may be given at the family's request. For more complete information regarding laboratory procedures, diagnosis, and treatment for sexual assault and abuse victims, refer to the CDC 2010 Guidelines for Treatment of Sexually Transmitted Diseases (see www.cdc.gov/std/treatment).[22]

SPECIAL CONSIDERATIONS REGARDING HIV/AIDS IN THE REPRODUCTIVE HEALTH SETTING

For many young women, reproductive health care clinics may be the only source of health care. Each patient should be asked "What do you do to protect yourself from infection with HIV (the virus that causes AIDS) and other sexually transmitted infections?" Providers may be able to determine readiness for behavior change by assessing this answer. The patient who answers, "I thought I would get some condoms while I'm here today," may be more receptive to behavioral change than the patient who answers, "Who, me?"

Although reproductive health physicians are more likely than other primary care physicians to ask about sex and drug behavior, many are reluctant to risk offending patients. It may be helpful to begin with, "I'm going to ask you some personal questions that I ask everyone, because I think it is so important to your health. Is that all right with you?"

Other Key Points. Avoid making assumptions about a patient's sexual and other behaviors based on appearances. In particular, avoid assumptions such as:

- Sexually experienced people know how to use safer sex techniques.
- People with good jobs and families don't use drugs.
- Single people have lots of partners and risky sex practices.
- Older people have few partners and infrequent sex.
- Married people are heterosexual and don't have sex with partners of the same sex.

Remember that terminology can sometimes get in the way of clarity with this type of risk assessment. For example, teens may not know the word "monogamous." Some may think "sexually active" means vigorous sex, or many partners. Some people who engage in same-sex behavior do not think of themselves as "homosexual," particularly in settings where acknowledging same-sex behavior or identity is stigmatized.

COUNSELING ABOUT SAFER SEX

Teach safer sex skills, including correct use of male and female condoms and other latex and plastic barriers, to all at-risk patients (Table 21–6). Advise all patients that a crucial time for diligent safer sex practices is the first few months of a new relationship. Delaying intercourse may allow the couple the opportunity to get screened for common STIs, including HIV, together. Include prevention skills for oral sex, because gonorrhea, syphilis, HSV-1, and (to a lesser extent) HIV transmission through unprotected oral sex is possible, especially with activities that expose the mouth to semen or blood.[23]

Customize teaching methods for individual patients. Use audiovisual, print, and electronic teaching aids appropriate to the patient's comfort, pleasure, age, language, culture, and learning style. Be sure to make your guidance specific to the patient and related to her particular issues, rather than giving vague, global advice:

- "Starting today, put condoms on the night stand beside the bed," rather than "always use condoms."

- "Maybe you should reconsider whether to date this person, who is also dating other women," rather than "Have fewer, safer partners."

- "Next time you're out with friends and might have sex, avoid getting high on drugs or alcohol," rather than "Have safer sex."

POSTEXPOSURE PROPHYLAXIS, SEX, AND DRUGS

In cases of isolated high-risk exposures to HIV—unprotected vaginal or anal intercourse, rape, receptive oral sex with ejaculation, or sharing injection equipment when the partner is known or suspected to be infected—consider giving postexposure prophylaxis for HIV (HIV-PEP). Although data on efficacy are limited, an increasing number of health care providers offer treatment to survivors of sexual assault and to other types of patients as well.[24] HIV-PEP should begin as soon as possible, and no later than 72 hours after the exposure. Treatment usually consists of a 1-month course of drugs combined from 2 or 3 antiretroviral drug groups, much like the combination therapy regimens used by persons with HIV. Discuss treatment protocol options with your local rape crisis

Table 21–6 Options for sexual intimacy and HIV and STI prevention

Safe	All unprotected sexual activities, when both partners are monogamous and known by testing to be free of HIV and other STIs; also sexual fantasies, massage, hugging, body rubbing, dry kissing, masturbation without contact with partner's semen, vaginal secretions, blood, or broken skin, erotic conversation, books, movies, videos, electronic images, erotic bathing, showering, eroticizing feet, hands, hips, abdomen, ears, other body parts
Low, but Potential Risk	All sexual activities, when both partners are monogamous, but have not been tested; includes wet kissing with no broken skin, cracked lips, or damaged mouth tissue; hand-to-genital touching or mutual masturbation on healthy, intact skin or with a latex or plastic barrier; vaginal or anal intercourse using latex or plastic condom correctly with adequate lubrication; oral sex on a man wearing a latex or plastic condom; oral sex on a woman using a latex or plastic barrier such as a female condom, dental dam, or plastic wrap
Unsafe in the absence of mutual monogamy and HIV testing of both partners	Blood contact of any kind, including menstrual blood; any vaginal or anal intercourse without a latex or plastic condom; oral sex on a woman without a latex or plastic barrier such as a female condom, dental dam, plastic wrap, or modified male condom (especially if she is having her period or has a vaginal infection with discharge); oral sex on a man without a latex or plastic condom, especially if associated with semen in the mouth; oral-anal contact; shared sex toys or douching equipment; any sex that causes tissue damage or bleeding, such as rough vaginal or anal intercourse, rape, or fisting

center, or call the Post-Exposure Prophylaxis Hotline operated by the National HIV/AIDS Clinicians' Consultation Center for guidance on individual cases. The hotline is based at the University of California at San Francisco, and can be reached toll-free 24 hours a day, 7 days a week at 1–888–448–4911. Treatment may cost $1,000 to $1,600, is often associated with side effects, and may not be covered by health insurance plans. Thus, the decision to undertake HIV-PEP should succeed a thorough discussion of all components of the risk-benefit assessment, including the risk associated with the exposure and the patient's individual concerns.

FACTORS AFFECTING SEXUAL TRANSMISSION

The likelihood of sexual HIV transmission is variable. A major determining factor is the HIV viral load in the infected partner's genital secretions (semen or vaginal fluid), which is directly proportional to the HIV viral load in his or her plasma.[25] Risk of sexual transmission may be increased under certain circumstances:

- During early HIV infection (the weeks after the infection is acquired), because HIV viral load, and thus infectivity, is very high
- During late or uncontrolled HIV infection, when viral multiplication is not suppressed by antiretroviral treatment
- When either partner, but especially the HIV-infected partner, has a concurrent STI including trichomoniasis, gonorrhea, genital herpes, bacterial vaginosis, or chlamydia
- When blood or blood secretions are involved, or when tears in the exposed mucous membranes are present
- With anal sex (especially for the receptive partner), relative to vaginal sex

The risk of sexual transmission from an infected partner may be decreased (but not eliminated) under the following circumstances:

- If the HIV-infected partner is on an effective antiretroviral drug regimen and serum HIV viral load is undetectable. This does *not*, however, guarantee that HIV is not present in genital secretions, so transmission is still possible.
- If either the infected or the uninfected male partner is circumcised

Advice for Patients Seeking Contraceptive Services

Until further data are available, it is prudent to advise all patients as follows:

- Use male or female latex or plastic condoms each time you suspect any risk of exposure to HIV, but choose to have vaginal or anal intercourse.
- Use latex or plastic condoms for men and latex or plastic vulvar barriers for women any time you suspect any risk of HIV but choose to have oral sex.
- Vaginal spermicides do not protect against HIV or other STIs.
- Any tissue damage to the vulva, vagina, anus, or penis could increase susceptibility to HIV. Avoid intercourse until lesions are healed.

HIV TESTING AND COUNSELING

Reproductive health care providers represent the most important access point for women to receive HIV testing. Thus, HIV testing should be a standard component of care.[26,27]

When To Offer Testing

Offer routine HIV testing to *all* women.[26] Certain situations outside of the prenatal setting call for the care provider's strong recommendation to seek testing, and extra effort to assure that patients have reasonable access to counseling and testing services:

- Known sexual exposure to an HIV-infected person

- Shared injection equipment with an HIV-infected person

- Possible recent occupational exposure

- Clinical settings with a ≥1% HIV seroprevalence

- Settings serving "populations at increased behavioral or clinical HIV risk," such as STI clinics, teen clinics with high rates of RTI, or correctional facilities, regardless of that setting's HIV seroprevalence

- Clinical signs or symptoms suggesting HIV infection (e.g., fever or illness of unknown origin, opportunistic infection without known reason for immune suppression)

- Diagnosis suggesting increased risk for HIV (such as another RTI or blood-borne infection)

- Patient's request

Prenatal testing.   Many women learn they have HIV when testing is done as part of routine prenatal care. Some prospective studies have indicated that pregnancy itself may also confer an increased risk of acquiring HIV infection.[27]

Counseling about pregnancy options is an especially important component of post-test counseling if the HIV diagnosis is made early in pregnancy; the patient may be overwhelmed by the news, and by the information to absorb. Pregnant women with HIV are faced with the same sorts of reproductive decisions as women without HIV, with similar percentages of terminated pregnancies and live births. For the HIV-infected woman who chooses to continue the pregnancy, consult appropriate guidelines for the use of antiretroviral therapy. Detailed guidelines are available at www.aidsinfo.nih.gov/guidelines.

Table 21–7 Components of counseling in the setting of HIV testing

Deciding whether to have the test
- Your right to decide whether to be tested
- Voluntary informed consent
- Who will see the results if test is done here, including state laws
- Other sites for testing; home testing options

Benefits of being tested
- Peace of mind; knowing, one way or the other
- If infected:
  - Options for HIV therapy, managing related problems
  - Prevent transmission to others
  - Make informed childbearing decisions
  - Diagnose illness or symptoms
  - Access assistance programs

Difficulties with being tested
- Learning you have a very serious illness
- Telling sex or injecting-drug-equipment-sharing partners (health care agencies can provide help with this task)

What results mean
- If antibody positive:
  - You are infected
  - You can pass the virus on to other people
  - Need to establish care with knowledgeable provider and undergo further assessment for disease staging
- If antibody negative or indeterminate:
  - You are not infected, or
  - You are infected, but antibodies are not yet detectable; infection may have been acquired up to 6 months previously

Reducing risk for HIV
- Develop a personalized risk-reduction plan today with counselor
- Offer condoms and other safer sex supplies
- Referral for drug, alcohol treatment

Test Counseling

Reproductive heath care providers should be prepared to explain to women how the test is done, what the routine screening procedure will and will not reveal, implications of anonymous vs. confidential testing, and instructions on how to obtain test results. A guide (Table 21–7) for providing this information and for giving negative and positive test results may be helpful.

Counseling and Testing Issues

Confidentiality. Confidential testing is name-linked, and information is protected to a degree determined by state law and, at the testing site, by formal policies and staff commitment to confidentiality.

Testing technology. HIV testing most frequently involves testing serum using a screening test called enzyme immunoassay (EIA) and a confirmatory test called Western blot. While both tests are very sensitive and specific, neither is perfect, so an HIV test is reported as positive only after obtaining positive results from at least two EIAs and one Western blot or other confirmatory test using the same test sample. As with any screening test, prevalence of the infection within the client's population is the major factor in determining a test's predictive value; the higher the prevalence, the greater the likelihood that a positive test result means that the person is truly infected. Always regard HIV test results in the context of the patient history and clinical picture, and re-evaluate when they are not in agreement.

New technologies have added options for testing other body fluids and for providing rapid test results. These newer technologies are FDA-approved and provide sensitivity and specificity comparable to traditional tests. Early reports are reassuring regarding acceptability of these options. Updated information on the types of tests available for HIV screening can be found at www.cdc.gov/hiv/rapid_testing. Some options include home testing—a finger-prick blood sample is mailed to the testing site, and the client obtains results by phone, along with counseling—and rapid screening tests, including those that use saliva instead of blood. *Definitive* positive results require a confirmatory test such as a Western Blot.

Documentation of HIV Test Results. Recording HIV test results is important for ongoing medical care, although problems with confidentiality may result. This dilemma can be addressed by maintaining HIV-related information in a separate chart, by using a code for HIV test results, or by removing HIV-related information before releasing the chart. This latter practice is required by law in some states. State and local professional associations may offer guidance for appropriate, lawful charting that does not compromise the patient, provider, or health care delivery. However, many states require reporting when HIV is detected; specific information is available at www.cdc.gov/hiv/topics/surveillance/reporting.htm.

CLINICAL CHARACTERISTICS OF HIV INFECTION IN WOMEN

The current standard of care for HIV is highly active antiretroviral therapy (HAART), a combination of oral antiretroviral agents that inhibit different targets of the virus. HAART regimens can be composed of drugs from two, three, or more classes, including nucleoside analog reverse transcriptase inhibitors (NRTI), non-nucleoside reverse transcriptase inhibitors (NNRTIs), protease inhibitors (PIs), integrase inhibitors,

CCR-5 inhibitors, and fusion inhibitors. HAART should be initiated and managed by—or in close consultation with—an experienced HIV clinician in order to prevent the development of resistance to single drugs or to entire classes of drugs. Having an experienced care provider has been shown to be a factor in prolonging life for persons with HIV. HIV mutation and resistance can occur quickly if the patient is not adherent with the regimen. While single daily dosing regimens and formulations that combine agents from several classes have emerged as the standard of care and have greatly simplified the approach to treatment, side effects still occur, and all regimens are expensive. The decision to initiate therapy is based on assessment of HIV viral load in the plasma, CD4 count, and presence of opportunistic infections. Viral load testing uses DNA or RNA detection assays to measure the actual amount of HIV in plasma, permitting an accurate determination of real-time viral activity and a rapid assessment of antiretroviral drug efficacy. For complete information on recommended regimens, see www.aidsinfo.nih.gov/guidelines.

Reproductive health care would ideally be managed in the primary care/HIV care setting also, but in some cases these are two providers in two different sites, so careful attention to shared information, shared decision making, and collaboration is essential. Advice on medical management of patients with HIV is available from the National HIV/AIDS Clinicians' Consultation Center based at the University of California at San Francisco. This no-cost "warmline" is staffed Monday through Friday from 6:00 a.m. to 5:00 p.m. Pacific Time, and voicemail is available 24 hours a day, 7 days a week. Call 1–800–933–3413.

Gynecologic Management

The keys to successful management of gynecologic infections in women with HIV are a high index of suspicion, prompt diagnosis, aggressive treatment (especially for immunocompromised women), and primary or secondary prophylaxis when appropriate. Table 21–8 outlines general stages of HIV infection and related concerns; a discussion of some specific conditions follows.

Table 21–8 Stages of HIV infection and reproductive health concerns

	Primary HIV Infection/Seroconversion	Symptom-Free	Early Symptoms	Discrete Illness/Cascade of Illness/Endstage
Duration	Average 1–8 weeks	Few months to many years	Few months to several years	Few months to several years
CD4 Cell Count x 106 /L Normal = 500–1600	Normal or slightly low	Typically > 350	Typically < 350	AIDS diagnosis at 200 or less
Viral Load copies/ml Normal = 500–1600	High	Variable	Rising (without HAART)	High (without HAART)
Characteristics	Self-limited flu-like illness can occur; HIV antibody not detectable 6–12 weeks post-infection,* but serum viral assays positive.		Fevers, night sweats, zoster, vulvovaginal candidiasis, oral thrush, hairy leukoplakia, seborrheic dermatitis, weight loss, fatigue, loss of appetite	Mild or severe multiple opportunistic bacterial, viral, fungal, parasitic infections; cancers, including Kaposi's sarcoma, lymphoma, cervical cancer; Neurologic illness including dementia, peripheral neuropathy
Reproductive Health Concerns	Nonspecific presentation if primary infection is symptomatic; sex partner(s) and offspring may be at risk with ongoing risk behavior. Assess contraception, safer sex practices.	Usually asymptomatic, though risk of transmission less than with primary infection. Offer anticipatory guidance on future pregnancy planning. Frequent Paps, aggressive management of abnormal findings. Assess contraception, safer sex practices.	Pregnancy likely to be normal except for transmission risk for offspring. Frequent Paps, aggressive management of abnormal findings. Assess contraception, safer sex practices.	Medications may interfere with hormonal contraception; assess drug interactions. Assist with short-range and long-range child care plans. Pregnancy may result in prematurity, low birthweight, premature rupture of membranes, other complications. Frequent Paps, aggressive management of abnormal findings. Assess contraception, safer sex practices.
Risk of Transmission to Offspring	Risk may increase above 25% baseline if primary infection occurs during pregnancy.	25% each pregnancy without treatment. Decreased to about 2% with effective HAART.	25% each pregnancy without treatment. Decreased to about 2% with effective HAART.	25% each pregnancy without treatment. Decreased to about 2% with effective HAART.

Source: Modified from Anderson (ed.) (2001).[28]

* Newer rapid tests may detect antibody to HIV earlier. See www.cdc.gov/hiv/topics/testing/rapid/index.htm for details and updated information.

Vulvovaginal candidiasis (VVC). VVC is common in HIV-infected women and may recur frequently when immune status deteriorates. Nonalbicans species may occur and may be less responsive to topical imidazole or oral azole therapy. First-line treatment is a 7-day course of one of the topical imidazole antifungal agents. If topical treatment proves unsatisfactory, consider oral fluconazole (a single dose, 150 mg orally). Boric acid may be useful for women who experience infection with resistant *Candida* species.

Human papillomavirus and cervical disease. Genital warts caused by certain types of HPV (types 6 and 11) may progress more rapidly with immune compromise. Women with HIV have significantly higher rates of Pap smear-detected abnormalities, dysplasia and progression to cervical cancer relative to HIV-uninfected women. Consider baseline colposcopy or cervicography, appropriate Pap smear intervals (see below), and prompt colposcopy and excision of any abnormal findings. One-year Pap smear intervals are appropriate for women with a history of normal results. Screen every 6 months for women who have symptomatic HIV, a CD4 < 200, or both. Shorten the interval to 4 to 6 months for ASCUS/ LGSIL findings and, following treatment of preinvasive lesions, every 3 to 4 months for a year, then at 6-month intervals. Finally, while neither the quadrivalent nor the bivalent HPV vaccine has been extensively studied in HIV-infected women, preliminary data and the fact that the vaccine is protein-based (no live virus) recommend consideration of its administration to HIV-infected women who qualify according to the ACIP guidelines.

Pelvic inflammatory disease (PID). In general, immunosuppressed women with PID do not appear to require more aggressive treatment than other women, but the approach should be individualized. Depending on the severity of PID and immune status, providers should consider parenteral therapy and hospitalization, based on factors considered in HIV-negative women.

Genital Herpes. In the presence of immune dysfunction, herpes lesions may be more extensive, more painful, atypical in location or appearance, and slower to heal. In a large study in Africa, suppressive therapy with twice daily oral acyclovir was associated with a reduction in plasma HIV viral load relative to placebo.[29] Benefits of suppressive therapy include reduction of symptomatic outbreaks, reduction in risk of HSV-2 transmission to sex partners (demonstrated in heterosexual couples), and, possibly, a favorable effect on HIV itself due to direct activity against HIV. Treatment of symptomatic episodes of genital herpes should be accordance with standard guidelines for HIV-infected persons.

Psychological Care and Support

Women with HIV often experience significant psychosocial stress, often related to the fact that they may be the primary caregivers for their families. They will often need guidance, support, and referral to assist with fundamental concerns including stable housing, economic stability, childcare, and addiction.

Reproductive Health Care

For HIV-infected women, the decision about whether to get pregnant is similar to that for uninfected women, and their desire for a child is often profound. Counseling for women who are pregnant or contemplating pregnancy includes important medical issues:

- Impact of HIV on pregnancy
- Impact of pregnancy on HIV
- Effect of antiretroviral medication and other drugs on woman and developing fetus
- Risk of perinatal transmission and options for reducing risk
- Risk of breastfeeding for HIV transmission
- Course of HIV in perinatally infected infants
- Access to HIV-experienced obstetric and pediatric care
- Access to antiretroviral medications

Counseling for pregnancy optimally includes a full understanding of the patient's personal goals, her support network, an understanding of stressors in her life, and her overall physical and emotional status. Once this groundwork is in place, guide the patient through specific questions to help her predict how she would feel, how others would feel, and what might happen.

HIV-infected women who do not wish to become pregnant are more likely to succeed with a contraceptive method they have chosen for themselves and feel comfortable using (Table 21–9). The goal is high contraceptive efficacy, low risk of woman-to-partner HIV transmission (if applicable), and low risk of partner-to-woman STI transmission. This goal is met by choices such as hormonal contraceptives or IUC, plus male condoms.

Thousands of U.S. women with HIV give birth each year. Generally, HIV-infected women who are immunocompetent have uneventful pregnancies with normal labor and delivery. Just as with any women with serious systemic illness, immunocompromised women may have complicated pregnancies, including prematurity, low birthweight, and premature rupture of membranes. However, the effects of HIV on preg-

Table 21–9 Contraception for the HIV-infected woman

Method	Possible Benefits	Possible Drawbacks
Oral Contraceptives	• Good effectiveness with consistent use • Less blood loss to avoid anemia	• Unclear interaction of steroids and immune function • Possible interaction with certain antibiotics, antiretrovirals, other drugs • Possible increased shedding of virus from genital tract • No RTI protection • No HIV protection for partner
Depo-Provera	Good low-maintenance effectiveness	• Unclear interaction of steroids and immune function • Possible increased shedding of virus from genital tract • Possible increase in cervical inflammation • No RTI protection • No HIV protection for partner
IUD	Good low-maintenance effectiveness	• Risk of infection during insertion interval • No RTI protection • No HIV protection for partner • Increased days of bleeding, possible anemia
Diaphragm	Some RTI protection for the cervix	• Increases vulnerability to UTIs for some users • Requires good technique
Male, Female Condom	Good RTI protection, HIV protection for partner	• Male condom requires partner cooperation; partner cooperation helpful with female condom • Requires good technique
Surgical Sterilization	Good low-maintenance efficacy for women who desire no more children	• No RTI protection • No HIV protection for partner

Sources: Adapted Cates W Jr. (2001)[3]

nancy are hard to differentiate from the effects of poverty, poor health care, or addiction. Pregnancy does not appear to speed HIV progression.

Risks of HIV Transmission in the Perinatal Period

Without HAART, each offspring of an infected woman in the U.S. faces approximately a 25% risk of being infected in utero, during birth, or while breastfeeding. With HAART, the risk falls to 2% or less (see below).

Reducing perinatal transmission risk. Strategies to reduce perinatal HIV transmission continue to evolve rapidly. HAART is recommended for all pregnant women with the goal of suppressing plasma HIV RNA to undetectable levels. Antiretroviral treatment is also recommended for HIV-exposed infants in their first weeks of life. HAART initiation for this purpose may be delayed until the second trimester.

Labor and delivery. In the absence of breastfeeding, an estimated 60% to 75% of perinatal HIV transmissions occur around the time of labor and delivery, and a number of strategies can reduce exposure of the neonate to maternal blood and secretions. In addition to intrapartum HAART, suggested approaches include vaginal disinfection, RTI treatment during pregnancy to lower viral shedding at term, avoidance of intrapartum invasive procedures, and cesarean delivery. Scheduled cesarean delivery before rupture of membranes is recommended for women whose HIV viral load at 36 weeks or later is above 1,000 copies/mL. Avoid delays in delivery once membranes have ruptured. The risk of perinatal HIV transmission can double when fetal membranes rupture more than 4 hours before delivery.

Breastfeeding. Advise women in the United States to bottle feed infants to reduce the risk of postnatal HIV transmission via breast milk. The precise risk of HIV transmission via breast milk is difficult to quantify and may be influenced by the woman's HIV status (with high viral loads during primary infection and late stage disease), her use of HAART, breastfeeding patterns, and other factors. Among infected women who breastfeed, approximately 10% to 15% of all vertical transmissions are associated with breastfeeding. (See Chapter 18 on Postpartum Contraception and Lactation.) Little is known about the impact of breastfeeding on the HIV-infected woman's nutritional status and overall health, or about the immunoprotective qualities of the breast milk produced by immunocompromised women.

ALPHABETICAL CATALOGUE OF REPRODUCTIVE TRACT INFECTIONS

ACUTE URETHRAL SYNDROME (dysuria-pyuria syndrome) is distinct from bacterial cystitis and typically results from a direct urethral infection with the sexually transmitted pathogens C. trachomatis or N. gonorrhoeae. Bacterial cystitis itself is not sexually transmitted per se; however, it can be sexually associated. "Honeymoon" cystitis—that is, cystitis that occurs after frequent vaginal intercourse—is believed to be caused by friction against the urethra during sexual intercourse. In this case, the underlying etiology is mechanical, and coital movements help vaginal organisms ascend into the bladder. Use of the diaphragm with spermicides and spermicidally coated condoms have been associated with a higher risk of acute urethral syndrome.

Prevalence. Urinary tract infections are second in prevalence only to upper respiratory infections. Depending on the population studied, as many as 10% to 25% of reproductive-age women report dysuria during the previous year. Among women with genital chlamydial infections, approximately 10% are infected at the urethra only.

Symptoms. Painful, urgent, and frequent urination, as well as dyspareunia, characterizes this syndrome. Occasionally, hematuria is the precipitating event for seeking clinical evaluation. Consider pyelonephritis in the presence of fever, or if costovertebral angle pain or tenderness are present.

Diagnosis. Women with >10 organisms (coliform bacteria or other uropathogens) per milliliter (ml) of urine have bacterial cystitis; however, a smaller number of organisms may also cause symptoms. Women with dysuria, frequency, pyuria ($\geq$10 white blood cells [WBCs] per 400x field on microscopic examination of urinary sediment), and a negative Gram stain of unspun urine have acute urethral syndrome, and chlamydia should be strongly suspected. A definitive diagnosis of the etiologic organism requires cultures or nucleic acid amplification testing (for gonorrhea and chlamydia) of the urethra or urine. Dysuria may also be caused by vulvovaginitis or genital herpes simplex virus infection.

Treatment. Bacterial cystitis can be treated with a variety of antibiotics that achieve a high concentration in urine. Initial episodes of bacterial cystitis can be treated with appropriate single-dose therapy such as sulfamethoxazole 1.6 g plus trimethoprim 320 mg (Bactrim or Septra). Fluoroquinolones (e.g., ciprofloxacin 250 mg twice a day, OR ofloxacin 200 mg twice a day) can be effective. Three days is the usual course. If bacteriuria is absent in the presence of pyuria, consider presumptive treatment for chlamydial infection.

Potential complications. Left untreated, bacterial infections of the lower genitourinary tract can ascend to the upper tract, leading to pyelonephritis.

Behavioral messages to emphasize. Understand how to take any prescribed oral medications. Drink copious fluids to flush the genitourinary system. If C. trachomatis or N. gonorrhoeae organisms are isolated or strongly suspected, arrange for treatment of sex partner(s). (See the sections on these specific infections.)

BACTERIAL VAGINOSIS (BV) is a clinical syndrome in which several species of vaginal bacteria (including Gardnerella vaginalis, Mycoplasma hominis, and various anaerobes) replace the normal H_2O_2-producing

Lactobacillus species and cause vaginitis symptoms. Bacterial vaginosis is a sexually associated condition, but it is not usually considered a specific STI; however, it does occur frequently in lesbians and may represent an STI in this group. Treatment of the male partner has not been found to be effective in preventing the recurrence of BV. Because of the increased risk for postoperative infectious complications associated with BV, some specialists recommend that before performing surgical abortion, providers treat women with symptomatic BV in addition to providing routine prophylaxis.

Symptoms. Excessive or malodorous discharge is a common finding. Erythema, edema, and pruritus of the external genitalia may be seen if the discharge is profuse.

Diagnosis. The clinical diagnosis of bacterial vaginosis is made if three of the following four criteria are present: increased amounts of homogenous discharge; elevated vaginal pH (greater than 4.5); fishy odor on addition of 10% KOH; and identification of clue cells (small coccobacillary organisms associated with epithelial cells) on saline wet mount (> 20% of vaginal epithelial cells). Alternatively, rapid tests that detect high numbers of *Gardnerella vaginalis* bacteria, or byproducts of anaerobic metabolism such as sialidase, are also available. Primarily used in research, a Gram stain of the vaginal discharge reveals the relative absence of lactobacilli with replacement of other anaerobic organisms. Cultures and polymerase chain reaction (PCR) for G. vaginalis, M. hominis, or Mobiluncus are not useful and should not be performed.

Treatment. Patients with symptomatic disease should be offered treatment. The three recommended regimens are metronidazole, 500 mg orally twice daily for 7 days; OR metronidazole gel, 0.75%, one full applicator (5 g) vaginally at bed time for 5 days; OR clindamycin cream, 2%, one full applicator (5 g) vaginally at bed time for 7 days. Other alternatives are oral clindamycin 300 mg two times a day for 7 days; clindamycin ovules 100 mg vaginally at bedtime for 3 days; tinidazole two grams orally once daily for 3 days; or tinidazole one gram orally once daily for 5 days. During the second and third trimester of pregnancy, 7-day oral regimens of metronidazole 500 mg two times a day or 250 mg three times a day, or clindamycin 300 mg two times a day, are options; systemic (oral) therapy is generally preferred.

Potential complications. Recurrent infections are common. Bacterial vaginosis is associated with an increased risk of PID, and may also cause cervicitis. Bacterial vaginosis is associated with an increased risk of adverse pregnancy outcomes, including preterm delivery and low birthweight.

Behavioral messages to emphasize. The use of condoms by male partners has been associated with a reduced risk of recurrence of bacterial vaginosis, and may be a useful adjunct to antibiotic treatment, especially for women with recurrent disease. Avoid douching, as this promotes loss of vaginal lactobacilli and likely exacerbates the problem. Avoid drinking alcohol until 24 hours after completing oral metronidazole therapy or 48 hours after completing tinidazole therapy.

CANDIDIASIS (vulvovaginal candidiasis (VVC)) is caused by Candida species—usually C. albicans—that are dimorphic fungi that grow as oval, budding yeast cells and as chains of cells (hyphae). Candida are normal flora of the skin, mouth, and vagina. VVC is not considered a STI per se; however, sex partners do exchange orogenital strains of Candida. Risk factors for VVC are incompletely understood, but include immunosuppressed states, glucose intolerance, and (in some women) antibiotic therapy.

Symptoms. Clinical presentation includes whitish vaginal discharge and erythema, edema, and pruritus of the external genitalia. Symptoms or signs alone do not distinguish the microbial etiology. Male sex partners may develop balanitis or cutaneous lesions on the penis.

Diagnosis. The presumptive criteria are typical clinical symptoms of vulvovaginitis and microscopic identification of yeast forms (budding cells) or pseudohyphae in KOH wet-mount preparations of vaginal discharge. VVC is definitively diagnosed when a vaginal culture is positive for C. albicans or other Candida species in a symptomatic woman. Because up to 40% of women are vaginally colonized with Candida species in the absence of VVC, cultures are not recommended unless chronic suppressive therapy is under consideration, in which case they are recommended to confirm both the etiology and ideally susceptibility to antifungal agents.

Treatment. Single-dose oral fluconazole, 150 mg, is a convenient therapy. In addition, many topical formulations provide effective candidiasis treatment. Examples include miconazole vaginal suppositories, 200 mg intravaginally at bedtime for 3 days; OR miconazole, 2%, vaginal cream, one full applicator (5 g) intravaginally at bedtime for 3 days (and applied externally for vulvitis); OR clotrimazole vaginal tablets, 100 mg intravaginally, daily for 3 days; OR butoconazole cream, 2%, 5 g intravaginally for 3 days. A variety of other effective treatment regimens exists. In general, more severe infections may need treatment of longer duration. Over-the-counter preparations for intravaginal administration of miconazole, clotrimazole, and butaconazole are available. Women with resistant VVC may benefit from treatment with boric acid, provided as 600 mg in a type O gelatin capsule administered vaginally once daily for 2 weeks (avoid in pregnancy).

Potential complications. Secondary excoriation may occur. Recurrent infections are common, particularly with antibiotic use, immunosuppression, or diabetes.

Behavioral messages to emphasize. Wear a sanitary pad to protect clothing. Change pads frequently. To reduce moisture in the area, avoid panty hose, tight fitting clothing, and noncotton panties. Store suppositories in a refrigerator. Continue taking medicine even during menses.

CERVICITIS is a term used to refer to the syndrome of cervical inflammation that can accompany infection with some STI, notably Chlamydia trachomatis, Neisseria gonorrhoeae, and Mycoplasma genitalium, and occasionally trichomoniasis and genital herpes. It is defined as the presence of endocervical mucopurulent discharge, easily induced bleeding, and/or edematous ectopy. Cervicitis can have noninfectious causes, including chemical trauma, and may also be promoted by progesterone-based hormonal therapy or bacterial vaginosis.

Prevalence. Based on extrapolation from local studies, cervicitis probably occurs more frequently than male urethritis. Up to 3 million cases per year may occur annually.

Symptoms. Cervical mucopurulent discharge may be exuded from the cervix and may be perceived as abnormal vaginal discharge, and cervical bleeding may manifest as intermenstrual bleeding.

Diagnosis. Diagnosis is made by visualizing either mucopus on a swab of endocervical secretions or friability (bleeding) on gentle passage of a cotton-tipped swab. In most cases, a microbial organism cannot be identified. A definitive etiologic diagnosis is made when either chlamydia or gonorrhea (or less commonly, another STI) is isolated.

Treatment. Presumptive treatment should be provided based on the individual patient's risk for chlamydial and/or gonococcal infections, and it should be directed at these organisms (particularly chlamydia). In women at low risk for these STI, the results of sensitive diagnostic tests for C. trachomatis or N. gonorrhoeae should determine the need for treatment. Chlamydia is treated with azithromycin 1 g orally in a single dose OR doxycycline 100 mg orally twice a day for 7 days. The section on Gonorrhea contains the range of recommended treatment regimens for this infection.

Potential complications. PID (with subsequent infertility) may complicate infection. In addition, neonatal chlamydial infections, such as ophthalmia or pneumonia, may be acquired during delivery if the mother has an infected cervix. If a pregnant woman is infected, she may be at risk for postpartum endometritis.

Behavioral messages to emphasize. If infection involves C. trachomatis or N. gonorrhoeae, sex partner(s) should be treated for these bacteria. Avoid sex until completion of the prescribed course of medication and/or for 1 week after treatment was started. Understand how to take prescribed oral medications. Return early if symptoms persist or recur. Use condoms to prevent future infections.

CHANCROID is a type of genital ulcer disease caused by Hemophilus ducreyi, a gram-negative bacillus. Chancroid is implicated as potentiating HIV transmission.

Prevalence. Chancroid occurs more frequently in the developing than in the developed world. However, chancroid is endemic in selected areas of the United States, and outbreaks have occurred in settings where sex is exchanged for drugs or money.

Symptoms. Women are frequently asymptomatic, but ulcers may occur internally and go unnoticed. Usually a single painful ulcer, surrounded by erythematous edges, appears in men. Ulcers may be necrotic or severely erosive with a ragged serpiginous border. Painful inguinal lymphadenopathy (bubo) presents in about half of the cases and may rupture in 25% to 60% of cases. Ulcers usually occur on the coronal sulcus, glans, or shaft of the penis.

Diagnosis. A painful ulcer, particularly if accompanied by a unilateral bubo, could suggest chancroid, but keep in mind that the overwhelming majority of genital ulcer disease in the United States is caused by herpes simplex virus. Because syphilis also causes genital ulcers (known as chancres), all new ulcers not known to be genital herpes should be examined with darkfield microscopy when adequate facilities exist. If chancroid is identified, perform serologic tests for syphilis and HIV. The diagnosis is definitive when H. ducreyi is recovered by culture or appropriate selective media.

Treatment. Azithromycin 1 g orally in a single dose OR ceftriaxone 250 mg IM in a single dose OR ciprofloxacin 500 mg orally twice a day for 3 days OR erythromycin base 500 mg orally four times a day for 7 days. Persons infected with HIV have higher rates of treatment failure with single-dose therapy. The susceptibility of H. ducreyi to this combination of antimicrobial agents varies throughout the world. Evaluate the results of therapy after a maximum of 7 days, and continue therapy until ulcers or lymph nodes have healed. Fluctuant lymph nodes should be aspirated through healthy, adjacent, normal skin. Incision and drainage or excision of nodes will delay healing and are contraindicated. Apply compresses to ulcers to remove necrotic material. All sex partners should be simultaneously treated.

Potential complications. Systemic spread is not known to occur. Lesions may become secondarily infected and necrotic. Buboes may rupture and suppurate, resulting in fistulae. Ulcers on the prepuce may cause paraphimosis or phimosis.

Behavioral messages to emphasize. Because genital ulcers can be a risk for HIV infection, get an HIV test at baseline treatment and again in 3 months. Sex partner(s) should be treated as soon as possible. Return for evaluation 3 to 5 days after therapy begins and thereafter return weekly for evaluation until the infection is entirely healed. The prepuce should remain retracted during therapy, except in the presence of preputial edema.

CHLAMYDIA is the common name for infections caused by Chlamydia trachomatis. Genital chlamydial infection is the leading cause of preventable infertility and ectopic pregnancy. Chlamydia is the most commonly reported infectious disease in the United States. An estimated 3 million new cases occur annually. Like viruses, chlamydiae are obligate intracellular parasites and can be isolated in the laboratory only by cell culture. Unlike viruses, C. trachomatis is susceptible to antibiotics. Because many chlamydial infections are asymptomatic and probably chronic, widespread screening is necessary to control this infection and its sequelae. CDC recommends that all sexually active women age 25 years or younger be screened annually for C. trachomatis (Table 21–3). For further information about the syndromes caused by C. trachomatis, see the sections on Cervicitis, Acute Dysuria Syndrome, Nongonococcal Urethritis, and Pelvic Inflammatory Disease (PID) in this chapter. The recommended regimens for all sites of uncomplicated chlamydial infection are azithromycin 1 g orally in a single dose OR doxycycline 100 mg orally twice a day for 7 days. Alternatives are ofloxacin 300 mg orally two times a day for 7 days OR levofloxacin 500 mg orally for 7 days OR erythromycin base 500 mg orally four times a day for 7 days OR erythromycin ethylsuccinate 800 mg orally four times a day for 7 days. During pregnancy, the recommended regimens are azithromycin 1 g orally in a single dose OR amoxicillin 500 mg orally three times daily for 7 days. Alternatives are erythromycin base 500 mg orally four times daily for 7 days OR erythromycin base 250 mg orally four times daily for 14 days OR erythromycin ethylsuccinate 800 mg orally four times a day for 7 days OR erythromycin ethylsuccinate 400 mg orally four times a day for 14 days. In general, erythromycin-based regimens are inferior to the other drugs listed and should be viewed as second-line therapy. If these regimens are used, a test-of-use at 1 month after treatment is required.

GENITAL HERPES is caused by herpes simplex virus (HSV) types 1 and 2 DNA viruses that cannot be distinguished clinically; however, initial infection with HSV type 1 (HSV-1) is typically less severe and causes less frequent (and sometimes no) recurrences relative to HSV type 2

(HSV-2) is more common in genital disease and is responsible for nearly all recurrent genital herpes.

Prevalence. Symptomatic primary (or initial) HSV infections affect an estimated 200,000 persons each year. Recurrent HSV infections are much more common. An estimated 45 million Americans are infected with genital HSV, though most infections are asymptomatic.[30] Persons without symptoms transmit most HSV infection.

Symptoms. Single or multiple vesicles, which are usually pruritic, can appear anywhere on the genitalia. Vesicles spontaneously rupture to form shallow ulcers that may be very painful. Lesions resolve spontaneously with minimal scarring. The first clinical occurrence is termed first episode infection (mean duration 12 days). Subsequent, usually milder, occurrences are termed recurrent infections (mean duration 4.5 days). The interval between clinical episodes is termed latency. Viral shedding from the cervix, vulva or penile skin occurs intermittently without clinical symptoms during latency. HSV-2 genital infections are more likely to recur than is HSV-1, thus identification of the type of infecting virus at initial infection has prognostic value.

Diagnosis. When typical genital lesions are present or a pattern of recurrence has developed, suspect herpes infection. An HSV tissue culture demonstrates the characteristic cytopathic effect following inoculation of a specimen from the cervix, the urethra, or the base of a genital lesion. Several type-specific HSV serologic assays may help in the diagnosis of unrecognized infection, in management of sex partners of those with HSV, or, in pregnant women, to diagnose HSV susceptibility or recent infection.

Treatment. No cure for HSV exists; however, antiviral drugs are helpful in reducing or suppressing symptoms. Oral administrations effective both in treating clinically symptomatic episodes and in suppressing or reducing recurrent outbreaks. Topical therapy is ineffective. Initial episodes can be treated with any of the following oral regimens, each given for 7–10 days:

Initial episodes can be treated with any of the following:

- Acyclovir
  - 400 mg three times a day OR
  - 200 mg capsules five times a day
- Famciclovir
  - 250 mg five times a day
- Valacyclovir
  - 1.0 g two times a day

Recurrent infections can be treated with any of the following oral regimens:

- Acyclovir
  - 400 mg three times a day for 5 days OR
  - 800 mg twice a day for 5 days OR
  - 800 mg three times a day for 2 days
- Famciclovir
  - 125 mg twice a day for 5 days
  - 1000 mg twice a day for 1 day
  - 500 mg PO x 1, then 250 mg BID for 2 days
- Valacyclovir
  - 500 mg twice a day for 3 days OR
  - 500 mg twice a day for 5 days OR
  - 1.0 g once a day for 5 days.

Daily prophylaxis with valacyclovir by HSV-infected persons reduces the risk of transmission to uninfected partners. Regimens given orally to prevent recurrences include the following:

- Acyclovir 400 mg twice a day OR
- Famciclovir 250 mg twice a day OR
- Valacyclovir
  - 500 mg once a day OR
  - 1.0 g once a day.

Famciclovir and valacyclovir offer more convenient dosing but are not more effective clinically at treating symptomatic disease than acyclovir; however, famciclovir is less effective at suppressing subclinical shedding. For persons infected with HIV, increased dosages and/or extended duration of therapy is recommended.

Potential complications. *Men and women:* HSV infection can cause neuralgia, meningitis, ascending myelitis, urinary retention, urethral strictures, and lymphatic suppuration. These outcomes are generally more common in women. *Women:* Pregnancy loss and preterm delivery have been associated with HSV infections, usually in primary infection occurring in the third trimester. *Neonates:* During vaginal delivery, virus from an active genital infection can cause neonatal herpes. This condition ranges in severity from clinically inapparent infections to local infections of the eyes, skin, or mucous membranes or to severely disseminated infection that may involve the central nervous system. Full-blown neonatal herpes has a high fatality rate, and survivors often have ocular or neurologic sequelae.

Behavioral messages to emphasize. Because both initial and recurrent lesions shed high concentrations of the virus, abstain from sexual activity while ulcers are present. However, most genital HSV transmission occurs during asymptomatic intervals. Condoms offer some protection from HSV acquisition. Prophylactic valacyclovir reduces HSV transmission risks. A recent study demonstrated that use of coitally dependent tenofovir gel significantly reduced the rate of HSV-2 acquisition (by 51%) in South African women; this finding was unexpected, and further study is required to define a potential role for this product in HSV-2 prevention. The risk of transmission to the neonate from an infected mother is highest among women with primary herpes infection (the first time they have been infected with either HSV-1 or HSV-2) during the third trimester, lower among women with nonprimary first episodes of the disease and least among women with recurrent herpes. At the onset of labor, describe any symptoms and examine for lesions. If no symptoms or signs are present, the infant may be delivered vaginally. Infants delivered through an infected birth canal should be cultured and followed carefully. Genital herpes (and other diseases causing genital ulcers) have been associated with an increased risk of acquiring HIV infections. Clinically evaluating asymptomatic partners has little value for preventing transmission of HSV; however, some recommend serologic screening of pregnant women to identify those at risk for HSV acquisition during pregnancy.

GONORRHEA is caused by Neisseria gonorrhoeae, a gram-negative bacterium seen as a diplococcus on Gram stain. About 650,000 new cases of gonorrhea occur each year, making it the second most commonly reported infectious disease in the United States.

Symptoms. Women are most commonly asymptomatic, but may have abnormal vaginal discharge, abnormal menses, or dysuria. Symptomatic men usually have dysuria, increased frequency of urination, and purulent urethral discharge. An estimated one-fourth of infected men can be asymptomatic. Pharyngeal gonorrhea can occasionally produce symptoms of pharyngitis, but most infections are asymptomatic.

Diagnosis. In men, presumptive diagnosis relies on microscopically identifying typical gram-negative intracellular diplococci on smear of urethral exudates. In women, Gram stain of endocervical secretions of infected women is positive only half the time and is not commonly performed. Definitive diagnosis, especially in women, requires recovery of bacteria either by culture or molecular testing (NAAT). NAAT can be performed on urine or on self-collected vaginal swab. Although the use of culture allows for antimicrobial susceptibility testing, increasing use of

NAAT has increased the number of women tested and offers a noninvasive method for diagnosis. A definitive diagnosis by culture is required if the specimen is extragenital or from a child or if is important for medicolegal reasons.

Treatment. In many areas of the United States, about one-fourth of men and two-fifths of women with gonococcal infections also have a coexisting chlamydial infection. For this reason, and to address concerns for increasing antibiotic resistance in gonorrhea, use both a single-dose antigonococcal drug AND an antichlamydial regimen, regardless of the chlamydia diagnostic test result. The recommended therapy for gonorrhea is ceftriaxone 250 mg IM once. If this is not available, cefixime 400 mg orally once may be used as an alternative. See the CDC's website on this topic for frequent updates (www.cdc.gov/std/treatment). See the Chlamydia section for discussion of treatment regimens. Pharyngeal gonorrhea may be more difficult to treat, and ceftriaxone 250 mg IM should be used if possible.

Potential complications. Up to 40% of untreated women with cervical gonorrhea develop PID and are at risk for its sequelae (see the section on PID), including involuntary sterility and pelvic abscesses. Men are at risk for epididymitis, urethral stricture, and sterility. Newborns are at risk for ophthalmia neonatorum, scalp abscess at the site of fetal monitors, rhinitis, or anorectal infection. All infected untreated persons are at risk for disseminated gonococcal infection.

Behavioral messages to emphasize. Sex partner(s) should be treated. Avoid sex until both you and partner(s) have been treated.

GRANULOMA INGUINALE (Donovanosis) is caused by Calymmatobacterium granulomatis (formerly known as Donovania granulomatis), a bipolar, gram-negative bacterium (Donovan body) that in a crush preparation appears in vacuolar compartments within histiocytes, white blood cells, or plasma cells.

Prevalence. Granuloma inguinale is rare in the United States. However, it is endemic in certain less developed countries including India, Papua New Guinea, Central Australia, and Southern Africa.

Symptoms. Initially, single or multiple subcutaneous nodules appear at the site of inoculation. Nodules erode to form granulomatous, heaped ulcers that are painless, bleed on contact, and enlarge slowly. Spread by autoinoculation is common.

Diagnosis. The typical clinical presentation is sufficient to suggest the diagnosis. Resolution of the lesions following specific antibiotic therapy supports the diagnosis. The patient's or partner's history of travel to endemic areas helps substantiate the clinical impression. A microscopic examination of biopsy specimens from the ulcer margin reveals the pathognomonic Donovan bodies. Tissue culture of C. granulomatis is not feasible.

Treatment. Recommended initial regimens are doxycycline 100 mg orally twice a day OR trimethoprim-sulfamethoxazole, 1 double-strength tablet twice a day until all lesions have completely healed (usually a minimum of 3 weeks). Alternatives are ciprofloxacin 750 mg orally twice a day OR erythromycin 500 mg orally four times a day OR azithromycin 1 mg orally once a week—all for at least 3 weeks.

Potential complications. Lesions may become secondarily infected. Fibrous, keloid-like formations may deform the genitalia. Pseudoelephantoid enlargement of the labia, penis, or scrotum occurs. Necrosis and destruction of the genitalia may result.

Behavioral messages to emphasize. Understand how to take prescribed oral medications. Return for evaluation 3 to 5 days after therapy begins. Assure examination of sex partner(s) as soon as possible. Return weekly or biweekly for evaluation until the infection is entirely healed.

HEPATITIS A is caused by hepatitis A virus (HAV), an RNA virus that is typically transmitted by the fecal-oral route. For this reason, HAV can be transmitted through oral-anal sex.

Symptoms. The majority of infections are symptomatic, causing fatigue, anorexia, nausea, vomiting, headache, fever, dark urine, jaundice, and moderate liver enlargement with tenderness.

Diagnosis. HAV infection is clinically indistinguishable from other forms of hepatitis. Routine viral hepatitis serology should be performed in such patients. Serum IgM antiHAV is almost always detectable at the onset of symptoms, and IgG antiHAV levels rise soon thereafter. Measurement of serum IgM antiHAV is the diagnostic test of choice.

Treatment/Prevention. No specific therapy exists; therapy is supportive. Vaccines made from recombinant genetic material are available. Specific vaccination and post-exposure prophylaxis strategies are of proven efficacy in preventing hepatitis A infection. Vaccinating all men who have sex with men, persons who use illicit drugs, and travelers to endemic areas against hepatitis A is currently recommended.

Potential complications. Long-term sequelae are rare. Rarely, acute fulminant hepatitis can occur, resulting in hepatic failure and death.

Behavioral messages to emphasize. HAV vaccination is strongly encouraged for target groups. Consult public health authorities regarding recommendations for post-exposure prophylaxis of household contacts and sex partners.

HEPATITIS B is caused by hepatitis B virus (HBV), a DNA virus with multiple antigenic components. In the United States, about 5% of the general population show evidence of past HBV infections. An estimated 120,000 new cases of HBV infection are transmitted sexually each year. Heterosexual intercourse is now the predominant mode of HBV transmission.

Symptoms. Most HBV infections are not clinically apparent. When present, symptoms include a serum sickness-like prodrome (skin eruptions, urticaria, arthralgias, arthritis), lassitude, anorexia, nausea, vomiting, headache, fever, dark urine, jaundice, and moderate liver enlargement with tenderness.

Diagnosis. HBV infection is clinically indistinguishable from other forms of hepatitis. A patient with the typical clinical symptoms and exposure to a patient with definitive or presumed HBV infection may be presumed to have HBV infection. Serodiagnosis of HBV infection is the best method for clinicians to reach a definitive diagnosis. Positive results of the following tests are reliable:

- Hepatitis B surface antigen (HBsAg): Acute HBV infection or, with no acute disease exposure, the chronic active state (infectious)

- HBe antigen: More infectious than if just HBsAg-positive, because the virus is actively replicating

- antiHBs (surface antibody): Past infection or immunization with present immunity

- antiHBc (core antibody): Past or current infection.

Treatment. No specific therapy exists. Provide supportive and symptomatic care. Vaccines made from recombinant genetic material are available. Specific vaccination and post-exposure prophylaxis strategies are of proven efficacy in preventing hepatitis B. Vaccinating all newborn infants and adolescents against hepatitis B is currently recommended. In addition, the Advisory Committee on Immunization Practices recommends HBV vaccination for all persons with recent STI and those who have a history of sexual activity with more than one partner in the previous 6 months. Subsidized HBV vaccine programs are available in many states.

Potential complications. Long-term sequelae include chronic, persistent, active hepatitis, cirrhosis, hepatocellular carcinoma, hepatic failure, and death. Rarely, the course may be fulminant with hepatic failure.

Behavioral messages to emphasize. HBV vaccination is strongly encouraged for all young, sexually active clients. The full vaccination regimen is necessary for maximum protection. If you have hepatitis B, you should be followed to document seroconversion to immunity or persistence of chronic carrier state.

HEPATITIS C is caused by hepatitis C virus (HCV), an RNA virus that is typically transmitted by the parenteral route (needle sharing or transfusion to contaminated blood). HCV has been detected in genital secretions, but is probably infrequently sexually transmitted unless exchange of blood or bloody secretions occurs.

Symptoms. The majority of infections is asymptomatic, but occasionally can present with fatigue, anorexia, nausea, vomiting, headache, fever, dark urine, jaundice, and moderate liver enlargement with tenderness.

Diagnosis. HCV infection is clinically indistinguishable from other forms of hepatitis. Routine viral hepatitis serology should be performed in such patients. Serum IgM antiHCV is almost always detectable at the onset of symptoms, and IgG antiHCV levels rise soon thereafter. Measurement of serum IgM antiHCV is the diagnostic test of choice in the setting of acute hepatitis.

Treatment/Prevention. No specific therapy exists; therapy is supportive. No vaccine is available. Patients should be educated about ways to avoid transmission through contaminated needles or by sharing such items as razors with household or sexual contacts who are infected.

Potential complications. Long-term sequelae include chronic, persistent, active hepatitis, cirrhosis, hepatocellular carcinoma, hepatic failure, and death. Rarely, the course may be fulminant with hepatic failure.

Behavioral messages to emphasize. Sex partners already in an established relationship do not need to change their sexual practices if one partner is found to be HCV-infected; the partner of unknown status should be screened. If you have HCV and are beginning a new sexual relationship, use safer sex precautions as applicable for routine STI protection (e.g., condoms).

HUMAN IMMUNODEFICIENCY VIRUS (HIV) See "Special Considerations Regarding HIV/AIDS in the Reproductive Health Setting."

HUMAN PAPILLOMAVIRUS (HPV) are common viruses that include over 100 types specific to the human genital tract. Two major clinical syndromes arise from these infections: genital warts and epithelial (notably, cervical) neoplasia. HPV vaccination should be a standard practice in reproductive health care. Genital warts are discussed below; cervical neoplasia is discussed in Chapter 22.

GENITAL WARTS (Condyloma acuminata) are caused by several of the many types of human papillomavirus (HPV), a small, slowly growing DNA virus belonging to the papovavirus group. Types 6 and 11 usually cause visible genital warts. Other HPV types in the genital region are associated with vaginal, anal, and cervical dysplasia.

Prevalence. Genital warts account for more than 1 million physician office visits annually, making condyloma the most common symptomatic viral RTI in the United States. The most sensitive measures of HPV indicate up to 80% of all sexually active young women are infected with this virus. Cases of condyloma have been correlated with earlier onset of sexual activity, multiple sex partners, and a higher frequency of casual relationships than in controls.

Symptoms. Single or multiple soft, fleshy, papillary or sessile, painless keratinized growths appear around the vulvovaginal area, penis, anus, urethra, or perineum. Women infected with condyloma may exhibit typical growths on the walls of the vagina or cervix and may be unaware of their existence. Regular genital self-examinations may be helpful in detecting such growths on the external genitalia of both women and men. From 60% to 90% of male partners of women with condyloma have HPV infection on the penis, although infection may not be visible to the naked eye.

Diagnosis. No evidence supports the use of HPV DNA tests in the routine diagnosis or management of visible genital warts. A diagnosis is made from the typical clinical signs on the external genitalia. Colposcopy is valuable for diagnosing flat warts, which are difficult to see. Exclude the possible diagnosis of condylomata lata by obtaining a serologic test for syphilis. A biopsy is usually unnecessary but would be required to make a definitive diagnosis. When neoplasia is a possibility, take a biopsy of any atypical lesions or persistent warts before initiating therapy.

Treatment. Several different treatment regimens can be used, depending on client preference, available resources, and the experience of the health care provider. None of the currently available treatments is superior to others or ideal for all patients. The currently available treatments for visible genital warts consist of two types: (1) patient-applied therapies and (2) provider-administered therapies.

Patient-applied therapies:

- *Podofilox* 0.5% solution or gel. Patients apply podofilox solution with a cotton swab, or a podofilox gel with a finger, to visible genital warts twice daily for 3 days, followed by 4 days of no therapy. This process may be repeated up to a total of four times. Podofilox should not be used during pregnancy.

- *Imiquimod* 5% cream. Patients should apply imiquimod cream with a finger, at bedtime, 3 times a week, for up to 16 weeks. They should wash with mild soap and water after 6 to 10 hours. Imiquimod should not be used during pregnancy.

Provider-administered therapies:

- *Cryotherapy* with liquid nitrogen or cryoprobe. Repeat applications every 1 to 2 weeks.

- *Trichloroacetic acid (TCA) or bichloroacetic acid (BCA)* 80% to 90%. Apply a small amount to only the warts and allow to dry, at which time a white "frosting" develops. Repeat weekly as needed.

- *Podophyllin resin* 10% to 25% in tincture of benzoin. A small amount of podophyllin should be applied to each wart and allowed to air dry. Avoid normal tissue. Wash off thoroughly in 1 to 4 hours to reduce local irritation. Podophyllin should not be used during pregnancy and is not recommended for vaginal use.

- Sinecatechins (green tea extract) 15% ointment. Apply TID for up to 16 weeks

- *Surgical removal.* Scissor or shaving excision, curette, or electrosurgery is possible.

HPV infection is an infectious condition even when asymptomatic. However, for most persons, it has a benign natural history, and some individuals may not be infectious for long periods of time. No therapy completely eradicates the virus, although the burden of HPV appears to decline in the years following initial infection. HPV has been demonstrated in adjacent tissue even after attempts to eliminate subclinical HPV by extensive laser vaporization of the anogenital area. The effect of genital wart treatment on HPV transmission and the natural history of HPV are unknown. Therefore, the goal of treatment is the temporary removal of visible genital warts and the amelioration of symptoms and signs, *not* the eradication of HPV.

Potential complications. Lesions may enlarge and destroy tissue. Giant condyloma, while histologically benign, may simulate carcinoma. In pregnancy, warts enlarge, are extremely vascular, and may obstruct the birth canal to necessitate a cesarean delivery. Neither routine HPV screening tests nor cesarean delivery for prevention of the transmission of HPV to the newborn is indicated. The perinatal transmission rate is unknown, although probably low. Persons with HIV disease can have rapidly growing genital warts. Women infected with HIV have an increased risk of progressive HPV-cervical disease.

Prevention. Two vaccines to prevent genital HPV infection are now available. One is a quadrivalent vaccine that protects against acquisition of type 6, 11, 16, and 18 (Gardasil) and the other is a bivalent vaccine that protects against types 16 and 18 (Cervarix). Large multicenter studies in young women indicate that both are nearly 100% effective in preventing infection with these HPV types and in preventing associated cervical neoplasia. Recommendations for immunization target pre-adolescent girls age 10 to 12 years, prior to the onset of sexual activity; however, the vaccines are approved and recommended for women up to 25 years (www.cdc.gov/nip/acip). Data on the efficacy of the quadrivalent HPV vaccines in protecting young men from vaccine-type HPV acquisition indicate similarly high levels of protection, and the vaccine may be offered to prevent genital warts in young men.

Behavioral messages to emphasize. Return for regular treatment until lesions have resolved. Once warts have responded to therapy, no special follow-up is necessary. Because most partners are probably already infected, examination of sex partners is not necessary. Most new HPV infections are acquired from sex partners who have no symptoms or signs of the infection. To reduce risks of sequelae from cervical cancer, regular Pap smears are crucial for all women with documented HPV infection, regardless of whether they have received HPV vaccine. HPV testing is useful in triaging women with Pap smears showing ASCUS and for primary screening of cervical neoplasia in women over 30 years. Smoking cessation will reduce the risk of HPV and neoplasia.

LYMPHOGRANULOMA VENEREUM (LGV) is caused by serovars L1, L2, or L3 of Chlamydia trachomatis. LGV infections are endemic in Asia and Africa and were thought to be relatively rare in the United States. However, beginning in 2003, outbreaks of rectal LGV (proctitis) were documented in several U.S. cities among men who reported unprotected receptive anal sex (most of whom were also HIV-infected).

Symptoms. The primary lesion of LGV is a 2 to 3 mm painless vesicle or nonindurated ulcer at the site of inoculation. Patients commonly fail to notice this primary lesion. Regional adenopathy follows a week to a month later and is the most common clinical symptom. A sensation of stiffness and aching in the groin, followed by swelling of the inguinal region, may be the first indications of infections for most patients. Adenopathy may subside spontaneously or proceed to the formation of abscesses that rupture to produce draining sinuses or fistulae. In patients who acquire the infection from receptive anal intercourse, proctitis can result and may be severe.

Diagnosis. LGV is often diagnosed clinically and may be confused with chancroid because of the painful adenopathy. LGV-specific serology has been validated for the classical form of the disease, in which the complement fixation test is sensitive, and 80% of patients have a titer of 1:16 or higher. Levels of 1:64 are considered diagnostic. However, these tests have not been well-validated for the diagnosis of LGV proctitis. Because the sequelae of LGV are serious and preventable, do not withhold treatment pending laboratory confirmation. A definitive diagnosis requires isolating C. trachomatis from an appropriate specimen and confirming the isolate as an LGV immunotype. However, these laboratory diagnostic capabilities are not widely available.

Treatment. Prescribe doxycycline 100 mg orally two times a day for 21 days OR erythromycin 500 mg orally four times a day for 21 days. Aspirate fluctuant lymph nodes as needed. Incision and drainage or excision of nodes will delay healing and are contraindicated.

Potential complications. Dissemination may occur with nephropathy, hepatomegaly, or phlebitis. Large polypoid swelling of the vulva (esthiomene), anal margin, or rectal mucosa may occur. The most common severe morbidity results from rectal involvement: perianal abscess and rectovaginal or other fistulae are early consequences, and rectal stricture may develop 1 to 10 years after infection.

Behavioral messages to emphasize. Return for evaluation 3 to 5 days after therapy begins. Assure examination of sex partner(s) as soon as possible. For all patients with LGV proctitis, knowledge of HIV status is essential given the epidemiology of the current outbreak.

MOLLUSCUM CONTAGIOSUM is caused by molluscum contagiosum virus, the largest DNA virus of the poxvirus group.

Prevalence. As an STI, molluscum contagiosum occurs infrequently, about 1 case for every 100 cases of gonorrhea. Outbreaks have been reported among groups at high risk for other RTI.

Symptoms. Lesions are 1 to 5 mm, smooth, rounded, firm, shiny flesh-colored to pearly-white papules with characteristically umbilicated centers. They are most commonly seen on the trunk and anogenital region and are generally asymptomatic. Exceptions to this occur in immunosuppressed patients (particularly HIV-positive with low CD4 counts), in whom the lesions can be diffuse or become bulky.

Diagnosis. Infection is usually diagnosed on the basis of the typical clinical presentation. Microscopic examination of lesions or lesion material reveals the pathognomonic molluscum inclusion bodies.

Treatment. Lesions may resolve spontaneously without scarring. However, they may be removed by curettage after cryoanesthesia. Treatment with caustic chemicals (podophyllin, trichloroacetic acid, silver nitrate) and cryotherapy (liquid nitrogen) have been successful. If every lesion is not extirpated, the condition may recur.

Potential complications. Secondary infection, usually with staphylococcus, may occur. Lesions rarely attain a size greater than 10 mm in diameter.

Behavioral messages to emphasize. Return for reexamination 1 month after treatment so any new lesions can be removed. Sex partner(s) should be examined.

MYCOPLASMA GENITALIUM is a bacterium that has recently been associated with urethritis in men and cervicitis and PID in women. No specific diagnostic test is currently available. Studies are underway to determine the prevalence in representative populations and the best approach to treatment.

PELVIC INFLAMMATORY DISEASE (PID) can be caused by varying combinations of N. gonorrhoeae, C. trachomatis, anaerobic bacteria, facultative gram-negative rods (such as E. coli), Mycoplasma hominis, and a variety of other microbial agents. Clinical PID is usually of polymicrobial etiology. N. gonorrhoeae and C. trachomatis may cause antecedent inflammation, which makes the tubes susceptible to invasion by anaerobic organisms.

Prevalence. PID accounts for nearly 180,000 hospitalizations every year in the United States. More than 1 million episodes occur annually. Among American women of reproductive age, 1 in 7 reports having received treatment for PID.

Symptoms. Based on retrospective reports, many women with PID have atypical or no symptoms. Women may have pain and tenderness involving the lower abdomen, cervix, uterus, or adnexae, occasionally with fever, chills, and elevated white blood cell (WBC) count and erythrocyte sedimentation rate (ESR). The condition is more likely if the patient has multiple sex partners or a history of PID or is in the first 5 to 10 days of her menstrual cycle. More specific criteria, such as endometrial biopsy, magnetic resonance imaging, or diagnostic laparoscopy, are warranted only in selected instances.

Diagnosis. Women who have the typical clinical symptoms are presumed to have PID if other serious conditions, such as acute appendicitis or ectopic pregnancy, can be excluded. The diagnosis of PID is often based on imprecise clinical findings. Maintain a low threshold for diagnosing PID, because even mild or moderate PID has the potential for reproductive sequelae. Use objective criteria to monitor response to antibiotics, especially if ambulatory treatment is given. Direct visualization of inflamed (edema, hyperemia, or tubal exudate) fallopian tube(s) during laparoscopy or laparotomy confirms the diagnosis of PID. Cultures of tubal exudate may help establish the microbiologic etiology.

Treatment. Because the causative organism is usually unknown at the time of the initial therapy, use treatment regimens that are active against the broadest possible range of pathogens. Antimicrobial coverage should include N. gonorrhoeae, C. trachomatis, anaerobes, gram-negative facultative bacteria, and streptococci.

Hospitalization and inpatient care: Since hospitalization is no longer synonymous with parenteral therapy, the decision to hospitalize is based on the clinician's discretion. Data show hospitalization did not improve short or long-term outcomes in women with symptomatic PID. Consider hospitalizing patients with acute PID when (1) surgical emergencies, such as appendicitis and ectopic pregnancy, are not definitely excluded; (2) severe illness precludes outpatient management; (3) the woman is unable to follow or tolerate an outpatient regimen; or (4) the woman has failed to respond to outpatient therapy. Special consideration may be given to adolescents both to preserve their fertility and to improve their adherence.

Combined drug therapy is recommended in all cases since the full bacterial etiology of PID is not clear and is generally polymicrobial.

Parenteral treatment: Two parenteral regimens are recommended for both inpatient and outpatient care:

- *Regimen A:* Either cefotetan 2.0 g IV every 12 hours, OR cefoxitin 2.0 g IV every 6 hours for at least 24 hours after the patient clinically improves PLUS doxycycline 100 mg orally or IV every 12 hours. Continue doxycycline 100 mg orally twice daily after discharge to complete at least 14 days of therapy.

- *Regimen B:* Clindamycin 900 mg, IV three times a day, PLUS gentamicin 2 mg per kilogram (kg) IV loading dose and maintenance 1.5 mg/kg IV every 8 hours. Continue oral therapy as above.

Oral treatment:

- Ceftriaxone 250 mg IM; OR Cefoxitin 2.0 g IM along with probenecid 1.0 g orally PLUS doxycycline 100 mg taken orally twice daily for 14 days.

Potential complications. Potentially life-threatening complications include ectopic pregnancy and pelvic abscess. Other sequelae are involuntary infertility, recurrent or chronic PID, chronic abdominal pain, pelvic adhesions, premature hysterectomy, and depression.

Behavioral messages to emphasize. For outpatient therapy, return for evaluation 2 to 3 days after initiation of therapy. Return for further evaluation 4 days after completing therapy. Refer sex partner(s) for evaluation and treatment (even if they are asymptomatic). Avoid sexual activity throughout the course of treatment. Understand how to take prescribed oral medications.

SYPHILIS is caused by Treponema pallidum, a spirochete with 6 to 14 regular spirals and characteristic motility.

Prevalence. Because of recent syphilis elimination efforts, primary and secondary syphilis currently are declining in the United States among women. Congenital syphilis is also on the wane. However, syphilis rates are increasing among men who have sex with men, and it remains an important STI, with serious sequelae if not treated. In heterosexual populations, southeastern states have the highest rates of both syphilis and congenital syphilis, although recent outbreaks have occurred in the Southwest.

Symptoms. *Primary:* The classical chancre is a painless, indurated ulcer, located at the site of exposure. The differential diagnosis for all genital lesions should include syphilis. *Secondary:* Patients may have a highly variable skin rash, mucous patches, condylomata lata (fleshy, moist tissue growths), lymphadenopathy, alopecia, or other signs. *Latent:* Patients are without clinical signs of infection.

Diagnosis. The 2010 CDC STD Treatment Guidelines discuss the types of serologic testing that are available. The clinical presentation by stage is as follows:

- *Primary:* Patients have typical lesion(s) and either a positive darkfield exam; a fluorescent antibody technique in material from a chancre, regional lymph node, or other lesion; or they have been exposed to syphilis within 90 days of lesion onset.

- *Secondary:* Patients have a typical clinical presentation and a strongly reactive serologic test; condyloma lata will be darkfield positive.

- *Latent:* Patients have serologic evidence of untreated syphilis without clinical signs.

- Primary and secondary syphilis are definitively diagnosed by demonstrating T. pallidum with darkfield microscopy or fluorescent antibody technique, but can be presumptively diagnosed in the setting of a compatible clinical presentation and reactive serology. A definitive diagnosis of latent syphilis cannot be made under usual circumstances.

Treatment. *Primary, secondary, or early syphilis of less than 1 year duration:* benzathine penicillin G 2.4 million units IM in a single dose. Alternative regimens include ceftriaxone 1 gram IV or IM daily for 8–10 days. The regimen of doxycycline 100 mg orally twice daily for 14 days is inferior, and not recommended unless no other alternatives are available.

Syphilis of indeterminate length or of more than 1 year duration: benzathine penicillin G 7.2 million units total; 2.4 million units IM, weekly, for 3 successive weeks.

Patients allergic to penicillin: Doxycycline 100 mg orally two times a day. [Note: Duration of therapy depends on the estimated duration of infection. If duration has been less than 1 year, treat the infection for 14 days; otherwise, treat for 28 days.]

Penicillin-allergic pregnant women or for doxycycline-intolerant patients only: Consult the 2010 Guidelines for Treatment of Sexually Transmitted Diseases.

Congenital syphilis or if the patient is simultaneously infected with syphilis and HIV: Refer to the 2010 Guidelines for Treatment of Sexually Transmitted Diseases.

Potential complications. Late syphilis and congenital syphilis, both complications of early syphilis, are preventable with prompt diagnosis and treatment. Sequelae of late syphilis include neurosyphilis (general paresis, tabes dorsalis, and focal neurologic signs), cardiovascular syphilis (thoracic aortic aneurism, aortic insufficiency), and localized gumma formation.

Behavioral messages to emphasize. Because genital ulcers may be associated with HIV infection, get an HIV test. Return for follow-up syphilis serologies at 3 and 6 months for early syphilis, and at 6 and 12 months for late latent disease. HIV-positive patients should return 1, 2, 3, 6, 9, and 12 months after therapy; pregnant partners should be followed monthly. Sex partner(s) should be evaluated and treated. Avoid sexual activity until treatment is completed.

TRICHOMONIASIS is caused by Trichomonas vaginalis, a motile protozoan with an undulating membrane and four flagella.

Prevalence. Trichomoniasis is the most common curable STI in the United States and worldwide. Each year an estimated 3 million U.S. women become infected.

Symptoms. Excessive, frothy, diffuse, yellow-green vaginal discharge is common, although clinical presentation varies from no signs or symptoms to erythema, edema, and pruritus of the external genitalia. Dysuria and dyspareunia are also frequent. The type of symptoms or signs alone does not distinguish the microbial etiology. Male sex partners may develop urethritis, balanitis, or cutaneous lesions on the penis; however, the majority of males infected with T. vaginalis are asymptomatic.

Diagnosis. Trichomoniasis is diagnosed when a vaginal culture or antigen test is positive for T. vaginalis OR typical motile trichomonads are identified in a saline wet mount of vaginal discharge. Liquid-based cervical cytology (Pap smear) is a specific means of making the diagnosis. Nucleic acid amplification tests are expected to become available in the near future.

Treatment. Metronidazole 2.0 g orally at one time. Alternative regimens are metronidazole 500 mg orally twice daily for 7 days or tinidazole 2 g orally at one time. Most treatment failures are due to failure to treat the index patient's sex partners; initial management should include retreatment of the patient and partners with single-dose metronidazole (2.0 g). Metronidazole-resistant T. vaginalis, although uncommon, can occur. Most treatment failures respond to higher doses of metronidazole therapy or to a single dose of tinidazole (2 g). Sex partners should be simultaneously treated with the same regimen as the index client.

Potential complications. Secondary excoriation may occur. Recurrent infections are common. Trichomoniasis has been associated with an increased risk of salpingitis, low birthweight, prematurity, and acquisition of HIV.

Behavioral messages to emphasize. Make sure sex partner(s) are treated. Use condoms to prevent future infections. Avoid drinking alcohol until 24 hours after completing metronidazole therapy or 48 hours after tinidazole.

URETHRITIS, INCLUDING NONGONOCOCCAL URETHRITIS (NGU) is caused by Chlamydia trachomatis about 30% of the time. Other sexually transmissible agents, which cause 10% to 45% of NGU, include Trichomonas vaginalis, Mycoplasma genitalium, and herpes simplex virus; Ureaplasma urealyticum may also contribute. The etiology of the remaining cases is unknown.

Prevalence. NGU appears more frequently than gonorrhea in both public STI clinics and private practices. More than 1 million cases annually are estimated to occur in men.

Symptoms. Men usually have dysuria, urinary frequency, and mucoid to purulent urethral discharge. Many men have asymptomatic infections.

Diagnosis. Men with typical clinical symptoms are presumed to have NGU when their gonorrhea tests are negative and they have either white blood cells (WBCs) on a Gram stain of urethral discharge or sexual exposure to an agent known to cause NGU. Asymptomatic men with negative gonorrhea tests are also presumed to have NGU if > 5 WBCs per oil immersion field appear on an intraurethral smear. Chlamydia testing is strongly recommended for a specific diagnosis. Gonococcal and nongonococcal urethritis may coexist in the same patient.

Treatment. When the etiology is C. trachomatis, or unknown, the following treatment is recommended: azithromycin 1 g orally in a single dose OR doxycycline 100 mg orally twice daily for 7 days. For patients who fail their first trial of antibiotics and whose partners have been treated, the persistent urethritis should be documented (either by visual examination of discharge or microscopy to quantify WBC). In this case, the patient should be treated with metronidazole 2.0 g orally as a single dose, and if not previously treated with azithromycin, treated with azithromycin 1.0 g orally as a single dose. For herpes simplex infections, see the sections of this chapter that deal specifically with these agents.

Potential complications. Urethral strictures or epididymitis may occur. If C. trachomatis is transmitted to female sex partners, the condition may result in mucopurulent cervicitis and PID. If C. trachomatis is transmitted to a pregnant woman, complications may include neonatal infections such as conjunctivitis or pneumonia.

Behavioral messages to emphasize. If chlamydial infection or other STI is diagnosed, sex partner(s) should be treated. Avoid sex until treatment is completed. Use condoms to prevent future infections.

VAGINITIS is a general term that refers to the syndrome of abnormal vaginal discharge and related patient complaints, which may include abnormal odor and vulvovaginal pruritus or nonspecific discomfort. Specific causes of vaginitis discussed in this catalogue include bacterial vaginosis (BV) and vulvovaginal candidiasis (VVC). Other causes of vaginitis that reproductive health clinicians might encounter include:

Desquamative inflammatory vaginitis (DIV) is a relatively uncommon, but probably under-diagnosed, form of vaginitis in which women complain of copious, purulent vaginal discharge, typically accompanied by vaginal pain or burning and dyspareunia. DIV may be more common in older (peri- or postmenopausal) women, though the epidemiology is poorly defined. Occasionally frank vestibulitis or excoriations will occur. On examination of vaginal fluid, the characteristic findings are elevated vaginal pH (usually 5.5 to 7.4), few lactobacilli, and numerous gram-positive cocci. Group B streptococcus may be involved in the pathogenesis of this condition. Treatment includes a relatively prolonged course of clindamycin 2% cream administered vaginally at bedtime, usually given for at least 14 days OR 10% hydrocortisone cream 5 g administered nightly at bedtime for at least 14 days. Longer courses of therapy are often required.

Irritant/chemical vaginitis occurs commonly, though few population-based data are available. Any substance that can elicit a mucosal inflammatory response, including douches, some spermicides, soaps or other cleansing agents, or other feminine-hygiene products, can be responsible if administered vaginally. This condition may result in vaginal discharge characterized by numerous WBC. When evaluating women for vulvo-vaginal complaints take a careful history of use of any vaginal products or of products applied directly to the vulva.

REFERENCES

1. Eng TR, Butler WT. The hidden epidemic confronting sexually transmitted diseases. Committee on Prevention and Control of Sexually Transmitted Diseases, IoMUS, Division of Health Promotion and Disease Prevention, 1996.
2. Centers for Disease Control and Prevention. Sexually Transmitted Disease Surveillance, 2008. Atlanta, GA: U.S. Department of Health and Human Services, 2009.
3. Cates W, Jr. Review of non-hormonal contraception (condoms, intrauterine devices, nonoxynol-9 and combos) on HIV acquisition. J Acquir Immune Defic Syndr. 2005;38 Suppl 1:S8–10.
4. Pilcher CD, Tien HC, Eron JJ, Jr., et al. Brief but efficient: acute HIV infection and the sexual transmission of HIV. J Infect Dis. 2004;189:1785–92.
5. UNAIDS and WHO. New data on male circumcision and HIV prevention: policy and programme implications; WHO/UNAIDS technical consultation male circumcision and HIV prevention: research implications for policy and programming montreux. Geneva: Joint United Nations Programme on HIV/AIDS and World Health Organization, 2007.
6. Padian NS, van der Straten A, Ramjee G, et al. Diaphragm and lubricant gel for prevention of HIV acquisition in southern African women: a randomised controlled trial. Lancet. 2007;370:251–61.
7. Ness RB, Keder LM, Soper DE, et al. Oral contraception and the recognition of endometritis. Am J Obstet Gynecol. 1997;176:580–5.
8. Morrison CS, Bright P, Wong EL, et al. Hormonal contraceptive use, cervical ectopy, and the acquisition of cervical infections. Sex Transm Dis. 2004;31:561–7.
9. Morrison CS, Richardson BA, Mmiro F, et al. Hormonal contraception and the risk of HIV acquisition. AIDS. 2007;21:85–95.
10. Cates W, Jr., Padian NS. The interrelationship of reproductive health and sexually transmitted diseases. In: Goldman M N, M., editors. Women and Health. San Diego, California: Academic Press, 2000.
11. Grimes DA. Intrauterine device and upper-genital-tract infection. Lancet. 2000;356: 1013–9.
12. Van Damme L, Ramjee G, Alary M, et al. Effectiveness of COL-1492, a nonoxynol-9 vaginal gel, on HIV-1 transmission in female sex workers: a randomised controlled trial. Lancet. 2002;360:971–7.
13. Karim QA, Karim SS, Frohlich JA, et al. Effectiveness and safety of tenofovir gel, an antiretroviral microbicide, for the prevention of HIV infection in women. Science. 2010;10:1126.
14. Martino JL, Vermund SH. Vaginal douching: evidence for risks or benefits to women's health. Epidemiol Rev. 2002;24:109–24.
15. Nowicki MJ, Laskus T, Nikolopoulou G, et al. Presence of hepatitis C virus (HCV) RNA in the genital tracts of HCV/HIV-1-coinfected women. J Infect Dis. 2005;192:1557–65.
16. Leigh BC. Alcohol and condom use: a meta-analysis of event-level studies. Sex Transm Dis. 2002;29:476–82.
17. Cates W, Jr. A risk-assessment tool for integrated reproductive health services. Fam Plann Perspect. 1997;29:41–3.
18. Screening for chlamydial infection: recommendations and rationale. Am J Prev Med. 2001;20:90–4.
19. Screening for gonorrhea: recommendation statement. Ann Fam Med. 2005;3:263–7.

20. Chou R, Huffman LH, Fu R, Smits AK, Korthuis PT. Screening for HIV: a review of the evidence for the U.S. Preventive Services Task Force. Ann Intern Med. 2005;143:55–73.
21. American College of Obstetrics and Gynecology and American Academy Pediatrics Guidelines for Perinatal Care, 5th ed. Washington, D.C.: American College of Obstetrics and Gynecology and American Academy Pediatrics, 2002.
22. Centers for Disease Control and Prevention. Sexually Transmitted Diseases Treatment Guidelines, 2010. MMWR. 2010;59:RR-12.
23. Royce RA, Sena A, Cates W, Jr., Cohen MS. Sexual transmission of HIV. N Engl J Med. 1997;336:1072–8.
24. Centers for Disease Control and Prevention. Antiretroviral postexposure prophylaxis after sexual, injection-drug use, or other nonoccupational exposure to HIV in the United States: recommendations from the U.S. Department of Health and Human Services. MMWR. 2005;54.
25. Gray RH, Wawer MJ, Brookmeyer R, et al. Probability of HIV-1 transmission per coital act in monogamous, heterosexual, HIV-1-discordant couples in Rakai, Uganda. Lancet. 2001;357:1149–53.
26. CENTERS FOR DISEASE CONTROL AND PREVENTION. Revised recommendations for HIV testing for adults, adolescents, and pregnant women in healthcare settings. MMWR. 2006;55 (RR-14).
27. Gray RH, Li X, Kigozi G, et al. Increased risk of incident HIV during pregnancy in Rakai, Uganda: a prospective study. Lancet. 2005;366:1182–8.
28. A guide to the clinical care of women with HIV. In: Anderson RJe, ed. Rockville, MD: HIV/AIDS Bureau, Health Resources and Services Administration, 2001.
29. Lingappa JR, Baeten JM, Wald A, et al. Daily aciclovir for HIV-1 disease progression in people dually infected with HIV-1 and herpes simplex virus type 2: a randomised placebo-controlled trial. Lancet. 2010;375:824–33.
30. CENTERS FOR DISEASE CONTROL AND PREVENTION. Seroprevalence of herpes simplex virus type 2 among persons aged 14–49 years—United States, 2005–2008. MMWR. 2010;59:456–9.

Female Genital Tract Cancer Screening

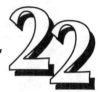

Michael S. Policar, MD, MPH

- Cervical and breast cancer screening guidelines have evolved rapidly in the past few years and include many significant and controversial modifications.

- According to guidelines issued by the American College of Obstetricians and Gynecologists (ACOG) in 2009,[1] cervical cytology screening should begin at age 21 and should be discontinued after total hysterectomy for benign disease or in women older than 65 to 70 years old who have a history of 3 or more normal cytology results in the prior 10 years.

- Women 21 to 29 years of age should have cervical cytology screening every 2 years. Women age 30 and older who have had 3 consecutively negative tests should receive cervical cytology every 3 years.

- Asymptomatic women under 21 years of age do not need routine cervical cytology or a pelvic examination at the time of a well-woman visit.[2]

- New USPSTF guidelines recommend that women who choose to have mammograms do so biennially (every other year).[3]

A reproductive health care visit represents an ideal opportunity to offer periodic health screening services, including screening for genital tract cancers. As early as the 1920s, the prevalent philosophy of the American medical community was that individuals of all ages should receive an annual physical examination and a battery of routine screening tests to detect early, asymptomatic disease.[4] Over the past two decades, however, the wisdom of this practice has been challenged, and research studies and health policy discussions have focused upon the optimal content of periodic health screening: which tests should or should not be performed, how often each screening test should be done, and whether each test should be performed routinely or limited to persons with cer-

Table 22-1 Recommendation grades used by the U.S. Preventive Services Task Force

Grade	Definition	Suggestions for Practice
A	The USPSTF recommends the service. There is high certainty that the net benefit is substantial.	Offer or provide this service.
B	The USPSTF recommends the service. There is high certainty that the net benefit is moderate or there is moderate certainty that the net benefit is moderate to substantial.	Offer or provide this service.
C	The USPSTF recommends against routinely providing the service. There may be considerations that support providing the service in an individual patient. There is at least moderate certainty that the net benefit is small.	Offer or provide this service only if other considerations support the offering or providing the service in an individual patient.
D	The USPSTF recommends against the service. There is moderate or high certainty that the service has no net benefit or that the harms outweigh the benefits.	Discourage the use of this service.
I	The USPSTF concludes that the current evidence is insufficient to assess the balance of benefits and harms of the service. Evidence is lacking, of poor quality, or conflicting, and the balance of benefits and harms cannot be determined.	Read the clinical considerations section of USPSTF Recommendation Statement. If the service is offered, patients should understand the uncertainty about the balance of benefits and harms.

tain risk factors. While many approaches to periodic health screening have been proposed, the recommendations of the United States Preventive Services Task Force (USPSTF) are considered the blueprint for the screening guidelines developed by most state Departments of Health, professional specialty societies, and health plans. The guidelines emphasize that the most important clinical contribution to maximizing a person's health status is by avoiding the development of disease through primary prevention, based on focused risk assessment and counseling interventions, rather than on periodic physical examination or laboratory testing. Using an evidence-based methodology, the USPSTF guidelines gauge the strength of each recommendation with a letter grade, which is assigned using a combination of the balance of net benefits and harms of the intervention and the level of certainty regarding net benefit, based upon the quality of the research studies used to develop the recommendation. Of note, in 2007 the USPSTF updated the definitions of the grades it assigns to recommendations and now includes "suggestions for practice" associated with each grade.[5]

In the past, the concept of an annual well-woman visit included a breast exam, cervical cytology, and bimanual pelvic exam performed yearly in women who had initiated sexual activity. However, owing in part to the changes in cancer screening recommendations listed below, many women will no longer require yearly visits for the purpose of receiving screening tests, irrespective of their choice of contraceptive method. As it relates to contraceptive practice, it is reasonable to recommend that women seek a check-up visit once every 1 to 3 years, depending upon her underlying health status, the risk level of her sexual behaviors, the recommended intervals of the screening tests that she requires, and her own personal preferences. If she chooses not to receive this service, "opportunistic prevention" can be offered by providing prevention guidance and screening tests at the time of problem-oriented visits.

Another issue that may arise at a health-screening visit is whether to provide comprehensive preventive health services or only those related to reproductive health. Increasingly, patients will have an established relationship with a primary care provider from whom they will receive some or all necessary preventive health services. If so, it is important for the reproductive health care provider to avoid duplication of tests already completed, and ideally, with the permission of the patient, to transmit the record of the reproductive health care visits to the primary care provider. In other cases, the only opportunity available to a woman to receive preventive health care services is during her reproductive health care visit. Consequently, if you are equipped to do so in your practice, it is appropriate to offer her the full range of recommended preventive interventions. Two helpful sources of age-specific disease prevention guidelines are the USPSTF (www.uspreventiveservicestaskforce. org) and "Preventing Cancer, Cardiovascular Disease, and Diabetes: A Common Agenda of the American Cancer Society, the American Diabetes Association, and the American Heart Association."[6]

Over the years, annual health screening also has been linked with the provision of prescription hormonal contraceptives. In many cases, a woman could get a prescription for combined hormonal contraceptives only when she underwent an annual well-woman visit. However, current thinking is that only those medical conditions that could impact contraceptive choice or safety should be the subject of routine or targeted screening before a prescription for hormonal contraception is given. For example, the 2004 WHO Selected Practice Recommendations for Contraceptive Use[7] do not recommend breast or genital tract examination, cervical cancer screening, STI assessment or lab test screening, hemoglobin determination, or routine lab tests as "contributing substantially to safe and effective use of a hormonal contraceptive method." These guidelines also specify that it is desirable to have a blood pressure measurement taken before initiation of combined hormonal contraceptives, progestin-only pills, progestin-only injections, and implants. No published domestic or international guidelines *require* genital tract cancer or sexually transmitted infection screening prior the provision of prescription contraceptives, based on the attitude that doing so is unnecessary for safe contraceptive use and that any unnecessary barriers to contraceptive services should be removed.[8] Furthermore, hormonal methods need not be restricted or withheld from a woman solely because she has an abnormal cytology result. There is no reason to believe that the use of any contraceptive method will hasten the progression of an existing cervical lesion. All too often, the unfortunate result of withholding contraceptives from a woman with an abnormal cytology or biopsy is unintended pregnancy, which makes diagnosis more difficult and often delays treatment.

CERVICAL CANCER SCREENING
THE NATURAL HISTORY OF CERVICAL CANCER

There is now widespread agreement that the cause of pre-invasive cervical lesions is an accumulation of DNA mutations in immature metaplastic cells as a consequence of persistent human papilloma virus (HPV) infection in concert with other carcinogenic cofactors. A convenient and accurate analogy to describe the development of pre-invasive cervical lesions is the requirement for plant growth: a seed, receptive soil, and fertilizer to promote growth.

The Seed: Infection with a High-Risk Type of HPV

Genital HPV infections are transmitted by skin-to-skin contact during sexual intercourse. Although more than 100 DNA-types of HPV have been identified, only a limited number are associated with premalignant and malignant epithelial lesions of the lower genital tract: HPV types 16 and 18 account for about 70% of cervical intraepithelial neoplasia (CIN) 2 or 3 lesions and cervical cancers, while the remaining 30% are due to HPV types 31, 33, 35, 39, 45, 51, 52, 56 and 58.[9] The high-risk HPV types exert their cancer-causing effects through a series of events leading to the degradation of the p53 tumor suppressor protein in infected cells, reducing the host's ability to reject cells with random DNA mutations. Infections due to HPV types 6 and 11, the cause of genital warts and most low-grade cervical lesions, are felt to exhibit no malignant potential.

The Soil: Squamous Metaplasia within the Transformation Zone

The cervix consists of two types of epithelium:

- *Squamous epithelium*, which covers the vagina and the portio vaginalis of the cervix

- *Columnar epithelium*, which covers the endocervical canal, and in younger women, the area around the external cervical os

At menarche, the vaginal pH drops into an acidic range and causes the fragile columnar epithelial cells around the cervical os to be replaced by squamous epithelium, a process referred to as squamous metaplasia. As this process proceeds over decades, the advancing edge of the squamous epithelium (referred to as the squamocolumnar junction) migrates centrally toward the cervical os and ultimately into the endocervical canal. The immature metaplastic cells found in younger women are particularly vulnerable to infection with HPV. Because squamous cell cancers and their precursors virtually always develop within the field of metaplasia (also called the transformation zone), both cytological and colposcopic evaluation focus upon this area.

The Fertilizer: An Oncogenic Cofactor

HPV infection alone is insufficient to initiate the development of a pre-invasive cervical lesion. A facilitating agent, or oncogenic co-factor, appears to be necessary to act in concert with HPV to initiate these premalignant changes. For example, cigarette smoking has been identified as a powerful cofactor,[10] doubling a smoker's risk of cervical cancer.

RISK FACTORS FOR CERVICAL CANCER

Epidemiological observations are consistent with the biological mechanism of cervical cancer. The following are primary epidemiological risk factors for the development of cervical cancer:

- Early onset of intercourse (defined as a sexual debut before 20 years old). Metaplasia is most active during adolescence, making a young woman more vulnerable to cell changes that result from HPV infection.

- High number of sex partners. The greater the number of sex partners, the greater the risk of acquiring a high-risk type of HPV.

- Male sex partner who has had other partners, especially if a previous partner had cervical cancer.

- Clinical history of condyloma acuminata. Infection with a low-risk type of HPV is a risk marker for co-infection with a high-risk type.[11]

- Infection with the human immunodeficiency virus (HIV) and other medical conditions associated with immunodeficiency. These illnesses decrease the ability of the immune system to recognize and reject abnormal cells.

Behavioral protective factors include virginity, long-term celibacy, life-long mutual monogamy, and long-term use of condoms. Factors that appear to have no effect on cervical cancer risk include history of herpes simplex virus infection or the circumcision status of the male partner. The effect of race and socioeconomic status are controversial. Studies show higher rates of cervical cancer among African American women and women of lower socio-economic status;[12] however, it is unclear whether the higher rates are related to poor access to medical care and, consequently, cervical cytology services, or other undetermined factors.

HPV infections are widespread among sexually active adults, costly to characterize virologically through HPV DNA testing, and cannot be eradicated with antiviral drugs. HPV infections are transient in a majority of infected individuals, but persistent infection with high-risk HPV types is necessary for the development of high-grade lesions and cancer. Rather than relying on a behavioral strategy that focuses on the sexual transmissibility of HPV, it makes more sense from a public health viewpoint to prevent cervical cancer and its precursors through screening programs that will detect and permit treatment of high-grade preinvasive lesions before life-threatening invasive cervical cancers have a chance to develop, as well as through HPV vaccination of young women before sexual debut.

PREVENTION OF CERVICAL CANCER WITH HPV VACCINATION

Vaccination against high-risk HPV infection holds promise for primary prevention of cervical cancer worldwide. The U.S. FDA has approved two HPV vaccines:

- A quadrivalent HPV (HPV4) vaccine (Gardasil), which includes antigens for HPV types 6, 11, 16, and 18 (approved in 2006)

- A bivalent HPV (HPV2) vaccine (Cervarix), which includes antigens for HPV types 16 and 18 (approved in 2009)

Both vaccines consist of three injected doses of genetically manufactured viral envelope proteins (virus-like particles), rather than the live or attenuated virus, to stimulate the production of anti-HPV antibodies. When given to previously uninfected women, both vaccines have high efficacy in preventing cervical pre-cancer lesions related HPV 16 and 18 infection. HPV4 also has high efficacy against genital warts induced by HPV 6 and HPV 11 and vaginal and vulvar pre-cancer lesions related to infection with HPV 16 and 18. At this time, the HPV vaccines do not appear to cause any serious long-term adverse effects but an important immediate problem in some women is severe pain at the injection site that can trigger a vasovagal fainting episode. For this reason, women receiving the vaccine should be monitored for a few minutes after the injection in order to prevent a fall. Because one third of high-grade preinvasive lesions contain high-risk HPV types not included in the vaccine, women who have been vaccinated are advised to continue to receive routine cervical cytology tests at currently recommended intervals. The CDC's Advisory Committee on Immunization Practices (ACIP) has published guidelines regarding the use of HPV vaccines.[13,14]

- Routine vaccination of females aged 11 or 12 years with 3 doses of either HPV2 or HPV4 is recommended. The vaccination series can be started beginning at age 9 years.

- Vaccination is recommended for females aged 13 through 26 years who have not been vaccinated previously or who have not completed the 3-dose series. If a female reaches age 26 years before the vaccination series is complete, remaining doses can be administered after age 26 years. Ideally, vaccine should be administered before potential exposure to HPV through sexual contact.

- Women should be advised that vaccination would have no therapeutic effect on an existing HPV infection, genital warts, or an abnormal cervical cytology.

- With increasing severity of abnormal cervical cytology findings, the likelihood of infection with HPV 16 or 18 increases, and benefits of vaccination decrease. Vaccination is still recommended for such women, because vaccination can provide protection against infection with HPV vaccine types not already acquired.

- Prevaccination assessments (e.g., cytology testing or screening for high-risk HPV DNA, type-specific HPV tests, or HPV antibody) to establish the appropriateness of HPV vaccination are not recommended at any age.

- Lactating women can receive HPV vaccine.

- HPV2 and HPV4 are not live vaccines and can be administered to women who are immunosuppressed (from disease or medications). However, the immune response and vaccine efficacy might be less than that in immunocompetent persons.

In October 2009, the U.S. Food and Drug Administration (FDA) licensed HPV4 for use in males aged 9 through 26 years for prevention of genital warts caused by HPV types 6 and 11. Modeling suggests that adding male HPV vaccination to a female-only HPV vaccination program is not the most cost-effective vaccination strategy for reducing the overall burden of HPV-associated conditions in males and females when vaccination coverage of females is more than 80%. Because the health burden of HPV infection is greater in females than males, and numerous models have shown vaccination of adolescent girls to be a cost-effective use of public health resources, improving coverage in females aged 11 and 12 years is a more effective and cost-effective strategy than adding male vaccination.[15]

SCREENING FOR CERVICAL CANCER

Cervical cytology screening (the Pap smear), more than any other screening test, has proven its cost-effectiveness over the years.[16] Based upon current screening patterns in the United States, early detection and treatment of pre-invasive cervical lesions prevents at least 70% of potential cervical cancers. In 2010, of the 11,270 American women[17] who develop new cases of cervical cancer[18]:

- One half have never had cervical cytology screening

- Ten percent had not been screened within the past 5 years

- The remaining forty percent had received a cytology test within the past 5 years, but either there was a falsely negative result, the patient was not managed correctly, or there was inadequate follow-up of the patient.

False-negative results occur in about 20% of cytology tests and occur either because the lesion exfoliated too few cells to be detected, there was a sampling error by the clinician, or there was an interpretive error in the cytopathology lab. In 1996, the U.S. FDA approved the technique of liquid-based cytology (LBC) with thin-layer preparation technique (Thin Prep Cytology Test, BD SurePath Cytology Test), which is intended to improve screening accuracy by increasing the number of cells sampled and by removing blood, mucus, and debris from the background of the smear. Early studies suggested that LBC improved screening accuracy over traditional practices;[19,20] however, a large randomized clinical trial from the Netherlands[21] and a meta-analysis of eight studies[22] concluded that liquid-based cervical cytology is neither more sensitive nor more specific for detection of high-grade cervical intraepithelial neoplasia compared with the conventional cytology test.

Controversy persists as to whether the additional cost associated with these tests justifies their use or, in contrast, if the increased cost of screening actually may lead to fewer cytology tests being performed.[23,24] However, a large majority of cytopathology labs in the United States have adopted this approach (and no longer offer processing of glass cytology tests) because it improves the efficiency of cytotechnicians, facilitates computerized screening or rescreening, and serves as a platform for evaluation of other pathogens in the cytology sample, specifically high-risk HPV, gonorrhea, and Chlamydia.

HPV Testing as an Adjunct to Cytological Screening

HPV-DNA tests for 13 high-risk HPV types can be used with cervical cytology in two ways:

- **Intermediary triage** of an abnormal cytology result. With this strategy, once the cytopathology laboratory determines that certain abnormal cytology findings are present, a "reflex" HPV-DNA test is performed. Management of these cytology findings with positive reflex HPV DNA test results is described in Table 22–3.

- **Co-screening,** in which an HPV DNA test and cytology are performed simultaneously in women 30 years old and older.

Early work concluded that co-screening improves the sensitivity of screening for high-grade squamous intraepithelial lesions (HSIL) or cancer to at least 92% when compared with a sensitivity of 80% for cytology alone.[25] However, some studies published more recently show similar rates of CIN 3 detection in women who are co-screened compared to those who receive cytology alone.[1] Of equal importance is the negative predictive value of this approach, since women who are both cytology negative and HPV negative have an extremely low risk of developing HSIL within the next 10 years. Either LBC or a conventional cytology can be used, but the later requires "co-collection" of an HPV DNA sample. The HPV DNA test utilized should test for high-risk HPV types only, as the presence of low-risk HPV types is not relevant to management. Additionally, co-screening is not recommended for women who are under 30 years old or who are immunocompromised. Most importantly, women who are HPV-DNA negative and who have a benign cytology result should not be rescreened before 3 years, since the risk of a new lesion is negligible and likelihood a false-positive test is significant. The combination of a negative cytology and a positive HPV test is followed with a repeat of both tests in 12 months.[26] If you intend to perform cervical cancer co-screening, it is critical to inform the patient in advance of sampling that she is being screened for HPV and that she need not have cervical rescreening earlier than 3 years if both tests are negative.

Technical Aspects of Cytological Screening

High accuracy in cytological screening depends on a good quality cervical sample, appropriately performed preparation, and competent cytopathology interpretation.

- Cytological screening may be performed whenever heavy menstrual bleeding is not present.

- Moisten the speculum with warm water or a small amount of lubricating gel applied away from the tip of the speculum. Since samples most easily contaminated by blood should be taken early in the sampling sequence, nucleic acid amplification tests (NAATs) for chlamydia and gonorrhea should be performed before the cytology sample.

- Liquid based cytology sampling:
  - Do not remove mucus, discharge, or blood from the cervix with a swab prior to collecting a LBC sample. This practice may remove a significant amount of cellular material, resulting in a scanty sample.
  - Use either a brush and spatula or a broom device that can be broken off and dropped into the solution, as instructed by the cytopathology lab used by your practice.
  - If using the brush, insert the brush into the cervix until only the bottom fibers are visible. Slowly rotate ¼ to ½ turn in one direction. Do NOT over-rotate as this may cause bleeding and loss of endocervical cells.
  - Vigorously twirl the brush and spatula in the liquid at least 10 times. Push the brush against the side of the vial to remove any mucus. Use the spatula to mechanically remove mucus and cells from the brush.

- Glass slide cytology sampling and preparation:
  - First sample the exocervix by rotating a wooden or plastic spatula 360° around the exocervix, then sample the endocervical canal using a brush-sampling device, or if one is not available, a saline-moistened cotton-tipped applicator.
  - Place the spatula sample on a glass slide, creating a thin layer that covers most of the slide's surface. Then gently roll the brush or swab on top of the first sample. Apply fixative immediately in order to avoid air-drying.
  - Unless specifically requested by the cytopathology laboratory, separate slides are not needed for each sample, nor is segmenting the slide into a section for the exocervical sample and another for the endocervical sample.
  - Sampling of the vaginal pool is not helpful and actually may decrease the quality of the sample by adding degenerating cells and other debris.

Cervical Cytology Screening Intervals

The national recommendations for cervical cancer screening intervals have evolved rapidly and include significant changes from earlier guidelines, often resulting in inconsistent, or even incorrect, practices among providers.[27] Before 2002, all women were advised to initiate cervical cancer screening with the onset of sexual activity, or at 18 years old (even if virginal), and to have an annual cytology screening unless they were at low risk for cervical cancer. As a consequence, most national women's health care organizations, including ACOG and the U.S. Title X Family Planning Program,[28] recommended that screening intervals be based upon a woman's risk factors for cervical cancer; that is, high-risk women were screened annually while low-risk women were screened less often, but no less than every 3 years.

Three major national organizations, ACOG (2009), the USPSTF (2002), and the American Cancer Society (2002), have issued recommendations regarding the periodicity of cervical cancer screening.[1,29,30] While there is a great deal of overlap among the guidelines, differences exist among them, which currently prevents the existence of a single "national standard" regarding periodicity. At this time, ACOG guidelines have been updated most recently, and the USPSTF and the American Cancer Society updates are expected in 2011. Clinicians (or entire practices) should adopt one of the guidelines, or develop a composite "practice specific" policy, which then is followed consistently for all women. The guidelines also specify that these recommendations apply to *asymptomatic* women who are being screened for cervical cancer, while those who are "under surveillance" for prior abnormal cytology results or who have undergone treatment for a pre-invasive cervical lesion should be followed under other protocols.

The guidelines are explicit in their categorization of when screening should start, when it can be discontinued, and how often it should be performed in between these points. In 2002, the American Cancer Society,[30] relying on new studies of the natural history of HPV infections and consequent pre-invasive cervical lesions, recommended that a woman delay her first screen until 3 years after her first episode of vaginal intercourse or to start screening at 21 years old, given the possibility that some women would not disclose their sexual history or that a provider might not ask about it. In 2006, the American Society for Colposcopy and Cervical Pathology (ASCCP) took the next step by recommending that women under 21 years of age should not receive HPV-DNA testing under any circumstances and also sharply differentiated the management of abnormal cytology and histology results in adolescents compared with adult women.[31] More recently, in 2009, the ACOG flatly recommended that cervical cancer screening should begin at 21 years of age, regardless of the age of onset of sexual activity.[1,32] The newest ACOG guidelines on this topic add further advice for the management of adolescents who had abnormal cytology screening results in the "old system" and how they should be transitioned to the new.

Evolution in thinking on this subject has occurred because of the realization that in younger women most HPV infections are transient and not dangerous at the time of infection. If persistent infection with a high-risk type of HPV does result in the development of a high-grade lesion, it typically does so over a period of years or even decades, allowing ample time for the discovery of a pre-invasive lesion once a woman starts screening at 21 years of age. In addition, invasive cervical cancer is exceedingly rare in adolescents, occurring at a rate of 1 to 2 cases per million women per year, and some of these cases do not appear to have been preventable by screening.

Beyond the fact that screening of adolescents has no apparent benefit, the harms of screening are becoming better understood. Numerous studies have shown the negative psychological effects of screening, disclosure of abnormal results, and treatment, including effects on sexual function. Even more concerning are the findings that pregnancy outcomes following LEEP show a significant increase in the rate of preterm birth.

These recommendations represent an important departure from the longstanding U.S. public health recommendation that women receive

Table 22–2 Cervical cytology screening intervals

Recent ACOG recommendations specify a lengthening of the cervical cancer screening interval in women 21 years of age and older:

- **21–29 years old**. Screen every 2 years.
- **30 years to 65–70 years old**. Screen every 3 years if she meets the following conditions:
  —3 consecutive negative cytology screening test results and no history of CIN 2–3, not HIV-infected, not immune compromised, and not exposed to DES in utero, *OR*
  —Negative test co-test results on both cervical cytology screening and HPV DNA testing.
- **Do not increase the screening interval** beyond annual screening for women with the following conditions:
  —HIV-positive
  —Immune compromised (e.g., a major organ transplant)
  —Exposed in utero to diethylstilbestrol (DES)
  —History of treatment for CIN 2 or 3
- Screening may be discontinued at age 65–70 after 3 consecutive negative screening tests in the prior decade. *Continue* routine cervical cytology examinations for:
  —Sexually active older women with multiple partners, because they have some risk for new HPV infection and CIN
  —Women with a previous history of abnormal cytology
- Discontinue routine screening after total hysterectomy if performed for benign indications and no history of high-grade CIN. *Continue* routine cervical cytology examinations if:
  —History of CIN 2 or 3 — or if a negative history cannot be documented. Continue screening even after a period of post-treatment surveillance.
  —There are no good data to support or refute discontinuing screening. The screening interval may then be extended.

annual cytology screening. Both clinician-initiated discussions and public educational campaigns will be necessary to re-educate consumers regarding these changes.[33] A number of studies have shown that most women believe that they need to have annual cytology tests, and many are suspicious that the recommendations for longer cytology screening intervals are economically, rather than clinically, motivated.[34] When a well-screened woman over 30 years old requests an annual cytology test, it may seem expedient for a clinician to acquiesce to her request and provide one. However, studies show that performing cytology tests more often than necessary can do more harm than good, since the hazards of a false-positive test will exceed the negligible benefit of the shorter screening interval. For example, in a study by Sawaya, in order to prevent a single case of cervical cancer in a cohort of 100,000 well-screened women between 45 to 59 years old by screening annually instead of every 3 years, an additional 209,324 cytology tests and 11,502 colposcopies would be required.[35] Providers are fearful of encountering a patient with an interval cancer and being sued for a missed diagnosis and also concerned that well-woman visits will be skipped if they are not tied to the need for a cytology test. There is also concern that sexually active adolescents will not receive annual Chlamydia screening and targeted screening for other sexually transmitted infections once they are informed that annual screening pelvic examinations and cytology tests are no longer recommended. While these are legitimate concerns, they must be addressed in ways other than requiring women to receive a test that may be unnecessary and potentially harmful should a false-positive result occur.

MANAGEMENT OF ABNORMAL CYTOLOGY RESULTS

The classification system recommended by the third Bethesda workshop (the 2001 Bethesda System) contained a number of modifications to include new screening technologies, as well as to remedy points of confusion between pathologists and clinicians. Cervical cytology reports conforming to the 2001 Bethesda System format include comments in each of the following categories, as applicable:

- Specimen type (conventional smear vs. liquid-based vs. other)
- Specimen adequacy (satisfactory or unsatisfactory for evaluation)
- General categorization (Negative, Epithelial cell abnormality, Other)
- Interpretation/Result
- Automated review and ancillary testing (including HPV reflex results, if done)
- Educational notes and suggestions (optional)

Negative, with Comments Regarding Specimen Adequacy

While the 2001 Bethesda System has eliminated the category of "satisfactory, but limited by ..." (SBLB), comments regarding suboptimal specimen quality still may be made. The finding that most often limits interpretation is a paucity of endocervical cells. Their presence confirms that in the process of sampling the transformation zone, the active squamocolumnar junction was included. Even with the best of sampling efforts, however, endocervical cells are absent in up to 10% of cytology tests obtained from premenopausal women and as many as 50% from postmenopausal women.[36] If a negative result is reported, take the next test in 1 year. Repeat cytology at 6 months if:

- The cervix cannot be clearly visualized or the endocervical canal sampled.

- A previous cytology report showed a glandular abnormality.

- A woman with a previously abnormal cytology result did not receive adequate follow-up.

- An HPV-DNA test within the past year turned positive.

- Previous screening was insufficient.

The proportion of cytology tests with this reading provides an important opportunity to monitor cytology technique. If the percentage of cytology results with no endocervical cells present exceeds 10%, remedial action is necessary. If clinician education regarding cytology test technique and a switch to brush sampling devices does not result in improvement, the laboratory's cytopathologist should be consulted in order to determine whether the problem lies with the laboratory or the provider and to define further steps necessary to rectify the problem.

Unsatisfactory for evaluation. Inadequate sampling, air drying, excessive red or white blood cells, or other factors make interpretation impossible. Because unsatisfactory smears have a greater likelihood of being abnormal,[37] repeat the smear, preferably when the woman is at mid-cycle and has not had intercourse or used vaginal products for at least 24 hours. Do not repeat the cytology test earlier than 6 weeks from the previous smear; repetitive sampling over short periods of time may increase the risk of falsely negative smears due to decreased exfoliation of abnormal cells and a greater likelihood of reparative changes. Unless a woman has a history of endometrial hyperplasia, progestin withdrawal is not necessary after this short course of estrogen exposure. If the proportion of unsatisfactory smears within a practice is greater than 5%, remedial action in consultation with the cytopathologist is recommended.

Negative for Intraepithelial Lesion or Malignancy: Organisms

Trichomonas vaginalis. While the cytology test is a relatively insensitive test for the detection of Trichomonas (it detects trichomonads in only about one-half of infected women), its specificity is as high as 98%.[38] Because the prevalence of trichomonas vaginal colonization in reproductive-aged women is about 5%, the positive predictive value of a cytology test reporting trichomonas is about 72%. When the cytology report indicates presence of Trichomonas, review the woman's medical record to determine whether the infection was recently treated. If it has been, no further action is required. If it has not been treated, offer treatment to avoid horizontal transmission to a new sexual partner and to prevent an uncomfortable case of symptomatic vaginal trichomoniasis. The practice of requiring microscopic saline suspension to confirm vaginal trichomonads is illogical because the sensitivity of this test is only 60%. Instead, if the saline suspension is negative and confirmation is desired, use a test with high sensitivity and specificity, such as a DNA test or Diamond's media culture. Repeat the cytology test after the next routine screening interval, unless the narrative report mentions obscuring inflammation and indicates the need to repeat the test after treatment.

Fungus morphologically consistent with Candida spp. In most cases, Candida detected on cytology is due to normal vaginal colonization with low levels of Candida, rather than frank vaginal candidiasis. Candida colonization is not dangerous to the affected woman or her sexual partner. Repeat the cytology test only if the inflammation due to the candidiasis is of sufficient severity that the cytopathologist recommends that repeated repeat test after treatment is complete.

Shift in flora suggestive of bacterial vaginosis. This reading refers to changes detected in the bacterial flora of the vagina in which the normal Lactobacillus are not abundant but coccobacilli are seen in numbers greater than normal. While this description was devised to suggest the possibility of bacterial vaginosis (BV), it is both an insensitive and nonspecific indicator of BV. The clinical diagnosis of BV is made solely on clinical findings (see Chapter 21 on Reproductive Tract Infections), and neither vaginal culture nor cytology findings have any role in the diagnosis of this condition. Management is controversial. Many clinicians feel that no further evaluation is necessary and that the next cytology test should be performed at the routine interval, while others feel that the woman should be informed that BV is inferred from findings on the smear and be offered clinical evaluation for BV.

Bacteria morphologically consistent with Actinomyces spp. Actinomyces israelii is an anaerobic bacterium capable of causing a rare, but severe, pelvic infection called pelvic actinomycosis, especially in long-term intrauterine contraceptive (IUC) users over 35 years of age. The vast majority of IUC users with "Actinomyces-like organisms (ALO)" on their cytology reports have an asymptomatic cervical colonization (not infection) that does not require either antibiotic therapy or removal of the IUC. However, IUC users with Actinomyces on their cytology should have a bimanual pelvic examination to determine whether they have evidence of pelvic infection if one was not performed at the time of the cytology test. If symptoms or physical findings suggest pelvic actinomycosis, remove the IUC and initiate intensive antibiotic therapy. Advise the woman to use another method of contraception. (See Chapter 7 on Intrauterine Contraception.)

Cellular changes consistent with herpes simplex virus (HSV). Although an insensitive indicator of cervical herpes simplex shedding, this cytology finding is quite specific to herpes infection. If the patient requests confirmation, a positive HSV-2 type-specific serology will confirm prior infection, but an HSV culture should be avoided, since viral shedding is intermittent and unpredictable. Unless inflammation interferes with the interpretation of the test, the next cytology test should be performed at the routine interval.

Negative for Intraepithelial Lesion or Malignancy: Other Non-Neoplastic Findings

Reactive cellular changes associated with inflammation. Nonspecific reactive inflammatory changes may be associated with benign metaplasia, mechanical or chemical irritation, post-traumatic repair, chlamydial or gonococcal endocervicitis, trichomoniasis, viral infection, invasive cervical cancer, or other unknown factors. Of these possibilities, the only infectious conditions amenable to antibiotic therapy are gonococcal and chlamydial endocervicitis and vaginal trichomoniasis. Women who recently have been evaluated for these organisms and found to be uninfected do not require further evaluation or antibiotic therapy. Evaluate women who have not been screened recently by performing gonorrhea and chlamydia tests and treating women who test positive. Empirically treating women with inflammatory cytology test results with topical antibiotic sulfa creams is of no value in either the treatment of cervical infection or the resolution of abnormal result and is to be avoided.[45] Rarely, the only cytology test finding in a woman with an invasive cervical carcinoma is the persistent finding of inflammation. Some experts recommend that women who have had consecutive cytology results with unexplained inflammation be evaluated by colposcopy, although the recommendation is not evidence-based; other experts contend that colposcopy is unnecessary because of the extremely low likelihood of detecting a cervical cancer in this circumstance.

Cytological changes associated with the use of an IUC detected on cytology are of a benign nature and do not require further investigation.

Atrophy. Atrophy is most common in postmenopausal women or those with estrogen-deficiency states. Treatment of the vaginal atrophy is indicated only if the woman has symptomatic atrophic vaginitis; it is not necessary for the asymptomatic woman. Cytology screening intervals do not need to be modified, and the woman does not need to be notified.

Endometrial cells, cytologically benign, in a woman 40 years of age or older. Endometrial cells found on cytology are an insignificant finding in premenopausal women with normal ovulatory cycling. However, because the endometrium normally is atrophic in postmenopausal women, the finding of endometrial cells may be the result of exfoliation from a focus of endometrial hyperplasia or adenocarcinoma. For this reason, consider the finding of endometrial cells in a postmenopausal woman as a danger sign and sample the endometrium. Because a premenopausal woman with chronic anovulation also is at risk for endometrial hyperplasia, manage the finding of endometrial cells in the same way.

Epithelial Cell Abnormalities: Squamous Cell

The atypical squamous cell (ASC) category refers to the finding of cells with nuclear atypia that are not normal, yet not diagnostic of squamous intraepithelial lesion (SIL). The majority of ASC-US smears are due to benign HPV infections, although 2.5% of women over 40 years old and 11% under 40 years old with this reading have CIN 2 or worse, and very rarely, invasive cancer.[40] The Colposcopy and Cervical Pathology (ASCCP) 2006 Consensus Guidelines[26] describe three acceptable options for the management of women with ASC-US results: follow with 6-month screening interval twice, perform a "reflex" HPV-DNA test to differentiate women who are at high risk for having or progressing to HSIL (also called intermediary triage), or perform colposcopy. Management recommendations for other abnormal cytology results from the American Society for ASCCP are contained in Table 22–3.

Epithelial Cell Abnormalities: Glandular Cell

Atypical glandular cells (AGC). AGC may result from HPV infection of glandular cells, adenocarcinoma-in-situ (AIS), adenocarcinoma, or in some cases, an SIL lesion. Because adenocarcinomas of the cervix are associated with a rate of false-negative cytology as high as 40%,[41] women with AGC require aggressive evaluation in order to exclude a cancer diagnosis. There is no role for observation (repeat cytology) in this situation.

Table 22–3 ASCCP consensus guidelines for management of women with cervical cytological abnormalities[47]

	Initial Intervention	Next Step	Following step
ASC-US	Either: • Repeat cytology at 6 mos	• Negative: repeat cytology at 6 mos →	• Negative: routine screening
—— Or ——	Or: • HPV DNA testing (reflex test)	• ≥ASC: colposcopy • Negative: repeat cytology at 12 mos → • Positive: colposcopy	• ≥ASC: colposcopy • Negative: routine screening • ≥ASC: colposcopy
LSIL *Post-menopausal*	Or: • Colposcopy (with ECS)	• No CIN, HPV pos: cytology at 6&12 mos or HPV testing at 12 mos → • No CIN, HPV unkn: cytology at 12 mos → • CIN: per ASCCP CIN guideline	• Negative: routine screening • ≥ ASC or HPV (+): repeat colposcopy
ASC-H	• Colposcopy	• No CIN 2,3: cytology at 6&12 mo or HPV testing at 12 mos → • CIN 2,3: per ASCCP CIN guideline	• Negative: routine screening • ≥ASC or HPV (+): colposcopy
LSIL *Not pregnant*	• Colposcopy (with ECS*)	• No CIN: cytology at 6&12 mos or HPV testing at 12 mos → • CIN/cancer: per ASCCP CIN guideline	• Negative: routine screening • ≥ASC or HPV (+): colposcopy
LSIL *Pregnant women*	Either • Colposcopy OR • Defer colposcopy ≥ 6 wks postpartum	• No CIN 2,3: postpartum follow-up • CIN 2,3: per ASCCP CIN guideline	

(continued)

Table 22-3 ASCCP consensus guidelines for management of women with cervical cytological abnormalities[47] —(cont'd)

	Initial Intervention	Next Step	Following step

HSIL	Either
	• Immediate LEEP (if CIN 2, 3 likely)
	• Colposcopy with ECS
		• No CIN 2,3
		  • Unsatisfactory: DEP
		  • Satisfactory (either):
		    • Colposcopy + cytology at 6 mos intervals for 1 yr →
		    • Pathologist review
		    • DEP**
		CIN 2,3: per ASCCP CIN guideline
			• Negative cytology x2: routine screening
			• HSIL: DEP
			• Other results: per ASCCP CIN guideline
			NOTES
			• If no cervical lesion, evaluate for VaIN*** with Lugol's solution

AGC: Atypical endometrial cells	• Endometrial biopsy+ ECS (in all cases)	No endometrial pathology: colposcopy	

AGC
All other sub-categories
	• Colposcopy + ECS
	AND
	• HPV testing
	AND
	• Endometrial sampling (if ≥35 yrs or at risk for endometrial neoplasia)
		• Cytology= AGC-favor neoplasia or AIS: DEP
		• Cytology= AGC –not specified (NOS):
		  • Bx= CIN *or*AIS: per ASCCP guideline
		  • No CIN *and* No AIS:
		    • HPV neg: cytology+HPV in 12 mos →
		    • HPV pos: cytology+HPV in 6 mos →
		    • HPV status unknown: cytology at 6 month intervals 4 times →
			• All tests negative: routine screening
			• Any > ASC or HPV positive: colposcopy

* **ECS** = endocervical sampling in non-pregnant women, either with endocervical curettage or cervical brush

** **DEP**= diagnostic excisional procedure, e.g., LEEP cone or cold-knife cone biopsy

*** **VaIN** =vaginal intraepithelial neoplasia

Table 22–4 Indications for colposcopy

- Cytology result with atypical squamous cells, cannot exclude HSIL (ASC-H), high-grade squamous intraepithelial lesion (HSIL), or suspicion of cancer
- Cytology with LSIL in a women > 21 years old, unless pregnant or post-menopausal
- Cytology with atypical glandular cells (AGC), unless AGC-atypical endometrial cells *and* positive endometrial sampling
- Cytology showing ASC-US in the following circumstances
  - Women who are unlikely or unwilling to return for follow-up
  - Repeat cytology test with ASC-US or worse performed during observation period
  - High-risk HPV DNA present at initial or subsequent testing
- Cervical leukoplakia (white lesion visible to the naked eye without the application of acetic acid) or other unexplained cervical lesion, regardless of cytology result
- Unexplained or persistent cervical bleeding regardless of cytology result

TREATMENT OF HISTOLOGICAL ABNORMALITIES

Since the early 1990s, management protocols have become much more conservative, due to the recognition that most LSIL lesions will regress without treatment, rather than progress to higher-grade lesions or cancer. Once a diagnosis of CIN 1 is made in a patient with a fully visible cervical lesion, she should be followed until there is evidence of CIN 2/3 or persistence of CIN 1 over the period of 2 years or more. The preferred approach to follow-up is either cytology alone at 6 and 12 months or HPV DNA testing at 12 months, although an acceptable alternative is colposcopy plus cytology at 12 months. If any of these alternatives is chosen, both the provider and the patient must be diligent with follow-up. Alternatively, if the patient is uncomfortable with being observed and requests treatment, or if she is a poor follow-up risk, immediate treatment is an acceptable choice.

There is universal agreement that high-grade SIL must be treated, because the risk of progression to cervical cancer is both more likely and more immediate.[31]

OVARIAN CANCER SCREENING

In the United States in 2010, 21,900 women were diagnosed with ovarian cancer, making this cancer the ninth most common among American women.[17] However, because of the low 5-year survival rates with this disease, especially in the later stages when it is more commonly diagnosed, it is the leading cause (53%) of gynecologic cancer deaths, accounting for 13,850 deaths in the United States. The average age at diagnosis is 60 years. A woman's lifetime risk of ovarian cancer is about 1 in 70.

Although some risk factors for ovarian cancer are well known, a majority of women diagnosed with this condition have none.[42] Geographic differences are marked; rates in Sweden and the United States are 13 to15 cases per 100,000 women per year, while the rate in Japan is 3 cases per 100,000 women per year. This difference in part may be related to dietary fat intake, which is higher in the United States and Scandinavia and lower in Japan. A long interval of ovulatory cycles also is associated with ovarian cancer; low parity, delayed childbearing, obesity, and infertility are weak risk factors.

Familial predisposition accounts for 5% to 10% of cases, and the risk of ovarian cancer is 5% if one first-degree relative had ovarian cancer and 7% if two or more first-degree relatives had the condition. A site-specific familial ovarian cancer syndrome has been described, which is mediated through a highly penetrant autosomal dominant gene; in these cases, the risk to a first-degree relative is up to 50%. In addition, women with BRCA mutations are at greater lifetime risk of ovarian cancer, about 50% for BRCA-1 and 15% for BRCA-2. Another genetic syndrome, called hereditary non-polyposis colon cancer (Lynch II syndrome), also is associated with increased risk. Because there is no accurate method to detect early ovarian cancer in these high-risk women, expert consensus guidelines recommend prophylactic oophorectomy for women who have two or more first-degree relatives with ovarian cancer and who have completed childbearing.[43]

Conversely, oral contraceptive use reduces the risk of ovarian cancer by as much as 80% in women age 40 to 59 years. Not only does longer duration of use provide more protection, but the effect lasts for as long as 15 years after oral contraceptives are discontinued.[44] There is a decreased risk of ovarian cancer in women who have chronic anovulation (i.e., polycystic ovary syndrome); protection also is seen with increasing parity and greater duration of lactation. Contraceptive sterilization is associated with a 40% to 50% reduction in the risk of ovarian cancer, and hysterectomy (without oophorectomy) with a 35% reduction.

OVARIAN CANCER SCREENING TECHNIQUES

Ovarian cancer typically is diagnosed during an evaluation of a symptomatic woman, but it may be detected as a mass found incidentally during pelvic examination or ultrasound. While early ovarian cancer has been long considered a "silent cancer," a recent study showed that 70% of women recalled having symptoms for 3 months or longer before their diagnosis.[45] Ovarian cancer can be associated with pelvic pain, abdominal discomfort and distention, bloating after meals, feeling full quickly, constipation, nausea, urinary frequency, and rarely, irregular vaginal bleeding. In advanced stages, ovarian cancer is often accompanied by fatigue, nonspecific gastrointestinal symptoms, poor appetite and weight loss, increased abdominal girth, or shortness of breath due to pleural effusion. Women who experience such symptoms daily for more than a few weeks should be evaluated. The best way to promptly diagnose ovarian cancer is for both the patient and her clinician to have a high index of suspicion when characteristic symptoms occur.

A number of techniques have been suggested to screen for the early stages of asymptomatic ovarian cancer: periodic bimanual pelvic examination, serum CA-125 measurement, and a transvaginal ultrasound study. Conducting a bimanual pelvic exam as part of an annual well-woman exam has been used as screening test for ovarian cancer for decades, but it is insensitive and has poor specificity. National guidelines contain inconsistent recommendations; ACOG recommends an annual pelvic exam to screen for ovarian cancer in women 21 years of age and older,[2] while the USPSTF does not.[46] However, recent ACOG guidelines state that a screening pelvic exam in asymptomatic women under 21 years old is not recommended. Consequently, in an asymptomatic adolescent seen for a well-woman visit or contraceptive services, current guidelines advise neither a pelvic exam nor a cervical cytology screen. In short, assuming that NAAT testing is available for Chlamydia screening (and gonorrhea screening, if indicated) from a urine sample or a self-administered vaginal sample, there is no need for a physical exam beyond a blood pressure check.

Screening with the serum tumor marker CA-125 will detect up to 80% of women with advanced non-mucinous ovarian cancers, but the test is only 50% to 70% sensitive for early-stage cancers and has poor specificity (many false-positive results), which may lead to unnecessary invasive and costly workups. Screening average-risk women with this test is not recommended because of the low prevalence of ovarian cancer and the test's moderate sensitivity and poor specificity. Vaginal-probe pelvic ultrasound also has been suggested as a screening test because of its high sensitivity (98%), but it has poor specificity and the highest cost of any of the screening modalities. The USPSTF recommends *against* routine screening for ovarian cancer with any of these modalities (D Recommendation), because the potential harms outweigh the potential benefits.[46]

However, guidelines from the U.S. National Institutes of Health state that these tests should be offered annually to women who have familial risk factors for ovarian cancer, starting at 25 to 30 years old.[43]

B REAST CANCER SCREENING

In 2010, breast cancer was the second leading cause of cancer deaths in women in the United States, accounting for 28% of all cancer cases and 15% of cancer deaths in women (about 40,000 deaths per year).[10] Incidence rates of breast cancer increased 1% per year since the 1970's, but from 1999 to 2006 decreased by 2% per year. Mortality also has been falling since 1990, as a result of earlier diagnosis and improved treatments.[47] A woman's lifetime risk of breast cancer, assuming she lives to old age, is about 1 in 9. Risk factors are helpful indicators of risk, but do not predict the development of breast cancer in the majority of cases. Of women with breast cancer, 21% of women age 30 to 54 years have risk factor(s), as do 29% of women between 55 and 84 years old[48] (Table 22–5). Given the multiplicity of breast cancer risk factors, and their relative contribution to breast cancer risk, it is challenging for a clinician to forecast an individual patient's likelihood of acquiring breast cancer. Two free internet-based programs are available to quickly calculate a patient's breast cancer risk:

- *The Breast Cancer Risk Assessment Tool*, sponsored by the National Cancer Institute, projects a woman's individualized risk for invasive breast cancer over a 5-year period and over her lifetime. It can be found at www.bcra.nci.nih.gov/brc/, or use www.cancer.gov/bcrisktool.

- *The Detailed Breast Cancer Risk Calculator* produces estimates using each of the Gail Model 1 and NSABP model-2. It is located at www.halls.md/breast/risk.htm.

BREAST CANCER SCREENING TECHNIQUES

Breast self-examination (BSE). The longstanding recommendation that all adult women practice monthly BSE has been abandoned as a national practice recommendation. In 2009, the USPSTF recommended against teaching BSE (Grade: D recommendation). Although BSE may provide women with a sense of empowerment and occasionally may result in earlier detection of a breast mass than might occur by coincidence, two very large randomized clinical trials have shown that breast cancer mortality and survival is no greater in women who practice BSE than in those who do not. The larger study, involving 266,000 women in Shanghai, China, concluded that BSE actually might cause more hazard than benefit, owing to the many false positives that result from BSE. From a public health standpoint, these studies suggest that financial and educational resources should not be used to implement population-based BSE programs. For individual women, the message in these studies is that a formal, timed regimen of BSE is no more effective in preventing death from breast cancer than the incidental discovery of unusual breast changes. Nonetheless, women still must be counseled to take note of changes in their breasts and when they occur and bring the finding to the attention of their clinician.

For women who continue to practice BSE, the optimal time for performing BSE is 1 to 7 days after the end of the menses. Performing the exam after a shower, while the skin still is wet, may improve accuracy. After inspecting her breasts while she is sitting or standing in front of a

Table 22–5 Risk characteristics of breast cancer

Factor	High-Risk Group	Low-Risk Group
Relative risk > 4.0		
Age	Old	Young
Country of birth	North America, Northern Europe	Asia, Africa
Two first-degree relatives with breast cancer diagnosed at an early age	Yes	No
History of cancer in one breast	Yes	No
Relative risk = 2.1–4.0		
Nodular densities on mammogram (postmenopausal)	Densities occupy >75% of breast volume	Parenchyma composed entirely of fat
One first-degree relative with breast cancer	Yes	No
Biopsy-confirmed atypical hyperplasia	Yes	No
High-dose radiation to chest	Yes	No
Oophorectomy before age 35	No	Yes
Relative risk = 1.1–2.0		
Socioeconomic status	High	Low
Place of residence	Urban	Rural
Race/ethnicity		
—Breast cancer at ≥40 years	Caucasian	Asian
—Breast cancer at < 40 years	Black	Asian
Religion	Jewish	Adventist, Mormon
Age at first full-term pregnancy	≥ 30 years	< 20 years
Age at menarche	< 12 years	> 14 years
Age at menopause	> 55 years	< 45 years
Obesity (postmenopausal)	Obese	Slender
Breastfeeding	None	Several years
—Breast cancer < 45 year		
Hormone replacement therapy > 10 years	Yes	No
Height	Tall	Short
History of primary cancer in endometrium, ovary, or colon	Yes	No
Alcohol consumption	Yes	No

Source: Hulka BS, et al. (1995),[59] with updates.

mirror, the woman should palpate each breast in turn, with her hand on the side of the breast being examined placed behind her head. The objective of BSE is to detect a significant change in the breasts from one month to the next, not necessarily the finding of a dominant nodule.

Clinical Breast Examination (CBE). While most consensus guidelines include clinical breast examination (CBE) as a component of the periodic health examination in adult women, there is disagreement regarding age of initiation and frequency of screening. The USPSTF concludes that the current evidence is insufficient to assess the additional benefits and harms of CBE beyond screening mammography in women 40 years or older, while the American Cancer Society recommends that CBE should be performed at least every 3 years from 20 to 39 years old and annually thereafter.[49] CBE is not a highly accurate screening test, having a sensitivity of only 54% and a false positive rate of 6%. However, one benefit of CBE is that about 5% to 15% of breast cancers missed on mammography are found on CBE, the combination thereby improving detection rates. Consequently, CBE should be considered as an adjunct to mammography and offered to all women starting no later than when they are 40 years old.

When performing CBE,[50] examine the breasts while the woman is sitting with her hands on her hips or behind her head. Repeat the exam while the woman is lying down. Examine each breast in vertical strips. Palpate with flat portion of your fingers rather than your fingertips. If a woman has very pendulous breasts, place your hand between her breast and chest wall, then palpate tissue between your hands. Be sure to include the axillary tail of the breast in the examination. Lymph node examination of the supraclavicular and axillary nodes is an integral component of the examination. Draw a diagram in the medical record indicating the position and size of abnormalities, noting that dominant nodules have measurable dimensions, while fibrocystic change does not.

MAMMOGRAPHY

When used as a screening test, the purpose of mammography is to detect preclinical breast cancer before a mass can be palpated clinically. Large-scale studies show that in women who receive at least biennial mammograms over a 10-year period, breast cancer mortality is reduced by an average of 24%, with the largest reduction in women 50 to 69 years old. The accuracy of mammography as a screening test has improved over the last two decades, resulting in a false-negative rate of 5% to 15% and a false-positive rate of 3% to 6%.

In 2009, the USPSTF published updated guidelines for breast cancer screening[3]:

- Every-other-year (biennial) screening mammography for women between the ages of 50 and 74 years. (Grade B recommendation)

- Against *routine* screening mammography in women aged 40 to 49 years. (Grade C recommendation). If performed, it should be done biennially.

These guidelines should not be interpreted to mean that mammograms should not be performed in the younger age group. Instead, the decision must be an individual one that "takes into account patient context, including the patient's values regarding specific benefits and harms." Clinicians should *routinely counsel* women regarding the pros and cons of mammography and leave the decision to the client. The American Cancer Society did not change its guidelines and continues to recommend annual mammography beginning at age 40.

Women with an increased risk of breast cancer should initiate mammographic screening before age 40. According to the guidelines of the American College of Radiology,[51] younger women should start mammograms at the following times:

- 10 years before the age of diagnosis of a first-degree relative with breast cancer, but not before the age of 30

- After the diagnosis of breast cancer

- Age 25 to 30 years if known or suspected carrier of the BRCA-2 breast cancer gene

- Age 20 to 25 years if known or suspected carrier of BRCA-1 breast cancer gene

- 6 to 12 months after radiation therapy if breast tissue is conserved, then every 6 to 12 months for 1 to 2 years, then annually

- A breast biopsy shows lobular carcinoma in situ (LCIS) or atypical ductal hyperplasia

Table 22–6 BI-RADS mammogram reporting system

Category	Assessment	Recommendation
0	Incomplete	Further diagnostic imaging studies needed until a final category can be assigned
1	Negative	Routine screening interval
2	Benign finding	Routine screening interval
3	Probably benign	Follow-up 4–6 months for 2 years (or longer) until stability can be demonstrated
4	Suspicious	Biopsy
5	Highly suspicious	Biopsy

- 8 years after radiation therapy to the chest or mediastinum, or by age 25, whichever occurs last

An international reporting system for mammogram results, developed by the American College of Radiologists and adopted internationally, is entitled BI-RADS (Breast Imaging Reporting and Data System).[52] The six categories of assessment and management of each are contained in Table 22–6. Women with assessments of BI-RADS 4 or 5 should be referred immediately for breast biopsy. Pay special attention to women with category "zero" results, as they will need to receive additional imaging studies, and those with category 3 results, since they will need further follow-up imaging studies at an interval specified by the radiologist. Women with BI-RADS category 3 results who are at increased risk of breast cancer should be referred to a breast specialist. When used as a diagnostic test in a woman with a breast abnormality, mammography can suggest malignancy at the location of the finding and exclude malignancy elsewhere in the same or opposite breast. In the presence of a dominant breast nodule, a negative diagnostic mammogram does not exclude the diagnosis of breast cancer. In this case, tissue sampling, either by fine-needle aspiration cytology or open biopsy, is the only definitive procedure to exclude cancer.

Useful algorithms describing the management of women with abnormal mammograms and other breast complaints or clinical findings have been developed by the California Department of Health Services and can be found at www.qap.sdsu.edu/screening/breastcancer/bda.[53]

REFERENCES

1. ACOG Committee on Practice Bulletins—Gynecology. ACOG Practice Bulletin no. 109: Cervical cytology screening. Obstet Gynecol. 2009;114:1409–20.
2. ACOG Committee on Practice Bulletins–Gynecology. Routine pelvic examination and cervical cytology screening. Obstet Gynecol. 2009;114:1190–93.
3. U.S. Preventive Services Task Force. Screening for Breast Cancer: U.S. Preventive Services Task Force Recommendation Statement. Ann Intern Med. 2009 15:716–26.
4. American Medical Association. Periodic health examination: a manual for physicians. Chicago: American Medical Association, 1940.
5. U.S. Preventive Services Task Force Grade Definitions. May 2008 [cited November 10, 2010]. Accessed at http://www.uspreventiveservicestaskforce.org/uspstf/grades.htm.
6. Eyre H, Kahn R, et.al. Preventing cancer, cardiovascular disease, and diabetes: a common agenda for the American Cancer Society, the American Diabetes Association, and the American Heart Association. CA Cancer J Clin. 2004;54:190–207.
7. World Health Organization, Selected practice recommendations for contraceptive use, 2nd edition 2004. Accessed at http://whqlibdoc.who.int/publications/2004/9241562846.pdf.
8. Stewart FH, Harper CC, Ellertson CE, Grimes DA, Sawaya GF, Trussell J. Clinical breast and pelvic examination requirements for hormonal contraception: Current practice vs. evidence. JAMA. 2001;285:2232–9.

9. Munoz N, Bosch FX, de Sanjose S, Herrero R, et al. Epidemiologic classification of human papillomavirus types associated with cervical cancer. N Eng J Med. 2003;348:518–27.
10. Winkelstein W, Jr. Smoking and cervical cancer—current status: a review. Am J Epidemiol. 1990;131:945–57.
11. Centers for Disease Control and Prevention, Workowski KA, Berman SM. Sexually transmitted diseases treatment guidelines, 2006. MMWR Recomm Rep. 2006;55(RR-11):1–94.
12. Centers for Disease Control. Black-white differences in cervical cancer mortality—United States, 1980–1987. MMWR 1990;39:245–8.
13. Markowitz LE, Dunne EF, Saraiya M, et al. Quadrivalent Human Papillomavirus Vaccine: Recommendations of the Advisory Committee on Immunization Practices (ACIP).MMWR Recomm Rep. 2007;56(RR-2):1–24.
14. Advisory Committee on Immunization Practices (ACIP). FDA Licensure of Bivalent Human Papillomavirus Vaccine (HPV2, Cervarix) for Use in Females and Updated HPV Vaccination. MMWR. 2010;59:626–9.
15. Advisory Committee on Immunization Practices (ACIP). FDA Licensure of Quadrivalent Human Papillomavirus Vaccine (HPV4, Gardasil) for Use in Males and Guidance from the Advisory Committee on Immunization Practices. MMWR. 2010;59:630–2.
16. Koss LG. The Papanicolaou test for cervical cancer detection. A triumph and a tragedy. JAMA. 1989;261:737–43.
17. Jemal A, Siegel R, Xu J, Ward E Cancer Statistics, 2010. CA Cancer J Clin. 2010 Jul 7. [Epub].
18. National Institutes of Health Cervical Cancer. NIH Consensus Statement 1996; 14:1–38.
19. Hessling JJ, et al. Effectiveness of thin-layer preparations vs. conventional cytologys in a blinded split-sample study. Extended cytologic evaluation. J Repro Med. 2001;46:880–6.
20. Wertlake P. Results of AutoCytology system-assisted and manual cytologic screen comparison. J Reprod Med. 1999;44:11–7.
21. Siebers AG, Klinkhamer PJ, Grefte JM, Massuger LF, Vedder JE, Beijers-Broos A, Bulten J, Arbyn M.Comparison of liquid-based cytology with conventional cytology for detection of cervical cancer precursors: a randomized controlled trial. JAMA. 2009;302:1757–64.
22. Arbyn M, Bergeron C, Klinkhamer P, Martin-Hirsch P, Siebers AG, Bulten J. Liquid compared with conventional cervical cytology: a systematic review and meta-analysis. Obstet Gynecol. 2008;111:167–77.
23. Hutchinson ML. Assessing the costs and benefits of alternative rescreening strategies [editorial]. Acta Cytol. 1996;40–8.
24. Sawaya GF, Grimes DA. New technologies in cervical cytology screening: A word of caution. Obstet Gynecol. 1999;94:304–7.
25. Wright TC Jr, Schiffman M, Solomon D, Cox JT, Garcia F, Goldie S, Hatch K, Noller KL, Roach N, Runowicz C, Saslow D. Interim guidance for the use of human papillomavirus DNA testing as an adjunct to cervical cytology for screening. Obstet Gynecol. 2004;103:304–9.
26. Wright Jr TC, L. Massad S, Dunton CJ, Spitzer M, Wilkinson EJ, Solomon D. ASCCP 2006 consensus guidelines for the management of women with abnormal cervical cancer screening tests. Am J Obstet Gynecol. 2007;197:346–55.
27. Yabroff KR, Saraiya M, Meissner HI, Haggstrom DA, Wideroff L, Yuan G, Berkowitz Z, Davis WW, Benard VB, Coughlin SS. Specialty differences in primary care physician reports of papanicolaou test screening practices: a national survey, 2006 to 2007. Ann Intern Med. 2009;151:602–11.

28. Department of Health and Human Services. Improving the quality of clinician cytology technique and management, client cytology education, and the evaluation of cytology laboratory testing: a resource guide for Title X family planning projects. Washington DC: U.S. Department of Health and Human Services, Public Health Service, Office of Population Affairs, Office of Family Planning, 1989:3–4, 59.

29. U.S. Preventive Services Task Force, Screening for Cervical Cancer, 2003 Accessed at http://www.uspreventiveservicestaskforce.org/uspstf/uspscerv.htm.

30. Saslow D, Roncowicz CD, et al. American Cancer Society Guideline for the Detection of Cervical Neoplasia and Cancer. CA Cancer J Clin. 2002;52:342–362.

31. Wright Jr TC, L. Massad S, Dunton CJ, Spitzer M, Wilkinson EJ, Solomon D. ASCCP 2006 consensus guidelines for the management of women with cervical intraepithelial neoplasia or adenocarcinoma in situ. Am J Obstet Gynecol. 2007;197:340–5.

32. American College of Obstetricians and Gynecologists. ACOG Committee opinion no. 463: Cervical cancer in adolescents: screening, evaluation, and management. Obstet Gynecol. 2010;116(2 Pt 1):469–72.

33. Rolnick SJ, LaFerla JJ, Jackson J, Akkerman D, Compo R. Impact of a new cervical Pap smear screening guideline on member perceptions and comfort levels. Prev Med. 1999;28:530–4.

34. Sirovich BE, Woloshin S, Schwartz LM. Screening for cervical cancer: will women accept less? Am J Med. 2005;118:151.

35. Sawaya GF, McConnell KJ, Kulasingam SL, Lawson HW, et al. Risk of cervical cancer associated with extending the interval between cervical-cancer screenings. N Engl J Med. 2003;349:1501–9.

36. Kivlahan C, Ingram E. Papanicolaou smears without endovervical cells. Are they inadequate? Acta Cytol. 1986;30:258–260.

37. Ransdell JS, Davey DD, Zalesky S. Clinicopathologic correlation of the unsatisfactory Papanicolaou smear. Cancer. 1997;81:139–43.

38. Krieger JN, Tam MR, Stevens CE, et al. Diagnosis of trichomoniasis: comparison of conventional wet mount examination with cytologic studies, cultures, and monoclonal antibody staining of direct specimens. JAMA. 1988;259:1223–7.

39. Reiter RC. Management of initial atypical cervical cytology: a randomized prospective study. Obstet Gynecol. 1986;237–40.

40. Kinney WK, Manos MM, Hurley LB, et al. Where's the high grade cervical neoplasia? The importance of minimally abnormal Papanicolaou diagnoses. Obstet Gynecol. 1998;91:973–6.

41. Hurt WG, Silverberg SG, Frable WJ, Belgrad R, Crooks LD. Adenocarcinoma of the cervix: histopathologic and clinical features. Am J Obstet Gynecol. 1977;129:304–15.

42. Whittemore AS, Harris R, Itnyre J. Characteristics relating to ovarian cancer risk. Collaborative analysis of 12 US case-control studies. II. Invasive epithelial ovarian cancers in white women. Am J Epidemiol. 1992;136:1184–1203.

43. National Institute of Health Consensus Development Panel on Ovarian Cancer, NIH consensus conference. Ovarian cancer. Screening, treatment, and follow up. JAMA. 1995;273:491–7.

44. Rosenberg L, Palmer JR, Zauber AG. A case control study of oral contraceptive use and invasive epithelial ovarian cancer. Am J Epidemiol. 1994;139:654–61.

45. American College of Obstetricians and Gynecologists Committee on Gynecologic Practice. The role of the generalist obstetrician-gynecologist in the early detection of ovarian cancer. ACOG Committee Opinion number 280. Obstet Gynecol. 2002;100:1413–5.

46. USPSTF. Screening for Ovarian Cancer, 2004. Accessed at http://www.uspreventive servicestaskforce.org/uspstf/uspsovar.htm.

47. Berry DA, Cronin KA, Plevritis SK, Fryback DG, et al. and Cancer Intervention and Surveillance Modeling Network (CISNET) Collaborators. Effect of screening and adjuvant therapy on mortality from breast cancer. N Engl J Med. 2005;353:1784–92

48. Hulka, BS, Stark AT. Breast cancer: cause and prevention. Lancet. 1995;346:883–7.

49. Smith RA, Cokkinides V. Eyre HJ. American Cancer Society guidelines for early detection of cancer 2006. CA Cancer J Clin. 2006;56:11–25.
50. Barton MB, Harris R, Fletcher S. Does this patient have breast cancer? The screening clinical breast exam: should it be done? How? JAMA. 1999;282:1270.
51. Lee CH, Dershaw DD, Kopans D Breast cancer screening with imaging: recommendations from the Society of Breast Imaging and the ACR on the use of mammography, breast MRI, breast ultrasound, and other technologies for the detection of clinically occult breast cancer. J Am Coll Radiol. 2010;7:18–27.
52. Liberman, A.F. Abramson, F.B. Squires et al. The Breast Imaging Reporting and Data System: positive predictive value of mammographic features and final assessment categories. Am Jour Radiol. 1998;171:35–40.
53. Cancer Clinical Services Quality Assurance Project. Breast diagnostic algorithms for primary care clinicians, 2005. Accessed at http://qap.sdsu.edu/screening/breastcancer/bda/index.html.

Pregnancy Testing and Assessment of Early Normal and Abnormal Pregnancy

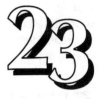

Mary Fjerstad, NP, MHS
Alison Edelman, MD, MPH

- Expedient scheduling for a pregnancy confirmation, as soon as the woman suspects she may be pregnant, is an essential family planning service.

- Early pregnancy diagnosis allows the woman to consider all her options for pregnancy care: parenthood, abortion, and adoption.

- With early pregnancy diagnosis, a woman planning to continue her pregnancy can begin to take prenatal precautions and medical care during the early, most vulnerable stages of fetal development.

- Early confirmation of pregnancy allows a woman considering abortion more time for counseling and decision making and more options surrounding care (medication or vacuum aspiration abortion). In addition, her abortion can be performed when it is safest— early in pregnancy.

- A negative test may be extremely reassuring to a woman who does not want to be pregnant.

ESSENTIAL PREGNANCY INFORMATION FOR EVERYONE

Certain situations provide key opportunities or a teachable moment to educate women regarding the prevention or planning of a pregnancy. Clinician visits to discuss negative pregnancy tests or to screen for sexually transmitted infection (STI) are a common and under-exploited opportunity for intervention. As many as one-quarter of all adolescent girls who conceive have previously had one or more visits to learn that their pregnancy test was negative.[1]

Once an unintended pregnancy occurs, the opportunity to prevent or prepare is lost. Integration of pregnancy prevention and preconception care into routine gynecological services is cost-effective and strongly recommended to assure systematic review of a medical history, completion of recommended screening tests and immunizations, and planning and preparing for pregnancy, including initiation of folic acid.[2]

EDUCATION AND COUNSELING

The issues surrounding personal fertility are complex, and a pregnancy diagnosis visit should provide the client an opportunity to clarify and articulate her feelings. Before conducting the pregnancy test or performing an examination, find out what the woman hopes her result will be. Realize that ambivalence is very common. When presenting the test results, elicit the client's reaction and allow time for her to express her feelings. Assess the woman's support system. Provide referrals if she feels counseling would be helpful. This is especially important if her support system is not adequate. Emphasize that a decision based on her test result does not need to be made that day. Encourage the woman to talk with her partner, family, or friends. Outline all the options available.

- Every woman who tests positive for a pregnancy should be provided information about all her pregnancy options, because she may change her mind after leaving your office.

- If the client is pregnant and plans to continue her pregnancy, educate her regarding healthy antenatal practices and be certain she has an appropriate resource for prenatal care. Review common pregnancy warning signs with her (Table 23–4).

- If the client plans to continue her pregnancy, but does not want to parent the child, refer her to a reputable resource that can help with adoption.

- If the client is pregnant but does not plan to continue her pregnancy, refer her for abortion services. While women should make this decision without undue pressure, it is important to understand that the sooner the decision is made and acted upon, the safer the procedure will be. (See Chapter 24 on Abortion.)

- If a woman is pregnant with an intrauterine contraceptive (IUC) in place, it should be removed immediately whether she is planning to continue her pregnancy or have an abortion. The IUC should be removed as soon as pregnancy is diagnosed. The passage of time may lead to retraction of IUC strings as the uterus increases in size. An IUC in situ increases the risk of septic abortion and other complications such as late miscarriage, preterm delivery, and placental abruption.[3]

- If the client is not pregnant and wishes she were, counsel her about her own fertility. If appropriate, refer her for fertility evaluation. Educate her regarding the importance of healthy preconception care including taking a daily vitamin that includes folic acid (0.4 mg daily) before and during the first trimester of pregnancy.[4]

- If the client is not pregnant, plans to continue being sexually active, and is happy with the negative test result, then birth control counseling is appropriate. A pregnancy scare can be a good bridge from risk-taking behavior to effective, ongoing contraceptive use.

- Offer STI testing to high-risk women.

Possible Early Pregnancy Exposure to Teratogens

At the first visit, briefly discuss a woman's use of prescription drugs, over-the-counter medications or herbs, and illegal substances, because the use of one or more of these substances is common.[5,6] Many of these products may be teratogenic; cessation of their use could prevent abnormalities or awareness of the risk posed by use could influence decisions regarding pregnancy continuation. The Organization of Teratology Information Services (www.otispregnancy.org) provides up-to-date resources and fact sheets about both maternal and paternal exposures to medications, herbal products, infectious agents, vaccines, medical conditions, illicit substances, and alcohol dependency.

Recent Contraceptive Practices

When making a visit for a pregnancy diagnosis, a client's contraceptive practice is an important topic for two reasons. First, some forms of contraception are associated with higher risk of ectopic pregnancy. Second, the discussion helps the woman understand why her method failed (if it did) in order to motivate her to change the way she uses the method or to change the method. This latter insight may be important now or only after her pregnancy is complete.

Domestic Violence Screening and Referral

A review of 13 studies found a prevalence of domestic violence against pregnant women ranging from 0.9% to 20.1%.[7] Homicide related to intimate partner violence is the leading cause of maternal mortality in the United States, accounting for 13% to 24% of all deaths in pregnancy.[8] **Because of the prevalence of domestic violence, and particularly** among women in the prenatal and postpartum period, clinicians providing gynecologic care, pregnancy screening, and prenatal care are in a unique position to screen for, recognize, and intervene. Women who have experienced domestic violence often report that a question by a health care worker was the first step in disclosure and recognition.[9]

Clinicians should be aware of community-based resources such as local domestic violence hotlines, shelters, advocacy organizations, and support groups for victims of domestic violence. National resources include the National Domestic Violence Hotline (1–800–799-SAFE) and the National Sexual Violence Center (1–877–739–3895). Internet sites include the National Domestic Violence Hotline (www.ndvh.org), the Family Violence Prevention Fund (http://endabuse.org), the National Coalition against Domestic Violence (www.ncadv.org), and local domestic violence hotlines (www.usdoj.gov/ovw/).

Pregnancy Care Referral

Encourage early entry into pregnancy care so gestational dating can be confirmed and baseline vital signs can be documented. If she selects pregnancy continuation, screening tests can be performed, including genetic testing, if indicated. If she selects pregnancy termination, expedient care is also important as earlier procedures are associated with less morbidity. If you do not provide prenatal or abortion care, provide a referral list to facilitate the patient's access to care. In making a referral, consider factors such as the patient's primary language, indications for high-risk perinatal care, accessibility of the clinic/hospital logistically and financially and any special delivery needs (e.g., need for cesarean section) or desires (e.g., epidural or natural delivery, postpartum sterilization).

There is often a delay of several weeks until the patient will have her first pregnancy care appointment, so review the signs and symptoms (i.e., severe pain or bleeding) that may signal problems during early pregnancy, and tell her whom to contact if a problem or emergency arises in the interim (Table 23–4).

PREGNANCY EVALUATION: HISTORY, SYMPTOMS, PHYSICAL EXAM, AND LABORATORY EVALUATION

Although confirmation of pregnancy is the most pressing issue for women presenting with the concern of a possible pregnancy, a general history and, if possible, a physical exam should also be performed as this may reveal additional health issues that need to be addressed and could also affect pregnancy care. A pregnancy evaluation has several goals:

1. Determine whether or not the woman is pregnant (see the section on Pregnancy Testing).

2. Identify possible problems that require further evaluation or urgent intervention, such as ectopic pregnancy, uncontrolled diabetes, or a need to immediately change a medication.

3. Assess gestational age accurately.

4. Help the patient make and implement her own plans for the pregnancy.

5. Screen for chlamydia, HIV, and syphilis as part of routine prenatal testing. Screening for gonorrhea is also indicated if the woman is at high risk because of high community prevalence or exposure to multiple partners. Screening for chlamydia and, if indicated, gonorrhea is recommended even if the patient is considering abortion, because these infections are statistically associated with an increased risk of postabortal infection.[10]

6. Document of Rh status and baseline hematocrit or hemoglobin

Confirm the pregnancy with a pregnancy test and estimate the gestational age by reviewing pregnancy signs and symptoms, obtaining the last menstrual period (LMP), and performing a pelvic exam. Women often know or suspect they might be pregnant, so a particularly useful question to ask is simply: why do you think you are pregnant now? As early as 2 weeks after conception, even before the first missed menstrual period, hormonal changes may make breasts tender, sore, fuller, or heavier. Fatigue, nausea, and urinary frequency may be noted at 4 weeks following the LMP (www.mayoclinic.com).

Along with documenting the LMP, discuss whether it was a normal versus a light or mistimed period. A light or mistimed period may mean that fertilization and implantation actually occurred before the LMP, and for this reason, the date of the previous menstrual period (PMP) should be determined. The date when pregnancy symptoms began can also help better corroborate the fertilization date.

Women may also report irregular light bleeding or spotting. This is common in a normal early pregnancy and is due to the trophoblastic tissue of the early pregnancy (blastocyst) invading into the endometrium.[11] However, heavy bleeding, particularly when accompanied by lower abdominal pain, may signal threatened spontaneous abortion.[12] Ectopic pregnancy may be completely asymptomatic, but presence of pain accompanied by spotting or moderate to severe bleeding should alert the clinician to the possibility of ectopic pregnancy,[13] discussed later in the chapter.

A pelvic exam can confirm pregnancy test results and correlate uterine enlargement with menstrual dates. The pelvic exam may also

Table 23–1 Possible reasons for discrepancy between uterine size and menstrual dates

Uterus Smaller Than Expected	Uterus Larger Than Expected
Fertilization later than dates suggest	Fertilization earlier than dates suggest
Ectopic pregnancy	Uterine leiomyomata (fibroids)
Incomplete or missed, spontaneous abortion	Twin gestation
Error in pregnancy test	Hydatidiform mole*
Uterine anomaly (e.g., unicollate uterus)	Normal variation between women at a given length of pregnancy
Normal variation between women at a given length of pregnancy	

* In 28% of molar pregnancies, uterine size is larger than expected; in 14%, the uterus is smaller than expected, and in the rest, the uterus is normal size for dates. [14]

help to screen for abnormal pregnancy (e.g., ectopic pregnancy), uterine abnormalities (e.g., fibroids, etc.), or sexually transmitted infection (STI). If the uterine size by bimanual examination does not correspond to the estimated length of gestation based on LMP, consider the possible reasons for the discrepancy (Table 23–1). Ultrasound evaluation is often helpful in this situation as it can both document pregnancy location and confirm gestational dating.

Rh screening is a standard recommendation for any pregnant woman. Women whose blood is typed as Rh D negative are typically administered anti-D immune globulin under the following circumstances:

- When undergoing spontaneous or induced abortion
- When experiencing vaginal bleeding or trauma
- Routinely at 28 weeks gestation
- After delivery

Administering anti-D immune globulin under these circumstances is to prevent the risk of Rh sensitization; however, the majority of these are caused from a fetal-maternal hemorrhage at the time of delivery, and Rh sensitization from first-trimester events are rare.[15] The recommendation to give anti-D immune globulin for first-trimester bleeding, miscarriage, or abortion varies between countries, but the American College of Obstetricians and Gynecologists (ACOG) recommends 50 mcg of anti-D immune globulin for these situations.[15–17] For bleeding, miscarriage, or abortion occuring after the first trimester, ACOG recommends the standard 300 mcg dose.

A hemoglobin or hematocrit can also be helpful at the time of initial evaluation to assess the need for iron or nutritional supplementation, to perform additional screening for thalassemias, to assess the cumulative extent of any bleeding, and to provide an important baseline for later comparison.

Definitions Used For Dating The Pregnancy

Menstrual age dates the pregnancy beginning from the first day of the LMP. Menstrual age is stated in days or weeks from the LMP. The normal pregnancy duration is 40 menstrual weeks. The term gestational age is often used interchangeably with menstrual age.[18] When the actual date of conception is known (e.g., as in assisted fertility), the pregnancy can be dated according to this date. Assuming that a woman ovulates mid-cycle, the conceptional age of a full-term pregnancy is 38 weeks. This chapter will refer to pregnancy dating with the terms *LMP* or *menstrual age*.

Timing Early Pregnancy Events

Following ovulation, fertilization of the ovum (egg) by sperm occurs within the fimbria of the fallopian tube (distal end). Over the next 2 days, the fertilized ovum remains unattached within the fallopian tube, using tubal fluids to sustain nutrition and energy for early cellular cleavage. After this stage, the solid ball of cells (the morula or embryo) leaves the oviduct and enters the uterine cavity. The endometrium is the multilayered mucosal lining of the uterine cavity. The decidua is the highly modified endometrium specialized for implantation and support of a pregnancy.[19] By 6 days after ovulation, the embryo, now a blastocyst, is ready to attach and implant. At this time, it finds an endometrial lining of sufficient depth, vascularity, and nutritional richness to sustain the early embryo and subsequent development of the placenta. By the end of the 3rd week (21 days LMP), the blastocyst begins to implant into the thickened endometrium. The tissue of the blastocyst is divided into two important layers. The *outer cell layer*, called the trophoblast, eventually forms the chorionic membranes and the placenta. As trophoblastic cells form placental tissue, the placental tissue produces human chorionic gonadotropin hormone (hCG). These are the molecules that are detected by a pregnancy test. The hCG secreted by the trophoblast prevents the regression of the corpus luteum and thus maintains a continued supply of progesterone for the maintenance of pregnancy until the placental tissue itself starts to produce increasing quantities of progesterone by 6 to 7 weeks after fertilization. Progesterone is essential for the maintenance of early pregnancy. The *inner cell layer* of the blastocyst develops into the embryo, amnion, umbilical cord, and primary and secondary yolk sacs.[20] Figure 23–1 below provides a visual representation of the landmarks of early pregnancy and the corresponding rise of hCG.

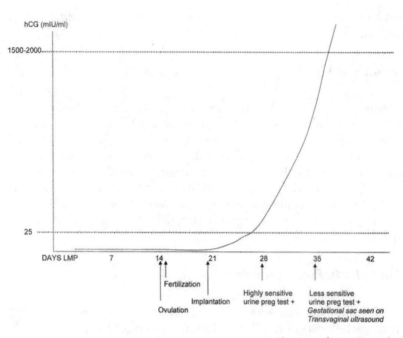

hCG (mIU/ml)

1500-2000

25

DAYS LMP   7   14   21   28   35   42

↑↑ Fertilization
Ovulation

↑ Implantation

↑ Highly sensitive
urine preg test +

↑ Less sensitive
urine preg test +
Gestational sac seen on
Transvaginal ultrasound

(Courtesy of Mary Fjerstad, NP)

Figure 23–1 Very early pregnancy timeline (based on 28-day cycle)

hCG LEVELS IN PREGNANCY, PREGNANCY TESTING, AND PITFALLS OF PREGNANCY TESTS

hCG LEVELS IN PREGNANCY

Pregnancy tests detect the hCG in a pregnant woman's urine, blood, or serum.

Serum or urine pregnancy tests today detect four independent molecules: intact hCG, hyperglycosylated hCG (H-hCG), and free β-subunit and pituitary hCG.[21,22] hCG is the accurate term used in this text to denote the types of hCG tested in pregnancy and replaces the formerly used term βhCG.

Elevated hCG can be detected in the woman's serum at low levels as early as 21 days LMP, very soon after implantation occurs. In general, serum levels of hCG reach 50 to 250 mIU/ml by the time of the first missed menstrual period; hCG reaches a peak of >100,000 mIU/ml at approximately 10 to 12 weeks LMP and then declines to a plateau that is maintained until delivery.[21] (See Figure 23–2.) Low levels of hCG may simply indicate that a normal pregnancy is earlier in gestation than men-

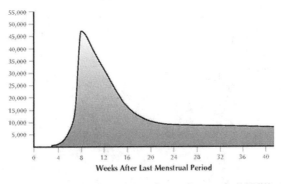

Source Braunstein (1976)[23] with permission.

Figure 23–2 hCG levels during normal pregnancy

strual dates suggest. These values can also vary significantly between individuals.

A single hCG value tells you only if a woman is pregnant, but it does not determine the pregnancy's viability or location. A single hCG value is meaningful in only two situations: when a sensitive test indicates that the woman is pregnant and when the hCG level is 1,500 to 2,000 mIU/ml or higher. This 1,500 to 2,000 mIU/ml level correlates with the ability to visualize a pregnancy via transvaginal ultrasound, also called the discriminatory zone.[24] (See Ultrasound section, below). Typically the pattern of hCG rise, fall, or plateau in combination with the clinical picture, sonogram (if performed), and risk factors for ectopic pregnancy is more important than a single value in determining the location and status of the pregnancy.

During the first 10 weeks of pregnancy, a hCG rise of 66% over 2 days or 48 hours is generally considered acceptable evidence of a viable intrauterine pregnancy; however, rates of increase over 48 hours can be as high as 228% and as low as 53%.[25] In ectopic pregnancies, values may plateau or increase at a slower than normal rate. One study demonstrated that almost 30% of women with ectopic pregnancies had initial patterns of hCG change that mimicked either an intrauterine pregnancy or a complete miscarriage.[26]

In abnormal pregnancies, hCG levels often increase abnormally, plateau, or decrease. Elevated levels are normal with a multiple gestation, reflecting the increased placental mass. Extremely high hCG production, with hCG levels as high as 2 million mIU/ml, can occur with a molar pregnancy, such as hydatidiform mole or gestational trophoblastic disease.[21] Abnormally low hCG levels often occur before a spontaneous abortion or with an ectopic pregnancy. The rate of rise of hCG in ectopic pregnancy generally is lower than for intrauterine pregnancies, but the

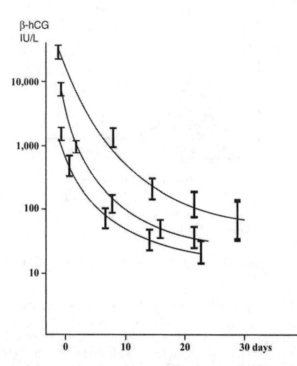

Disappearance curves of serum hCG in three groups of women. Semilogarithmic scale. Upper curve represents women (n=36) who had elective vacuum aspiration abortion at 7–13 weeks LMP. Middle curve represents women (n=35) with spontaneous abortion at 6–15 weeks LMP treated with uterine aspiration. Lower curve represents women (n=35) with ectopic pregnancies diagnosed 2.5–11.0 weeks after LMP and removed surgically.

Source: Steier et al. (1984)[28] with permission.

Figure 23–3 Disappearance curve of hCG after abortion, miscarriage and surgical treatment of ectopic pregnancy

curves overlap.[27] (hCG patterns in ectopic pregnancy will be discussed in more detail later in the chapter in the section, Managing Problems in Early Pregnancy.)

Following the clinical course of a stable patient when the location and status of the pregnancy are unknown is both art and science because interruption of a desired pregnancy that is viable and intrauterine should be avoided, yet it is also imperative to prevent evolution of ectopic pregnancy to the point of rupture.

hCG LEVELS AFTER PREGNANCY COMPLETION

After a pregnancy ends in delivery or by abortion, hCG levels gradually decrease. Figure 23–3 represents the hCG disappearance curve following uterine aspiration at 7 to 13 weeks (upper curve), miscarriage at 6 to 15 weeks (middle curve), and surgical treatment of ectopic pregnancy (bottom curve).[28] The initial decrease in hCG after full-term delivery is quite rapid, so that a hCG level following the delivery will have dropped to less than 50 mIU within 2 weeks, and hCG will be undetectable after 3 to 4 weeks.[23]

If first-trimester vacuum aspiration or medication abortion successfully ended the pregnancy, hCG clears normally from the bloodstream as expected and the hCG level declines steadily, halving at least every 48 hours after vacuum aspiration and after medication abortion, or halving within 2 to 4 days of taking misoprostol.[29–31] When patients have medication abortion, hCG continues to increase following mifepristone but then declines precipitously after administration of misoprostol.[32] However, since hCG levels are near their peak[33] at about 10 to 12 weeks LMP, hCG levels may still be high enough 2 weeks following an abortion that pregnancy tests—both blood-based and urine—will still be positive. Sensitive pregnancy tests, including commonly-used office or home use urine test kits are likely to be positive between 16 to 60 days.[28,34]

By the first follow-up visit, 6 to 18 days after taking mifepristone, hCG levels drop to 20% of the initial value (measured on the day of mifepristone intake) in 98.5% of successful medication abortions.[35] However, it is possible for some successful medication abortion patients to have hCG levels decline with a lengthy plateau. Patients who require uterine evacuation intervention less than 15 days after medication abortion due to prolonged bleeding or pain generally have higher absolute and relative hCG values than women with normal courses whose hCG values drop sharply. Unfortunately, due to overlap of hCG levels between those with a successful medication abortion and those who require uterine aspiration, no clinical decisions regarding uterine evacuation can be made based on hCG levels alone.[32,36]

In the case of a continuing pregnancy, hCG levels will demonstrate an upward trend: over 2 days, a mean rise of 124% and a minimum rise of 53%.[25] If an ectopic pregnancy continues to evolve after medication or vacuum aspiration abortion, hCG values can behave erratically; these patterns are discussed in more detail in the section, Managing Problems in Early Pregnancy.

Research has demonstrated the expected fall of hCG following successful medication abortion. The outcome of medication abortion can be followed by quantitative hCG instead of ultrasound, and this may save a woman from returning to the clinic for an in-person examination, especially if she travels great distance to receive mifepristone and plans to self-administer the misoprostol at home. Draw a quantitative hCG on the day the woman receives mifepristone in the clinic; the level is expected to drop by 50% within 4 days of receiving mifepristone if the pregnancy aborted.[30] If hCG is tested 6 to 18 days after receiving mifepristone, a drop of 80% has a very strong predictive value in confirming successful medication abortion.[35]

PREGNANCY TEST OPTIONS
HIGHLY SENSITIVE URINE PREGNANCY TESTS, LESS SENSITIVE URINE PREGNANCY TESTS, SERUM QUANTITATIVE hCG TESTS

Understand every test available and used in your setting: sensitivity of the test, correct procedure for performing the test, and number of minutes required for the test to register positive or negative results. (Brand names of pregnancy tests will not be discussed in this chapter because the names frequently change.)

HIGHLY SENSITIVE URINE PREGNANCY TESTS

- For home or clinic use
- Clinical Laboratory Improvement Amendment (CLIA) waived

Cross-reactions with other hormones are not a problem for highly-sensitive urine pregnancy tests. Most have a stated sensitivity of 25 mIU/ml. The over-the-counter (OTC) pregnancy tests sold for home use and those used in clinics are essentially the same.

Specificity and sensitivity. Highly-sensitive urine pregnancy tests are intended to provide accurate qualitative (positive/negative) results with hCG levels as low as 5 to 50 mIU/ml. Tests can be positive as early as the day of the first missed menses, depending on the sensitivity of the test. One study reported that 98% of women have a positive pregnancy test within 28 days LMP.[37] On the other hand, another study reported that, even using an extremely sensitive test (0.13 mIU/ml), among 142 women with self-reported onset of LMP, 10% of clinical pregnancies were undetectable on the first day of missed menses. Implantation can occur after the first day of the next expected menses.[38] Early pregnancies produce quite a variable range of hCG levels, and the time at which a pregnancy is detected accurately by different pregnancy tests varies widely. Moreover, few clinic pregnancy tests or home tests have been calibrated against the three critical forms of hCG: intact hCG, H-hCG, and free β-subunit.[22]

Accuracy. A study of 18 different OTC pregnancy tests demonstrated hCG levels from 23 to 2,438 mIU/ml in well-dated pregnancies 28 to 30 days LMP.[39] Thus for a test to detect 95% of pregnancies at the time of missed menses, it would need to consistently detect an hCG of at least 12.4 mIU/ml. This study found that most tests were consistently accurate at a urine hCG of 100 mIU/ml and that some brands had technical or design problems.[39] Manufacturer's claims that a pregnancy test can detect pregnancy "as early as the day of the missed menstrual period" are based on data that are almost 30 years old that assumed that urine hCG concentrations were the same as serum hCG concentrations. In fact, the average urine hCG concentration is generally less than half of the corresponding serum hCG concentration, depending on the time of pregnancy and specificity of the test.[22]

Uses. Highly-sensitive urine pregnancy tests can be used to confirm or rule out pregnancy. These tests are appropriate for screening prior to procedures, such as biopsy or x-ray, or prior to prescribing a drug that would be contraindicated during pregnancy. They are also appropriate in screening for possible ectopic pregnancy. Only 1% of ectopic pregnancies would be missed (false negative) with a urine test sensitivity of 50 mIU/ml.[23] A false-negative test is rare even 30 days after successful medication abortion. Patients are more likely to have a false-positive or inconclusive test (25% of results are false-positive or inconclusive in women 30 days after a successful medication abortion).[40] (See section on hCG Levels After Pregnancy Completion.)

LESS-SENSITIVE URINE PREGNANCY TESTS

- Most are designated as CLIA moderate complexity although some are CLIA-waived.

Specificity and sensitivity. The sensitivity of these pregnancy tests range from 200 to 2,000 mIU/ml. Be aware of the sensitivity of the less-sensitive urine pregnancy test used in your setting.

Uses. Less-sensitive tests have a fairly narrow range of use. They are not appropriate to "rule out" pregnancy, because early pregnancy, ectopic pregnancy, impending spontaneous abortion and, in rare cases, even later pregnancies (16 to 20 weeks) may be missed due to their low hCG levels. Less-sensitive tests can be used to confirm pregnancy ≥6 weeks LMP or to document the disappearance of hCG after abortion. However, even for this use, a less-sensitive test (sensitivity 1,500–2,000 mIU/ml) had a 60.8% false-positive rate 2 weeks after successful medication abortion.[41] This study, however, found that a *negative* less-sensitive test result is reassuring of medication abortion success. Put another way, a negative pregnancy test after medication abortion is reassuring, but a positive test may not mean much. Although rare, it is also possible for less-sensitive pregnancy test to have false-negative results (at the follow-up, the woman is still pregnant but the test result is negative).[40,41,42] Therefore, a negative pregnancy test following abortion should be reassuring *only* if it is concordant with a history of bleeding, passage of tissue, abatement of pregnancy symptoms, and clinical assessment.

Home Pregnancy Testing.

Home pregnancy test kits offer the advantages of privacy, anonymity, and convenience. Moreover, they are popular; over the years, the number of women using home pregnancy tests has remained constant; there were 230 million over-the-counter pregnancy tests sold in 2009.[43] Because home pregnancy tests are easily accessible, a woman may identify pregnancy early and thus be more able to be an active manager of her own health care.

Accuracy. Test accuracy can be affected by the technique and experience of the user, and by the user's ability to follow the test instructions precisely.[44] The most common error with home pregnancy tests is a negative result because the test was performed too early in pregnancy.

In addition, a woman using a home pregnancy test may have difficulty understanding the directions packaged in the test kit. In an evaluation of instructions from thirteen OTC urine pregnancy tests, the reading level required to understand the instructions ranged from a 7th to a 14th grade reading level.[45]

Uses. A positive result helps to facilitate early entry into care and possibly an earlier change to healthy behaviors. Further clinical evaluation is needed to confirm the pregnancy, determine the length of gestation, identify location (intra- or extrauterine), and viability. If the home test result is negative, clinical evaluation also may be needed to determine the cause of menstrual delay or other symptoms that have prompted the test, especially if normal menses do not resume.

Serum Quantitative hCG Radioimmunoassay (RIA) or Immunometric Assay

A quantitative serum hCG test is designed to provide a *level* or number of hCG mIU/ml; thus, the rise or fall of the hCG level may provide important information about the status of the pregnancy.

Use of a serum *quantitative* hCG test only to confirm early pregnancy does not have any advantages over *qualitative* (yes/no) highly-sensitive urine tests. Highly-sensitive urine pregnancy kits are equally specific for hCG and provide immediate results at much lower cost. Only certain clinical situations justify the additional expense of serum hCG testing.

Specificity and sensitivity. Serum quantitative hCG tests provide accurate results with levels as low as 5 mIU/ml. Thus they reliably detect pregnancy soon after implantation around 21 days LMP. Tests are usually "batched" because of expense; test processing requires 1 to 2 hours. Be sure to specify *quantitative* hCG when ordering this test. In addition, it is optimal but not essential to use the same laboratory for serial hCG tests to limit inter-assay variation between laboratories. However, virtually all laboratories now use the Third International Standard for hCG quantitation, which limits this variation. Given that some patients often have to travel significant distances for repeat hCG tests, it may be difficult to have all samples sent to the same laboratory. In this case, as long as the patient is stable, and the clinician has confirmed that all laboratories are using the Third International Standard, it is acceptable to use different laboratories for hCG testing.

Uses. Serial testing of serum hCG can be used to check the increasing or decreasing trend of hCG levels to assist in the diagnosis of an ectopic pregnancy, evolving spontaneous abortion, or possible retained products of conception. A single result alone is not usually meaningful. Rather, the pattern of hCG in conjunction with other diagnostic tests, such as sonography, clinical evaluation of the patient, and consideration of risk factors leads to a diagnosis of normal or abnormal intrauterine pregnancy or ectopic pregnancy. A single hCG result alone *is* significant when the level is 1,500–2,000, mIU/ml; at this level, if an intrauterine pregnancy is not visualized on transvaginal ultrasound, begin a work-up to diagnose or rule out ectopic pregnancy. Very high levels of hCG can be associated with molar pregnancy or multiple pregnancies, such as twins.

PITFALLS OF PREGNANCY TESTING

Correctly interpreting pregnancy test results is not always entirely straightforward:

1. hCG levels change drastically over the course of pregnancy, especially during the first 8 to 10 weeks (Figure 23–2).

2. **To detect a potentially viable pregnancy, the hCG Reference Service recommends that pregnancy tests should be performed no earlier than day 31 since the start of the last LMP.**[21]

3. Tests may be performed incorrectly, thus leading to an incorrect reading and interpretation. For example, if a test is not read when the designated number of minutes elapses but sits for several hours, a negative test may turn faintly positive.

4. Both positive and negative test results must be interpreted in relation to (1) the sensitivity, specificity, and characteristics of the test being used and (2) the clinical evaluation, including ultrasound examination when appropriate.

5. If pregnancy test results are discordant with other clinical signs, consider the possible reasons for the discrepancy. Plan appropriate follow-up or further evaluation to protect the patient against possible consequences of an incorrect test result.

6. Very early pregnancy loss, or a *biochemical* pregnancy, refers to an embryo that fails to implant in the uterus or is rejected by the uterus. hCG levels reach a peak 2 weeks after conception (28 days after start of LMP) at approximately 10 to 100 mIU/ml,

then rapidly drop. A normal or heavier than usual menstrual period follows. Women may have a positive pregnancy test in the last week of their menstrual cycle, but if the test is repeated a few days or a week later, the test is negative; transient hCG may extend to 5 days after the time of the missed menses.[39]

7. Any test result can be wrong. Laboratory errors do occur, including specimen mix-up and incorrectly performed test procedures. For accurate results, instructions for the kit must be followed meticulously and timed with a stopwatch. Use control solutions to verify accuracy. Observe test-kit and reagent expiration dates.

8. Know exactly what kind of pregnancy test was performed and what sensitivity the test has. Without this information, it is not possible to assess the clinical significance of a negative result or to evaluate the possibility of a false-positive result.

9. Do not base clinical management on the results of a *home* pregnancy test. Although home kits have excellent theoretical accuracy, their use even by trained personnel may not reliably provide the sensitivity or specificity needed for optimal clinical management.[46,47] Be careful about accepting the results of a urine pregnancy test performed in another facility, especially in critical clinical situations such as ectopic pregnancy.

10. False-negative results can occur. With *less-sensitive* urine pregnancy tests, false-negative results frequently occur because the test is performed too early or too late in pregnancy. Menstrual cycle length and thus timing of ovulation can vary monthly for women.[37] hCG levels vary from individual to individual in pregnancy; in women with well-dated pregnancies, hCG levels ranged from 23 to 2,438 mIU/ml 28 to 30 days after the onset of the last known menstrual period.[38] At the time of the first missed menses, some of these women with hCG levels on the lower range would have had negative urine pregnancy tests. Abnormal pregnancy and urine that is too diluted may be responsible for false-negative results.

A false-negative result can also occur with a *highly-sensitive* urine pregnancy test if the test is performed too early in the cycle, before implantation occurs. In this situation, the result is a "true" negative, which could be misleading if not repeated a few days later.

If a false-negative result is suspected because the test is performed too early, repeat the test in a few days to a week, depending on the clinical situation. If a false-negative result is suspected for other reasons, order a serum quantitative hCG.

11. It is rare but known in the literature that urine and serum pregnancy tests may yield false-negative results when hCG is present at extreme concentrations. Known as the *high-dose hook effect*, the *secondary* antibody binding sites become saturated with free hCG so that the *primary* antibody complex is unable to bind, preventing detection of the antigen.[11,48] In one case of molar pregnancy, only after multiple dilutions of the serum was a hCG of 1.5 million mIU/ml detected.[49] In another case of complete molar pregnancy, the hCG level was 3,704,085 mIU/ml.[50] If you suspect a molar pregnancy, notify the laboratory so that they can perform dilutions, if necessary.

The important thing to remember is that laboratory test results should be questioned if they are discordant with clinical findings.

12. False-positive urine and serum pregnancy test results are not common, but they can cause perplexing dilemmas:

— False-positive results with highly-sensitive urine pregnancy tests are very rare, but laboratory error is always possible. A false-positive result could occur if the woman has had treatment involving hCG injection within the preceding 14 days. Faint false-positive results have been reported with urine samples contaminated by blood or recent use of Chinese herbal medication.[51] If you suspect a false-positive result, obtain a serum quantitative hCG.

— When a positive pregnancy test is not confirmed by the presence of a pregnancy in the uterus, do not assume the test result is false. The pregnancy may be too early to be seen sonographically; ectopic pregnancy should also be kept in the differential diagnosis.

— In very rare cases, pregnancy test results are positive even though the patient is not pregnant, because hCG actually is present and originating from a source other than pregnancy. hCG levels persist after a recent pregnancy or after hCG treatment. Low levels of hCG (5 to 30 mIU) may be associated with tumors of the pancreas, ovaries, breast, and many other sites.[52] Some normal postmenopausal women also have low levels of circulating hCG-like substance of pituitary origin.[53,54] In addition, patients with end-stage renal disease may produce hCG, which registers as false-positive pregnancy tests due to decreased urinary clearance as well as regulatory disturbances.[55]

— Phantom hCG or heterophilic antibodies can cause a *serum* hCG to be positive (typically at low levels) but urine tests to be negative. These antibodies are present only in the blood and at high enough levels to interfere with serum hCG radioimmunoassay in a small number of women (1/3,300).[21,56,57] In these cases, hCG is falsely detected due to interfering antibodies found in human serum. While uncommon, false-positive or phantom hCG tests have led to the misdiagnosis of ectopic pregnancy, or to the erroneous assumption of post-gestational choriocarcinoma positive hCG tests. Since these interfering antibodies are present only in blood, perform a urine pregnancy test as a confirmatory hCG measurement when clinically indicated to rule out the false-positive serum hCG results due to heterophilic antibodies.[22]

13. For follow-up after molar pregnancy or choriocarcinoma, use serum quantitative hCG testing. The hCG protein produced by tumor cells may be abnormal and in some cases may be missed by other test methods. If persistent hCG levels are found, the condition must be managed by an expert, and hCG levels in both blood and urine should be checked, because false-positive blood results are possible.[57,58]

ULTRASOUND IN VERY EARLY PREGNANCY

Targeted ultrasound in the outpatient setting when a woman has a positive pregnancy test has several purposes:

1. Identifying that the pregnancy is intrauterine, thereby virtually ruling out an ectopic pregnancy

2. Dating the pregnancy

Unfortunately, when sonography is performed very early in pregnancy, corroboration of pregnancy and its location (intra- or extra-uterine) cannot always be confirmed. When a patient's highly-sensitive urine pregnancy test is positive but no intrauterine pregnancy is visualized by transvaginal sonography, there are several possible explanations:

- Elevated hCG due to reasons other than pregnancy

- Very early intra-uterine pregnancy; too early for gestational sac to be visualized (<4.5 weeks)

- Abnormal pregnancy—intrauterine pregnancy not growing at the normal rate; may be an anembryonic pregnancy or impending spontaneous pregnancy loss

- Ectopic pregnancy

In addition, certain things can delay the visualization of a normal gestational sac including body habitus (i.e., obesity), fibroids, uterine anom-

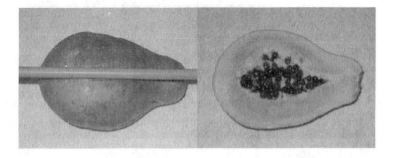

Figure 23–4 Papaya (cut) resembling the shape of the uterus shown in the longitudinal view

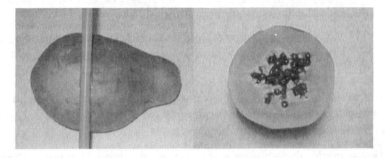

Figure 23–5 Papaya (cut) resembling the shape of the uterus shown in the transverse view

alies, or an acutely retroverted uterus. Abnormal or delayed growth of a pregnancy can also prevent visualization at the expected time.

EARLIEST ULTRASOUND VISUALIZATION OF PREGNANCY

The first indication of pregnancy by transvaginal ultrasound is the gestational sac. A true gestational sac can be challenging to distinguish from a *pseudosac,* which can be present with an ectopic pregnancy. A pseudosac is the sloughing of decidua that produces a fluid collection in the endometrial cavity.[59] Approximately 10% of patients with ectopic pregnancy have a pseudosac visualized on ultrasound.[60]

Visualization of the uterus with transvaginal ultrasound should be performed in a systematic fashion and include evaluation both in the longitudinal and transverse views. **You must train yourself to look at the uterus and its contents in the longitudinal and transverse views.** Avoid the temptation of focusing only on the gestational sac because other important findings can be missed with this approach (e.g., twins, ectopic pregnancy, uterine anomalies, fluid in the cul-de-sac, ovarian mass). The longitudinal view captures the uterus in its long axis, making it possible to visualize the cervix and endometrial cavity up to the fundus and to orient the viewer in the pelvis. The papaya in Figure 23–4 resembles a uterus in the longitudinal plane.

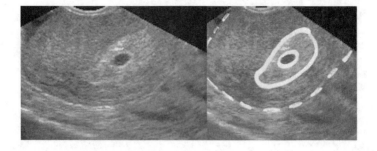

Figure 23–6A and Figure 23–6B. Intrauterine gestational sac with choriodecidual reaction. The double decidual reaction is seen in which the ring closest to the sac is bright white (echogenic), somewhat faded in the middle of the reaction, and then brighter again at the edge of the choriodecidual reaction. In view B, the inner and outer rings of the reaction are outlined with solid white lines and the uterus is outlined with a broken white line. (Courtesy of Mary Fjerstad, NP)

The adnexae, uterus, and cul-de-sac should then be viewed in the transverse position. The image of the papaya shown in Figure 23–5 represents the uterus in the transverse plane.

Transvaginal ultrasound allows for visualization of the entire pelvis: identification of the uterus, ovaries, presence or absence of ovarian cysts, and presence or absence of fluid in the cul-de-sac.

When the clinician or sonographer visualizes all the characteristics of a true gestational sac in the uterus, the likelihood of ectopic pregnancy is remote. In contrast, presence of an actual pseudosac is a harbinger of ectopic pregnancy. Therefore it is vital to assess the sac in multiple planes (longitudinal and transverse) to be assured that the sac has *all* the characteristics of a true sac.

The following are characteristics of a normal gestational sac:

1. A true gestational sac is a three-dimensional round or oval structure, implanted off-center to the midline, and normally grows about 1 mm/day.[24] (See Figures 23–7 and 23–8.)

2. Completely surrounded by a multi-layered echogenic choriodecidual reaction, known as the double decidual reaction. The appearance is of a multi-layered fluffy white cloud surrounding the gestational sac, whiter near the sac and at the outer edge of the reaction. Another description of the appearance of the choriodecidual reaction is that of an orange rind or halo (see Figure 23–6A and 6B and 23–8).

In contrast, the illustration (Figure 23–9) and ultrasound images (Figure 23–10) and (Figure 23–11) demonstrate pseudosacs.

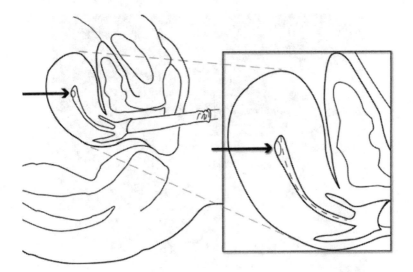

Figure 23–7   Illustration of eccentric implantation. The pregnancy implants into the thickened endometrium or decidua. In effect, it burrows into the endometrial lining; it does not float in the endometrial cavity. That's why the gestational sac is off-center to the midline of the endometrial cavity (arrow). (Courtesy of Mary Fjerstad, NP)

Small amounts of free pelvic fluid can be seen in intrauterine pregnancies, as well as in ectopic pregnancies. The presence of a moderate to large amount of fluid in the cul-de-sac has a 96% specificity for diagnosing ectopic pregnancy. In 15% of confirmed ectopic pregnancies, sonolucent fluid in the cul-de-sac was the *only* extrauterine finding.[62] One study found that visualization of any free fluid had 63% sensitivity and 80% specificity in diagnosing ectopic pregnancy in patients presenting to the emergency department.[63] In other words, ectopic pregnancy itself was not visualized directly in the adnexa, but fluid in the cul-de-sac was the only visual sonographic clue of ectopic pregnancy, along with absence of intrauterine gestational sac. In the ultrasound image (Figure 23–12), free fluid in the cul-de-sac is seen.

Visualization of the Yolk Sac Within the Gestational Sac

The yolk sac is derived from embryonic tissue, therefore a pseudosac will not produce a yolk sac. When a yolk sac is seen within an intrauterine sac, it confirms that it is a true intrauterine gestational sac with virtually great accuracy because the sensitivity for diagnosing intrauterine gestations greater than 5.5 weeks approaches 100%.[64] (See Figure 23–13.)

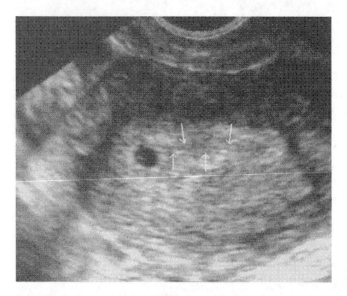

Figure 23–8 Longitudinal view of an intrauterine gestational sac, choriodecual reaction and endometrial cavity line. Note the thin black line that extends longitudinally through the endometrial cavity, sometimes referred to as the endometrial cavity line (arrows). The gestational sac is adjacent to, but does not displace, the endometrial cavity line, thereby demonstrating an eccentric implantation.[61] In addition, the double decidual reaction (multi-layered echogenicity) surrounding the gestational sac is seen. (Courtesy of Mary Andrews, NP)

CORRELATION OF HCG, ULTRASOUND FINDINGS AND CLINICAL PICTURE

When an intrauterine pregnancy cannot be visualized by transvaginal ultrasound, the clinician must evaluate the ultrasound findings, the pregnancy test results, knowledge of expected hCG values, and the patient's clinical picture in conjunction with risk factors of ectopic pregnancy.

The landmarks for timing of findings by transvaginal ultrasound are as follows:

Table 23–2 Timing of landmarks in early pregnancy (with transvaginal ultrasound based on 28-day cycle)[18]

20–32 days gestation from LMP	positive highly-sensitive urine pregnancy test
35 days LMP (5 weeks)	gestational sac can usually be visualized
40 days LMP (5½ weeks)	yolk sac virtually always is seen
48 days LMP (6½ weeks)	embryonic pole with cardiac motion is seen

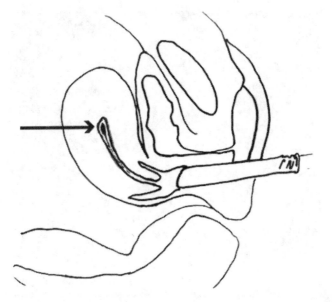

Figure 23–9 Illustration of a pseudosac. This is a fluid collection within the endometrium; the fluid collection can be large or small, irregular shaped or round (at least when viewed in one plane), but it is not implanted in the decidual lining; it is midline in the cavity, not eccentric to the midline. (Courtesy of Mary Fjerstad, NP)

Since the amount of hCG in early pregnancy directly correlates with the quantity of pregnancy tissue growing, the level of hCG at which a gestational sac *should* be seen on transvaginal ultrasound has been determined. The level of hCG at which the gestational sac of a normal intrauterine pregnancy should seen on ultrasound is called the "discriminatory zone." The accepted discriminatory zone of hCG is 1,500 to 2,000 mIU/ml with transvaginal ultrasound.[24]

The sensitivity of less-sensitive urine pregnancy tests discussed in this chapter is 1,500 to 2,000 mIU/ml. When one of these tests is positive, an intrauterine gestational sac can be seen with transvaginal ultrasound. However, false-negative pregnancy tests can occur and if diagnosis of ectopic pregnancy is being considered, a confirmatory quantitative serum hCG test should be performed as well.

When a pregnancy is not visualized on ultrasound, knowledge of the discriminatory zone and pregnancy test results is useful in managing patients; is this a very early pregnancy or should there be a higher index of suspicion for ectopic pregnancy? If a patient has a positive highly-sensitive urine pregnancy test, she reports regular menses, her LMP was < 5 weeks ago and the less-sensitive urine pregnancy test is negative, the following is true: 1) she is very early in pregnancy, 2) it is too early in pregnancy to expect to be able to visualize a pregnancy by ultrasound,

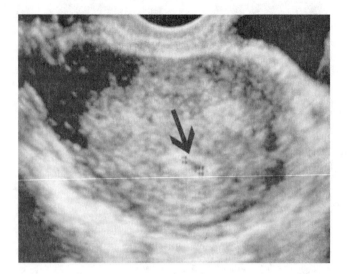

Figure 23–10 Pseudosac Note that the choriodecidual reaction is not multi-layered; it is a thin, homogenous echogenic rim. Note also that the fluid-filled sac (arrow) is mid-line in the uterine cavity, not eccentrically implanted as would be a true gestational sac. Also note that the fluid-filled sac is irregularly shaped. Another view taken at the same session demonstrates that the sac lost all semblance of roundness when it was viewed in a different plane (Figure 23–11). (Courtesy of Mary Fjerstad, NP)

3) it is too early to determine the location of the pregnancy, and 4) although the pregnancy may be ectopic, the most likely possibility is that it is intrauterine, since only approximately 2% of pregnancies are reported to be ectopic.[65]

- If an intrauterine gestational sac is not seen on transvaginal ultrasound and the correctly recalled LMP *is earlier than 5 weeks ago*, the patient is not at high risk for ectopic pregnancy and is deemed to be compliant, she can be given information about the signs and symptoms of ectopic pregnancy with warnings to seek emergency care should they occur, and told to return in 3 to 7 days for a repeat ultrasound or hCG testing. Most likely, an intrauterine pregnancy will be seen on transvaginal ultrasound at that time. If no intrauterine pregnancy is visualized at the follow-up scan, even if the less-sensitive pregnancy test is negative, the patient should be worked up for ectopic pregnancy.

- If, on the other hand, *both the highly-sensitive and the low-sensitivity urine pregnancy tests are positive*, regardless of the patient's LMP, then visualization of intrauterine gestation by transvaginal sonogram is expected. Because the low-sensitivity urine pregnancy test is positive, the patient's hCG is at the level of the discriminatory zone. If no gestational sac is visualized in the uterus,

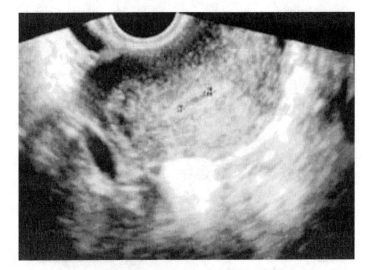

Figure 23–11 Another view of the pseudosac This image is of the same patient at the same session as Figure 23–10, showing the sac in a different plane. In this plane, the sac is flattened and doesn't resemble a normal round or oval gestational sac at all. These two images emphasize the importance of performing a systematic scan in both the longitudinal and transverse planes and the importance of recognizing red flags when the sac does not match all the characteristics of a normal gestational sac. This patient had an ectopic pregnancy. (Courtesy of Mary Fjerstad, NP)

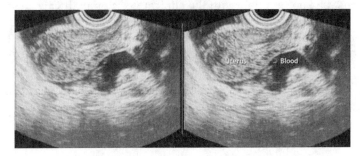

Figure 23–12 Free fluid in the cul-de-sac (Courtesy of Matthew Reeves, MD)

this patient should be presumed to have an ectopic pregnancy, which, if the patient is asymptomatic, may be determined by following serial serum quantitative hCG tests or by referral for a diagnostic ultrasound.

- If patients have *risk factors for ectopic pregnancy, bleeding, pain or free fluid* in the cul-de-sac visualized by sonogram, especially if the 2,000 mIU/ml test is positive and there is no intrauterine gestational sac visualized by transvaginal ultrasound, they should be presumed to have an ectopic pregnancy until proven otherwise. Any patient with acute symptoms of ectopic pregnancy

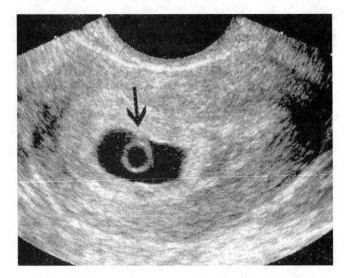

Figure 23–13 Yolk sac appears within the intrauterine gestational sac (arrow).

should be immediately referred to the emergency department for definitive treatment. The patient should also be told to not eat or drink anything prior to her evaluation, because a surgical intervention may be necessary.

It must be kept in mind with the clinical decision pathways described above that both false-positive and false-negative results can occur with clinic-based low-sensitivity (1,500–2,000 mIU/ml) pregnancy tests. For potentially critical situations, especially in women with highly desired pregnancies, the safest course is to order a quantitative serum hCG test for confirmation of the hCG level.

Ectopic pregnancy will be discussed in more detail below, Managing Problems in Early Pregnancy.

MANAGING PROBLEMS IN EARLY PREGNANCY

Consider the possibility of pregnancy whenever a reproductive-aged woman has symptoms such as abdominal pain, abnormal bleeding, or irregular or missed menstrual periods. The patient's history, as well as her own assessment of pregnancy risk, may be helpful. A highly-sensitive pregnancy test is a prudent precaution to take when considering a diagnosis in a reproductive-aged female, no matter what the woman's history indicates. An old adage in gynecology and obstetrics is that every reproductive-aged woman is presumed pregnant and this pregnancy may be ectopic until proven otherwise.

Table 23–3 Efficacy of misoprostol treatment for early pregnancy loss (misoprostol 800 mcg administered vaginally with a second dose administered on day 3 if expulsion was incomplete)

Success with one treatment of misoprostol	71%
Success with misoprostol repeated in 48 hours	84%
Efficacy according to types of pregnancy loss:	
Embryonic or fetal death	88%
Anembryonic pregnancy	81%
Incomplete or inevitable abortion	93%

Source: Zhang et al. (2005)[68] with permission

EARLY PREGNANCY LOSS

Spontaneous Abortion

A meta-analysis found that approximately 15% of clinically recognized pregnancies end spontaneously in early pregnancy.[66] The diagnosis of spontaneous abortion may be made on the basis of a pelvic examination, abnormal bleeding, or ultrasound findings. If the cervix is dilated and products of conception are visible in the cervix or vagina, then an abortion is inevitable. An ultrasound evaluation may help determine whether the uterine cavity is already empty. If ectopic pregnancy has been excluded and bleeding is not heavy, women have a choice of several options for management, including expectant management, medical treatment (misoprostol), or vacuum aspiration. A prospective observational trial of 30 women having spontaneous abortion found success rates for expectant management are 82.1% at 2 weeks and 100% by 30 days.[67] As long as the woman is stable, success rates of expectant management increase with time and patience. In a randomized trial of 652 women using misoprostol for early pregnancy loss, misoprostol 800 mcg administered vaginally was 84% successful by day 8.[68] The success of misoprostol treatment varied with the *type* of early pregnancy loss (see Table 23–3). Education and informed consent require an explanation of the advantages and disadvantages of uterine aspiration, medical treatment, and expectant management; respect the patient's preference as you both weigh all medical considerations. (See Chapter 24, Abortion.)

Vacuum aspiration is indicated if bleeding is so heavy that it results in hemodynamic instability or is life-threatening.

If the pregnancy is wanted and the patient's condition is stable, you can delay intervention while further evaluating whether the pregnancy may be viable. Serial quantitative hCG levels and an ultrasound evaluation are likely to confirm the diagnosis. When the woman desires to continue her pregnancy, take time for a careful and thorough evaluation.

Intervention on the basis of an initial exam or ultrasound will seem abrupt and shocking as the woman first begins to acknowledge the possibility of her loss and grief.

Anembryonic Pregnancy

Anembryonic pregnancy, formerly known as *blighted ovum*, refers to a pregnancy in which the gestational sac developed normally but the embryo never materialized, or an embryo developed but was then reabsorbed.[19] Figure 23–14a demonstrates the classic empty amnion sign; this is the most obvious form of anembryonic pregnancy. Trophoblastic tissue continues to function, causing continued growth of the gestational sac, although at a slower than normal rate.[33] An anembryonic pregnancy is diagnosed when a transvaginal ultrasound reveals a mean sac diameter (MSD) of 8 to 10 mm or greater with no visible yolk sac, or an MSD exceeding 16 to 18 mm with no detectable cardiac activity or embryo.[33,67]

Anembryonic pregnancy may be indistinguishable by sonogram from incomplete abortion, but there is no sign of external bleeding in anembryonic pregnancy.[19] Although the MSD of 16 mm has been cited as the measurement at which an abnormal pregnancy is suspected, if the pregnancy is highly desired, it is best not to intervene at a rigid set of measurements. When the MSD is in the borderline range, correlate with serial hCG levels or a follow-up ultrasound. If the pregnancy is nonviable, the hCG levels will decline or the follow-up ultrasound will show no sac growth or no development of a yolk sac or embryo.

As with spontaneous or missed abortion, an anembryonic pregnancy may be managed expectantly, with vacuum aspiration, or with misoprostol alone.[68,69]

Embryonic or Fetal Demise

Early pregnancy loss is confirmed when no embryonic heartbeat is seen on transvaginal ultrasound and either 1) the sonogram demonstrates an embryo that measures more than 5 mm in length[70] or 2) the gestational age is known with certainty and is at least 7 weeks.[19] Most of the time, when the embryo is visible at all, cardiac activity is detectable, but that may not be the case, especially when only a fetal pole is seen. When the embryonic length is more than 5 mm and duration of gestation is at least 7 weeks and cardiac activity is absent, embryonic demise is highly likely. However, if it is a desired pregnancy, be cautious and certain of the diagnosis prior to uterine evacuation with either vacuum aspiration or misoprostol. The scan should be performed using the highest transducer frequency possible, and if possible, ask a second independent clinician to confirm the sonographic findings.[71] Since this is not an emer-

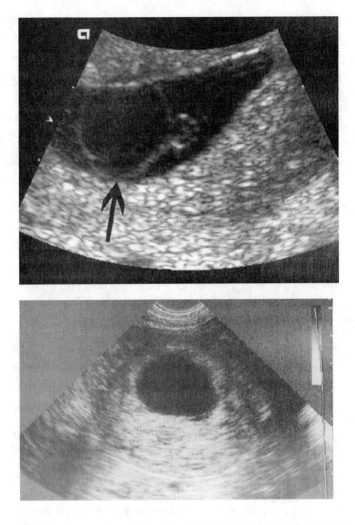

Figure 23–14 A and B Anembryonic pregnancies. The amnion can be seen but there is no yolk sac or embryonic structure within it (arrow figure a). (Courtesy of Matthew Reeves, MD)

gency, a follow-up ultrasound may be repeated in 1 week to avoid the risk of terminating a normal desired pregnancy. If the embryonic heart rate is less than 80 beats per minute, subsequent demise is very likely within 1 to 2 weeks.[72] Embryonic or fetal demise may be managed by vacuum aspiration or by medical treatment with misoprostol; these treatments are more effective than expectant management for embryonic or fetal demise. A randomized controlled trial of 131 women found that in cases of early embryonic or fetal demise, the success rate of misoprostol was 86.7% by day 7, whereas expectant management had a success rate of 28.9%.[73]

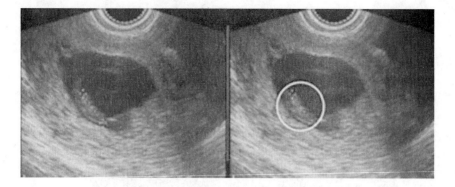

Figure 23–15 Embryonic demise. The embryo (marked) has not grown in proportion to the size of the gestational sac. The caliper placement represents measurement of early embryonic length. (Courtesy Matthew Reeves, MD)

Figure 23–15 shows early embryonic demise. There is no cardiac activity (which can only be assessed in real-time, not on a still image).

ECTOPIC PREGNANCY

During the history-taking of a pregnant woman, assess the risk factors for ectopic pregnancy, although more than half of identified ectopic pregnancies occur in women without known risk factors.[74]

Risk Factors For Ectopic Pregnancy

Certain risk factors are strongly associated with ectopic pregnancy. The factors most strongly associated include etiologies that cause fallopian tube damage or pathology. A meta-analysis reported that history of previous ectopic pregnancy was the strongest risk factor associated with ectopic pregnancy.[75] A later nested case-control study of 367 women with ectopic pregnancies reported that women with an ectopic pregnancy were almost 3 times as likely to have had a prior ectopic pregnancy when compared with controls.[13] A woman with a previous ectopic pregnancy has about a 10% to 15% chance of recurrence, depending on type of treatment she underwent for the previous ectopic pregnancy. Laparotomy versus laparoscopy does not affect the risk of recurrence; however salpingostomy is associated with a greater risk of repeat ectopic pregnancy than are salpingectomy or treatment with methotrexate.[76,77]

A history of tubal surgery, including tubal sterilization and reconstructive tubal surgery, increases risk of ectopic pregnancy. It is very rare for a woman who has had a tubal ligation or who has an intrauterine contraceptive (IUC) in place to become pregnant, but should pregnancy occur, an estimated 25% to 50% of such pregnancies are ectopic.[27] More specifically, as many as half of pregnancies occurring in women with a levonorgestrel IUC in place may be ectopic, whereas the rate in women with a copper IUC in place is approximately 1 in 16.[78] Though these rates are high, the absolute risk of developing an ectopic pregnancy in a woman using an IUC for contraception is very low, because the IUC is a very effective means of contraception, and any pregnancy is unlikely to occur. (See Chapter 7 on Intrauterine Contraceptives.)

Women who become pregnant after transabdominal tubal sterilization have a 9-fold increased risk of ectopic pregnancy; bipolar coagulation carries a greater risk than other transabdominal methods, such as postpartum bilateral salpingectomy.[79,80] However the 10-year cumulative probability of ectopic pregnancy after these procedures is low, at 7.3 per 1,000 procedures.[80]

Previous genital tract infection can be a cause of tubal pathology, but largely depends on extent of disease. One recent study showed that a history of outpatient treatment for cervical infection with chlamydia or gonorrhea, or current infection with chlamydia or gonorrhea, did not increase risk of ectopic pregnancy.[13] It is theorized that most cervical infections that are treated on an outpatient basis do not go on to develop into pelvic inflammatory disease (PID) and damage the fallopian tubes; therefore, risk of ectopic pregnancy is not increased.[81] However, repeated chlamydial infections, even if asymptomatic, can cause microscopic tubal scarring and adhesions, which prevent or impede migration of the fertilized ovum to the uterus. A retrospective cohort study of 11,000 Wisconsin women found that compared to a woman who had only one reported case of chlamydial infection, women with two reported infections were 4 times as likely to be hospitalized for an ectopic pregnancy. Women with 3 or more reported chlamydial infections were 11 times as likely to be hospitalized for ectopic pregnancy.[82]

Other factors that are weakly associated with ectopic pregnancy include dose-dependent smoking, age over 35, and infertility.[83]

The most important specific question to ask when considering the possibility of ectopic pregnancy is "Is there an intrauterine pregnancy?"[11] If the answer is "yes" then an ectopic pregnancy is virtually ruled out because the possibility of a heterotopic pregnancy, discussed later in the chapter, is so rare. If the answer is "no," meaning there is no *definitive* intrauterine pregnancy, then further evaluation is warranted.

A woman who has clinical evidence of a possible ruptured ectopic pregnancy, such as hypotension or postural hypotension, fainting, falling hemoglobin or hematocrit, severe abdominal pain, guarding, or rebound tenderness requires immediate referral for emergency management where surgery is available if needed. Unfortunately, this classic presentation of pain, abnormal vaginal bleeding, and palpable adnexal mass is present in only 45% of patients with ectopic pregnancy.[84] Physical examination and vital signs are variable and unreliable indicators of ectopic pregnancy; vital signs of patients with ruptured ectopic pregnancies may even be normal. Hemodynamic variables do not correlate well with blood loss in patients with ectopic pregnancy; for instance, paradoxic bradycardia is common.[11]

A highly-sensitive urine pregnancy test is almost certain to be positive (false-negative rate is less than 1%)[23] but less-sensitive urine pregnancy tests (1,500–2,000 mIU/ml) are not sensitive enough to detect the lower hCG levels associated with ectopic gestation in about 50% of cases.[85]

The clinician considers the possibility of ectopic pregnancy because the woman has less serious and nonspecific symptoms such as bleeding in early pregnancy, uterine enlargement that does not correlate with dates (uterus is too small), an ultrasound that fails to demonstrate an intrauterine gestation, or an early uterine aspiration abortion that fails to recover identifiable products of conception from the uterine cavity. Often the patient is completely asymptomatic. These situations may allow time for further outpatient evaluation if the patient is willing and able to monitor her own symptoms carefully, has access to emergency intervention, and is by all indications early in her pregnancy. Warn the patient to watch for ectopic pregnancy danger signs (Table 23–4) while the evaluation is pending, and to return immediately for emergency care if danger signs occur.

Table 23–4 Early pregnancy danger signs

Possible Ectopic Pregnancy
Sudden intense pain, persistent pain, or cramping in the lower abdomen, usually localized to one side or the other
Irregular bleeding or spotting with abdominal pain when period is late or after an abnormally light period
Fainting or dizziness persisting more than a few seconds. These may be signs of internal bleeding. (Internal bleeding is not necessarily associated with vaginal bleeding.).

Possible Miscarriage
Late last period and bleeding heavy, possibly with clots or clumps of tissue; cramping more severe than usual
Period is prolonged and heavy—5 to 7 days of "heaviest" days
Abdominal pain or fever

Contact your clinician immediately or go to a hospital emergency room if you develop any of these signs.

Source: Stewart et al. (1987)[86] with permission.

Further Steps In Evaluation

Further steps in evaluation of ectopic pregnancy may include the following:

1. **Quantitative serum hCG assay**

   An initial level can be compared with the hCG level 2 days (48 hours) later if the diagnosis is still uncertain.

   There is no single predictable hCG pattern in ectopic pregnancy. Table 23–5 depicts the expected range of hCG rise with viable intrauterine pregnancy, the fall expected with complete spontaneous abortion, and the various patterns seen in ectopic pregnancy.

   The rate of rise of hCG in ectopic pregnancy generally is lower than for intrauterine pregnancies, and the drop is usually not as steep as it is for complete spontaneous abortion. In the majority

Table 23–5 Rise or decline in sequential quantitative hCG values in early viable intrauterine pregnancy, complete spontaneous abortion, and ectopic pregnancy

Type of Pregnancy	
Early viable intrauterine pregnancy	
Mean rise in hCG in 2 days, % increase	124
Minimum expected rise in hCG in 2 days, % increase[a]	53
Complete spontaneous abortion	
Range of minimum expected decline in hCG, % decrease[b]	21-35
Ectopic pregnancy[c]	
% of women who experienced a **rise** in hCG (Group A)	60
• % of pregnancies in Group A whose first two hCG values were consistent with intrauterine pregnancy	35
• Median rise in hCG in 2 days, % increase	75
% of women who experienced a **decline** in hCG (Group B)	40
• % of pregnancies in Group B whose first two hCG values were consistent with complete spontaneous abortion	20
• Median decline in hCG in 2 days, % decrease	27
Group A and Group B combined	
• % of pregnancies with first two hCG values out of range for normal intrauterine pregnancy or complete spontaneous abortion	71
• % of pregnancies with first two hCG values consistent with range for normal intrauterine pregnancy	21
• % of pregnancies with first two hCG values consistent with range for complete spontaneous abortion	8

Sources: Barnhart et al (2004), Seeber and Barnhart (2006), Silva et al (2006) with permission.

[a] hCG will increase at this rate or faster in 99% of early viable intrauterine pregnancies.

[b] The rate of decrease depends on the initial hCG value.

[c] 287 women presented to ER with pain or bleeding; initial hCG was <5,000, pregnancy not visualized with transvaginal ultrasound. The first two hCG tests were taken at least 24 hours but no more than 7 days apart.

of patients with ectopic pregnancy (71%), the first two hCG levels either will not increase as expected for intrauterine pregnancy or will not fall as sharply as expected with completed spontaneous abortion.[87] But the rising and falling curves of hCG overlap in ectopic, normal intrauterine, and spontaneously aborting pregnancies. The main point is that there is no characteristic hCG pattern for ectopic pregnancy; in 20% of ectopic pregnancies, the first two hCG values rise as expected in intrauterine pregnancy.[87,81] In 8% of ectopic pregnancies, the hCG decline is as fast or faster than the decline seen with complete spontaneous abortion.[87] Until the location and status of the pregnancy are confirmed, hCG should be followed until one of the following assessment pathways leads you to a diagnosis:

- The hCG curve is outside of that expected. (This is typically determined by 2 hCG levels taken 48 hours apart. If a woman is asymptomatic with no adnexal mass noted on exam or ultrasound and has a highly desired pregnancy, more levels may be desired to confirm or rule out ectopic pregnancy.)

- Ultrasound confirms presence of intrauterine or ectopic pregnancy.

- The patient becomes symptomatic.

- The hCG values fall to non-pregnant levels.

- Tissue evaluated from uterine evacuation confirms presence or absence of products of conception.

2. **Tissue evaluation and pathology report**

   If no intrauterine pregnancy is visualized by transvaginal ultrasound when the hCG is 1,500– to 2,000 mIU/ml (the discriminatory cut-off), especially if the pregnancy is not desired, experts advocate evacuating the contents of the uterus to differentiate a spontaneous abortion from an ectopic pregnancy.[83] If a uterine evacuation is performed, products of conception should be identified in the fresh tissue aspirate; this confirms an intrauterine pregnancy and virtually rules out ectopic pregnancy. Visual examination of the fresh specimen has been found to be as accurate as a pathology examination in determining that the abortion was complete although tissue examinations by both the surgeons and the pathologists had poor validity for identifying abnormal abortion outcomes.[88] The histological result (pathology report) is sometimes inconsistent with the diagnosis of the provider who cared for the patient and examined the fresh tissue specimen, and this may result in unnecessary further investigation and treatment.[89] Nonetheless, if products of conception are not identified by examination of the fresh tissue aspirate, send the tissue for microscopic tissue evaluation with a rapid pathology report by phone. Placental villi identified in the evacuated specimen can in most instances rule out an ectopic pregnancy.[90]

If products of conception are not identified in the examination of the fresh tissue aspirate, draw the first quantitative hCG immediately after the procedure. If the first hCG is not higher than 1700 mIU/ml, draw a serum hCG again in 24 to 72 hours to be sure that the hCG drops at least 50%.[91] If an ectopic pregnancy is still evolving, hCG levels typically will not plummet—they will typically plateau or rise.[76]

3. **Ultrasound evaluation**

   The diagnosis of ectopic pregnancy can be made conclusively if a gestational sac and fetal heartbeat are detected outside of the uterine cavity. Unless an intrauterine gestation (gestational sac with yolk sac) can be identified with certainty or an extrauterine gestation is visible, ultrasound results do not provide a definitive diagnosis. An intrauterine pregnancy *should* be visualized on transvaginal ultrasound by the time the 1,500 to 2,000 mIU/ml pregnancy test is positive (or the serum quantitative hCG is ≥1,700 mIU/ml).

   If after completing these diagnostic steps, ectopic pregnancy cannot be excluded, additional evaluation or treatment will be needed. Refer the patient immediately for surgical management if she becomes symptomatic during the process of evaluation or medical treatment.

Further Steps In Treatment

Early diagnosis is very important in ectopic pregnancy. Although early diagnosis and intervention have helped to reduce ectopic pregnancy mortality, ectopic pregnancy is still the leading cause of pregnancy-related death during the first trimester.[92] Also, early diagnosis allows more time for conservative management, which also may help to preserve the woman's future fertility. Further steps in treatment may include the following:

1. **Treatment with methotrexate**

   Asymptomatic, early ectopic pregnancy may be treated with methotrexate[81,93,94] to induce dissolution of trophoblast tissue. Success rates reported with a single- or multiple-dose treatment with methotrexate range from 88.9 to 96%.[81]

   Methotrexate is more effective in earlier gestation. Relative contraindications to medical versus surgical treatment of ectopic pregnancy are gestational sac >3.5 cm and embryonic cardiac activity.[81] One study found that the single best predictor for success was initial hCG level; lower hCG levels were directly correlated with successful methotrexate treatment, ranging from 98% success rate when hCG was <1,000 mIU/ml to 68% success rate was hCG was >15,000 mIU/ml.[94]

2. **Surgery**

   Surgical treatment of ectopic pregnancy (salpingostomy or salpingectomy) is required if the ectopic pregnancy has ruptured, the patient is clinically not a candidate for medical treatment, medical treatment with methotrexate has failed, or a patient is unable to comply with the intensive follow-up for outpatient medical management.[76] In addition, some patients and clinicians may prefer surgical management. Laparoscopy is now preferred over laparotomy because there is less operating time, less blood loss during the procedure, fewer hospital days, and quicker convalescence.[76]

3. **Expectant management**

   Although expectant management is not a standard option, pioneer studies revealed that the natural course of many early tubal ectopic pregnancies will be spontaneous tubal abortion or reabsorption. These small studies described expectant management of patients with small ectopic pregnancies that lacked cardiac activity or declining hCG activity.[95,96] However, a Cochrane Review of 35 randomized controlled trials concluded that clear criteria for intervention versus expectant management have not yet been defined.[97] If you choose to manage the patient expectantly, note that ectopic pregnancies have ruptured at very low hCG levels. One retrospective study of 693 ectopic pregnancies found that 11% of women with a ruptured tube had serum hCG levels less than 100 mIU/ml.[98]

HETEROTOPIC PREGNANCY

Heterotopic pregnancy is the simultaneous occurrence of two or more implantation sites, most commonly a concomitant intrauterine pregnancy and an ectopic pregnancy.[76] The incidence of heterotopic pregnancy in the general population is reported as 1:4,000.[83] The risk increases in patients treated with fertility drugs and reproductive technologies. The risk of heterotopic pregnancy in women undergoing assisted reproductive techniques is as high as 1%.[99]

Clinicians should be aware of the possibility of heterotopic pregnancy if, following vacuum aspiration or medication abortion, miscarriage, or

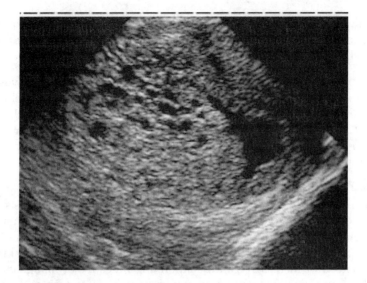

Figure 23–16 Molar pregnancy. The "snow storm" appearance of a molar pregnancy is the result of multiple small cystic spaces. The larger cysts are visible as sonolucent spaces while the smaller cysts create echogenic areas due to the multiple interfaces between the cysts. (Courtesy Matthew Reeves, MD).

progressing intrauterine pregnancy, women exhibit the signs and symptoms of ectopic pregnancy, or hCG levels increase or plateau.

MOLAR PREGNANCY

Hydatidiform mole (molar pregnancy) is an abnormal conception with excessive trophoblastic proliferation. Molar pregnancies are classified as either complete (genetic material exclusively of paternal origin, no fetus present) or partial (one maternal and two paternal contributions-usually two sperm fertilize a normal oocyte, fetus often present).[100] Patients with molar pregnancies typically present in the first trimester with abnormal bleeding and very high levels of hCG[101] (see Pitfalls of Pregnancy Testing). Uterine size is often greater than expected with a complete mole due to hydropic trophoblastic tissue. However, many patients with hydatidiform mole are entirely asymptomatic in the first trimester and do not have the classical signs such as vaginal bleeding, increased uterine volume and theca lutein cysts.[102]

Two studies found that ultrasound correctly identified 40% to 60% of molar pregnancies during the first or early second trimester, when trophoblastic change is not as proliferative.[103,104] See Chapter 24, Abortion, for a more complete discussion of confirmation of molar pregnancy.

Although molar pregnancies are initially benign, their high hCG levels can cause medical sequelae including hyperemesis gravidarum, hyperthyroidism, hypertension, or large theca lutein cysts.

Trophoblastic tissue of molar pregnancies may become invasive, which can lead to malignant conditions such as gestational trophoblastic disease and choriocarcinoma. These conditions are more likely with complete (20%) than partial (<5%) moles.[101] The standard of care for treatment is uterine evacuation with close surveillance of post-evacuation serum hCG for gestational trophoblastic disease.

Gestational trophoblastic disease is highly curable if detected early. If there is delay in diagnosis or treatment, widespread metastasis can occur; occasionally patients with metastatic disease still die.[105] This risk for metastasis is why hCG levels are monitored following treatment for a molar pregnancy for approximately 6 to 12 months until negative. Levels that plateau or increase post-evacuation are indicative of malignancy.[101] As the occurrence of a new pregnancy during this monitoring can mask malignancy or confuse the clinical picture, use of effective contraception during this time period is strongly recommended.

REFERENCES

1. Zabin LS, Emerson MR, Ringers PA, Sedivy V. Adolescents with negative pregnancy test results. An accessible at-risk group. JAMA. 1996;275:113–117.
2. ACOG. ACOG technical bulletin. Preconceptual care. Number 205-May 1995. American College of Obstetricians and Gynecologists. In J Gynaecol Obstet. 1995:201–207.
3. Kim SK, Romero R, Kusanovic, JP, Erez, O, Vaisbuch, E, Mazaki-Tovi S, Gotsch F, Mittal P, Chaiworapongsa T, Pacora P, Oggé, G, Gomez R, Yoon BH, Yeo L, Lamont RF, Hassan SS. The prognosis of pregnancy conceived despite the presence of an intrauterine device (IUD). J. Perinat. Med. 2010;38:45–63.
4. Erickson JD. Folic acid and prevention of spina bifida and anencephaly. 10 years after the U.S. Public Health Service recommendation. MMWR Recomm Rep. Sep 13 2002;51(RR-13):1–3.
5. Werler MM, Mitchell AA, Hernandez-Diaz S, Honein MA and the National Birth Defects Prevention Study. Use of over-the-counter medications during pregnancy. Am J Obstet Gynecol. 2005;193:771–777.
6. Schwarz EB, Maselli J, Morton M, Gonzales R. Prescription of teratogenic medications in United States ambulatory practices. Am J Med. 2005;118:1240–1249.
7. Gazmararian JA, Lazorick S, Spitz AM, Ballard TJ, Saltzman LE, Marks JS. Prevalence of violence against pregnant women. JAMA. 1996 275:1915–1920.
8. Plichta SB. Intimate partner violence and physical health consequences: policy and practice implications. J Interpers Violence. 2004;19:1296–323.
9. Rodriguez M, Quiroga S, Bauer H. Breaking the silence: battered women's perspectives on medical care. Arch Fam Med. 1996;5:153–158.
10. Sawaya GF, Grady D, Kerlikowske K, Grimes DA. Antibiotics at the time of induced abortion: the case for universal prophylaxis based on a meta-analysis. Obstet Gynecol. 1996;87:884–890.
11. Promes SB, Nobay F. Pitfalls in first-trimester bleeding. Emerg Med Clinics N Am. 2010;28: 219–234.

12. Hasan R, Baird DD, Herring AH, Olshan AF, Jonsson Funk ML, Hartmann K. Association between first-trimester vaginal bleeding and miscarriage. Obstet Gynecol. 2009; 115:860–7.
13. Barnhart KT, Sammel MD, Gracia CR, et al. Risk factors for ectopic pregnancy in women with symptomatic first-trimester pregnancies. Fertil Steril. 2006;86:36–43.
14. Soto-Wright V, Bernstein M, Goldstein DP, Berkowitz RS. The changing clinical presentation of complete molar pregnancy. Obstet Gynecol. 1995;86:775–779.
15. ACOG. ACOG practice bulletin: prevention of Rh D alloimmunization. Number 4, 1999.
16. World Health Organization: Safe abortion guidelines: Technical and policy guidelines for health systems. Geneva: WHO. 2003, p. 24.
17. RCOG guideline. The use of Anti-D immunoglobulin for Rh prophylaxis. May 2002:4.
18. Filly, RA, Hadlock FP. Sonographic determination of menstrual age. In: Callen PW, (ed). Ultrasonography in obstetrics and gynecology, 4th ed. Philadelphia: W.B. Saunders Company; 2000. pp.146–147.
19. Gupta, N, Angtuaco TL. Embryosonology in the first trimester of pregnancy. Ultrasound Clinics. 2007;2:175–185.
20. Goldstein SR, Reeves, MF. Clinical assessment and ultrasound in early pregnancy. In: Paul, M, Lichtenberg ES, Borgatta L, Grimes DA, Stubblefield PG, Creinin MD (editors). Management of unintended and abnormal pregnancy: Comprehensive abortion care. Chichester UK: Wiley-Blackwell; 2009. p. 65–66.
21. hCG Reference Service [Internet]: Albuquerque New Mexico: hCG Reference Service; c2000 [updated 2002). Available from: http://www.hcglab.com/sources.htm
22. Davies S, Byrn F, Cole LA. Human chorionic gonadotropin testing for early pregnancy viability and complications. Clin Lab Med. 2003;23:257–264.
23. Braunstein G. hCG testing: a clinical guide for the testing of human chorionic gonadotropin. Abbott Park, IL: Abbott Diagnostics, 1992.
24. Timor Tritsch IE, Rottem S. (Eds.) Transvaginal sonography. 2nd ed. New York: Elsevier Science Publishing Co., Inc, 1995.
25. Barnhart KT, Sammel MD, Rinaudo PF, et al. Symptomatic patients with an early viable intrauterine pregnancy; hCG curves redefined. Obstet Gynecol. 2004;104:50–5.
26. Dart RG, Mitterando J, Dart LM. Rate of change of serial b-human chorionic gonadotropin values as a predictor of ectopic pregnancy in patients with indeterminate transvaginal ultrasound findings. Ann Emerg Med. 1999;34:703–10.
27. Barnhart, Kurt. Ectopic Pregnancy. N Engl J Med. 2009;361:379–87.
28. Steier JA, Bergsjo P, Myking OL. Human chorionic gondaotropin in maternal plasma after induced abortion, spontaneous abortion, and removed ectopic pregnancy. Obstet Gynecol. 1984;64:391–394.
29. Aral K, Gurkan Zorlu C, Gokmen O. Plasma human chorionic gonadotropin levels after induced abortion. Adv Contracept. 1996;12:11–14.
30. Schaff EA, Fielding SL, Eisinger S, Stadalius L. Mifepristone and misoprostol for early abortion when no gestational sac is present. Contraception. 2001;63:251–254.
31. Walker K, Schaff E, Fielding S et al. Monitoring serum chorionic gonadotropin levels after mifepristone abortion. Contraception.2001;64:271–3.
32. Rørbye C, Morgaard M, Nilas L. Prediction of late failure after medical abortion from serial beta hCG measurements and ultrasonography. Hum Reprod. 2004;19:85–89
33. Callen PW. Ultrasonography in obstetrics and gynecology. 4th ed. Philadelphia: WB Saunders Company, 2000. p.1023.
34. Marrs RP, Kletzky OA, Howard WF, Mishell DR, Jr. Disappearance of human chorionic gonadotropin and resumption of ovulation following abortion. Am J Obstet Gynecol. 1979;135:731–736.
35. Fiala C, Safar P, Bygdeman M, Gemzell-Danielsson K. Verifying the effectiveness of medical abortion; ultrasound versus hCG testing. Europ J Obstet Gynecol Reprod Biol. 2003;109:190–195.

36. Parashar P, Iversen OE, Midbøe G, Myking O. Bjørge L. Medical abortion in the first trimester: the use of serum hCG and endometrial thickness as markers of completeness. Eur J Contracept Reprod Health Care. 2007;12:366–71.
37. Chard T. Pregnancy tests: a review. Hum Reprod.1992;7:701–710.
38. Wilcox AJ, Baird DD, Dunson D, McChesney R, Weinberg CR. Natural limits of pregnancy testing in relation to the expected menstrual period. JAMA. 2001;286:1759–61.
39. Cole LA, Khanlian SA, Sutton JM, Davies S, Rayburn WF. Accuracy of home pregnancy tests at the time of missed menses. Am J Ob Gyn. 2004;190:100–105.
40. Perriera LK, Reeves MF, Chen BA, Hohmann HL, Hayes J, Creinin MD. Feasibility of telephone follow-up after medical abortion. Contraception. 2010;81:143–149.
41. Godfrey EM, Anderson A, Fielding SL. Clinical utility of urine pregnancy assays to determine medical abortion outcome is limited. Contraception. 2007;75:378–382.
42. Clark, Wesley, Hillary Bracken, Jini Tanenhaus, Suzanne Schweikert, E. Steve Lichtenberg, Beverly Winikoff. Alternatives to a routine follow-up visit for early medical abortion. Obstet Gynecol. 2010;115:264–272.
43. Self-Diagnostics, US, Market Size and Forecast, Segment Performance, Retail Challens and Companies and Brands: Sales data entirely from Information Resources, Inc., InfoScan® Reviews Information (FDMx-Excludes Walmart). February, 2010.
44. Tomlinson C, Marshall J, Ellis JE. Comparison of accuracy and certainty of results of six home pregnancy tests available over-the-other. Current Medical Research and Opinion. 2008;24:1645–1649.
45. Wallace LS. Making sense of home pregnancy test instructions. J Womens Health. 2009;18:363–368.
46. Doshi ML. Accuracy of consumer performed in-home tests for early pregnancy detection.
47. Hicks JM, Iosefsohn M. Reliability of home pregnancy-test kits in the hands of laypersons. N Engl J Med. 1989;320:320–321.
48. Kazemi MR, Vargas JE, Lo JC. Hyperthyroidism and a negative hCG test in molar pregnancy (Letter to the editor). Am J Med. 2004;117:889–890.
49. Tabas JA, Strehlow M, Isaacs E. A false negative pregnancy test in a patient with hydatidiform molar pregnancy (correspondence). N Engl J Med. 2003;249:2172–2173.
50. Cole LA. Human chorionic gonadotropin tests. Expert Review of Molecular Diagnostics. 2009;9:1–28.
51. IPAS. Pregnancy test trouble shooting guide. Product Literature. Chapel Hill, North Carolina: IPAS, 300 Market Street Suite 200; 2003.
52. Bandi ZL, Schoen I, Waters M. An algorithm for testing and reporting serum choriogonadotropin at clinically significant decision levels with use of "pregnancy test" reagents. Clin Chem. 1989;35:545–551.
53. Cole LA.Background hCG in non-pregnant individuals: need for more sensitive point-of-care and over-the-counter pregnancy tests. Clin Biochem. 2009;42:168–75
54. Cole LA, Khanlian SA, Muller CY. Detection of perimenopause or postmenopause human chorionic gonadotropin: an unnecessary source of alarm. Am J Obstet Gynecol 2008;198:275.e1–275.e7.
55. Fahy BG, Gouzd VA, Atallah JN. Pregnancy tests with end-stage renal disease. J Clin Anesthesia. 2009;20:609–613.
56. Knight AK, Bingemann T, Cole L, Cunningham-Rundles C. Frequent false positive beta human chorionic gonadotropin tests in immuglobulin A deficiency. Clin Exp Immunol. 2005;141:333–337.
57. Rotmensch S, Cole LA. False diagnosis and needless therapy of presumed malignant disease in women with false-positive human chorionic gonadotropin concentrations. Lancet. 2000;355:712–715.
58. Cole LA, Shahabi S, Butler SA, et al. Utility of commonly used commercial human chorionic gonadotropin immunoassays in the diagnosis and management of trophoblastic diseases. Clin Chem. 2001;47:308–315.

59. Paul M, Schaff E, Nichols M. Early medical abortion: the roles of clinic assessment, human chorionic gonadotropin assays and ultrasonography in medical abortion practice. Am J Obstet Gynecol. 2000;183(2Suppl):S34–43.

60. Bhatt, S, Ghazale H, Cogra VS. Sonographic evaluation of ectopic pregnancy. Radiol Clin N Am. 2007;45:549–560.

61. Yeh, H. Efficacy of the intradecidual sign and fallacy of the double decidual sign in the diagnosis of early intrauterine pregnancy. (Letter to the editor). Radiology. 1999;210:579–582.

62. Della-Giustina D, Denny M. Ectopic pregnancy. Emerg Med Clinics North Am. 2003;21:565–584.

63. Mahony BS, Filly RA, Nyberg DA, Callen PW. Sonographic evaluation of ectopic pregnancy. J Ultrasound Med. 1985;4:221–228.

64. Gracia CR and Barnhart KT. Diagnosing ectopic pregnancy: decision analysis comparing six strategies. Obstet Gynecol. 2001;97: 464–470.

65. Centers for Disease Control. Current trends in ectopic pregnancy: United Sates, 1990–92. MMWR. 1995;44;46–8.

66. Sotiriadis A, Makrydimas G, Paptheodorou S, Ioannidis J. Expectant, medical or surgical management of first-trimester miscarriage: a meta-analysis. Obstet Gynecol 2005;105:1104–1113.

67. Pauletta, Joana, Nuno Clode, Luís M. Graça. Expectant management of incomplete abortion in the first trimester. International Journal of Gynecology and Obstetrics. 2009;106:35–38.

68. Zhang J, Giles JM, Barnhart K, Creinin MD, Westhoff C, Frederick MM. A comparison of medical management with misoprostol and surgical management for early pregnancy failure. N Engl J Med. 2005;353:761–769.

69. Grønlund A, Grønlund L, Clevin L, Andersen B, Palmgren N, Lidegaard Ø. Management of missed abortion: comparison of medical treatment with either mifepristone + misoprostol or misoprostol alone with surgical evacuation. A multi-center trial in Copenhagen county, Denmark. Acta Obstet Gynecol Scand. 2002;81:1060–1065.

70. Fender L, Twining P. Imaging in Obstetrics and Infertility. In:Adam A, Dixon AK (editors).Grainger & Allison's diagnostic radiology: a textbook of medical imaging, 5th edition. Philadelphia: Churchill Livingstone; 2008.

71. Laing, FC, Frates MC. Ultrasound evaluation during the first trimester of pregnancy. In: Callen, PW, (ed). Ultrasonography in obstetrics and gynecology. Philadelphia: W.B. Saunders Company; 2000. p. 130–131.

72. Doubilet PM, Benson CB. Atlas of Ultrasound in Obstetrics and Gynecology 2003. Hagerstown, MD: Lippincott Williams & Wilkins; 2003.

73. Bagratee JS, Khullar V, Regan L, Moodley J, Kagoro H. A randomized controlled trial comparing medical and expectant management of first trimester miscarriage. Human Reproduction 2004;19:266–71.

74. Murray H, Baakdah H, Bardell T, Tulandi T. Diagnosis and treatment of ectopic pregnancy. CMAJ. 2005;173:905–12.

75. Ankum WM, BOL BW, van der Veen F, Bossuyt PM. Risk factors for ectopic pregnancy: a meta-analysis. Fertil Steril. 1996;65:1093–1099.

76. Kulp JL, Barnhart KT. Ectopic Pregnancy. In: Paul M, Lichtenberg SE, Borgatta L, Grimes DA, Stubblefield PG, Creinin MD (editors). Management of unintended and abnormal pregnancy: Comprehensive Abortion Care. (1st ed, pp 280–292.). Chichester, UK: Wiley-Blackwell; 2009.

77. Yao M, Tulandi T. Current status of surgical and nonsurgical management of ectopic pregnancy. Fertil Steril. 1997;67:421– 433.

78. Furlong LA. Ectopic regnancy risk when contraception fails: a review. J Reprod Med. 2002;47:881–885.

79. Mol BW, Ankum WM, Bossuyt PM, van der Veen F. Contraception and the risk of ectopic pregnancy: a meta-analysis. Contraception. 1995;52:337–341.

80. Peterson HB, Zhisen X, Hughes JM, Wilcox LS, Taylor LR, Trussell J. The risk of ectopic pregnancy after tubal sterilization. U.S. Collaborative Review of Sterilization Working Group. N Engl J Med. 1997;336:762–767.

81. Mukul LV, Teal SB. Current management of ectopic pregnancy. Ostet Gynecol Clin N Am. 2007;34:403–419.

82. Hillis SD, Owens LM, Marchbanks PA, Amsterdam LF, MacKenzie WR. Recurrent chlamydial infections increase the risks of hospitalization for ectopic pregnancy and p elvic inflammatory disease. Am J Obstet Gynecol. 1997;176:103–107.

83. Seeber BE, Barnhart KT. Clinical expert series: suspected ectopic pregnancy. Obstet Gynecol. 2006;107:399–413.

84. Gurel S. Ectopic pregnancy. Ultrasound Clin. 2008:3:331–343.

85. ACOG. ACOG technical bulletin. Ectopic pregnancy: The American College of Obstetricians and Gynecologists; March 1989. p.126.

86. Stewart F, Guest F, Stewart G, Hatcher R. Understanding your body. Every woman's guide to gynecology and health. New York: Bantam Books, 1987. p. 128, Figure 8.3.

87. Silva C, Sammel MD, Zhou L, Gracia C, Hummel AC and Barnhart K. Human chorionic gonadotripin profile for women with ectopic pregnancy. Obstet Gynecol. 2006;107:605–610.

88. Paul M, Leckle, E, Mitchell C, Rogers A, Fox M. Is pathology examination useful after surgical abortion? Obstet Gynecol. 2002;99:567–571.

89. Heath V, Chadwick V, Cooke I, Manek S, MacKenzie IZ. Should tissue from pregnancy termination and uterine evacuation routinely be examined histologically? Br J Obstet Gynecol. 2000;107:727–730.

90. Dart R, Dart L, Mitchell P, O'Rourke N. The utility of a dilatation and evacuation procedure in patients with symptoms suggestive of ectopic pregnancy and indeterminate transvaginal ultrasonography. Acad Emerg Med. 1999;6:1024–1029.

91. Edwards J, Creinin MD. Surgical abortion for gestations of less than 6 weeks. In: Creinin MD, Edwards J, (eds). Early abortion: surgical and medical options. Obstet Gynecol Fertil. 1997;20:11–19.

92. Centers for Disease Control and Prevention. Ectopic pregnancy—United States, 1990–1992. MMWR. 1995;44:46–48.

93. Thurman AR, Cornelius M, Korte JE, et al. An alternative monitoring protocol for single-dose methotrexate therapy in ectopic pregnancy. Am J Obstet Gynecol. 2010;202:139.e1–6.

94. Lipscomb GH, Gomez IG, Givens VM, et al. Yolk sac on transvaginal ultrasound as a prognostic indicator in the treatment of ectopic pregnancy with single-dose methotrexate. Am J Obstet Gynecol. 2009;200:338.e1–338.e4.

95. Banerjee S, Aslam N, Woelfer B, Lawrence A, Elson J, Jurkovic D. Expectant management of early pregnancies of unknown location: a prospective evaluation of methods to predict spontaneous resolution of pregnancy. Bri J Obstet Gynaecol. 2001;108:158–163.

96. Korhonen J, Stenman U, Ylostalo P. Low-dose oral methotrexate with expectant management of ectopic pregnancy. Obstet Gynecol.1996;88:775–8.

97. Hajenius PJ, Mol F, Mol BWJ, Bossuyt PMM, Ankum WM, Van der Veen F. Interventions for tubal ectopic pregnancy. Cochrane Database of Systematic Reviews 2007, Issue 1. Art. No.: CD000324.

98. Saxon D, Falcone T, Mascha EJ, Marino T, Yao M, Tulandi T. A study of ruptured tubal ectopic pregnancy. Obstet Gynecol. 1997;90:46–49.

99. Beyer DA, Dumesic DA. Heterotopic pregnancy: an emerging diagnostic challenge. OBG Management. 2002;14:36–46.

100. Sebire NJ, Seckl MJ. Gestational trophoblastic disease. In: Paul M, Lichtenberg ES, Borgatta L, Grimes DA, Stubblefield PG, Creinin MD (editors.) Management of unintended and abnormal pregnancy; comprehensive abortion care. Chichester, UK: Wiley-Blackwell; 2009. P. 294–295.

101. Soper JT, Mutch DG, Schink JC for the American College of Obstetricians and Gynecologists. Diagnosis and treatment of gestational trophoblastic disease: ACOG practice bulletin No. 53. Gynecol Oncol 2004;93:574–585.

102. Mangili G, Garavaglia E, Cavoretto P, et al. Clinical presentation of hydatidiform mole in northern Italy: has it changed in the last twenty years? Am J Obstet Gynecol 2008;198:302.e1–302.e4.

103. Fowler DJ, Lindsay I, Seckl MJ, Sebire NJ. Routine pre-evacuation ultrasound diagnosis of hydatidiform mole: experience of >1000 cases from a regional referral centre. Ultrasound Obstet Gynecol. 2006;27:56–60.

104. Johns JN, Greenwold S, Buckley E, Jauniaux E. A prospective study of ultrasound screening for molar pregnancies in missed miscarriages. Ultrasound Obstet Gynecol. 2005; 25:493–7.

105. El-Helw LM, Hancock BW. Treatment of metastatic gestational trophoblastic neoplasia. Lancet Oncol. 2007;8:715–24.

Abortion

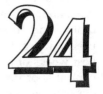

Maureen Paul, MD, MPH
Tara Stein, MD, MPH

- Access to legal, safe abortion is a critical part of women's primary reproductive health care.

- Address expeditiously any woman's request for pregnancy confirmation and provide her with information about all her options, including prompt services or referral if she is considering abortion.

- Approximately 90% of all abortions in the United States occur during the first trimester; more than 60% take place at or before 8 weeks following the onset of the woman's last normal menstrual period.

- Medication methods (most commonly mifepristone followed by misoprostol) are effective and safe options for women seeking abortion during the early weeks of pregnancy.

Women have abortions for many interrelated reasons. In a recent large U.S. survey,[1] women most frequently cited financial concerns, relationship problems, or work, school, or family responsibilities as reasons for their decision to have an abortion. Approximately 12% of the women reported concerns about their own health or that of the embryo-fetus as reasons for the abortion, and 1% reported that they were ending a pregnancy that resulted from coerced sex. In other studies, women who presented for second-trimester abortions were more likely to have had a delayed diagnosis of pregnancy and to have encountered logistical difficulties in accessing services, such as finding a provider, obtaining public insurance, or arranging transportation.[2,3] A woman's decision to terminate her pregnancy is based on her unique situation, and it often involves complex moral considerations regarding her responsibilities to herself and others. Each woman deserves to feel respected and supported as she makes her decision; it is not appropriate or logical to treat abortion as a regrettable human "failure."

In the past, many clinicians delayed scheduling an abortion until 7 weeks following the onset of a woman's last menstrual period (LMP), because pregnancy tests lacked the sensitivity to confirm early pregnancy and uterine aspiration resulted in slightly higher rates of incomplete abortion. Today, highly sensitive pregnancy tests (see Chapter 23 on Pregnancy Testing and Management of Early Pregnancy), ultrasonography, and improved abortion methods allow clinicians to diagnose pregnancy and offer safe and effective abortion options during the earliest weeks of pregnancy. Several excellent reviews describe the various clinical abortion techniques in more detail.[4-11] This chapter provides an overview for clinicians who evaluate and refer women for abortion services, as well as those who offer early medication or aspiration abortion in their practices.

LEGAL STATUS OF ABORTION

On January 22, 1973, the U.S. Supreme Court decided *Roe v. Wade* [410 U.S. 113 (1973)], the landmark case that legalized abortion nationwide. The *Roe* Court recognized the decision to carry or terminate a pregnancy as part of a fundamental constitutional right to privacy, thereby affording it high protection. Holding that the government could not interfere with a woman's choice to have an abortion unless it had a "compelling" reason to do so, the Justices attempted to balance the interests involved by establishing a "trimester framework":[12]

1. In the first trimester, the abortion decision and procedure must be left to the judgment of the pregnant woman and her physician, largely unimpeded by governmental regulations.

2. In the second trimester, each state may choose to regulate abortion procedures in ways that are reasonably related to the pregnant woman's health.

3. In the third trimester, if and when a fetus reaches viability, the state may elect to promote its interest in potential human life by prohibiting abortion, as long as it provides an exception for abortions necessary to protect the woman's life or health.

As legal abortion became one of the most commonly performed procedures in the United States, abortion opponents introduced legislation at the local, state, and national levels to reduce access to abortion services. Passage of the Hyde Amendment in 1976 restricted federal funding for abortion, thereby curtailing access for poor women,[13,14] and numerous states regulated minors' access to abortion through provisions for parental involvement. Under *Roe*, the Supreme Court upheld such limitations on poor women's and young women's access to abortion, but it generally struck down other kinds of abortion restrictions.[12]

The Supreme Court's 1992 landmark decision in *Planned Parenthood of Southeastern Pennsylvania v. Casey* [505 U.S. 833 (1992)] greatly encouraged additional regulation of abortion by replacing *Roe's* trimester framework with a standard that allowed state restrictions on abortion as long as they did not impose an "undue burden" on a woman's ability to seek abortion. Under this less protective standard, the Supreme Court has upheld mandatory waiting periods, biased counseling provisions, and burdensome design requirements for facilities that provide abortion services; such laws have proliferated in recent years. Although the *Casey* Court weakened considerably the legal standard used to test the constitutionality of abortion restrictions, it affirmed women's fundamental right to choose abortion before fetal viability and upheld the requirement that any ban on abortion where the fetus is viable must provide an exception to safeguard a woman's life or health.[12]

In the 1990s, after the *Casey* decision failed to overturn *Roe*, abortion opponents launched a concerted campaign to restrict methods of abortion. These efforts remained largely unsuccessful until 2007 when the U.S. Supreme Court, made increasingly conservative by two George W. Bush appointees, considered the federal Partial-Birth Abortion Ban Act of 2003 [18 U.S.C. 1531 (2003)]. In a sweeping 5–4 ruling, the Court upheld this federal abortion ban, which criminalizes certain safe second-trimester abortion procedures even when a physician believes that such a procedure is necessary to preserve a woman's health. This decision invited further abortion restrictions by crediting an asserted state interest in promoting respect for "embryonic and fetal life" [Gonzales v. Carhart, 550 U.S. 124, 163 (2007)], while dismissing decades of Supreme Court precedent that held women's health paramount.[15,16]

Election of the prochoice President Barack Obama in 2008 represented a positive shift for women's health. Early in his administration, President Obama helped to restore critical reproductive health services worldwide by rescinding the "global gag rule", a regulation that had prohibited U.S. support for foreign non-governmental organizations that engaged in abortion-related activities.[17] Following the murder of Kansas abortion provider, Dr. George Tiller, in May 2009, the Department of Justice revitalized the Task Force on Violence Against Reproductive Health Care Providers that had remained largely dormant under the preceding Bush administration. This Task Force aims to uphold the 1993 Freedom of Access to Clinic Entrances (FACE) Act [18 U.S.C. 248 (1994)] and other laws by coordinating efforts to prevent, investigate and prosecute acts of violence and harassment against abortion providers.[12] Notwithstanding these efforts and others, however, reversing the long-standing erosion of women's reproductive rights remains a formidable challenge, reinforced as it is by a growing number of abortion restrictions, an anti-abortion movement determined to overturn *Roe* altogether, and existing life-long appointments of conservative judges to the federal courts, including the Supreme Court, and to some state courts.[18]

THE PUBLIC HEALTH IMPACT OF LEGAL ABORTION

The *Roe v. Wade* decision ushered in a new era in women's health, producing immediate public health benefits. Rates of abortion complications and deaths plummeted because abortion was more readily available closer to home, earlier in pregnancy, and at lower cost.[19] Abortion practices became safer after studies in the 1970s revealed that vacuum aspiration carried less morbidity than sharp curettage, local anesthesia was safer than general anesthesia, abortions performed in freestanding clinics were safer than those performed in hospitals, and dilation and evacuation (D&E) was safer than the second-trimester labor induction methods used at the time.

In order to maintain the important public health benefits brought by the *Roe v. Wade* decision, abortion must remain not only safe and legal, but also available to women who need it. In addition to increasing restrictions on abortion, the shortage of trained providers limits women's access to services.[20] More than 60% of U.S. abortion doctors are at least 50 years old,[21] and many have begun to retire. Between 2000 and 2008 the number of facilities providing abortion services declined from 1,819 to 1,793, leaving 87% percent of U.S. counties without an abortion provider.[22] Consequently, many women travel long distances to obtain their abortion; indeed, 1 in 5 women who have an abortion travel 50 miles or more for the service.[20] This travel burden not only adds to the time a woman will be away from work and her family, but also may compound the costs of abortion to include transportation and lodging. Important efforts are ongoing to address this provider shortage by integrating abortion into mainstream medical education and expanding the range of practitioners who can provide services.

CHARACTERISTICS OF WOMEN WHO OBTAIN ABORTIONS

Through its voluntary abortion surveillance program, the Centers for Disease Control and Prevention (CDC) currently collect abortion statistics from 47 states, the District of Columbia, and New York City.[23] Historically, the annual numbers of legal abortions reported by the CDC have been about 15% lower than those based on independent national surveys by the Guttmacher Institute. In 1998, however, this discrepancy widened to 30% to 35%, in part because the CDC discontinued its practice of including estimates from states that do not report to the voluntary program (including California, which accounted for about 23% of abortions in 1997).[23,24]

According to the Guttmacher Institute, the annual number of legal induced abortions rose dramatically following the *Roe* decision to reach 1.5 million in 1980 (Table 24–1). The number remained remarkably stable throughout the 1980s, peaking at 1.6 million in 1990, and then trended downward to reach 1.2 million in 2004[25] and 2008.[22] The abortion rate (number of abortions per 1,000 women aged 15–44 years) showed a similar trend, falling from 27.4 in 1990 to 19.7 in 2004[25,26] and 19.6 in 2008[22] (Table 24–1).[25,26]

About 90% of abortions take place in the first trimester, a figure that has remained fairly stable over time; however, the proportion of abortions occurring at 8 weeks or less has increased from 38% in 1973 to 61% in 2004 and 62% in 2007[23] (Table 24–1). Moreover, very early abortions (6 weeks' gestation or less) have become more common, rising from 14% of all abortions in 1992 to 33% in 2007. In contrast, the small percentage of abortions (about 5%) performed at or after 16 weeks' gestation has remained largely unchanged.[23]

Not surprisingly, most women who have abortions are young and unmarried (Table 24–1). In 2008, women in their twenties had more than half of all reported abortions in the United States. Teenagers obtained 18% of abortions that year, a dramatic decrease from nearly 33% in 1973. Eighty-five percent of women who obtained abortions in 2008 were unmarried. In addition, the majority of women (60% in 2008) already had at least one child.[26–28]

Reflecting growing health disparities, poor women bear a disproportionate share of the burden of unintended pregnancy and its consequences. Women living below the U.S. poverty line have rates of unintended pregnancy (112 per 1,000 women) and abortion (44 per 1,000 women) several-fold higher than those in higher income categories.[29] Between 1994 and 2001 rates of unintended pregnancy and abortion fell among many U.S. population subgroups (including teenagers), but rose among economically disadvantaged women. During this time, the rate of unintended births increased from 20 to 22 per 1,000 women overall and from 40 to 58 per 1,000 for women living below poverty.[29]

Women's ability to manage their fertility depends on many factors, including access to affordable and effective contraception.[30,31] About half of the unintended pregnancies and abortions in the United States occur in contraceptive non-users. Common reasons for non-use among women having abortions include a perceived low risk of pregnancy, concerns or ambivalence about contraception, and problems accessing contraception. Although 54% of women obtaining abortions report that they used contraception during the month that they became pregnant, they may rely

Table 24–1 Percent distribution of legal abortions by characteristics of woman—United States, selected years, 1973 to 2008

	1973	1980	1990	2000	2004	2008
Characteristics	%	%	%	%	%	%
Age (years)						
≤ 19	32.8	29.6	22.6	18.6	16.9	17.6
20–24	32.3	35.4	33.1	32.7	33.2	33.4
25–29	17.4	19.6	22.4	23.0	23.3	24.4
≥ 30	17.5	15.4	21.9	25.7	26.6	24.6
Race and Hispanic ethnicity						
Non-Hispanic white	N/A	N/A	52.9	36.5	34.2	36.1
Hispanic	N/A	N/A	12.1	19.8	22.0	24.9
Black	N/A	N/A	31.4	37.2	37.1	29.6
Other	N/A	N/A	4.0	7.0	7.8	9.4
Marital Status						
Married	29.0	20.6	17.7	15.2	13.8	14.8
Unmarried	71.0	79.4	82.3	84.8	86.2	85.2
No. Prior Live Births						
None	55.2	57.9	48.5	40.5	40.5	39.1
1	15.4	19.6	24.7	27.5	27.5	26.5
≥ 2	29.4	22.5	26.9	32.0	32.0	34.5
Weeks of Gestation						
≤ 8	38.2	51.0	51.3	57.1	61.3	n/a
9–10	29.7	26.6	25.8	20.5	17.8	n/a
11–12	17.5	12.9	12.1	10.5	9.6	n/a
13–15	6.0	5.1	6.4	6.6	6.7	n/a
16–20	7.2	3.5	3.6	4.0	3.5	n/a
≥ 21	1.4	0.9	0.8	1.3	1.1	n/a
# Reported Abortions	744,610	1,553,890	1,608,620	1,312,990	1,222,100	1,212,350
Abortion rate*	16.3	29.3	27.4	21.3	19.7	19.6
Abortion ratio**	19.3	30	28.0	24.5	22.9	22.4

n/a = not available.

Adapted from Henshaw SK, Kost K. (2008)[25] and Jones RK, et al.[27]

* Abortions per 1,000 women aged 15-44 years

**Abortions per 1,000 live births

on less-effective methods or use methods inconsistently or incorrectly.[29,32] Providers of abortion care can help address this situation by informing women about contraceptive options (including long-acting methods), offering them the method of their choice, and helping them overcome any barriers to effective use.

EVALUATION AND PREPARATION OF PATIENTS FOR ABORTION

DECIDING WHETHER TO CONTINUE A PREGNANCY

The process of deciding whether to continue a pregnancy commonly begins as soon as a woman suspects she is pregnant. Some women will have made a firm decision by the time they seek pregnancy confirmation; others may need to explore their options further. Providing prompt and convenient pregnancy confirmation services has important benefits, including the following:

- Allows the woman ample time to consider her options
- Facilitates the initiation of prenatal care
- Increases the likelihood that a woman will be eligible for the full range of early abortion options
- Decreases both the risks and the costs of complications
- Expedites the diagnosis of pregnancy abnormalities, such as ectopic pregnancy

Clinicians can facilitate a woman's decision-making by providing her with accurate and unbiased information about her pregnancy and helping her to explore her feelings in a supportive and nonjudgmental setting.[33] Basic factual information and discussion will meet the needs of most women; some patients may desire more extensive education, evaluation, or counseling to ensure that they are making an informed decision. Depending on the scope of services that your practice provides, you may need to refer patients for financial assistance, further counseling, first- or second-trimester abortions, prenatal care, adoption services, or other necessary care.

PRE-ABORTION EVALUATION

Because most women who request abortion are young and healthy, the pre-abortion medical evaluation is usually straightforward. The main goals of the evaluation include the following:

- Confirm pregnancy and estimate gestational age.
- Identify possible problems that require further evaluation or intervention, such as ectopic gestation.

- Identify medical or gynecologic conditions that might influence the choice of abortion methods.

History-Taking

Ask the patient about her recent menstrual history, including the regularity of her menstrual cycle and the onset of her last normal menstrual period. Recording her contraceptive history, including recent use of hormonal methods, helps to establish the accuracy of gestational dating based on LMP. Inquire as well about future contraceptive plans, so that the patient can start a contraceptive method immediately after her abortion if she so chooses.

The medical history should include the following:

- Any relevant obstetric and gynecologic history, including outcomes of prior pregnancies, complications of previous abortions, history of uterine abnormalities (e.g., large leiomyomata [fibroids], bicornuate uterus), and any surgery involving the cervix or uterus (e.g., conization of the cervix, cesarean delivery)

- Acute or chronic illnesses that may require more evaluation or adjunctive therapy

- Allergies to latex, local anesthetics, antiseptic solutions, analgesics, antibiotics, antiprogestins, prostaglandins, or other medications

- Current drug use (prescription, illicit, or over-the-counter), including asthma medications, anticoagulants or systemic corticosteroids

This history may affect the provider's recommendations for abortion method, pre-abortion testing, pain control, or follow-up. Rarely, with medically complicated patients, it may be appropriate to perform the abortion in a hospital setting where staff and resources are readily available to manage any serious problems that may arise.

Clinical Examination

Perform a targeted physical assessment that includes vital signs and a pelvic examination to determine uterine size and position and to confirm gestational age based on the woman's LMP. Note any findings, such as large uterine fibroids or cervical stenosis, that may indicate the need for further evaluation or influence the selection of an abortion method. If a pregnant woman has an intrauterine contraceptive in place, remove it expeditiously to prevent the risk of septic abortion.

Ultrasonography

Although many abortion providers in the United States use ultrasound routinely for gestational dating,[21] the National Abortion Federation guidelines do not require it before first trimester abortion as long as the gestational age estimate by LMP and uterine size reasonably concur.[34] In many cases, clinical assessment of gestational age by history of LMP and pelvic examination, combined with a protocol for ultrasound as needed, suffices for provision of safe early abortion.[35-37] Consider ultrasound evaluation if the patient is unsure of her LMP, if you suspect pregnancy beyond 9 weeks, if you detect an adnexal mass or suspect ectopic pregnancy, or to evaluate further some other pelvic finding. Ultrasound dating is the standard of care for second-trimester abortion in the United States.[34]

Laboratory Tests

Routine laboratory evaluation prior to abortion is minimal and includes a urine pregnancy test (unless ultrasound is performed to confirm the pregnancy and gestational age) and Rh typing. Additional testing may be necessary as determined by the women's history or physical examination findings. These tests may include:

- Hemoglobin or hematocrit
- Screening for reproductive tract infection

  (Some U.S. providers routinely screen for chlamydia at the abortion visit, whereas others prefer to treat all patients prophylactically without screening.[21] If chlamydia or gonorrhea is suspected or identified, initiate treatment prior to or at the time of the abortion.)

- Serial serum quantitative hCG levels to monitor a possible ectopic pregnancy or evaluate a missed or incomplete spontaneous abortion

  (In addition, some clinicians may choose to follow serial hCG levels to confirm successful completion of a medication abortion in lieu of performing an ultrasound.[37])

PATIENT EDUCATION AND INFORMED CONSENT

A woman seeking abortion will need information about the methods available to her; how they are done; their safety, success rates, risks, costs, time required; and follow-up care. Although the patient may want her partner or other supportive persons involved in the information session, offer her a chance to talk privately with you in case she has any confidential concerns, as well as to screen for domestic violence or coer-

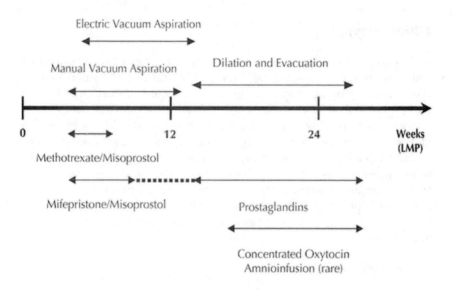

Figure 24–1 Options for terminating pregnancy, by duration of pregnancy

cion. Providers must follow any state regulations regarding the information provided to patients, as well as those governing parental notification or consent for minors seeking abortion.[12] Once the woman has the information she needs to make a decision and has all her questions answered, ask her to sign the appropriate consent forms before the abortion.

More than any other factor, the gestational age of the pregnancy determines which abortion method the woman may choose (Figure 24–1). A patient may opt for a vacuum aspiration abortion throughout the first trimester or a medication abortion during the first 63 days (9 weeks) of pregnancy, although the efficacy of some medication abortion regimens extends beyond this point as well. After the first trimester, abortion methods include dilation and evacuation (D&E) or medical induction. A woman's options may be limited by other factors, such as cost or lack of skilled D&E providers in her community.[22]

Abortion has no evidence-based contraindications *per se*, although some medical conditions or problems, such as severe anemia or abnormal uterine anatomy, may affect which abortion method or clinical setting would be safest for the woman. Mostly the choice between a medication or aspiration abortion depends on the woman's preferences. In helping the patient decide between medication abortion and aspiration, explain the important features of each method (Table 24–2), emphasizing that both methods are highly effective. Most women will express a clear preference and be highly satisfied with the method they choose.[38]

The main advantages of vacuum aspiration are its speed and predictability and the option for sedation or general anesthesia. The drawbacks

Table 24-2 Characteristics of early abortion methods

Vacuum Aspiration Abortion	Medication Abortion
Highly effective	Highly effective
Procedure brief	Abortion process usually takes 1–3 days to complete (sometimes longer)
Involves invasive procedure	Avoids invasive procedure (aspiration) if successful
Allows option of sedation or general anesthesia	Avoids anesthesia
Usually requires only 1 visit	Often involves at least 2 visits
Lighter perceived bleeding	Heavier perceived bleeding
Requires clinical setting	May occur in privacy of home

are the procedure's invasiveness and the small risk of uterine perforation. Reasons commonly cited for choosing medication abortion include that it is non-invasive and more "natural" and that it affords women greater privacy and control over the abortion process.[39,40] Disadvantages of medication methods include the length of time required to complete the abortion process and the longer period of bleeding and cramping that commonly accompanies passage of the pregnancy.

CLINICAL PROVISION OF ABORTION METHODS

FIRST-TRIMESTER MEDICATION ABORTION

Since the introduction of mifepristone in Europe more than two decades ago, its use for abortion has risen gradually each year. The U.S. Food and Drug Administration (FDA) approved mifepristone for abortion in September of 2000, and by 2008 medication abortion accounted for 17% of all abortions (about 25% of early abortions) that occurred in U.S. nonhospital facilities that year.[22] Most members of the National Abortion Federation, including Planned Parenthood affiliates, currently offer early medication abortion services, and many private doctors, including obstetrician-gynecologists and family practice physicians, provide abortion care within their primary care offices.[41] In several states, advanced practice clinicians (nurse practitioners, nurse midwives, physician assistants) provide some or all aspects of early medication abortion care in accordance with state laws.[42,43] Efforts are ongoing to expand women's access to medication abortion by training diverse types of practitioners.

Substantial research supports the effectiveness of medication abortion during the first 7–9 weeks of pregnancy, depending on the regimen used. These regimens include mifepristone-misoprostol, methotrexate-misoprostol, and misoprostol alone. Use of mifepristone-misoprostol predominates in the United States, but the other regimens represent critical alternatives where mifepristone is unaffordable or unavailable.

Medications Used for Early Abortion

Mifepristone

Mifepristone is sold in the United States under the brand name Mifeprex®. Mifepristone is a 19-norsteroid with a high affinity for progesterone receptors; it also binds to glucocorticoid receptors and, to a lesser extent, androgen receptors. The drug blocks the action of progesterone, which is necessary to establish and maintain placental attachment. Mifepristone also softens the cervix and stimulates synthesis of prostaglandins by cells of the early decidua.[6]

Millions of women worldwide have used the combination of mifepristone and misoprostol for abortion through 63 days (9 weeks) with an impressive safety record.[44,45] However some limitations apply to the use of mifepristone. It should not be used in women with known or suspected ectopic pregnancy. In addition, the FDA drug label for mifepristone advises against its use in the following circumstances:

- Intrauterine contraception in place (must be removed before treatment)

- Chronic adrenal failure

- Current long-term systemic corticosteroid therapy

- History of allergy to mifepristone, misoprostol, or other prostaglandin

- Hemorrhagic disorders or concurrent anti-coagulant therapy

- Inherited porphyrias

Methotrexate

Methotrexate is a folic acid analogue that competitively inhibits dihydrofolate reductase, an enzyme necessary for DNA synthesis. Methotrexate causes abortion by its action on the rapidly dividing cells of the early placenta; when combined with misoprostol, it is effective in inducing abortion through 49 days (7 weeks) of gestation.[46] Methotrexate is FDA approved for treatment of choriocarcinoma and certain other types of cancer, severe psoriasis, and rheumatoid arthritis. Use of methotrexate for treatment of ectopic pregnancy[47] or early medication abortion is not included in the FDA drug label, but these uses are supported by published evidence accumulated over many years.

Before mifepristone became available in the United States, clinicians commonly employed a regimen of methotrexate and vaginal misoprostol for early medication abortion. Methotrexate regimens are still used in Canada because mifepristone is not commercially available there. The efficacy of methotrexate-misoprostol through 7 weeks of gestation compares favorably to mifepristone regimens, but it is associated with a longer duration until complete abortion.[48] Single-dose methotrexate therapy for medication abortion or ectopic pregnancy has little, if any, systemic toxicity, but it should not be administered to women with chronic renal or hepatic disease. Methotrexate is a known teratogen when used in high doses; the teratogenic risk associated with single-dose methotrexate is unknown but warrants caution.[6]

Misoprostol

Misoprostol is a prostaglandin E1 analogue that softens the cervix and stimulates uterine contractions, thereby facilitating expulsion of the pregnancy. Although misoprostol alone can induce abortion, protocols that combine it with mifepristone are more effective.[49] Sold in the United States as a generic drug, as well as under the brand name Cytotec®, misoprostol is a widely available, inexpensive medication marketed for prevention of gastrointestinal ulcer disease. The FDA has approved an early abortion regimen using mifepristone in combination with misoprostol.

Misoprostol can cause mild, short-term systemic prostaglandin effects, including nausea, vomiting, diarrhea, and temporary elevation of body temperature—side effects that women commonly report with all medication abortion regimens. It can be administered orally (swallowed), vaginally, buccally (tucked between cheek and gum), or sublingually (placed under the tongue), and the pharmacokinetics of the drug differ by route of administration. An oral dose of misoprostol results in rapid, high peak blood levels with relatively weak stimulation of the uterus, while a vaginal, buccal, or sublingual dose produces overall lower blood levels but a more sustained uterine effect.[50-52] Prenatal exposure to misoprostol has been associated with major congenital anomalies, primarily of the skull and limbs, but the absolute risk is low (estimated to be about 1%).[52,53]

Facility and Staffing Considerations

As a medical treatment that relies on good patient education, support, and follow-up, medication abortion is well-suited to the scope of practice of primary care providers, including nurse practitioners, nurse midwives, and physician assistants. The FDA stipulates that medication abortion providers must be able to assess the duration of pregnancy, diagnose ectopic pregnancy, and provide or refer for vacuum aspiration or emergency treatment when necessary; personal expertise in ultrasound or aspiration is not required. These capabilities do not differ from those needed by any clinician caring for reproductive-aged women who may present for diagnosis or evaluation of early pregnancy. Laws in many states, however, restrict the extent to which nonphysicians can practice medication abortion,[12] so checking state-specific requirements before initiating the service is important. The Abortion Access Project (www.abortionaccess.org) may be helpful in providing information and identifying lawyers familiar with the regulations in each state.

Providing medication abortion does not require specialized facilities; a typical medical office with space for private consultation, physical examination, equipment and medication for handling an allergic reaction, and arrangements for a urine pregnancy test and Rh typing suffices. In addition, the office must have a protocol for backup or referral, 24-hour emergency telephone service, and trained staff. Other practical issues to consider include state laws or regulations, if any, specific to facilities that provide abortion services, as well as any requirements for information provision, waiting periods, or parental consent or notification for minors seeking abortion care. Several organizations can provide additional information about these issues, including the National Abortion Federation (www.prochoice.org).

In the United States, mifepristone is not available through pharmacies; rather, it is sold directly to licensed physicians who meet the aforementioned FDA qualifications after they sign and return a Prescriber's Agreement provided by the drug's distributor. Prescribers agree to report adverse events and to give each patient a Medication Guide to read and a Patient Agreement to read and sign. Information and forms necessary to enroll as a mifepristone provider are available at www.earlyoptionpill.com.

Information Provision

A woman undergoing medication abortion needs detailed information about the medications she will take, when and how to take them, what to expect during the process, possible side effects and complications, and what to do if she has questions or concerns (Table 24–3). Most U.S. abortion providers use an alternative evidence-based mifepristone regimen in preference to the original protocol delineated on the product label for mifepristone. Such "off-label" use of therapeutic medications is both legally permitted and common, allowing clinicians to offer patients new and improved treatments based on updated scientific research. Patients using an evidence-based alternative regimen should sign additional forms that provide information about the regimen, how it differs from the FDA protocol, and its benefits and risks.

Table 24–3 Patient education for early medication abortion

1. Discuss the woman's decision to have an abortion and confirm that her decision is certain and voluntary.

2. Discuss the treatment alternatives (medication abortion or vacuum aspiration) and explain the benefits and risks of each method.

3. Describe the medication regimens available and their FDA status. For mifepristone-misoprostol abortion, explain the differences between the FDA-approved regimen and newer evidence-based regimens.

4. Explain what to expect in regard to bleeding and cramping. These symptoms typically intensify during expulsion of the pregnancy (usually 2–4 hours) and then gradually subside. Passage of clots is common during expulsion. Lighter bleeding or spotting typically lasts about 2 weeks, but may be longer.

5. Explain that the patient is unlikely to see products of conception unless she is close to 9 weeks' gestation, in which case the embryo will be very small and often obscured by blood clots.

6. Discuss known side effects of the medication abortion regimen including mild gastrointestinal symptoms; short-term fever, warmth or chills; or oral ulcers (methotrexate only).

7. Explain that the drugs used for medication abortion may increase the risk of birth defects if the pregnancy were to continue. **Emphasize that aspiration abortion is advised if the medication abortion method fails.**

8. Discuss possible complications including failed abortion, incomplete abortion, hemorrhage, or infection. Emphasize that atypical infections have occurred rarely after use of mifepristone combined with misoprostol (see text).

9. Provide instructions about how to administer the misoprostol. Depending on the regimen used, routes of administration can include oral (swallowed), buccal (tucked between cheek and gum), sublingual (under the tongue), or vaginal (inserted deep into the vagina after washing hands). A drawing or picture of buccal or sublingual placement may be helpful, because these terms are unfamiliar to most women. Also explain how to use pain medications.

10. Explain the time commitment and expected number of visits.

11. Provide 24-hour emergency contact information and emphasize warning signs that may require evaluation, including the following:

    a. Prolonged or heavy bleeding (≥2 soaked maxipads per hour for 2 consecutive hours);

    b. Fever (≥100.4° F) lasting more than 4 hours or beginning in the days after misoprostol administration;

    c. Abdominal pain or discomfort or 'feeling sick' (including weakness, nausea, vomiting or diarrhea, with or without fever) more than 24 hours after using misoprostol.

12. Provide information about available contraceptive methods and when to initiate the chosen method, if any.

13. Address issues of confidentiality.

14. Review all required consent forms, which must be signed before administration of the medication regimen.

Mifepristone-Misoprostol Regimens

Although use of mifepristone alone results in abortion in some cases, the addition of misoprostol increases efficacy. The early abortion regimen approved by the FDA in 2000 (Table 24–4) was based on studies conducted more than a decade ago that used 600 mg of mifepristone orally at the first visit, followed 2 days later by 400 mcg of misoprostol orally at the second visit. The patients then returned in approximately 2 weeks for a follow-up visit to assess whether the pregnancy had passed. The success rate (complete abortion without the need for aspiration) of this regimen ranged from 92% to 96% in women with pregnancies of 49 days' duration or less but fell significantly thereafter.[54,55]

Subsequent studies conducted in the United States and internationally led to the development of improved evidence-based mifepristone regimens that were more effective and convenient with fewer side effects (Table 24–4). In brief, key research findings underpinning these new protocols included the following:

- Mifepristone, 200 mg, is as effective as a 600 mg dose when combined with misoprostol in various regimens.[56,57]

- Self-administration of misoprostol at home is safe, effective, and highly acceptable to women.[58]

- Compared with the oral route of misoprostol used in the original FDA-approved regimen, administration of misoprostol 800 mcg vaginally or buccally following mifepristone extends high efficacy through 63 days of gestation,[59–63] and most studies report a lower incidence of side effects as well. Sublingual misoprostol 800 mcg also yields high success rates through 63 days but produces more side effects compared with the vaginal route;[64,65] studies assessing efficacy and side effects with lower doses are ongoing.

- Shorter dosing intervals between mifepristone and misoprostol (24 hours for buccal or sublingual administration and 6–24 hours for vaginal administration) do not affect efficacy significantly.[63,66–68]

During the first few years following FDA approval of mifepristone, the evidence-based regimen of mifepristone 200 mg followed by 800 mcg vaginal misoprostol became common practice in the United States.[6] However, emerging reports of serious infections in a small number of women using this regimen, including a few deaths from clostridial infections,[69,70] prompted many U.S. clinicians to adopt protocols using alternative routes of misoprostol administration (although an association between these infections and vaginal misoprostol was never confirmed). Currently, the regimen of mifepristone 200 mg followed by buccal misoprostol 800 mcg predominates in the United States, with reported success rates of 96% to 98% through 9 weeks of gestation.[63,71]

Table 24-4 Selected clinical protocols for early medication abortion

Visit	Mifepristone: FDA-Approved Regimen (≤49 days)	Mifepristone: Alternative Evidence-Based Regimens (≤63 days)	Methotrexate Regimen (≤49 days)
One	*Day 1* Give 600 mg mifepristone orally	*Day 1* Give 200 mg mifepristone orally Provide appropriate number of misoprostol* tablets to take home with instructions for administration: • 4 tablets (800 mcg) vaginally in 6–48 hrs, OR • 4 tablets (800 mcg) buccally** in 24–48 hours, OR • 4 tablets (800 mcg) sublingually** in 24–48 hours	*Day 1* Administer methotrexate 50 mg/m² body surface area IM or 50 mg orally Provide 4 tablets (800 mcg) misoprostol with instructions for vaginal administration at home in 3–7 days
	Administer Rh₀(D)-immune globulin 50 mcg to Rh₀(D)-negative women. Provide analgesics and instructions for their use.		
Two	*Day 3* Administer 2 tablets (400 mcg) misoprostol orally	*Day 3–14 (at least 24 hrs after misoprostol administration)* Assess outcome • If abortion complete, offer contraceptive counseling • If abortion has not occurred, offer repeat dose of misoprostol unless patient prefers aspiration • If ongoing viable pregnancy, follow-up in about 1 week • If persistent non-viable pregnancy, follow-up may occur in about 4 weeks	*Day 5–9 (at least 24 hrs after misoprostol insertion)* Assess outcome • If abortion complete, offer contraceptive counseling • If abortion has not occurred, provide repeat dose of vaginal misoprostol (800 mcg) unless patient prefers aspiration • If ongoing viable pregnancy, follow-up at about Day 14 • If persistent non-viable pregnancy, follow-up in about 4 weeks

Table 24-4 Selected clinical protocols for early medication abortion—Continued

Visit	Mifepristone: FDA-Approved Regimen (≤49 days)	Mifepristone: Alternative Evidence-Based Regimens (≤63 days)	Methotrexate Regimen (≤49 days)
Three	*Day 14* Assess outcome. Schedule aspiration abortion if ongoing viable pregnancy	*Day 14–21 (only needed if viable pregnancy on previous visit)* Schedule aspiration abortion if viable pregnancy persists	*Day 14 (only needed if viable pregnancy on previous visit)* Schedule aspiration abortion if viable pregnancy persists
Four	Approximately 4–5 weeks after initiation of treatment for patients who are awaiting resolution of a non-viable pregnancy. Offer aspiration if non-viable pregnancy persists		

* Each tablet contains 200 mcg of misoprostol.

**With buccal or sublingual misoprostol, instruct the patient to swallow any residual pill fragments after 30 minutes.

Methotrexate-misoprostol regimens. Prior to the availability of mifepristone in the United States, U.S. researchers developed other regimens for early medication abortion using methotrexate and misoprostol. Because these drugs are widely available and inexpensive, they offer an important alternative when mifepristone is unaffordable or unavailable. Used in combination with vaginal misoprostol 800 mcg, methotrexate is 92% to 96% successful in terminating pregnancy through 49 days of gestation.[6,48,72] However, 15% to 25% of women may need to wait up to a month for expulsion of the gestational sac to occur.[46,48,73] During this delay, they will no longer feel pregnant if the pregnancy has stopped growing.

Most protocols use intramuscular methotrexate at a dose of 50 mg per square meter of body surface, but a 50 mg dose taken orally (dissolved in orange juice to disguise the taste) is comparably effective[73,74] (Table 24–4). Three to 7 days after methotrexate treatment, the woman inserts misoprostol 800 mcg vaginally. She may repeat the misoprostol dose if bleeding does not occur after 24 hours or if she has not aborted by the time of the 1-week follow-up visit. Most women will abort successfully by 4 weeks following initiation of treatment.

Misoprostol-only regimens. Although misoprostol alone is not as effective as combined mifepristone regimens,[49] it remains an important alternative in countries where mifepristone is not available or abortion is illegible or inaccessible.[75] Researchers have studied a variety of early-abortion regimens using misoprostol alone; most involve multiple doses and therefore higher rates of side effects than occur with mifepristone regimens.[6] According to a recent systematic review, success rates range from 84% to 96% in studies using 800 mcg vaginal misoprostol (usually premoistened before insertion) every 24 hours for two to three doses in pregnancies through 63 days' gestation.[76] A similar dose of sublingual misoprostol is about 85% effective when given at 3-hour intervals, although side effects are increased compared with the vaginal route.[77]

Anecdotal evidence suggests that some women in the United States are using misoprostol to self-induce abortion.[78] This practice may grow as word spreads through informal information networks, and women may present for follow-up treatment after self-administration. Women who seek care due to problems, such as heavy bleeding or incomplete abortion, may not acknowledge use of misoprostol unless the provider specifically requests this information. In addition to following guidelines for problem management and referral used for other medication abortion patients (see below), (1) treat or refer for management of side effects, particularly if the woman used large doses of misoprostol; (2) strongly advise aspiration abortion if the pregnancy is ongoing to avoid the potential teratogenic effects of misoprostol; and (3) help the woman obtain the information, family planning care, and other health services that she may need on an ongoing basis.

Follow-up After Medication Abortion

No matter which drug combination or regimen they use, women undergoing medication abortion are likely to experience cramping and bleeding. In most cases, pain can be managed with non-steroidal anti-inflammatory drugs (NSAIDs), such as ibuprofen, or acetaminophen with codeine phosphate (300 mg/30 mg). NSAIDs do not interfere with the effectiveness of misoprostol.[79] Although bleeding may seem abundant to those experiencing it, the amount of bleeding is rarely clinically significant. One study that used mifepristone with oral or vaginal misoprostol through 63 days' gestation found median blood losses ranging from 83 ml to 89 ml,[80] compared with the 50 ml typically lost during menses or the nearly 500 ml typically given in a blood donation. Although the range of bleeding varies widely among women, meaningful changes in hemoglobin seldom occur.[80] Bleeding is usually heaviest during expulsion of the pregnancy; lighter flow or spotting lasts about 2 weeks on average, but may be longer.[81] Use of combined oral contraceptives does not alter bleeding patterns after medication abortion.[81,82]

Providing patients with parameters for excessive bleeding enhances safety. Advise the patient to call if she soaks 2 or more large pads per hour for 2 consecutive hours. If the patient feels otherwise well, monitoring periodically by telephone for another 2 hours is acceptable. Patients whose bleeding does not slow after this interval warrant prompt in-person evaluation. Some providers treat excessive bleeding with another dose of misoprostol or an ergot alkaloid such as methylergonovine maleate (Methergine®) before resorting to aspiration. Heavy bleeding that prompts a woman to contact her clinician may occur in the several days following misoprostol administration or it may be delayed for 3 to 5 weeks.[83] Bleeding heavy enough to require aspiration occurs in less than 1% of patients, and less than 1 in 1,000 women will need a blood transfusion for excessive bleeding.[6,84]

Side effects common with all medication abortion regimens include nausea, headache, vomiting, diarrhea, dizziness, fever, and chills.[6] These side effects typically subside within a few hours and seldom require treatment. Temperature elevation (100.4° F or more) that lasts more than 4 hours or that begins in the days after misoprostol administration, however, warrants clinical assessment.

A disadvantage of medication abortion is that it often involves two to three office visits (Table 24–4), depending on the regimen used. With the alternative evidence-based mifepristone-misoprostol regimens commonly used in the United States, two office visits currently are typical:

the first to evaluate the patient and provide the medications, and a second follow-up visit to assess whether the pregnancy has ended. Newer data suggest that the second office visit may be replaced by telephone follow-up combined with a sensitive urine pregnancy test at home 30 days after mifepristone is given.[85] Additional office visits may be necessary if the FDA-approved regimen is used, if state regulations require a separate counseling visit before the patient has an abortion, or if the medication abortion fails. If a growing pregnancy persists for 2 to 3 weeks after treatment, aspiration abortion is strongly recommended because of the potential risk of birth defects following exposure to misoprostol. If the pregnancy has stopped growing but has not completely passed out of the uterus, the woman may choose to have another course of misoprostol, an aspiration procedure, or simply wait for expulsion to occur.

Clinical methods used to confirm abortion include a history of bleeding with evidence of uterine involution on follow-up examination, appropriately falling serum quantitative hCG determinations, or ultrasonography. Although most medication abortion researchers in the United States relied on ultrasonography to assess gestational age and clinical outcomes, many providers offer safe medication abortion services without routine use of ultrasound.[36,37,86,87] Whatever method you choose to follow patients, remember these important guidelines:

- If a woman has a gestational sac on initial ultrasound examination and no sac on follow-up, then her abortion is complete. Aspiration for a thickened endometrial stripe or "debris" in the uterus is not indicated unless the patient is bleeding heavily or has symptoms or signs of infection.[88]

- If you are following serum hCGs in lieu of sonography to determine treatment success, draw an initial quantitative hCG test on the day of mifepristone or methotrexate administration and a second test about 24 hours after she uses misoprostol. If the hCG values fall by at least 50% at 24 hours, then the abortion is most likely complete.[6] Alternatively, a decline of at least 80% 1 week after mifepristone usually indicates success.[37,89] Rapidly rising hCG values typically signal a continuing pregnancy, while a slow rise, plateau, or slow fall may indicate ectopic pregnancy.[47] (See Chapter 23, Pregnancy Testing and Management of Early Pregnancy.)

- Absent or minimal bleeding after taking misoprostol may indicate treatment failure.

- hCG may not clear from the body for a month or more after complete abortion, and pregnancy testing during this time may yield misleading results. Although a negative urine pregnancy test result 1 to 2 weeks following treatment is reassuring, a positive test does not necessarily mean that the pregnancy is continuing.[90] (see Chapter 23, Pregnancy Testing and Management of Early Pregnancy)

FIRST-TRIMESTER VACUUM ASPIRATION ABORTION

Introduced in the United States in 1967, vacuum aspiration (suction curettage) is the method used for virtually all first-trimester instrumental abortions in the United States.[23] Aspiration is a safe and simple way to empty the uterus completely and quickly using modest cervical dilation and a hand-held syringe (manual vacuum aspiration) or an electric vacuum pump. Most states limit abortion provision to physicians; however, in a few states without such restrictions, advanced practice clinicians have provided aspiration abortions for years with an impressive safety record.[91]

Vacuum aspiration using local cervical anesthesia with or without oral NSAIDs or mild intravenous sedation can be provided safely and appropriately in a medical office setting equipped with the same emergency back-up equipment and supplies needed to provide injectable medications (drugs and resuscitation equipment to manage an allergic reaction, seizure, or cardiac arrest). In addition, the office should have available the medications needed to treat uterine bleeding and a plan for transferring a woman to a surgical facility in the rare event that she needs an evaluation for uterine perforation. The availability of portable and inexpensive manual vacuum aspirators has facilitated abortion provision in primary care settings that do not have electric pumps, as well as resource-poor settings worldwide. Research indicates that manual vacuum aspiration (MVA) is as effective and safe as electric vacuum aspiration;[92,93] although pain is comparable,[94,95] women prefer the quietness of the MVA device.[95-97]

As the first step in an aspiration procedure, perform a bimanual examination to determine the size and position of the uterus. Insert a short-bladed speculum, such as a Moore Graves design, to draw the cervix close to the perineum for adequate visualization and straighten a flexed uterus. Although vaginal cleansing with an antiseptic solution is common practice, its efficacy in preventing postabortal infection has not been established.[98,99] Of greater importance for infection prevention is the use of a *no-touch technique*, i.e., not touching the parts of instruments, including the tips of dilators or cannulae, that will enter the sterile uterine cavity.[100]

Administer a local anesthetic such as lidocaine amide to the cervix to reduce pain. The total amount of lidocaine administered should not exceed 200 mg (20 cc of 1% lidocaine or 40 cc of 0.5% lidocaine). Inject

2–3 cc of the anesthetic into the lip of the cervix before placing a tenaculum to keep the cervix stabilized, and then administer the remaining solution at two to four sites either directly into the cervical stroma or paracervically. Limited evidence suggests that deep injections (approximately 3 cm) are more effective than superficial injections.[101]

Using Pratt or Denniston dilators, stretch the cervix gently and incrementally as needed to accommodate an aspiration cannula of appropriate size for the gestation (Figure 24-2). Typically, the diameter of the cannula in millimeters corresponds to the duration of the pregnancy in weeks (for example, a 7 mm cannula to evacuate a pregnancy at 7 weeks). Insert a cannula through the dilated cervix and connect it to either a manual vacuum syringe or an electric vacuum pump. Remove the products of conception by a combination of rotary and back-and-forth motions (Figure 24-2). Detection of a "gritty" sensation as the cannula moves across the endometrial surface typically indicates that the uterus is empty.

Examining the removed tissue helps to confirm complete evacuation. If the products of conception are not readily apparent, suspending the tissue in water, saline, or white vinegar and checking with backlighting may facilitate the evaluation.[100] If pregnancy tissue is still not identified, a postprocedure sonogram may confirm retained products or assist in

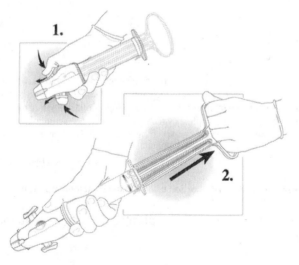

A. Prepare the manual vacuum aspirator (MVA) by pushing the valve buttons down and forward until they lock into place (1). Pull the plunger back until the arms snap outward and catch on the cylinder base (2).

Figure 24–2 Performing an early abortion using a manual vacuum aspirator. Figure continues on the next page.

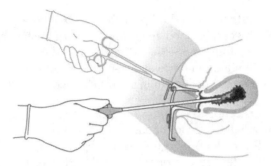

B. After washing the cervix with antiseptic solution, administering paracervical anesthesia and applying a tenaculum, open the cervix as needed with mechanical dilators to allow for insertion of an appropriately sized cannula. In general, the diameter of the cannula should approximate the gestational age in weeks (e.g., use a 7-mm cannula to evacuate a 7-week pregnancy).

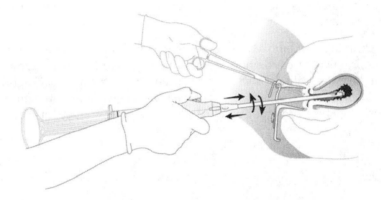

C. While applying traction to the tenaculum, advance the cannula into the upper uterine cavity. Attach the prepared aspirator to the cannula, release the vacuum by pressing the buttons, and evacuate the contents of the uterus using a combination of rotary and back-and-forth motions. Signs of complete evacuation include contraction of the uterus and detection of a gritty sensation as the cannula moves across the endometrial surface, with no further tissue passing through the cannula.

©Ipas/Illustration by Stephen C. Edgerton

Figure 24–2 Performing an early abortion using a manual vacuum aspirator.

the diagnosis of uncommon complications such as a missed ectopic pregnancy.

SECOND-TRIMESTER DILATION AND EVACUATION

After the first trimester, the most common method for abortion in the United States is dilation and evacuation (D&E), a procedure that combines aspiration with the use of forceps.[23] Most women prefer D&E to medical induction methods that typically entail hospitalization, higher costs, and a prolonged period of labor.[102] Although D&E requires surgical expertise, it is safer than older *instillation methods* of induction that involved infusion or injection of prostaglandins, hypertonic saline, or urea into the amniotic cavity.[103,104] The comparative safety of D&E and modern induction methods has not been established, although one limited study reported a higher complication rate with misoprostol induction than with D&E, based solely on the greater need for curettage to remove retained placenta.[105]

Using preoperative sonography to obtain an accurate estimation of gestational age enhances the safety of D&E abortion, and intraoperative sonography may be helpful as well. Because the cervix requires more dilation for a second-trimester D&E than for a first-trimester aspiration to permit evacuation of the larger products of conception, preoperative cervical preparation using osmotic dilating devices, misoprostol, or a combination is recommended (see Adjunctive Techniques). After administering anesthesia, the clinician removes the osmotic dilators and empties the uterus using appropriate instruments. In the United States, the federal abortion ban [18 U.S.C. 1531 (2003)] effectively prohibits intentionally extracting the fetus as intact as possible unless surgical techniques or a preoperative medication such as digoxin is used to assure fetal demise before extraction.[12]

SECOND-TRIMESTER INDUCTION ABORTION

Second-trimester induction abortion involves administration of medications that cause the uterus to contract and eventually expel the fetus and placenta. Although induction is used commonly in many European countries, it accounts for only a small proportion of abortions after the first trimester in the United States.[23] Modern induction agents have largely replaced older instillation methods, conferring a considerable safety advantage.

Misoprostol alone, when administered in multiple doses, is effective for second-trimester abortion. Based on current evidence, the recommended regimen for pregnancies between 13 and 22 weeks' gestation is 400 mcg of misoprostol administered vaginally every 3 hours for up to five doses.[106] With misoprostol-alone regimens, the median time to abortion is 10 to 19 hours, and 70% to 90% of women will abort within 24 hours.[107] Pretreatment with mifepristone enhances efficacy and shortens the time required to induce abortion by about 50%.[108] The Royal College of Obstetricians and Gynaecologists (RCOG) in the United Kingdom has endorsed the mifepristone-misoprostol combination for abortion at 15 weeks' gestation or more when providers with specialized skills for D&E are not available.[8] The regimen recommended by RCOG includes mifepristone 200 mg orally followed 36 to 48 hours later by misoprostol 800 mcg vaginally, then misoprostol 400 mcg orally every 3 hours to a maximum of four oral doses. Success rates as high as 97% have been reported with this protocol.[109] Other less favorable and less frequently used methods include vaginal administration of dinoprostone, a prostaglandin approved by the FDA for second-trimester abortion, and intravenous administration of high-dose oxytocin.[110,111]

All second-trimester induction methods have side effects specific to the medications used. Although retained placenta requiring curettage was common with older induction methods, its frequency has decreased to less than 10% with use of mifepristone or misoprostol induction regimens.[107,108]

A DJUNCTIVE TECHNIQUES

Clinicians use several adjunctive techniques to facilitate abortion procedures, including pretreatment with osmotic dilators and administration of perioperative uterotonic agents. Use of osmotic dilators decreases the risk of cervical laceration or perforation,[112,113] although the minimal risk of uterine injury in first-trimester abortion may not justify their routine use. The Society of Family Planning recommends cervical preparation routinely before second-trimester D&E abortion and advises consideration in women with risk factors (e.g., adolescents, those with pregnancies in the late first trimester, or those in whom the clinician anticipates difficulty dilating the cervix).[114,115]

Osmotic dilating devices. Two types of osmotic dilating devices are currently available in the United States: *Laminaria japonica* or *digitata* consist of sterile stalks of dried seaweed, and Dilapan-S is a synthetic polyacrylonitrile (plastic) rod. The clinician places osmotic dilators so they extend through the endocervical canal and dilate both the internal and external os. The devices absorb fluid and expand, exerting radial pressure on the cervix to dilate it, and they stimulate release of prostaglandins to soften the cervix as well. Laminaria tents reach maximum dilation in 12 to 24 hours, so they are most commonly inserted the day before a D&E procedure. In contrast, Dilapan-S devices dilate quickly, achieving most of their effect within 4 to 6 hours, so their use often allows clinicians to complete second-trimester D&E abortions in a shorter time frame than in the past. Many clinicians use a combination of osmotic dilators, and several serial insertions may be necessary for procedures later in pregnancy.[115]

Misoprostol. Treatment with misoprostol prior to D&E abortion causes cervical softening and dilation (called ripening) that can reduce the need for additional mechanical dilation or make it easier. Vaginal insertion of misoprostol has greater efficacy and fewer side effects than oral administration.[116,117] Numerous studies suggest that an optimal regimen for first-trimester cervical preparation is 400 mcg administered vaginally 3 hours prior to the procedure.[114,118] This regimen is as effective as overnight laminaria for first-trimester cervical preparation.[116] The same dose of misoprostol administered sublingually 2 to 4 hours before aspiration abortion primes the cervix as well as vaginal misoprostol, but with a higher incidence of side effects.[117–119] Although less well studied, buccal misoprostol has pharmacokinetics similar to vaginal misoprostol[50] and may represent an effective alternative route of administration.[114–120] Mifepristone is also an excellent cervical ripener, but it requires a long preparation time (24 to 48 hours).[121]

Experienced providers may use misoprostol safely in lieu of osmotic dilators before early second-trimester abortions or in combination with osmotic dilators for later D&E procedures.[115–122] Optimal regimens for these uses are not yet well-defined.[123] One randomized trial of women having abortions at 13 to 16 weeks of pregnancy found that overnight preparation with 3 to 6 laminaria resulted in more dilation and faster procedure times than misoprostol 400 mcg administered vaginally 3 to 4 hours before evacuation.[124] However, most procedures were completed without difficulty, and women expressed a strong preference for a 1-day procedure. Misoprostol has the potential problem of inducing contractions that can result in unscheduled delivery of the fetus, so it may not be acceptable for home administration after the first trimester. Side effects include nausea, vomiting, diarrhea, and fever or shivering. Although uterine rupture has been reported following misoprostol use in the second trimester, primarily in women who had a scar from prior uterine surgery, these cases are rare and do not contraindicate its use.[115]

Uterotonic agents. Agents such as vasopressin, oxytocin, prostaglandins, and ergotamines (e.g., methylergonovine maleate or Methergine®) strengthen uterine contractility, and they may constrict blood vessels as well. Prophylactic use of uterotonic agents in second trimester abortions may help reduce blood loss.[125] Adding vasopressin or oxytocin to the cervical anesthetic solution provides a simple means of administration, as does direct injection of Methergine®, dilute vasopressin, or oxytocin into the cervix at the end of the procedure. Many providers give patients oral Methergine® to use at home for a few days, particularly following second-trimester abortions.[126]

MANAGING POSTABORTION COMPLICATIONS

Take seriously any complaint or problem after an abortion procedure. Inform all abortion patients to watch for warning signs (Table 24–3), and tell them how to contact you in case they have questions or problems. Prompt recognition and management can be critical in preventing the rare serious outcome.

THE SAFETY OF ABORTION

Modern methods of abortion are remarkably safe. Since the nationwide legalization of abortion in the United States, abortion-related mortality has decreased by 90%, with most of the decline occurring from 1973 to 1976.[127] The risk of dying from a modern legal abortion is less than 1 in 100,000 procedures, which represents the lowest mortality risk of all pregnancy outcomes. Pregnancy-related death rates are twice as high for spontaneous abortion and 12 times higher for continuing pregnancy and childbirth.[128] In the largest study of legally induced first-trimester abortions reported to date, minor complications occurred in 8 per 1,000 cases and complications warranting hospitalization in 0.7 per 1,000.[129] The single greatest factor influencing the safety of abortion is gestational age. Abortions are safer when performed early in pregnancy, which emphasizes the importance of access for women seeking abortion.[127]

Medication abortion using mifepristone regimens has proven safe and effective. A review of reports from the 202 Planned Parenthood sites that provided early medication abortions using mifepristone and vaginal misoprostol during 2001 to early 2004 found an overall success rate of 99.7%. Only 206 adverse events were reported among 95,163 patients—a rate of 2 adverse events per 1,000 abortions.[84] Heavy bleeding was the most common complication, occurring in 2 per 1,000 treatments, and few women required blood transfusions (0.5 transfusions per 1,000 abortions). Infections requiring parenteral antibiotics occurred at a rate of 0.2 per 1,000 mifepristone abortions. In a subsequent report, the low rate of serious infections decreased even further with a switch from vaginal to buccal administration of misoprostol combined with universal antibiotic prophylaxis.[130]

In the decade following FDA approval of mifepristone, nearly 1.5 million North American women have used mifepristone in combination with misoprostol for early abortion; 10 fatalities have been reported in this cohort, for a mortality rate of less than 1 per 100,000 abortions.[131-132] One woman died from hemorrhage resulting from a ruptured ectopic pregnancy,[133] and 9 women died of pelvic infection complicated by septic shock. The causative agent in 8 cases of infection was *Clostridium sordellii*, a toxin-producing bacterium that has been associated with rare, serious infections following childbirth, spontaneous abortion (miscarriage), gynecological procedures, and other clinical events.[69,70,134] The CDC identified *Clostridium perfringens* as the pathogen in 1 case of infection. The clinical manifestations of *Clostridium sordellii* toxic shock infections differ from those typically seen in women with endometritis[69] (see below). Intensive investigations by health authorities have not established a causal relationship between the medications used for early abortion and these adverse events, and contamination of mifepristone and misoprostol tablets has been ruled out. Updated labeling for mifepristone reminds providers to remain aware of the possibility of unrecognized ectopic pregnancy or infection throughout the treatment period.

IMMEDIATE AND SHORT-TERM COMPLICATIONS

Abortion complications, while not common, include the following immediate and short-term problems:

Bleeding. Regardless of whether they have undergone medication or aspiration methods, almost all women have at least some bleeding during and after an abortion. Typically, bleeding persists for at least several days, with light bleeding or spotting continuing for as long as 2 to 4 weeks. In medication abortion patients, the absence of bleeding after misoprostol administration may indicate unsuccessful abortion.

Promptly evaluate the source of bleeding that is excessive or prolonged. The most common causes of hemorrhage after aspiration or D&E abortion are uterine atony and retained placental or fetal tissue. Atony, which typically occurs immediately after the procedure, almost always responds to uterotonic agents and uterine massage. Women with retained tissue may present with heavy bleeding several days to a few weeks following the abortion (see Incomplete Abortion, below). After a medication abortion, less than 1 in 100 women require aspiration or curettage to stop bleeding, and less than 1 in 1,000 require transfusion.[6] Bleeding that requires treatment is often not due to immediate hemorrhage but rather persistent or delayed bleeding that occurs 3 to 5 weeks following mifepristone administration.[83] Medication abortion patients and providers, therefore, need to remain vigilant for bleeding even if findings appear normal on the follow-up examination.

Incomplete abortion. When part of the pregnancy tissue remains in the uterus, the abortion procedure is *incomplete*. This problem occurs following approximately 0.3% to 2% of aspiration procedures.[135] Retained pregnancy tissue is likely to cause continued bleeding and cramping that prompt women to seek care. Treatment with misoprostol or vacuum aspiration is appropriate. Medication abortion regimens take a longer time to empty the uterus than does aspiration, and an ultrasound examination may show residual tissue after the pregnancy sac has passed. This normal finding does not require intervention unless the patient is bleeding excessively or has symptoms or signs of an infection.[88]

Continuing pregnancy. In less than 1% of cases, an attempt to terminate pregnancy fails altogether.[6,84,135] A woman with a continuing pregnancy may have ongoing symptoms of pregnancy and a soft or enlarged uterus. Ultrasound or hCG testing may help to identify this problem. (See Chapter 23, Pregnancy Testing and Management of Early Pregnancy.) Providing or referring the patient for an effective means to terminate the pregnancy is appropriate treatment.

Meticulous tissue examination after an aspiration abortion minimizes the risk of a continuing pregnancy. Failure to visualize products of conception in the aspirate warrants further investigation for a continuing intrauterine or ectopic pregnancy. Failed aspiration abortion occurs more often in women with uterine abnormalities, such as a bicornuate uterus or a cavity distorted by fibroids. Treatment options include medication abortion (if the patient is still within an eligible gestational age limit) or respiration using ultrasound guidance as needed. Ongoing pregnancy due to failed medication abortion potentially involves an increased risk for fetal malformation, so encourage the patient to consider carefully before deciding to continue the pregnancy to term.[6]

Intrauterine blood clots (hematometra). Intrauterine blood clots can occur immediately or as long as a few days after an aspiration abortion; their presence may cause severe cramping and pain. Sometimes called the *postabortal* or *redo syndrome*, this problem occurs after approximately 0.02% of first-trimester vacuum aspiration abortion procedures.[135] Typical findings on the pelvic examination include a large, tense, and tender uterus with little or no bleeding from the cervix. A simple vacuum aspiration remedies the problem; pain and cramping resolve within a few minutes.

Cervical, uterine, or abdominal organ trauma. External cervical tears can occur if the tenaculum detaches from the cervix. Management options include applying pressure and observing, applying ferric subsulfate (Monsel's) solution, or, rarely, placing suture. A small midline uterine perforation in the first trimester can be managed safely with careful observation for 2 to 4 hours, and hospitalization is not necessary unless evidence arises of internal bleeding, abdominal pain, or rebound tenderness. More severe cervical or uterine trauma, including perforation with damage to nearby abdominal organs or vessels, is rare.[135] Depending on their severity, these complications may require exploratory surgery to identify and repair the uterus or abdominal organ injury, or even hysterectomy. Providers typically prepare the cervix with osmotic dilating devices or misoprostol before second-trimester abortion to decrease the risk of uterine trauma.[113] Avoiding routine use of a uterine sound or sharp curette during aspiration abortion also may reduce the risk.[135]

Uterine rupture has been reported with use of misoprostol for induction of labor at term and rarely in conjunction with mifepristone or other uterotonic agents in second-trimester medical abortion. Most cases occur in women with a previous uterine scar.[136]

Infection. Infection rates reported in U.S. studies following first-trimester aspiration abortion range from 0.1% to 0.5%; rates are slightly higher, 0.4% to 2%, following second-trimester D&E or induction.[135] A systematic review of infectious complications reported in studies that used various medication regimens for first- and second-trimester abortion found an overall infection rate of 0.9%.[137]

Measures to minimize the risk of postabortal infection include screening for pre-existing reproductive tract infections (with treatment before or at the time of the abortion) or administering prophylactic antibiotics at the time of the abortion,[138] using a no-touch technique, and emptying the uterus completely during aspiration or D&E. Antibiotic regimens used commonly by U.S. providers include doxycycline 100 to 200 mg taken as a single dose, or 100 mg taken twice daily for 3 to 7 days.[21,139] Because pregnant patients may experience nausea and vomiting, many clinicians wait until after the procedure to begin the antibiotics. Although some providers use additional antibiotic prophylaxis for women who may be at increased risk for subacute bacterial endocarditis, the American Heart Association does not recommend prophylaxis for genitourinary procedures.[140]

Common symptoms of postabortal pelvic infection include persistent cramping, abdominal pain, fever, discharge, and malaise. Treatment of uncomplicated pelvic infection includes broad spectrum antibiotics and aspiration of retained tissue, if present. Hospitalization for intravenous antibiotic therapy is warranted in patients with severe illness or suspected pelvic abscess and in those who are immunocompromised, unable to tolerate oral medications, or fail to respond to outpatient therapy.

The few patients who developed toxic shock from *Clostridium sordellii* infection presented with atypical findings, including flu-like symptoms and absence of fever.[69] Suspect an atypical infection if a patient manifests the following symptoms or signs in the days following misoprostol use for medication abortion:

- Nausea, vomiting, diarrhea, weakness with or without abdominal pain
- Tachycardia or hypotension
- Lack of fever with little tenderness on pelvic examination
- High hemoglobin or hematocrit value
- Marked leukocytosis (unusually high white blood cell count)

If you suspect atypical infection, refer the patient immediately to the emergency room with a copy of the mifepristone Medication Guide, which has been updated to reflect information about these infections. Because hospital personnel may know little about medication abortion or *Clostridium sordellii* or *perfringens*, call the emergency room to explain why you are making the referral.

LONG-TERM HEALTH OUTCOMES

Women who seek abortion services may ask about possible long-term health effects. Public debate about long-term effects has been used inappropriately as a rationale for limiting women's access to legal abortion services. Reassuring expert reviews of this topic have been published.[141] The study of long-term health outcomes is methodologically challenging; as new research findings are published, pay attention to the quality of study design and the criteria for determining causality. Conclusions in three key areas are briefly summarized below.

Future Reproductive Health and Fertility

First-trimester aspiration abortion is not associated with a measurable increased risk for impaired fertility or ectopic pregnancy.[141-142] Although occasional European reports have suggested an increased risk of preterm birth after first-trimester vacuum aspiration,[143] several large, well-designed cohort studies have found no association.[144-145] Increased risks for spontaneous abortion or preterm delivery and low birthweight infant have been reported after second-trimester D&E abortion, but adequate preparation of the cervix before the procedure may mitigate these risks.[142,146] Research to date has found no association between mifepristone-misoprostol abortion and the risk of subsequent ectopic pregnancy,[147] preterm delivery, or low birthweight infant.[148]

Psychological Health

The contention that induced abortion causes lasting psychological harm is misleading and unsubstantiated. Although research on abortion and mental health is methodologically limited, recent systematic reviews of the literature by the American Psychological Association and others confirm that no causal association is evident between induced abortion and mental health problems.[149-151] So-called *abortion trauma syndrome* (purportedly characterized by such symptoms as persistent guilt and sadness) has been described in materials distributed by lay groups, but no such syndrome is defined in peer-reviewed scientific literature or in the professional diagnostic codes.[152] The syndrome is the conclusion of self-selected groups of women, in some cases linked to religious groups. If abortion caused incapacitating emotional responses frequently, this association would be evident because abortion is such a common procedure. (About 1 in 3 women in the United States will have at least one induced abortion during their reproductive years.[28])

Temporary feelings of loss or sadness may follow what is sometimes a difficult decision to terminate a pregnancy,[153] but these normal reactions do not constitute mental health problems. Psychiatric problems following abortion are rare,[154–155] and they are more likely to occur among women with preexisting mental health conditions.[149,151,154,156] Many studies document benefits from induced abortion, such as enhanced self-esteem.[153,154,157] Relief is a predominant emotion after abortion, and long-term follow-up studies confirm that most women remain satisfied with their decision to have had an abortion.[153–158] Recent studies show no significant differences in psychological responses among women having medication abortions and those having aspiration abortions.[159–161]

Breast Cancer

The question of whether induced abortion has any effect on the risk of subsequent breast cancer has received intense scrutiny. Epidemiologic research on this topic is complex because of study design problems that could lead to spurious association. For example, recall bias may explain some of the positive associations found in case-control studies that compare abortion histories of healthy women with those of women who have breast cancer, because healthy women are less likely than women with cancer to report sensitive events such as prior abortion. Large, prospective studies that collect data on reproductive events *before* the diagnosis of breast cancer have found no association between induced abortion and breast cancer.[162–163] A recent comprehensive reanalysis of the worldwide research on abortion and breast cancer, including 53 studies from 16 countries, confirms this conclusion.[164] Moreover, numerous authoritative organizations, including the National Cancer Institute and the American College of Obstetricians and Gynecologists (ACOG), have concluded that no evidence supports a true association between induced abortion and subsequent breast cancer risk.[165–166]

POSTABORTION CONTRACEPTION

Fertility returns quickly following abortion. Ovulation, and with it the possibility of another pregnancy, may occur as soon as 10 days after abortion. Helping a woman initiate an effective method of contraception is an essential task in providing abortion care, and it should not be deferred to a follow-up visit. If the unplanned pregnancy occurred while the woman was using a contraceptive method, help her identify any personal, situational, or method-related factors that may have contributed to the contraceptive failure. Also, explain the availability of emergency contraception and, if possible, provide a supply she can have on hand at home in case of future need.

The woman may start a hormonal method of contraception immediately after an aspiration or D&E abortion or as soon as she wishes after using misoprostol in medication abortion regimens. Many providers initiate the hormonal method on the same day as the abortion, or any time within the first 7 days for oral contraceptives and injectables, or any time within the first 5 days for the patch or ring. Intrauterine contraception can be inserted safely at the conclusion of an aspiration procedure or at the time pregnancy expulsion is confirmed following medication abortion.

REFERENCES

1. Finer LB, Frahwirth LF, Dauphinee LA, Singh S, Moore AM. Reasons U.S. women have abortions: quantitative and qualitative perspectives. Perspect Sex Reprod Health. 2005;37:110–8.
2. Drey EA, Foster DG, Jackson RA, Lee SJ, Cardenas LH, Darney PD. Risk factors associated with presenting for abortion in the second trimester. Obstet Gynecol. 2006;107:128–35.
3. Kiley JW, Yee LM, Niemi CM, Feinglass JM, Simon MA. Delays in request for pregnancy termination: comparison of patients in the first and second trimesters. Contraception. 2010;81:446–51.
4. Paul M, Lichtenberg ES, Borgatta L, Grimes DA, Stubblefield PG, Creinin MD, editors. Management of unintended and abnormal pregnancy: Comprehensive abortion care. Oxford: Blackwell-Wiley; 2009.
5. Kottke MJ, Zieman M. Management of abortion. In: Rock JA, Jones HW III, (editors). TeLinde's operative gynecology. 10th ed. Philadelphia: Lippincott Williams & Wilkins; 2008. p. 776–97.
6. American College of Obstetricians and Gynecologists (ACOG). Medical management of abortion. ACOG Practice Bulletin No. 67. Obstet Gynecol. 2005;106:871–82.
7. Stubblefield PG, Carr Ellis S, Borgatta L. Methods for induced abortion. Obstet Gynecol. 2004;104:174–85.
8. Royal College of Obstetricians and Gynaecologists. The care of women requesting induced abortion. London: Royal College of Obstetricians and Gynaecologists; 2004.
9. Glick E. Surgical abortion. Reno, NV: West End Women's Medical Group, 1998.
10. Edwards J, Carson SA. New technologies permit safe abortion at less than six weeks' gestation and provide timely detection of ectopic gestation. Am J Obstet Gynecol. 1997;176:1101–6.
11. Baird DT, Grimes DA, Van Look PFA. Modern methods of inducing abortion. Oxford; Cambridge, Ma: Blackwell Science, 1995.
12. Jones BS, Dalven J. Abortion law and policy in the USA. In: Paul M, Lichtenberg ES, Borgatta L, Grimes DA, Stubblefield PG, Creinin MD, (editors). Management of unintended and abnormal pregnancy: Comprehensive abortion care. Oxford: Blackwell-Wiley; 2009. p. 36–47.
13. Fried MG. The economics of abortion access in the US: restrictions on government funding for abortion is the post-Roe battleground. Conscience. 2005–2006;26:11–5.
14. Henshaw SK, Joyce TJ, Dennis A, Finer LB, Blanchard K. Restrictions on Medicaid funding for abortions: a literature review. New York: Guttmacher Institute, 2009.
15. Stewart FH, Shields WC, Hwang AC. The federal abortion ban: a clinical and moral dilemma and international policy setback. Contraception. 2004;69:433–5.

16. Weitz TA, Yanow S. Implications of the Federal Abortion Ban for women's health in the United States. Reprod Health Matters. 2008;16(31 Suppl):99–107.

17. Crane BB, Dusenberry J. Power and politics in international funding for reproductive health: the US Global Gag Rule. Reprod Health Matters. 2004;12:128–37.

18. Joffe C. Dispatches from the abortion wars: The costs of fanaticism to doctors, patients, and the rest of us. Boston: Beacon Press, 2010.

19. Cates W, Jr., Grimes DA, Schulz KF. The public health impact of legal abortion: 30 years later. Perspect Sex Reprod Health. 2003;35:25–8.

20. American College of Obstetricians and Gynecologists. Abortion access and training. ACOG Committee Opinion No. 424, January 2009.

21. O'Connell K, Jones HE, Simon M, Saporta V, Paul M, Lichtenberg ES; National Abortion Federation Members. First-trimester surgical abortion practices: a survey of National Abortion Federation members. Contraception. 2009;79:385–92.

22. Jones RK, Kooistra K. Abortion incidence and access to services in the United States, 2008. Perspect Sex Reprod Health. 2011;43:41–50.

23. Pazol K, Zane SB, Parker WY, Hall LR, Gamble SB, Hamdan S., Berg C, Cook DA. Centers for Disease Control and Prevention (CDC). Abortion surveillance – United States, 2007. MMWR Surveill Summ. 2011;60:1–40.

24. Gamble SB, Strauss LT, Parker WY, Cook DA, Zane SB, Hamdan S. Abortion surveillance – United States, 2005. MMWR Surveill Summ. 2008;57:1–32.

25. Henshaw SK, Kost K. Trends in the characteristics of women obtaining abortions, 1974 to 2004. New York: Guttmacher Institute, 2008.

26. Jones RK, Kost K, Singh S, Henshaw SK, Finer LB. Trends in abortion in the United States. Clin Obstet Gynecol. 2009;52:119–29.

27. Jones RK, Finer LB, Singh S. Characteristics of U.S. abortion patients, 2008 [Internet]. New York: Guttmacher Institute; May 2010 [cited 2010 Sept 22]. Available from: http://www.guttmacher.org/pubs/US-Abortion-Patients.pdf.

28. Guttmacher Institute. Facts on induced abortion in the United States [Internet]. New York: Guttmacher Institute; [updated 2011 Jan; cited 2011 Mar 23]. Available from: http://www.guttmacher.org/pubs/fb_induced_abortion.html.

29. Finer LB, Henshaw SK. Disparities in rates of unintended pregnancy in the United States, 1994 and 2001. Perspect Sex Reprod Health. 2006;38:90–6.

30. Trussell J, Wynn LL. Reducing unintended pregnancy in the United States. Contraception. 2008;77:1–5.

31. Dehlendorf C, Rodriguez MI, Levy K, Borrero S, Steinauer J. Disparities in family planning. Am J Obstet Gynecol. 2010;202:214–20.

32. Jones RK, Darroch JE, Henshaw SK. Contraceptive use among U.S. women having abortions in 2000–2001. Perspect Sex Reprod Health. 2002;34:294–303.

33. Baker A, Beresford T. Informed consent, patient education, and counseling. In: Paul M, Lichtenberg ES, Borgatta L, Grimes DA, Stubblefield PG, Creinin MD (editors). Management of unintended and abnormal pregnancy: Comprehensive abortion care. Oxford: Blackwell-Wiley; 2009. p. 48–62.

34. National Abortion Federation. 2010 Clinical Policy Guidelines [Internet]. Washington: National Abortion Federation; 2011 [cited 2011 Mar 15]. Available from: http://www.prochoice.org/pubs_research/publications/clinical_policy_html.

35. Fielding SL, Schaff EA, Nam NY. Clinicians' perception of sonogram indication for mifepristone abortion up to 63 days. Contraception. 2002;66:27–31.

36. Kaneshiro B, Edelman A, Sneeringer RK, Ponce de Leon RG. Expanding medical abortion: can medical abortion be effectively provided without the routine use of ultrasound? Contraception. 2011;83:194-201.

37. Clark W, Panton T, Hann L, Gold M. Medication abortion employing routine sequential measurements of serum hCG and sonography only when indicated. Contraception. 2007;75:131–5.

38. Henshaw RC, Naji SA, Russell IT, Templeton AA. Comparison of medical abortion with surgical vacuum aspiration: women's preferences and acceptability of treatment. BMJ. 1993:307:714–7.
39. Winikoff B. Acceptability of medical abortion in early pregnancy. Fam Plann Perspect. 1995;27:142–8, 185.
40. Fielding SL, Edmunds E, Schaff EA. Having an abortion using mifepristone and home misoprostol: a qualitative analysis of women's experiences. Perspect Sex Reprod Health. 2002;34:34–40.
41. Prine LW, Lesnewski R. Medication abortion and family physicians' scope of practice. J Am Board Fam Pract. 2005;18:304–6.
42. Hwang AC, Koyama A, Taylor D, Henderson JT, Miller S. Advanced practice clinicians' interest in providing medical abortion: results of a California survey. Perspect Sex Reprod Health. 2005;37:92–7.
43. Yarnall J, Swica Y, Winikoff B. Non-physician clinicians can safely provide first trimester medical abortion. Reprod Health Matters. 2009;17:61–9.
44. Jones RK, Henshaw SK. Mifepristone for early medical abortion: experiences in France, Great Britain and Sweden. Perspect Sex Reprod Health. 2002;34:154–61.
45. Fiala C, Gemzel-Danielsson K. Review of medical abortion using mifepristone in combination with a prostaglandin analogue. Contraception. 2006;74:66–86.
46. Creinin MD, Vittinghoff E, Keder L, Darney PD, Tiller G. Methotrexate and misoprostol for early abortion: a multicenter trial. I. Safety and efficacy. Contraception. 1996;53:321–7.
47. Barnhart K. Clinical Practice. Ectopic Pregnancy. N Engl J Med. 2009;361:379–87.
48. Weibe E, Dunn S, Guilbert E, Jacot F, Lugtig L. Comparison of abortions induced by methotrexate or mifepristone followed by misoprostol. Obstet Gynecol. 2002;99: 813–9.
49. Jain JK, Dutton C, Harwood B, Meckstroth KR, Mishell DR Jr. A prospective randomized, double-blinded, placebo-controlled trial comparing mifepristone and vaginal misoprostol to vaginal misoprostol alone for elective termination of pregnancy. Hum Reprod. 2002;17:1477–82.
50. Meckstroth KR, Whitaker AK, Bertisch S, Goldberg AB, Darney PD. Misoprostol administered by epithelial routes: drug absorption and uterine response. Obstet Gynecol. 2006;108:582–90.
51. Tang OS, Ho PC. The pharmacokinetics and different regimens of misoprostol in early first-trimester medical abortion. Contraception. 2006;74:26–30.
52. Tang OS, Gemzell-Danielsson K, Ho PC. Misoprostol: Pharmacokinetic profiles, effects on the uterus and side-effects. Int J Gynaecol Obstet. 2007;99 Suppl 2: S160–7.
53. da Silva Dal Pizzol T, Knop FP, Mengue SS. Prenatal exposure to misoprostol and congenital anomalies: systematic review and meta-analysis. Reprod Toxicol. 2006;22: 666–71.
54. Spitz IM, Bardin CW, Benton L, Robbins A. Early pregnancy termination with mifepristone and misoprostol in the United States. N Engl J Med. 1998;338:1241–7.
55. Peyron R, Aubeny E, Targosz V, Silvestre L, Renault M, Elkik F, et al. Early termination of pregnancy with mifepristone (RU 486) and the orally active prostaglandin misoprostol. N Engl J Med. 1993;328:1509–13.
56. World Health Organisation Task Force on Post-Ovulatory Methods of Fertility Regulation. Comparison of two doses of mifepristone in combination with misoprostol for early medical abortion: a randomized trial. BJOG. 2000;107:524–30.
57. Shannon CS, Winikoff B, Hausknecht R, Schaff E, Blumenthal PD, Oyer D, et al. Multicenter trial of a simplified mifepristone medical abortion regimen. Obstet Gynecol. 2005;105:345–51.
58. Schaff EA, Stadalius LS, Eisinger SH, Franks P. Vaginal misoprostol administered at home after mifepristone (RU486) for abortion. J Fam Pract. 1997;44:353–60.

59. el-Refaey H, Rajasekar D, Abdalla M, Calder L, Templeton A. Induction of abortion with mifepristone (RU 486) and oral or vaginal misoprostol. N Engl J Med. 1995;332:983–7.

60. Schaff EA, Fielding SL, Westhoff C. Randomized trial of oral versus vaginal misoprostol at one day after mifepristone for early medical abortion. Contraception. 2001;64:81–5.

61. Schaff EA, Fielding SL, Westhoff C. Randomized trial of oral versus vaginal misoprostol 2 days after mifepristone 200 mg for abortion up to 63 days of pregnancy. Contraception. 2002;66:247–50.

62. Middleton T, Schaff E, Fielding SL, Scahill M, Shannon C, Westheimer E, et al. Randomized trial of mifepristone and buccal or vaginal misprostol for abortion through 56 days of last menstrual period. Contraception. 2005;72:328–32.

63. Winikoff B, Dzuba IG, Creinin MD, Crowden WA, Goldberg AB, Gonzales J, et al. Two distinct oral routes of misoprostol in mifepristone medical abortion: a randomized trial. Obstet Gynecol. 2008;112:1303–10.

64. Tang OS, Chan CC, Ng EH, Lee SW, Ho PC. A prospective, randomized, placebo-controlled trial on the use of mifepristone with sublingual or vaginal misoprostol for medical abortions of less than 9 weeks gestation. Hum Reprod. 2003;18:2315–8.

65. Hamoda H, Ashok PW, Flett GM, Templeton A. A randomised controlled trial of mifepristone in combination with misoprostol administered sublingually or vaginally for medical abortion up to 13 weeks of gestation. BJOG. 2005;112:1102–8.

66. Raghavan S, Comendant R, Digol I, Ungureanu S, Friptu V, Bracken H, et al. Two-pill regimens of misprostol after mifepristone medical abortion through 63 days' gestational age: a randomized controlled trial of sublingual and oral misoprostol. Contraception. 2009;79:84–90.

67. Schaff EA, Fielding SL, Westhoff C, Ellertson C, Eisinger SH, Stadallus LS, et al. Vaginal misoprostol administered 1, 2, or 3 days after mifepristone for early medical abortion: A randomized trial. JAMA. 2000;284:1948–53.

68. Creinin MD, Fox MC, Teal S, Chen A, Schaff EA, Meyn LA; MOD Study Trial Group. A randomized comparison of misoprostol 6 to 8 hours versus 24 hours after mifepristone for abortion. Obstet Gynecol. 2004;103:851–9.

69. Fischer M, Bhatnagar J, Guarner J, Reagan S, Hacker JK, Van Meter SH, et al. Fatal toxic shock syndrome associated with Clostridium sordellii after medical abortion. N Engl J Med. 2005;353:2352–60.

70. Cohen AL, Bhatnagar J, Reagan S, Zane SB, D'Angeli MA, Fischer M, et al. Toxic shock associated with Clostridium sordellii and Clostridium perfringens after medical and spontaneous abortion. Obstet Gynecol. 2007;110:1027–33.

71. Fjerstad M, Sivin I, Lichtenberg ES, Trussell J, Cleland K, Cullins V. Effectiveness of medical abortion with mifepristone and buccal misoprostol through 59 gestational days. Contraception. 2009;80:282–6.

72. Kahn JG, Becker BJ, MacIsaac L, Amory JK, Neuhaus J, Olkin I, et al. The efficacy of medical abortion: a meta-analysis. Contraception. 2000;61:29–40.

73. Creinin MD, Vittinghoff E, Schaff E, Klaisle C, Darney PD, Dean C. Medical abortion with oral methotrexate and vaginal misoprostol. Obstet Gynecol. 1997;90:611–6.

74. Wiebe ER. Oral methotrexate compared with injected methotrexate when used with misoprostol for abortion. Am J Obstet Gynecol. 1999;181:149–52.

75. Miller SE, Lehman T, Campbell M, Hemmerling A, Anderson SB, Rodriguez H, et al. Misoprostol and declining abortion-related morbidity in Santo Domingo, Dominican Republic: a temporal association. BJOG. 2005;112:1291–6.

76. Moreno-Ruiz NL, Borgatta L, Yanow S, Kapp N, Wiebe ER, Winikoff B. Alternatives to mifepristone for early medical abortion. Int J Gynaecol Obstet. 2007;96:212–8.

77. von Hertzen H, Piaggio G, Huong NT, Arustamyan K, Cabezas E, Gomez M, et al; WHO Research Group on Postovulatory Methods of Fertility Regulation. Efficacy of two intervals and two routes of administration of misoprostol for termination of early pregnancy: a randomised controlled equivalence trial. Lancet. 2007;369: 1938–46.

78. Rosing MA, Archbald CD. The knowledge, acceptability, and use of misoprostol for self-induced medical abortion in an urban US population. J Am Med Womens Assoc. 2000;55:183–5.

79. Creinin MD, Shulman T. Effect of nonsteroidal anti-inflammatory drugs on the action of misoprostol in a regimen for early abortion. Contraception. 1997;56:165–8.

80. Tang OS, Lee SW, Ho PC. A prospective randomized study on the measured blood loss in medical termination of early pregnancy by three different misoprostol regimens after pretreatment with mifepristone. Hum Reprod. 2002;17:2865–8.

81. Davis A, Westhoff C, de Nonno L. Bleeding patterns after early abortion with mifepristone and misoprostol or manual vacuum aspiration. J Am Med Womens Assoc. 2000;55 Suppl 3:141–4.

82. Tang OS, Gao PP, Cheng L, Lee SW, Ho PC. A randomized double-blind placebo-controlled study to assess the effect of oral contraceptive pills on the outcome of medical abortion with mifepristone and misoprostol. Hum Reprod. 1999;14:722–5.

83. Allen RH, Westhoff C, DeNonno L, Fielding SL, Schaff EA. Curettage after mifepristone-induced abortion: frequency, timing, and indications. Obstet Gynecol. 2001;98:101–6.

84. Henderson JT, Hwang AC, Harper CC, Stewart FH. Safety of mifepristone abortions in clinical use. Contraception. 2005;72:175–8.

85. Perriera LK, Reeves MF, Chen BA, Hohmann HL, Hayes J, Creinin MD. Feasibility of telephone follow-up after medical abortion. Contraception. 2010;81:143–9.

86. Clark W, Bracken H, Tanenhaus J, Schweikert S, Lichtenberg ES, Winikoff B. Alternatives to a routine follow-up visit for early medical abortion. Obstet Gynecol. 2010;115:264–72.

87. Rossi B, Creinin MD, Meyn LA. Ability of the clinician and patient to predict the outcome of mifepristone and misoprostol medical abortion. Contraception. 2004;70:313–7.

88. Cowett AA, Cohen LS, Lichtenberg S, Stika CS. Ultrasound evaluation of the endometrium after medical termination of pregnancy. Obstet Gynecol. 2004;103:871–5.

89. Fiala C, Safar P, Bygdeman M, Gemzell-Danielsson K. Verifying the effectiveness of medical abortion; ultrasound versus hCG testing. Eur J Obstet Gynecol Reprod Biol. 2003;109:190–5.

90. Godfrey EM, Anderson A, Fielding SL, Meyn L, Creinin MD. Clinical utility of urine pregnancy assays to determine medical abortion outcome is limited. Contraception. 2007;75:378–82.

91. Weitz T, Anderson P, Taylor D. Advancing scope of practice for advanced practice clinicians: more than a matter of access. Contraception. 2009;80:105–7.

92. Goldberg AB, Dean G, Kang MS, Youssof S, Darney PD. Manual versus electric vacuum aspiration for early first-trimester abortion: a controlled study of complication rates. Obstet Gynecol. 2004;103:101–7.

93. Wen J, Cai QY, Deng F, Li YP. Manual versus electric vacuum aspiration for first-trimester abortion: a systematic review. BJOG. 2008;115:5–13.

94. Bird ST, Harvey SM, Beckman LJ, Nichols MD, Rogers K, Blumenthal PD. Similarities in women's perceptions and acceptability of manual vacuum aspiration and electric vacuum aspiration for first trimester abortion. Contraception. 2003;67:207–12.

95. Dean G, Cardenas L, Darney P, Goldberg,A. Acceptability of manual versus electric aspiration for first trimester abortion: a randomized trial. Contraception. 2003;67: 201–6.

96. Bird ST, Harvey SM, Nichols MD, Edelman A. Comparing the acceptability of manual vacuum aspiration and electric vacuum aspiration as methods of early abortion. J Am Med Womens Assoc. 2001;56:124–6.

97. Edelman A, Nichols MD, Jensen J. Comparison of pain and time of procedures with two first-trimester abortion techniques performed by residents and faculty. Am J Obstet Gynecol. 2001;184:1564–7.

98. Lundh C, Meirik O, Nygren KG. Vaginal cleansing at vacuum aspiration abortion does not reduce the risk of postoperative infection. Acta Obstet Gynecol Scand. 1983;62:275–7.

99. Varli IH, Lindelius A, Bergstrom A. Is preoperative vaginal cleansing necessary for control of infection after first trimester vacuum curettage? Acta Obstet Gynecol Scand. 2005;84:650–3.

100. Meckstroth K, Paul M. First trimester aspiration abortion. In: Paul M, Lichtenberg ES, Borgatta L, Grimes DA, Stubblefield PG, Creinin MD, (editors). Management of unintended and abnormal pregnancy: Comprehensive abortion care. Oxford: Wiley-Blackwell; 2009. p. 135–56.

101. Renner RM, Jensen JT, Nichols MD, Edelman AB. Pain control in first-trimester surgical abortion: a systematic review of randomized controlled trials. Contraception. 2010;81:372–88.

102. Grimes DA, Smith SM, Witham AD. Mifepristone and misoprostol versus dilation and evacuation for midtrimester abortion: a pilot randomised controlled trial. BJOG. 2004;111:148–53.

103. Grimes DA, Schulz KF, Cates W Jr, Tyler CW Jr. Mid-trimester abortion by dilatation and evacuation: a safe and practical alternative. N Engl J Med. 1977;296:1141–5.

104. Grimes DA, Schulz KF. Morbidity and mortality from second-trimester abortions. J Reprod Med. 1985;30:505–14.

105. Autry AM, Hayes EC, Jacobson GF, Kirby RS. A comparison of medical induction and dilation and evacuation for second-trimester abortion. Am J Obstet Gynecol. 2002;187:393–7.

106. Ho PC, Blumenthal PD, Gemzell-Danielsson K, Gomez Ponce de Leon R, Mittal S, Tang OS. Misoprostol for the termination of pregnancy with a live fetus at 13 to 26 weeks. Int J Gynaecol Obstet. 2007;99 Suppl 2:S178–81.

107. Kapp N, von Hertzen H. Medical methods to induce abortion in the second trimester. In:Paul M, Lichtenberg ES, Borgatta L, Grimes DA, Stubblefield PG, Creinin MD, (editors). Management of unintended and abnormal pregnancy: Comprehensive abortion care. Oxford: Wiley-Blackwell; 2009. p. 178–92.

108. Kapp N, Borgatta L, Stubblefield P, Vragovic O, Moreno N. Mifepristone in second-trimester medical abortion: a randomized controlled trial. Obstet Gynecol. 2007;110: 1304–10.

109. Ashok PW, Templeton A, Wagaarachchi PT, Flett GM. Midtrimester medical termination of pregnancy: a review of 1002 consecutive cases. Contraception. 2004;69:51–8.

110. Winkler CL, Gray SE, Hauth JC, Owen J, Tucker JM. Mid-second-trimester labor induction: concentrated oxytocin compared with prostaglandin E2 vaginal suppositories. Obstet Gynecol. 1991;77:297–300.

111. Nuthalapaty FS, Ramsey PS, Biggio JR, Owen J. High-dose vaginal misoprostol versus concentrated oxytocin plus low-dose vaginal misoprostol for midtrimestrer labor induction: a randomized trial. Am J Obstet Gynecol. 2005;193:1065–70.

112. Schulz KF, Grimes DA, Cates W Jr. Measures to prevent cervical injury during suction curettage abortion. Lancet. 1983;1:1182–5.

113. Grimes DA, Schulz KF, Cates WJ Jr. Prevention of uterine perforation during curettage abortion. JAMA. 1984;251:2108–11.

114. Allen RH, Goldberg AB; Board of Society of Family Planning. Cervical dilation before first-trimester surgical abortion (<14 weeks' gestation). Contraception. 2007;76:139–56.

115. Fox MC, Hayes JL; Society of Family Planning. Cervical preparation for second-trimester surgical abortion prior to 20 weeks of gestation. SFP Guidance 20071. Contraception. 2007;76:486–95.
116. MacIsaac L, Grossman D, Balistreri E, Darney P. A randomized controlled trial of laminaria, oral misoprostol, and vaginal misoprostol before abortion. Obstet Gynecol.1999;93 (5 Pt 1):766–70.
117. Carbonell Esteve JL, Mari JM, Valero F, Llorente M, Salvador I, Varela L, et al. Sublingual versus vaginal misoprostol (400 microg) for cervical priming in first-trimester abortion: a randomized trial. Contraception. 2006;74:328–33.
118. Kapp N, Lohr PA, Ngo TD, Hayes JL. Cervical preparation for first trimester surgical abortion. Cochrane Database Syst Rev. 2010; 2:CD007207.
119. Tang OS, Mok KH, Ho PC. A randomized study comparing the use of sublingual to vaginal misoprostol for pre-operative cervical priming prior to surgical termination of pregnancy in the first trimester. Hum Reprod. 2004;19:1101–4.
120. Panchal HB, Godfrey EM, Patel A. Buccal misoprostol for cervical ripening prior to first trimester abortion. Contraception. 2010;81:161–4.
121. Ashok PW, Flett GM, Templeton A. Mifepristone versus vaginally administered misoprostol for cervical priming before first-trimester termination of pregnancy: a randomized, controlled trial. Am J Obstet Gynecol. 2000;183:998–1002.
122. Nucatola D, Roth N, Saulsberry V, Gatter M. Serious adverse events associated with the use of misoprostol alone for cervical preparation prior to early second trimester surgical abortion (12–16 weeks). Contraception. 2008;78:245–8.
123. Patel A, Talmont E, Morfesis J, Pelta M, Gatter M, Momtaz MR, et al.; Planned Parenthood Federation of America Buccal Misoprostol Waiver Group. Adequacy and safety of buccal misoprostol for cervical preparation prior to termination of second-trimester pregnancy. Contraception. 2006;73:420–30.
124. Goldberg AB, Drey EA, Whitaker AK, Kang MS, Meckstroth KR, Darney PD. Misoprostol compared with laminaria before early second-trimester surgical abortion: a randomized trial. Obstet Gynecol. 2005;106:234–41.
125. Schulz KF, Grimes DA, Christensen DD. Vasopressin reduces blood loss from second-trimester dilatation and evacuation abortion. Lancet. 1985;2:353–6.
126. O'Connell K, Jones HE, Lichtenberg ES, Paul M. Second-trimester surgical abortion practices: a survey of National Abortion Federation members. Contraception. 2008:78:492–9.
127. Bartlett LA, Berg CJ, Shulman HB, Zane SB, Green CA, Whitehead S, et al. Risk factors for legal induced abortion-related mortality in the United States. Obstet Gynecol. 2004;103:729–37.
128. Grimes DA. Estimation of pregnancy-related mortality risk by pregnancy outcome, United States, 1991 to 1999. Am J Obstet Gynecol. 2006;194:92–4.
129. Hakim-Elahi E, Tovell HM, Burnhill MS. Complications of first-trimester abortion: a report of 170,000 cases. Obstet Gynecol. 1990;76:129–35.
130. Fjerstad M, Trussell J, Sivin I, Lichtenberg ES, Cullins V. Rates of serious infection after changes in regimens for medical abortion. N Engl J Med. 2009;361:145–51.
131. Meites E, Zane S, Gould C. Fatal Clostridium sordellii infections after medical abortions [letter]. N Engl J Med. 2010;363:1382-3.
132. Sinave C, Le Templier G, Blouin D, Leveille F, Deland E. Toxic shock syndrome due to *Clostridium sordellii*: a dramatic postpartum and postabortion disease. Clin Infect Dis. 2002;35:1441–3.
133. Shannon C, Brothers LP, Philip NM, Winikoff B. Ectopic pregnancy and medical abortion. Obstet Gynecol. 2004;104:161–7.
134. Ho CS, Bhatnagar J, Cohen AL, Hacker JK, Zane SB, Reagan S, et al. Undiagnosed cases of fatal Clostridium-associated toxic shock in Californian women of childbearing age. Am J Obstet Gynecol. 2009;201:459.e1–7. Epub 2009 Jul 22.

135. Lichtenberg ES, Grimes DA. Surgical complications: Prevention and management. In: Paul M, Lichtenberg ES, Borgatta L, Grimes DA, Stubblefield PG, Creinin MD, (editors). Management of unintended and abnormal pregnancy: Comprehensive abortion care. Oxford: Blackwell-Wiley; 2009. p. 224–51.

136. Goyal V. Uterine rupture in second-trimester misoprostol-induced abortion after cesarean delivery: a systematic review. Obstet Gynecol. 2009;113:1117–23.

137. Shannon C, Brothers LP, Philip NM, Winikoff B. Infection after medical abortion: a review of the literature. Contraception. 2004;70:183–90.

138. Sawaya GF, Grady D, Kerlikowske K, Grimes DA. Antibiotics at the time of induced abortion: the case for universal prophylaxis based on a meta-analysis. Obstet Gynecol. 1996;87 (5 Pt 2):884–90.

139. Lichtenberg ES, Shott S. A randomized clinical trial of prophylaxis for vacuum abortion: 3 versus 7 days of doxycycline. Obstet Gynecol. 2003;101:726–31.

140. Wilson W, Taubert KA, Gewitz M, Lockhart PB, Baddour LM, Levison M, et al.; American Heart Association Rheumatic Fever, Endocarditis, and Kawasaki Disease Committee; American Heart Association Council on Cardiovascular Disease in the Young; American Heart Association Council on Clinical Cardiology; American Heart Association Council on Cardiovascular Surgery and Anesthesia; Quality of Care and Outcomes Research Interdisciplinary Working Group. Prevention of infective endocarditis: Guidelines from the American Heart Association. Circulation. 2007;116: 1736–54.

141. Hogue CJR, Boardman LA, Stotland N. Answering questions about long-term outcomes. In: Paul M, Lichtenberg ES, Borgatta L, Grimes DA, Stubblefield PG, Creinin MD (editors). Management of unintended and abnormal pregnancy: Comprehensive abortion care. Oxford: Blackwell-Wiley; 2009. p. 252–63.

142. Atrash HK, Hogue CJ. The effect of pregnancy termination on future reproduction. Baillieres Clin Obstet Gynaecol. 1990;4:391–405.

143. Moreau C, Kaminski M, Ancel PY, Bouyer J, Escande B, Thiriez G, et al.; EPIPAGE Group. Previous induced abortions and the risk of very preterm delivery: results of the EPIPAGE study. BJOG. 2005;112:430–7.

144. Zhou W, Sorensen HT, Olsen J. Induced abortion and subsequent pregnancy duration. Obstet Gynecol.1999;94:948–53.

145. Raatikainen K, Heiskanen N, Heinonen S. Induced abortion: not an independent risk factor for pregnancy outcome, but a challenge for health counseling. Ann Epidemiol. 2006;16:587–92.

146. Kalish RB, Chasen ST, Rosenzweig LB, Rashbaum WK, Chervenak FA. Impact of midtrimester dilation and evacuation on subsequent pregnancy outcome. Am J Obstet Gynecol. 2002;187:882–5.

147. Virk J, Zhang J, Olsen J. Medical abortion and the risk of subsequent adverse pregnancy outcomes. N Engl J Med. 2007;357:648–53.

148. Chen A, Yuan W, Meirik O, Wang X, Wu SZ, Zhou L. Mifepristone-induced early abortion and outcome of subsequent wanted pregnancy. Am J Epidemiol. 2004;160:110–7.

149. American Psychological Association, Task Force on Mental Health and Abortion. Report of the APA task force on mental health and abortion [Internet]. Washington: American Psychological Association; 2008 [cited 2010 Apr 30]. Available from: http://www.apa.org/pi/women/programs/abortion/mental-health.pdf.

150. Charles VE, Polis CB, Sridhara SK, Blum RW. Abortion and long-term mental health outcomes: a systematic review of the evidence. Contraception. 2008;78:436–50

151. Major B, Applebaum M, Beckman L, Dutton MA, Russo NF, West C. Abortion and mental health: evaluating the evidence. Am Psychol. 2009;64:863–90.

152. Stotland NL. The myth of the abortion trauma syndrome. JAMA. 1992;268:2078–9.

153. Major B, Cozzarelli C, Cooper L, Zubek J, Richards C, Wilhite M, et al. Psychological responses of women after first-trimester abortion. Arch Gen Psychiatry. 2000;57: 777–84.

154. Adler NE. Abortion and the null hypothesis. Arch Gen Psychiatry. 2000;57:785–6.
155. Urquhart DR, Templeton AA. Psychiatric morbidity and acceptability following medical and surgical methods of induced abortion. Br J Obstet Gynaecol. 1991;98: 396–9.
156. Gilchrest AC, Hannaford PC, Frank P, Kay CR. Termination of pregnancy and psychiatric morbidity. Br J Psychiatry. 1995;167:243–8.
157. Henshaw R, Naji S, Russell I, Templeton A. Psychological responses following medical abortion (using mifepristone and gemeprost) and surgical vacuum aspiration: a patient-centered, partially randomised prospective study. Acta Obstet Gynecol Scand. 1994;73:812–8.
158. Kero A, Hogberg U, Lalos A. Wellbeing and mental growth–long-term effects of legal abortion. Soc Sci Med. 2004;58:2559–69.
159. Ashok PW, Hamoda H, Flett GM, Kidd A, Fitzmaurice A, Templeton A. Psychological sequelae of medical and surgical abortion at 10–13 weeks gestation. Acta Obstet Gynecol Scand. 2005;84:761–6.
160. Lowenstein L, Deutsch M, Gruberg R, Solt I, Yagil Y, Nevo O, et al. Psychological distress symptoms in women undergoing medical vs. surgical termination of pregnancy. Gen Hosp Psychiatry. 2006;28:43–7.
161. Sit D, Rothschild AJ, Creinin MD, Hanusa BH, Wisner KL. Psychiatric outcomes following medical and surgical abortion. Hum Reprod. 2007;22:878–84.
162. Melbye M, Wohlfahrt J, Olsen JH, Frisch M, Westergaard T, Helweg-Larsen K, et al. Induced abortion and the risk of breast cancer. N Engl J Med. 1997;336:81–5.
163. Michels KB, Xue F, Colditz GA, Willet WC. Induced and spontaneous abortion and incidence of breast cancer among young women: a prospective cohort study. Arch Intern Med. 2007;167:814–20.
164. Beral V, Bull D, Doll R, Peto R, Reeves G; Collaborative Group on Hormonal Factors in Breast Cancer. Breast cancer and abortion: collaborative reanalysis of data from 53 epidemiological studies, including 83,000 women with breast cancer from 16 countries. Lancet. 2004;363:1007–16.
165. National Cancer Institute. Abortion, miscarriage, and breast cancer risk [Internet]. Washington: National Cancer Institute; [updated 2010 Jan; cited 2010 Apr 30]. Available from: http://www.cancer.gov/cancertopics/factsheet/Risk/abortion-miscarriage.
166. American College of Obstetricians and Gynecologists. Induced abortion and breast cancer risk. ACOG Committee Opinion No. 434, June 2009.

Perimenopause, Menopause and Postmenopause: Health Promotion Strategies

Anita L. Nelson, MD

- The diagnosis of perimenopause is a clinical one. Its onset is heralded by changes in menstrual cyclicity, onset of vasomotor or related symptoms, or reduced fertility.

- Hormone levels fluctuate rapidly and erratically during perimenopause. Therefore, measuring gonadotropins or sex steroids is not only unnecessary to make the diagnosis, but may lead to a misdiagnosis.

- Many perimenopausal women need effective contraception. Hormonal methods provide significant noncontraceptive benefits to many women at this time of life.

- The most important health message for perimenopausal and postmenopausal women is to adopt and maintain healthy lifestyles.

- Clinicians should identify women who are at increased risk for breast cancer (using the Gail model) and postmenopausal women at increased risk for fracture (using the FRAX model), so those women may be given therapies to reduce their chances of developing those serious diseases.

- Postmenopausal hormone therapy is given to treat specific symptoms. In healthy, newly menopausal women, short-term use is not associated with any of the increased risks seen in the overall population of women who participated in studies of the Women's Health Initiative, except perhaps for the risk for venous thromboembolism.

- Other nonhormonal therapies by prescription are effective in reducing vasomotor symptoms and in reducing osteoporosis fracture risk, but most of the herbal therapies have been shown to be no more effective than placebo.

Most women entering menopause today are reasonably healthy. Health challenges during the perimenopausal and postmenopausal years are important because there are so many women (baby boomers) now moving into and through these years that the public health implications and the financial implications are enormous. From both the medical and societal perspectives, this is uncharted water. Never in history has there been an expectation that women would spend one third of their lives after menopause. Health habits established during the perimenopausal and the early postmenopausal years can determine the woman's health status and quality of life for her elderly years when serious health problems (and costs) are greatest.

PERIMENOPAUSE

Perimenopause starts when a woman first experiences menstrual irregularities or other symptoms that reflect her diminishing ovarian reserve. Perimenopause ends 12 months after her final menstrual period (menopause), when she becomes, by definition, postmenopausal.

PERIMENOPAUSAL PHYSIOLOGY

Each woman travels her own unique course through perimenopause, but the changes she experiences reflect both changes in the ovary and dysfunction in the hypothalamic pituitary ovarian axis.[1] Women who experienced regular cycling in their 20s and 30s often notice subtle changes in their menstrual cycles starting in their late 30s and early 40s. At first, there may be a reduction in the interval between their menstrual periods and, later, an irregular and longer spacing between menses, as more cycles are anovulatory. Menses can become irregular, heavy, and prolonged enough to require evaluation, intervention, and occasionally, surgical therapy.

Entering puberty, each woman has about 900,000 ovarian follicles; she exits her reproductive years at menopause with only a few thousand. Every day, follicles are recruited regardless of whether a woman is cycling, using hormonal contraceptives, or is pregnant. The follicles that are most responsive to follicle stimulating hormone (FSH) are recruited early in a woman's reproductive life. Most follicles undergo atresia; only a few hundred ever advance to become dominant follicles with potential for ovulation. The earliest manifestation of functional ovarian changes begins by age 35 to 37 when fewer follicles are left. In general, those remaining follicles are less responsive and require higher levels of FSH to recruit them. FSH levels are able to rise because the remaining follicles produce lower levels of estradiol and inhibin B and do not provide as much negative feedback to the hypothalamus and the pituitary. (See Chapter 2 on The Menstrual Cycle.) Starting in the mid-30s, the reservoir of primordial follicles available for recruitment starts to deplete at an accelerated rate.[2]

FSH levels (especially on cycle day 3) have been used to assess a woman's fertility potential:

- FSH levels below 10 on cycle day 3 indicate good ovarian reserve.

- FSH levels greater than 25 indicate virtually no potential for ovulation, even with ovulation induction.

- Intermediate values (between 10–25) indicate reduced fertility.

Other markers have been found to be useful in assessing ovarian reserve in women, particularly in those with infertility. Anti-müllerian hormone (AMH) and inhibin B are the most commonly used tests because they decline as menopause approaches.[3,4] AMH can be drawn at any time in the menstrual cycle and predicts, within 5 years, the onset of menopause. Inhibin B must be drawn in the follicular phase.[5] Low antral follicle count seen on ultrasound also predicts low ovarian reserve.[5–7]

Fertility per cycle starts to decline in women by age 35 to 40, usually even before any menstrual disorders or hot flashes develop. In Hutterite populations with unregulated fertility, 11% of women had their last pregnancy before age 34, and 33% completed childbearing before age 40; only about 13% had any pregnancies after age 45.[8] In donor insemination programs, women under age 31 had annual pregnancy rates of 74%; women over age 35 had rates of 54%.[9]

Years before menopause, a woman can begin to experience dramatic fluctuations in gonadotropins and estrogen, replacing the expected pattern of GnRH pulses and the orderly, predictable pattern of estradiol production. Collectively, these fluctuations have been characterized as "hormonal chaos."[10] The *fluctuations* in estrogen levels are responsible for vasomotor symptoms and for the disturbances seen in bleeding patterns experienced by some perimenopausal women. In particular, as estrogen levels *drop*, the woman may experience hot flashes and unscheduled spotting and bleeding. As more of the cycles are anovulatory in the last few years approaching menopause, cycle length increases. For healthy U.S. women, mean cycle lengths in the 4 years prior to menopause have been reported to be 30.48, 35.02, 45.15, and 80.22 days.[11] However, contrary to prevailing opinion, newer studies have revealed that the heavy, prolonged bleeding episodes during these years do not occur during anovulatory cycles, but rather are more likely to occur during ovulatory ones.[12]

Although perimenopause is a useful term to describe the years during which women experience these hormonal changes, the diagnosis of perimenopause is a clinical one. Just as the changes that occur following the woman's first period are fully expected and do not need testing of go-nadotropin or sex steroid levels for confirmation, the changes that occur approaching the final menses are expected and testing is needed only when history and physical exam suggest other etiologies (e.g., tuberculosis, thyroid dysfunction). Because sex steroid and gonadotropin levels vary so dramatically from day to day, their measurement using blood, saliva or any other body fluid is not necessary and may even lead to an incorrect diagnosis. In one longitudinal study of woman's hormone levels for 180 days, the irregular patterns of FSH and estrone showed days when the FSH was so very high and the estrogen was so low that together they were consistent with the diagnosis of menopause, but the woman was still capable of ovulation.[10] Unexpected ovulation in a woman who has been told she was menopausal could have serious consequences.

PERIMENOPAUSAL HEALTH PROMOTION: LIFESTYLE ISSUES

Most women in their perimenopausal years consider themselves to be in reasonably good health; however, often they need to be encouraged to adopt or maintain long-term healthy lifestyles prior to menopause to optimize their health later in life.

Obesity is a major health problem in the United States. It has been calculated that if current U.S. trends continue, obesity's negative effects will cancel out all the gains made in the past decades from smoking cessation.[13] Among women aged 20 to 39, 27.5% are obese (BMI ≥ 30) and 22% are overweight (BMI 25–29.9). Among women aged 40 to 59, 34.3% are obese and 28% are overweight. That leaves only one third of women in this transitional age group with normal weight. Among women over age 60, the weight groups shift slightly, and 33% are obese and 35% are overweight; however, just as with younger women, less than one in three women has a normal weight. African American women have greater obesity rates; over 50% in the over 40 age group are obese, and only about 20% have normal weight. Among Hispanic women over 40, an even greater proportion is overweight and few women have normal weight.[14] Obesity has been associated with worse menopausal symptoms, psychological and sexuality scores, general health care, and quality of life.[15]

A decrease in ovulatory cycling may make it more challenging for women in their 40s and 50s to lose weight. During the luteal phase, a woman's resting metabolic rate increases. Without that increase in metabolism in the second half of the menstrual cycle, more of a woman's caloric intake is stored as fat and less is burned for energy. Other factors are also important. In one interesting study of midlife and older women, respondents said they would eat more than they wanted because they strongly object to letting food go to waste. Family responsibilities and preferences were also major barriers to physical activity and heart-healthy eating.[16]

Encourage a weight-loss diet that your patient can maintain. Reduced caloric diets result in clinically meaningful weight loss independent of the macronutrient they emphasize.[17] Promote exercise, not only to contribute to weight control and to improve cardiovascular health, but also to enhance bone remodeling and to strengthen muscles for balance. A recent analysis found that women in this age group may need at least one hour of exercise a day to avoid weight gain if they do not diet.[18] Unfortunately, as many as 70% to 80% of older U.S. women do not even exercise 45 minutes, 3 times a week.[19]

Screen for signs of stress and depression. Also screen for smoking and passive smoking exposure. In a recent study evaluating the relative health burdens of social and behavioral risk factors, the greatest burden of disease in the United States came from poverty, smoking, and low educational status (lack of a high-school diploma).[20] Smoking addiction can be medically treated.

REPRODUCTIVE CARCINOMA DURING THE PERIMENOPAUSAL YEARS

Recommendations for reproductive system cancer screening have undergone significant changes in recent years, as the pathophysiology of the different cancers has become better understood (cervical and ovarian cancers), as the effectiveness of prior screening strategies has been re-evaluated (breast cancer), and as risk factors for disease have increased (endometrial carcinoma). The specific recommendations for routine screening for female genital tract cancers are described in detail in Chapter 22.

In general, screening protocols are different for women who are identified as being at low risk compared with women who are at higher risk for developing a given cancer. For example, the screening recommendations for women who are known to be persistently infected with high-risk human papilloma virus (HPV) are different from those for women who are not so infected. Women who are BRAC-1 or BRAC-2 mutation carriers who have not completed childbearing need more sensitive and more comprehensive testing; these women need screening with MRI for breast cancer and at least annual pelvic ultrasound studies to identify ovarian, and possibly, fallopian tube carcinoma.[21] A woman with hereditary nonpolyposis colorectal carcinoma may need annual endometrial biopsies starting at age 35 and until she undergoes a prophylactic hysterectomy.

Care for women with extremely high risk for developing cancer is best provided by specialists. Care for women with moderately increased risk and those with risks of the general population can well be provided by generalists. However, it is important to identify these two groups. A patient's perception of her own risks is often incorrect. In general, women tend to overestimate the impact of breast cancer. A 2009 poll revealed that 40% of women estimated that the risk of developing breast cancer between age 40 and 50 was somewhere between 20% and 50%. In reality, the risk of developing breast cancer during those years is only 1.4%.

Clinicians need to systematically review the patient's personal and family history to identify women who are at moderate risk because very effective medical therapies can profoundly reduce their chance of developing breast cancer. Use the Gail model to calculate each woman's individual 5-year and lifetime risk of breast cancer. Calculations can be made by entering the answers to the questions asked on Table 25–1 into a computer model available at www.bcra.nci.nih.gov/brc/start.htm. This model can be downloaded to local computers. Offer chemoprophylaxis to women whose 5-year risk of developing breast cancer is greater than 1.66%. Strongly encourage those with a 5-year risk in excess of 5% to use chemopreventative agents.[22]

Two different selective estrogen receptor modulators (SERMs)—tamoxifen and raloxifene—are currently used to treat women with elevated 5-year risks for developing breast cancer:

- *Tamoxifen* is the preferred agent for premenopausal women. Its use decreases both invasive and in situ disease by almost 50%.The risk of developing estrogen/progesterone receptor pos-

Table 25–1 Breast cancer risk assessment questions to calculate a woman's risk for next 5 years and over her lifetime

1. Does the woman have a medical history of any breast cancer or of ductal carcinoma in situ (DCIS) or lobular carcinoma in situ (LCIS)?

2. What is the woman's age?

3. What was the woman's age at the time of her first menstrual period?

4. What was the woman's age at the time of her first live birth of a child?

5. How many of the woman's first-degree relatives—mother, sisters, daughters—have had breast cancer?

6. Has the woman ever had a breast biopsy?

    A. How many breast biopsies (positive or negative) has the woman had?

    B. Has the woman had at least one breast biopsy with atypical hyperplasia?

7. What is the woman's race/ethnicity?

National Cancer Institute (2010).[145]

itive cancers were even more dramatically diminished by tamoxifen. Tamoxifen also works well in postmenopausal women but is associated with an increased risk of endometrial carcinoma in that age group.[23,24] However, for postmenopausal women who have had a hysterectomy, tamoxifen may be an appropriate choice.

- *Raloxifene* carries FDA approval for prevention of breast cancer in postmenopausal women with osteoporosis. Raloxifene was compared with tamoxifen in the STAR study and was found to be as effective as tamoxifen in reducing the risk of invasive breast cancer. In contrast to tamoxifen, raloxifene did not reduce the risk of ductal carcinoma in situ (DCIS) or lobular carcinoma in situ (LCIS).[25] Raloxifene is not used for adjuvant therapy for women following conservative surgery, whereas tamoxifen is very helpful in this approach.[26]

Both raloxifene and tamoxifen increase the risk of venous thromboembolism, so patients taking either of these drugs need to advise their doctors that they need prophylaxis against venous thromboembolism if they ever need surgery or are immobilized.[27] Despite the proven ability of these SERMs to prevent breast cancer, a recent study found that in 2005 only 0.08% of U.S. women age 40 to 79 took tamoxifen to prevent breast cancer.

Other agents are being studied for their ability to prevent breast cancer in moderate-risk women. Another SERM, lasofoxifene, has been found to have promise.[28] Aromatase inhibitors, such as letrozole (which has shown clinical superiority to tamoxifen as adjuvant therapy to prevent ductal carcinoma recurrence) is another obvious candidate. One study concluded that bisphosphonates are associated with a reduced risk of breast cancer.[29]

PERIMENOPAUSAL BLEEDING CONTROL AND CONTRACEPTIVE OPTIONS

The topics of bleeding control and contraception are combined because they have an obvious synergy—hormonal birth control often treats bleeding. Excessive bleeding is a significant problem during the perimenopause period. Most women undergoing surgical therapies for heavy or prolonged bleeding (such as endometrial ablation and hysterectomy) are over 40 years of age. Some of these women have pelvic pathology (leiomyoma, atypical hyperplasia, adenomyosis), but the majority have only functional problems, better suited to medical management. A full list of treatments for excessive menstrual bleeding is provided in Chapter 20 on Menstrual Disorders, but we will summarize here various contraceptive methods that can be used to control the menstrual challenges that are so common during perimenopause.

Many women in their perimenopausal years are still at least intermittently at risk for pregnancy and need effective contraception. Nearly one third of pregnancies that occur in women over age 40 are terminated.[30] Unfortunately, studies show that women in their early 40s are twice as likely as women in their late 30s to report not using contraceptives.[31] In addition, hormonal contraception is often used to help women control other disturbing perimenopausal symptoms, including vasomotor symptoms and vulvovaginal atrophy.

Combined Hormonal Contraceptives

Healthy, normal weight, nonsmoking women can use combined hormonal contraceptives (pills, patches, and vaginal rings) until menopause. These methods will control the endometrium and maintain predictable cyclic bleeding. For women with adenomyosis, these methods also reduce the amount of blood loss and the pain experienced with menstruation (see Chapter 20). The progestin in combined hormonal contraceptive methods reduces a woman's risk of developing endometrial hyperplasia or endometrial and ovarian carcinoma, without increasing her risk of developing breast cancer.[32] However, if the woman is obese (as are over one third of U.S. women in their 40s), ACOG reminds us to recognize that both age and obesity are independent risk factors for venous thromboembolism and that estrogen-containing methods of contraceptives should be used by these women "with caution."[33]

Pills, patch or ring methods can provide excellent control of vasomotor symptoms. However, some women experience hot flashes during hormone-free days. For those women, reduce or eliminate the number of the hormone-free days. You can select a pill formulation with fewer placebo pills or have her start her next active pills in a conventional 28-day pack on the first day of each scheduled bleeding days. Alternatively, eliminate the hormone-free days with extended cycle use of either combination pills or vaginal contraceptive rings. There are many FDA-approved hormonal methods of birth control with variations in formulations to allow more individualized therapies.

An interesting question arises with the use of combined hormonal contraceptive methods that effectively treat a woman's perimenopausal or menopausal symptoms: how can you tell when she becomes menopausal and no longer needs the higher doses of hormones found in those contraceptives? The effects of the pill, patch, or ring will be completely gone 14 days after product cessation, so her FSH and estradiol levels will reflect her own status. However, because of the "hormonal chaos" that is perimenopause, testing these women is still fraught with the same problems presented by testing any other perimenopausal woman—the results may falsely diagnose menopause. Therefore, hormonal contraceptive methods may be continued until about age 50 to 52 unless the woman's risks with these methods exceed the benefits she is enjoying. If the risks are related to estrogen, switch her to a progestin-only method. Another option is to stop the hormonal birth control method, provide a barrier method and follow her clinically as you would any woman undergoing natural menopause (see discussion to follow).

Progestin-Only Methods

These methods as a group can be used by virtually every perimenopausal woman. There are very few medical contraindications to use of progestin-only methods. Only women with recent history (≤5 years) of breast cancer carry a category 4 rating by the U.S. MEC guidelines for progestin-only pills.[34] Women with medical problems that are increasingly common in these years (such as hypertension, diabetes, obesity, and tobacco smoking) are all candidates for most progestin methods. Another benefit that progestin-only methods provide is to protect the endometrium from unopposed estrogen stimulation. Contraceptive efficacy of progestin-only pills is the same in the typical-use efficacy of combined hormonal pills. The progestin-releasing IUD and implant provide top-tier pregnancy protection. The only major potential issue that progestin-only products raise is their impact on the menstrual cycle. None provides the predictable cyclic bleeding that is delivered by combined hormonal methods. The blood loss associated with the use of progestin-only methods is much healthier than the blood loss from anovulatory cycling that women in this age group experience. The progestin-only methods provide some relief from vasomotor symptoms, but less than do combined hormonal methods.

The levonorgestrel intrauterine contraceptive (LNg IUC) is the most effective medical treatment for heavy menstrual bleeding. In clinical trials, 85% of women with idiopathic heavy menstrual bleeding had normalization of monthly blood loss (<80 ml) and at least a 50% reduction in their blood loss. By 6 months of use, the LNg IUC users had a 71% reduction in median blood loss.[35] Longer use of the LNg IUC is associated with increasing rates of amenorrhea. By 5 years of use, 50% of users have no spotting or bleeding. Replacing the first LNg IUC with a new unit maintains the pattern of bleeding that the woman had established with her first unit.[36] Another very significant advantage of the LNg IUC in perimenopausal women is that estrogen therapy can be added to treat peri/postmenopausal symptoms without increasing her risk of endometrial cancer. A woman's uterus is protected by the LNg IUC from unopposed estrogen stimulation.[37,38] Use of the LNg IUC may be extended to at least 7 years if the woman is using it only for endometrial protection.

The contraceptive implant [ENG rod] provides top-tier contraceptive efficacy and is extremely convenient to use. The only contraindications to its use are current or recent breast cancer and use of drugs that increase cytochrome-P450 activity.[34] The etonogestrel-containing rod also provides progestin to control estrogen stimulation of the endometrium. However, unpredictable bleeding patterns with this implant may be less well tolerated by perimenopausal women than by younger women. In part, this may be because of enhanced clinician concern about unscheduled spotting and bleeding in perimenopausal women (reflected in high rates of biopsy for women with abnormal bleeding) and, in part, it may be the woman's own dislike of irregular bleeding, which may have bothered her prior to implant placement.

Depo-Provera (DMPA) can be used by perimenopausal women for both contraception and for treatment of excessive bleeding. After about 2 injections, nearly one half of women have no spotting or bleeding. The effect of DMPA may linger for months after the last injection. In postmenopausal estrogen-deficient women, DMPA provides some protection from loss of bone mineral density, but in perimenopausal women, it may diminish bone mineral density. Estrogen can be added to DMPA to help control vasomotor symptoms; however, routine use of estrogen is not needed for bone health because women who use DMPA just before menopause do not undergo the rapid loss of bone mineral density following menopause.[39]

Progestin-only pills are tremendously underutilized, especially in this patient population, for whom their safety and noncontraceptive benefits are particularly important. For example, in the short term, progestin-only pills are less expensive than intrauterine contraceptives and implants and are more rapidly reversible than injections. Taken daily, they can help reduce menstrual blood loss without increasing the frequency of bleeding episodes in perimenopausal women.

NONHORMONAL METHODS

The copper intrauterine contraceptive (IUC) provides convenient and excellent long-term pregnancy protection. Evidence also suggests that women who use the copper IUC are at lower risk of developing endometrial carcinoma. Placement of new copper IUC in a perimenopausal woman who only needs a few years of contraception and who may already be experiencing irregular or prolonged bleeding may not be a first-line choice. However, copper IUC users who are happy with their method in their perimenopausal years but are approaching their 10th year of use are excellent candidates for extended use of their IUCs. One recent report has shown that one copper IUC may be used for up to 20 years without any evidence of reduced efficacy; in that study, there were no pregnancies between years 8 and 20 of use.[40]

Barrier methods may seem to be very appropriate for women at this time in their lives when pregnancy risks are reduced and coital frequency may be somewhat diminished compared with earlier years. However, couples need to be asked about any erectile dysfunction, because the male condom may amplify that problem; many men lose their erection with condom placement. Women in the perimenopausal years may have pelvic relaxation, making the diaphragm more difficult to use. The female condom, the cervical Hat, and the contraceptive sponge may still be good barrier options. Coitus interruptus is a reasonable behavioral option for couples, especially those experienced in its use. However, fertility awareness methods are far less applicable in perimenopausal women whose cycle lengths are rapidly changing, unless the TwoDay Method is used to identify at-risk days. (See Chapter 16 on Fertility Awareness-based Methods.)

The benefits of sterilization are markedly reduced because women will need protection for only a few more years, while the risks of the procedure increase as women age.

PERIMENOPAUSAL SYMPTOMS

At least 15% to 40% of menstruating women in their 40s experience hot flashes, which are often as disturbing as those that occur after menopause. As mentioned above, women (and men) tend to become symptomatic when their estrogen levels decline rapidly. Absolute estrogen levels in themselves do not explain hot flashes: there is no difference in average estrogen levels between symptomatic and asymptomatic women.[41] The dropping estradiol levels can also be associated with poor sleep, hot flashes, higher anxiety, and depression, even in cycling reproductive-age women.

Healthy, nonsmoking perimenopausal women with persistent or severe vasomotor symptoms can be treated with combined hormonal contraceptives[42] or with postmenopausal doses of estrogen and progestin treatments, although the latter can worsen the menstrual abnormalities that often accompany perimenopause. As noted above, if a woman becomes symptomatic during the hormone-free week of combined hormonal contraceptive use, she can try reducing or eliminating the hormone-free days. Other approaches include combining postmenopausal estrogen therapy with a progestin-only contraceptive method such as DMPA or the LNg IUC. Nonhormonal treatment options, such as those discussed below for postmenopausal women, are also helpful for treating symptomatic perimenopausal women.

MENOPAUSE

Menopause means permanent cessation of menses following or in association with loss of ovarian activity. Menopause can be diagnosed in women in the following circumstances:

- Women who have had surgical removal of their ovaries

- Women with intact ovaries and uterus who have been amenorrheic for 1 year with no other cause

- Women who had a hysterectomy with ovarian preservation when estradiol production has decreased to a menopausal level

After menopause, women are no longer at risk for pregnancy since they have no more recruitable follicles, but this lack of follicles also results in decreased ovarian production of estrogen.

The median age of menopause in U.S. women is 51.3 years. Approximately 1% of women undergo menopause before age 40; at the other extreme, 2% of women are still menstruating at age 55. Menopause before age 30 (*premature ovarian insufficiency*) can be associated with chromosomal abnormalities (e.g., gonadal dysgenesis), so a genetic evaluation is appropriate in this situation. Premature ovarian insufficiency is a risk factor for significant medical problems, including osteoporosis and cardiovascular disease, and can be a personal tragedy for the woman who has not yet completed her desired childbearing, so accurate diagnosis is essential. *Premature menopause* (<40 years old) and *early menopause* (<45 years old) are strongly influenced by family history, but otherwise, the age of menopause does not follow a clear familial pattern and is generally not predictable. Women who smoke, have type-1 diabetes, live at high altitudes, or are undernourished or vegetarian undergo menopause at younger ages than do women without these risk factors.

HEALTH RISKS IN POSTMENOPAUSE

Most women, including those over age 50, are not well informed about their long-term health risks. In a 1997 telephone survey of U.S. women, 34% reported that breast cancer is the greatest health problem confronting women, while less than 8% reported that cardiovascular disease or stroke was a major concern.[43] Since then, there has been an improvement in American women's awareness of cardiovascular disease risk with 57% now recognizing cardiovascular disease as the leading cause of death. Sadly, only 53% said they would call 911 if they had chest pain.[44]

These misperceptions of real health hazards can be dangerous. Health care provider recommendations for smoking cessation, exercise, and dietary changes may be ignored because they have little impact on the woman's breast cancer susceptibility and because they may require profound, and often challenging, lifestyle modifications. On the other hand, women may be reluctant to use postmenopausal hormone therapy even in the short term, because they harbor inflated estimates of their baseline risks of developing breast cancer. Inform women of their true health risks, design appropriate interventions, and make referrals as needed.

Cardiovascular Health

Because cardiovascular disease (CVD) is such an enormous health problem,[45] it is important to identify risk factors for CVD. Many women have risk factors for CVD. In the United States, 25% of women are sedentary, 20% smoke, 52% over age 45 have hypertension, and 40% over age 55 have elevated cholesterol.[43] For women over 65, the picture is even more bleak: over 75% have hypertension and nearly 1 in 5 has diabetes. Rapid menopausal transition itself has been identified as a risk factor for atherosclerosis.[46]

Models are available to estimate a woman's 10-year risk of coronary artery disease (CAD) based on 5 major risk factors—family history of premature cardiovascular disease, low levels of high-density lipoprotein cholesterol (HDL-C <50mg/dL), age >55, smoking, and hypertension—plus calculation of the Framingham Risk score.[47,48] Women over 50 with one risk factor are considered to be at increased lifetime risk.[49] The prevalence of diabetes is important because diabetic women enter menopause with the same probabilities for heart attack and stroke as similarly aged men and should be treated *a priori* as if they have CAD.[45] Blood pressure control is critical in forestalling premature myocardial infarction (MI) and stroke; the upper limit for normal blood pressure in healthy women is 120 mmHg systolic and 80 mmHg diastolic. Statins have been shown to improve life expectancy in women with dyslipidemia, as well as those women with normal lipids but elevated C-reactive protein levels.[50] A recent study demonstrated that aerobic exercise reduced weight, total body fat and both intraperitoneal fat and subcutaneous fat in previously sedentary women.[51] However, because 59% of women over 55 have arthritis, recommendations for exercise need to be realistic.

Osteoporosis and Fracture

The rapid bone loss that women experience during the first 5 years of menopause has long been attributed to estrogen deficiency. Estrogen is known to suppress osteoclast activity and to slow bone reabsorption and turnover. It now appears that decreased levels of inhibin also contribute to that rapid loss.[52] Whatever the cause of bone loss, the outcome of concern is fracture. The most common fractures among women under age 65 are wrist or forearm fractures, which usually result when women extend their arms to brace their fall. Later in life, women frequently experience spontaneous vertebral crush fractures, which not only create painful spinal deformities, but also result in the loss of mobility and height, increased respiratory problems, and abdominal protrusion, which leads to dyspepsia. The most serious fracture site is the hip. Hip fractures generally occur later in life when women lose their sense of balance and are not able to block their falls. Women with osteopenia have twice the risk for hip fracture compared with women with normal bone mineral density (BMD), and women with osteoporosis have a nearly 9-fold increased risk.[53] The impacts of hip fracture can be devastating. A 70-year-old woman who suffers a hip fracture faces an 8% to 18% increase in her risk of dying within a year of the event. Quality of life is generally profoundly diminished. After the hip fracture, only 50% of the 70-year-old survivors completely heal; 25% are dependent on family members for care, and the remaining 25% are living in nursing homes. Older women have even worse outcomes. Hip fracture is the second most common reason older women need nursing home care.

Fracture Prevention Measures

Bone health measures should begin early in life. Weight-bearing exercise in moderation is critical to initiate the skeletal modeling and remodeling process. Smoking cessation is important, as is moderation in alcohol use. Later in life, other factors start to influence bone health. A critical as weight control is, it is important to know that weight loss by menopausal women reduces their bone mineral density.

All women 50 years and older should be evaluated for risk factors for osteoporosis. Offer prophylactic measures to all menopausal women, even women who enter menopause with robust bone. Therapies to prevent osteoporosis are most effective when initiated early in menopause, because the goal is to preserve the maximum bone density and strength to prevent future fractures.[54,55] Adequate calcium intake at all ages is needed to provide the building blocks to construct new bone. Menopausal women not using postmenopausal hormone therapy require 1,200 mg of calcium a day; those taking postmenopausal hormone therapy may need 1,000 mg. The typical American diet is deficient in calcium (see Table 25–2). Most women require daily supplements, which should be taken in divided doses; only 500 or 600 mg of calcium can be absorbed at any time. Calcium should be taken with food to maximize its absorption.

Because of extensive use of sunscreen for skin cancer prevention, vitamin D deficiencies are now widespread. People who live above latitude 52° require vitamin D supplementation from at least October to March, because the ultraviolet B radiation is filtered by the earth's atmosphere during those winter months. Elderly women and women who are housebound or unable to synthesize vitamin D may routinely need greater vitamin D supplementation, but studies show that even in Miami, many reproductive-aged women had vitamin D deficiency at the

Table 25–2 Dietary sources of calcium

Food	Serving	Calcium (mg)	% Daily Value
Cheddar cheese, shredded	1.5 oz.	306	31%
Milk, nonfat	8 fl oz.	302	30%
Yogurt, plain, low fat	8 oz.	300	30%
Milk, reduced fat (2% milk fat)	8 fl oz.	297	30%
Milk, whole (3.25% milk fat)	8 fl oz.	291	29%
Cottage cheese, 1% milk fat	2 cups	276	28%
Mozzarella, part skim	1.5 oz.	275	28%
Tofu, firm, with calcium	1.5 cups	275	28%
Orange juice, calcium fortified	6 fl oz.	200–260	20–26%
Salmon, pink, canned, solids with bone	3 oz.	181	18%
Tofu, soft, with calcium	0.5 cups	138	14%
Frozen yogurt, vanilla, soft serve	0.5 cup	103	10%
Turnip greens, boiled	0.5 cup	99	10%
Kale, cooked	1 cup	94	9%
Ice cream, vanilla	0.5 cup	85	8.5%
Soy beverage, calcium fortified	8 fl oz.	80–500	8–50%
Chinese cabbage, raw	1 cup	74	7%
Tortilla, corn, ready to bake/fry	1 medium	42	4%
Sour cream, reduced fat, cultured	2 tbsp.	32	3%
Broccoli, raw	0.5 cup	21	2%
Cream cheese, regular	1 tbsp.	12	1%

Adapted from Bone health and osteoporosis: a report of the Surgeon General (2004).[146]

end of winter. Smoking worsens the state of vitamin D in postmenopausal women. The latest RDA for vitamin D is 600 IU/day up to age 70 and 800 IU/day for ages 71 and older.[151]

As women age, other issues need to be addressed. To help prevent older women from falling, recommend home safety improvements such as removing loose rugs, rerouting wiring out of their pathways, installing lights over all stairways, and ensuring that porches, tubs and showers, and stairways have guardrails. (See Table 25–3.) Home safety guides are offered in English, Spanish, and Chinese at www.cdc.gov/pubs/ncipc.aspx. Recommend vision correction. If possible, avoid prescribing treatments that create ambulation problems such as hypotension or dizziness. A classic unfortunate combination of drugs is a sleeping aid with a diuretic. Hip protectors may be important in certain clinical situations.

Table 25–3 Home safety measures for fall prevention

Lighting
    Provide ample lighting
    Have easy-to-locate light switches for rooms and stairs
    Use night lights to illuminate pathways from bedroom to bathroom and kitchen
    Provide light on all stairways

Obstructions
    Remove clutter, low lying objects
    Remove raised door sills to ensure smooth transition

Floors and carpets
    Provide nonskid rugs on slippery floors
    Repair/replace worn, buckled, or curled carpet
    Use nonskid floor wax

Furniture
    Arrange furniture to ensure clear pathways
    Remove or avoid low chairs and armless chairs
    Adjust bed height if too high or low

Storage
    Install shelves and cupboards at accessible height
    Keep frequently used items at waist height

Bathroom
    Install grab bars in tub, shower, and near toilet
    Install chair in shower and tub
    Elevate low toilet seat or install safety frame

Stairways and halls
    Install handrails on both sides of stairs
    Remove or tape down throw rugs and runners
    Repair loose and broken steps
    Install nonskid treads on steps

Adapted from Home Safety Checklists (2010).[147]

Screening for bone mineral density (BMD) for osteoporosis is recommended for all women 65 years and older. Younger postmenopausal women should undergo BMD testing if they have 1 major or 2 minor risk factors for osteoporosis.[56] See Table 25–4 for recommendations for assessing BMD from the North American Menopausal Society.

Until recently, the most common tool to assess fracture risk has been to assess the woman's BMD by measuring calcium content at several different sites along her spine and her hips with a DEXA scan. For a postmenopausal woman, the BMD at each site measured by the DEXA is compared with the BMD of healthy young women to calculate the woman's T-score. The T-scores are used to stratify women into different

Table 25–4 Candidates for screening bone mineral density: North American Menopause Society recommendations

Routine screening recommended

All women over 65, regardless of clinical risk factors

Postmenopausal women with medical causes of bone loss (e.g., steroid use, hyperparathyroidism), regardless of age

Postmenopausal women with a fragility fracture (e.g., fracture from a fall from standing height or less)

Testing should be considered for postmenopausal women age 50 and over with one or more of the following risk factors:

Fracture after menopause (not skull, facial bone, ankle, finger and toe)

Body weight <127 lbs.; BMI <21

History of hip fracture in a parent

Current smoker

Rheumatoid arthritis

Alcohol intake of more than 2 units per day (one unit = 12 oz beer; 4 oz wine; 1 oz liquor)

North American Menopause Association (2010).[148]

risk groups. Women whose T-score is at least 2.5 standard deviations below normal are diagnosed as having *osteoporosis*. Women whose T-score is between 1.0 and 2.5 standard deviations below normal are diagnosed as having *osteopenia*. Every standard deviation in bone mineral density below normal is associated with more than a doubling risk of fracture.

Medical therapies for people with osteoporosis have shown significant efficacy in reducing the risk of fracture.[57] While treatment of people with osteoporosis is clearly justified, more fractures occur to people who have osteopenia than occur to people with osteoporosis, because there are so many more postmenopausal women with osteopenia. However, most people who have osteopenia will not suffer fracture, so universal treatment of all those with osteopenia is not warranted. It is clear that osteopenic women who are slender (<127 lbs or BMI <20) and those who have suffered a prior fracture have fracture risks similar to individuals with osteoporosis and should be treated. The challenge has been to identify which of the remaining osteopenic individuals are at high enough risk of fracture to justify treatment.

There is now agreement among most organizations that treatment should be given to individuals whose 10-year risk for fracturing a hip is at least 3% and those whose chance of fracturing any other major bone is at least 20%.[58–61] A woman's individual risk of fracture can now be calculated for women in different countries and of different ethnicities using the WHO Fracture Risk Assessment tool (FRAX). The FRAX algorithm requires selective information from the woman's personal and family

Table 25–5 WHO Fracture Risk Assessment Tool (FRAX)*

Age
Sex
Weight
Height
Parent hip fracture
Current smoking
Glucocorticoids
Rheumatoid arthritis
Secondary osteoporosis
Alcohol 3 or more units per day
BMD (g/cm²) at femur and spine or BMI

* www.shef.ac.uk/FRAX/index.htm

Adapted from the FRAX- WHO Assessment Fracture Risk Tool (2010).[149]

history (see Table 25–5). The FRAX calculator is available at www.nof.org. It combines the risk factor information from Table 25–5 with either the woman's bone mineral density (BMD) or (for women without access to DEXA scan) with her body mass index (BMI) to estimate her 10-year risk for hip fracture and for her 10-year risk for other major bone fractures.[60] It is expected that the DEXA machines will routinely incorporate the FRAX personal risk factors and include the 10-year fracture rates as part of the DEXA report, once appropriate FRAX filters can be put in place.

Women should be periodically screened using the FRAX calculator (using BMD or BMI) to determine their 10-year fracture risks.[58] Women with low fracture risks should be advised to include adequate amounts of calcium (at least 1,200 mg/day) and vitamin D (400–800 IU/day) in their diet (including supplements), to engage in regular weight-bearing and muscle-strengthening exercise to reduce the risk of falls and fractures and to avoid tobacco smoking and excessive alcohol intake. There is some evidence that after one year of exercise, there may be slowing of bone loss. Aerobic exercise, resistance exercise and walking are all more effective than no prescribed program.[62] Women who are identified to be at higher risk of fracture (>3% 10-year risk of hip fracture or >20% 10-year probability of major fracture) should be treated with one of the current FDA-approved therapies. As mentioned, in addition to the individuals identified by the FRAX model, women who are slender and those who have suffered prior fractures need to be treated.

For osteoporosis and osteopenia due to age-related estrogen deficiency, therapies for fracture prevention include bisphosphonates (alen-

Table 25–6 Recommended treatments for fracture prevention

Agent	Preferred Patient Population
Calcium and Vitamin D	All women age 50 and older
Postmenopausal hormone therapy (HT)	Younger women with menopausal symptoms
SERMs	Young women not candidates for HT or bisphosphonates
Bisphosphonates	First line therapy, especially older women
RANKL antibodies	Osteoporotic women unable to use bisphosphonates
Parathyroid hormone	High risk patients, glucocorticoid-induced osteoporosis

Source: Modified from Miller (2010).[150]

dronate, ibandronate, risedronate, or zoledronate), SERMs (raloxifene and lasofoxifene) and postmenopausal estrogen or estrogen/progestin therapies. Significant osteoporosis and osteoporosis caused by other medical conditions should be managed by specialists. See Table 25–6 for general treatment recommendations.

Bisphosphonates. Selected bisphosphonates (alendronate) have been shown to provide ongoing fracture risk reduction for up to 10 years. They reduce vertebral fracture rates by about 40%[57] and hip fracture risks by 50%.[63] Other bisphosphonates (Risedronate) have more modest effects on fracture reduction when used by women with osteoporosis.[64] Another bisphosphonate (etidronate) reduces vertebral but no other fractures.[65] It is important to be familiar with the different formulations to choose therapies that meet specific areas of concern for individual patients.

One advantage to bisphosphonate therapy is that considerable protection lingers for over 12 months after its cessation. This has prompted some experts to recommend some different bisphosphonate holidays for different risk groups of users.[66] The frequently documented poor utilization of oral bisphosphonates is worrisome because it can lead to bone weakness. Once-a-week and once-a-month oral dosing has been developed to try to facilitate better drug utilization. Once-a-year infusions are available, especially for those who cannot or do not take the oral therapies as directed. Acute phase response with a flu-like symptoms is quite frequent with the first infusion (42%) but declines over subsequent uses.[67] Atypical femur fractures (subtrochanteric and diaphyseal femur fractures often heralded by thigh pain), which are very rare events (occurring in less than 1% of hip fractures), tend to occur most in people who have had prolonged treatment with bisphosphonates for osteoporosis.[68] Occasional treatment holidays determined by risk group may be helpful to reduce this risk. Concerns about osteonecrosis of the jaw with alendronate are found almost exclusively with high doses given intravenously to treat metastatic lesions in the bone, not with doses used for fracture prevention. Atrial fibrillation with use of bisphosphonates has turned out to be a very rare event not related to only one formulation. Bisphosphonates have not been associated with increased risk of esophageal or gastric cancer.

RANKL antibodies. Denosumab, a new agent, is a human monoclonal antibody to the receptor activator of nuclear factor-kB ligand (RANKL). This antibody blocks the binding of the receptor activator to the receptor (RANK), which inhibits the development and activity of osteoclasts, which, in turn, decrease bone resorption. It is administered subcutaneously every 6 months for 36 months. Tested in osteoporotic women age 60 to 90, it reduced vertebral fractures by 68%, hip fractures by 40%, and non-vertebral fractures by 20%. No increases were noted in cancer, infection, cardiovascular disease, delayed fractured healing or hypocalcemia for patients who are predisposed to hypocalcemia.[69] Monitoring calcium, phosphorus, and magnesium levels is recommended. The effects of this agent wear off rapidly after treatment cessation.

SERMs. Raloxifene reduces the risk of vertebral fractures and nonvertebral fractures, but not the risk of hip fractures. Lasofoxifene is a newer SERM that in the long run has ability to reduce nonvertebral but not vertebral fractures.[28] Since some SERMs (raloxifene on-label and tamoxifen off-label) also offer significant protection from breast cancer, their use may be best reserved for women under 65. The effects of SERMs rapidly disappear after drug cessation.[70] New SERMs and SERM-estrogen combination therapies are being developed.[71]

Estrogen. Many, but not all, postmenopausal estrogen products are approved for the prevention of menopausally-related osteoporosis.[72,73] Interestingly, estrogen is the only treatment that has demonstrated its ability to significantly reduce the risk of hip fracture in a general population; all other products have been tested only in high-risk populations. Estrogen users in the Women's Health Initiative (WHI) study demonstrated reductions in vertebral and hip fractures that were comparable in magnitude to the reductions in fractures seen with other agents.[74] The FDA advises that estrogen be used for osteoporosis prevention or treatment only in women who use hormonal therapy for other indications and in other women who cannot use other antiresorptive therapies. Estrogen may be best suited for bone protection in recently menopausal women.

Breast Cancer

Postmenopausal women are very concerned about breast cancer. It is the most common nonskin cancer and the second most common cause of cancer deaths. The risk of breast cancer increases with age and weight in postmenopausal women. Screening recommendations are in flux:

- Self-breast examination is best recommended for women who are motivated. Routine use is no longer recommended.[75]
- Clinical breast examination is essential.[76,77]
- The schedule for routine mammography for low-risk women has been reassessed, balancing new estimates of the potential benefits of frequent testing (early cancer detection) against the harm done (unnecessary biopsies and costs). (See Chapter 22 on Female Genital Tract Cancer Screening.) As new technologies for screening are developed, they will be incorporated into practice.

As discussed above for perimenopausal women, continue to periodically calculate your patient's risk of developing breast cancer in the next 5 years by using the Gail model. Younger menopausal women with no prior personal history of breast cancer who have a 5-year risk greater than 1.66% should be offered chemoprevention with SERMs. Women over age 66 typically have that level of risk. Routine therapy for them should be individualized to consider other factors that influence life expectancy. Clinicians should strongly encourage the use of chemoprevention in women with a 5-year risk of at least 5%.

POSTMENOPAUSAL SYMPTOMS

Because women age as they move into menopause, it is often difficult to distinguish which symptoms are due to ovarian senescence from those which are due to aging itself. The most common symptom of the menopausal syndrome is the hot flash, but many symptomatic women report being troubled by fatigue, moodiness, depression, difficulty sleeping, decreased libido and orgasmic response, anxiety, changes in memory and cognition, weight gain, joint pain, scalp hair loss, hair growth or acne on face, skin changes, palpitations, nausea, headaches, and urinary tract infections.

Hot flashes affect 68% to 90% of recently menopausal women in the United States. Hot flashes can be quite uncomfortable and embarrassing. During a flash, women radiate heat from all parts of their bodies; toe temperatures have been observed to increase by up to 7° Fahrenheit.[78] One explanation of why some women become symptomatic while others do not may lie with differences between women in the function of their hypothalamic thermoregulatory zones. This zone represents a range of fluctuations in body temperature that the hypothalamus will tolerate without making any adjustments. When body temperatures exceed the limits of that zone, however, a person responds rapidly. The woman's heart rate increases and she will vasodilate (flush), then she will start to perspire to radiate off heat. In some women, the loss of estrogen with menopause narrows that thermoregulatory zone, so even minor fluctuations in temperature will trigger symptomatic hot flashes. In other women, the zone is much wider and they do not experience any vaso-motor symptoms.[85] Other factors have recently been implicated in the pathophysiology of the hot flash. Serum leptin levels (especially in obese women) have been associated with the occurrence and duration of hot flashes independent of estradiol levels.[79] Abnormal vascular reactivity has been suggested to be an underlying factor common to both hot flashes and later cardiovascular disease.[80]

At night, hot flashes can disrupt a woman's normal sleep cycle. It has been suggested that even if a woman is not completely awakened, the quality of her sleep may be diminished by hot flashes. Studies with laboratory polysomnographs have not always supported this hypothesis. Some researchers have reported no decrease in sleep quality between postmenopausal women and premenopausal women or between symptomatic women and asymptomatic women, although the postmenopausal women reported increased dissatisfaction with their sleep.[81,82] The 2005 NIH State-of-the-Science Conference Statement concluded that there is moderate evidence that menopause is the cause of sleep disturbances in some women, but it is unclear whether difficulty sleeping is due solely to vasomotor symptoms.[83]

Chronic sleep deprivation has been linked to mood disturbances, irritability, anxiety, and tearfulness.[84] The prevalence of mood symptoms in premenopausal women is 8% to 37%; in perimenopause 11% to 21% of women experience mood disorder; and in postmenopause (natural or surgical), 8% to 37% of women report such a problem.[83] Sleep disruptions also can significantly reduce a woman's concentration and memory. In one study of reproductive-age women who were tested prior to bilateral oophorectomy and again 2 months postoperatively, those given placebo demonstrated significantly decreased scores in immediate and delayed recall of paired association compared with those given hormonal therapies.[85] The biological plausibility of this functional impairment is supported by blood perfusion studies, which clearly demonstrated significantly reduced blood flow to the brain during the 20 to 30 minutes that each hot flash lasted.[86]

TREATMENTS FOR MENOPAUSAL SYMPTOMS

Vasomotor Symptoms

Hormonal Therapy and Estrogen-Based Therapies

Estrogen is the most effective therapy for vasomotor symptoms, because it reduces both the frequency and the intensity of the hot flashes. In clinical trials, low-dose formulations of postmenopausal hormone therapies have been shown to be as effective as higher-dose formulations in alleviating vasomotor symptoms.[87] In fact, we do not know what the lowest effective dose of estrogen is because in the latest clinical dosing trial, the dose that was expected to fail (0.3 mg conjugated equine estrogen [CEE]) was found to reduce hot flashes as well as the historical standard dose (0.625 mg CEE). That same lower dose (0.3 mg) of estrogen also increased bone mineral density and relieved vaginal atrophy as well as the conventional dose did. It should be noted that the terminology used to discuss this therapy has changed: it is now called postmenopausal hormone therapy (not hormone *replacement* therapy) underscoring the fact that it is being offered as therapy targeted to treat specific problems.

Risks and benefits. Evaluating all of the available data, a recent Endocrine Society Scientific Statement concluded that menopausal hormone therapy was associated with a 40% reduction in mortality in women in trials in which participants had a mean age of 60 years or less or women within 10 years of menopausal onset.[88]

The risks associated with postmenopausal hormone therapy have been clarified since the publication of the initial results of the Women's Health Initiative (WHI). In the randomized, placebo-controlled trials (RTCs) of the WHI, the risks of recently menopausal women (aged 50 to 59) have subsequently been shown to be distinctly different (much lower) than the risks reported for the entire study population, which included women in their 70s.[89] (See Table 25–7.) For example, women in the estrogen/progestin arm who entered the study in their 50s had *no* statistically significant increase in coronary heart disease,[90] stroke,[89] invasive breast cancer,[91] or total mortality[89] compared with placebo users. The estrogen-only arm of the study, which followed subjects for longer than the combined hormonal arm did, found that for women starting estrogen therapy near the time of menopause, there was no increase in the risk of coronary heart disease or stroke,[89] VTE,[92] invasive breast cancer,[93] or total mortality.[89] In fact, all the relative risk point estimates for each of the outcomes except VTE were below 1.0 for the younger women (on the protective side). Another study found that women aged 50 to 59 in the estrogen-only arm in the WHI not only had *no* increased risk for coronary heart disease (CHD) overall, but actually had *decreased* risks for many of the subgroups of CHD, including lower risk for myocardial infarction, coronary death, coronary artery by-pass grafting (CABG), percutaneous coronary intervention (PCI), and angina.[94] No statistically significant weight gain has been reported in hormone therapy users.

In more detailed reanalyses of the breast cancer data from the RCT arms of WHI, the overall results with short-term use have been similarly reassuring. Women who had no postmenopausal hormone exposure prior to entry into the WHI showed no statistically significant increase in breast cancer for the full 5.2 years of the estrogen/progestin arm.[95] No data are available for younger HT users and breast cancer. Of the women

Table 25–7 Women's Health Initiative hazard ratios for use of postmenopausal hormone therapy by age group (95% CI)

	CCE/MPA Ages		CCE Alone Ages	
	50–79	50–59	50–79	50–59
Coronary heart disease	1.23 (0.99 – 1.53)[1]	1.29 (0.79 – 2.12)[1]	0.95 (0.78 – 1.16)[1]	0.63 (0.36 – 1.09)[1]
Stroke	1.31 (1.03 – 1.68)[1]	1.41 (0.75 – 2.65)[1]	1.33 (1.05 – 1.68)[1]	0.89 (0.47 – 1.69)[1]
Invasive breast cancer	1.24 (1.01 – 1.54)[2]	1.20 (0.80 – 1.82)[2]	0.80 (0.62 – 1.04)[5]	0.72 (0.43 – 1.21)[5]
Venous thromboembolism	2.11 (1.58 – 2.82)[3]		1.33 (0.99 – 1.79)[4]	1.22 (0.62 – 2.42)[4]
Total mortality	1.00 (0.83 – 1.19)[1]	0.69 (0.44 – 1.07)[1]	1.04 (0.88 – 1.22)[1]	0.71 (0.46 – 1.11)

Sources:

[1] Rossouw JE, et al. (2007)[89]
[2] Chlebowski RT, et al. (2003)[91]
[3] Roussouw JT, et al. (2002)[95]
[4] Anderson GL, et al. (2004)[92]
[5] Stefanick ML, et al. (2006)[93]

who did develop breast cancer while participating in WHI, those who were using estrogen and progestin were found to have more advanced lesions than those who used placebo. Long-term follow-up (average 11 years) has shown that they also had more breast-cancer related deaths than women who developed breast cancer on placebos. The absolute number of deaths during this follow-up period was small: 25 (0.03%) of the HT group versus 12 (0.01%) of the placebo group.[96] One study suggested that women who develop mastalgia with initiation of hormone therapy had a 48% higher risk of breast cancer development that those who did not.[97]

On the other hand, women in the estrogen-only arm of the WHI study had *no* statistically significant increase in breast cancer overall for the full 7.8 years of study exposure, regardless of their previous hormone exposure.[93] Breaking down the various types of breast cancer into more detail, it has been found that estrogen-only arm showed a statistically significant 30% *reduction* in two of the most common postmenopausal breast cancers—localized disease and ductal carcinoma. Risks for all the other subtypes of breast cancer were reduced in the estrogen-only group except for a small (not statistically significant) increase in the risk of lobular carcinoma.[93] Longer term (11 years) follow-up shows that, overall, women in the estrogen arm had a statistically lower level risk of developing breast cancer. These findings are supported by the Nurse's Health Study, which found no risk of increase for any type of breast cancer from use of estrogen-only therapy, with use extending for up to 15 years of use.[98]

Other studies have reported that the impact that hormone therapy has on the risk of breast cancer may vary depending upon the prevalence of other risk factors.[99] Hormonal therapy does tend to increase breast density, making detection of a small lesion more challenging, and is associated with the requirement for more follow-up testing.[91,93] However, stopping hormones 2 to 3 weeks prior to performing a woman's mammogram allows her breasts to return to their normal density.[100,101]

The risks of probable dementia and mild cognitive impairment were increased for older women (over age 75) when they used hormones.[102] VTE risk has been an important topic with the WHI, which showed a statistically significant risk of VTE in the hormone therapy arm, but the confidence interval from VTE in the estrogen-alone arm indicated there was no statistically significant increased risk (the values ranged both above and below 1, which indicates no effect). (For an explanation of confidence intervals, see Explaining Risk to Patients in Chapter 11, Combined Oral Contraceptives.) When VTE risk is added to stroke risk, however, the estrogen-only arm showed an increased risk. Since the WHI publication, researchers have demonstrated in case-controlled studies that transdermal estrogen users have half the VTE risk as oral estrogen users.[88-90]

These studies also suggest that select progestins may also contribute to VTE risks and recommend the use of micronized progestins and pregnanes, because non-pregnane progestins were associated with a quadrupled risk of VTE.

Other health benefits and risks have emerged from further analysis of the WHI data. The women in the hormonal arms had significantly *lower* rates of developing diabetes compared with placebo users; the relative risk was 0.77 (95% CI, 0.67–0.93). Women using estrogen and progestin had a notable reduction in insulin resistance compared with their baseline levels.[103] Continuous (but not sequential) combined hormone therapy decreases the risk of endometrial carcinoma.[104]

Most of the risks seen in the WHI have now been shown to be reversible. Three years after stopping treatment with estrogen and progestin, the increased cardiovascular risks seen in the complete population during the trial were no longer detectable. The risk of invasive breast cancer declined.[105] This is the same pattern seen in prior studies, in which the risk of breast cancer returned to the woman's age-adjusted baseline risk within 4 years of stopping her estrogen and progestin therapies.[106]

In addition to studying over 27,000 women in the randomized, controlled trial (RCT), the WHI also studied a very large group of postmenopausal women in its observational arm. Compared with nonusers, women in the observational arm who used estrogen and progestin or estrogen only had no statistically significant increase in the risk of coronary heart disease, stroke and VTE. Interestingly, all their reported risks were below those seen in the WHI RCTs, which have been cited as support for the hypothesis that estrogen has a two-phase effect. Initial exposure to estrogen by women with established atherosclerotic disease can destabilize arterial plaque and cause an increase in cardiovascular events. In women without atherosclerosis, positive effects on lipids normalize (or reduce) a woman's risk for cardiovascular disease.[107] To test that hypothesis more directly, the experiences of women in both the RTC and the observational study of the WHI have been analyzed. The outcomes of this analysis were similar to those seen in the overall RTC results because women of all ages (not just the younger women) were included and because no adjustments were made for years of use.[107,108] Although the authors did not include a discussion of this aspect of the data, it was interesting to note that the outcomes of the women in the placebo groups who had early postmenopausal hormonal therapy were better than those in the placebo group with no prior hormonal therapy. In the RTCs, the incidence of many adverse outcomes was higher in placebo users who had never used hormone therapy: coronary heart disease (7.07 vs. 4.28), invasive breast cancer (3.73 vs. 2.67), and global index (21.57 vs. 17.20). The same differences were reported in the large observational study where coronary heart disease was reported to be 4.33 in never users vs. 3.42 in prior users.[108,109]

Other investigators have studied risks with hormone therapy use from other data sources. In one study, more than 10 years of hormone therapy use was associated with an increase in a woman's risk of lung cancer.[109] Evidence from WHI suggests that this risk may be associated with long-term smoking rather than with estrogen-progestin regimens. Case-control studies suggest that the risk of developing ovarian cancer may be slightly increased in current hormone therapy users. One study found that current use of hormone therapy—regardless of duration of use, formulation, estrogen dose, regimen, progestin type and type of administration—was associated with a 36% increase in ovarian cancer. This small risk disappeared within 2 to 4 years of discontinuation.[110]

Formulations. Hormone therapy comes in many different formulations of estrogen and many different delivery systems.[111] Conjugated equine estrogens (CEE) have been used as oral and vaginal topical agents for over 50 years. CEE was the estrogen that was studied in the WHI (albeit at higher doses than used today). Progestin (usually medroxyprogesterone acetate [MPA]) is usually added to protect the endometrium in women with uteri.

Estradiol is available in oral, patch, and gel formulations. Some patches combine estradiol with different progestins, including norgestimate and levonorgestrel. Oral and vaginal preparations of micronized progesterone provide endometrial protection, as do oral preparation of MPA and norethindrone acetate. As noted, case-control studies and clinical trials have reported that transdermally administered estradiol products were associated with half the VTE risk seen with oral CEE.[112–114] Transdermal delivery systems have been recommended by some as a preferred approach because many of the serum markers for cardiovascular disease (e.g., C-reactive protein) and some markers for thrombosis are less elevated by transdermal estrogen than they are by orally ingested estrogen formulations. While these findings may be exciting, caution must be used in interpreting the significance of surrogate markers in the absence of differences in clinical outcomes (e.g., myocardial infarction).

Androgens

Androgens have a favorable impact on hot flashes. However, there are no longer any commercially available FDA-approved products containing androgens. Because of concerns over hepatic safety, the FDA rejected an application for an androgen-eluting patch designed to increase libido, but clinical studies are continuing. It is known that androgens such as testosterone, especially when combined with estrogen, are helpful for osteoporosis. Androgens are converted in the bone into estrogens where they can slow bone resorption by the osteoclasts. Androgens also stimulate osteoblasts (the cells that lay down new bone matrix). Many women request testosterone that requires pharmaceutical compounding, but be cautious in granting such prescriptions, because there is no oversight for the quality or safety of the products produced by compounding pharmacists.

Dehydroepiandrosterone (DHEA) is a pro-drug. After menopause, all estrogens and all androgens come from peripheral conversion of DHEA, which is primarily produced in the adrenal gland. Over-the-counter DHEA has been marketed (unregulated) for years as a food supplement, despite the fact that the only source of DHEA in nature is the adrenal gland of primates, which is rarely considered a dietary delicacy. More recent research has demonstrated that low-dose DHEA may be administered vaginally.[115] The impact of DHEA has been demonstrated in earlier studies;[116] FDA-approved formulations may offer benefits to women in the future.

Tibolone

Tibolone is an interesting mixture with estrogenic, progestogenic, and androgenic properties. Although tibolone has been used for decades by women outside the United States, the FDA has declined to approve it because of concerns about breast cancer and thrombosis.

Bio-identical Hormones

There is growing concern about the accuracy of claims made by many of the manufacturers of so-called "bio-identical" hormones. The FDA has sent letters to many of the major manufacturers warning them to re-evaluate their claims and to include patient information about potential risks of their products. In general, there is no need to have to turn to compounding pharmacies to provide women estradiol and progesterone, because there are FDA-approved prescription versions of these compounds.

Nonhormonal Therapies

The only therapies that may have efficacy comparable to estrogen in treating vasomotor symptoms are high doses of gabapentin or pregabalin. In one comparative study of gabapentin up to 2,400 mg/day versus CEE 0.625 mg/day, hot flash frequency was reduced by 71% with gabapentin and by 72% with estrogen.[117] Studies with lower-dose gabapentin (300 mg TID) showed about a 50% reduction in hot flashes.[118,119] Another study in which gabapentin doses were increased to 2,700 mg a day showed only a 54% reduction in vasomotor symptoms.[120] Gabapentin often causes nausea and other gastrointestinal side effects, so doses should be titrated slowly until the desired effect is achieved.

Low-dose selective serotonin receptor inhibitors (SSRIs) and selective serotonin norepinephrine receptor inhibitors (SNRIs) have been demonstrated to be more effective than placebo in reducing the frequency, but not the severity, of hot flashes.[121] SSRIs and SNRIs are often the first-line therapy for women who do not want to use hormones and for women with contraindications to hormone use. A recent meta-analysis showed that, as a class, SSRIs reduce hot flashes by 1 episode a day.[121] It found that there were differences between formulations: sertraline had no effect; fluoxetine had a modest effect. The most effective agents in this class were desvenlafaxine 100 mg/day, venlafaxine 75 mg/day, paroxetine 10 to 20mg/day, or paroxetine controlled-release 12.5 to 25 mg/day. For women being treated for breast cancer, remember that paroxetine reduces metabolism of tamoxifen.[121]

Adding SSRIs to gabapentin does not improve outcome; if the patient gets insufficient relief from one class of treatments, she should be switched to another class; a second agent should not be added.[122]

Clonidine. Applying one clonidine patch (0.05 to 0.1 mg) each week reduced hot flashes by 46% in one clinical trial, but 40% of women discontinued clonidine because of side effects such as dizziness and dry mouth.[123] Overall, clonidine reduces hot flashes about 20% to 65%, and appears to be most effective in women with tamoxifen-induced hot flashes.[124] Transdermal clonidine therapy is preferred over oral clonidine. Clonidine is particularly attractive for women with hypertension requiring medical therapy, because clonidine may be used to help control both blood pressure and hot flashes. Clonidine raises the sweating threshold in symptomatic, but not asymptomatic, postmenopausal women.[125] Users are more likely to report difficulty sleeping.[126]

Bellergal-S. Bellergal-S is a combination of belladonna alkaloids, ergotamine tartrate, and phenobarbital. As an autonomic system stabilizer, Bellergal-S inhibits the sympathetic-parasympathetic pathway. Early studies showed a 66% reduction in menopausal symptoms with Bellergal-S compared with a 24% reduction with placebo.[127] A more recent study showed that all benefits were seen at 2 and 4 weeks of treatment, but that by 8 weeks, there was no difference in the frequency of hot flashes experienced by women using Bellergal-S and those given placebos.[128] Bellergal-S often sedates, which may be helpful if it is used only at night. There is some potential for addiction. Bellergal-S should not be prescribed to women with hypertension, because it contains the potent vasoconstrictor ergotamine.

A structured review of all randomized control studies utilizing non-hormonal therapies concluded that the studies of herbal agents, including red clover, phytoestrogens, ginseng, evening primrose, dong quai and vitamin E, showed that none of those medications was superior to placebo in reducing the frequency or intensity of vasomotor symptoms.[121] In a recent study of black cohosh, the placebo was found to be more effective than the black cohosh.[129] Acupuncture has been reported to significantly reduce the severity, but not the frequency, of nocturnal hot flashes when compared with placebo.[130]

Lifestyle Measures

The following recommendations should be offered to symptomatic women:

- Smoking cessation reduces hot flashes and is a top priority for good overall health.

- A woman may notice that certain triggers (such as spicy foods, computer screens, or chocolate) spark her symptoms. Have her avoid those triggers.

- Layered clothing may help. Removing a jacket during a hot flash may reduce heat discomfort, and the jacket can be put back on if a postflash chill occurs.

- Control room temperature and, more importantly, humidity. This helps some women reduce discomfort during hot flashes.

- Relaxation techniques and self-hypnosis reduce the number hot flashes by up to 50%.[131,132]

- Exercise may alter the frequency or intensity of hot flashes,[133] and it improves sleep quality (and cardiac and bone health).

VULVOVAGINAL ATROPHY

Urogenital atrophy is the most inevitable consequence of menopause. The vagina, the trigone of the bladder, and the urethra have the highest concentrations of estrogen receptors in the body. Overall, vaginal dryness is a problem reported by 4% to 22% of premenopausal women and 17% to 30% of postmenopausal women.[83]

The most common complaints that result from urogenital atrophy are dyspareunia and vaginal infections. Women with low estrogen levels (especially those who do not engage in vaginal intercourse) experience a thinning of the vaginal epithelium. As its rugation flattens, the vagina becomes considerably less elastic. There is breakdown of the collagen, smooth muscle, and elastin in the vagina. The underlying local vessels and lymphatic supply disappear, resulting in decreased transudation during sexual arousal.[134] Vaginal dryness has been reported as a *frequent* sexual problem by 44% of postmenopausal women compared with 14% of premenopausal women.[135] The introduction of treatments for erectile dysfunction has increased the number of postmenopausal women complaining of dyspareunia due to vulvovaginal atrophy.

Atrophy of the vagina also decreases natural defenses against infection. Vaginal fluid loses its protective acidity; the rise in vaginal pH (pH = 6.5–7.5) results from the loss of glycogen—needed support for the growth of Lactobacillus.

After menopause, constriction of the estrogen-sensitive vaginal tissues in the vulva and vagina causes the urethral meatus to rotate downward, closer to the vagina. Dysuria in postmenopausal women can be due to the increased incidence of cystitis, to the thinned tissue surrounding the urethral tissue, or to the development of urethral caruncles. Caruncles form when tissues surrounding the urethral meatus contract and evert the distal portion of the urethral tissue, creating the classic appearance of a red, tender, fleshy halo surrounding the meatus. This tissue may not be sufficiently epithelialized to tolerate external exposure and can be irritated by urination or wiping, although many women with caruncles are asymptomatic. Topical estrogen cream can be used to reverse these changes in symptomatic women.

If dyspareunia due to vulvar vaginal atrophy is the woman's primary complaint, water-soluble and silicone-based lubricants can reduce friction during coitus. If this fails, low-dose vaginal estrogen therapy, 1/2 applicator of estrogen 2 times a week, achieves the same favorable results as the traditional, higher-dose therapies.[136,137] In addition, studies now show that early high-dose therapy is not needed to "prime the pump." Estrogen products are available for vaginal use as creams, suppositories, and vaginal estrogen rings. Response is relatively rapid; within 6 weeks, the vagina becomes more elastic because of thickening (rugation) of the vaginal walls. Return of adequate lubrication may take longer (months) because blood vessels and lymphatics need time to regrow.

Measurable amounts of estrogen are rapidly absorbed through the vaginal wall and enter the systemic circulation. Depending upon which estrogen is being monitored, systemic estrogen levels rise but generally remain in the postmenopausal range.[138] Absorption may provide some bone protection, but absorption also raises issues of estrogen exposure that could affect the endometrium or the risk of breast cancer recurrence among breast cancer survivors.

The North American Menopause Society has advised that women with an intact uterus may use vaginal estrogen therapy without having to add a progestin.[72] Recent studies (usually 1–2 years in duration) support that conclusion.[139] However, since in practice, patients do not have baseline biopsies performed, it may still be prudent to periodically provide progestin challenges to high-risk women. At a minimum, any bleeding that occurs to women using unopposed estrogen therapy demands immediate evaluation to rule out endometrial hyperplasia or cancer. Studies have shown that placing estrogen creams only in the outer third of the vagina helps women's symptoms but minimizes endometrial stimulation.[140] The prohormone DHEA is being investigated for treatment of vaginal atrophy.[141,142]

Urinary incontinence and pelvic relaxation are also very common problems for postmenopausal women. WHI demonstrated that estrogen therapy is not helpful to treat stress incontinence. However, if surgical therapies are pursued, preoperative topical application of estrogen to the vagina may improve healing. Modest (5%–10%) weight loss has been shown to improve urinary incontinence in overweight and obese women.[143] Pessaries are being more frequently utilized to treat symptoms associated with pelvic relaxation.

S UMMARY

Emphasize lifestyle changes to promote long-term health for all perimenopausal and postmenopausal women. Recommend exercise, weight control, stress management, accident prevention, and social connectedness.

- *Vasomotor symptoms:* Women with disturbing vasomotor symptoms deserve treatment. Estrogens at low doses are the most effective therapy, but SSRIs, SNRIs, gabapentin, pregabalin, and clonidine offer varying levels of symptomatic relief. Unfortunately, none of the herbal products has been shown to be superior to placebo in reducing hot flashes.

- *Vulvovaginal atrophy:* For women with vulvovaginal atrophy, small doses of topical estrogen therapy are effective.

- *Bone health:* Exercise and calcium with vitamin D are also essential for bone health. Identify women who have an increased risk of fracture in the next 10 years and treat them prophylactically. Recommend home safety measures to reduce the risk for falls.

- *Breast cancer:* Identify women at moderate risk of breast cancer and provide them chemoprevention. Screen women in the general population with annual breast exams and periodic mammography.

- *Cardiovascular risk:* For women with risk factors for CVD (such as hypertension, diabetes, obesity, hyperlipidemia, or elevated C-reactive protein), directed therapies are most appropriate. Blood pressure normalization extends years of life. In appropriate candidates, ACE inhibitors not only reduce stroke and myocardial infarction risk, but also protect against renal failure. Statins combined with diet and exercise help reduce cardiovascular events in women with dyslipidemia.

- *Diabetes:* For diabetic women, good glucose control with diet and oral hypoglycemic agents or insulin is the healthiest approach and improves longevity as well as quality of life (delayed onset of blindness, renal failure, etc.).

In a long-term study, dispositional optimism was shown to be associated with a decreased risk of cardiovascular disease.[144] Mental exercise and social connectedness are key recommendations for the mental activity and psychological health of the patient. Advise all women to keep healthy, get involved, stay alert, get enough sleep, use tools to compensate for mental decline, and keep in contact with others to maintain long-term vivaciousness and quality of life.

REFERENCES

1. Buyuk, E, Nejat, E, Neal-Perry G. Determinants of Female Reproductive Senescence: Differential Roles for the Ovary and the Neuroendocrine Axis Semin Reprod Med. 2010;28:370–9.
2. Faddy MJ, Gosden RG, Gougeon A, Richardson SJ, Nelson JF. Accelerated disappearance of ovarian follicles in mid-life: implications for forecasting menopause. Human Reproduction. 1992;7:1342–6.
3. Sowers M. Eyvazzadeh A., McConnel D, et al. Anti-mullerian hormone and inhibin B in the definition of ovarian aging and the menopause transition. J Clin Endocrinol Metab. 2008;93:3478–83.
4. Hagan CP, Aksglaede L, Sorenson K, et al.Serum levels of anti-Mullerian hormone as a marker of ovarian function in 926 healthy females from birth through adulthood and in 172 Turner syndrome patients. J Clin Endocrinol Metab, in press.
5. Van Disseldorp J, Lambalk CB, Kwee J, et al. Comparison of inter- and intra-variability of anti-Mullerian hormone and antral follicle counts. Hum Reprod. 2010;25:221–227.
6. Gougeon A, Chain GB. Morphometric studies of small follicles in ovaries of women at different ages. J Reprod Fertil. 1987;81:433–442.
7. Broekmans JM, de Zielgler D, Howles CM, Gougeon A, Trew G, Olivennes F. The antral follicle count: practical recommendations for better standardization. Fertil Steril. 2010;94:1044–51.
8. Tietze C. Reproductive span and rate of reproduction among Hutterite women. Fertil Steril. 1957;8:89–97.
9. van Noord-Zaadstra BM, Looman CW, Alsbach H, Habbema JD, te Velde ER, Karbaat J. Delaying childbearing: effect of age on fecundity and outcome of pregnancy. BMJ. 1991;302:1361–5.
10. Santoro N, Brown JR, Adel T, Skurnick JH. Characterization of reproductive hormonal dynamics in the perimenopause. J Clin Endocrinol Metab. 1996;81:1495–501.
11. Ferrell RJ, Simon JA, Pincus SM, Rodriguez G, O'Connor KA, Holman DJ, Weinstein M. The length of perimenopausal menstrual cycles increases later and to a greater degree than previously reported. Fertil Steril. 2006;86:619–624.
12. Hale GE, Manconi F, Luscombe G, Fraser IS. Quantitative measurements of menstrual blood loss in ovulatory and anovulatory cycles in middle- and late-reproductive age and the menopausal transition. Obstet Gynecol. 2010;115(2 Pt 1):249–56.
13. Stewart ST, Cutler DM, Rosen AB. Forecasting the effects of obesity and smoking on U.S. life expectancy. N Engl J Med. 2009;361:2252–60.
14. Flegal KM, Carroll MD, Ogden CL, Curtin LR. Prevalence and trends in obesity among US adults, 1999–2008. JAMA. 2010;303:235–41.

15. Castelo-Branco C, Palacios S, Ferrer-Barriendos J, Cancelo M, Quereda F, Alberich X. Impact of anthropometric parameters on quality of life during menopause. Fertil Steril. 2009;92:1947–52

16. Folta SC. Factors related to cardiovascular disease risk reduction in midlife and older women; a qualitative study. Prev Chronic Dis. 2008;5:A06.

17. Sacks FM, Bray GA, Carey VJ, Smith SR, Ryan DH, Anton SD, et al. Comparison of weight-loss diets with different compositions of fat, protein, and carbohydrates. N Engl J Med. 2009;360:859–73.

18. Lee IM, Djoussé L, Sesso HD, Wang L, Buring JE. Physical activity and weight gain prevention. JAMA. 2010;303:1173–9.

19. Buchner DM. Physical activity and quality of life in older adults. JAMA. 1997; 277:64–6.

20. Muennig, P, Fiscella K, Tancredi D, Franks P. The relative Health burden of selected social and behavioral risk factors in the United States: implications for policy. Am J Publ Health. 2010;100:1758–64.

21. American College of Obstetricians and Gynecologists. ACOG Practice Bulletin No. 103: Hereditary breast and ovarian cancer syndrome. Obstet Gynecol. 2009;113: 957–66.

22. Visvanathan K, Lippman SM, Hurley P, Temin S. American Society of Clinical Oncology clinical practice guideline update on the use of pharmacologic interventions including tamoxifen, raloxifene, and aromatase inhibition for breast cancer risk reduction. Gynecol Oncol. 2009;115:132–4.

23. Fisher B, Costantino JP, Wickerham DL, Redmond CK, Kavanah M, Cronin WM, et al. Tamoxifen for prevention of breast cancer: report of the National Surgical Adjuvant Breast and Bowel Project P-1 Study. J Natl Cancer Inst. 1998;90:1371–88.

24. Cuzick J, Forbes J, Edwards R, Baum M, Cawthorn S, Coates A, Hamed A, Howell A, Powles T; IBIS investigators. First results from the International Breast Cancer Intervention Study (IBIS-I): a randomised prevention trial. Lancet. 2002;360:817–24.

25. Cummings SR, Eckert S, Krueger KA, Grady D, Powles TJ, Cauley JA, et al. The effect of raloxifene on risk of breast cancer in postmenopausal women: results from the MORE randomized trial. Multiple Outcomes of Raloxifene Evaluation. JAMA. 1999;281(23):2189–97. Erratum in: JAMA. 1999;282:2124.

26. Study of Tamoxifen and Raloxifene (STAR). Available from: http://www.cancer.gov/newscenter/pressreleases/STARresultsApr172006 (accessed 05–03–10).

27. Chlebowski RT, Breast cancer risk reduction: strategies for women at increased risk. Annu Rev Med. 2002;53:519–40.

28. Cummings SR, Ensrud K, Delmas PD, LaCroix AZ, Vukicevic S, Reid DM, et al. PEARL Study Investigators. Lasofoxifene in postmenopausal women with osteoporosis. N Engl J Med. 2010;362:686–96.

29. Newcomb PA, Trentham-Dietz A, Hampton JM. Bisphosphonates for osteoporosis treatment are associated with reduced breast cancer risk. Br J Cancer. 2010;102: 799–802.

30. Henshaw SK. Unintended pregnancy in the United States. Fam Plann Perspect. 1998; 30:24–29, 46.

31. Upson K, Reed SD, Prager SW, Schiff MA. Factors associated with contraceptive nonuse among US women ages 35–44 years at risk of unwanted pregnancy. Contraception. 2010;81:427–35.

32. Marchbanks PA, McDonald JA, Wilson HG, Folger SG, Mandel MG, Daling JR, et al. Oral contraceptives and the risk of breast cancer. N Engl J Med. 2002;346:2025–32.

33. ACOG Committee on Practice Bulletins-Gynecology. ACOG practice bulletin. No. 73: Use of hormonal contraception in women with coexisting medical conditions. Obstet Gynecol. 2006;107:1453–72.

34. Centers for Disease Control and Prevention. U.S. Medical Eligibility Criteria for Contraceptive Use, 2010. MMWR 2010;59. Available from: http://www.cdc.gov/mmwr/pdf/rr/rr59e0528.pdf.

35. Kaunitz AM, Bissonnette F, Monteiro I, Lukkari-Lax E, Muysers C, Jensen JT. Levonorgestrel-releasing intrauterine system or medroxyprogesterone for heavy menstrual bleeding: a randomized controlled trial. Obstet Gynecol. 2010;116:625–32.

36. Heikinheimo O, Inki P, Kunz M, Gemzell-Danielsson K. Predictors of bleeding and user satisfaction during consecutive use of the levonorgestrel-releasing intrauterine system. Hum Reprod. 2010;25:1423–7.

37. Varila E, Wahlström T, Rauramo I. A 5-year follow-up study on the use of a levonor-gestrel intrauterine system in women receiving hormone replacement therapy. Fertil Steril. 2001;76:969–73.

38. Raudaskoski TH, Lahti EI, Kauppila AJ, Apaja-Sarkkinen MA, Laatikainen TJ. Trans-dermal estrogen with a levonorgestrel-releasing intrauterine device for climacteric complaints: clinical and endometrial responses. Am J Obstet Gynecol. 1995;172(1 Pt 1):114–9.

39. Cundy T, Cornish J, Roberts H, Reid IR. Menopausal bone loss in long-term users of depot medroxyprogesterone acetate contraception. Am J Obstet Gynecol. 2002;186: 978–83.

40. Sivin I. Utility and drawbacks of continuous use of a copper T IUD for 20 years. Con-traception. 2007;75(6 Suppl):S70–5.

41. Freedman RR. Menopausal hot flashes. In: Lobo RA, Kelsey J, Marcus R, eds. Meno-pause: Biology and Pathobiology. San Diego: Academic Press, 2000:219.

42. Kaunitz AM. Oral contraceptive use in menopause. Am J Obstet Gynecol. 2001;185(2 Suppl):S32–7.

43. Mosca L, Jones WK, King KB, Ouyang P, Redberg RF, Hill MN. Awareness, percep-tion, and knowledge of heart disease risk and prevention among women in the United States. American Heart Association Women's Heart Disease and Stroke Cam-paign Task Force. Arch Fam Med. 2000;9:506–15.

44. Mosca L, Mochari-Greenberger H, Dolor RJ, Newby LK, Robb KJ. Twelve-year follow-up of American women's awareness of cardiovascular disease risk and bar-riers to heart health. Circ Cardiovasc Qual Outcomes. 2010 120–7.

45. Centers for Disease Control and Prevention (CDC). Major cardiovascular disease (CVD) during 1997–1999 and major CVD hospital discharge rates in 1997 among women with diabetes-United States. MMWR. 2001;50:948–54.

46. Johnson BD, Dwyer KM, Stanczyk FZ, Bittner V, Berga SL, Braunstein GD, Azziz R, Yang Y, Hale GE, Bairey M. The relationship of menopausal status and rapid meno-pausal transition with carotid intima-media thickness progression in women: a report from the Los Angeles Atherosclerosis Study. J Clin Endocrinol Metab. 2010;95:4432–40.

47. Mosca L, Appel LJ, Benjamin EJ, Berra K, Chandra-Strobos N, Fabunmi RP, et al. American Heart Association. Evidence-based guidelines for cardiovascular disease prevention in women. Circulation. 2004;109:672–93.

48. Executive Summary of The Third Report of The National Cholesterol Education Pro-gram (NCEP) Expert Panel on Detection, Evaluation, and Treatment of High Blood Cholesterol In Adults (Adult Treatment Panel III). JAMA. 2001;285:2486–97.

49. Mosca L, Banka CL, Benjamin EJ, et al. Evidence-based guidelines for cardiovascular disease prevention in women: 2007 update. J Am Coll Cardiol. 2007;49:1230–50.

50. Ridker PM, Danielson E, Fonseca FA, Genest J, Gott AM, Kastelein JJ, et al. Rosuva-statin to prevent vascular events in men and women with elevated C-reactive pro-tein. N Engl J Med. 2008;359:2195–207.

51. Friedenreich CM, Woolcott CG, McTiernan A, Terry T, Brant R, et al. Adiposity changes after a 1-year aerobic exercise intervention among postmenopausal women: a randomized controlled trial. Int J Obes. 2011;35:427–35.

52. Ebeling PR, Gagnon C, Sims NA, Mumm S, McAuley SA, Poulton J, KW Ng. Lack of sustained response to teriparatide in a patient with adult hypophosphatasia. J Clin Endocrinol Metab. 2010;95:1007–12.

53. Siris ES, Miller PD, Barrett-Connor E, Faulkner KG, Wehren LE, Abbott TA, et al. Identification and fracture outcomes of undiagnosed low bone mineral density in postmenopausal women: results from the National Osteoporosis Risk Assessment. JAMA. 2001;286:2815–22.
54. Lindsay R, Cosman F. Estrogen in prevention and treatment of osteoporosis. Ann N Y Acad Sci. 1990;592:326–333;discussion 334–45.
55. Torgerson DJ, Bell-Syer SE. Hormone replacement therapy and prevention of non-vertebral fractures: a meta-analysis of randomized trials. JAMA. 2001;285:2891–7.
56. Lim LS, Hoeksema LJ, Sherin K. Screening for Osteoporosis in the Adult U.S. Population. ACPM Position Statement on Preventive Practice. Am J Prev Med. 2009;36(4).
57. Cranney A, Guyatt G, Griffith L, Wells G, Tugwell P, Rosen C; Osteoporosis Methodology Group and The Osteoporosis Research Advisory Group. Meta-analyses of therapies for postmenopausal osteoporosis. IX: Summary of meta-analyses of therapies for postmenopausal osteoporosis. Endocr Rev. 2002;23:570–8.
58. Lim LS, Hoeksema LJ, Sherin K; ACPM Prevention Practice Committee. Screening for osteoporosis in the adult U.S. population: ACPM position statement on preventive practice. Am J Prev Med. 2009;36:366–75.
59. Management of osteoporosis in postmenopausal women: 2010 position statement of the North American Menopause Society. Menopause. 2010;17:25–54; quiz 55–6.
60. Kanis JA, McCloskey EV, Johansson H, Strom O, Borgstrom F, Oden A. How to decide who to treat. Best Pract Res Clin Rheumatol. 2009;23:711–26.
61. Dawson-Hughes B, Tosteson A, Melton III L, Baim S., Favus M. Khosla S, Lindsay R. Implications of absolute fracture risk assessment for osteoporosis practice guidelines in the USA. International Osteoporosis Foundation and National Osteoporosis Foundation. 2007.
62. Bonaiuti D, Shea B, Iovine R, Negrini S, Welch V, Kember HHCG, Wells GA, Tugwell P, Cranney A. Exercise for preventing and treating osteoporosis in postmenopausal women. Cochrane Database of Systematic Reviews. 2002, Issue 2: CD000333
63. Black DM, Cummings SR, Karpf DB, Cauley JA, Thompson DE, Nevitt MC, et al. Randomised trial of effect of alendronate on risk of fracture in women with existing vertebral fractures. Fracture Intervention Trial Research Group. Lancet. 1996;348: 1535–41.
64. Wells, GA, Cranney A, Peterson J, B Goucher M, Shea B, Welch V, Coyle D, Tugwell P. Etidronate for the primary and secondary prevention of osteoporotic fractures in postmenopausal women. Cochrane Database of Systematic Reviews. 2008, Issue 1. CD 003376.
65. Wells, GA, Cranney A, Peterson J, B Goucher M, Shea B, Welch V, Coyle D, Tugwell P. Alendronate for the primary and secondary prevention of osteoporotic fractures in postmenopausal women. Cochrane Database of Systematic Reviews. 2008, Issue 1. CD 001155.
66. Watts NB, Diab DL. Long-term use of bisphosphonates in osteoporosis J Clin Endocrinol Metab. 2010;95:1555–65.
67. Reid IR, Gamble GD, Mesenbrink P, Lakatos P, Black DM. Characterization of and risk factors for the acute-phase response after zoledronic acide. J Clin Endocrinol Metab. 2010;95:4380–7.
68. Black DM, Kelly MP, Genant HK, et al. Bisphosphonates and fractures of the subtrochanteric or diaphyseal femur. N Engl J Med. 2010;362:1761–71.
69. Cummings SR: San Martin J, McClung MR, Siris ES, Eastall R, Reid IR, Delmas PD, et al. Denosumab for prevention of fractures in postmenopausal women with osteoporosis. N Engl J Med. 2009;36:756–65.
70. Neele SJ, Evertz R, De Valk-De Roo G, Roos JC, Netelenbos JC. Effect of 1 year of discontinuation of raloxifene or estrogen therapy on bone mineral density after 5 years of treatment in healthy postmenopausal women. Bone. 2002;30:599–603.

71. Lobo RA, Pinkerton JV, Gass ML, Dorin MH, Ronkin S, Pickar JH, Constantine G. Evaluation of bazedoxifene/conjugated estrogens for the treatment of menopausal symptoms and effects on metabolic parameters and overall safety profile. Fertil Steril. 2009;92:1025–38.

72. Valimaki MJ, Laitinen KA, Tahtela RK, Hirvonen EJ, Risteli JP. The effects of transdermal estrogen therapy on bone mass and turnover in early postmenopausal smokers: a prospective, controlled study. Am J Obstet Gynecol. 2003;189:1213–20.

73. Farquhar C, Marjoribanks J, Lethaby A, Suckling JA, Lamberts Q. Long term hormone therapy for perimenopausal and postmenopausal women. Cochrane Database of Systematic Reviews 2009, Issue 2. CD004142.

74. Writing Group for the Women's Health Initiative Investigators. Risks and Benefits of Estrogen Plus Progestin in Healthy Postmenopausal Women: Principal Results From the Women's Health Initiative Randomized Controlled Trial. JAMA. 2002;288:321–333.

75. Thomas DB, Gao DL, Ray RM, Wang WW, Allison CJ, Chen FL, et al. Randomized trial of breast self-examination in Shanghai: final results. J Natl Cancer Inst. 2002;94:1445–57.

76. U.S. Preventive Services Task Force. Screening for breast cancer: U.S.Preventive Services Task Force recommendation statement. Ann Intern Med. 2009;151:716–26, W-236. Erratum in: Ann Intern Med. 2010;152:199–200.

77. Chiarelli AM, Majpruz V, Brown P, Thériault M, Shumak R, Mai V. The contribution of clinical breast examination to the accuracy of breast screening. J Natl Cancer Inst. 2009;101:1236–43.

78. Molnar GW. Body temperatures during menopausal hot flashes. J Appl Physiol. 1975; 38:499–503.

79. Alexander C, Cochran CH, Gallicchio L, Miller SR, Flaws JA, Zacur H. Serum leptin levels, hormone levels and hot flashes in midlife women. Fertil Steril. 2010;94:1037–43.

80. Thurston RC, Sutton-Tyrrell K, Everson-Rose SA, Hess R, Matthews KA. Hot flashes and subclinical cardiovascular diseae: findings from the Study of Women's Health across the Nation Heart Study. Circulation. 2008;1818:1234–40.

81. Young T, Rabago D, Zgierska A, Austin D, Laurel F. Objective and subjective sleep quality in premenopausal, perimenopausal, and postmenopausal women in the Wisconsin Sleep Cohort Study. Sleep. 2003;26:667–72.

82. Freedman RR. Pathophysiology and treatment of menopausal hot flashes. Semin Reprod Med. 2005;23:117–125.

83. National Institutes of Health. National Institutes of Health State-of-the-Science Conference statement: management of menopause-related symptoms. Ann Intern Med. 2005;142(12 Pt 1):1003–1013.

84. Baker A, Simpson S, Dawson D. Sleep disruption and mood changes associated with menopause. J Psychosom Res. 1997;43:359–69.

85. Phillips SM, Sherwin BB. Effects on memory function in surgically menopausal women. Psychoneuroendocrinology. 1992;17:485–95.

86. Greene RA. Estrogen and cerebral blood flow: a mechanism to explain the impact of estrogen on the incidence and treatment of Alzheimer's disease. Int J Fertil Womens Med. 2000;45:253–7.

87. Utian WH, Shoupe D, Bachmann G, Pinkerton JV, Pickar JH. Relief of vasomotor symptoms and vaginal atrophy with lower doses of conjugated equine estrogens and medroxyprogesterone acetate. Fertil Steril. 2001;75:1065–79.

88. Santen RJ, Allred DC, Ardoin SP, Archer DF, Boyd N, Braunstein GD, et al. Postmenopausal hormone therapy: an Endocrine Society scientific statement. J Clin Endocrinol Metab. 2010;95:S1–66.

89. Rossouw JE, Prentice RL, Manson JE, Wu L, Barad D, Barnabei VM, et al. Postmenopausal hormone therapy and risk of cardiovascular disease by age and years since menopause. JAMA. 2007;297:1465–77. Erratum in: JAMA. 2008;299:1426.

90. Manson JE, Hsia J, Johnson KC, Rossouw JE, Assaf AR, Lasser NL,et al. Women's Health Initiative Investigators. Estrogen plus progestin and the risk of coronary heart disease. N Engl J Med. 2003;349:523–34.
91. Chlebowski RT, Hendrix SL, Langer RD, Stefanick ML, Gass M, Lane D, et al. WHI Investigators. Influence of estrogen plus progestin on breast cancer and mammography in healthy postmenopausal women: the Women's Health Initiative Randomized Trial. JAMA. 2003;289:3243–53.
92. Anderson GL, Limacher M, Assaf AR, Bassford T, Beresford SA, Black H, et al. Women's Health Initiative Steering Committee. Effects of conjugated equine estrogen in postmenopausal women with hysterectomy: the Women's Health Initiative randomized controlled trial. JAMA. 2004;291:1701–12.
93. Stefanick ML, Anderson GL, Margolis KL, Hendrix SL, Rodabough RJ, Paskett ED, et al. WHI Investigators. Effects of conjugated equine estrogens on breast cancer and mammography screening in postmenopausal women with hysterectomy. JAMA. 2006;295:1647–57.
94. North American Menopause Society. Estrogen and progestogen use in postmenopausal women: 2010 position statement of The North American Menopause Society. Menopause. 2010;17:242–55.
95. Rossouw JE, Anderson GL, Prentice RL, LaCroix AZ, Kooperberg C, Stefanick ML, Jackson RD, et al. Writing Group for the Women's Health Initiative Investigators. Risks and benefits of estrogen plus progestin in healthy postmenopausal women: principal results From the Women's Health Initiative randomized controlled trial. JAMA. 2002;288:321–33.
96. Chebowski RT, Hendrix SL, Langer RD, Stefanick ML, Gass M, et al. Influence of estrogen plus progestin on greast cancer and mammography in healthy postmenopausal women: the Women's Health Initiative Randomized Trial. JAMA. 2003;289: 3243–53.
97. Crandall C, Aragaki A, Chlebowski R, McTiernan A, Anderson G, Hendrix S, Cochrane B, Kuller L, Cauley J. New-onset breast tenderness after initiation of estrogen plus progestin therapy and breast cancer risk. Arch Intern. 2009;169:1684–91.
98. Chen WY, Manson JE, Hankinson SE, Rosner B, Holmes MD, Willett WC, Colditz GA. Unopposed estrogen therapy and the risk of invasive breast cancer. Arch Intern Med. 2006;166:1027–32.
99. Lumachi F, Frigo A, Basso U, Tombolan, V, Eermani M. Estrogen therapy and risk of breast cancer in postmenopausal women: a case-control study and results of a multivariate analysis. Menopause. 2010;17:524–528.
100. Greendale GA, Reboussin BA, Slone S, Wasilauskas C, Pike MC, Ursin G. Postmenopausal hormone therapy and change in mammographic density. J Natl Cancer Inst. 2003;95:30–7.
101. Crandall C, Guan M, Laughlin G, Ursin G, Stanczk F, Ingles S, Barrett-Connor E, Greendale G. Increases in serum estrone sulfate level are associated with increased mammographic density during menopausal hormone therapy. Cancer Epidemiol Biomarkers Prev. 2008 17:1674–1681.
102. Shumaker SA, Legault C, Kuller L, Rapp SR, Thal L, Lane DS, et al. Women's Health Initiative Memory Study. Conjugated equine estrogens and incidence of probable dementia and mild cognitive impairment in postmenopausal women: Women's Health Initiative Memory Study. JAMA. 2004;291:2947–58.
103. Margolis KL, Bonds DE, Rodabough RJ, Tinker L, Phillips LS, Allen C, et al. Women's Health Initiative Investigators. Effect of oestrogen plus progestin on the incidence of diabetes in postmenopausal women: results from the Women's Health Initiative Hormone Trial. Diabetologia. 2004;47:1175–87.
104. Jaakkola S, Lyytinen H, Pukkala E, Ylikorkala O. Endometrial cancer in postmenopausal women using estradiol-progestin therapy. Obstet Gynecol. 2009;114:1197–204.

105. Heiss G, Wallace R, Anderson GL, Aragaki A, Beresford SA, Brzyski R, et al. WHI Investigators. Health risks and benefits 3 years after stopping randomized treatment with estrogen and progestin. JAMA. 2008;299:1036–45.
106. Schairer C, Lubin J, Troisi R, Sturgeon S, Brinton L, Hoover R. Menopausal estrogen and estrogen-progestin replacement therapy and breast cancer risk. JAMA. 2000;283:485–91.
107. Prentice RL, Langer RD, Stefanick ML, Howard BV, Pettinger M, Anderson GL, Barad D, Curb JD, Kotchen J, Kuller L, Limacher M, Wactawski-Wende J; Women's Health Initiative Investigators. Combined analysis of Women's Health Initiative observational and clinical trial data on postmenopausal hormone treatment and cardiovascular disease. Am J Epidemiol. 2006;163:589–99.
108. Prentice RL, Manson JE, Langer RD, Anderson GL, Pettinger M, Jackson RD, Johnson KC, Kuller LH, Lane DS, Wactawski-Wende J, Brzyski R, Allison M, Ockene J, Sarto G, Rossouw JE. Benefits and risks of postmenopausal hormone therapy when it is initiated soon after menopause. Am J Epidemiol. 2009;170:12–23.
109. Slatore CG, Chien JW, Au DH, Satia JA, White E. Lung cancer and hormone replacement therapy: association in the vitamins and lifestyle study. J Clin Oncol. 2010;28:1540–6.
110. Mørch LS, Løkkegaard E, Andreasen AH, Krüger-Kjaer S, Lidegaard O. Hormone therapy and ovarian cancer. JAMA. 2009;302:298–305.
111. Marshall DD, Iglesia C. A guide to lotions and potions for treating vaginal atrophy. OBG Management. 2009;21:29–37.
112. Canonico M, Fournier A, Carcaillon L, Olié V, Plu-Bureau G, Oger E, et al. Postmenopausal hormone therapy and risk of idiopathic venous thromboembolism: results from the E3N cohort study. Arterioscler Thromb Vasc Biol. 2010;30:340–5.
113. Straczek C, Oger E, Yon de Jonage-Canonico MB, Plu-Bureau G, Conard J, Meyer G, et al. Estrogen and Thromboembolism Risk (ESTHER) Study Group. Prothrombotic mutations, hormone therapy, and venous thromboembolism among postmenopausal women: impact of the route of estrogen administration. Circulation. 2005;112:3495–500.
114. Canonico M, Oger E, Plu-Bureau G, Conard J, Meyer G, Lévesque H,et al. Estrogen and Thromboembolism Risk (ESTHER) Study Group. Hormone therapy and venous thromboembolism among postmenopausal women: impact of the route of estrogen administration and progestogens: the ESTHER study. Circulation. 2007;115:840–5.
115. Labrie F, Calvo E, Morissette J, Martel C, Labrie C, Bernard B, Bernerd F et al. Pangenomic changes induced by DHEA in the skin of postmenopausal women. J Steroid Biochem Mol Biol. 2008;112:186–93.
116. Labrie F, Diamond P, Cusan L, Gomez JL, Belander A, Candas B. Effect of 12-month dehydroepiandrosterone replacement therapy on bone, vagina, and endometrium in postmenopausal women. J Clin Endocrinol Metab. 1997;82:3498–505.
117. Reddy SY, Warner H, Guttuso T Jr, Messing S, DiGrazio W, Thornburg L, Guzick DS. Gabapentin, estrogen, and placebo for treating hot flushes: a randomized controlled trial. Obstet Gynecol. 2006;108:41–8.
118. Butt DA, Lock M, Lewis JE, Ross S, Moineddin R. Gabapentin for the treatment of menopausal hot flashes: a randomized controlled trial. Menopause. 2008;15:310–8.
119. Pandya KJ, Morrow GR, Roscoe JA, Zhao H, Hickok JT, Pajon E,et al. Gabapentin for hot flashes in 420 women with breast cancer: a randomised double-blind placebo-controlled trial. Lancet. 2005;366:818–24.
120. Guttuso T Jr, Kurlan R, McDermott MP, Kieburtz K. Gabapentin's effects on hot flashes in postmenopausal women: a randomized controlled trial. Obstet Gynecol. 2003;101:337–45.
121. Martin KA, Manson JE. Approach to the patient with menopausal symptoms. J Clin Endocrinol Metab. 2008;93:4567–75.

122. Loprinzi CL, Kugler JW, Barton DL, Dueck AC, Tschetter LK, Nelimark RA, et al. Phase III trial of gabapentin alone or in conjunction with an antidepressant in the management of hot flashes in women who have inadequate control with an antidepressant alone: NCCTG N03C5. J Clin Oncol. 2007;25:308–12.
123. Laufer LR, Erlik Y, Meldrum DR, Judd HL. Effect of clonidine on hot flashes in postmenopausal women. Obstet Gynecol. 1982;60:583–6.
124. Clayden JR, Bell JW, Pollard P. Menopausal flushing: double-blind trial of a non-hormonal medication. Br Med J. 1974;1:409–12.
125. Freedman RR, Dinsay R. Clonidine raises the sweating threshold in symptomatic but not in asymptomatic postmenopausal women. Fertil Steril. 2000;74:20–3.
126. Pandya KJ, Raubertas RF, Flynn PJ, Hynes HE, Rosenbluth RJ, Kirshner JJ, et al. Oral clonidine in postmenopausal patients with breast cancer experiencing tamoxifen-induced hot flashes: a University of Rochester Cancer Center Community Clinical Oncology Program study. Ann Intern Med. 2000;132:788–93.
127. Lebherz TB, French L. Nonhormonal treatment of the menopausal syndrome. A double-blind evaluation of an autonomic system stabilizer. Obstet Gynecol. 1969;33:795–9.
128. Bergmans MG, Merkus JM, Corbey RS, Schellekens LA, Ubachs JM. Effect of Bellergal Retard on climacteric complaints: a double-blind, placebo-controlled study. Maturitas. 1987;9:227–34.
129. Pockaj BA, Gallagher JG, Loprinzi CL, Stella PJ, Barton DL, Sloan JA, et al. Phase III double-blind, randomized, placebo-controlled crossover trial of black cohosh in the management of hot flashes: NCCTG Trial N01CC1. J Clin Oncol. 2006;24:2836–41.
130. Huang MI, Nir Y, Chen B, Schnyer R, Manber R. A randomized controlled pilot study of acupuncture for postmenopausal hot flashes: effect on nocturnal hot flashes and sleep quality. Fertil Steril. 2006;86:700–710.
131. Freedman RR, Woodward S. Behavioral treatment of menopausal hot flushes: evaluation by ambulatory monitoring. Am J Obstet Gynecol. 1992;167:436–9.
132. Wijma K, Melin A, Nedstrand E, Hammar M. Treatment of menopausal symptoms with applied relaxation: a pilot study. J Behav Ther Exp Psychiatry. 1997;28:251–61.
132. Taylor M. Alternatives to conventional hormone replacement therapy. Contemp Ob/GYN. 1999 May:23–50.
133. Karacan S. Effects of long-term aerobic exercise on physical fitness and postmenopausal symptoms with menopausal rating scale. Sci. Sports. 2009;25:39–46.
134. Society of Obstetricians and Gynaecologists of Canada. The detection and management of vaginal atrophy. Number 145, May 2004. Int J Gynaecol Obstet. 2005; 88:222–8.
135. Rosen RC, Taylor JF, Leiblum SR, Bachmann GA. Prevalence of sexual dysfunction in women: results of a survey study of 329 women in an outpatient gynecological clinic. J Sex Marital Ther. 1993;19:171–88.
136. Bachmann G, Bouchard C, Hoppe D, Ranganath R, Altomare C, Vieweg A, et al. Efficacy and safety of low-dose regimens of conjugated estrogens cream administered vaginally. Menopause. 2009;16:719–27.
137. Freedman M, Kaunitz AM, Reape KZ, Hait H, Shu H. Twice-weekly synthetic conjugated estrogens vaginal cream for the treatment of vaginal atrophy. Menopause. 2009;16:735–41.
138. Dorr MB, Nelson AL, Mayer PR, Ranganath RP, Norris PM, Helzner EC, Preston RA. Plasma estrogen concentrations after oral and vaginal estrogen administration in women with atrophic vaginitis. Fertil Steril. 2010 May 11. [Epub ahead of print]
139. Simon JA, Ibe C. Vulvovaginal atrophy: current and future therapies (CME). J Sex Med. 2010;7:1042–50
140. Cicinelli E, Di Naro E, De Ziegler D, Matteo M, Morgese S, Galantino P, et al. Placement of the vaginal 17beta-estradiol tablets in the inner or outer one third of the vagina affects the preferential delivery of 17beta-estradiol toward the uterus or peri-

urethral areas, thereby modifying efficacy and endometrial safety. Am J Obstet Gynecol. 2003;189:55–8.

141. Labrie F, Luu-The V, Bélanger A, Lin SX, Simard J, Pelletier G, Labrie C. Is dehydroepiandrosterone a hormone? J Endocrinol. 2005;187:169–96.

142. Labrie F, Diamond P, Cusan L, Gomez JL, Bélanger A, Candas B. Effect of 12-month dehydroepiandrosterone replacement therapy on bone, vagina, and endometrium in postmenopausal women. J Clin Endocrinol Metab. 1997;82:3498–505.

143. Wing R, Creasman J, West D, Richter H, Meyers D, Burgio K, Franklin F, Gorin A, Vitrringhoff E, et al. Improving urinary incontinence in overweight and obese women through modest weight loss. Obstetrics & Gynecol 2010;116:284–292.

144. Giltay EJ, Kamphuis MH, Kalmijn S, Zitman FG, Kromhout D. Dispositional optimism and the risk of cardiovascular death: the Zutphen Elderly Study. Arch Intern Med. 2006;166:431–6.

145. National Cancer Insititute. Available from: http://www.cancer.gov/bcrisktool/. Accessed October 18, 2010.

146. Bone health and osteoporosis: a report of the Surgeon General. Rockville, MD: U.S. Dept. of Health and Human Services, Public Health Service, Office of the Surgeon General; Washington, D.C.: 2004. p.35. Available from: http://www.surgeongeneral.gov/library/bonehealth/ppt_html.html. Accessed September 3, 2010.

147. Home Safety Checklists. Fall Prevention Project, Pima Council on Aging. Available at: www.cdc.gov/ncipc/duip/fallsmaterial.htm. Accessed October 14, 2010.

148. Management of osteoporosis in postmenopausal women: 2010 position statement of The North American Menopause Society. Menopause: The Journal of the North American Menopause Society. Vol 17 No 1: 25–54.

149. WHO Assessment Fracture Risk Tool. World Health Organization Collaborating Centre for Metabolic Bone Diseases. Available at: www.shef.ac.ukk/FRAX/index.htm. Accessed October 14, 2010.

150. Miller PD, Derman RJ. What is the best balance of benefits and risks among anti-resorptive therapies for postmenopausal osteoporosis? Osteoporos Int. 2010;21:1793–802.

LATE REFERENCE

151. Ross AC, Manson JE, Abrams SA, et al. The 2011 report on dietary reference intakes for calcium and vitamin D from the Institute of Medicine: what clinicians need to know. J Clin Endocrinol Metab. 2011;96:53–8.

Contraceptive Efficacy

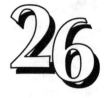

James Trussell, PhD

- Pregnancy rates during *perfect use* reflect how effective methods can be in preventing pregnancy when used *consistently and correctly* according to instructions.

- Pregnancy rates during *typical use* reflect how effective methods are for the average person who does not always use methods correctly or consistently.

- Pregnancy rates during typical use of adherence-dependent methods generally vary widely for different groups using the same method, primarily due to differences in the propensity to use the method perfectly.

- Additional empirically-based estimates of pregnancy rates during perfect use are needed.

A general explanation of the sources of evidence and the logic underlying the summary table on contraceptive efficacy (Table 3–2) is provided in Chapter 3 on Choosing a Contraceptive. This chapter more completely explains the derivation of the estimates of the first-year probabilities of pregnancy during typical use (column 2) and perfect use (column 3) in Table 3–2, reproduced as Table 26–1.[1-3] The chapter also contains tables summarizing the literature on contraceptive efficacy for each method. These are arranged in the order in which they appear in summary Table 26–1. In these tables, all studies were conducted in the United States unless otherwise noted. In the epidemiology literature, the term *efficacy* refers to how well an intervention (in this case a contraceptive method) works in clinical trials and the term *effectiveness* refers to how well it works in actual practice. We use both sorts of evidence in this chapter, but in this chapter, in Chapter 3 and throughout the book, we use these terms interchangeably in the common everyday sense of how well a method works. Finally, the chapter explains the derivation of the estimates of the proportion of women continuing use of each method for one year; this is the complement of the proportion discontinuing use within the first year for method-related reasons (one of which is contraceptive failure).

NO METHOD

Our estimate of the percentage of women becoming pregnant among those not using contraception is based on populations in which the use of contraception is rare, and on couples who report that they stopped using contraceptives because they want to conceive. Based on this evidence, we conclude that 85 of 100 sexually active couples would experience an accidental pregnancy in the first year if they used no contraception. Available evidence in the United States suggests that only about 40% of married couples who do not use contraception (but who still wish to avoid pregnancy) become pregnant within 1 year.[4,5] However, such couples are almost certainly self-selected for low fecundity or low frequency of intercourse. They do not use contraception because, in part, they are aware that they are unlikely to conceive. The probability of pregnancy of 85%, therefore, is our best guess of the fraction of women now using reversible methods of contraception who would become pregnant within 1 year if they were to abandon their current method but not otherwise change their behavior. Couples who have unprotected intercourse for a year without achieving pregnancy are, by definition, infertile (but by no means are they necessarily sterile—see Chapter 3). Table 26–2 summarizes the studies of the risk of pregnancy among women who are neither using contraception nor breastfeeding.

TYPICAL USE OF SPERMICIDES, WITHDRAWAL, FERTILITY AWARENESS-BASED METHODS, DIAPHRAGM, MALE CONDOM, ORAL CONTRACEPTIVE PILLS, AND DEPO-PROVERA

Our estimates of the probability of pregnancy during the first year of typical use for withdrawal, fertility awareness-based methods, the male condom, the pill, and Depo-Provera are weighted averages of estimates derived from the 1995 and the 2002 National Surveys of Family Growth (NSFG) and for spermicides and the diaphragm from the 1995 NSFG, all corrected for underreporting of abortion.[6,7] Since the overwhelming majority of women using fertility awareness-based methods in the NSFG use calendar rhythm (see Table 3–1), the probability of failure during typical use of the newer methods shown in Table 3–1 would be expected to be lower.

The correction for underreporting of abortion may produce estimates that are too high because women in abortion clinics (surveys of whom provided the information for the correction) tend to over-report use of a contraceptive method at the time they became pregnant. Moreover, women in personal interviews for the NSFG also might over-report use of a contraceptive method at the time of a conception leading to a live birth. Evidence for this suspicion is provided by uncorrected first-year probabilities of pregnancy of 3.7% for the IUC and 2.3% for Norplant (methods with little or no scope for user error) in the 1995 NSFG; these probabilities are much higher than rates observed in clinical trials of these methods, and for this reason we did not base the typical-use estimates for the IUC on the NSFG.[8] We would naturally expect over-reporting of contraceptive use in both the NSFG and surveys conducted in abortion clinics, because the woman (couple) can then blame the pregnancy on contraceptive "failure."

Thus, biases in opposite directions affect these estimates. Pregnancy rates based on the NSFG alone would tend to be too low because induced abortions (and contraceptive failures leading to induced abortions) are underreported but would tend to be too high because contraceptive failures leading to live births are over-reported. We reason that the former bias is the more important one.

The NSFG does not ask for brand of pill; thus combined and progestin-only pills cannot be distinguished. However, since use of the combined pill is far more common than use of the progestin-only pill, the results from the NSFG overwhelmingly reflect typical use of combined pills. The efficacy of progestin-only pills may be lower than that for combined pills since progestin-only pills are probably less forgiving of nonadherence to the dosing schedule.

PERFECT USE OF THE SPONGE AND DIAPHRAGM

Our estimates of the probabilities of pregnancy during the first year of perfect use of the sponge and diaphragm correspond with results of a reanalysis of data from two clinical trials in which women were randomly assigned to use the diaphragm or sponge or to use the diaphragm or cervical cap.[9] The results indicate that among parous women who use the sponge perfectly, 19.4% to 20.5% will experience a pregnancy within the first year. The corresponding range for nulliparous women is 9.0% to 9.5%. In contrast, parous users of the diaphragm do not appear to have higher pregnancy rates during perfect use than do nulliparous users; 4.3% to 8.4% of all women experience an accidental pregnancy during the first year of perfect use of the diaphragm. Our estimates in the third column of Table 26–1 (and Table 3–2 in Chapter 3 on Choosing a Contraceptive) are obtained from the midpoints of these ranges.

TYPICAL USE OF THE SPONGE

Here we also draw on results of the same clinical trial in which women were randomly assigned to the sponge or diaphragm. The proportion becoming pregnant during the first year of typical use for parous users of the sponge (27.4%) was about twice as high as for nulliparous users of that method (14.0%). There was no such differential for the diaphragm, where the proportion becoming pregnant in the first year of typical use for parous users (12.4%) was marginally lower than that for nulliparous users (12.8%).[10] Rather than using the estimates of failure during typical use from the clinical trial directly, we extrapolated what the estimate would be if based on all users of the sponge from the estimate for the diaphragm based on the NSFG. Specifically, we set the estimates for nulliparous users of the sponge equal to the estimate for all users of the diaphragm based on the 1995 NSFG (12%). We doubled the estimates for nulliparous users of the sponge to obtain the estimate for parous users.

PERFECT AND TYPICAL USE OF THE FEMALE CONDOM

The typical-use estimate for the female condom is based on the results of a 6-month clinical trial of the Reality female condom (now called the fc female condom); 12.4% of women in the United States experienced a pregnancy during the first 6 months of use.[10] The 12-month probability of pregnancy for users of Reality in the United States was projected from the relation between the pregnancy rates in the first 6 months and the pregnancy rates in the second 6 months for users of the diaphragm, sponge and cervical cap.[10] The probability of pregnancy during 6 months of perfect use of Reality by U.S. women who met the adherence criteria stipulated in the study protocol was 2.6%. Those who reported fewer than 4 acts of intercourse during the month prior to any follow-up visit, who did not use Reality at every act of intercourse, who ever reported not following the Reality instructions, or who used another method of contraception were censored at the beginning of the first interval where nonadherence was noted.[11] Under the assumption that the probability of pregnancy in the second 6 months of perfect use would be the same, the probability of pregnancy during a year of perfect use would be 5.1%. There have been no efficacy trials of the second version of the female condom, the fc2 female condom.

PERFECT USE OF WITHDRAWAL AND SPERMICIDES

Our estimate of the proportion becoming pregnant during a year of perfect use of withdrawal is a guess based on the reasoning that the risk of pregnancy resulting from pre-ejaculatory fluid is modest. Although three studies found no motile sperm in the pre-ejaculate,[12-14] the most recent study did not replicate this result, perhaps because the samples were examined within 2 minutes of production.[15] In that study, 37% of subjects produced pre-ejaculatory samples that contained motile sperm, and the sperm concentration and the percentage of motile sperm were similar in an individual's pre-ejaculatory and ejaculatory specimens. However, the actual number of sperm in the pre-ejaculate was low.

Our estimate of the proportion becoming pregnant during a year of perfect use of spermicides is based on a recent NIH trial of 5 spermicides.[16] We assumed that the pregnancy rate per cycle during perfect use would be constant, extrapolated a 1-year probability from the 6-cycle probability reported for each method, and took as our estimate the median (18%) of those 5 estimates. Our estimate is considerably higher than would be expected from the extensive literature on the contraceptive efficacy of spermicides.

Six studies outside the United States,[17-22] in addition to several U.S. studies reviewed earlier,[1] have yielded very low probabilities of pregnancy during the first year of typical use of spermicides, much lower than any estimates for barriers with spermicides. The efficacy literature on spermicides is dominated by studies of suppositories, foams, and film; high spermicide efficacy is documented only in these studies. There are few studies of creams and gels used alone, and those with the lowest pregnancy rates are more than 30 years old (Table 26–3). We consider it likely that the spermicide studies suffer from flaws in analysis or design that are not apparent in the brief published descriptions. For example, an FDA advisory committee was openly skeptical of one German study:[17] "the way in which the survey was designed and the manner in which the various incentives were offered" (physicians reportedly received a fee for completing survey data forms) "would clearly make the data resulting from the survey unacceptable to any scientific group or regulatory agency."[23,24]

The first clinical trial of Emko vaginal foam is also one of the few studies to compute separate pregnancy rates for cycles in which the product was used at every act of intercourse and for cycles in which unprotected intercourse occurred.[25] The design of that trial was also quite sophisticated. Women were randomly assigned to six groups. Each group used three different spermicidal products for three cycles each. The six groups represented all possible permutations of orders of use of the three products. If the pregnancy rate for three cycles of consistent use (not perfect use, which requires both consistent *and* correct use) of Emko vaginal foam is extrapolated, then the implied proportion becoming pregnant in the first year of consistent use is 8.9%.

A recent randomized clinical trial comparing the efficacy of a film and a foaming tablet—the first trial of spermicides conducted according to modern standards of design, execution, and analysis—supports the conclusion that the contraceptive efficacy of spermicides is considerably lower than was previously thought.[26] In that trial, 6-month probabilities of pregnancy during consistent use were 28% for the tablet and 24% for the film, probabilities that were nearly identical to those during typical use in that trial and about the same as the 12-month probability of pregnancy during typical use of spermicides in the 1995 NSFG.

PERFECT USE OF FERTILITY AWARENESS-BASED METHODS

The perfect-use estimates for fertility awareness-based methods are based on empirical estimates of 4.8% for the Standard Days method, 3.5% for the TwoDay method, 3.2% for the ovulation method, and 0.4 per 100 woman-years for the symptothermal method.[27-30] Published "method failure" rates for other variants of natural family planning are incorrect (see Chapter 3).

PERFECT USE OF THE MALE CONDOM

Our estimate of the proportion becoming pregnant during a year of perfect use of the male condom is based on results from the only three studies of the male condom meeting modern standards of design, execution, and analysis.[31-33] In each study, couples were randomly assigned to use either a latex condom or a polyurethane condom. All three studies reported efficacy during consistent use but only one reported efficacy during perfect use;[32] in that study the 6-cycle probability of pregnancy during perfect use (0.7%) was 70% of that (1%) during typical use. We assumed that in the other two studies the 6-cycle probability of pregnancy during perfect use would also be 70% of the 6-cycle probability during typical use, assumed that the pregnancy rate per cycle during perfect use would be constant, extrapolated a 1-year probability from the 6-cycle probability reported for the latex condom in each trial, and took as our estimate the median (2%, also the mean) of those 3 estimates. This estimate is consistent with an estimate based on studies of condom breakage and slippage.[34] Under the assumption that 1.5% of condoms break or slip off the penis and that women have intercourse twice a week, then about 1.5% of women would experience condom breaks during the half-week that they are at risk of pregnancy during each cycle. The per-cycle probability of conception would be reduced by 98.5%, from 0.1358 to only 0.0020, if a condom failure results in no protection whatsoever against pregnancy, so that about 2.6% of women would become pregnant each year.[35] Unfortunately, breakage and slippage rates did not accurately predict pregnancy rates during consistent use in one clinical trial of the latex and polyurethane male condom,[31] and estimates of condom breakage and slippage during intercourse or withdrawal vary substantially across studies in developed countries,[34] from a low of 0.6% among commercial sex workers in Nevada's legal brothels[34] to a high of 7.2% among monogamous couples in North Carolina.[36]

PERFECT USE OF ORAL CONTRACEPTIVE PILLS, DEPO-PROVERA, AND IMPLANON, AND TYPICAL USE OF IMPLANON

Although the lowest reported pregnancy rate for the combined pill during typical use is 0% (Table 26–11), recent studies indicate that pregnancies do occur, albeit rarely, during perfect use. Hence we set the perfect-use estimate for the pill at the very low level of 0.3%. The lowest reported pregnancy rate for the progestin-only pill exceeds 1% (see Table 26–10). It is likely that the progestin-only pill is less effective than the combined pill during typical use, since the progestin-only pill is probably less forgiving of nonadherence to the dosing schedule. Whether the progestin-only pill is also less effective during perfect use is unknown.

The perfect-use estimate for Depo-Provera is the weighted average of the results from the seven trials of the 150 mg IM dose (90-day or 3-month) and the two trials of the 104 mg SC dose shown in Table 26–12. These trials yield an estimate of efficacy during perfect rather than typical use because either women late for an injection were discontinued or all pregnancies reported occurred during actual use (after one injection but before the next was scheduled). In the two trials of DMPA-SC, there were no reported pregnancies during perfect use in either study.[37,38] It is possible that DMPA-SC has higher efficacy than DMPA-IM during perfect use, but the company that markets both products has made no such claim.

No clinical study has reported an Implanon failure (see Table 26–14). However, pregnancies during use of Implanon have been reported.[39] We arbitrarily set the perfect-use and typical-use failure rates for Implanon at 0.05%.

TYPICAL AND PERFECT USE OF EVRA AND NUVARING

The typical- and perfect-use estimates for the Evra patch and NuvaRing were set equal to those for the pill. It is possible that the patch and ring will prove to have better efficacy than the pill during typical use, because of better adherence with the dosing schedule. However, such superior efficacy has not been demonstrated in randomized trials. While in one trial the failure rate was lower among women randomly assigned to use the Evra patch (1.2%) than among those assigned to use the pill (2.2%), the difference was not statistically significant (p=0.6).[40] In a subsequent paper that argues that better adherence to the dosing schedule leads to better contraceptive efficacy of the patch than the pill during typical use, the authors acknowledge that it would require a trial with 24,143 subjects to demonstrate such superiority and conclude that "studies of this size to compare effectiveness may not be practical."[41] Women were randomly assigned to the NuvaRing or the pill in two studies. In one, the pregnancy rates were identical (1.2 per 100 woman-years of exposure).[42] In the second, the pregnancy rates did not differ significantly (0.25 versus 0.99 per 100 woman-years of exposure).[43]

TYPICAL AND PERFECT USE OF INTRAUTERINE CONTRACEPTIVES (IUCS)

The estimate for typical use of the ParaGard (Copper T 380A) IUC is taken directly from the large study for that method shown in Table 26–13. The estimate for Mirena (LNg-IUC) is the weighted average of the results from the three studies shown in Table 26–13. The estimate for perfect use of the Copper T 380A was obtained by removing the pregnancies that resulted when the device was not known to be in situ,[44] on the perhaps-questionable assumption that these pregnancies should be classified as user failures and the empirically-based assumption that expulsions are so uncommon that the denominator of the perfect-use pregnancy rate is virtually the same as the denominator for the typical-use rate (Table 26–13). The perfect-use estimate for the LNg-IUC was derived analogously. No differences in the typical-use and perfect-use estimates for LNg-IUC are apparent due to the fact that only one significant digit is shown.

TYPICAL AND PERFECT USE OF STERILIZATION

The weighted average of the results from the nine vasectomy studies in Table 26–16 analyzed with life-table procedures is 0.02% becoming pregnant in the year following the procedure. In eight of these studies, pregnancies occurred after the ejaculate had been declared to be sperm-free. This perfect-use estimate of 0.02% is undoubtedly too low, because clinicians are understandably loath to publish articles describing their surgical failures and journals would be reluctant to publish an article documenting poor surgical technique. The difference between typical-use and perfect-use pregnancy rates for vasectomy would depend on the frequency of unprotected intercourse after the procedure had been performed but before the ejaculate had been certified to be sperm-free. We arbitrarily set the typical- and perfect-use estimates to 0.15% and 0.10%, respectively. For female sterilization (except for Essure and Adiana), there is no scope for user error. The typical- and perfect-use estimates are the pooled results from the U.S. Collaborative Review of Sterilization, a prospective study of 10,685 women undergoing tubal sterilization.[45] We are less concerned about publication bias with female than with male sterilization because the largest studies of female sterilization are based on prospective, multicenter clinical trials, not retrospective reports from one investigator.

CONTRACEPTIVE CONTINUATION

Contraceptives will be effective at preventing unintended pregnancy only if women or couples continue to use them once they have initiated use. The proportions of women continuing use at the end of the first year for withdrawal, fertility awareness-based methods, the male condom, the pill, and Depo-Provera were obtained from the 2002 NSFG and for spermicides, the sponge, and the diaphragm were obtained from the 1995 NSFG.[5,8] Only method-related reasons for discontinuation (changing methods or termination of contraceptive use while still at risk for unintended pregnancy) were counted. Other reasons for discontinuing use of a method (such as attempting to get pregnant or not having intercourse) are not counted in the discontinuation rate because these reasons are unrelated to the method and do not apply to women seeking to avoid pregnancy and at risk of becoming pregnant. For the female condom, we adjusted the continuation rate for the male condom to reflect a higher pregnancy rate.

We set the continuation rates for the Evra patch and NuvaRing equal to that for the pill. We set the continuation rate for Implanon equal to that for Norplant, which was derived from the 1995 NSFG.[8]

Discontinuation rates of the two IUCs (for reasons related to the contraceptive) are based on clinical trials. The estimate for the Copper T 380A IUC was taken directly from the large study for that method shown in Table 26–13. The estimate for the LNg-IUC is the weighted average from the three studies shown in Table 26–13.

EMERGENCY CONTRACEPTION
See Chapter 6.

THE LACTATIONAL AMENORRHEA METHOD (LAM)

LAM is a highly effective, temporary method of contraception. If the infant is being fed only its mother's breastmilk (or is given supplemental nonbreastmilk feeds only to a minor extent) and if the woman has not experienced her first postpartum menses, then breastfeeding provides more than 98% protection from pregnancy in the first 6 months following a birth.[46,47] Four prospective clinical studies of the contraceptive effect of LAM demonstrated cumulative 6-month life-table perfect-use pregnancy rates of 0.5%, 0.6%, 1.0%, and 1.5% among women who relied solely on LAM.[48-51]

REFERENCES

1. Trussell J, Kost K. Contraceptive failure in the United States: a critical review of the literature. Stud Fam Plann. 1987;18:237–83.
2. Trussell J, Hatcher RA, Cates W, Stewart FH, Kost K. Contraceptive failure in the United States: an update. Stud Fam Plann. 1990;21:51–4.
3. Trussell J. Contraceptive failure in the United States. Contraception. 2004;70:89–96.
4. Grady WR, Hayward MD, Yagi J. Contraceptive failure in the United States: estimates from the 1982 National Survey of Family Growth. Fam Plann Perspect. 1986;18:200–9.
5. Vaughan B, Trussell J, Kost K, Singh S, Jones R. Discontinuation and resumption of contraceptive use: results from the 2002 National Survey of Family Growth. Contraception. 2008;78:271–83.
6. Kost K, Singh S, Vaughan B, Trussell J, Bankole A. Estimates of contraceptive failure from the 2002 National Survey of Family Growth. Contraception. 2008;77:10–21.
7. Trussell J. Estimates of contraceptive failure from the 1995 National Survey of Family Growth. Contraception. 2008;78:85.
8. Trussell J, Vaughan B. Contraceptive failure, method-related discontinuation and resumption of use: results from the 1995 National Survey of Family Growth. Fam Plann Perspect. 1999;31:64–72, 93.
9. Trussell J, Strickler J, Vaughan B. Contraceptive efficacy of the diaphragm, the sponge and the cervical cap. Fam Plann Perspect. 1993;25:100–5, 135.
10. Trussell J, Sturgen K, Strickler J, Dominik R. Comparative contraceptive efficacy of the female condom and other barrier methods. Fam Plann Perspect. 1994;26:66–72.
11. Farr G, Gabelnick H, Sturgen K, Dorflinger L. Contraceptive efficacy and acceptability of the female condom. Am J Public Health. 1994;84:1960–4.
12. Ilaria G, Jacobs JL, Polsky B, Koll B, Baron P, MacLow C, Armstrong D, Schlegel PN. Detection of HIV-1 DNA sequences in pre-ejaculatory fluid. Lancet. 1992;340:1469.
13. Pudney J, Oneta M, Mayer K, Seage G, Anderson D. Pre-ejaculatory fluid as potential vector for sexual transmission of HIV-1. Lancet. 1992;340:1470.
14. Zukerman Z, Weiss DB, Orvieto R. Does preejaculatory penile secretion originating from Cowper's gland contain sperm? J Assist Reprod Genet. 2003;20:157–9.
15. Killick SR, Leary C, Trussell J, Guthrie KA. Sperm content of pre-ejaculatory fluid. Hum Fertil. 2011;14:48–52.

16. Raymond EG, Chen PL, Luoto J. Contraceptive effectiveness and safety of five nonoxynol-9 spermicides: a randomized trial. Obstet Gynecol. 2004;103:430–9.
17. Brehm H, Haase W. Die alternative zur hormonalen kontrazeption? Med Welt. 1975;26:1610–7. German.
18. Dimpfl J, Salomon W, Schicketanz KH. Die spermizide barriere. Sexualmedizin. 1984;13:95–8. German.
19. Florence N. Das kontrazeptive vaginal-suppositorium: ergebnisse einer klinischen fünfjahresstudie. Sexualmedizin. 1977;6:385–6. German.
20. Godts P. Klinische prüfung eines vaginalem antikonzipiens. Ars Medici. 1973;2:589–93. German.
21. Iizuka R, Kobayashi T, Kawakami S, Nakamura Y, Ikeuchi M, Chin B, Mochimaru F, Sumi K, Sato H, Yamaguchi J, Ohno T, Shiina M, Maeda N, Tokoro H, Suzuki T, Hayashi K, Takahashi T, Akatsuka M, Kasuga Y, Kurokawa H. Clinical experience with the Vaginal Contraceptive Film containing the spermicide polyoxyethylene nonylphenyl ether (C-Film study group). Jpn J Fertil Steril. 1980;25:64–8. (In Japanese; translation supplied by Apothecus Inc.)
22. Salomon W, Haase W. Intravaginale kontrazeption. Sexualmedizin. 1977;6:198–202. German.
23. Over-the-Counter Contraceptives and Other Vaginal Drug Products Review Panel (Elizabeth B. Connell, Chairman). Encare Oval. Memorandum to Food and Drug Administration Commissioner Donald Kennedy, February 9, 1978.
24. Stewart FH, Stewart G, Guest FJ, Hatcher RA. My body, my health: the concerned woman's guide to gynecology. New York: John Wiley & Sons; 1979.
25. Mears E. Chemical contraceptive trial: II. J Reprod Fertil. 1962;4:337–43.
26. Raymond E, Dominik R, The Spermicide Trial Group. Contraceptive effectiveness of two spermicides: a randomized trial. Obstet Gynecol. 1999;93:896–903.
27. Arévalo M, Jennings V, Sinai I. Efficacy of a new method of family planning: the Standard Days method. Contraception. 2002;65:333–8.
28. Arévalo M, Jennings V, Nikula M, Sinai I.Efficacy of the new TwoDay Method of family planning. Fertil Steril. 2004;82:885–92.
29. Trussell J, Grummer-Strawn L. Contraceptive failure of the ovulation method of periodic abstinence. Fam Plann Perspect. 1990;22:65–75.
30. Frank-Herrmann P, Heil J, Gnoth C, Toledo E, Baur S, Pyper C, Jenetzky E, Strowitzki T, Freundl G. The effectiveness of a fertility awareness based method to avoid pregnancy in relation to a couple's sexual behaviour during the fertile time: a prospective longitudinal study. Hum Reprod. 2007;22:1310–9.
31. Frezieres RG, Walsh TL, Nelson AL, Clark VA, Coulson AH. Evaluation of the efficacy of a polyurethane condom: results from a randomized controlled clinical trial. Fam Plann Perspect. 1999;31:81–7.
32. Walsh TL, Frezieres RG, Peacock K, Nelson AL, Clark VA, Bernstein L. Evaluation of the efficacy of a nonlatex condom: results from a randomized, controlled clinical trial. Perspect Sex Reprod Health. 2003;35:79–86.
33. Steiner MJ, Dominik R, Rountree RW, Nanda K, Dorflinger LJ. Contraceptive effectiveness of a polyurethane condom and a latex condom: a randomized controlled trial. Obstet Gynecol. 2003;101:539–47.
34. Albert AE, Warner DL, Hatcher RA, Trussell J, Bennett C. Condom use among female commercial sex workers in Nevada's legal brothels. Am J Public Health. 1995;85:1514–20.
35. Kestelman P, Trussell J. Efficacy of the simultaneous use of condoms and spermicides. Fam Plann Perspect. 1991;23:226–7, 232.
36. Steiner M, Piedrahita C, Glover L, Joanis C. Can condom users likely to experience condom failure be identified? Fam Plann Perspect. 1993;25:220–3, 226.
37. Jain J, Jakimiuk AJ, Bode FR, Ross D, Kaunitz AM. Contraceptive efficacy and safety of DMPA-SC. Contraception. 2004;70:269–75.

38. Kaunitz AM, Darney PD, Ross D, Wolter KD, Speroff L. Subcutaneous DMPA vs. Intramuscular DMPA: a 2-year randomized study of contraceptive efficacy and bone mineral desity. Contraception. 2009;80:7–17.

39. Graesslin O, Korver T. The contraceptive efficacy of Implanon: a review of clinical trials and marketing experience. Eur J Contracept Reprod Health Care. 2008;13 Suppl 1:S4–12.

40. Audet MC, Moreau M, Koltun WD, Waldbaum AS, Shangold G, Fisher AC, Creasy GW. Evaluation of contraceptive efficacy and cycle control of a transdermal contraceptive patch vs. an oral contraceptive. JAMA. 2001;285:2347–54.

41. Archer DF, Cullins V, Creasy GW, Fisher AC. The impact of improved compliance with a weekly contraceptive transdermal system (Ortho Evra® on contraceptive efficacy. Contraception. 2004;69:189–95.

42. Oddsson K, Leifels-Fischer B, de Melo NR, Wiel-Masson D, Benedetto C, Verhoeven CH, Dieben TO. Efficacy and safety of a contraceptive vaginal ring (NuvaRing) compared with a combined oral contraceptive: a 1-year randomized trial. Contraception. 2005;71:176–82.

43. Ahrendt HJ, Nisand I, Bastianelli C, Gómez MA, Gemzell-Danielsson K, Urdl W, Karskov B, Oeyen L, Bitzer J, Page G, Milsom I. Efficacy, acceptability and tolerability of the combined contraceptive ring, NuvaRing, compared with an oral contraceptive containing 30 microg of ethinyl estradiol and 3 mg of drospirenone. Contraception. 2006;74:451–7.

44. Sivin, I. (Center for Biomedical Research, Population Council). Email to : James Trussell (Office of Population Research, Princeton University). 1992.

45. Peterson HB, Xia Z, Hughes JM, Wilcox LS, Tylor LR, Trussell J. The risk of pregnancy after tubal sterilization: findings from the U.S. Collaborative Review of Sterilization. Am J Obstet Gynecol. 1996;174:1161–70.

46. Kennedy KI, Rivera R, McNeilly AS. Consensus statement on the use of breast-feeding as a family planning method. Contraception. 1989;39:477–96.

47. Kennedy KI, Labbok MH, Van Look PFA. Lactational amenorrhea method for family planning. Int J Gynaecol Obstet. 1996;54:55–7.

48. Kazi A, Kennedy KI, Visness CM, Khan T. Effectiveness of the lactational amenorrhea method in Pakistan. Fertil Steril. 1995;64:717–23.

49. Labbok MH, Hight-Laukaran V, Peterson AE, Fletcher V, von Hertzen H, Van Look PFA. Multicenter study of the Lactational Amenorrhea Method (LAM): I. Efficacy, duration, and implications for clinical application. Contraception. 1997;55:326–36.

50. Pérez A, Labbok MH, Queenan JT. Clinical study of the lactational amenorrhoea method for family planning. Lancet. 1992;339:968–70.

51. Ramos R, Kennedy KI, Visness CM. Effectiveness of lactational amenorrhea in prevention of pregnancy in Manila, the Philippines: non-comparative prospective trial. BMJ. 1996;313:909–12.

Table 26–1 Percentage of women experiencing an unintended pregnancy during the first year of typical use and the first year of perfect use of contraception and the percentage continuing use at the end of the first year. United States.

Method (1)	% of Women Experiencing an Unintended Pregnancy within the First Year of Use		% of Women Continuing Use at One Year[3] (4)
	Typical Use[1] (2)	Perfect Use[2] (3)	
No method[4]	85	85	
Spermicides[5]	28	18	42
Fertility awareness-based methods	24		47
Standard Days method[6]		5	
TwoDay method[6]		4	
Ovulation method[6]		3	
Symptothermal method[6]		0.4	
Withdrawal	22	4	46
Sponge			36
Parous women	24	20	
Nulliparous women	12	9	
Condom[7]			
Female (fc)	21	5	41
Male	18	2	43
Diaphragm[8]	12	6	57
Combined pill and progestin-only pill	9	0.3	67
Evra patch	9	0.3	67
NuvaRing	9	0.3	67
Depo-Provera	6	0.2	56
Intrauterine contraceptives			
ParaGard (copper T)	0.8	0.6	78
Mirena (LNg)	0.2	0.2	80
Implanon	0.05	0.05	84
Female sterilization	0.5	0.5	100
Male sterilization	0.15	0.10	

Emergency Contraception: Emergency contraceptive pills or insertion of a copper intrauterine contraceptive after unprotected intercourse substantially reduces the risk of pregnancy.[9] (See Chapter 6.)

Lactational Amenorrhea Method: LAM is a highly effective, *temporary* method of contraception.[10] (See Chapter 18.)

Source: See text

(continued)

Table 26–1 Percentage of women experiencing an unintended pregnancy during the first year of typical use and the first year of perfect use of contraception and the percentage continuing use at the end of the first year. United States–*(cont'd)*

Notes:

[1] Among *typical* couples who initiate use of a method (not necessarily for the first time), the percentage who experience an accidental pregnancy during the first year if they do not stop use for any reason other than pregnancy. Estimates of the probability of pregnancy during the first year of typical use for spermicides and the diaphragm are taken from the 1995 National Survey of Family Growth corrected for underreporting of abortion; estimates for fertility awareness-based methods, withdrawal, the male condom, the pill, and Depo-Provera are taken from the 1995 and 2002 National Survey of Family Growth corrected for underreporting of abortion. See the text for the derivation of estimates for the other methods.

[2] Among couples who initiate use of a method (not necessarily for the first time) and who use it *perfectly* (both consistently and correctly), the percentage who experience an accidental pregnancy during the first year if they do not stop use for any other reason. See the text for the derivation of the estimate for each method.

[3] Among couples attempting to avoid pregnancy, the percentage who continue to use a method for 1 year.

[4] The percentages becoming pregnant in columns (2) and (3) are based on data from populations where contraception is not used and from women who cease using contraception in order to become pregnant. Among such populations, about 89% become pregnant within 1 year. This estimate was lowered slightly (to 85%) to represent the percentage who would become pregnant within 1 year among women now relying on reversible methods of contraception if they abandoned contraception altogether.

[5] Foams, creams, gels, vaginal suppositories, and vaginal film.

[6] The Ovulation and TwoDay methods are based on evaluation of cervical mucus. The Standard Days method avoids intercourse on cycle days 8 through 19. The Symptothermal method is a double-check method based on evaluation of cervical mucus to determine the first fertile day and evaluation of cervical mucus and temperature to determine the last fertile day.

[7] Without spermicides.

[8] With spermicidal cream or jelly.

[9] ella, Plan B One-Step and Next Choice are the only dedicated products specifically marketed for emergency contraception. The label for Plan B One-Step (one dose is 1 white pill) says to take the pill within 72 hours after unprotected intercourse. Research has shown that that all of the brands listed here are effective when used within 120 hours after unprotected sex. The label for Next Choice (one dose is 1 peach pill) says to take one pill within 72 hours after unprotected intercourse and another pill 12 hours later. Research has shown that that both pills can be taken at the same time with no decrease in efficacy or increase in side effects and that they are effective when used within 120 hours after unprotected sex. The Food and Drug Administration has in addition declared the following 19 brands of oral contraceptives to be safe and effective for emergency contraception: Ogestrel (1 dose is 2 white pills), Nordette (1 dose is 4 light-orange pills), Cryselle, Levora, Low-Ogestrel, Lo/Ovral, or Quasence (1 dose is 4 white pills), Jolessa, Portia, Seasonale or Trivora (1 dose is 4 pink pills), Seasonique (1 dose is 4 light-blue-green pills), Enpresse (one dose is 4 orange pills), Lessina (1 dose is 5 pink pills), Aviane or LoSeasonique (one dose is 5 orange pills), Lutera or Sronyx (one dose is 5 white pills), and Lybrel (one dose is 6 yellow pills).

[10] However, to maintain effective protection against pregnancy, another method of contraception must be used as soon as menstruation resumes, the frequency or duration of breastfeeds is reduced, bottle feeds are introduced, or the baby reaches 6 months of age.

Table 26-2 Summary of studies of pregnancy rates among women neither contracepting nor breastfeeding[a]

Reference	N for Analysis	Life-Table 12-Month % Pregnant	Characteristics of the Sample	LFU (%)[g]	Comments
Grady et al., 1986	1,028	43.1	All married	20.6[r]	1982 NSFG; estimate far too low; see text
Sivin and Stern, 1979	420	78.1	48% nulliparous	?	Following removal of copper–medicated IUD for planned pregnancy
Vessey et al., 1978	779	82	All nulligravid	?	Britain; Oxford/FPA study following cessation of method use for planned pregnancy; conceptions leading to a live birth
Tatum, 1975	553	84.6		17.2	Following removal of copper–medicated IUD for planned pregnancy
Sivin, 1987	96	87	All parous	?	Chile, Dominican Republic, Finland, Sweden, United States; following removal of Norplant for planned pregnancy
Tietze and Lewit, 1970	378	88.2	89% aged 15–29	19.0	Following removal of nonmedicated IUD for planned pregnancy
Sheps, 1965	397	88.8	All married Hutterites	?	Conceptions leading to the first live birth following marriage among women reporting no fetal losses before the first conception
Vessey et al., 1978	1,343	89	All parous	?	Britain; Oxford/FPA study following cessation of method use for planned pregnancy; conceptions leading to a live birth
Belhadj et al., 1986	110	94.0[c]	All parous; aged 18–36	9.1	Brazil, Chile, Dominican Republic, Singapore, United States; following removal of medicated IUD for planned pregnancy

Notes:

[a] Updated from Trussell and Kost (1987), Table 1.

[c] Calculated by James Trussell from data in the article.

[g] Most of these studies incorrectly report the loss to follow-up probability as the number of women lost at any time during the study divided by the total number of women entering the study. Thus, these are the probabilities presented in the table. However, the correct measure of LFU would be a gross life-table probability. When available, gross 12-month probabilities are denoted by the letter "g."

[r] Nonresponse rate for entire survey.

For table references, see reference section.

Table 26–3 Summary of studies of contraceptive failure: spermicides[a]

Reference	Method Brand	N for Analysis	Life-Table 12-Month % Pregnant	Risk of Pregnancy — Pearl Index Pregnancy Rate			Characteristics of the Sample	LFU (%)[g]	Comments
				Index	Total Exposure	Maximum Exposure			
Edelman, 1980	S'positive	200		0.0	2,682 Mo.	?		?	Study conducted by Jordan-Simner, Inc., as reported by Edelman
Squire et al., 1979	Semicid Suppository	326	0.3				69% aged 20–34; 55% married; "well educated"; "highly motivated"; 24% prior use of oral contraceptives	0.0[c]	89% reported exclusive use of foam
Soloman and Haase, 1977	Patentex (Encare) Oval	1,652		0.3[c]	34,506 Cy.	54 Mo.	13% aged 15–20, 48% aged 21–30, 33% aged 31–40, 6% aged 41–45, 42% nulliparous	?	Subjects who used for less than one year excluded? Germany
Iizuka et al., 1980	Vaginal Contraceptive Film (C-Film)	168		0.6	2,161 Mo.	?	All women had been pregnant before; 20% aged <25, 64% aged 25–34,17% aged 35+	?	Japan
Brehm and Haase, 1975	Patentex (Encare) Oval	10,017		0.9[c]	63,759 Cy.	?	18% aged <21, 20% aged >35; 46% parity 0	?	Germany; FDA rejected this study because of flawed design (see text)
Florence, 1977	a-gen 53	103		1.2[c]	2,255 Cy.	61 Mo.	17% aged 17–20, 51% aged 21–30, 20% aged 31–40,12% aged 41+	?	Belgium
Dimpfl et al., 1974	Pantentex (Encare) Oval	482	1.5				22% aged <21,25% aged >31; 44% parity 0; 60% married	?	Denmark, Germany, Poland, Switzerland
Bushnell, 1965	Emko Vaginal Foam	130		1.8	2,737 Mo.	57 Mo.	Aged 17–51; 76% aged 20–35	?	

(continued)

Table 26-3 Summary of studies of contraceptive failure: spermicides[a]—*(cont'd)*

Reference	Method Brand	N for Analysis	Life-Table 12-Month % Pregnant	Pearl Index Pregnancy Rate — Index	Pearl Index Pregnancy Rate — Total Exposure	Pearl Index Pregnancy Rate — Maximum Exposure	Characteristics of the Sample	LFU (%)[g]	Comments
Godts, 1973	a-gen 53	56		1.9[c]	1,344 Cy.	32 Mo.	21% aged 18–20, 46% aged 21–30, 18% aged 31–40, 14% aged 41+; all gravid	?	
Carpenter and Martin, 1970	Emko Pre-fil Vaginal Foam	1,778		3.4[c]	17,200 Cy.	18 Cy.	69% aged 21–35; 24% ≥12 years education; 44% no previous contraceptive experience	14.2[c]	All women agreed to exclusive use of foam
Brigato et al., 1982	Vaginal Contraceptive Film (C-Film)	37		3.9[c]	924 Mo.	?		?	Italy
Wolf et al., 1957	Preceptin Vaginal Gel	112		4.2[c]	1,145 Mo.	?	All aged 13–40; mean age = 25[i]; all married	6.9[c]	
Bernstein, 1971	Emko Pre-fil Vaginal Foam	2,932		4.3[c]	28,332 Cy.	20 Cy.	70% aged 21–35; 39% ≥12 years education	16.1[c]	All women agreed to exclusive use of foam
Tyler, 1965	Delfen Vaginal Foam	672		6.0	9,486 Cy.	≥16 Mo.	Rates for full applicator doses and half doses combined	?	
Apothecus, 1992	Vaginal Contraceptive Film (C-Film)	761		6.5	6,501 Mo.	?			Belgium, Netherlands, Britain, Germany, Switzerland, Denmark, Sweden, Israel, Egypt; results never published; quality of study unknown

(continued)

Table 26-3 Summary of studies of contraceptive failure: spermicides–(cont'd)

Reference	Method Brand	N for Analysis	Life-Table 12-Month % Pregnant	Pearl Index Pregnancy Rate			Characteristics of the Sample	LFU (%)[g]	Comments
				Index	Total Exposure	Maximum Exposure			
Kleppinger, 1965	Delfen Vaginal Foam	138		7.5	1,116 Mo.	19 Mo.	53% aged 21–30; 27% postpartum	0.0[c-g]	
Dubrow and Kuder, 1958	Delfen Vaginal Cream	338		7.6	633 Mo.	12 Mo.	Mean age = 25; 93% ≤12 years education; 39% black; 45% Puerto Rican t	59.5[c]	
Dubrow and Kuder, 1958	Preceptin Vaginal Gel	835		8.1	3,728 Mo.	23 Mo.	Mean age = 25; 93% ≤12 years education; 39% black; 45% Puerto Rican t	45.1[c]	
Wolf et al., 1957	Delfen Vaginal Cream	875		8.9[c]	5,232 Mo.	30 Mo.	All aged 13–40; mean age = 25; all married	13.0[c]	
Frankman et al., 1975	Vaginal Contraceptive Film (C-Film)	237		9.0	1,866 Mo.	23 Mo.		?	Sweden; data included in Apothecus (1992)
Rovinsky, 1964	Delfen Vaginal Cream	251		9.1	2,915 Mo.	67 Mo.	70% aged 20–34; 55% Puerto Rican; 10% ≥13 years education	28.0[c]	
Raymond et al., 2004	100 mg suppository (Encare)	299	10.0[d]				44% aged 18–25	22	Random assignment to 100 mg suppository, 52.5 mg gel, 100 mg gel, 150 mg gel or 100 mg film
Raymond et al., 2004	100 mg film (Ortho Options Contraceptive Film)	295	11.9[d]				43% aged 18–25	24	Random assignment to 100 mg film, 52.5 mg gel, 100 mg gel, 150 mg gel or 100 mg suppository

(continued)

Table 26-3 Summary of studies of contraceptive failure: spermicides[a]—(cont'd)

				Risk of Pregnancy					
			Life-Table	Pearl Index Pregnancy Rate					
Reference	Method Brand	N for Analysis	12-Month % Pregnant	Index	Total Exposure	Maximum Exposure	Characteristics of the Sample	LFU (%)[g]	Comments
Vessey et al., 1982		?		11.9	303 Yr.	?	All white; at recruitment aged 25–39 and married; at enrollment, all women had been using the diaphragm, IUD, or pill successfully for at least 5 months	0.3[t,v]	Britain; Oxford/FPA study
Jones and Forrest, 1992		267	13.4				Aged 15–44[t]	21[r]	NSFG 1988; probablity when standardized and corrected for estimated underreporting of abortion = 30.2[s]
Raymond et al., 2004	150 mg gel (Ortho Options Conceptrol)	300	14.0[d]		43% aged 18–25	21	Random assignment to 150 mg gel, 52.5 mg gel, 100 mg gel, 100 mg film or 100 mg suppository		
Vaughan et al., 1977		596	14.9[s]				Aged 15–44; all married[t]	19.0[r]	NSFG 1973
Trussell and Vaughan, 1999		164	15.3				Aged 15–44[t]	21[r]	NSFG 1995
Raymond et al., 2004	100 mg gel (Ortho Options Conceptrol)	295	15.5[d]				46% aged 18–25	25	Random assignment to 100 mg gel, 52.5 mg gel, 150 mg gel, 100 mg film or 100 mg suppository
Trussell, 2008		272	16.4				Aged 15–44[t]	21[r]	NSFG 1995; probability when corrected for estimated underreporting of absorption = 28.2

(continued)

Table 26-3 Summary of studies of contraceptive failure: spermicides[a]—(cont'd)

Reference	Method Brand	N for Analysis	Life-Table 12-Month % Pregnant	Risk of Pregnancy Pearl Index Pregnancy Rate			Characteristics of the Sample	LFU (%)[g]	Comments
				Index	Total Exposure	Maximum Exposure			
Fu et al., 1999		?	16.6					21[r]	NSFG 1995; probability when standardized and corrected for estimated underreporting of abortion = 29.0[s]
Grady et al., 1983		1,106	17.5[s,c]				Aged 15–44; all married[t]	18.2[r]	NSFG 1973 and 1976
Schirm et al., 1982		1,106	17.9[s]				Aged 15–44; all married[t]	18.2[r]	NSFG 1973 and 1976
Mears, 1962	Emko Aerosol Foam (nonoxynol 10–11)	425		18.0[c]	722 Cy.	3 Cy.	Pearl index of 9.3 among consistent and 48.4 among inconsistent users	>20[c,t]	Britain; postal trial; random assignment to foam, foaming tablet, or pessary with crossover design
Kasabach, 1962	Koromex A Jelly	242		21.0[c]	2,058 Mo.	24 Mo.	36% aged 25–35; all married; 68% "had a high school education"; all parous	19.3[c]	
Bracher and Santow, 1992		89	21.5				27% aged <20, 56% aged 20–29, 17% aged 30+; 49% parity 0; 87% married or cohabiting	25[r]	Australian Family Survey; first use of method
Grady et al., 1986		284	21.8[s]				Aged 15–44; all married[t]	20.6[r]	NSFG 1982
Raymond et al., 2004	52.5 mg gel (Advantage S)	296	22.2[d]				43% aged 18–25	20	Random assignment to 52.5 mg gel, 100 mg gel, 150 mg gel, 100 mg film or 100 mg suppository

(continued)

Table 26–3 Summary of studies of contraceptive failure: spermicides[a]—(cont'd)

Reference	Method Brand	N for Analysis	Life-Table 12-Month % Pregnant	Pearl Index Pregnancy Rate — Index	Pearl Index Pregnancy Rate — Total Exposure	Maximum Exposure	Characteristics of the Sample	LFU (%)[g]	Comments
				Risk of Pregnancy					
Dingle and Tietze, 1963	Lactikol	170		23.5	1,789 Mo.	36 Mo.	Median age = 24.5	3.2[t]	
Frank, 1962	Koromex A Jelly	824		24.8[c]	5,767 Mo.	12 Mo.	72% aged 21–35	17.0[c]	
Raymond et al., 1999	Vaginal Contraceptive Film	369	24.9[d]				Aged 18–35; 17% nulligravid	5.8	Mexico, Ecuador, Guatemala, Ghana, United States; random assignment to Vaginal Contraceptive Film or Conceptrol foaming tablets
Raymond et al., 1999	Conceptrol foaming tablets	365	28.0[d]				Aged 18–35; 16% nulligravid	7.3	Mexico, Ecuador, Guatemala, Ghana, United States; random assignment to Conceptrol foaming tablets or Vaginal Contraceptive Film
Tietze and Lewit, 1967	Emko Vaginal Foam	779	28.3				86% < age 30; all married; 47% ≥ high school completion; 75% nonwhite	6.9[g]	
Dingle and Tietze, 1963	Durafoam	421		28.5	2,985 Mo.	36 Mo.	Median age = 26.1	3.2[t]	

(continued)

Table 26–3 Summary of studies of contraceptive failure: spermicides[a]—(cont'd)

Reference	Method Brand	N for Analysis	Life-Table 12-Month % Pregnant	Pearl Index Pregnancy Rate — Index	Pearl Index Pregnancy Rate — Total Exposure	Pearl Index Pregnancy Rate — Maximum Exposure	Characteristics of the Sample	LFU (%)[g]	Comments
Mears, 1962	Genexol Pessary (nonoxynol 10–11)	425		30.3	730 Cy.	3 Cy.		>20[c,t]	Britain; postal trial; random assignment to foam, foaming tablets, or pessary with crossover design
Tietze and Lewit, 1967	Cooper Creme and Creme Jel, Koromex A, Lactikol Creme and Jelly, Lanesta Gel	806	36.8				79% < age 30; all married; 53% ≥ high school completion; 75% nonwhite	3.4[g]	
Mears, 1962	Volpar Foaming Tablets (phenyl mercuric acetate)	425		48.2[c]	728 Cy.	3 Cy.	Pearl index of 44.4 among consistent and 64.1 among inconsistent users	>20[c,t]	Britain; postal trial; random assignment to foam, foaming tablet, or pessary with crossover design
Mears and Please, 1962	Staycept Cream (hexyl resorcinol)	678		49.6[c]	707 Cy.	3 Cy.	Pearl index of 31.4 among consistent and 132.0 among inconsistent users	>41[c,t]	Britain; postal trial: random assignment to cream, foaming tablet, or pessary with crossover design
Mears and Please, 1962	Genexol Pessary (quinine)	678		52.2	647 Cy.	3 Cy.		>41[c,t]	Britain; postal trial: random assignment to cream, foaming tablet, or pessary with crossover design
Smith et al., 1974	Vaginal Contraceptive Film (C-Film)	63[c]		55.7[c]	194[c] Mo.	<15[c]	Aged 16–35	9.5[c]	Britain; trial terminated for ethical reasons

(continued)

Table 26–3 Summary of studies of contraceptive failure: spermicides[a]—(cont'd)

			Risk of Pregnancy					
		Life-Table	Pearl Index Pregnancy Rate					
Reference	Method Brand	N for Analysis	12-Month % Pregnant	Index	Total Exposure	Maximum Exposure	Characteristics of the Sample	LFU (%)[g]	Comments
Mears and Please, 1962	Volpar Foaming Tablets (phenyl mercuric acetate)	678		59.0[c]	705 Cy.	3 Cy.	Pearl index of 47.8 among consistent and 106.7 among inconsistent users	>41[c,t]	Britain; postal trial; random assignment to cream, foaming tablet, or pessary with crossover design

Notes:

[a] Updated from Trussell and Kost (1987), Table 2.

[c] Calculated by James Trussell from data in the article.

[d] 6-month probability; 12-month probability not available.

[g] Most of these studies incorrectly report the loss to follow-up probability (LFU) as the number of women lost at any time during the study divided by the total number of women entering the study. Thus, these are the probabilities presented in the table. However, the correct measure of LFU would be a gross life-table probability. When available, gross 12-month probabilities are denoted by the letter "g."[r] Nonresponse rate for entire survey.

[s] Standardized: Vaughan et al., (1977) (1973 NSFG)—intention (the average of probabilities for preventers and delayers); Grady et al., (1983) (1973 and 1976 NSFG)—intention. Our calculation (the average of probabilities for preventers and delayers); Schirm et al., (1982) (1973 and 1976 NSFG)—intention, age, and income; Grady et al., (1986) (1982 NSFG)—intention, age, poverty status, and parity; Jones and Forrest, (1992) (1988 NSFG)—age, marital status, and poverty status; Fu et al., (1999) (1995 NSFG)—age, union status, poverty status.

[t] Total for all methods in the study.

[v] The authors report that LFU for "relevant reasons (withdrawal of cooperation or loss of contact)" was 0.3% per year in the 1982 study. In the 1982 study, women had been followed for 9.5 years on average; if 0.3% are LFU per year, then 2.8% would be LFU in 9.5 years. LFU including death and emigration is about twice as high as LFU for "relevant reasons."

For table references, see reference section.

Table 26–4 Summary of studies of contraceptive failure: fertility awareness methods[a]

Reference	Method	N for Analysis	Life-Table 12-Month % Pregnant	Pearl Index Pregnancy Rate — Index	Total Exposure	Maximum Exposure	Characteristics of the Sample	LFU (%)[g]	Comments
Frank-Hermann et al., 2007	Symptothermal method	900	1.6				88% aged < 35	?	Germany
Trussell and Grummer Strawn, 1990	Ovulation	725	3.2				Mean age = 30; proven fertility; agreed to use OM alone; cohabiting; 765 of 869 learned OM to satisfaction of teachers; 725 entered effectiveness study	?	Reanalysis of W.H.O. (1981) trial; probability based on 13 cycles of *perfect* use
Arévalo, et al., 2004	TwoDay	450	3.5				23% aged 18–24; 29% aged 25–29; 26% aged 30–34; 22% aged 35–39; all parous	4.4	Guatemala, Peru, and the Philippines
Rice et al., 1981	Calendar + BBT	723	8.2				Aged 19–44; 9% aged 19–24, 54% aged 25–34, 37% aged 35–44; all parity 1+	3.4[c]	United States, France, Colombia, Canada, Mauritius
Dolack, 1978	Ovulation	329		10.5[c]	3,354 Cy.	?	Aged 19–48; mean age = 28; 40% had used oral contraceptives prior to study	18.0[c]	
Arévalo et al., 2002	Standard Days	478	12.0					7.1	Bolivia, Peru, Philippines
Johnston et al.,	CervicalMucus + BBT + Other Signs	268	13.3[c]				73% aged 22–32; all married or de facto married; 48% ≥12 years education (n = 460)	33.9[c,t]	Australia; probability based on 13 cycles
Wade et al., 1981	Cervical Mucus + BBT + Calendar	239	13.9[c]				Aged 20–39; 78% married	11.4[c-g]	Random assignment to OM or CM + BBT + Cal
Johnston et al., 1978	Calendar + BBT + Other Signs	192	14.3				73% aged 22–32; all married or de facto married; 48% ≥12 years education (n = 460)	33.9[c,t]	Australia; probability based on 13 cycles
Tietze et al., 1951	Calendar	409		14.4	7,267 Mo.	>60 Mo.	57% aged 25–34	13.4[c,t]	

(continued)

Table 26–4 Summary of studies of contraceptive failure: fertility awareness methods[a]—(cont'd)

Reference	Method	N for Analysis	Life-Table 12-Month % Pregnant	Pearl Index Pregnancy Rate			Characteristics of the Sample	LFU (%)[g]	Comments
				Index	Total Exposure	Maximum Exposure			
Vessey et al., 1982	Rhythm	?		15.5	161 Yr.	?	All white; at recruitment aged 25–39 and married; at enrollment, all women had been using the diaphragm, IUD, or pill successfully for at least 5 months	0.3[t,v]	Britain; Oxford/FPA study
Klaus et al., 1979	Ovulation	?	15.8[n]				67% aged 18–34; 52% ≥13 years education; some use of concurrent methods	2.9[n]	Probability based on only 12 cycles
Johnston et al., 1978	Cervical Mucus + BBT + Other Signs + Other Methods	94	16.0				78% aged 22–32; all married or de facto married; 53% ≥12 years education ("other" not limited to rhythm)	33.9[c,t]	Australia; probability based on 13 cycles
Grady et al., 1986	Rhythm	167	16.1[s]				Aged 15–44; all married[t]	20.6[r]	NSFG 1982
Ball, 1976	Ovulation	124		16.8[c]	1,626 Cy.	22 Cy.	Aged 20–39	1.6[c]	Australia
Bracher and Santow, 1992	Rhythm	137	17.9				14% aged <20, 75% aged 20–29, 11% aged 30+; 46% parity 0; 92% married or cohabiting	25[r]	Australian Family Survey; first use of method
Kambic et al., 1981, 1982	Ovulation or Cervical Mucus + BBT	235	18.2[n]				81% aged 20–34; 83% married; approx. 30% used barrier methods concurrently[t]	6.5[n]	
Grady et al., 1983	Rhythm	412	18.3[s,c]				Aged 15–44; all married[t]	18.2[r]	NSFG 1973 and 1976

(continued)

Table 26-4 Summary of studies of contraceptive failure: fertility awareness methods[a]—(cont'd)

Reference	Method	N for Analysis	Life-Table 12-Month % Pregnant	Pearl Index Pregnancy Rate			Characteristics of the Sample	LFU (%)[g]	Comments
				Index	Total Exposure	Maximum Exposure			
Johnston et al., 1978	Ovulation + Other Methods	71	18.8				80% aged 22–32; all married or de facto married; 49% ≥12 years education ("other" not limited to rhythm)	33.9[c,t]	Australia; probability based on 13 cycles
Vaughan et al., 1977	Rhythm	220	19.1[s]				Aged 15–44; all married[t]	19.0[r]	NSFG 1973
Trussell, 2008		249	19.6				Aged 15–44[t]	21[r]	NSFG 1995; probability when corrected for estimated underreporting of abortion = 22.6
W.H.O., 1981	Ovulation	725	19.6				Mean age about 30; proven fertility; agreed to use OM alone; 54% desired no more children; 765 of 869 learned OM to satisfaction of teachers; 725 entered effectiveness study	?	New Zealand, India, Ireland, Philippines, El Salvador; probability based on 13 cycles
Trussell and Vaughan, 1999		250	19.8				Aged 15–44[t]	21[r]	NSFG 1995
Fu et al., 1999		?	20.2					21[r]	NSFG 1995; probability when standardized and corrected for estimated underreporting of abortion = 25.3[s]

(continued)

CONTRACEPTIVE TECHNOLOGY

Table 26–4 Summary of studies of contraceptive failure: fertility awareness methods[a]—(cont'd)

Reference	Method	N for Analysis	Life-Table 12-Month % Pregnant	Risk of Pregnancy Pearl Index Pregnancy Rate			Characteristics of the Sample	LFU (%)[g]	Comments
				Index	Total Exposure	Maximum Exposure			
Jones and Forrest, 1992	Rhythm	289	20.9				Aged 15–44[t]	21[r]	NSFG 1988; probability when standardized and corrected for estimated underreporting of abortion = 31.4[s]
Kost et al., 2008		236	23.0				Aged 15–44[t]	27.5[r]	NSFG 2002; probability when corrected for estimated underreporting of abortion = 25.3
Bartzen, 1967	BBT	335		21.3[c]	4,824 Cy.	58 Mo.	Aged 19–45; mean age = 28	11.6[c]	
Schirm et al., 1982	Rhythm	412	23.7[s]				Aged 15–44; all married[t]	18.2[r]	NSFG 1973 and 1976
Marshall, 1976	Ovulation + BBT	84		23.9[c]	1,195 Cy.	32 Mo.	67% aged 20–34	1.2[c]	Britain
Johnston et al., 1978	Ovulation	586	26.4				69% aged 22–32; all married or de facto married; 44% ≥12 years education	33.9[c,t]	Australia; probability based on 13 cycles

(continued)

Table 26–4 Summary of studies of contraceptive failure: fertility awareness methods[a]—(cont'd)

Reference	Method	N for Analysis	Risk of Pregnancy				Characteristics of the Sample	LFU (%)[g]	Comments
			Life-Table 12-Month % Pregnant	Pearl Index Pregnancy Rate					
				Index	Total Exposure	Maximum Exposure			
Wade et al., 1981	Ovulation	191	37.2[c]				Aged 20–39; 74% married	13.8[c,g]	Random assignment to OM or CM + BBT + Cal

Notes:

[a] Updated from Trussell and Kost (1987), Table 3.

[c] Calculated by James Trussell from data in the article.

[g] Most of these studies incorrectly report the loss to follow-up probability (LFU) as the number of women lost at any time during the study divided by the total number of women entering the study. Thus, these are the probabilities presented in the table. However, the correct measure of LFU would be a gross life-table probability. When available, gross 12-month probabilities are denoted by the letter "g."

[n] Only net probabilities for this study.

[r] Nonresponse rate for entire survey.

[s] Standardized: Vaughan et al., (1977) (1973 NSFG)—intention (the average of probabilities for preventers and delayers); Grady et al., (1983) (1973 and 1976 NSFG)—intention. Our calculation (the average of probabilities for preventers and delayers); Schirm et al., (1982) (1973 and 1976 NSFG)—intention, age, and income; Grady et al., (1986) (1982 NSFG)—intention, age, poverty status, and parity; Jones and Forrest, (1992) (1988 NSFG)—age, marital status, and poverty status; Fu et al., (1999) (1995 NSFG)—age, union status, poverty status.

[t] Total for all methods in the study.

[v] The authors report that LFU for "relevant reasons (withdrawal of cooperation or loss of contact)" was 0.3% per year in the 1982 study. In the 1982 study, women had been followed for 9.5 years on average; if 0.3% are LFU per year, then 2.8% would be LFU in 9.5 years. LFU including death and emigration is about twice as high as LFU for "relevant reasons."

For table references, see reference section.

Table 26-5 Summary of studies of contraceptive failure: withdrawal

Reference	N for Analysis	Risk of Pregnancy					LFU (%)[g]	Comments
		Life-Table 12-Month % Pregnant	Pearl Index Pregnancy Rate					
			Index	Total Exposure	Maximum Exposure	Characteristics of the Sample[w]		
Vessey et al., 1982	?		6.7	674 Yr.	?	All white; at recruitment aged 25–39 and married; at enrollment, all women had been using the diaphragm, IUD, or pill successfully for at least 5 months	0.3[t,v]	Britain; Oxford/FPA study
Bracher and Santow, 1992	94	14.2				25% aged <20, 66% aged 20–29, 9% aged 30+; 57% parity 0; 92% married or cohabiting	25[r]	Australian Family Survey; first use of method
Westoff et al., 1961	~74		16.7	1,287 Mo.	?	All married; all white	5.7[r]	FGMA study
Cliquet et al., 1977	2,316	17.3				All aged 30–34 living in Belgium; 93% living as married[t]	22[r]	Belgium; 1971 National Survey on Family Development (NEGO II)
Trussell, 2008	438	18.7				Aged 15–44[t]	21[r]	NSFG 1995; probability when corrected for underreporting of abortion = 28.4
Kost et al., 2008	848	18.8				Aged 15–44[t]	27.5[r]	NSFG 2002; probability when corrected for underreporting of abortion = 18.4
Trussell and Vaughan, 1999	440	18.8				Aged 15–44[t]	21[r]	NSFG 1995

(continued)

Table 26–5 Summary of studies of contraceptive failure: withdrawal—*(cont'd)*

Reference	N for Analysis	Life-Table 12-Month % Pregnant	Risk of Pregnancy — Pearl Index Pregnancy Rate			Characteristics of the Sample[w]	LFU (%)[g]	Comments
			Index	Total Exposure	Maximum Exposure			
Fu et al., 1999	?	20.1					21[r]	NSFG 1995; probability when standardized and corrected for estimated underreporting of abortion = 27.1[s]
Debusschere, 1980	3,561	20.8				Aged 16–44 living in Flanders; 85% married[t]	40[r]	Belgium; 1975–1976 National Survey on Family Development (NEGO III)
Peel, 1972	62		21.9	1,640 Mo.	60 Mo.	All married	2.9[t]	Britain; Hull Family Survey

Notes:

[a] Updated from Trussell and Kost (1987), Table 1.

[c] Calculated by James Trussell from data in the article.

[g] Most of these studies incorrectly report the loss to follow-up probability (LFU) as the number of women lost at any time during the study divided by the total number of women entering the study. Thus, these are the probabilities presented in the table. However, the correct measure of LFU would be a gross life-table probability. When available, gross 12-month probabilities are denoted by the letter "g."

[r] Nonresponse rate for entire survey.

[s] Fu et al., (1999) (1995 NSFG) — age, union status, poverty status.

[t] Total for all methods in the study.

[v] The authors report that LFU for "relevant reasons" (withdrawal of cooperation or loss of contact)" was 0.3% per year in the 1982 study. In the 1982 study, women had been followed for 9.5 years on average; if 0.3% are LFU per year, then 2.8% would be LFU in 9.5 years. LFU including death and emigration is about twice as high as LFU for "relevant reasons."

[w] Unless otherwise noted, characteristics refer to females.

For table references, see reference section.

Table 26–6 Summary of studies of contraceptive failure: cervical cap and other female barrier methods with spermicide[a]

Reference	Method Brand	N for Analysis	Life-Table 12-Month % Pregnant	Risk of Pregnancy Pearl Index Pregnancy Rate			Characteristics of the Sample	LFU (%)[g]	Comments
				Index	Total Exposure	Maximum Exposure			
Shihata and Trussell, 1991	FemCap	106	4.8					0.0[g]	Probability based on 13 cycles
Denniston and Putney, 1981	Prentif Cavity-rim	110	8.0[b,n]				98% aged 20–35; 70% nulliparous	20.9[c]	
Cagen, 1986	Prentif Cavity-rim	620	8.1[n]				87% aged 20–34; 80% always used spermicide and 14% never did	38.5[c]	LFU = "no response"
Koch, 1982	Prentif Cavity-rim	372	8.4				76% aged 20–29; 65% college graduates	8.0[c]	Women advised also to use condom for the first several cap uses
Mauck et al., 1996	Lea's Shield	79	8.7[b]				Mean age = 29.6; mean education = 14.2 years; 19% nulliparous	6.4[b,g]	
Richwald et al., 1989	Prentif Cavity-rim	3,433	11.3				Mean age 29.0; 91% white non-Hispanic; 80% unmarried; almost 60% college graduates; 64% one or more previous pregnancies; 6.1% failure rate among perfect users, 11.9% among imperfect users	18[g]	Women advised to use extra spermicide or use condoms during first 2 months of use; 15 sites; 14 in Los Angeles, 1 in Santa Fe
Mauck et al., 1999	FemCap	355	13.5[d]				Mean age = 29.1; 23% nulligravid	3.7[c]	Random assignment to FemCap or Ortho All-Flex diaphragm

(continued)

Table 26-6 Summary of studies of contraceptive failure: cervical cap and other female barrier methods with spermicide[a]—*(cont'd)*

Reference	Method Brand	N for Analysis	Life-Table 12-Month % Pregnant	Pearl Index	Total Exposure	Maximum Exposure	Characteristics of the Sample	LFU (%)[g]	Comments
Powell et al., 1986	Prentif Cavity-rim and Vimule	477	16.6				67% aged 25–34 "about half" unmarried; 97% high school graduates; 17% using the pill when fitted for cap	43.8[c]	Canada; back-up methods encouraged (including the emergency contraceptive pills used by 23 women in cases of cap dislodgement)
Bernstein et al., 1986	Prentif Cavity-rim	687[c]	17.4				95% aged ≤35, 16% married, 96% ≥ high school completion	26.3[c-g]	Random assignment to the diaphragm or cervical cap
Kassell and McElroy, 1981	Prentif Cavity-rim	90		18.1[c]	731 Mo.	12 Mo.	Mean age = 23.6; mean education = 14.7 years	10.0[c]	
Boehm, 1983	Prentif Cavity-rim	47		18.1[c]	397 Mo.	12 Mo.		31.6	All women reported exclusive use of cap
Lehfeldt and Sivin, 1984	Prentif Cavity-rim	130	19.1				37% aged 16–25; 72% college graduates; 91% nulliparous	7.2[g]	All women agreed to exclusive use of cap

(continued)

Table 26–6 Summary of studies of contraceptive failure: cervical cap and other female barrier methods with spermicide[a]—*(cont'd)*

| | | | | Risk of Pregnancy | | | | | |
| | | | Life-Table 12-Month | | Pearl Index Pregnancy Rate | | | LFU | |
Reference	Method Brand	N for Analysis	% Pregnant	Index	Total Exposure	Maximum Exposure	Characteristics of the Sample	(%)[g]	Comments
Smith and Lee, 1984	Prentif Cavity-rim and Vimule	33	27.0				80% aged 20–29; clients at university student health service	1.5– 4.6[c]	Regular users for whom the cap (with spermicide) was the sole method used "during the fertile portion of the cycle"

Notes:

[a] Updated from Trussell and Kost (1987), Table 4.

[b] 6-month net probability; 12-month probability not available.

[c] Calculated by James Trussell from data in the article.

[g] Most of these studies incorrectly report the loss to follow-up (LFU) probability as the number of women lost at any time during the study divided by the total number of women entering the study. Thus, these are the probabilities presented in the table. However, the correct measure of LFU would be a gross life-table probability. When available, gross 12-month probabilities are denoted by the letter "g."

[n] Only net probabilities available for this study.

For table references, see reference section.

Table 26–7 Summary of studies of contraceptive failure: sponge[a]

Reference	N for Analysis	Life-Table 12-Month % Pregnant	Characteristics of the Sample	LFU (%)[g]	Comments
Jones and Forrest, 1992	227	14.5	Aged 15–44[t]	21[r]	NSFG 1988
Edelman et al., 1984	722	17.0	89% aged 20–34, 28% married; 77% ≥13 years education; 94% white, 49% never-married; 38% used oral contraceptives prior to entering study	33.2[c,g]	Random assignment to the diaphragm or sponge
McIntyre and Higgins, 1986	723	17.4	89% aged 20–34, 28% married; 77% ≥13 years education; 94% white, 49% never-married; 38% used oral contraceptives prior to entering the study	33.2[c,g]	A reanalysis of data used by Edelman et al. (1984); random assignment to the diaphragm or sponge; much higher probability for parous women
Trussell and Vaughan, 1999	111	18.4	Aged 15–44[t]	21[r]	NSFG 1995
Bounds and Guillebaud, 1984	126	24.5	92% aged 20–34; all married/consensual union; "most" ≥13 years education; 99% white	1.7[g]	Britain; random assignment to the diaphragm or sponge

Notes:

[a] Updated from Trussell and Kost (1987), Table 4.

[c] Calculated by James Trussell from data in the article.

[g] Most of these studies incorrectly report the loss to follow-up (LFU) probability as the number of women lost at any time during the study divided by the total number of women entering the study. Thus, these are the probabilities presented in the table. However, the correct measure of LFU would be a gross life-table probability. When available, gross 12-month probabilities are denoted by the letter "g."

[r] Nonresponse rate for entire survey.

[t] Total for all methods in the study.

For table references, see reference section.

Table 26-8 Summary of studies of contraceptive failure: diaphragm with spermicide[a]

Reference	N for Analysis	Life-Table 12-Month % Pregnant	Risk of Pregnancy — Pearl Index Pregnancy Rate — Index	Total Exposure	Maximum Exposure	Characteristics of the Sample	LFU (%)[g]	Comments
Stim, 1980	1,238		1.1[c]	911 Yr.	4 Yr.	Median age = 24	19.5	Fit-free diaphragm without spermicides; continuous wearing with brief daily removal for cleaning but not within 6 hours after intercourse; 1,238 women given device, with follow-up of 997
Lane et al., 1976	2,168	2.1[c]				61% aged 21–34; 71% unmarried; 92% white	1.2[c-g]	Probability downward biased due to improper exposure allocated to women LFU
Vessey and Wiggins, 1974	4,052		2.4	5,909 Mo.	>60 Mo.	All white; at recruitment aged 25–39 and married; all had been using the diaphragm for at least 5 months at enrollment; no previous pill use	1.0[v]	Britain; Oxford/FPA study
Vessey et al., 1982	?		5.5	2,582 Yr.	24 Mo.	All white and aged 25–34; all married at recruitment; at enrollment, all women had been using the diaphragm, IUD, or pill successfully for at least 5 months	0.3[t,v]	Britain; Oxford/FPA study
Mauck et al., 1999	403	7.9[d]				Mean age = 28.8; 25% nulligravid	4.2[c]	Ortho All-Flex diaphragm; random assignment to Ortho All-Flex diaphragm or FemCap

(continued)

Table 26-8 Summary of studies of contraceptive failure: diaphragm with spermicide[a]—(cont'd)

Reference	N for Analysis	Life-Table 12-Month % Pregnant	Risk of Pregnancy — Pearl Index Pregnancy Rate — Index	Total Exposure	Maximum Exposure	Characteristics of the Sample	LFU (%)[g]	Comments
Trussell, 2008	165	8.0				Aged 15–44[t]	21[r]	NSFG 1995; probability when corrected for estimated underreporting of abortion = 11.5
Trussell and Vaughan, 1999	166	8.1				Aged 15–44[t]	21[r]	NSFG 1995
Loudon et al., 1991	269		8.7	2,350 Mo.	12 Mo.	Mean age = 28.6; 57% gravidity 0; 68% married or cohabiting; 54% already using the diaphragm at start of trial	>3.7	Britain; random assignment of spermicide: either C-Film or jelly
Fu et al., 1999	?	9.2					21[r]	NSFG 1995; probability when standardized and corrected for estimated underreporting of abortion = 15.9s
Dubrow and Kuder, 1958	873		9.3	5,814 Mo.	48 Mo.	Mean age = 25; 39% black; 45% Puerto Rican; 93% ≤12 years education[t]	38.0[c]	
Jones and Forrest, 1992	472	10.4				Aged 15–44[t]	21[r]	NSFG 1988; probability when standardized and corrected for estimated underreporting of abortion = 22.0s
Hall, 1973	347	10.6				Approximately 75% aged 20–24; 47% black; 38% Hispanic; all postpartum	16.0	

(continued)

CONTRACEPTIVE TECHNOLOGY

Table 26-8 Summary of studies of contraceptive failure: diaphragm with spermicide[a]—*(cont'd)*

Reference	N for Analysis	Life-Table 12-Month % Pregnant	Risk of Pregnancy Pearl Index Pregnancy Rate Index	Total Exposure	Maximum Exposure	Characteristics of the Sample	LFU (%)[g]	Comments
Bounds and Guillebaud, 1984	123	10.9				90% aged 20–34; all married/consensual union; "most" ≥13 years education; 96% white	0.0	Britain; random assignment to the diaphragm or sponge
Edelman et al., 1984	717	12.5				88% aged 20–34; 55% never married; 76% ≥13 years education; 94% white; 39% used oral contraceptives prior to entering study	37.8[c,g]	Random assignment to the diaphragm or sponge
McIntyre and Higgins, 1986	717	12.9				88% aged 20–34; 55% never married; 76% ≥13 years education; 94% white; 39% used oral contraceptives prior to entering study	37.8[c,g]	A reanalysis of data used by Edelman et al. (1984); random assignment to the diaphragm or sponge
Vaughan et al., 1977	166	13.1[s]				Aged 15–44; all married[t]	19.0[r]	NSFG 1973
Dingle and Tietze, 1963	189		14.3	2,012 Mo.	36 Mo.	Median age = 22.8	3.2[t]	
Grady et al., 1983	349	14.3[c,s]				Aged 15–44; all married[t]	18.2[r]	NSFG 1973 and 1976
Bernstein et al., 1986	707[c]	16.7				96% aged ≤35; 17% married; 97% ≥ high school completion	33.5[c,g]	Random assignment to the diaphragm or cervical cap
Barnhart et al., 2007	297	17.0				Mean age = 28.4	15.5[c]	

(continued)

Table 26–8 Summary of studies of contraceptive failure: diaphragm with spermicide[a]—*(cont'd)*

Reference	N for Analysis	Life-Table 12-Month % Pregnant	Pearl Index Pregnancy Rate — Index	Pearl Index Pregnancy Rate — Total Exposure	Pearl Index Pregnancy Rate — Maximum Exposure	Characteristics of the Sample	LFU (%)[g]	Comments
Grady et al., 1986	257	17.0[s]				Aged 15–44; all married[t]	20.6[r]	NSFG 1982
Tietze and Lewit, 1967	1,197	17.9				86% aged <30; all married; 60% ≥ high school completion; 50% white	7.2[g]	
Schirm et al., 1982	349	18.6[s]				Aged 15–44; all married[t]	18.2[r]	NSFG 1973 and 1976
Kovacs et al., 1986	324	20.9[t]				28% aged 24–26	52.2	Australia
Bracher and Santow, 1992	219	21.0				12% aged <20; 77% aged 20–29, 11% aged 30+; 56% parity 0; 87% married or cohabiting	25[r]	Australian Family Survey; first use of method
Bounds et al., 1995	80	21.2				Mean age = 29.6; 60% nulliparous	1.3	Britain; probability during consistent use = 12.3; random assignment to diaphragm with spermicide or diaphragm only
Smith et al., 1995	110	24.1				Mean age = 28.8	26.0	Britain; fit-free diaphragm without spermicide; continuous wearing with brief daily removal for cleaning but not within 6 hours after intercourse

(continued)

Table 26–8 Summary of studies of contraceptive failure: diaphragm with spermicide[a]—(cont'd)

Reference	N for Analysis	Life-Table 12-Month % Pregnant	Pearl Index Pregnancy Rate Index	Total Exposure	Maximum Exposure	Characteristics of the Sample	LFU (%)[g]	Comments
			Risk of Pregnancy					
Bounds et al., 1995	84	28.6				Mean age = 29.5; 55% nulliparous	0.0[g]	Britain; diaphragm without spermicide; probability during consistent use = 19.3; random assignment to diaphragm only or diaphragm with spermicide

Notes:

[a] Updated from Trussell and Kost (1987), Table 5.

[c] Calculated by James Trussell from data in the article.

[d] 6-month probability; 12-month probability not available.

[g] Most of these studies incorrectly report the loss to follow-up (LFU) probability as the number of women lost at any time during the study divided by the total number of women entering the study. Thus, these are the probabilities presented in the table. However, the correct measure of LFU would be a gross life-table probability. When available, gross 12-month probabilities are denoted by the letter "g."

[r] Nonresponse rate for entire survey.

[s] Standardized: Vaughan et al., (1977) (1973 NSFG)—intention (the average of probabilities for preventers and delayers); Grady et al., (1983) (1973 and 1976 NSFG)—intention. Our calculation (the average of probabilities for preventers and delayers); Schirm et al., (1982) (1973 and 1976 NSFG)—intention, age, and income; Grady et al., (1986) (1982 NSFG)—intention, age, poverty status, and parity; Jones and Forrest, (1992) (1988 NSFG)—age, marital status, and poverty status; Fu et al., (1999) (1995 NSFG)—age, union status, poverty status.

[t] Total for all methods in the study.

[v] The authors report that LFU for "relevant reasons (withdrawal of cooperation or loss of contact)" was 0.3% per year in the 1982 study and "about 10 per 1,000" per year in the 1974 study. In the 1982 study, women had been followed for 9.5 years on average; if 0.3% are LFU per year, then 2.8% would be LFU in 9.5 years. LFU including death and emigration is about twice as high as LFU for "relevant reasons."

For table references, see reference section.

Table 26-9 Summary of studies of contraceptive failure: male condom[a]

Reference	N for Analysis	Life-Table 12-Month % Pregnant	Pearl Index Pregnancy Rate — Index	Pearl Index Pregnancy Rate — Total Exposure	Pearl Index Pregnancy Rate — Maximum Exposure	Characteristics of the Sample[w]	LFU (%)[g]	Comments
Potts and McDevitt, 1975	397	2.1[b]				77% males ≥ age 40; all married	4.8[c]	Britain; postal trial of spermicidally lubricated condom
Steiner et al., 2003	436	3.3[d]				72% living with partner	5.8	Kimono Select latex condom; random assignment to Kimono Select latex or eZ-on plastic condom
Peel, 1972	96		3.9	3,689 Mo.	60 Mo.	All married	2.9[t]	Britain; Hull Family Survey
Frezieres et al., 1999	383	4.1[d]				Mean age of male and female subjects = 27 [1 1[u]]	3.9[c]	Avanti plastic condom; random assignment to Avanti plastic or Ramses latex condom
Glass et al., 1974	2,057	4.2				All white; at recruitment aged 25–39 and married; at enrollment, all women had been using the diaphragm, IUD, or pill successfully for at least 5 months	<1.0[v]	Britain; Oxford/FPA study
Vessey et al., 1988	?		4.4	10,000c Yr.	24 Mo.	All white; at recruitment aged 25–39 and married; at enrollment, all women had been using the diaphragm, IUD, or pill successfully for at least 5 months	?	Britain; Oxford/FPA study
John, 1973	85		5.7[c]	261 Yr.	>7 Yr.	?	?	Britain; retrospective study

(continued)

Table 26-9 Summary of studies of contraceptive failure: male condom[a]—(cont'd)

Reference	N for Analysis	Life-Table 12-Month % Pregnant	Risk of Pregnancy			Characteristics of the Sample[w]	LFU (%)[g]	Comments
			Pearl Index Pregnancy Rate					
			Index	Total Exposure	Maximum Exposure			
Vessey et al., 1982	?		6.0	4,317 Yr.	24 Mo.	All white and aged 25–34; all married at recruitment; at enrollment all women were using the diaphragm, IUD, or pill successfully for at least 5 months	0.3v	Britain; Oxford/FPA study
Frezieres et al., 1999	384	6.2[d]				Mean age of male and female subjects = 27	2.9c	Ramses latex condom; random assignment to Ramses latex or Avanti plastic condom
Jones and Forrest, 1992	1,728	7.2				Aged 15–44[t]	21r	NSFG 1988; probability when standardized and corrected for estimated underreporting of abortion = 15.8s
Walsh et al., 2003	415	7.9[d]				74% > high school education[t]	0.7	Trojan-Enz or LifeStyles latex condom; random assignment to Trojan-Enz latex or LifeStyles latex condom or Tactylon plastic condom
Bracher and Santow, 1992	262	8.1				16% aged <20, 65% aged 20–29, 19% aged 30+; 48% parity 0; 83% married or cohabiting	25r	Australian Family Survey; first use of method
Trussell, 2008	2,909	8.6				Aged 15–44[t]	21r	NSFG 1995; probability when corrected for estimated underreporting of abortion = 17.8
Trussell and Vaughan, 1999	2,925	8.7				Aged 15–44[t]	21r	NSFG 1995

(continued)

Table 26–9 Summary of studies of contraceptive failure: male condom[a]—(cont'd)

Reference	N for Analysis	Life-Table 12-Month % Pregnant	Risk of Pregnancy — Pearl Index Pregnancy Rate — Index	Total Exposure	Maximum Exposure	Characteristics of the Sample[w]	LFU (%)[g] Comments
Steiner et al., 2003	442	9.2[d]				73% living with partner	5.1 eZ-on plastic condom; random assignment to eZ-on plastic or Kimono Select latex condom
Schirm et al., 1982	1,223	9.6[s]				Aged 15–44; all married[t]	18.2[r] NSFG 1973 and 1976
Grady et al., 1983	1,223	9.7[s,c]				Aged 15–44; all married[t]	18.2[r] NSFG 1973 and 1976
Fu et al., 1999	?	9.7					21[r] NSFG 1995; probability when standardized and corrected for estimated underreporting of abortion = 14.[s]
Vaughan et al., 1977	696	10.1[s]				Aged 15–44; all married[t]	19.0[r] NSFG 1973
Walsh et al., 2003	415	10.8[d]				74% > high school education[t]	0.7 Tactylon plastic condom; random assignment to Tactylon plastic or Trojan-Enz latex or LifeStyles latex condom
Grady et al., 1986	526	13.8[s]				Aged 15–44; all married[t]	20.6[r] NSFG 1982
Westoff et al., 1961	~212		13.8[c]	10,062 Mo.	?	All married	5.7[r] FGMA study

(continued)

Table 26-9 Summary of studies of contraceptive failure: male condom[a]—(cont'd)

Reference	N for Analysis	Life-Table 12-Month % Pregnant	Risk of Pregnancy Pearl Index Pregnancy Rate Index	Risk of Pregnancy Pearl Index Pregnancy Rate Total Exposure	Risk of Pregnancy Pearl Index Pregnancy Rate Maximum Exposure	Characteristics of the Sample[w]	LFU (%)[g]	Comments
Kost et al., 2008	3,845	13.9				Aged 15–44[t]	27.5[r]	NSFG 1995; probability when corrected for estimated underreporting of abortion = 17.4

Notes:

[a] Updated from Trussell and Kost (1987), Table 6.

[b] 24-month probability; 12-month probability not published.

[c] Calculated by James Trussell from data in the article.

[d] 6-month probability; 12-month probability not available.

[g] Most of these studies incorrectly report the loss to follow-up probability (LFU) as the number of women lost at any time during the study divided by the total number of women entering the study. Thus, these are the probabilities presented in the table. However, the correct measure of LFU would be a gross life-table probability. When available, gross 12-month probabilities are denoted by the letter "g."

[r] Nonresponse rate for entire survey.

[s] Standardized: Vaughan et al., (1977) (1973 NSFG)—intention (the average of probabilities for preventers and delayers); Grady et al., (1983) (1973 and 1976 NSFG)—intention. Our calculation (the average of probabilities for preventers and delayers); Schirm et al., (1982) (1973 and 1976 NSFG)—intention, age, and income; Grady et al., (1986) (1982 NSFG)—intention, age, poverty status, and parity; Jones and Forrest, (1992) (1988 NSFG)—age, marital status, and poverty status; Fu et al., (1999) (1995 NSFG)—age, union status, poverty status.

[t] Total for all methods in the study.

[v] The authors report that LFU for "relevant reasons (withdrawal of cooperation or loss of contact)" was 0.3% per year in 1982 study. In the 1982 study, women had been followed for 9.5 years on average; if 0.3% are LFU per year, then 2.8% would be LFU in 9.5 years. LFU including death and emigration is about twice as high as LFU for "relevant reasons."

[w] Unless otherwise noted, characteristics refer to females.

For table references, see reference section.

Table 26–10 Summary of studies of contraceptive failure: progestin-only pill[a]

Reference	Method Brand	N for Analysis	Life-Table 12-Month % Pregnant	Pearl Index Pregnancy Rate — Index	Total Exposure	Maximum Exposure	Characteristics of the Sample	LFU (%)[g]	Comments
Collaborative Study Group, 1998	Desogestrel 75 mcg (Cerazette)	979	0.41		728 Yr.	13 Cy.	Mean age = 29.6 years. ~ 1/3 breast feeding		Finland, Germany, Netherlands, Norway, Sweden, United Kingdom; random assignment to desogestrel 75 mcg or levonorgestrel 30 mcg
Broome and Fetherby, 1990	Femulen, Micronor, Microval, Neogest	358		0.2	18,125 Mo.	150 Mo.		?	At a minimum, 14,103 months (78% of the total exposure) capture use beyond the first year; 46% of women used for >4 years and 13% used for >8 years. Retrospective chart review; England
Bisset et al., 1990	Femulen, Micronor, Neogest, Microval	1,042		1.01	24,942 Mo.	?			United Kingdom. Retrospective chart review; cases with no followup excluded
Postlethwaite, 1979	Femulen (Ethynodiol diacetate 0.5 mg)	309	1.1[c]				Aged 17–48	21.0[c]	Britain

(continued)

CONTRACEPTIVE TECHNOLOGY

Table 26-10 Summary of studies of contraceptive failure: progestin-only pill—*(cont'd)*

			Life-Table 12-Month % Pregnant	Risk of Pregnancy					
				Pearl Index Pregnancy Rate					
Reference	Method Brand	N for Analysis		Index	Total Exposure	Maximum Exposure	Characteristics of the Sample	LFU (%)[g]	Comments
Shroff et al., 1987	Femulen (Ethynodiol diacetate 0.5 mg)	425	1.1[n]				72% aged 16–34; 25% nulligravid	12.7[c]	Britain; authors employed by manufacturer
Board, 1971	Micronor (Norethindrone 0.35 mg)	154		1.3	1,882 Mo.	19 Mo.		?	
Collaborative Study Group, 1998	Levonorgestrel 30 mcg (Microval)	327		1.55	258 Yr.	13 Cy.	Mean age = 29.6 years. ~ 1/3 breast feeding	?	Finland, Germany, Netherlands, Norway, Sweden, United Kingdom; random assignment to levonorgestrel 30 mcg or desogestrel 75 mcg
Keifer, 1973	Micronor (Norethindrone 0.35 mg)	151		1.68	2,141 Mo.	26 Mo.	Aged 18–45; 84% aged 21–35; 74% previous oral contraceptive users; at least 32% current users at start	4.6[c]	
Vessey et al., 1985	Micronor (Norethindrone 0.35 mg)	?		1.98[c]	404 Yr.	12 Mo.	All white and aged 25–34; all married at recruitment; at enrollment, all women had been using the diaphragm, IUD, or pill successfully for at least 5 months	0.3[t,v]	Britain; Oxford/FPA study

(continued)

Table 26–10 Summary of studies of contraceptive failure: progestin-only pill[a]—(cont'd)

Reference	Method Brand	N for Analysis	Life-Table 12-Month % Pregnant	Risk of Pregnancy Pearl Index Pregnancy Rate Index	Risk of Pregnancy Pearl Index Pregnancy Rate Total Exposure	Risk of Pregnancy Pearl Index Pregnancy Rate Maximum Exposure	Characteristics of the Sample	LFU (%)[g]	Comments
Korba and Paulson, 1974	Ovrette (Norgestrel 0.075 mg)	2,202		2.19[c]	29,006 Mo.	67 Mo.		?	Authors employed by manufacturer
McQuarrie et al., 1972	Micronor (Norethindrone 0.35 mg)	318		2.64[c]	3,453 Cy.	27 Mo.	Aged 16–42; mean age = 26; all white	2.2[c]	
Nelson, 1973	Megestrol acetate (0.5 mg)	342		2.7	3,552 Mo.	41 Mo.		14.6[c]	
Jubhari et al., 1974	Quingestanol acetate (0.3 mg)	382	2.9[n]				Mean age = 23; "predominantly white, single and nulliparous"	14.0	
Hawkins and Benster, 1977	Norethisterone (0.35 mg)	200	6.8				Mean age = 25; postpartum women, 71% within 3 months of delivery[t]	5.2[c]	Britain
Hawkins and Benster, 1977	Megestrol acetate (0.5 mg)	174	8.7				Mean age = 25; postpartum women, 71% within 3 months of delivery[t]	8.4[c]	Britain
Sheth et al., 1982	Levonorgestrel (0.30 mg)	128	9.5[n]				Mean age = 25.7	2.1[t]	Yugoslavia, India
Hawkins and Benster, 1977	Chlormadinone acetate (0.5 mg)	182	9.6				Mean age = 26; postpartum women, 71% within 3 months of delivery[t]	3.3[c]	Britain

(continued)

Table 26-10 Summary of studies of contraceptive failure: progestin-only pill[a]—(cont'd)

Reference	Method Brand	N for Analysis	Risk of Pregnancy					LFU (%)[g]	Comments
			Life-Table 12-Month % Pregnant	Pearl Index Pregnancy Rate					
				Index	Total Exposure	Maximum Exposure	Characteristics of the Sample		
Sheth et al., 1982	Norethisterone (0.35 mg)	130	13.2[n]				Mean age = 25.6	2.1[t]	Yugoslavia, India

Notes:

[a] Updated from Trussell and Kost (1987), Table 8.

[c] Calculated by James Trussell from data in the article.

[g] Most of these studies incorrectly report the loss to follow-up (LFU) probability as the number of women lost at any time during the study divided by the total number of women entering the study. Thus, these are the probabilities presented in the table. However, the correct measure of LFU would be a gross life-table probability. When available, gross 12-month probabilities are denoted by the letter "g."

[n] Only net probabilities available for this study.

[t] Total for all methods in the study.

[v] The authors report that LFU for "relevant reasons (withdrawal of cooperation or loss of contact)" was 0.3% per year in the 1982 study. In the 1985 study, women had probably been followed for 12.5 years on average; if 0.3% are LFU per year, then 3.7% would be LFU in 12.5 years. LFU including death and emigration is about twice as high as LFU for "relevant reasons."

For table references, see reference section.

Table 26–11 Summary of studies of contraceptive failure: combined oral contraceptives, vaginal rings, and patches[a]

Reference	Method Brand	N for Analysis	Risk of Pregnancy — Life-Table 12-Month % Pregnant	Risk of Pregnancy — Pearl Index Pregnancy Rate — Index	Risk of Pregnancy — Pearl Index Pregnancy Rate — Total Exposure	Risk of Pregnancy — Pearl Index Pregnancy Rate — Maximum Exposure	Characteristics of the Sample	LFU (%)[g]	Comments
Teichmann et al., 2009	Lybrel	323		0.0	3,072 Cy.		Aged 18–49; mean age = 27.6	<2.8[c]	Random assignment to Lybrel or Alesse
Preston, 1972	Norlestrin 2.5 (80% dose)	378	0.0[c]				Aged 15–46; 46% aged 25–34; 36% white; 64% on pill at start	9.5	Author employed by manufacturer; pill not marketed
Ledger, 1970	Ortho-Novum 1/80	144	0.0[c]				All aged 14–43; mean age = 24; mostly graduate students or wives of students	14.0[c]	
Woutersz, 1981	Lo/Ovral	1,700		0.12	22,489 Cy.	53 Cy.	65% aged 20–29; 55% on pill at start	23.8	Author employed by manufacturer
Korba and Heil, 1975	Ovral	6,806		0.19	127,872 Cy.	110 Cy.	Mean age = 25; 26% white; approximately 80% had not used other oral contraceptives within 3 months	?	Mexico, Puerto Rico, United States; author employed by manufacturer
Lammers andoOp ten Berg, 1991	Mercilon	1,684		0.20	25,970 Cy.	36 Cy.	23% aged <20, 51% aged 20–29, 14% aged 30–34; 12% aged 35+	?	Authors employed by manufacturer; Belgium, Denmark, Finland, France, Hungary, Netherlands, Norway, Poland, Sweden, Switzerland, West Germany, Yugoslavia
Ellis, 1987	Ortho-Novum 7/7/7	619		0.22	909[c] Yr.	?	Mean age = 24.5; 40.5% nulligravid	?	United States, Canada, France

(continued)

Table 26-11 Summary of studies of contraceptive failure: combined oral contraceptives, vaginal rings, and patches[a]—*(cont'd)*

Reference	Method Brand	N for Analysis	Risk of Pregnancy	Pearl Index Pregnancy Rate			Characteristics of the Sample	LFU (%)[g]	Comments
			Life-Table 12-Month % Pregnant	Index	Total Exposure	Maximum Exposure			
Ahrendt et al., 2006	NuvaRing			0.24	408.8 Yr.			2.2[e]	Austria, Belgium, Denmark, France, Germany, Italy, Norway, Spain, Sweden, Switzerland; random assignment to Yasmin or NuvaRing
Morigi and Pasquale, 1978	Modicon	1,168		0.24[c]	16,345 Cy.	53 Cy.	Aged 13–54; 85% aged 19–36; 61% previous use of oral contraceptives	?	Mexico, Puerto Rico, Canada, United States; author employed by manufacturer
Hughes, 1978	Ovamin	453	0.24[c]				Aged 16–40; % new users not stated	11.9[c]	Britain
Vessey et al., 1982	50 μg estrogen	?		0.25	10,400 Yr.	24 Mo.	All white and aged 25–34; all married at recruitment; at enrollment, all women had been using the diaphragm, IUD, or pill successfully for at least 5 months	0.3[t,v]	Britain; Oxford/FPA study
Runnebaum et al., 1992	Ortho-Cyclen	59,701		0.27[c]	342,348 Cy.	6 Cy.	Mean age = 24.0; 32% parous	?	Germany
Kaunitz et al., 1999	Ortho-Novum 7/7/7	321	0.30				Mean age = 27.8; 65% used hormonal contraception in prior month	6.9[c]	Trial design discontinued subjects who did not adhere to dosing schedule

(continued)

Table 26–11 Summary of studies of contraceptive failure: combined oral contraceptives, vaginal rings, and patches[a]—*(cont'd)*

| | | | | Risk of Pregnancy | | | | | |
| | | | Life-Table 12-Month % Pregnant | Pearl Index Pregnancy Rate | | | | | |
Reference	Method Brand	N for Analysis		Index	Total Exposure	Maximum Exposure	Characteristics of the Sample	LFU (%)[g]	Comments
Bannemerschult et al., 1997	Alesse	805		0.30	4,400 Cy.	6 Cy.	Mean age = 25.6	0.6[c]	Germany; some women who did not return for follow-up visits were excluded
Royal College, 1974		23,611		0.34	?	48 Mo.	75% aged 20–34; all married/living as married; 62% on pill at start (20% new users)	32.0[c]	Britain
Woutersz, 1983	Nordette	1,130		0.35	11,064 Cy.	31 Cy.	71% aged 20–30; 48% no use of hormones and not pregnant within 60 days of start	8.1[c]	Author employed by manufacturer
Vessey et al., 1982	<50 µg estrogen	?		0.38	3,158 Yr.	24 Mo.	All white and aged 25–34; all married at recruitment; at enrollment, all women had been using the diaphragm, IUD, or pill successfully for at least 5 months	0.3[t,v]	Britain; Oxford/FPA study
Kaunitz, 2000	Ortho-Novum 7/7/7	2,675	0.39[d]				Mean age = 28.5[t]	6.0[c]	Random assignment to Ortho-Novum 7/7/7 or Cyclessa; 2.5% of subjects discontinued for noncompliance
Parsey and Pong, 2000	Yasmin	326		0.41	3,201 Cy.	13 Cy.	Mean age = 26.4	?	

(continued)

Table 26-11 Summary of studies of contraceptive failure: combined oral contraceptives, vaginal rings, and patches[a]—*(cont'd)*

			Risk of Pregnancy						
			Life-Table 12-Month	Pearl Index Pregnancy Rate					
Reference	Method Brand	N for Analysis	% Pregnant	Index	Total Exposure	Maximum Exposure	Characteristics of the Sample	LFU (%)[g]	Comments
Hernádi et al., 2009	Yaz	1,101	0.5				Aged 18–35 at recruitment; mean age = 24.7	1.9[c]	Czech Republic, Italy, Hungary, Slovak Republic, Latvia, Belgium
Kaunitz, 2000	Cyclessa	2,643	0.51[d]				Mean age = 28.5[t]	5.8[c]	Random assignment to Cyclessa or Ortho-Novum 7/7/7; 2.4% of subjects discontinued for non-compliance
Anderson et al., 2003	Seasonale	456	0.55					8.6	Random assignment to Seasonale or Nordette; noncompliant patients excluded
Gauthier et al., 1992	Ortho Tri-Cyclen	661	0.57[b]				Mean age = 27.9; 24% nulligravid	?	France; 2 authors employed by manufacturer
Åkerlund et al., 1993	Mercilon	485		0.57[c]	4,543 Cy.	12 Mo.	Mean age = 23.8	?	Denmark, Norway, Sweden; random assignment to Mercilon or Marvelon; cycles excluded if the pill-taking period was less than 18 or more than 33 days or if the pill-free period was less than 5 or more than 9 days

(continued)

Table 26–11 Summary of studies of contraceptive failure: combined oral contraceptives, vaginal rings, and patches[a]—*(cont'd)*

Reference	Method Brand	N for Analysis	Life-Table 12-Month % Pregnant	Pearl Index Pregnancy Rate — Index	Pearl Index Pregnancy Rate — Total Exposure	Pearl Index Pregnancy Rate — Maximum Exposure	Characteristics of the Sample	LFU (%)[g]	Comments
Anderson et al., 2006	Seasonique	1,006	0.6				Mean age = 27.4	14.8	
Preston, 1974 and 1972	Norlestrin 2.5 (60% dose)	1,192		0.63[c]	14,536 Cy.	>18 Cy.	Aged 14–47; 35% aged 25–34; 47% white; 56% on pill at start	13.7	Author employed by manufacturer; pill not marketed
Roumen et al., 2001	NuvaRing	1,145		0.64[c]	12,109 Cy.	13 Cy.	Mean age = 28.2	?	Austria, Belgium, Denmark, Finland, France, Germany, Israel, Netherlands, Norway, Spain, Sweden, United Kingdom
Archer et al., 1999	Alesse	1,708	0.69[b]				Mean age = 27.2	12.1	Cycles in which 3 or more consecutive active pills were missed and all subsequent cycles from that subject were excluded from the analysis
Smallwood et al., 2001	Evra patch	1,664	0.7				Mean age = 28.7	?	Australia, Austria, Belgium, France, Israel, Netherlands, Sweden, Switzerland, United Kingdom, United States

(continued)

Table 26–11 Summary of studies of contraceptive failure: combined oral contraceptives, vaginal rings, and patches[a]—(cont'd)

Reference	Method Brand	N for Analysis	Life-Table 12-Month % Pregnant	Pearl Index Pregnancy Rate (Risk of Pregnancy)			Characteristics of the Sample	LFU (%)[g]	Comments
				Index	Total Exposure	Maximum Exposure			
Palacios et al., 2010	Natazio	1,377		0.73	23,368 Cy.	20 Cy.	Mean age = 30	0.002[c]	Austria, Germany, Spain
London et al., 1992	Triphasil (Tri-Levlen)	2,124		0.80	11,306 Cy.	6 Cy.	Mean age = 25.5	?	Random assignment to Triphasil or Ortho Tri-Cyclen
Åkerlund et al., 1993	Marvelon (Ortho-Cept, Desogen)	497		0.83[c]	4,688 Cy.	12 Mo.	Mean age = 23.1	?	Denmark, Norway, Sweden; random assignment to Marvelon or Mercilon; cycles excluded if the pill-taking period was less than 18 or more than 33 days or if the pill-free period was less than 5 or more than 9 days
Corson, 1990	Lo/Ovral	737		0.94[c]	9,727 Cy.	24 Cy.	Mean age = 24.3	?	Random assignment to Lo/Ovral or Ortho-Cyclen
London et al., 1992	Ortho Tri-Cyclen	2,110		0.94	11,006 Cy.	6 Cy.	Mean age = 25.6	?	Random assignment to Ortho Tri-Cyclen or Triphasil
Preston, 1974 and 1972	Norlestrin 2.5 (40% dose)	1,393		0.94[c]	15,265 Cy.	>18 Cy.	Aged 13–42; 27% aged 25–34; 39% white; 49% on pill at start	16.3	Author employed by manufacturer; pill not marketed

(continued)

Table 26–11 Summary of studies of contraceptive failure: combined oral contraceptives, vaginal rings, and patches[a]—(cont'd)

Reference	Method Brand	N for Analysis	Life-Table 12-Month % Pregnant	Pearl Index	Total Exposure	Maximum Exposure	Characteristics of the Sample	LFU (%)[g]	Comments
Ahrendt et al., 2006	Yasmin	484		0.99	404.8 Yr.	13 Cy.		3.3[c]	Austria, Belgium, Denmark, France, Germany, Italy, Norway, Spain, Sweden, Switzerland; random assignment to Yasmin or NuvaRing
The Mircette Study Group, 1998	Mircette	1,226		1.02	14,050 Cy.	13 Cy.	Mean age = 28.3	6.8[c]	
Endrikat et al., 1995	Mercilon	219		1.04[c]	2,496 Cy.	12 Cy.	Mean age = 25.0	?	Austria, France; random assignment to Mercilon or Meliane; cycles excluded if more than two pills were missed or pill-taking was irregular
Oddsson et al., 2005	Microgynon	518	1.07				Mean age = 27.2; 53% nulligravid	6.4[c]	Random assignment to Microgynon or NuvaRing; Belgium, Brazil, Chile, Denmark, Finland, France, Germany, Italy, Norway, Spain, Sweden
Ellsworth, 1986	Triphasil	1,264		1.09	8,349 Cy.	34 Cy.	All < age 38	?	17 U.S. centers

(continued)

Table 26–11 Summary of studies of contraceptive failure: combined oral contraceptives, vaginal rings, and patches[a]—*(cont'd)*

Reference	Method Brand	N for Analysis	Risk of Pregnancy Life-Table 12-Month % Pregnant	Risk of Pregnancy Pearl Index Pregnancy Rate Index	Total Exposure	Maximum Exposure	Characteristics of the Sample	LFU (%)[g]	Comments
Corson, 1990	Ortho-Cyclen	736		1.11[c]	9,351 Cy.	24 Cy.	Mean age = 24.6	?	Random assignment to Ortho-Cyclen or Lo/Ovral
Dieben et al., 2002	NuvaRing	2,322	1.18				Mean age = 28.2	?	United States, Canada, Europe; Pearl index for United States = 1.75; European results published separately by Roumen et al. (2001)
Teichmann et al., 2009	Alesse	318		1.19	3,270 Cy.	12 Cy.	Aged 18–48; mean age = 27.2	<2.2[c]	Random assignment to Alesse or Lybrel
Oddsson et al., 2005	NuvaRing	512	1.2				Mean age = 27.0; 57% nulligravid	6.4[c]	Random assignment to NuvaRing or Microgynon; Belgium, Brazil, Chile, Denmark, Finland, France, Germany, Italy, Norway, Spain, Sweden
Bachmann et al., 2004	Yaz	1,018	1.26				Mean age = 24.7	4.6	Argentina, Austria, Brazil, Poland, United States

(continued)

Table 26-11 Summary of studies of contraceptive failure: combined oral contraceptives, vaginal rings, and patches[a]—(cont'd)

Reference	Method Brand	N for Analysis	Risk of Pregnancy Life-Table 12-Month % Pregnant	Pearl Index Pregnancy Rate Index	Pearl Index Pregnancy Rate Total Exposure	Pearl Index Pregnancy Rate Maximum Exposure	Characteristics of the Sample	LFU (%)[g]	Comments
Audet et al., 2001	Evra patch	811	1.3				Mean age = 28.0	3.9[c]	Random assignment to Evra patch or Triphasil
Anderson et al., 2003	Nordette	226	1.45					9.3	Random assignment to Nordette or Seasonale; noncompliant patients excluded
Preston, 1974 and 1972	Norlestrin 1.0 (60% dose)	1,872		1.47[c]	20,341 Cy.	>18 Cy.	Aged 14–44; 30% aged 25–34; 42% white; 55% on pill at start	13.1	Author employed by manufacturer; pill not marketed
Preston, 1974	Norlestrin 1.0 (20% dose)	276		1.59[c]	2,449 Cy.	?		?	Author employed by manufacturer; pill not marketed
Archer et al., 2006	Lybrel	2,134		1.6	?	13 Cy.	Mean age = 28.8	10.5[c]	Subjects discontinued if they missed ≥3 consecutive pills or ≥ 5 pills in any pill pack
Audet et al., 2001	Triphasil	605	1.8				Mean age = 27.8	7.9[c]	Random assignment to Triphasil or Evra patch
Nakajima et al., 2007	Loestrin 24 Fe	705		1.82	?	6 Cy.	Aged 18–45; mean age = 28.9	8.4	Random assignment to Loestrin 24 Fe or Loestrin Fe
Vaughan et al., 1977		2,434	2.0[s]				Aged 15–44; all married[t]	19.0[r]	NSFG 1973
Bracher and Santow, 1992		1,830	2.2				42% aged <20, 49% aged 20–29, 9% aged 30+; 67% parity 0; 45% married or cohabiting	25[r]	Australian Family Survey, first use of method

(continued)

Table 26–11 Summary of studies of contraceptive failure: combined oral contraceptives, vaginal rings, and patches[a]—*(cont'd)*

Reference	Method Brand	N for Analysis	Life-Table 12-Month % Pregnant	Risk of Pregnancy — Pearl Index Pregnancy Rate			Characteristics of the Sample	LFU (%)[g]	Comments
				Index	Total Exposure	Maximum Exposure			
Schirm et al., 1982		4,487	2.4[s]				Aged 15–44; all married[t]	18.2[r]	NSFG 1973 and 1976
Grady et al., 1983		4,487	2.5[c,s]				Aged 15–44; all married[t]	18.2[r]	NSFG 1973 and 1976
Bounds et al., 1979	Microgynon-30	55	2.6[c]				Aged 16–39; mean age = 26; 62% used oral contraceptives as last contraceptive before study	5.5[c]	Britain; probability based on only 12 cycles
Kroll et al., 2010	LoSeasonique	2,185		2.74	20,937 Cy.	4 91-day Cy.	Mean age = 26.7	13.9	
Nakajima et al., 2007	Loestrin Fe	181		2.98	?	6 Cy.	Aged 18–45; mean age = 28.5	8.6	Random assignment to Loestrin Fe or Loestrin 24 Fe
Grady et al., 1986		856	2.9[s]				Aged 15–44; all married[t]	20.6[r]	NSFG 1982
Jones and Forrest, 1992		3,041	5.1				Aged 15–44; all married[t]	21[r]	NSFG 1988; probability when standardized and corrected for estimated under-reporting of abortion = 7.3s
Preston, 1974	Norlestrin 1.0 (40% dose)	313		5.80[c]	1,570 Cy.	?		?	Author employed by manufacturer; pill not marketed
Bounds et al., 1979	Loestrin-20	55	5.9[c]				Aged 16–39; mean age = 26; 65% used oral contraceptives as last contraceptive before study	5.5[c]	Britain; probability based on only 12 cycles
Trussell, 2008		2,127	6.7				Aged 15–44[c]	21[r]	NSFG 1995; probability when corrected for estimated underreporting of abortion = 8.8

(continued)

Table 26–11 Summary of studies of contraceptive failure: combined oral contraceptives, vaginal rings, and patches[a]—(cont'd)

Reference	Method Brand	N for Analysis	Risk of Pregnancy				Characteristics of the Sample	LFU (%)[g]	Comments
			Life-Table 12-Month % Pregnant	Pearl Index Pregnancy Rate					
				Index	Total Exposure	Maximum Exposure			
Trussell and Vaughan, 1999		2,130	6.9				Aged 15–44[t]	21[r]	NSFG 1995
Fu et al., 1999		?	7.3					21[r]	NSFG 1995; probability when standardized and corrected for estimated underreporting of abortion = 8.1[s]
Kost et al., 2008		2,451	7.7				Aged 15–44[t]	27.5[r]	NSFG 2002; probability when corrected for estimated underreporting of abortion = 8.7
Preston, 1974	Norlestrin 2.5 (20% dose)	178		10.45[c]	871 Cy.	?		?	Author employed by manufacturer; pill not marketed

Notes:

[a] Updated from Trussell and Kost (1987), Table 8.

[b] 12-cycle probability; 12-month probability not available.

[c] Calculated by James Trussell from data in the article.

[d] 6-cycle probability.

[g] Most of these studies incorrectly report the loss to follow-up (LFU) probability as the number of women lost at any time during the study divided by the total number of women entering the study. Thus, these are the probabilities presented in the table. However, the correct measure of LFU would be a gross life-table probability. When available, gross 12-month probabilities are denoted by the letter "g."

[r] Nonresponse rate for entire survey.

[s] Standardized: Vaughan et al., (1977) (1973 NSFG)—intention (the average of probabilities for preventers and delayers); Grady et al., (1983) (1973 and 1976 NSFG)—intention. Our calculation (the average of probabilities for preventers and delayers); Schirm et al., (1982) (1973 and 1976 NSFG)—intention, age, and income; Grady et al., (1986) (1982 NSFG)—intention, age, parity; Jones and Forrest, (1992) (1988 NSFG)—age, marital status, and poverty status; Fu et al., (1999) (1995 NSFG)—age, union status, poverty status.

[t] Total for all methods in the study.

[v] The authors report that LFU for "relevant reasons (withdrawal of cooperation or loss of contact)" was 0.3% per year in the 1982 study. In the 1982 study, women had probably been followed for 9.5 years on average; if 0.3% are LFU per year, then 2.8% would be LFU in 9.5 years. LFU including death and emigration is about twice as high as LFU for "relevant reasons."

For table references, see reference section.

Contraceptive Technology

Table 26-12 Summary of studies of contraceptive failure: injectables[a]

Reference	Method Brand	N for Analysis	Life-Table 12-Month % Pregnant	Characteristics of the Sample	LFU (%)[g]	Comments
Kaunitz et al., 2009	Depo-Provera SC 104 mg (90-Day)	266	0.0[c]	Mean age = 25.9	?	Random assignment to Depo-Provera SC or Depo-Provera IM
Kaunitz et al., 2009	Depo-Provera 150 mg (90-Day)	268	0.0[c]	Mean age = 25.8	?	Random assignment to Depo-Provera IM or Depo-Provera SC
Jain et al., 2004	Depo-Provera SC 104 mg (90-Day)	1,779	0.0	Mean age = 30.6		Brazil, Bulgaria, Canada, Chile, Estonia, Indonesia, Latvia, Lithuania, Mexico, Norway, Pakistan, Peru, Poland, Romania, Russia, United Kingdom, United States
W.H.O., 1988	Depo-Provera 25 mg + Estradiol Cypionate 5 mg (30-Day)	1,168	0.0	Aged 18–35; mean age = 26; proven fertility	11.4[g]	Egypt, Thailand, Mexico, Guatemala, Cuba, Indonesia, Pakistan, U.S.S.R., Philippines, Italy, Hungary, Chile
W.H.O., 1986	Depo-Provera 150 mg (90-Day)	607	0.0	Mean age = 27.7[t]	8.6[g]	7 developing countries
Mishell et al., 1968	Depo-Provera 150 mg (90-Day)	100	0.0[c]	59% aged 21–30	24.0[c]	Injection immediately postpartum
Howard et al., 1982	Norigest 200 mg (56-Day)	383	0.0[c]		6.5[n]	Britain
Kaunitz et al., 1999	Lunelle	782	0.0	Mean age = 27.3; 44% used hormonal contraception in prior month	8.6[c]	Trial design discontinued subjects who did not adhere to dosing schedule
Hall et al., 1997	Cyclofem (Lunelle)	3,183	0.0		12.9[c]	Brazil, Chile, Colombia, Peru. Perfect use analysis since trial design discontinued women who were late for injections
W.H.O., 1983	Depo-Provera 150 mg (90-Day)	1,587	0.1	Mean age = 27.4[t]	8.1	87% of women from 9 developing countries

(continued)

Table 26–12 Summary of studies of contraceptive failure: injectables[a]—(cont'd)

Reference	Method Brand	N for Analysis	Life-Table 12-Month % Pregnant	Characteristics of the Sample	LFU (%)[g]	Comments
W.H.O., 1988	Norigest 50 mg + Estradiol Valerate 5 mg (30-Day)	1,152	0.18	Aged 18–35; mean age = 26.7; proven fertility	10.5[g]	Egypt, Thailand, Mexico, Guatemala, Cuba, Indonesia, Pakistan, U.S.S.R., Philippines, Italy, Hungary, Chile
Sangi-Haghpeykar et al., 1996	Depo-Provera 150 mg (3-Month)	536	0.2	25% nulligravid; mean age = 24.4; primarily low income	5.4[c]	
Scutchfield et al., 1971	Depo-Provera 150 mg (90-Day)	650	0.2[c]	66% aged 20–34; 50% married	6.8[n]	
Schwallie and Assenzo, 1973	Depo-Provera 150 mg (90-Day)	3,857	0.3	86% aged 20–39	18.6	Primarily United States; also Chile, Jamaica, Mexico; authors employed by manufacturer
W.H.O., 1983	Norigest 200 mg (60-789 Day)	789	0.4	Mean age = 27.4[t]	7.1	87% of women from 9 developing countries
W.H.O., 1986	Depo-Provera 100 mg (90-Day)	609	0.4	Mean age = 27.7[t]	8.2[g]	7 developing countries
W.H.O., 1983	Norigest 200 mg (84-Day)	796	0.6	Mean age = 27.4[t]	7.4	87% of women from 9 developing countries
W.H.O., 1977	Depo-Provera 150 mg (84-Day)	846	0.7	87% aged 20–34	6.2	10 developing countries
Schwallie and Assenzo, 1972	Depo-Provera 300 mg (180-Day)	991	2.3[n]	88% aged 20–39	28.9	United States, Chile; authors employed by manufacturer
Fu et al., 1999	Depo-Provera 150 mg	?	2.8		21[r]	NSFG 1995; probability when standardized and corrected for estimated underreporting of abortion = 2.6[s]
Trussell, 2008	Depo-Provera 150 mg (90-Day)	209	2.9	Aged 15–44[t]	21[r]	NSFG 1995; probability when corrected for estimated underreporting of abortion = 5.4

(continued)

Table 26-12 Summary of studies of contraceptive failure: injectables[a]—*(cont'd)*

Reference	Method Brand	N for Analysis	Life-Table 12-Month % Pregnant	Characteristics of the Sample	LFU (%)[g]	Comments
Trussell and Vaughan, 1999	Depo-Provera 150 mg (90-Day)	209	3.2	Aged 15–44[t]	21[r]	NSFG 1995
W.H.O., 1977	Norigest 200 mg (84-Day)	832	3.6	84% aged 20–34	5.8	10 developing countries
Kost et al., 2008	Depo-Provera 150 mg (90-Day)	715	7.5	Aged 15–44[t]	27.5[r]	NSFG 2002; probability when corrected for estimated underreporting of abortion = 6.7

Notes:

[a] Updated from Trussell and Kost (1987), Table 9.

[c] Calculated by James Trussell from data in the article.

[g] Most of these studies incorrectly report the loss to follow-up (LFU) probability as the number of women lost at any time during the study divided by the total number of women entering the study. Thus, these are the probabilities presented in the table. However, the correct measure of LFU would be a gross life-table probability. When available, gross 12-month probabilities are denoted by the letter "g."

[n] Only net probabilities available for this study.

[r] Nonresponse rate for entire survey.

[s] Fu et al., (1995 NSFG)—age, union status, poverty status.

[t] Total for all methods in the study.

For table references, see reference section.

Table 26–13 Summary of studies of contraceptive failure: intrauterine contraceptives[a]

Reference	Method Brand	N for Analysis	Life-Table 12-Month % Pregnant	Characteristics of the Sample	LFU (%)[g]	Comments
Luukkainen et al., 1987	LNg20	1,821	0.1	15% aged 17–25, 60% aged 26–35, 25% aged 36–40; 7% parity 0, 27% parity 1, 50% parity 2, 16% parity 3+	5.7[c]	Denmark, Finland, Hungary, Norway, Sweden
Sivin et al., 1990 Singapore, United States	LNg20	1,124	0.2	Mean age = 26.6; mean parity = 2.4	5.7[s,x]	Brazil, Chile, Dominican Republic, Egypt,
Sivin et al., 1990	TCu380A Slimline	698	0.3	Mean age = 28.5; mean parity = 2.7; 47.4% prior IUD use	6.0	Randomized trial of TCu380A and TCu380A Slimline. Egypt, Chile, Sweden, Dominican Republic, Brazil
Sivin et al., 1990	TCu380A	298	0.4	Mean age = 28.1; mean parity = 2.6; 49.0% prior IUD use	9.7	Randomized trial of TCu380A and TCu380A Slimline. Egypt, Chile, Sweden, Dominican Republic, Brazil
Cox and Blacksell, 2000	LNg20	692	0.6	All parous	?	United Kingdom
Sivin and Stern, 1979	TCu380A	3,536	0.8	72% aged 20–29; 64% nulliparous	18.3[n]	
Gibor and Mitchell, 1980	Progestasert	6,261	2.0[n]		?	Authors employed by manufacturer; United States (51%), Canada (5%), and at least 11 other countries
Trussell and Vaughan, 1999		59	3.7	Aged 15–44[t]	21[r]	NSFG 1995
Bracher and Santow, 1992		408	3.9	10% aged <20, 68% aged 20–29, 22% aged 30+; 25% parity 0; 87% married or cohabiting	25[r]	Australian Family Survey, first use of method

(continued)

Table 26–13 Summary of studies of contraceptive failure: intrauterine contraceptives[a]—(cont'd)

Reference	Method Brand	N for Analysis	Life-Table 12-Month % Pregnant	Characteristics of the Sample	LFU (%)[g]	Comments
Vaughan et al., 1977		576	4.2[s]	Aged 15–44; all married[t]	19.0[r]	NSFG 1973
Schirm et al., 1982		1,070	4.6[s]	Aged 15–44; all married[t]	18.2[r]	NSFG 1973 and 1976
Grady et al., 1983		1,070	4.8[c,s]	Aged 15–44; all married[t]	18.2[r]	NSFG 1973 and 1976
Grady et al., 1986		235	5.9[s]	Aged 15–44; all married[t]	20.6[r]	NSFG 1982

Notes:

[a] Updated from Trussell and Kost (1987), Table 7.

[c] Calculated by James Trussell from data in the article.

[g] Most of these studies incorrectly report the loss to follow-up (LFU) probability as the number of women lost at any time during the study divided by the total number of women entering the study. Thus, these are the probabilities presented in the table. However, the correct measure of LFU would be a gross life-table probability. When available, gross 12-month probabilities are denoted by the letter "g."

[n] Only net probabilities available for this study.

[r] Nonresponse rate for entire survey.

[s] Standardized: Vaughan et al., (1977) (1973 NSFG)—intention (the average of probabilities for preventers and delayers); Grady et al., (1983) (1973 and 1976 NSFG)—intention. Our calculation (the average of probabilities for preventers and delayers); Schirm et al., (1982) (1973 and 1976 NSFG)—intention, age, and income; Grady et al., (1986) (1982 NSFG)—intention, age, poverty status, and parity.

[t] Total for all methods in the study.

[x] Irving Sivin, personal communication to James Trussell, August 13, 1992.

For table references, see reference section.

Table 26–14 Summary of studies of contraceptive failure: implants[a]

| | | | Risk of Pregnancy | | | | | | |
| | | | Life-Table | Pearl Index Pregnancy Rate | | | | | |
Reference	Method Brand	N for Analysis	12-Month % Pregnant	Index	Total Exposure	Maximum Exposure	Characteristics of the Sample	LFU (%)[g]	Comments
Harvey, et al., 2009	Implanon	976		0	1,196.9 Yr.	3 Yr.	43% nulligravid	21.4[c]	Australia; retrospective chart review
Graesslin and Korver 2008; Darney et al., 2009	Implanon	923		0	24,100 Cy.	4 Yr.	Aged 18–40	2.2	Asia, Chile, Europe, United States
Lipetz et al., 2009	Implanon	493		0	808.4 Yr.	3 Yr.		3.2[c]	Wales; review of case notes for cost study
Flores	Implanon	417		0	958.5 Yr.	3 Yr.	Mean age = 25.8	18.9	Mexico City
Arribas-Mir, et al., 2009	Implanon	372		0	893.4 Yr.	3 Yr.	Mean age = 27.2; 42.7% nulliparous	4.3	Grenada, Spain
Lakha and Glasier, 2006	Implanon	324		0	?	4 Yr.	Mean age = 26	14.5[c]	Edinburgh; 33 women did not return for implant removal until at least 1 month after 3 years of use; the longest duration of use was 4 years and 8 days
Zheng et al., 1999a	Implanon	200		0	644.6 Yr.	4 Yr.		1.0[c]	
Smith and Reuter, 2002	Implanon	190		0	?	?		≥37.4	England; audit and postal survey

(continued)

Table 26-14 Summary of studies of contraceptive failure: Implants[a] —(cont'd)

Reference	Method Brand	N for Analysis	Risk of Pregnancy						LFU (%)[g]	Comments
			Life-Table 12-Month % Pregnant	Pearl Index Pregnancy Rate						
				Index	Total Exposure	Maximum Exposure	Characteristics of the Sample			
Thamkhantho, et al., 2008	Implanon	163		0	88.7 Yr.	1 Yr.			45.4	Bangkok; of the 89 women who returned for the 1-year follow-up none was LFU thereafter
Rai et al., 2004	Implanon	147		0	?	30 Mo.			30.6	London; retrospective chart review
Agarwal and Robinsom, 2005	Implanon	106		0	?	3 Yr.	Aged 15–43; 37% nulliparous		19[c]	Luton, England; 2 clients retained device for 3 and 8 months after its expiration date, respectively but neither became pregnant
Zheng et al., 1999b	Implanon	100		0	341.6 Yr.	4 Yr.			3.0[c]	China
Gezginc et al., 2007	Implanon	80		0	?	?	Mean age = 33		?	Turkey
Booranabunyat and Taneepanichskul, 2004	Implanon	53		0	306 Mo.	6 Mo.	Aged 35–48		0.0	Bangkok

(continued)

Table 26-14 Summary of studies of contraceptive failure: Implants[a]—*(cont'd)*

Reference	Method Brand	N for Analysis	Risk of Pregnancy					Characteristics of the Sample	LFU (%)[g]	Comments
			Life-Table 12-Month % Pregnant	Pearl Index Pregnancy Rate						
				Index	Total Exposure	Maximum Exposure				
Yildizbas et al., 2007	Implanon	41	0	0	20.5 Yr.	6 Mo.		Aged 18–40	0.0	Turkey

Notes:

[a] Updated from Trussell and Kost (1987), Table 9.

[c] Calculated by James Trussell from data provided by Sivin (1992).

[g] Proportion LFU in the first year (number of women LFU in the first year divided by the number entering the study); gross 12-month life-table probabilities denoted by the letter "g."

[r] Nonresponse rate for entire survey.

[s] Fu et al., (1999) (1995 NSFG)—age, union status, poverty status.

[t] Total for all methods in the study.

For table references, see reference section.

CONTRACEPTIVE TECHNOLOGY

Table 26–15 Summary of studies of contraceptive failure: female sterilization[a]

Reference	Procedure	N for Analysis	Life-Table 12-Month % Pregnant	Pearl Index Pregnancy Rate Index	Pearl Index Pregnancy Rate Total Exposure	Pearl Index Pregnancy Rate Maximum Exposure	Characteristics of the Sample	LFU (%)[g]	Comments
Engel, 1978	Laparoscopy	182	0.0[c]				"No failures" presumably some women followed for at least 12 months	?	
Valle and Battifora, 1978	Laparoscopy	165	0.0[c]				"Failure rate after 2 years follow-up is zero" all aged 22–38; 80% had at least 12 months follow-up	?	
Vessey et al., 1983	Procedures other than laparotomy and laparoscopy	345		0.0	331 Yr.	12 Mo.	All white; at recruitment aged 25–39 and married; at enrollment, all women had been using the diaphragm, IUD, or pill successfully for at least 5 months	0.3[v]	Britain; Oxford/FPA study
Chi et al., 1980	Culdoscopy: Pomeroy	392	0.0				Mean age = 32[t]	?	IFRP (19 countries)
Loffer and Pent, 1977	Laparoscopy	1,717		0.0[c]		>6 Mo.	Duration of follow-up not reported	?	
Chi et al., 1987	Minilaparotomy: Pomeroy	445	0.0[c]				Median age = 32	31.6	IFRP (19 countries)
Peterson et al., 1996	Postpartum partial salpingectomy	1,637	0.06				43% aged 18–27, 38% aged 28–33, 18% aged 34+	8.8	U.S. Collaborative Review of Sterilization

(continued)

Table 26-15 Summary of studies of contraceptive failure: female sterilization[a]—*(cont'd)*

Reference	Procedure	N for Analysis	Life-Table 12-Month % Pregnant	Risk of Pregnancy — Pearl Index Pregnancy Rate — Index	Risk of Pregnancy — Pearl Index Pregnancy Rate — Total Exposure	Risk of Pregnancy — Pearl Index Pregnancy Rate — Maximum Exposure	Characteristics of the Sample	LFU (%)[g]	Comments
Cooper et al., 2003	Essure implant	449	0.0[c]				Mean age = 31.9	2.2[c]	United States, Australia
Kerin et al., 2003	Essure implant	198	0.0				Mean age = 35	?	United States, Australia, Belgium, Spain
Arjona et al., 2008	Essure implant	1,612	0.0[c]				Mean age = 36.6	?	Spain; 3 women became pregnant before the 3-month followup
Vleugals and Voersema, 2005	Essure implant	161	0.0[c]				Mean age = 37.4	?	The Netherlands
Peterson et al., 1996	Unipolar coagulation	1,432	0.07				20% aged 18–27, 39% aged 28–33, 42% aged 34+	5.0	U.S. Collaborative Review of Sterilization
Dominik et al., 2000	Filshie Clip	1,063	0.11					31.3[c]	Dominican Republic, Guatemala, Haiti, Malaysia, Mexico, Panama, Venezuela
Sokal et al., 2000	Filshie Clip	1,378	0.17				Mean age = 31	18.1[c]	Brazil, Dominican Republic, Indonesia, Kenya, Mexico, Panama, Peru, Thailand

(continued)

Table 26-15 Summary of studies of contraceptive failure: female sterilization[a]—(cont'd)

| | | | Life-Table 12-Month | Risk of Pregnancy — Pearl Index Pregnancy Rate | | | | | |
| | | | | Index | Total Exposure | Maximum Exposure | | | |
Reference	Procedure	N for Analysis	% Pregnant				Characteristics of the Sample	LFU (%)[g]	Comments
Sokal et al., 2000	Tubal Ring	1,355	0.17				Mean age = 31	17.6[c]	Brazil, Dominican Republic, Indonesia, Kenya, Mexico, Panama, Peru, Thailand
Bhiwandiwala et al., 1982	Rocket Clip	630	0.18[u]					42.1[c,t]	IFRP (27 countries)
Peterson et al., 1996	Bipolar coagulation	2,267	0.23				31% aged 18–27, 35% aged 28–33, 35% aged 34+	10.5	U.S. Collaborative Review of Sterilization
Chi et al., 1980	Minilaparotomy	3,988	0.24				Mean age = 32[t]	?	IFRP (19 countries)
Bhiwandiwala et al., 1982	Electro-coagulation	6,542	0.26[u]					42.1[c,t]	IFRP (27 countries)
Vessey et al., 1983	Laparotomy: all procedures	743		0.28	716 Yr.	12 Mo.	All white; at recruitment aged 25–39 and married; at enrollment, all women had been using the diaphragm, IUD, or pill successfully for at least 5 months	0.3[t,v]	Britain; Oxford/FPA study
Mumford et al., 1980	Minilaparoscopy: Pomeroy	2,022	0.3[u]					?	IFRP (23 countries)
Chi et al., 1980	Electro-coagulation	3,594	0.32[c]					?	IFRP (19 countries)

(continued)

Table 26–15 Summary of studies of contraceptive failure: female sterilization[a]—(cont'd)

Reference	Procedure	N for Analysis	Life-Table 12-Month % Pregnant	Pearl Index Pregnancy Rate			Characteristics of the Sample	LFU (%)[g]	Comments
				Index	Total Exposure	Maximum Exposure			
Bhiwandiwala et al., 1982	Tubal Ring	5,046	0.47[u]					42.1[c,t]	IFRP (27 countries)
Mumford et al., 1980	Minilaparoscopy: Ring	1,324	0.51[u]					?	IFRP (23 countries)
Vessey et al., 1983	Laparoscopy: Tubal Diathermy	776		0.53	755 Yr.	12 Mo.	All white; at recruitment aged 25–39 and married; at enrollment, all women had been using the diaphragm, IUD, or pill successfully for at least 5 months	.3[v]	Britain: Oxford/FPA study
Chi et al., 1981	Tubal Ring	4,106	0.54[c]					?	IFRP (19 countries)
Peterson et al., 1996	All methods combined	10,685	0.55				33% aged 18–27, 35% aged 28–33, 32% aged 34+	10.8	U.S. Collaborative Review of Sterilization
Chi et al., 1980	Laparoscopy: Rocket Clip	457	0.59				Mean age = 32[t]	?	IFRP (19 countries)
Peterson et al., 1996	Rubber band	3,329	0.59				30% aged 18–27, 36% aged 28–33, 34% aged 34+	12.1	U.S. Collaborative Review of Sterilization
Mumford et al., 1980	Laparoscopy: Rings	4,262	0.60[u]					?	IFRP (23 countries)

(continued)

Table 26–15 Summary of studies of contraceptive failure: female sterilization[a]—(cont'd)

Reference	Procedure	N for Analysis	Life-Table 12-Month % Pregnant	Risk of Pregnancy Pearl Index Pregnancy Rate Index	Total Exposure	Maximum Exposure	Characteristics of the Sample	LFU (%)[g]	Comments
Vessey et al., 1983	Laparoscopy: Rings, Clips, etc.	379		0.60	334 Yr.	12 Mo.	All white; at recruitment aged 25–39 and married; at enrollment, all women had been using the diaphragm, IUD, or pill successfully for at least 5 months	0.3[t,v]	Britain; Oxford/FPA study
Dominik et al., 2000	Hulka Clip	1,062	0.69					33.1[c]	Dominican Republic, Guatemala, Haiti, Malaysia, Mexico, Panama, Venezuela
Peterson et al., 1996	Interval partial salpingectomy	425	0.73				28% aged 18–27, 32% aged 28–33, 40% aged 34+	7.3	U.S. Collaborative Review of Sterilization
Chi et al., 1987	Minilaparotomy: Rings and Clips	1,146	1.07	0.79	1,143 Yr.	12 Mo.	Median age = 32 years	13.5	IFRP (19 countries)
Vancaillie et al., 2008	Adiana implant	570					Median age = 31	3.0[c]	United States, Mexico, Australia; 3 women became pregnant before bilateral occlusion was confirmed
Yoon et al., 1977	Falope Ring	902		1.33[c]	3,617[c] Mo.	12 Mo.		21.0[c]	
Peterson et al., 1996	Spring Clip	1,595	1.82				44% aged 18–27, 30% aged 28–33, 26% aged 34+	16.4	U.S. Collaborative Review of Sterilization

(continued)

Table 26-15 Summary of studies of contraceptive failure: female sterilization[a]—(cont'd)

Reference	Procedure	N for Analysis	Life-Table 12-Month % Pregnant	Pearl Index Pregnancy Rate — Index	Pearl Index Pregnancy Rate — Total Exposure	Pearl Index Pregnancy Rate — Maximum Exposure	Characteristics of the Sample	LFU (%)[g]	Comments
Hulka et al., 1976	Spring Clip	1,079	2.3[2]					9.5[c]	United States, UK, Jamaica, Thailand, Singapore, El Salvador (defective clips)
Chi et al., 1981	Spring Clip	1,699	4.19[c]					?	IFRP (19 countries) (defective clips)
Chi et al., 1980	Culdoscopy: Tantalum Clip	498	8.19				Mean age = 32[t]	?	IFRP (19 countries)

Notes:

[a] Updated from Trussell and Kost (1987), Table 10.

[c] Calculated by James Trussell from data in the article.

[g] Most of these studies incorrectly report the loss to follow-up (LFU) probability as the number of women lost at any time during the study divided by the total number of women entering the study. Thus, these are the probabilities presented in the table. However, the correct measure of LFU would be a gross life-table probability. When available, gross 12-month probabilities are denoted by the letter "g."

[t] Total for all methods in the study.

[u] Study did not report whether the cumulative life-table probability was net or gross.

[v] The authors report that LFU for "relevant reasons (withdrawal of cooperation or loss of contact)" was 0.3% per year in the 1983 study. In the 1983 study, women had probably been followed for 10 years on average; if 0.3% are LFU per year, then 3.0% would be LFU in 10 years. LFU including death and emigration is about twice as high as LFU for "relevant reasons."

For table references, see reference section.

CONTRACEPTIVE TECHNOLOGY

Table 26-16 Summary of studies of contraceptive failure: vasectomy[a]

Reference	N for Analysis	Life-Table 12-Month % Pregnant	Pearl Index Pregnancy Rate — Index	Pearl Index Pregnancy Rate — Total Exposure	Pearl Index Pregnancy Rate — Maximum Exposure	Characteristics of the Sample	LFU (%)[g]	Comments
Moss, 1992	6,220	0.0[c]					?	1 pregnancy 10 years after vasectomy
Schmidt, 1988	5,000	0.0[c]					?	Presumably 0 pregnancies
Alderman, 1988	5,331	0.0[c]				5,331 of 8,879 had at least 2 post-op semen tests	?	Canada; 4 pregnancies, 4.5–8.6 years after vasectomy
Philip et al., 1984	16,039	0.0[c]				16,039 of 16,796 provided requested post-op semen samples	?	Britain; 6 pregnancies, 1.3–3 years after vasectomy; 3 pregnancies in first year among 757 men who did not supply post-op semen samples
Kase and Goldfarb, 1973	500	0.0[c]				2% ≥ aged 41	?	1 pregnancy 15 months after vasectomy
Vessey et al., 1982	?		0.08	2,500 Yr.	24 Mo.	Females all white; females at recruitment aged 25–39 and married; at enrollment, all women had been using the diaphragm, IUD, or pill successfully for at least 5 months	0.3[v]	Britain; Oxford/FPA study
Margaret Pyke Center, 1973	1,000	0.1[c]				24% ≥ age 41	?	Britain; 1 pregnancy in first year
Klapproth and Young, 1973	1,000	0.2[c]				35% ≥ age 41	10.0?	2 pregnancies, 3 and 4 months after vasectomy

(continued)

Table 26–16 Summary of studies of contraceptive failure: vasectomy[a]—(cont'd)

Reference	N for Analysis	Life-Table 12-Month % Pregnant	Risk of Pregnancy — Pearl Index Pregnancy Rate			Characteristics of the Sample	LFU (%)[g]	Comments
			Index	Total Exposure	Maximum Exposure			
Marshall and Lyon, 1972	200	0.5[c]				Age 25–60; "majority" aged 35–39	?	1 pregnancy 3 months after vasectomy
Jamieson et al., 2004	544	0.74					6.1	U.S. Collaborative Review of Sterilization; women interviewed after husbands' vasectomy

Notes:

[a] Updated from Trussell and Kost (1987), Table 10.

[c] Calculated by James Trussell from data in the article.

[g] Most of these studies incorrectly report the loss to follow-up (LFU) probability as the number of women lost at any time during the study divided by the total number of women entering the study. Thus, these are the probabilities presented in the table. However, the correct measure of LFU would be a gross life-table probability. When available, gross 12-month probabilities are denoted by the letter "g."

[t] Total for all methods in the study.

[v] The authors report that LFU for "relevant reasons (withdrawal of cooperation or loss of contact)" was 0.3% per year in the 1982 study. In the 1982 study, women had probably been followed for 9.5 years on average; if 0.3% are LFU per year, then 2.8% would be LFU in 9.5 years. LFU including death and emigration is about twice as high as LFU for "relevant reasons."

For table references, see reference section.

TABLE REFERENCES

Aérvalo M, Jennings V, Nikula M, Sinai I. Efficacy of the new TwoDay Method of family planning. Fertil Steril. 2004;82:885–92.

Agrawal A, Robinson C. An assessment of the first 3 years' use of Implanon in Luton. J Fam Plann Reprod Health Care. 2005;31:310–2.

Ahrendt HJ, Nisand I, Bastianelli C, Gómez MA, Gemzell-Danielsson K, Urdl W, Karskov B, Oeyen L, Bitzer J, Page G, Milsom I. Efficacy, acceptability and tolerability of the combined contraceptive ring, NuvaRing, compared with an oral contraceptive containing 30 microg of ethinyl estradiol and 3 mg of drospirenone. Contraception. 2006;74:451–7.

Åkerlund M, Røde A, Westergaard J. Comparative profiles of reliability, cycle control and side effects of two oral contraceptive formulations containing 150 μg desogestrel and either 30 μg or 20 μg ethinyl oestradiol. Brit J Obstet Gynaecol. 1993;100:832–8.

Alderman PM. The lurking sperm: a review of failures in 8879 vasectomies performed by one physician. JAMA. 1988;259:3142–4.

Anderson FD, Hait H, the Seasonale-301 Study Group. A multicenter, randomized study of an extended cycle oral contraceptive. Contraception. 2003;68:89–96.

Anderson FD, Gibbons W, Portman D, the Seasonique:℠ Study Group. Safety and efficacy of an extended-regimen oral contraceptive utilizing continuous low-dose ethinyl estradiol. Contraception. 2006;73:229–34.

Apothecus Pharmaceutical Corporation. VCF®: Vaginal Contraceptive Film®. East Norwich NY: Apothecus Inc, 1992.

Archer DF, Jensen JT, Johnson JV, Borisute H, Grubb GS, Constantine GD. Evaluation of a continuous regimen of levonorgestrel/ethinyl estradiol: phase 3 study results. Contraception. 2006;74:439–45.

Archer DF, Maheux R, DelConte A, O'Brien FB. North American levonorgestrel study group (NALSG). Efficacy and safety of a low-dose monophasic combination oral contraceptive containing 100 μ levonorgestrel and 20 μ ethinyl estradiol (Alesse). Am J Obstet Gynecol. 1999;181 Suppl 1:S39–44.

Arévalo M, Jennings V, Sinai I. Efficacy of a new method of family planning: the Standard Days Method. Contraception. 2002;65:333–8.

Arjona JE, Miño M, Cordón J, Povedano B, Pelegrin B, Castelo-Branco C. Satisfaction and tolerance with office hysteroscopic tubal sterilization. Fertil Steril. 2008;90:1182–6.

Arribas-Mir L, Rueda-Lozano D, Agrela-Cardona M, Cedeno-Benavides T, Olvera-Porcel C, Bueno-Cavanillas A. Insertion and 3-year follow-up experience of 372 etonogestrel subdermal contraceptive implants by family physicians in Granada, Spain. Contraception. 2009;80:457–62.

Audet MC, Moreau M, Koltun WD, Waldbaum AS, Shangold G, Fisher AC, Creasy GW. Evaluation of contraceptive efficacy and cycle control of a transdermal contraceptive patch vs an oral contraceptive. JAMA. 2001;285:2347–54.

Bachmann G, Sulak PJ, Sampson-Landers C, Benda N, Marr J. Efficacy and safety of a low-dose 24-day combined oral contraceptive containing 20 micrograms ethinylestradiol and 3 mg drospirenone. Contraception. 2004;70:191–8.

Ball M. A prospective field trial of the ovulation method of avoiding conception. Eur J Obstet Gynecol Reprod Biol. 1976;6:63–6.

Bannemerschult R, Hanker JP, Wunsch C, Fox P, Albring M, Brill K. A multicenter, uncontrolled clinical investigation of the contraceptive efficacy, cycle control, and safety of a new low dose oral contraceptive containing 20 μg ethinyl estradiol and 100 μg levonorgestrel over six treatment cycles. Contraception. 1997;56:285–90.

Barnhart KT, Rosenberg MJ, MacKay HT, Blithe DL, Higgins J, Walsh T, Wan L, Thomas M, Creinin MD, Westhoff C, Schlaff W, Archer DF, Ayers C, Kaunitz A, Das S, Moench TR. Contraceptive efficacy of a novel spermicidal microbicide used with a diaphragm: a randomized controlled trial. Obstet Gynecol. 2007;110:577–86.

Bartzen PJ. Effectiveness of the temperature rhythm system of contraception. Fertil Steril. 1967;18:694–706.

Belhadj H, Sivin I, Diaz S, Pavez M, Tejada AS, Brache V, Alvarez F, Shoupe D, Breaux H, Mishell DR, McCarthy T, Yo V. Recovery of fertility after use of the levonorgestrel 20 mcg/d or copper T 380 Ag intrauterine device. Contraception. 1986;34:261–7.

Bernstein GS. Clinical effectiveness of an aerosol contraceptive foam. Contraception. 1971;3:37–43.

Bernstein GS, Clark V, Coulson AH, Frezieres RG, Kilzer L, Moyer D, Nakamura RM, Walsh T. Use effectiveness study of cervical caps. Final report. Washington (DC): National Institute of Child Health and Human Development, 1986 July Contract No.: 1-HD-1–2804.

Bhiwandiwala PP, Mumford SD, Feldblum PJ. A comparison of different laparoscopic sterilization occlusion techniques in 24,439 procedures. Am J Obstet Gynecol. 1982;144:319–31.

Bisset AM, Dingwall-Fordyce I, Hamilton MIK. The efficacy of the progestogen-only pill as a contraceptive method. Br J Family Plann. 1990;16:84–7.

Board JA. Continuous norethindrone, 0.35 mg, as an oral contraceptive agent. Am J Obstet Gynecol. 1971;109:531–5.

Boehm D. The cervical cap: effectiveness as a contraceptive. J Nurse Midwifery. 1983;28:3–6.

Booranabunyat S, Taneepanichskul S. Implanon use in Thai women above the age of 35 years. Contraception. 2004;69:489–91.

Bounds W, Guillebaud J. Randomised comparison of the use-effectiveness and patient acceptability of the Collatex (Today) contraceptive sponge and the diaphragm. Br J Fam Plann. 1984;10:69–75.

Bounds W, Guillebaud J, Dominik R, Dalberth BT. The diaphragm with and without spermicide: a randomized, comparative efficacy trial. J Reprod Med.1995;40:764–74.

Bounds W, Vessey M, Wiggins P. A randomized double-blind trial of two low dose combined oral contraceptives. Brit J Obstet Gynaecol. 1979;86:325–9.

Bracher M, Santow G. Premature discontinuation of contraception in Australia. Fam Plann Perspect. 1992;24:58–65.

Brehm H, Haase W. Die alternative zur hormonalen kontrazeption? Med Welt. 1975;26:1610–7. German.

Brigato G, Pisano G, Bergamasco A, Pasqualini M, Cutugno G, Luppari T. Vaginal topical chemical contraception with C-Film. Ginecol Clinica. 1982;3:77–80. (In Italian; translation supplied by Apothecus Inc.)

Broome M, Fotherby K. Clinical experience with the progestogen-only pill. Contraception. 1990;42:489–95.

Bushnell LF. Aerosol foam: a practical and effective method of contraception. Pac Med Surg. 1965;73:353–5.

Cagen R. The cervical cap as a barrier contraceptive. Contraception. 1986;33:487–96.

Carpenter G, Martin JB. Clinical evaluation of a vaginal contraceptive foam. Adv Plann Parent. 1970;5:170–5.

Chi IC, Laufe LE, Gardner SD, Tolbert MA. An epidemiologic study of risk factors associated with pregnancy following female sterilization. Am J Obstet Gynecol. 1980;136:768–73.

Chi IC, Mumford SD, Gardner SD. Pregnancy risks following laparoscopic sterilization in nongravid and gravid women. J Reprod Med. 1981;26:289–94.

Chi IC, Siemens AJ, Champion CB, Gates D, Cilenti D. Pregnancy following minilaparotomy tubal sterilization: an update of an international data set. Contraception. 1987;35:171–8.

Cliquet RL, Schoenmaeckers R, Klinkenborg L. Effectiveness of contraception in Belgium: results of the second national fertility survey, 1971 (NEGO II). J Biosoc Sci. 1977;9:403–16.

Collaborative Study Group on the Desogestrel-containing Progestogen-only Pill. A double-blind study comparing the contraceptive efficacy, acceptability and safety of two progestogen-only pills containing desogestrel 75 micrograms/day or levonorgestrel 30 micrograms/day. Eur J Contracept Reprod Health Care. 1998;3:169–178.

Cooper JM, Carignan CS, Cher D, Kerin JF. Microinsert nonincisional hysteroscopic sterilization. Obstet Gynecol. 2003;102:59–67.

Cox M, Blacksell S. Clinical performance of the levonorgestrel intra-uterine system in routine use by the UK Family Planning and Reproductive Health Research Network: 12-month report. Br J Fam Plann. 2000;26:143–7.

Darney P, Patel A, Rosen K, Shapiro LS, Kaunitz AM. Safety and efficacy of a single-rod etonogestrel implant (Implanon): results from 11 international clinical trials. Fertil Steril. 2009;91:1646–53.

Debusschere R. Effectiviteit van de anticonceptie in Vlaanderen: resultaten van het NEGO-III-onderzoek 1975–1976. Bevolking en Gezin. 1980;1:5–28. German.

Denniston GC, Putney D. The cavity rim cervical cap. Adv Plann Parent. 1981;16:77–80.

Dieben TOM, Roumen JME, Apter D. Efficacy, cycle control and user acceptability of a novel combined contraceptive vaginal ring. Obstet Gynecol. 2002;100:585–93.

Dimpfl J, Salomon W, Schicketanz KH. Die spermizide barriere. Sexualmedizin. 1984;13:95–8. German.

Dingle JT, Tietze C. Comparative study of three contraceptive methods: vaginal foam tablets, jelly alone, and diaphragm with jelly or cream. Am J Obstet Gynecol. 1963;85:1012–22.

Dolack L. Study confirms values of ovulation method. Hospital Progress. 1978;59:64–6,72–3.

Dominik R, Gates D, Sokal D, Cordero M, Lasso de la Vega J, Remes Ruiz A, Thambu J, Lim D, Louissaint S, Galvez RS, Uribe L, Zighelboim I. Two randomized controlled trials comparing the Hulka and Filshie Clips for tubal sterilization. Contraception. 2000;62:169–75.

Dubrow H, Kuder K. Combined postpartum and family-planning clinic. Obstet Gynecol. 1958;11:586–90.

Edelman DA. Nonprescription vaginal contraception. Int J Gynecol Obstet. 1980;18:340–4.

Edelman DA, McIntyre SL, Harper J. A comparative trial of the Today contraceptive sponge and diaphragm. Am J Obstet Gynecol. 1984;150:869–76.

Ellis JW. Multiphasic oral contraceptives: efficacy and metabolic impact. J Reprod Med. 1987;32:28–36.

Ellsworth HS. Focus on triphasil. J Reprod Med. 1986;31:559–64.

Endrikat J, Jaques MA, Mayerhofer M, Pelissier C, Müller U, Düsterberg B. A twelve-month comparative clinical investigation of two low-dose oral contraceptives containing 20 μg ethinylestradiol/75 μg gestodene and 20 μg ethinylestradiol/150 μg desogestrel, with respect to efficacy, cycle control and tolerance. Contraception. 1995;52:229–35.

Engel T. Laparoscopic sterilization: electrosurgery or clip application? J Reprod Med. 1978;21:107–10.

Flores JB, Balderas ML, Bonilla MC, Vazquez-Estrada L. Clinical experience and acceptability of the etonogestrel subdermal contraceptive implant. Int J Gynaecol Obstet. 2005;90:228–33.

Florence N. Das kontrazeptive vaginal-suppositorium: ergebnisse einer klinischen fünfjahresstudie. Sexualmedizin. 1977;6:385–6. German.

Frank R. Clinical evaluation of a simple jelly-alone method of contraception. Fertil Steril. 1962;13:458–64.

Frank-Herrmann P, Heil J, Gnoth C, Toledo E, Baur S, Pyper C, Jenetzky E, Strowitzki T, Freundl G. The effectiveness of a fertility awareness based method to avoid pregnancy in relation to a couple's sexual behaviour during the fertile time: a prospective longitudinal study. Hum Reprod. 2007;22:1310–9.

Frankman O, Raabe N, Ingemansson CA. Clinical evaluation of C-Film, a vaginal contraceptive. J Int Med Res. 1975;3:292–6.

Frezieres RG, Walsh TL, Nelson AL, Clark VA, Coulson AH. Evaluation of the efficacy of a polyurethane condom: results from a randomized controlled clinical trial. Fam Plann Perspect. 1999;31:81–7.

Fu H, Darroch JE, Haas T, Ranjit N. Contraceptive failure rates: new estimates from the 1995 National Survey of Family Growth. Fam Plann Perspect. 1999;31:56–63.

Gezginc K, Balci O, Karatayli R, Colakoglu MC. Contraceptive efficacy and side effects of Implanon. Eur J Contracept Reprod Health Care. 2007;12:362–5.

Gibor Y, Mitchell C. Selected events following insertion of the Progestasert system. Contraception. 1980;21:491–503.

Glass R, Vessey M, Wiggins P. Use-effectiveness of the condom in a selected family planning clinic population in the United Kingdom. Contraception. 1974;10:591–8.

Godts P. Klinische prüfung eines vaginalem antikonzipiens. Ars Medici. 1973;28:584–93. German.

Grady WR, Hayward MD, Yagi J. Contraceptive failure in the United States: estimates from the 1982 National Survey of Family Growth. Fam Plann Perspect. 1986;18:200–9.

Grady WR, Hirsch MB, Keen N, Vaughan B. Contraceptive failure and continuation among married women in the United States, 1970–75. Stud Fam Plann. 1983;14:9–19.

Graesslin O, Korver T. The contraceptive efficacy of Implanon: a review of clinical trials and marketing experience. Eur J Contracept Reprod Health Care. 2008;13 Suppl 1:S4–12.

Hall P, Bahamondes L, Diaz J, Petta C. Introductory study of the once-a-month, injectable contraceptive Cyclofem in Brazil, Chile, Colombia, and Peru. Contraception. 1997;56:353–9.

Hall RE. Continuation and pregnancy rates with four contraceptive methods. Am J Obstet Gynecol. 1973;116:671–81.

Harvey C, Seib C, Lucke J. Continuation rates and reasons for removal among Implanon users accessing two family planning clinics in Queensland, Australia. Contraception. 2009;80:526–32.

Hawkins DF, Benster B. A comparative study of three low dose progestogens, chlormadinone acetate, megestrol acetate and norethisterone, as oral contraceptives. Br J Obstet Gynaecol. 1977;84:708–13.

Hernádi L, Marr J, Trummer D, De Leo V, Petraglia F. Efficacy and safety of a low-dose combined oral contraceptive containing drospirenone 3 mg and ethinylestradiol 20 mcg in a 24/4-day regimen. Contraception. 2009;80:18–24.

Howard G, Blair M, Chen JK, Fotherby K, Muggeridge J, Elder MG, Bye PG. A clinical trial of norethisterone oenanthate (Norigest) injected every two months. Contraception. 1982;25:333–43.

Hughes I. An open assessment of a new low dose estrogen combined oral contraceptive. J Int Med Res. 1978;6:41–5.

Hulka JF, Mercer JP, Fishburne JI, Kumarasamy T, Omran KF, Phillips JM, Lefler HT, Lieberman B, Lean TH, Pai DN, Koetsawang S, Castro VM. Spring clip sterilization: one-year follow-up of 1,079 cases. Am J Obstet Gynecol. 1976;125:1039–43.

Iizuka R, Kobayashi T, Kawakami S, Nakamura Y, Ikeuchi M, Chin B, Mochimaru F, Sumi K, Sato H, Yamaguchi J, Ohno T, Shiina M, Maeda N, Tokoro H, Suzuki T, Hayashi K, Takahashi T, Akatsuka M, Kasuga Y, Kurokawa H. Clinical experience with the Vaginal Contraceptive Film containing the spermicide polyoxyethylene nonylphenyl ether (C-Film study group). Jpn J Fertil Steril. 1980;25:64–8. (In Japanese; translation supplied by Apothecus Inc.)

Jain J, Jakimiuk AJ, Bode FR, Ross D, Kaunitz AM. Contraceptive efficacy and safety of DMPA-SC. Contraception. 2004;70:269–75.

Jamieson DJ, Costello C, Trussell J, Hillis SD, Marchbanks PA, Peterson HB; for the US Collaborative Review of Sterilization Working Group. The risk of pregnancy after vasectomy. Obstet Gynecol. 2004;103(5 Pt 1):848–850. Erratum in: Obstet Gynecol. 2004;104:200.

John APK. Contraception in a practice community. J R Coll Gen Pract. 1973;23:665–75.

Johnston JA, Roberts DB, Spencer RB. A survey evaluation of the efficacy and efficiency of natural family planning services and methods in Australia: report of a research project. Sydney: St. Vincent's Hospital; 1978.

Jones EF, Forrest JD. Contraceptive failure rates based on the 1988 NSFG. Fam Plann Perspect. 1992;24:12–9.

Jubhari S, Lane ME, Sobrero AJ. Continuous microdose (0.3 mg) quingestanol acetate as an oral contraceptive agent. Contraception. 1974;9:213–9.

Kambic R, Kambic M, Brixius AM, Miller S. A thirty-month clinical experience in natural family planning. Am J Public Health 1981;71:1255–8. Erratum in: Am J Public Health. 1982;72:538.

Kasabach HY. Clinical evaluation of vaginal jelly alone in the management of fertility. Clin Med. 1962;69:894–7.

Kase S, Goldfarb M. Office vasectomy review of 500 cases. Urology. 1973;1:60–2.

Kassell NC, McElroy MP. Emma Goldman Clinic for Women study. In: King L, (ed). The cervical cap handbook for users and fitters. Iowa City: Emma Goldman Clinic for Women; 1981. p. 11–9.

Kaunitz AM. Efficacy, cycle control, and safety of two triphasic oral contraceptives: Cyclessa (desogestrel/ethinyl estradiol) and Ortho-Novum 7/7/7 (norethindrone/ethinyl estradiol): a randomized clinical trial. Contraception. 2000;61:295–302.

Kaunitz AM, Darney PD, Ross D, Wolter KD, Speroff L. Subcutaneous DMPA vs. Intramuscular DMPA: a 2-year randomized study of contraceptive efficacy and bone mineral denisty. Contraception. 2009;80:7–17.

Kaunitz AM, Garceau RJ, Cromie MA, Lunelle Study Group. Comparative safety, efficacy, and cycle control of Lunelle monthly contraceptive injection (medroxyprogesterone acetate and estradiol cypionate injectable suspension) and Ortho-Novum 7/7/7 oral contraceptive (norethindrone/eithinyl estradiol triphasic). Contraception. 1999;60:179–87.

Keifer W. A clinical evaluation of continuous Norethindrone (0.35 mg). In: Ortho Pharmaceutical Corporation. A clinical symposium on 0.35 mg. Norethindrone: continuous regimen low-dose oral contraceptive. Proceedings of a symposium, New York City, February 22, 1971. Raritan: Ortho Pharmaceutical Corporation, 1973;9–14.

Kerin JF, Cooper JM, Price T, Herendael BJ, Cayuela-Font E, Cher D, Carignan CS. Hysteroscopic sterilization using a micro-insert device: results of a multicentre Phase II study. Hum Reprod. 2003;18:1223–30.

Klapproth HJ, Young IS. Vasectomy, vas ligation and vas occlusion. Urology. 1973;1:292–300.

Klaus H, Goebel JM, Muraski B, Egizio MT, Weitzel D, Taylor, RS, Fagan MU, Ek K, Hobday K. Use-effectiveness and client satisfaction in six centers teaching the Billings ovulation method. Contraception. 1979;19:613–29.

Kleppinger RK. A vaginal contraceptive foam. Penn Med J. 1965;68:31–4.

Koch JP. The Prentif contraceptive cervical cap: a contemporary study of its clinical safety and effectiveness. Contraception. 1982;25:135–59.

Korba VD, Heil CG. Eight years of fertility control with norgestrel-ethinyl estradiol (Ovral): an updated clinical review. Fertil Steril. 1975;26:973–81.

Korba VD, Paulson SR. Five years of fertility control with microdose norgestrel: an updated clinical review. J Reprod Med. 1974;13:71–5.

Kost K, Singh S, Vaughan B, Trussell J, Bankole A. Estimates of contraceptive failure from the 2002 National Survey of Family Growth. Contraception. 2008;77:10–21.

Kovacs GT, Jarman H, Dunn K, Westcott M, Baker HWG. The contraceptive diaphragm: is it an acceptable method in the 1980s? Aust NZ J Obstet Gynaecol. 1986;26:76–9.

Kroll R, Reape KZ, Margolis M. The efficacy and safety of a low-dose, 91-day, extended-regimen oral contraceptive with continuous ethinyl estradiol. Contraception. 2010;81:41–8.

Lakha F, Glasier AF. Continuation rates of Implanon in the UK: data from an observational study in a clinical setting. Contraception. 2006;74:287–9.

Lampe L, Andersson K, Atterfeldt P, Johansson EDB, Nilsson S, Nygren KG, Odlind V, Olsson SE, Rybo G, Sikström B, Nielsen NC, Buch A, Osler M, Steier A, Ulstein M. Effective contraception with the levonorgestrel-releasing intrauterine device: 12-month report of a European multicenter study. Contraception. 1987;36:169–79.

Lane ME, Arceo R, Sobrero AJ. Successful use of the diaphragm and jelly by a young population: report of a clinical study. Fam Plann Perspect. 1976;8:81–6.

Ledger WJ. Ortho 1557-O: a new oral contraceptive. Int J Fertil. 1970;15:88–92.

Lehfeldt H, Sivin I. Use effectiveness of the Prentif cervical cap in private practice: a prospective study. Contraception. 1984;30:331–8.

Lipetz C, Phillips C, Fleming C. Actual cost of providing long-acting reversible contraception: a study of Implanon cost. J Fam Plann Reprod Health Care. 2009;35:75–9.

Loffer FD, Pent D. Risks of laparoscopic fulguration and transection of the fallopian tube. Obstet Gynecol. 1977;49:218–22.

Loudon NB, Barden ME, Hepburn WB, Prescott RJ. A comparative study of the effectiveness and acceptability of the diaphragm used with spermicide in the form of C-film or a cream or jelly. Br J Fam Plann. 1991;17:41–4.

Luukkainen T, Allonen H, Haukkamaa M, Holma P, Pyörälä T, Terho J, Toivonen J, Batar I, Lampe L, Andersson K, Atterfeldt P, Johansson EDB, Nilsson S, Nygren KG, Odlind V, Olsson SE, Rybo G, Sikström B, Nielsen NC, Buch A, Osler M, Steier A, Ulstein M. Effective contraception with the levonorgestrel-releasing intrauterine device: 12-month report of a European multicenter study. Contraception. 1987;36:169–79.

Margaret Pyke Centre. One thousand vasectomies. Br Med J. 1973;4:216–21.

Marshall J. Cervical-mucus and basal body-temperature method of regulating births: field trial. Lancet. 1976;2:282–3.

Marshall S, Lyon RP. Variability of sperm disappearance from the ejaculate after vasectomy. J Urol. 1972;107:815–7.

Mauck C, Callahan M, Weiner DH, Dominik R, FemCap investigators' group. A comparative study of the safety and efficacy of FemCap, a new vaginal barrier contraceptive, and the Ortho All-Flex diaphragm. Contraception. 1999;60:71–80.

Mauck C, Glover LH, Miller E, Allen S, Archer DF, Blumenthal P, Rosenzweig BA, Dominik R, Sturgen K, Cooper J, Fingerhut F, Peacock L, Gabelnick HL. Lea's Shield®: a study of the safety and efficacy of a new vaginal barrier contraceptive used with and without spermicide. Contraception. 1996;53:329–35.

McIntyre SL, Higgins JE. Parity and use-effectiveness with the contraceptive sponge. Am J Obstet Gynecol. 1986;155:796–801.

McQuarrie HG, Harris JW, Ellsworth HS, Stone RA, Anderson AE. The clinical evaluation of norethindrone in cyclic and continuous regimens. Adv Plann Parent. 1972;7:124–30.

Mears E. Chemical contraceptive trial: II. J Reprod Fertil. 1962;4:337–43.

Mears E, Please NW. Chemical contraceptive trial. J Reprod Fertil. 1962;3:138–47.

The Mircette Study Group. An open-label, multicenter, noncomparative safety and efficacy study of Mircette, a low-dose estrogen-progestin oral contraceptive. Am J Obstet Gynecol. 1998;179 Suppl:S2–8.

Mishell DR, El-Habashy MA, Good RG, Moyer DL. Contraception with an injectable progestin. Am J Obstet Gynecol. 1968;101:1046–53.

Morigi EM, Pasquale SA. Clinical experience with a low dose oral contraceptive containing norethisterone and ethinyl oestradiol. Curr Med Res Opin. 1978;5:655–62.

Moss WM. A comparison of open-end versus closed-end vasectomies: a report on 6220 cases. Contraception. 1992;46:521–5.

Mumford SD, Bhiwandiwala PP, Chi IC. Laparoscopic and minilaparotomy female sterilisation compared in 15,167 cases. Lancet. 1980;2:1066–70.

Nakajima ST, Archer DF, Ellman H. Efficacy and safety of a new 24-day oral contraceptive regimen of norethindroneacetate 1 mg/ethinyl estradiol 20 μ (Loestrin® 24 Fe). Contraception. 2007;75:16–22.

Nelson JH. The use of the mini pill in private practice. J Reprod Med. 1973;10:139–43.

Oddsson K, Leifels-Fischer B, de Melo NR, Wiel-Masson D, Benedetto C, Verhoeven CH, Dieben TO. Efficacy and safety of a contraceptive vaginal ring (NuvaRing) compared with a combined oral contraceptive: a 1-year randomized trial. Contraception. 2005;71:176–82.

Palacios S, Wildt L, Parke S, Machlitt A, Römer T, Bitzer J. Efficacy and safety of a novel oral contraceptive based on oestradiol (oestradiol valerate/dienogest): a Phase III trial. Eur J Obstet Gynecol Reprod Biol. 2010;149:57–62.

Parsey KS, Pong A. An open-label, multicenter study to evaluate Yasmin, a low-dose combination oral contraceptive containing drospirenone, a new progestogen. Contraception. 2000;61:105–11.

Peel J. The Hull family survey: II. Family planning in the first five years of marriage. J Biosoc Sci. 1972;4:333–46.

Peterson HB, Xia Z, Hughes JM, Wilcox LS, Tylor LR, Trussell J. The risk of pregnancy after tubal sterilization: findings from the U.S. Collaborative Review of Sterilization. Am J Obstet Gynecol. 1996;174:1161–70.

Philp T, Guillebaud J, Budd D. Complications of vasectomy: review of 16,000 patients. Br J Urol. 1984;56;745–8.

Postlethwaite DL. Pregnancy rate of a progestogen oral contraceptive. Practitioner. 1979;222:272–5.

Potts M, McDevitt J. A use-effectiveness trial of spermicidally lubricated condoms. Contraception. 1975;11:701–10.

Powell MG, Mears BJ, Deber RB, Ferguson D. Contraception with the cervical cap: effectiveness, safety, continuity of use, and user satisfaction. Contraception. 1986;33:215–32.

Preston SN. A report of a collaborative dose-response clinical study using decreasing doses of combination oral contraceptives. Contraception. 1972;6:17–35.

Preston SN. A report of the correlation between the pregnancy rates of low estrogen formulations and pill-taking habits of females studied. J Reprod Med. 1974;13:75–7.

Rai K, Gupta S, Cotter S. Experience with Implanon in a northeast London family planning clinic. Eur J Contracept Reprod Health Care. 2004;9:39–46.

Raymond EG, Chen PL, Luoto J. Contraceptive effectiveness and safety of five nonoxynol-9 spermicides: a randomized trial. Obstet Gynecol. 2004;103:430–9.

Raymond E, Dominik R, the spermicide trial group. Contraceptive effectiveness of two spermicides: a randomized trial. Obstet Gynecol. 1999;93:896–903.

Rice FJ, Lanctôt CA, Garcia-Devesa C. Effectiveness of the sympto-thermal method of natural family planning: an international study. Int J Fertil. 1981;26:222–30.

Richwald GA, Greenland S, Gerber MM, Potik R, Kersey L, Comas MA. Effectiveness of the cavity-rim cervical cap: results of a large clinical study. Obstet Gynecol. 1989;74:143–8.

Roumen FJME, Apter D, Mulders TMT, Dieben TOM. Efficacy, tolerability and acceptability of a novel contraceptive vaginal ring releasing etonogestrel and ethinyl oestradiol. Hum Reprod. 2001;16:469–75.

Rovinsky JJ. Clinical effectiveness of a contraceptive cream. Obstet Gynecol. 1964;23:125–31.

Royal College of General Practitioners. Oral contraceptives and health. New York: Pitman Publishing Corporation; 1974.

Salomon W, Haase W. Intravaginale kontrazeption. Sexualmedizin. 1977;6:198–202. German.

Sangi-Haghpeykar H, Poindexter AN, Bateman L, Ditmore JR. Experiences of injectable contraceptive users in an urban setting. Obstet Gynecol. 1996;88:226–33.

Schirm AL, Trussell J, Menken J, Grady WR. Contraceptive failure in the United States: the impact of social, economic, and demographic factors. Fam Plann Perspect. 1982;14:68–75.

Schmidt SS. Vasectomy. JAMA. 1988;259:3176.

Schwallie PC, Assenzo JR. Contraceptive use-efficacy study utilizing Depo-Provera administered as an injection once every six months. Contraception. 1972;6:315–27.

Schwallie PC, Assenzo JR. Contraceptive use-efficacy study utilizing medroxyprogesterone acetate administered as an intramuscular injection once every 90 days. Fertil Steril. 1973;24:331–9.

Scutchfield FD, Long WN, Corey B, Tyler CW. Medroxyprogesterone acetate as an injectable female contraceptive. Contraception. 1971;3:21–35.

Sheps MC. An analysis of reproductive patterns in an American isolate. Popul Stud. 1965;19:65–80.

Sheth A, Jain U, Sharma S, Adatia A, Patankar S, Andolsek L, Pretnar-Darovec A, Belsey MA, Hall PE, Parker RA, Ayeni S, Pinol A, Foo CLH. A randomized, double-blind study of two combined and two progestogen-only oral contraceptives. Contraception. 1982;25:243–52.

Shihata AA, Trussell J. New female intravaginal barrier contraceptive device: preliminary clinical trial. Contraception. 1991;44:11–9.

Shroff NE, Pearce MY, Stratford ME, Wilkinson PD. Clinical experience with ethynodiol diacetate 0.5 mg daily as an oral contraceptive. Contraception. 1987;35:121–34.

Sivin I, El Mahgoub S, McCarthy T, Mishell DR, Shoupe D, Alvarez F, Brache V, Jimenez E, Diaz J, Faundes A, Diaz MM, Coutinho E, Mattos CER, Diaz S, Pavez M, Stern J. Long-term contraception with the Levonorgestrel 20 mcg/day (LNg-IUS) and the Copper T 380Ag intrauterine devices: a five-year randomized study. Contraception. 1990;42:361–78.

Sivin I, Shaaban M, Odlind V, Olsson SE, Diaz S, Pavez M, Alvarez F, Brache V, Diaz J. A randomized trial of the Gyne T 380 and Gyne T 380 Slimline intrauterine copper devices. Contraception. 1990;42:379–89.

Sivin I, Stern J. Long-acting, more effective copper T IUDs: a summary of U.S. experience, 1970–1975. Stud Fam Plann. 1979;10:263–81.

Smallwood GH, Meador ML, Lenihan JP, Shangold GA, Fisher AC, Creasy GW, and the ORTHO EVRA/EVRA 002 Study Group. Efficacy and safety of a transdermal contraceptive system. Obstet Gynecol. 2001;98:799–805.

Smith A, Reuter S. An assessment of the use of Implanon in three community services. J Fam Plann Reprod Health Care. 2002;28:193–6.

Smith C, Farr G, Feldblum PJ, Spence A. Effectiveness of the non-spermicidal fit-free diaphragm. Contraception. 1995;51:289–91.

Smith GG, Lee RJ. The use of cervical caps at the University of California, Berkeley: a survey. Contraception. 1984;30:115–23.

Smith M, Vessey MP, Bounds W, Warren J. C-Film as a contraceptive. Br Med J. 1974;4:291.

Sokal D, Gates D, Amatya R, Dominik R, and the Clinical investigator team. Two randomized controlled trials comparing the tubal ring and Filshie Clip for tubal sterilization. Fertil Steril. 2000;74:525–33.

Steiner MJ, Dominik R, Rountree RW, Nanda K, Dorflinger LJ. Contraceptive effectiveness of a polyurethane condom and a latex condom: a randomized controlled trial. Obstet Gynecol. 2003;101:539–47.

Stim EM. The nonspermicidal fit-free diaphragm: a new contraceptive method. Adv Plan Parent. 1980;15:88–98.

Squire JJ, Berger GS, Keith L. A retrospective clinical study of a vaginal contraceptive suppository. J Reprod Med. 1979;22:319–23.

Tatum HJ. Comparative experience with newer models of the copper T in the United States. In: Hefnawi F, Segal SJ, (eds). Analysis of intrauterine contraception. Amsterdam (Netherlands): North Holland, 1975. p. 155–63.

Teichmann A, Apter D, Emerich J, Greven K, Klasa-Mazurkiewicz D, Melis GB, Spaczynski M, Grubb G, Constantine GD, Spielmann D. Continuous daily levonorgestrel/ethinyl estradiol vs. 21-day, cyclic levonorgestrel/ethinyl estradiol: efficacy, safety and bleeding in a randomized, open-label trial. Contraception. 2009;20:504–11.

Thamkhantho M, Jivasak-Apimas S, Angsuwathana S, Chiravacharadej G, Intawong J. One-year assessment of women receiving sub-dermal contraceptive implant at Siriraj Family Planning Clinic. J Med Assoc Thai. 2008;91:775–80.

Tietze C, Lewit S. Comparison of three contraceptive methods: diaphragm with jelly or cream, vaginal foam, and jelly/cream alone. J Sex Res. 1967;3:295–311.

Tietze C, Lewit S. Evaluation of intrauterine devices: ninth progress report of the cooperative statistical program. Stud Fam Plann. 1970;1:1–40.

Tietze C, Poliakoff SR, Rock J. The clinical effectiveness of the rhythm method of contraception. Fertil Steril. 1951;2:444–50.

Trussell J. Estimates of contraceptive failure from the 2002 National Survey of Family Growth. Contraception. 2008;78:85.

Trussell J, Grummer-Strawn L. Contraceptive failure of the ovulation method of periodic abstinence. Fam Plann Perspect. 1990;22:65–75.

Trussell J, Hatcher RA, Cates W, Stewart FH, Kost K. Contraceptive failure in the United States: an update. Stud Fam Plann. 1990;21:51–4.

Trussell J, Kost K. Contraceptive failure in the United States: a critical review of the literature. Stud Fam Plann. 1987;18:237–83.

Trussell J, Vaughan B. Contraceptive failure, method-related discontinuation and resumption of use: results from the 1995 National Survey of Family Growth. Fam Plann Perspect. 1999;31:64–72, 93.

Tyler ET. Current developments in systemic contraception. Pac Med Surg. 1965;93:79–85.

Valle RF, Battifora HA. A new approach to tubal sterilization by laparoscopy. Fertil Steril. 1978;30:415–22.

Vancaillie TG, Anderson TL, Johns DA. A 12-month prospective evaluation of transcervical sterilization using implantable polymer matrices. Obstet Gynecol. 2008;112:1270–7.

Vaughan B, Trussell J, Menken J, Jones EF. Contraceptive failure among married women in the United States, 1970–1973. Fam Plann Perspect. 1977;9:251–8.

Vessey M, Huggins G, Lawless M, McPherson K, Yeates D. Tubal sterilization: findings in a large prospective study. Br J Obstet Gynaecol. 1983;90:203–9.

Vessey M, Lawless M, Yeates D. Efficacy of different contraceptive methods. Lancet. 1982;1:841–2.

Vessey MP, Lawless M, Yeates D, McPherson K. Progestogen-only oral contraception. Findings in a large prospective study with special reference to effectiveness. Br J Fam Plann. 1985;10:117–21.

Vessey MP, Villard-Mackintosh L, McPherson K, Yeates D. Factors influencing use-effectiveness of the condom. Br J Fam Plann. 1988;14:40–3.

Vessey M, Wiggins P. Use-effectiveness of the diaphragm in a selected family planning clinic population in the United Kingdom. Contraception. 1974;9:15–21.

Vessey MP, Wright NH, McPherson K, Wiggins P. Fertility after stopping different methods of contraception. Br Med J. 1978;1:265–7.

Vleugels MPH, Veersema S. Hysteroscopic sterilization in the outpatient department without anasthesis. Gynecol Surg. 2005;2:155–8.

Wade ME, McCarthy P, Braunstein GD, Abernathy JR, Suchindran CM, Harris GS, Danzer HC, Uricchio WA. A randomized prospective study of the use-effectiveness of two methods of natural family planning. Am J Obstet Gynecol. 1981;141:368–76.

Walsh TL, Frezieres RG, Peacock K, Nelson AL, Clark VA, Bernstein L. Evaluation of the efficacy of a nonlatex condom: results from a randomized, controlled clinical trial. Perspect Sex Reprod Health. 2003;35:79–86.

Westoff CF, Potter RG, Sagi PC, Mishler EG. Family growth in metropolitan America. Princeton: Princeton University Press; 1961.

Wolf L, Olson HJ, Tyler ET. Observations on the clinical use of cream-alone and gel-alone methods of contraception. Obstet Gynecol. 1957;10:316–21.

World Health Organization. A multicentered phase III comparative clinical trial of depot-medroxyprogesterone acetate given three-monthly at doses of 100 mg or 150 mg: I. Contraceptive efficacy and side effects. Contraception. 1986;34:223–35.

World Health Organization. A multicentered phase III comparative study of two hormonal contraceptive preparations given once-a-month by intramuscular injection: I. Contraceptive efficacy and side effects. Contraception. 1988;37:1–20.

World Health Organization. A prospective multicentre trial of the ovulation method of natural family planning. II. The effectiveness phase. Fertil Steril. 1981;36:591–8.

World Health Organization. Multinational comparative clinical evaluation of two long-acting injectable contraceptive steroids: norethisterone oenanthate and medroxyprogesterone acetate. Contraception. 1977;15:513–33.

World Health Organization. Multinational comparative clinical trial of long-acting injectable contraceptives: norethisterone enanthate given in two dosage regimens and depot-medroxyprogesterone acetate. Final report. Contraception. 1983;28:1–20.

Woutersz TB. A low-dose combination oral contraceptive: experience with 1,700 women treated for 22,489 cycles. J Reprod Med. 1981;26:615–20.

Woutersz TB. A new ultra-low-dose combination oral contraceptive. J Reprod Med. 1983;28:81–4.

Wyeth Laboratories. NORPLANT® SYSTEM Prescribing Information. Philadelphia (PA): Wyeth Laboratories; 1990 Dec 10.

Yildizbas B, Sahin HG, Kolusari A, Zeteroglu S, Kamaci M. Side effects and acceptability of Implanon: a pilot study conducted in eastern Turkey. Eur J Contracept Reprod Health Care. 2007;12:248–52.

Yoon IB, King TM, Parmley TH. A two-year experience with the Falope ring sterilization procedure. Am J Obstet Gynecol. 1977;127:109–12.

Zheng SR, Zheng HM, Qian SZ, Sang GW, Kaper RF. A long-term study of the efficacy and acceptability of a single-rod hormonal contraceptive implant (Implanon) in healthy women in China. Eur J Contracept Reprod Health Care. 1999a;4:85–93.

Zheng SR, Zheng HM, Qian SZ, Sang GW, Kaper RF. A randomized multicenter study comparing the efficacy and bleeding pattern of a single-rod (Implanon) and a six-capsule (Norplant) hormonal contraceptive implant. Contraception. 1999b;60:1–8.

Appendix 1

Webpages with Active Links to Many Other Websites

Boston Women's Health Book Collective . . . . www.ourbodiesourselves.org

CDC National Prevention Network . . . . cdcnpin.org

Contraceptive Technology . . . . www.contraceptivetechnology.org

Department of Health and Human Services . . . . www.healthfinder.gov

Princeton University . . . . www.princeton.edu/main

Appendix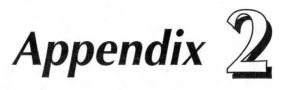

Network of Professional Organizations

Advocates for Youth
www.advocatesforyouth.org

AIDS Clinical Trials Information
Service (ACTIS)
www.aidsinfo.nih.gov

Alan Guttmacher Institute (AGI)
www.guttmacher.org

Alliance for Microbicide Development
www.microbicide.com

American Association of Sex Educators,
Counselors, and Therapists
www.aasect.org

American College Health Association
www.acha.org

American College of Obstetricians and
Gynecologists (ACOG)
www.acog.org

American Public Health Association
(APHA)
www.apha.org

American Social Health Association
(ASHA)
www.ashastd.org

American Society for Reproductive
Medicine (ASRM)
www.asrm.org

Association of Reproductive Health
Professionals (ARHP)
www.arhp.org

California Family Health Council
www.cfhc.org

Catholics for Choice
www.cath4choice.org

Centre for Development and
Population Activities (CEDPA)
www.cedpa.org

Centers for Disease Control and
Prevention (CDC)
www.cdc.gov/netinfo.htm

CDC Division of HIV/AIDS Prevention
www.cdc.gov/hiv/contactus.htm

Coalition Advancing Multipurpose
Innovations (CAMI)
www.cami-health.org

Columbia University School of Public
Health
www.mailman.columbia.edu/popfam

Committee on Population, National Academy of Sciences
www7.nationalacademies.org/cpop

Contraceptive Research and Development Program (CONRAD)
www.conrad.org

Contraceptive Technology Communications, Inc.
P.O. Box 49007
Atlanta, GA 30359
www.contraceptivetechnology.org

East-West Center Program on Population
www.eastwestcenter.org/Research/Research-program-overview/population-and-health

Education and Training Resource Associates (ETR)
www.etr.org

Engender Health
www.engenderhealth.org

Family Violence Prevention Fund
www.endabuse.org

FHI 360
www.fhi.org

Ford Foundation
www.fordfound.org

Ibis Reproductive Health
www.ibisreproductivehealth.org

Institute for Reproductive Health
www.irh.org

International Partnership for Microbicides
www.ipm-microbicides.org

International Planned Parenthood Federation (IPPF)
www.ippfwhr.org

International Union for the Scientific Study of Population (IUSSP)
www.iussp.org

IPAS
www.ipas.org

John Snow, Inc.
www.jsi.com

Johns Hopkins University School of Public Health
www.jhuccp.org

Kaiser Family Foundation
www.kff.org

National Abortion Federation (NAF)
www.prochoice.org

National Abortion and Reproductive Rights Action League (NARAL)
www.prochoiceamerica.org

National Association of Nurse Practitioners Women's Health (NPWH)
www.npwh.org

National Family Planning and Reproductive Health Association (NFPRHA)
www.nfprha.org

National Institute of Child Health and Human Development (NICHD)
www.nichd.nih.gov/about/cpr/cpr.htm

Office on Women's Health
www.womenshealth.gov

Pathfinder International
www.pathfind.org

Planned Parenthood Federation of America (PPFA)
www.plannedparenthood.org

Population Action International (PAI)
www.populationaction.org

Population Association of America (PAA)
www.populationassociation.org

Population Council
www.popcouncil.org

Population Institute
www.populationinstitute.org

Population Reference Bureau (PRB)
www.prb.org

Princeton University
http://opr.princeton.edu

Program for Appropriate Technology in Health (PATH)
www.path.org

Program for International Training and Health (INTRAH)
www.intrahealth.org

Religious Institute on Sexual Morality, Justice, and Healing
www.religiousinstitute.org

Reproductive Health Technologies
  Project (RHTP)
www.rhtp.org

Rockefeller Foundation
www.rockefellerfoundation.org

Sexuality Information and Education
  Council of the United States
  (SIECUS)
www.siecus.org

United Nations Population Information
  Network
www.un.org/popin

United Nations Population Fund
  (UNFPA)
www.unfpa.org/

University of Michigan School of
  Public Health
www.sph.umich.edu

University of North Carolina
  Population Center
www.cpc.unc.edu

U.S. Agency for International
  Development (USAID)
www.maqweb.org

William and Flora Hewlett Foundation
www.hewlett.org

World Bank
www.worldbank.org

World Health Organization
www.who.int

Appendix 3

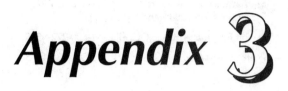

Pharmaceutical Company Websites and Toll-free Phone Numbers

Ansell Healthcare: condoms	1-800-232-1309	www.ansell.com
Apothecus: VCF	1-800-227-2393	www.apothecus.com
Bayer Healthcare: OCs, progestin IUC	1-888-237-5394	www.bayerhealthcare.com
Bristol-Myers Squibb Company: OCs, ERT	1-800-321-1335	www.bms.com
Church & Dwight: condoms	1-800-524-1328	www.churchdwight.com
Danco Laboratories: mifepristone	1-877-432-7596	www.earlyoptionpill.com
GlaxoSmithKline: antivirals, antibiotics	1-888-825-5249	www.gsk.com
Mayer Laboratories: condoms, sponge	1-800-426-6366	www.mayerlabs.com
Merck Pharmaceutical: OCs, vaginal ring, implant	1-800-444-2080	www.merck.com
Okamoto: condoms	1-800-283-7546	www.okamotousa.com
Ortho-McNeil Pharmaceutical: OCs, patch, diaphragm, IUC	1-800-526-7736	www.ortho-mcneil.com
Parke Davis (Pfizer): OCs	1-800-223-0432	www.pfizer.com
Pharmacia (Pfizer): injectables, ERT	1-800-323-4204	www.pfizer.com

Smart Practice: non-allergenic gloves	1-800-522-0800	www.smartpractice.com
Teva Pharmaceuticals: Plan B One-Step, copper IUD, OCs	1-800-222-0190	www.tevapharm-na.com
3M Pharmaceuticals: wart treatment, BV treatment	1-800-328-0255	www.3m.com/us/healthcare
Watson Pharmaceuticals: OC, ella	1-800-272-5525	www.watsonpharm.com
Wyeth Ayerst (Pfizer): OCs	1-800-438-1985	www.pfizer.com

Appendix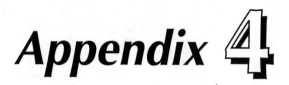

Hotlines and Websites

Topic	Organization	Hotline	Website
Abortion	Abortion Clinics OnLine		www.gynpages.com
	NARAL Pro-Choice America		www.naral.org
	National Abortion Federation	1-800-772-9100	www.prochoice.org
	Ibis Reproductive Health		www.medicationabortion.org
Adoption	Adopt a Special Kid-America	1-888-680-7349	www.adoptaspecialkid.org
	Adoptive Families	1-800-372-3300	www.adoptivefamilies.com
AIDS (*see HIV/AIDS*)			
AIDS Advocacy	Gay Men's Health Crisis	1-800-AIDS-NYC	www.gmhc.org
	Project Inform	1-800-822-7422	www.projinf.org
Alcoholism	Alcoholics Anonymous		www.aa.org
	Al-Anon & Alateen Family Groups	1-888-4AL-ANON	www.al-anon.org
	American Council on Alcoholism	1-800-527-5344	www.aca-usa.org
	Center on Addiction and the Family		www.coaf.org
	Co-Dependents Anonymous		www.codependents.org
	National Organization on Fetal Alcohol Syndrome	1-800-66-NOFAS	www.nofas.org
Anxiety (*see also Depression*)	Anxiety Disorders Association of America		www.adaa.org
	Freedom from Fear	1-866-615-6464	www.freedomfromfear.org
	NIMH Panic Disorder Information Line		www.nimh.nih.gov/health/topics/panic-disorder
Breast Cancer (*see also Cancer*)	National Alliance of Breast Cancer Organizations	1-800-ACS-2345	www.nabco.org
	Reach to Recovery (mastectomy patients)	1-800-221-2141	www.cancer.org
	Y-Me National Breast Cancer Organization		www.y-me.org
Breastfeeding	International Lactation Consultant Association	1-919-861-5577	www.ilca.org
	La Leche League International		www.lalecheleague.org
	The Linkages Project		www.linkagesproject.org

(continued)

CONTRACEPTIVE TECHNOLOGY

Topic	Organization	Hotline	Website
Cancer (see also specific cancers)	American Cancer Society	1-800-ACS-2345	www.cancer.org
	American Childhood Cancer Foundation	1-800-366-2223	www.candlelighters.org
	National Cancer Institute's Cancer Information	1-800-4-CANCER	http://cancer.gov
Child Abuse	Childhelp USA National Child Abuse Hotline	1-800- 4-A-CHILD	www.childhelpusa.org
	KidsPeace National Center for Kids Overcoming Crisis	1-800-25-PEACE	www.kidspeace.org
	National Center for Missing & Exploited Children	1-800-THE-LOST	www.ncmec.org
	Prevent Child Abuse America	1-312-663-3520	www.preventchildabuse.org
Contraception	Association of Reproductive Health Professionals	1-202-466-3825	www.arhp.org/topics/contraception
	EngenderHealth	1-212-561-8000	www.engenderhealth.org
	Planned Parenthood Federation of America	1-800-230-PLAN	www.plannedparenthood.org
	World Health Organization		www.who.int/health_topics/contraception/en/
Depression	Depression and Bipolar Support Alliance	1-800-826-3632	www.dbsalliance.org
	International Foundation for Research and Education on Depression	(1) 1-800-784-2433 (2) 1-800-442-HOPE	www.ifred.org
Domestic Violence	Family Violence Prevention Fund (for clinicians)	1-415-252-8900	http://endabuse.org/programs/healthcare
	Family Violence Prevention Fund (for women)	1-415-252-8900	http://endabuse.org
	National Domestic Violence Hotline	1-800-799-SAFE	www.thehotline.org
	National Resource Center on Domestic Violence	1-800-537-2238	www.pcadv.org
Drug Abuse	Alcohol & Drug Helpline	1-800-821-HELP	www.wellplace.com
	Narcotics Anonymous World Services	1-818-773-9999	www.na.org
Eating Disorders	National Association of Anorexia Nervosa and Associated Disorders (ANAD)	1-630-577-1330	www.anad.org
	National Eating Disorders Association	1-800- 931-2237	www.nationaleatingdisorders.org
Emergency Contraception	Emergency Contraception Website		http://not-2-late.com or ec.princeton.edu
	Planned Parenthood Federation of America	1-800-230-PLAN	www.ppfa.org/ec

(continued)

Topic	Organization	Hotline	Website
Endometriosis	Endometriosis Association	1-800-992-ENDO	www.EndometriosisAssn.org
Family/parenting	American Academy of Family Physicians	1-800-274-AAFP	www.aafp.org
	American Academy of Pediatrics		www.aap.org
Fitness	Aerobics and Fitness Association of America		www.afaa.com
Headaches	National Headache Foundation	1-888-NHF-5552	www.headaches.org
Hepatitis	Hepatitis B Coalition	1-651-647-9009	www.immunize.org
Herpes	National Herpes Hotline (ASHA)	1-919-361-8488	www.ashastd.org
HIV/AIDS	AIDSinfo	1-800-HIV-0440	www.aidsinfo.nih.gov/
	American Red Cross		www.cdc.gov/hiv/
	CDC National HIV/AIDS Hotline	1-415-544-9400	www.iasusa.org
	International AIDS Society-USA		www.unaids.org
	UNAIDS		
Hospice	National Hospice and Palliative Care Organization	1-800-658-8898	www.nhpco.org
HPV	National HPV and Cervical Cancer Prevention Hotline	1-919-361-4848	www.ashastd.org
Hypertension	American Heart Association	1-800-AHA-USA-1	
Infertility	Resolve National Infertility Helpline	1-703-506-3266	www.resolve.org
Interstitial Cystitis	Interstitial Cystitis Association	1-800-HELP-ICA	www.ichelp.org
Lactational Amenorrhea Method	The Linkages Project		www.linkagesproject.org
Menopause	North American Menopause Society	1-440-442-7550	www.menopause.org
Natural Family Planning	FertilityUK		www.fertilityUK.org

(continued)

Topic	Organization	Hotline	Website
Osteoporosis	National Osteoporosis Foundation	1-800-223-9994	www.nof.org
Ovarian Cancer (see also Cancer)	National Ovarian Cancer Coalition	1-888-OVARIAN	www.ovarian.org
Pregnancy, crisis (see also Adoption)	America's Pregnancy Helpline	1-888-942-6466	www.thehelpline.org
Pregnancy, delivery and postpartum	Bradley Method	1-800-4-A-BIRTH	www.bradleybirth.com
	Depression After Delivery, Inc.		www.depressionafterdelivery.com
	Lamaze International	1-800-368-4404	www.lamaze.org
	Postpartum Support International	1-800-944-4PPD	www.postpartum.net
Q & A	Go Ask Alice		www.goaskalice.columbia.edu
Sexual Assault	Rape Abuse & Incest National Network	1-800-656-HOPE	www.rainn.org
Sexually Transmitted Infections	American Social Health Association	1-800-227-8922	www.ashastd.org
	CDC Sexually Transmitted Disease Hotline	1-800-232-4636	www.cdc.gov/std.html
Smoking	American Cancer Society	1-800-ACS-2345	www.cancer.org
	American Lung Association	1-800-LUNGUSA	www.lungusa.org
Teens	Planned Parenthood - For Teens	1-800-230-PLAN	www.plannedparenthood.org/info-for-teens
Urinary Incontinence	National Association for Continence	1-800-BLADDER	www.nafc.org
Women's Health	Office of Women's Health (DHHS)	1-800-994-9662	www.womenshealth.gov

Index

A

Abdominal pain, 324(f)
Abortion, **695–727**
· aspiration, 716–718
· breast cancer and, 727
· characteristics of women seeking, 700(t)
· clinical examination, 702
· clinical management of, 705–720
· complications, 723–726
· contraception and post-abortion care, 727–728
· D&E method of, 718–719
· decision making about, 701
· early medication, 711(t), 712(t)
· first-trimester, 705–717
· health effects of, 726–727
· incomplete, 723
· induction method, 719
· laboratory tests for, 703
· legal status of, 696–698
· medication method for, 705–716, 711(t), 712(t), 723
· method selection and, 703–705
· methods of, 705–720, 711(t)–712(t)
· pre-abortion history, 702
· pre-abortion procedures, 701–703
· psychological health and, 726–727
· public health impact of, 698
· safety of, 722–723
· second-trimester adjunct techniques for, 720–721
· second-trimester dilation and evacuation, 718–719

Abortion—*continued*
· second-trimester induction of, 719–720
· statistics for, 698–701, 700(t)
Abortion services, **705–720**
Absolute risk, 274
Abstinence, 101–111
· counseling regarding, 107–109
· dangers/side effects/benefits, 67(t)
· definitions of, 102
· effectiveness of, 106
· indications for, 104–106
· levels of, 102–103, 104(t)
· noncoital sex and, 102
· planned *vs.* spontaneous, 110
· postpartum, 492
· and sexual rights/expression, 106–107
· sexuality education and, 109–110
· user instruction for, 110–111
Academy of Breastfeeding Medicine, 494–495, 504
Access to medical care, 70
Accutane, 53–54
ACHES system, 276(t), 323, 324(f)
ACIP (Advisory Committee on Immunization Practices), 627
Acne
· COCs and, 267–268, 317
· implants and, 196
· Ortho TriCyclen for, 254
ACOG. *See* American College of Obstetricians and Gynecologists
Acquired immune deficiency syndrome (AIDS). *See* HIV/AIDS

ACTH (adenocorticotropic hormone), 31

Actinomyces spp., 635–636

Actinomyces-like organisms (ALO), 180, 636

Activin, 33

Acupuncture, as treatment for dysmenorrhea, 554

Acute urethral syndrome, 595–596

Adenocarcinoma, 284, 637

Adenocarcinoma-in-situ (AIS), 637

Adenocorticotropic hormone (ACTH), 31

Adenomas, 282

Adenomyosis, 555

Adiana, 436–438, 442, 444, 449, 452, 456, 458, 527

Adolescents (adolescence)
· COCs and, 296
· patches and, 349
· vaginal ring and, 359–360

Advisory Committee on Immunization Practices (ACIP), 627

AGC. *See* Atypical glandular cells

Age, efficacy and, 57

AIS (adenocarcinoma-in-situ), 637

Alcohol, 281, 503, 559, 576, 598, 617, 644, 653, 753

Alendronate, 755

Allergic reactions
· DMPA and, 216–217, 225
· male condoms and, 376, 381–382

Allergies, medical eligibility criteria, 98

ALO. *See Actinomyces*-like organisms

Amenorrhea, 534–541
· COCs and, 311, 312
· DMPA and, 213
· implants and, 198, 201
· primary, 536–537
· secondary, 537–541

American Cancer Society, 631

American College of Obstetricians and Gynecologists (ACOG), 621, 631, 642

American Society for Colposcopy and Cervical Pathology (ASCCP), 631, 637

AMH (anti-müllerian hormone), 739

Anal sex
· condom use, 377
· initiation of, 103

Analytical pitfalls, 58

Androgen, 539

Androgens, 33, 763–764
· in COCs, 254
· male contraceptives and, 525

Anemias
· COCs and, 268–269
· medical eligibility criteria, 97

Anesthesia
· tubal ligation and, 457
· vasectomy and, 468, 469

Anovulation, as phase in menstrual cycle, 39

Anovulatory menorrhagia, 264

Anterior pituitary, 31, 33

Anticonvulsants, 242, 306, 307(t)

Antifibrinolytic therapy, 549, 550

Anti-müllerian hormone (AMH), 739

Anti-nausea treatment, 137

Antiprogestins, 115(t)

Anti-retroviral drugs, 242

Antiretrovirals (ARVs), 306, 307

Antisperm antibodies, 463

Areola sensitivity, 485–486

ARVs (antiretrovirals), 306, 307

ASC (atypical squamous cell), 637

ASC-H

ASCCP. *See* American Society for Colposcopy and Cervical Pathology

ASC-H, 638(t)

ASC-US. *See* Atypical squamous cell of undetermined significance

Asherman's syndrome, 537

Aspiration abortion, 705(t), 716–718

Asthma, 269

Atrophy, cervical, 637

Attributable risk, 274

Atypical glandular cells (AGC), 579(t), 637, 639(t)
Atypical squamous cell (ASC), 637
Atypical squamous cell of undetermined significance (ASC-US), 637, 638(t)
Avanti, 522

B

Bacterial vaginosis (BV), 596–598, 635
Bariatric surgery, 84, 302–303
Barrier methods. *See also* Diaphragms; Female condoms; Male condoms; Sponges, contraceptive
· advantages, 398–399
· breastfeeding and, 483, 494–495
· cervical cap, 522
· characteristics of, 393(t)
· disadvantages/cautions, 399–401
· effectiveness, 396–397
· failure rates, 809(t)–811(t)
· guidelines for use, 403–404
· lubricants with, 402
· mechanism of action, 392, 394–395
· medical eligibility criteria for, 82(t)–98(t)
· perimenopause and, 747
· postpartum use, 491–492
· problems, managing, 404–405
· providing, 401–403
· research on, 521–522
· spermicide with, 397
Basal body temperature (BBT), 495
BD SurePath Cytology Test, 628
Bellergal-S, 765
Benign breast conditions, COCs and reduction in, 267
Benzalkonium chloride, 392, 520
Bethesda System classification, 633
Billings Ovulation Method, 418–420, 428–429
Bioavailability, 253
Bio-identical hormones, 764
Biphasic formulations, 256–257

BI-RADS. *See* Breast Imaging Reporting and Data System
Bisphosphonates, 743, 755–756
Black cohosh, 766
Bleeding control, perimenopausal, 743–746
Bleeding problems
· abortion and, 723
· IUCs and, 154
Blood clots, intrauterine, 724
Blood loss
· with abortion, 723
· COCs and decreased, 263–264
· levonorgestrel system and, 65
· LNg IUC and, 153
BMD. *See* Bone mineral density
Bone density. *See also* Osteopenia; Osteoporosis
· COCs and, 269–270
· DMPA and, 216, 219–222
· implants and, 200
Bone mineral density (BMD), 269–270, 752, 753(t)
Brain, and menstrual cycle, 30–31, 33
BRCA1, 266
· and ovarian cancer, 641
· tubal sterilization and, 441
BRCA2, 266
· and ovarian cancer, 641
· tubal sterilization and, 441
Breast cancer
· abortion and, 727
· COCs and, 63, 285
· DMPA and, 219
· postmenopausal hormone therapy and, 742, 743, 761
· risk assessment questions, 742(t)
· risk characteristics of, 644(t)
Breast cancer screening, 643–647
· mammography, 645–647, 646(t)
· techniques, 643, 645
Breast conditions, COCs and, 267, 317–318
Breast Imaging Reporting and Data System (BI-RADS), 646(t), 647

Combined oral contraceptives
(COCs)—*continued*
· reproductive tract
infections/disorders, 91–94
· schistosomiasis, 94
· and sexual behavior, 14–16
· side-effect management, 311–319
· smoking-/hypertension-related
deaths and, 280(t)
· societal benefits of, 271–272
· special populations, 296–303
· TSS, history of, 95
· tuberculosis, 95
· user instructions, 319–326
· UTIs, 95
· vaginal ring and, 361
· venous thromboemoblism and,
275–279, 276(t)
Condoms. *See also* Female condoms;
Male condoms
· allergies, 98
· anemias, 97
· cardiovascular disease, 85–89
· depressive disorders, 91
· drug interactions, 98
· endocrine conditions, 95
· gastrointestinal conditions, 96–97
· HIV/AIDS, 94
· hormonal
contraception/IUCs/barrier
methods, 82(t)–98(t)
· improving effectiveness of, 52(f)
· malaria, 95
· medical eligibility criteria for,
82(t)–98(t)
· neurologic conditions, 90
· as ongoing contraception, 134(t)
· personal characteristics and
reproductive history, 82(t)–84(t)
· postpartum use, 491, 494
· pregnancy rate with, 50(t)
· promotion of, 377–378
· reported use, 46, 47
· reproductive tract
infections/disorders, 91–94

Condoms—*continued*
· schistosomiasis, 94
· and sexual behavior, 14
· testing of, 374
· TSS, history of, 95
· tuberculosis, 95
· UTIs, 95
Condyloma acuminata, 625
Confidence interval (CI), 274–275
Conjugated equite estrogens (CEE),
759, 763
Contact lens effects, 318
Continuation, contraceptive, 787,
791(t)–792(t)
Continuing use, 50(t)–51(t), 53
Contraceptive patch, **343–355.** 524
· advantages, 345–346
· allergies, 98
· anemias, 97
· cardiovascular disease, 85–89
· dangers/side effects/benefits, 66(t)
· depressive disorders, 91
· description, 343–344
· disadvantages/cautions, 346–348
· dislodged/detached, 352
· drug interactions, 98, 353
· effectiveness, 344
· endocrine conditions, 95
· follow-up, 352–353
· forgotten/missed, 352, 353(f),
353(t)
· gastrointestinal conditions, 96–97
· HIV/AIDS, 94
· hormonal
contraception/IUCs/barrier
methods, 82(t)–98(t)
· improving effectiveness of, 52(f)
· malaria, 95
· mechanism of action, 344
· medical eligibility criteria for,
82(t)–98(t)
· neurologic conditions, 90
· as ongoing contraception, 134(t)
· personal characteristics and
reproductive history, 82(t)–84(t)

Contraceptive patch—*continued*
- · postpartum use, 490, 493
- · pregnancy rate with, 50(t)
- · problems, managing, 352–353
- · providing, 349–352
- · reported use, 47
- · reproductive tract
    infections/disorders, 91–94
- · schistosomiasis, 94
- · skin reactions, 352
- · timing issues, 350–351
- · TSS, history of, 95
- · tuberculosis, 95
- · user instructions, 353–355
- · UTIs, 95

Contraceptive research and
development, **513–529**
- · chemical barriers and microbicides,
    520–522
- · drug development process, 519(t)
- · future, 528–529
- · history, 515–518, 516(t)
- · hormonal methods, 523–524
- · improving use-effectiveness, 528
- · IUCs, 526–527
- · mechanical barrier methods,
    521–522
- · men, methods for, 525–526
- · need for, 513–515
- · publication of, 58
- · sterilization methods, 527–528
- · systemic methods, 524–525
- · women, methods for, 523–525

Contraceptive selection, 45–71
- · benefits, non-contraceptive, 65,
    66(t)–67(t), 68
- · efficacy/effectiveness, 47–60,
    50(t)–51(t), 52(f)
- · medical eligibility criteria and, 80
- · personal considerations, 68–71
- · reported use, 47(t)
- · risks, in perspective, 62(t)
- · risks, major health, 66(t)–67(t)
- · safety concerns, 61–65, 66(t)–67(t)

Contraceptive selection—*continued*
- · stages of reproductive life and,
    69(t)
- · and unintended pregnancy, 50(t)
Contraceptive sponges. *See* Sponges,
contraceptive
Contraceptives, sexuality and, 12–20
Copper T380A IUC (ParaGard), 50(t),
148–149, 149(f), 526
- · breastfeeding and, 494
- · effectiveness, 151
- · failure rate, 437
- · menstrual disturbances, 154
- · placement instructions, 164–168,
    165(f)–168(f), 165(t)–168(t)
- · postpartum use, 492
Copper-releasing IUCs
- · advantages/indications, 127
- · allergies, 98
- · anemias, 97
- · cardiovascular disease, 85–89
- · cautions, 130
- · depressive disorders, 91
- · drug interactions, 98
- · effectiveness, 123
- · endocrine conditions, 95
- · gastrointestinal conditions, 96–97
- · HIV/AIDS, 94
- · hormonal
    contraception/IUCs/barrier
    methods, 82(t)–98(t)
- · malaria, 95
- · mechanism of action, 121
- · medical eligibility criteria for,
    82(t)–98(t)
- · neurologic conditions, 90
- · perimenopause and, 746
- · personal characteristics and
    reproductive history, 82(t)–84(t)
- · postpartum use, 492
- · reproductive tract
    infections/disorders, 91–94
- · schistosomiasis, 94
- · side effects, 127
- · treatment regimen, 135

Copper-releasing IUCs SP(O2)·
advantages/indications—*continued*
· TSS, history of, 95
· tuberculosis, 95
· usage, 787
· UTIs, 95
Corpus luteum, 484
COX-2 inhibitors, 524–525
Cramping, 155
Creams, spermicidal, 395
CVD. *See* Cardiovascular disease
Cyclofem, 523–524
Cytochrome P-450 enzyme, 304–307
Cytological screening
· HPV testing as adjunct to, 629
· intervals for, 630–633
· technical aspects of, 629–630

D

Dalkon Shield, 57, 517
Danazol, 116, 555
D&E. *See* Dilation and evacuation
Dehydroepiandrosterone (DHEA), 764
Dementia, 761
Depo-Provera (DMPA), 209
· advantages, 212–214
· adverse effects, 214–217
· allergies, 98
· anemias, 97
· bone density and, 219–222
· breastfeeding and, 218–219, 496–498, 499
· cancer risk and, 219
· cardiovascular disease, 85–89
· continuation rates, 211–212
· dangers/side effects/benefits, 66(t)
· depressive disorders, 91
· disadvantages, 217–218
· drug interactions, 98
· effectiveness, 210–212
· endocrine conditions, 95
· gastrointestinal conditions, 96–97
· HIV/AIDS, 94

Depo-Provera (DMPA)—*continued*
· hormonal
contraception/IUCs/barrier
methods, 82(t)–98(t)
· immune function and, 515
· malaria, 95
· mechanism of action, 210
· medical eligibility criteria for, 82(t)–98(t)
· neurologic conditions, 90
· perfect use, 785
· perimenopausal bleeding control, 746
· personal characteristics and
reproductive history, 82(t)–84(t)
· postpartum use, 490, 494
· precautions, 218
· pregnancy rate with, 50(t)
· problems, managing, 224–225
· providing, 223–224
· reproductive tract
infections/disorders, 91–94
· schistosomiasis, 94
· STIs and, 222–223
· as treatment for dysmenorrhea, 554
· TSS, history of, 95
· tuberculosis, 95
· user instructions, 225–229
· UTIs, 95
Depo-subQ provera 104 (DMPA-SC
104), 209, 211, 213–215, 523, 555
Depression
· COCs and, 316
· DMPA and, 216
· medical eligibility criteria, 91
DES (diethylstilbestrol), 116
Desogestrel, 193, 200, 238, 241, 254
DEXA. *See* Dual-energy X-ray
absorptiometry
Dextronorgestrel, 254
DHEA (dehydroepiandrosterone), 764
Diabetes, 762
· COCs and, 286–287, 299
· IUCs and, 160
· POPs and, 241

Diamond, Lisa, 7
Diaphragms
· allergies, 98
· anemias, 97
· cardiovascular disease, 85–89
· characteristics, 393(t)
· dangers/side effects/benefits, 67(t)
· depressive disorders, 91
· drug interactions, 98
· endocrine conditions, 95
· failure rates, 813(t)–817(t)
· fitting, 403
· gastrointestinal conditions, 96–97
· HIV/AIDS, 94
· hormonal
  contraception/IUCs/barrier
  methods, 82(t)–98(t)
· improving effectiveness of, 52(f)
· malaria, 95
· medical eligibility criteria for,
  82(t)–98(t)
· neurologic conditions, 90
· as ongoing contraception, 134(t)
· perfect use, 781
· personal characteristics and
  reproductive history, 82(t)–84(t)
· postpartum use, 490
· pregnancy rate with, 50(t)
· reproductive tract
  infections/disorders, 91–94
· research on, 522
· schistosomiasis, 94
· with spermicides, 813(t)–817(t)
· TSS, history of, 95
· tuberculosis, 95
· UTIs, 95
Diarrhea, 318, 322
Diazepam, 307
Dienogestrel, 254
Diethylstilbestrol (DES), 116
Dihydroxyprogesterone
acetophenide, 210
Dilapan, 720
Dilating devices, 720

Dilation and evacuation (D&E),
718–719
Dimethyl sulfoxide (DMSO), 528
DMPA. *See* Depo-Provera
DMPA-SC 104. *See* Depo-subQ
provera 104
Domestic violence, 70
Drospirenone, 254, 287–288, 294, 308
Drug development process, 517, 519(t)
Drug interactions
· ECPs and, 130
· medical eligibility criteria, 98
Drug-drug interactions, 303–308, 326
Dual method use, 378, 809(t)–811(t)
Dual-energy X-ray absorptiometry
(DEXA), 752, 754
Dysmenorrhea, 552–555
· COCs and decreased, 263
· implants and, 197
· primary, 553–554
· secondary, 554–555
Dyspareunia, 767
Dysuria, 767

E

Early menopause, 748
EC. *See* Emergency contraception
ECPs. *See* Emergency contraception
pills
Ectopic pregnancy
· COCs and reduction of, 263
· DMPA and, 210
· ECPs and, 128
· implants and, 197, 202
· IUCs and, 150, 152
· POPs and, 241
· surgical sterilization and, 438
· tubal sterilization and, 445–446
EE. *See* Ethinyl estradiol
Efficacy, contraceptive, 47–60
· comparison, 52(f)
· continuing use, 50(t)–51(t), 53
· counseling about, 59–60
· inherent, 56

Efficacy—*continued*
· over lifetime, 55
· over time, 54–55
· perfect use, 50(t)–51(t), 53
· quality of published evidence and, 57–59
· simultaneous use of methods, 54
· typical use, 49–53, 50(t)–51(t)
· user characteristics and, 56–57
EGF (epidermal growth factor), 34
Electrocoagulation, 451(f), 453, 455
ella, 113, 116, 136
Emergency contraception (EC), **113–137**
· advantages/indications, 126–127
· barriers to use, 116–117
· breastfeeding and, 500
· cautions with, 129–130
· counseling for, 132–133
· effectiveness, 123–126
· initiating ongoing contraception after, 134(t)
· IUCs and, 152
· mechanism of action, 121–123
· pills (*See* Emergency contraception pills)
· and pregnancy probability by cycle day, 131(f)
· promotion of awareness/use, 118–120
· providing, 130–136
· research on, 524
· side effects, 127–129
· treatment regimen, 135
· user instructions, 136–137
Emergency contraception pills (ECPs), 113–114, 115(t), 396
· advantages/indications, 126–127
· barriers to use, 116–117
· cautions, 129–130
· counseling for, 132–133
· effectiveness, 124–126
· and initiating ongoing contraception, 134(t)
· mechanism of action, 121–123

Emergency contraception pills (ECPs)—*continued*
· population impact of, 117–118
· promotion of awareness/use, 118–120
· providing, 132–133, 135–136
· side effects, 127–129
· treatment regimen, 135
· user instructions, 136–137
Emergency contraception services, 135
Emko, 783
Endocrine conditions, 95
Endometrial ablation, 443–444, 551–552
Endometrial cancer, 214, 266, 267
Endometrial cells, 637
Endometriosis, 554
· COCs and, 269
· DMPA and, 214
· implants and, 194, 197
Endometrium, 35, 237
Enovid, 252, 256, 259, 515
Epidermal growth factor (EGF), 34
Epithelial cell abnormalities, 637
Erythromycin, 527–528
'Escape ovulation,' 258, 260
Essure, 436–438, 442, 444, 445, 449, 451, 452, 456, 458, 527
Estradiol, 31, 33, 535, 744, 763
· breastfeeding and, 499
· implants and, 195
Estranes, 255(t)
Estrogen
· in birth control pills, 256
· breastfeeding and, 499
· implants and, 193, 197, 200, 202
· menopause and, 739
· osteoporosis and, 756
· perimenopause and, 747
Estrogen dermatitis, 240
Estrogen therapy, 541
Estrostep, 268
ET. *See* Estrogen therapy

Fertility awareness-based (FAB)
  methods—*continued*
· reported use, 47
· reproductive tract
    infections/disorders, 99
· safety issues, 423
· sex selection issues, 423
Fibrocycstic breast changes, 267
FibroPlant-LNg, 526–527
Film, spermicidal, 395
Filshie clip, 437, 455–456
First-day start, 291, 320
First-generation progestins, 253
First-trimester abortion
· aspiration, 716–718
· medication, 705–716
Foam, spermicidal, 395
Folate, in COCs, 270
Follicle-stimulating hormone (FSH),
  31, 33–34, 38, 535, 738–740
· breastfeeding and, 484
· DMPA and, 210
Follicular phase, 36, 38
Follistatin, 33
Fourth-generation progestins, 254
Fracture Risk Assessment tool
  (FRAX), 753, 754, 754(t)
Fractures
· fall prevention and, 752(t)
· postmenopause and, 749–756
Fraud, 57
Freedom of Access to Clinic Entrances
  (FACE) Act, 697
Frequency of intercourse, 57, 70
FSH. *See* Follicle-stimulating hormone
Funding, 518, 519
Fungus, 635

G

Gabapentin, 764
Gail model, 757
Galen, 29
Gallbladder disease, 282
GAPDH-2, 526

Gardasil, 626
Gastrointestinal conditions
· COCs and, 318
· medical eligibility criteria, 96–97
Gay, lesbian, bisexual, transgendered
  and questioning (GLBTQ), 103
Gels, spermicidal, 395
Gender, and sexual attitudes, 3, 4
Genital herpes, 602–605
Genital warts, 608–611
Gestodene, 254
GLBTQ (gay, lesbian, bisexual,
  transgendered and questioning), 103
Glucose intolerance
'Global gag rule,' 697
Glucose intolerance, 286–287
Glyceraldehyde-3-phosphate
  dehydrogenase, 526
Glycodelin, 121–122
Gonadotropin-releasing hormone
  (GnRH), 31, 33–34, 486, 536, 555
Gonanes, 255(t)
Gonorrhea, 180, 604–605, 628, 630
Gossypol, 526
Granuloma inguinale, 605–606
GyneFix, 526

H

Half-life, 253
Headaches, 324(f)
· COCs and, 299–300, 315–316
· patches and, 348
· vaginal ring and, 359
Heart valve abnormalities, 159
Heavy menstrual bleeding (HMB),
  547–552
· etiologies, 547–548
· treatments, 549–552, 550(t)
Hematometra, 724
Hemorrhagic stroke, 281
Hepatic neoplasms, 282
Hepatitis A, 606
Hepatitis B, 376, 607–608
Hepatitis C, 608

Herpes simplex virus (HSV), 582, 636
High-grade squamous intraepithelial lesions (HSIL), 637, 639(t)
Hirsutism, 267–268, 317
HIV/AIDS
· abstinence and, 107–108
· breastfeeding and, 483, 501, 504
· cervical cancer and, 625
· COCs and, 283, 301–302
· coitus interruptus and, 412
· and contraceptive choice, 574–575
· contraceptive selection and, 80
· DMPA and, 223
· hormonal contraception and, 515
· IUCs and, 159
· male condoms and, 374–380
· medical eligibility criteria, 94
· microbicide treatments for, 521
· RTIs and, 573–574
· safer sex, counseling about, 584, 585(t)
· stages of HIV infection, 591(t)
· testing/counseling, 587–589, 588(t)
· transmission, factors affecting, 573, 574, 586
· in women, 589–595, 594(t)
· worldwide impact of, 514
HMB. See Heavy menstrual bleeding
Hormonal contraceptives
· breastfeeding and, 495–500, 499
· HIV use and, 515
· medical eligibility criteria for, 82(t)–98(t)
· research on, 524
Hormonal therapies (HTs), 758–764
Hot flashes, 269, 747, 757–758
HPV. See Human papilloma virus
HSG. See Hysterosalpingogram
HSIL. See High-grade squamous intraepithelial lesions
HSV. See Herpes simplex virus
HTs. See Hormonal therapies
Hulka-Clemens clip, 455
Human immunodeficiency virus (HIV). See HIV/AIDS

Human papilloma virus (HPV), 608–609
· abstinence and, 107–108
· cervical cancer and, 63, 624–626
· COCs and, 283–284
· diaphragm and, 399
· perimenopause and, 741
· testing, 629, 637
· vaccination, 626–628
Human studies, 517, 519(t)
Hyde Amendment, 696
17-Hydroxy compounds, 499
Hyperkalemia, 308
Hyperlipidemia, 319
Hyperprolactinemia, 535
Hypertension, 254, 279, 280(t), 281, 299
Hypertriglyceridemia, 319
Hypothalamic amenorrhea, 535
Hypothalamus, 31, 485–486, 542
Hysterectomy, 443
Hysterosalpingogram (HSG), 438, 458

I

ICSI (intracytoplasmic sperm injection), 465
IDE (investigational device exemption), 517
ILCA (International Lactation Consultant Association), 504
Imperfect use, 56–57
Implanon, 193–203, 523
· dangers/side effects/benefits, 66(t)
· perfect use, 785
· postpartum use, 490, 494
· pregnancy rate with, 50(t)
· typical use, 785
Implants, contraceptive, **193–203**
· advantages, 196–198
· allergies and, 98
· anemias and, 97
· cardiovascular disease, 85–89
· contraindications, 200
· depressive disorders, 91

Lactational infertility, 485–486
Lactogenesis, 200
LAM. *See* Lactational Amenorrhea Method
Laparoscopy, 458
Laparoscopy tubal sterilization, 450, 450(f), 451(f), 453, 454(t), 455
Lasofoxifene, 743
Latex allergies, 358, 522
Latex condoms, 373(t)
LB (Levonorgestrel Butanoate), 523
LBC (liquid based cytology), 628
Leg pain, 324(f)
Leiomyoma, 269, 287
Leptin, 524
Leukemia inhibitory factor (LIF), 525
Levonorgestrel, 113, 114, 122, 194, 238, 254, 294
Levonorgestrel Butanoate (LB), 523
Levonorgestrel-releasing IUCs (LNg-IUCs), 148–150, 149(f)
· allergies, 98
· amenorrhea and, 537
· anemias, 97
· breastfeeding and, 496, 498
· cardiovascular disease, 85–89
· depressive disorders, 91
· drug interactions, 98
· effectiveness, 151
· endocrine conditions, 95
· failure rate, 437
· gastrointestinal conditions, 96–97
· health benefits of, 153
· HIV/AIDS, 94
· hormonal contraception/IUCs/barrier methods, 82(t)–98(t)
· malaria, 95
· medical eligibility criteria for, 82(t)–98(t)
· menstrual disturbances, 154–155
· neurologic conditions, 90
· perimenopause and, 745
· personal characteristics and reproductive history, 82(t)–84(t)

Levonorgestrel-releasing IUCs (LNg-IUCs)—*continued*
· placement instructions, 168–178, 169(t), 171(t)–178(t)
· reproductive tract infections/disorders, 91–94
· schistosomiasis, 94
· as therapy for heavy menstrual bleeding, 551
· TSS, history of, 95
· tuberculosis, 95
· UTIs, 95
LFU (loss-to-follow-up), 59
LGV. *See* Lymphogranuloma venereum
LH. *See* Luteinizing hormone
Libido, 285–286, 316–317
LIF (leukemia inhibitory factor), 525
Ligation and excision (vasectomy), 471
Lipids, 319
Lippes Loop, 515
Liquid based cytology (LBC), 628
Liver, 302–304
Liver cancer, 63, 282
LNg-IUC. *See* Levonorgestrel-releasing IUCs
Lonidamine, 526
Lo Ovral, 254
Loss-to-follow-up (LFU), 59
Low-grade squamous intraepithelial lesions (LSIL), 638(t), 640
Lubricants, oil-based, 402
Lubrication, condom use and, 381, 381(t)
Lunelle, 209–210, 523
Luteal phase, 40
Luteinizing hormone (LH), 31, 33, 38, 535
· breastfeeding and, 484–486
· DMPA and, 210
Lymphogranuloma venereum (LGV), 611–612

M

Male condoms, **371–384**
· advantages/indications, 374–375
· anal intercourse, use during, 377
· characteristics, 373(t)
· dangers/side effects/benefits, 66(t)
· disadvantages/cautions, 375–376
· effectiveness, 374
· failure rates, 818(t)–821(t)
· follow-up, 381–382
· history, 372
· improving effectiveness of, 52(f), 380, 381
· and lubricants, 381(t)
· mechanism of action, 372–374
· options, 372, 373
· oral intercourse, use during, 377
· perfect use, 784–785
· pregnancy rate with, 50(t)
· problems, managing, 381–382
· promotion of, 377–378
· providing, 378–380
· reported use of, 46–47
· research on, 522
· special issues, 376–377
· STI protection, 374–378
· storage of, 384
· user instructions, 382–384
Male sterilization. *See* Vasectomy
Mammography, 645–647, 646(t)
Manual vacuum aspiration (MVA), 716–718, 717(f)–718(f)
Mastalgia, 317–318
Masturbation, 106
Maternal death
· abortion and, 722
· COCs and reduction of, 263
· Mechanical barrier methods, 521-522
Mechanical occlusion, 455–457
Meclizine, 133
Medicaid, 448
Medical care, access to, 70
Medical eligibility criteria, **75–99**
· allergies, 98

Medical eligibility criteria—*continued*
· anemias, 97
· cardiovascular disease, 85–89
· categories, 77–80
· clarifications, 79–80
· contraceptive method initiation and continuation, 79
· depressive disorders, 91
· drug interactions, 98
· endocrine conditions, 95
· fertility awareness-based methods, 78–79
· gastrointestinal conditions, 96–97
· guidance updates, 80–81
· HIV/AIDS, 94
· hormonal contraception/IUCs/barrier methods, 82(t)–98(t)
· malaria, 95
· methodology, 76–77
· neurologic conditions, 90
· personal characteristics and reproductive history, 82(t)–84(t)
· reproductive tract infections/disorders, 91–94
· rheumatic diseases, 89–90
· schistosomiasis, 94
· screening for presence of conditions, 79
· for smoking and COC use, 78(t)
· surgical sterilization procedures, 53–54, 99
· TSS, history of, 95
· tuberculosis, 95
· UTIs, 95
Medical Eligibility Criteria for Contraceptive Use (WHO), 75–81
Medication abortion, 705–716
· clinical protocols for, 709–714, 711(t), 712(t)
· patient education for early, 709(t)
Medications, breastfeeding and, 504
Medroxyprogesterone acetate (MPA), 499, 541
Melanocytes, 317

Melanoma, 287
Melasma, 284, 317
Meloxicam, 114, 116
Menfegol, 392
Menopause, 536, 748. *See also*
Perimenopause
· defined, 748
· hormone therapy effect on, 758–764
· vasomotor symptoms, 758–766
· vulvovaginal atrophy and, 766–768
Menstrual changes
· DMPA and, 224–225
· ECPs and, 128–129
· POPs and, 239
Menstrual cycle, **29–42**
· brain and, 30–31, 33
· contraception and, 41–42
· DMPA and, 214–215
· events in, 37(f)
· phases of, 36, 38–41
· POPs and, 240
· pregnancy probability by day of, 131(f)
· regularity of, 57
· regulation of, 32(f)
· reproductive system and, 33–35
· terminology, 534(t)
· vaginal patch and, 350
Menstrual disorders, **533–563**
· amenorrhea, 534–541
· bleeding disorders, 534–552
· dysmenorrhea (painful menses), 552–555
· heavy/prolonged menstrual bleeding, 547–552
· infrequent menses, 541–547
· intermenstrual bleeding, 552
· other medical conditions, exacerbation of, 562–563
· postcoital bleeding, 552
· premenstrual dysphoric disorder (PMDD), 556–558, 561–562
· premenstrual syndrome (PMS), 556–561
· primary amenorrhea, 536–537

Menstrual disorders—*continued*
· secondary amenorrhea, 537–541
Menstrual migraines, 265, 300
Menstrual problems
· IUCs and, 154–155
· tubal sterilization and, 442
Menstruation, as phase in menstrual cycle, 40–41
Merck, 193, 194
Mesigyna, 210
Mestranol, 256
Methergine, 714, 721
Method failure rates, 59
Methotrexate, 706–707, 711(t), 712(t), 713
MI. *See* Myocardial infarction
Microbicides, 520–521
Mifepristone, 114, 524, 705–710, 711(t), 712(t), 719–723
Migraine headaches, 265, 300
Minilaparoscopy, 454(t), 458
Minilaparotomy, 450, 451, 451(f), 493
Minipills. *See* Progestin-only pills
Mircette, 254
Mirena IUC, 254, 526
· blood loss and, 65
· pregnancy rate with, 50(t)
Misoprostol, 707, 711(t), 712(t), 713–714, 720–721, 723
Mittelschmerz, 265
Molluscum contagiosum, 612–613
Monophasic formulations, of COCs, 256
Mood disorders (mood swings)
· COCs and, 316, 326
· menopause and, 758
Mosaicism, 536
MPA. *See* Medroxyprogesterone acetate
Müllerian agenesis, 537
Multiphasic formulations, of COCs, 256–257
Mycoplasma genitalium, 613
Myocardial infarction (MI), 61, 279–280

Myomas, 214

N

N-9. *See* Nonoxynol-9
National Health and Social Life
  Survey (NHSLS), 5, 9
National Survey of Family Growth
  (NSFG), 19
National Survey of Sexual Health and
  Behavior (NSSHB), 5
Natural membrane condoms, 372, 373,
  373(t)
Natural rubber latex condoms, 372,
  373, 381(t)
Natural Sensation Female Panty
  Condom, 522
Nausea
  · ECPs and, 127, 137
  · patches and, 348
NDA. *See* New drug application
Nesterone, 524
NETA. *See* Norethindrone acetate
Neurologic conditions, 90
New drug application (NDA),
  517–518, 519(t)
Nexplanon, 194
Next Choice, 114, 116, 117, 120, 125,
  129, 136
NHSLS (National Health and Social
  Life Survey), 5
Nipple sensitivity, 485–486
NNRTIs (non-nucleoside reverse
  transcriptase inhibitors), 307
Nomegestrol, 254
Nomegestrol acetate, 194
Noncoital sex, 102
Noncontraceptive benefits, 65–68,
  66(t)–67(t)
Nonlatex condoms, 522
Non-nucleoside reverse transcriptase
  inhibitors (NNRTIs), 307
Nonoxynol-9 (N-9), 373, 391, 392, 395,
  396, 520–521
19-Nor compounds, 499

Nordette, 254
Norelgestromin/EE patch, 524
Norethindrone, 114, 238, 239, 241, 253,
  294, 499
Norethindrone acetate (NETA), 253,
  541
Norethindrone ethanate, 210
Norethynodrel, 253
Norgestimate, 254, 317
Norgestrel, 114, 239, 241, 254, 499
Norplant, 194, 199, 201, 254, 517, 523
No-scalpel vasectomy (NSV), 468, 469,
  470(f)
NovaSure, 444
NSFG (National Survey of Family
  Growth), 19
NSSHB (National Survey of Sexual
  Health and Behavior), 5
NSV. *See* No-scalpel vasectomy
Nucleoside reverse transcriptase
  inhibitors (NRTIs), 307
NuvaRing®, 355
  · dangers/side effects/benefits, 66(t)
  · pregnancy rate with, 50(t)
  · typical and perfect use, 785–786

O

Obesity
  · DMPA and, 212
  · infrequent menses and, 544–545
  · patches and, 348
  · perimenopause and, 740–741
Occlusion methods
  · electrocoagulation, 453, 455
  · female, 453–457, 454(t)
  · male, 469, 471
  · mechanical, 455–457
OCs. *See* Oral contraceptives
Oil-based lubricants, 402
Ongoing contraception, 134(t)
Oral contraceptives (OCs)
  · as emergency contraceptives, 115(t)
  · first, 515
  · perfect use, 785

Oral contraceptives (OCs) SP(O2)· as
  emergency
  contraceptives—*continued*
  · postpartum use, 490
  · reported use, 46, 47
Oral dose, 707
Oral sex
  · condom use during, 377
  · initiation of, 103
Organ transplantation, 303
Organ trauma, 724–725
Organon, 193
Orlistat, 308
Ortho All-Flex diaphragm, 522
Ortho Evra®, 344, 347, 350–351
Ortho TriCyclen, 254, 268
Osmotic dilating devices, 720
Osteopenia, 753
Osteoporosis
  · defined, 753
  · postmenopause and, 749–756
OTC drugs. *See* Over-the-counter
  drugs
Ovabloc, 527
Ovarian cancer
  · COCs and, 265–266
  · screening, 641–642
  · tubal sterilization and, 441
Ovarian cysts
  · COCs and, 265
  · implants and, 199
  · POPs and, 241
Ovarian enzyme deficiency, 536
Ovaries, 33–34
  · breastfeeding and, 484
  · tubal sterilization and, 442–443
Ovcon, 252, 253
Over-the-counter (OTC) drugs,
  118–120
Ovulation, as phase in menstrual
  cycle, 38
Ovulation Method, 50(t)
Oxytocin, 502, 721

P

Pain
  · IUCs and, 155
  · tubal ligation and management of,
    457
Panty condoms, 522
Papanicolaou (Pap) smear, 155–156,
  628. *See also* Cervical cancer
  screening
Paracervical block, 181
ParaGard. *See* Copper T380A IUC
Parkland method, 456
Partner violence, 70
Patch. *See* Contraceptive patch
PATH female condom, 394, 522
Pattern
  · of childbearing, 70
  · of sexual activity, 69–70
PC6 (pro-protein convertase 6), 525
PCOS. *See* Polycystic ovarian
  syndrome
PE (pulmonary embolism), 275
Pearl index, 58–59
Pelvic infection, postabortal, 725
Pelvic inflammatory disease (PID),
  613–614
  · copper IUDs and, 130
  · DMPA and, 214
  · IUCs and, 156–157
Pelvic pain, implants and, 197
Perfect use, 49, 50(t)–51(t), 52–53
Perforation, uterine, 157
Perimenopause, **738–747**
  · bleeding control during, 743–746
  · COCs and, 297
  · contraceptive options for, 743–746
  · defined, 738
  · diagnosis, 739–740
  · health promotion, 740–741
  · nonhormonal methods during,
    746–747
  · physiology of, 738–740
  · reproductive carcinoma during,
    741–743

Q

Quick Start, 289–291, 320
Quinacrine, 527

R

RA (rheumatoid arthritis), 298
Radiation treatments, 536
Raloxifene, 743
RANKL antibodies, 756
Rape, 116–117, 132
Reality (female condom), 50(t), 392, 394(t), 522
Reddy (female condom), 522
Redo syndrome, 724
Regret
· female sterilization and, 444–446
· vasectomy and, 464–465
Relative risk, 273
Reproductive history
· fertility awareness-based methods, 99
· medical eligibility criteria, 82(t)–84(t)
Reproductive life, stages of, 69(t)
Reproductive tract cancers, 219
Reproductive tract infections (RTIs), 571–583. *See also* HIV/AIDS
· assessment/diagnosis, 576–578, 577(t)
· 'biological sexism' of, 572–573
· catalogue of, 595–619
· cervical cancer and, 63
· contraceptive choice and, 574–576, 575(t)
· fertility awareness-based methods, 99
· HIV and, 573, 574
· medical eligibility criteria, 91–94
· patient counseling, 578–579
· during pregnancy, 579, 580(t), 581(t), 582
· prevalence of, 572
· prevention, 574

Reproductive tract infections (RTIs)—*continued*
· risk factors, 574–576
· sexual assault and, 582–583
· transmission, 573, 574
Research and development. *See* Contraceptive research and development
Rheumatic diseases, 89–90
Rheumatoid arthritis (RA), 298
Rifampicin, 242
Rifampin, 130
Ring, vaginal. *See* Vaginal ring
Risedronate, 755
RISUG, 528
Roe v. Wade, 696, 698
RTIs. *See* Reproductive tract infections

S

Safety, contraceptive, 61–65, 66(t)–67(t)
· counseling about, 64–65
· major health risks, 62–63
· side effects, 63–64
· tubal sterilization and, 440–441
· Saf-T-Coil, 515
Saint John's Wort, 242, 308
Salpingectomy, 438
Same-Day Start method, 289–291
Schistosomiasis, 94
Seaweed, dried, 720
Secondary abstainers, 103, 104(t), 106
Secondary amenorrhea, 537–541
Second-generation progestins, 254
Second-trimester abortion, 718–719
Seizures, 213
Selective estrogen receptor modulators (SERMs), 742, 743, 756
Selective norepinephrine receptor inhibitors (SNRIs), 765
Selective serotonin reuptake inhibitors (SSRIs), 765
Severe leg pain, 324(f)

Sex hormone binding globulin
(SHBG), 268, 301
Sex therapy, 109
Sexual activity, onset of, 6–7
Sexual behavior, 3–12
· motivations for, 7–9
· pattern of, 69–70
· same-gender, 7
· 'typical,' 4–7
Sexual desire, 11–12
Sexual enjoyment, influence of COCs
on, 270, 286
Sexual expression, 106–107
Sexual fluidity, 7
Sexual problems, 9–11, 10(t)
Sexual rights, 106–107
Sexual violence, 4(t)
Sexuality, **1–22,** 443, 488–490
· contraceptives' influence on, 12–20
· helping clients with issues related
to, 20–22
· reproductive health professionals
and, 1–3
· in social context, 3–12
Sexuality education programs,
109–110
Sexually transmitted infections (STIs)
· abstinence and, 102, 107–108
· COCs and, 273, 282–283
· contraceptive selection and, 80
· contraceptives and, 65
· copper IUDs and, 130
· DMPA and, 222–223
· implants and, 199
· IUCs and, 180
· male condoms and, 374–378
· microbicide treatments for, 521
· POPs and, 241
· tubal sterilization and, 447
· vaginal barriers/spermicides and,
398–399
· vasectomy and, 467
· worldwide impact of, 514
SHBG. *See* Sex hormone binding
globulin

SHUG, 528
Shunts, heart valve, 159
Sickle cell disease
· COCs and, 269
· DMPA and, 214
· POPs and, 240
Side effects, 63–64, 66(t)–67(t)
SIL (squamous intraepithelial lesion),
637
Silastic band, 455
SILCS diaphragm, 522
Silk Parasol Panty Condom, 522
Simultaneous use of methods, 54
Sino-Implant (II), 523
Sinoplant I, 194
Sinoplant II, 194
Skin reactions
· COCs and, 317
· patches and, 347–348, 352
SLE (systemic lupus erythematosus),
302
Sleep cycle, hot flashes and, 758
Smoking
· breastfeeding and, 503
· cardiovascular disease and, 61
· cervical cancer and, 625
· COCs and, 277, 279, 280(t), 281,
300–301, 325
· medical eligibility criteria for COC
use and, 78(t)
SNRIs (selective norepinephrine
receptor inhibitors), 765
Soranus, 29
Spermatozoa, 38–39
Spermicidal condoms, 373–374
Spermicides
· advantages, 398–399
· allergies, 98
· anemias, 97
· with barrier methods, 809(t)–811(t)
· breastfeeding and, 494–495
· cardiovascular disease, 85–89
· characteristics of, 393(t)
· dangers/side effects/benefits, 67(t)
· depressive disorders, 91

Ulipristal acetate (UPA), 121, 124–125, 130
Unintended pregnancy(-ies), 514, 791(t)–792(t)
· contraceptive failure and, 45–47
· number of, 45
Uniplant, 194
UPA. *See* Ulipristal acetate
Upper-genital-tract infection, 180
Urethritis, 617–618
Urinary tract infection (UTI)
· medical eligibility criteria, 95
· vaginal barriers and, 405
U.S. Preventive Services Task Force (USPSTF), 622, 642
· periodicity of cervical cancer screening, 631
· recommendation grades, 622(t)
User characteristics, 56–57
Uterine bleeding, 198
Uterine fibroids, 269, 287
Uterine rupture, 724–725
Uterotonic agents, 721
Uterus
· abortion and trauma to, 724–725
· absence of, 536–537
UTI. *See* Urinary tract infection

V

VA feminine condom, 522
Vagina
· abnormal bleeding, 202–203
· irritation, 521
· lubrication, 502
· menopause and, 766–768
· vaginal ring and, 359, 363
Vaginal barriers. *See* Barrier methods
Vaginal ring, **355–365**
· advantages, 356–358
· allergies, 98
· anemias, 97
· breastfeeding and, 498
· cardiovascular disease, 85–89
· depressive disorders, 91

Vaginal ring—*continued*
· description, 355
· disadvantages/cautions, 358–360
· disconnected/broken, 363
· drug interactions, 98
· effectiveness, 356
· endocrine conditions, 95
· expelled, 362–363
· follow-up, 362–364
· gastrointestinal conditions, 96–97
· HIV/AIDS, 94
· improving effectiveness of, 52(f)
· inserting NuvaRing, 364(f)
· malaria, 95
· mechanism of action, 355
· medical eligibility criteria for, 82(t)–98(t)
· neurologic conditions, 90
· as ongoing contraception, 134(t)
· personal characteristics and reproductive history, 82(t)–84(t)
· postpartum use, 490, 493
· problems, managing, 362–364
· prolonged use, 363
· providing, 360–362
· reproductive tract infections/disorders, 91–94
· research on, 524
· schistosomiasis, 94
· TSS, history of, 95
· tuberculosis, 95
· user instructions, 364–365
· UTIs, 95
· vaginal symptoms and, 363
Vaginitis, 618–619
V-Amour, 522
Vasectomy, 435, **460–474**
· advantages, 461
· approaches to, 468–470
· counseling guidelines for, 466–468
· disadvantages/cautions, 461–462
· effectiveness, 460–461
· failure rates, 851(t)–852(t)
· follow-up, 472
· improving effectiveness of, 52(f)

ARE YOU CONNECTED?

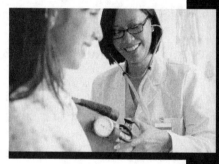

Committed Providers

Trusted Medical Education

Rigorous Science

Convener of Experts

Multidisciplinary Network

Association of
Reproductive
Health
Professionals

Connect Today at
www.arhp.org/join

Annual CE Conferences

CONTRACEPTIVE TECHNOLOGY

National Conferences Presented by the Authors of
Contraceptive Technology

3 Locations: Spring in *Boston* and *San Francisco,* and Fall in *Atlant.*

Designed for MDs, NPs, CNMs, PAs, RNs and Health Educators, these conferences focus on new and future contraception and provide an evidenc based approach to managing a variety of women's health issues, including

- **STDs** • **sexuality concerns** • **vaginitis** • **menopause symptoms** •
abnormal pap smear • **GYN complications**
- **general primary care concerns**

Clinical panels, case study sessions and hands-on skills labs promote dynamic, interactive exchanges between the audience and the expert faculty. Special Preconference Sessions take an in-depth look at key issues in women's health care.

Long considered the premier conference on contraception and reproductive health care, this is a conference you don't want to miss!

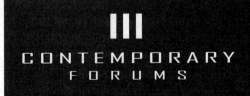

CONTEMPORARY
FORUMS

A REED ELSEVIER COMPANY

For more information contact:
www.ContemporaryForums.co
800-377-7707
info@cforums.com

ARDENT MEDIA, INC.

AN INVITATION TO YOU FROM ARDENT MEDIA

Ardent Media invites you to link your health related web site to www.ardentmediainc.com and/or www.contraceptivemedia.com. Please email info@ardentmediainc.com for inquiries.

Ardent Media seeks to expand its offerings in the health field, including mental and psychological health. As our name implies, we are open to publishing and distributing information in electronic form as well as print.

We are seeking material in formats such as internet web sites, video, audio and CD-ROM in addition to book and booklet material.

If you or your organization has produced material and is seeking distribution, or is planning to write or produce such material, please contact us.

We prefer that you fax or write us a description of your material prior to sending it. Please email us at info@ardentmediainc.com, write us at Box 286, Cooper Station P.O. New York, N.Y., 10276-0286 or Fax us at (212) 861-0998. Thank You.

Contraceptive Technology

❑ CD-ROM

Registration is required to activate your CD-ROM.
If you have already purchased, please include your receipt or proof of purchase.
If purchasing, please include the order form in the back of this
book along with your payment.
(See other side of this form for address.)

or

❑ New Media Survey

ABOUT YOU

1. Educational degree: _____
   Note: If you're a student, list degree you're studying for and expected date of graduation.

2. Describe your current position: _____

3. Circle your most important site of work:

   Managed care organization   **Private practice**   **Health department**
   Family planning clinic   **Hospital**   **Other** _____

4. Circle the number of women you have provided personal contraceptive or STI services in the past year:

   None   1-10   11-100   101-500   501-5000   More than 5000

5. I use a ❑ PDA or ❑ laptop while counseling patients. *(please check one or both)*
   PDA device type: _____

6. Name and address:

   Name _____
   Organization/Institution _____
   Address _____
   _____
   City _____ State _____ Zip _____
   Fax _____
   Email _____
   Website URL_____
   ❑ I am interested in linking my health related website to yours.

   (Please complete the Form found on the back of this page.)

Thank you for taking the time to help us serve you better!

Please photocopy or clip out both pages of this form and mail to:

Ardent Media Inc.
Box 286 Cooper Station P.O.
New York, New York 10276-0286
Please mail it along with your order.

Contraceptive Technology

❏ CD-ROM

*If you have already purchased, please include your receipt or proof of purchase.
If purchasing, please include the order form in the back of this
book along with your payment.
(See other side of this form for address.)*

or

❏ New Media Survey

As our thank you for completing this form and the ABOUT YOU form on the adjoining page, you will receive a special prepublication discount on future new media published by us.

In addition, the most helpful surveys will receive a free copy of *Safety Sexual* upon publication.

1. Would you be interested in having access to an electronic version of *Safely Sexual* or *Contraceptive Technology* if it were offered on the Internet, PDA or on a CD-ROM?
   ❏ **CT** ❏ **Safely Sexual** ❏ **CD-ROM** ❏ **PDA** ❏ **Internet**

2. Would you be interested in receiving electronic updates of *Contraceptive Technology* and/or *Safely Sexual* with new developments in the field?
   ❏ **CT** ❏ **Safely Sexual** ❏ **Both**

3. How often would you like to receive electronic updates?
   ❏ Every 3 months   ❏ Every 6 months   ❏ Other _____

4. What would you consider a fair price for an update as often as you specified above of a chapter or the entire *CT* book?
   Chapter $_____   Book $ _____

5. Would you be interested primarily in receiving electronic updates of specific chapters of CT? If yes, please specify your top 5 choices in order of preference by chapter number.
   1 _____   2 _____   3 _____   4 _____   5 _____

6. Let us know if you are interested in a CT and Safely Sexual CD-ROM or PDA:
   ❏ I am interested in a CD-ROM of ❏ *CT* ❏ *Safely Sexual* to printout information for patients.
   ❏ I am interested in a CD-ROM of ❏ *CT* ❏ *Safely Sexual* with additional information.
   Such as: ❏ audio ❏ video ❏ color graphics
        ❏ selected readings or source material
   ❏ I am interested in approximately __ copies of a ❏ **CD-ROM** ❏ **PDA** for ❏ *CT* ❏ *Safely Sexual*.
   ❏ I am part of a network of __ users and would like information on a net work license or bulk purchase of __ copies of a ❏ *CT* ❏ *SS* on ❏ **CD-ROM** ❏ **PDA**.
   ❏ I am interested in a ❏ CD-ROM ❏ PDA with high-end capabilities such as searching with Boolean logic, word proximity, and key words or phrases for ❏ *CT* ❏ *SS*.

7. What could we do to improve the book and electronic media to make it more useful to you?

8. What type of PDA do you have? _____

Please use additional sheet re: above questions 1-7 with your specific suggestions.

Please complete the other side of this form.

ARDENT MEDIA INC
is pleased to announce the birth of:
CONTRACEPTIVE TECHNOLOGY

in PDF format on CD-ROM

Contraceptive Technology (CT) books also include a CD-ROM with the complete text of CT in direct electronic conversion. Jump links are included so that you can go directly from the table of contents to any chapter or any topic listed in the subheads in the contents. Electronic links are included to the 300 Web sites recommended by the authors so that you can go online with your electronic version of CT and access instantly a wealth of helpful information to complement CT. This electronic format also enables you to quickly perform a keyword search of the entire book, including tables and footnotes, to help speed up the process of finding the information you need. As well, you will be able to quickly print out patient instructions for those you counsel, or other content for your own use.

Please read this overview BEFORE opening your CD-ROM.

Please save your receipt if you have purchased or when you do purchase the CD-ROM or book/CD combo. Your purchase information will be needed to register your product.

Each CD-ROM is for a single-user only unless you purchase a network license. The CD-ROM is protected and you must register it to receive a password to unlock and view the electronic document. In addition, you must have the CD-ROM in your drive to view the electronic document. You may register your CD-ROM at www.contraceptivemedia.com.

If you are considering the purchase of additional CD-ROMs, but are not sure if it is right for the needs of your organization, we ask that you fill out and send in the New Media Survey in the back of this book. Please include your specific needs and we will help you meet those needs.

For organizations with multiple computer users, we can provide either bulk quantity CD-ROMs at a discount, or you can purchase a network license if your computers are networked. Please fill out the New Media Survey in the back of this book, describe your needs and send it to us so that we can provide a solution. If your organization desires the ability to cut and paste for use within the network, a network license must be purchased as this function is not supported on single-user CD-ROMs.

You may use the CD-ROM on your computer or workstation but may not copy it or reproduce it through a LAN or other network.

If you or your organization wish to print out, reproduce or distribute any of the content on the CD for a purpose other than individual counseling or use (for example, for a class, workshop or seminar with multiple participants) please send us the New Media Survey near the back of this book or fill out the Survey describing your permissions request and we will contact you with a solution to obtain the written permission you need for a network license, other license, or provide you bulk CDs at a discount.

Hardware requirements:
PC or Mac with CD-ROM Drive

Software requirements:
PC; Win 95 or greater
Mac; OS 7 or greater

IMPORTANT: Access to the internet is required to register online.

Please carefully read the complete Single-User Purchaser Agreement for the CD-ROM at http://www.contraceptivemedia.com/terms before opening the CD-ROM package. CD-ROMs are returnable only if defective, and will be replaced in that event. By clicking on "I Agree" when you register, you are agreeing to be bound by the terms of the Purchaser Agreement.

ACCESSING THE CD ON A PC:
Place the CD in the CD Drive. A menu with instructions should automatically start. If you do not see a menu come up, navigate to your CD drive and click on CDRUN.EXE. Follow the on screen instructions to register and activate the CD-ROM.

ACCESSING THE CD ON A MAC:
Place the CD in the CD Drive. A menu with instructions should automatically start. If you do not see a menu come up, navigate to your CD drive and click on MACRUN.APP. Follow the on screen instructions to register and activate the CD-ROM.

Please visit our new web site to order or for more information:
contraceptivemedia.com

Thank you for helping *Contraceptive Technology* enter the electronic era.

Forthcoming Early 2012

by the authors of *Contraceptive Technology*
from ARDENT MEDIA INC.

The full table of contents and a sample chapter of *Safely Sexual*
are yours to examine on the CD-ROM in the back of
Contraceptive Technology

SAFELY SEXUAL

Written for the general public, *Safely Sexual* is the
practical guide to planning a safer sexual lifestyle,
preventing unplanned pregnancy, and protecting against HIV
and other sexually transmitted infections. It is perfect for distribution
to clients of family planning clinics and practitioners.

Includes 16 page color photo section of pills

> *"Just as Contraceptive Technology is considered the family planning
> 'bible' for clinicians, I have no doubt that Safely Sexual and its
> approaches will become a heavily relied upon resource for consumers."*
>
> *Vanessa Cullins, MD, MPH, MBA*
> *Vice President for Medical Affairs*
> *Planned Parenthood Federation of America*

250 pages, 5.5" x 8.25"

$19.95 - ISBN 0-9664902-8-2 - *Safely Sexual* Paperback
with CD-ROM & eBook
$29.95 - ISBN 0-9664902-9-0 - *Safely Sexual* Hardback
with CD-ROM & eBook
(including PDF of chapters and license to print out for counseling)

Visit our new website for further information: **contraceptivemedia.com**

Safely Sexual Table of Contents

ARDENT MEDIA INC.
Box 286 Cooper Station P.O.
New York, New York 10276-0286

Please Print Clearly

ORDER FORM
Ardent Media Inc Federal ID # 13-3984679

Forthcoming EARLY 2012
Safely Sexual

Description	Unit Price	Quantity	Total
Paperback Single-User CD-ROM and eBook version 5.5" x 8.25" - 250 pages ISBN 0-9664902-8-2	$19.95		
Hardback Single-User CD-ROM and eBook version 5.5" x 8.25" - 250 pages ISBN 0-9664902-9-0	$29.95		

Name _____
Address _____

City _____
State _____ Zip _____
Telephone _____
Fax _____
Email _____
Method of Payment: ❏ Purchase Order enclosed (Institutions only)
    ❏ Check ❏ Money Order ❏ MasterCard ❏ Visa
Credit Card #: _____
Expiration Date _____
Name on Card _____
    (Please Print Above)
Signature _____

Contact Ardent Media for discount information on bulk orders at our fax 212-861-0998, phone 212-861-1501 or write to our New York address listed on this page. Please see reverse side for more information on bulk discounts.

Prices are subject to change without notice. All sales final. No returns. Our standard returns policy applies for bookstores.

Subtotal	
10% Postage and handling (minimum $8.00) *International shipping additional (minimum $12.00)*	
NY residents add sales tax (NYC 8.875%)	
TOTAL DUE (US funds only)	

You may also order online at contraceptivemedia.com

ARDENT MEDIA INC
Ordering Information
1-877-CT2-3360

Credit card orders (VISA or Mastercard) or institutional purchase orders may be placed toll-free 9AM-5PM EST weekdays at the above telephone number.

Credit card orders (VISA or Mastercard) or institutional purchase orders may be faxed toll free 24 hours to 1-800-711-3724.

or

Please photocopy or clip the Order Form on the opposite side and mail with your check, money order, credit card information, or purchase order to: ARDENT MEDIA INC Box 286, Cooper Station P.O., New York, NY 10276-0286

or

Visit our new website
www.contraceptivemedia.com

Bulk Purchase Discounts: Safely Sexual. Minimum quantity for bulk discount is 25 copies. Please state if you are a nonprofit organization and the number of copies you are interested in purchasing. Bulk discount orders are nonreturnable. *Note:* Any of the ISBNs listed for *Safely Sexual* may be combined to qualify for the 25copy minimum: for example, 15 paperbacks and 10 hardbacks. Please contact us about bulk discounts at 212-861-1501, fax 212-861-0998 or email to info@ardentmediainc.com

---

Note to Book sellers:
All returns require written permission and label from the publisher. Write to the address above or fax to the number above for permission.

ARDENT MEDIA INC.
Box 286 Cooper Station P.O.
New York, New York 10276-0286

Please Print Clearly

Name _____

Address _____

_____

City _____ Zip- _____

State _____

Telephone _____

Fax _____

Email _____

Method of Payment: ☐ Purchase Order enclosed (Institutions only)

☐ Check ☐ Money Order ☐ MasterCard ☐ Visa

Credit Card #: _____

Expiration Date _____

Name on Card _____

(Please Print Above)

Signature _____

Contact Ardent Media for discount information on bulk orders (*Contraceptive Technology*: 25 copies or more) at our fax 212-861-0998, phone 212-861-1501 or write to our New York address listed on this page. Please see reverse side for more information on bulk discounts.

Prices are subject to change without notice. All sales final. No returns. Our standard returns policy applies for bookstores.

ORDER FORM

Ardent Media Inc Federal ID # 13-3984679

Forthcoming Fall 2011
Contraceptive Technology- New 20th Edition
Treatment of STDs • Medical Eligibility Criteria

Description	Unit Price	Quantity	Total
Hardback with Single-User CD-ROM and eBook version ISBN 978-1-59708-005-7	$119.95		
Paperback with Single-User CD-ROM and eBook version ISBN 978-1-59708-004-0	$99.95		

Subtotal	
10% Postage and handling (minimum $8.00) *International shipping additional (minimum $12.00)*	
NY residents add sales tax (NYC 8.875%)	
TOTAL DUE (US funds only)	

Note: Please send the New Media Form along with your order.

You may also order online at contraceptivemedia.com

ARDENT MEDIA INC
Ordering Information
1-877-CT2-3360

Credit card orders (VISA or Mastercard) or institutional purchase orders may be placed toll-free 9AM-5PM EST weekdays at the above telephone number.

Credit card orders (VISA or Mastercard) or institutional purchase orders may be faxed toll free 24 hours to 1-800-711-3724.

or

Please photocopy or clip the Order Form on the opposite side and mail with your check, money order, credit card information, or purchase order to: ARDENT MEDIA INC Box 286, Cooper Station P.O., New York, NY 10276-0286

or

Visit our new website
www.contraceptivemedia.com

This 20th edition of *Contraceptive Technology* is current until publication of the 21th edition scheduled for Fall 2014. Please write or fax ARDENT MEDIA to be notified of the publication of the 21th edition and receive a prepublication discount offer. Please state if you are a nonprofit organization and the number of copies you are interested in purchasing. Also check our website listed above for further information, sign up for email notification and prepublication discount offer.

Bulk Purchase Discounts: Contraceptive Technology. For discounts on orders of 25 copies or more please call 212-861-1501, fax 212-861-0998 or write the address above. Please state if you are a nonprofit organization and the number of copies you are interested in purchasing. Bulk discount orders are nonreturnable. *Note:* Any of the ISBNs listed for *Contraceptive Technology,* may be combined to qualify for the 25 copy minimum: for example, 15 paperbacks, and 10 hardbacks.

Note to Book sellers:
All returns require written permission and label from the publisher. Write to the address above or fax to the number above for permission.